Women's Health

A Textbook for Physiotherapists

Women's Health

A Textbook for Physiotherapists

Edited by

RUTH SAPSFORD AUA, DipPhty
Department of Physiotherapy,
Mater Misericordiae Hospital, Brisbane, Australia

JOANNE BULLOCK-SAXTON PhD, BPhty (Hons)
Department of Physiotherapy,
The University of Queensland, Brisbane, Australia

SUE MARKWELL BPhty
Departments of Gastroenterology and Physiotherapy,
Royal Brisbane Hospital, Brisbane, Australia

WB Saunders Company Ltd

London • Philadelphia • Toronto • Sydney • Tokyo

WB Saunders Company Ltd
An imprint of Harcourt Brace and Company Limited

This book is printed on acid free paper

A catalogue record for this book is available from the British Library

ISBN 0–7020–2209–8

Design by Landmark Design Associates

Printed in China

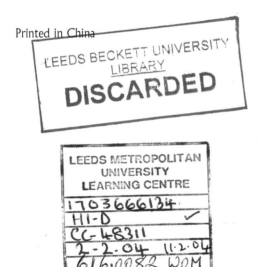

Contents

Contributors

Catherine Bagley BPhty
Physiotherapist, Mater Misericordiae Mothers' Hospital, Brisbane, Australia

Robyn Box MPhty
PhD candidate, Department of Physiotherapy, The University of Queensland, Brisbane, Australia

Joanne Bullock-Saxton PhD, BPhty (Hons)
Senior Lecturer, Department of Physiotherapy, The University of Queensland, Brisbane, Australia.

Karen Coombes BPhty
Physiotherapist, Prince Charles Hospital, Brisbane, Australia

Kate Copeland BPhty, BBus(Health Admin), AFACHSE
Health Administrator, Queensland Department of Health, Brisbane, Australia

Rachel Darken MBBS, DPM
Psychiatrist; Medical Co-ordinator, Medical Board of Queensland, Brisbane, Australia

Mellissa Hewitt-Locke BPhty
Private Practitioner, Sunnybank Medical Clinic, Brisbane, Australia

Katrina Horsley BPhty, MBA, AFACHSE
Director of Physiotherapy, Royal Women's Hospital, Brisbane, Australia

Jane Howard MBBS, LRCP, MRCS, DRCOG, GCEd, FACSHP
Medical Director, Family Planning Queensland, Brisbane, Australia

Helen Kerr MBBS, MRCP, DCH, MRCGP
General Practitioner, The University of Queensland Health Service, Brisbane, Australia

Yvonne Kirkegard MBBS
General Practitioner, The Lilian Cooper Centre, Brisbane, Australia

Judy Larsen BPhty
Director, St Andrew's Hydrotherapy Centre, Brisbane, Australia

Lurlene Livingstone DipPhty
Private Practitioner, Wesley Medical Centre, Brisbane, Australia

Sue Markwell BPhty
Physiotherapist, Departments of Gastroenterology and Physiotherapy, Royal Brisbane Hospital, Brisbane, Australia

Zoe McLachlan DipPhty
Chief Physiotherapist, Mercy Hospital for Women, Melbourne, Australia

Vivienne O'Connor MBChB, GCMedEd, FRACOG, FRCOG
Senior Lecturer, Department of Obstetrics and Gynaecology, The University of Queensland, Brisbane, Australia

Hildegard Reul-Hirche DipPhty
Physiotherapist, Royal Brisbane Hospital, Brisbane, Australia

Ruth Sapsford AUA, DipPhty
Physiotherapist, Mater Misericordiae Hospital, Brisbane, Australia

Robyn Sharpe BPhty
Physiotherapist, Royal Women's Hospital, Brisbane, Australia

Jan Hána, Park Kampa, 'Sitting Act' 1965

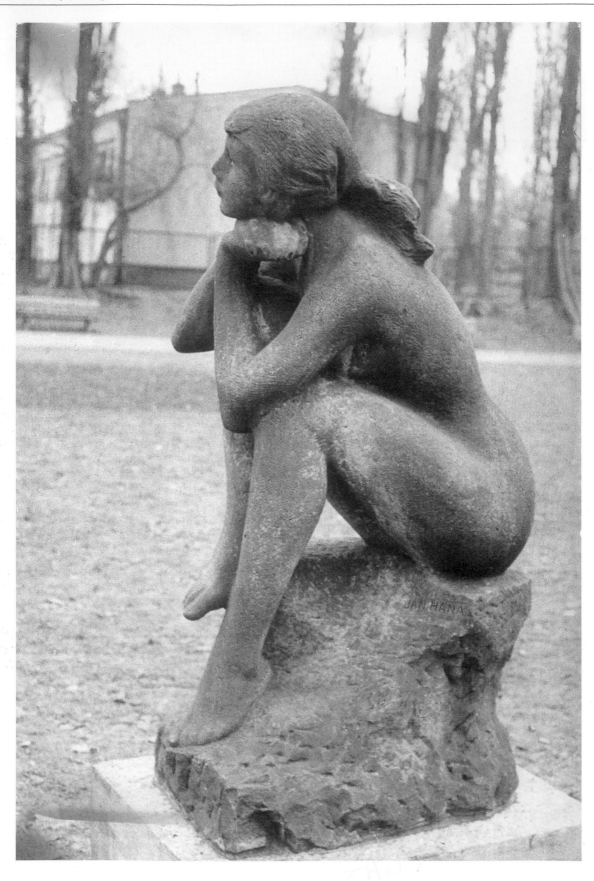

Preface

A focus on health issues relevant to females has been increasing over the last two decades, reflecting an awareness of the special health problems that women may experience. Increasing life expectancy, especially among women in the Western world, provides further impetus to the provision of education and care to ensure quality of that life.

Physiotherapy practice is essentially concerned with the optimal function of the neuromusculoskeletal systems. From adolescence through to old age, there are factors about being female which will influence optimal function. The musculoskeletal system must be considered as an integral part of each person as a whole. All physiotherapists involved in the treatment and education of women, therefore, need to be aware of these influences. This text approaches the issue of how 'being female' may impact on physiotherapy practice. We have attempted to consider briefly the physiological and psychological changes of each life stage (adolescence, child-bearing years and over 40 and beyond) and the health issues that arise from them. While information is categorized into life stages for the convenience of the text, many of the health issues discussed are spread over several decades.

Adolescence, for instance, is a time of skeletal growth, development of secondary sex characteristics, menarche, consideration of sexual issues and, in some cases, pregnancy. The child-bearing years can encompass a large time frame. The focus in this section relates to physiological, psychological, exercise and musculoskeletal considerations in this year of a woman's life. Particular attention is paid to the role of physiotherapy education and treatment during this period. In the time around the menopause and beyond, there are many other physiological factors at play, as well as the possibility of a late pregnancy, increased risk of injury and the increased incidence of particular pathology. Physiotherapy intervention in this life stage is considered in relation to the varied needs of women. In addition, this latter section encompasses issues associated with the elderly and the aged.

It has been apparent to us, in the drawing together of this text, that there is a great deal of skill in the profession in dealing with the issues of 'being female'. It is also clear that we are involved in a growing area of health education, prevention and management. Much research is required to continue to advance the knowledge and practice of physiotherapy. Many of the book's authors are experienced full-time clinicians in women's health who have incorporated relevant features of their own ideas and practice into the text. Clinical observations frequently provide a stimulus for research. The challenge is for clinical and academic teams to explore these initiatives and to advance the profession.

We have encouraged the use of case presentations to reinforce or illustrate some points and we hope that the readers find these of interest.

Ruth Sapsford AUA, DipPhty
Joanne Bullock-Saxton PhD, BPhty(Hons)
Sue Markwell BPhty

Preface

1

Women's Health and the Physiotherapist

KATE COPELAND

Since 1975, the International Year of Women, there has been an increased focus on women's health. Society in general and clinical practice in particular have undergone much change in the meantime. This textbook, prepared for undergraduate and practising physiotherapists, reflects these changes.

The focus of this book is on women's health throughout the lifecycle. For physiotherapists, undergraduate physiotherapy education has gradually changed from a focus on obstetrics and gynaecology to the broader issues encompassed by women's health. This has been supported by greater access to graduate learning opportunities and post-graduate studies.

Within the literature, contributions by physiotherapists to both clinical education and public awareness have included books written by Noble (1978, 1983), Williams and Booth (1985), Mitchell (1987), Chiarelli (1987), Simons (1987), Wilder (1988), Sundin (1989), Polden and Mantle (1990), Polden and Whiteford (1992) and Chiarelli and Markwell (1992). A major contribution to the advancement of the physiotherapist's role in women's health was provided by *Women's Health Through Lifestages – the Physiotherapist's Contribution* edited by Collins in 1987.

Despite these writings, no comprehensive textbook has emerged to guide the undergraduate learning experience and clinical development for physiotherapists working in women's health. A trio of physiotherapists with a broad range of clinical interests in women's health identified the need for such a text and set about making it a reality.

The intended audience for this book therefore includes the undergraduate physiotherapy student and those physiotherapists in clinical practice who require an overview of the current role of physiotherapy in women's health. Many sections will also indicate current and projected trends for the future.

Structured as it is in a life continuum, the book makes it equally easy to turn to a specific chapter to seek information or to read from beginning to end and follow the women's health lifecycle from puberty to old age.

Why Women's Health?

A question commonly asked is 'Why focus on women's health?'. Two particular responses to this are:

1. over 50% of the population is female and this alone is sufficient reason to focus on women's health issues;
2. there is a mutual dependence between women's activities, roles, anatomy and physiology and their health – a complex and rewarding field for further investigation.

More than 50% of the world's population is female

Since just over half of the population is female, physiotherapists and other health professionals need a broad understanding of the impact and implications of being female on the lifecycle and on specific health issues which can arise.

Physiotherapy has traditionally been a female-dominated profession and although this is changing, many practitioners developed an increased knowledge and awareness of women's health issues when they themselves encountered similar problems. As Broom (1991, p. 2) commented, 'As with many more women, pregnancy and childbirth marked turning points in my experience of my own body and in my understanding of the importance of reproductive health to women's autonomy'.

The impact on one's health of being female is felt throughout the entire life continuum. Health professionals need a thorough knowledge and understanding not only of anatomy and physiology but also of psychosocial influences. Many physiotherapists develop a special interest in a particular aspect of health care such as sports physiotherapy, paediatrics or cardiorespiratory care. Regardless of their area of practice, all physiotherapy practitioners need a thorough knowledge of current women's health care issues and management.

Inter-relationship of women's activities, roles, anatomy and physiology and health

It is important to recognize the mutual dependence of women's activities, roles, anatomy and physiology and the effects that these have on health.

Women have particular health needs which are related to their biological function, their roles in society and their participation in the workforce.

During the 1970s and 1980s, the women's movement led to an increased awareness of issues including equal pay, equal opportunity, childcare, women's health status and social equity. These issues represent areas where women have felt discriminated against, poorly served by society and powerless. In this book, women's concerns about their health and the health system have been viewed within the wider context of a range of social concerns.

It is recognized that there have been major changes in family life over the past 20 years. A recent report highlighted the fact that changes such as increased women's workforce participation, greater cultural diversity, increased mobility, higher divorce rates and repartnering, longer dependency by student or unemployed children and the effects of higher rates of unemployment on family life have all affected the demand for health and community services. It noted in particular that the traditional role of women as unpaid family carers and community volunteers could no longer be taken for granted when health and community services are being planned and provided (Council of Australian Governments (COAG), 1995).

Issues which need to be considered when women's health is examined include the unique influences of:

- the reproductive cycle and the bearing of children;
- the multiple roles managed by women (raising children, nurturing family members, caring for young, sick, disabled and elderly);
- the association between health status and broader cultural and socioeconomic factors;
- the increasing participation in the paid workforce.

During the consultation process for the preparation of the National Women's Health Policy in Australia (Commonwealth Department of Community Services and Health, 1989), the major issues identified were:

- reproductive health and sexuality;
- health of ageing women;
- emotional and mental health;
- violence against women;
- occupational health and safety;
- health needs of women as carers;
- health effects of sex role stereotyping on women.

Women want a health system that is affordable, accessible and responsive to their particular needs.

Women's Health – Two Decades of Change

Two global initiatives which focused international attention on the health and well-being of women were International Women's Year 1975, followed by the United Nations Decade for Women 1976–85.

One of the most impressive developments in health services in recent years has been a growing recognition of the need to provide services for women. Such services must take account of women's changing role in society. With increasing participation in the workforce, women are experiencing new health problems and new and different services are required to assist them in dealing with these.

It must be recognized that formulation of policy does not take place in a vacuum. A number of developments in general health and social policy provided the context for the development of the more broadly based health policies for women such as the National Women's Health Policy (1989) in Australia.

Moving from treatment of illness to promotion of health

On 12 September 1978 the Alma-Ata Declaration reaffirmed the World Health Organization (WHO) definition of health – 'Health is the state of complete physical, mental, and social well-being and not merely the absence of disease or infirmity' (WHO, 1978) – and created the framework for the International Declaration for Primary Health Care.

In the late 1970s, the WHO made it clear that a reorientation of health-care philosophy within a social justice framework was needed. The 'social health' perspective takes account of the interaction between social and economic factors and health or illness and often includes a rethinking of health service delivery. This led to the emphasis on primary health care and the stated need to co-ordinate with wider public policies to improve health significantly.

The term 'Health for all' was coined following international activities concerned with improving global health status. Whilst this is the target, a range of associated issues were identified by the WHO for urgent examination within individual countries. These included:

- equity in health;
- health promotion;
- the need to develop primary health care and to enhance prevention activity in primary health-care settings;
- co-operation between relevant agencies of government and the community, including the business sector;
- the need to increase consumer participation in decision making.

These issues paralleled the concerns identified repeatedly by women in Australia and overseas as fundamental to their own well-being. It also led to a growing recognition that the role of physiotherapy should be much broader than the provision of treatment to women with health problems. It meant that there should be improved access to health services for women who were marginalized by culture, language, isolation or poverty. Creating a paradigm shift from the treatment of illness to the maximization of health had its first tentative beginnings.

In 1981, the WHO produced a report on the formulation of global strategies to achieve 'Health for all by the year 2000', proposing that health systems develop appropriate infrastructures, starting with primary health care services.

Primary health care is often defined as the first level of contact by consumers with the health system. It combines personal care with local efforts in health promotion, the prevention and treatment of illness and rehabilitation. Also included are a wide spectrum of activities such as:

- provision of clean water and disposal of sewage;
- promotion of good nutrition;
- ensuring safe environments;
- access to health education;
- medical and nursing care.

Primary health care is the responsibility of individuals, consumers operating in groups and a range of health-care professionals. To be successful, primary health care must be accessible, affordable, appropriate and acceptable to the local community and the services should be planned and operated with significant community participation.

It was recognized that much of the health-care system actually concentrated on illness and so a reorientation was clearly needed. This led to the development of the concept of health promotion.

Defining health promotion

One aspect of confusion has been the similarities and differences between health education and health promotion.

The WHO (1986) identified health promotion as 'the process of enabling people to increase control over and to improve their health'. It has further been identified as '. . . a unifying concept for those who recognize the need for change in the ways and conditions of living, in order to promote better health' (WHO, 1987).

Bates and Winder (1984) identified health promotion as 'Any combination of health education and related organizational, political and economic interventions designed to facilitate behavioural and environmental adaptations that will improve or protect health'.

Health education and health promotion have a symbiotic relationship. Richardson (1994, p. 106) notes that:

> Health promotion is concerned with building a system which is conducive to health through health policies which seek to achieve environmental change and through endeavours which seek to produce changes in organizations in the interest of the health of their workers. Health education is an essential prerequisite of all health promotion programmes enabling critical choices to be made by the individual and through education of health professionals.

Health education is one way to place control in the hands of the individual.

For many years, physiotherapists have been aware of the need to work with individuals and groups to develop their personal skills in overcoming, managing or dealing with health problems and have been providers of health education. Less evident, at an individual or collective level, has been physiotherapy involvement in organizational, political and economic interventions.

Edmonds (1988) commented that sometimes the deeply caring motivation of some health professionals tends to emerge as judgemental and directive. Evans (1984, p. 74) was very critical of earlier attempts at health education. He wrote:

> Indeed all of what presently passes for 'health education', other than rather banal exhortations to eat a balanced diet and get more exercise and sleep, include recommendations to see one's doctor, dentist or other provider more frequently, and to comply with their instructions. In any other context this would be recognized, not as education, but as marketing of professional services.

Many health professionals, health educators and health promoters have devoted their lives to ensuring that health education and health promotion can create real change in the health of individuals, groups, communities and societies.

Ritchie (1991) provides an insightful review of 25 years of health education, identifying and outlining four clearly identifiable stages. Having traced the evolution of health education, some ideas on future directions are also provided.

- **Stage 1: education through health information provision.** During the 1960s, the traditional classroom model was used to 'teach' patients to act according to a set of instructions.
- **Stage 2: education through varied audiovisual channels.** Aware that 'providing factual information was not producing compliance' (Ritchie, 1991, p. 158), some health educators took steps to enable patients to receive information more effectively. The use of various visual and auditory methods improved attention but 'there were still many who were not perceiving what they were hearing or seeing in the manner the providers intended and many who were therefore unlikely to act on the information being given to them'.
- **Stage 3: education incorporating adult learning principles.** This evolved from evidence of the effectiveness of active participation of the learner. However, praise for people who took responsibility and changed in a positive way led to a reasonable viewpoint that defaulters should bear the blame for their inaction. 'The faulty premise (was) that the receipt of correct information would automatically lead to behaviour change, ... and failure to change was seen as a voluntary choice' (Ritchie, 1991).
- **Stage 4: education for health within the Ottawa Charter framework (p. 159).** Health education could now be put into context as one component of a broad approach, including improving the knowledge and skills of individuals and improving the social and environmental conditions in which they lived.

It can be seen that some of the responsibility has moved from the health professions to the individual with the provision of education, but social and economic environments also require change.

'The challenge then is for those of us committed to education for health to enter this fifth stage in the knowledge that we as educators are lifelong learners ourselves', concludes Ritchie (1991, p. 162). For physiotherapists this is evidenced by the importance of continuing professional development, the increased demand for postgraduate courses, the growth and recognition of fellowship of the professional colleges and the widespread recognition that knowledge is infinite.

In 1990, Polden and Mantle, in their textbook *Physiotherapy in Obstetrics and Gynaecology*, wrote of their deep conviction that:

> Thorough and effective physiotherapy is essential in this field and that physiotherapists should carry out the work. There are few specialist tutors for undergraduate physiotherapists, so students often receive a rudimentary introduction to obstetrics and gynaecology and obstetric placements that give students practical experience are not compulsory and are few in number (p. xiv).

Ottawa Charter for Health Promotion

Mention has been made of the Ottawa Charter framework. For those who may be unfamiliar with this development, a brief explanation is in order. In 1986, the First International Conference on Health Promotion was held in Ottawa. Five specific areas of action for health promotion were developed and articulated at this conference and are known as the Ottawa Charter for Health Promotion. The areas outlined were:

1. developing healthy public policy;
2. developing personal skills;
3. strengthening community action;
4. creating supportive environments;
5. reorienting health services.

These five broad categories identify the need for all sectors to work together to improve everyone's health and well-being. Saltman (1991, p. 51) interpreted the areas outlined in the Ottawa Charter into a hierarchy of action strategies to improve women's health.

1. **'An individual approach, involving the development of personal skill'.** This strategy identified that individual women would be able to increase control over their health and make informed choices through the provision of information, health education and programmes to enhance their life skills.
2. **'A community approach, involving the development of local strategies to support the processes and empowering strategies which assist individual women'.** This strategy uses health promotion to create social change and thereby affect the community, rather than individual women.
3. **'An ecological approach, acknowledging the complex inter-relationships between the health of women and the environments in which they live and work'.** This strategy acknowledges both the strong links between domestic and work environments and the relationships between industry and the communities from which the workforce is drawn.
4. **'A health sector approach, which acknowledges the integral role health services can play at all levels of health care'.** This strategy validates the role of health professionals furthering health promotion and the health of the community, as well as the individual and the treatment of sickness. Saltman refers specifically to the general practitioner but this concept is equally valid for all health professionals.
5. **'An organizational approach which takes health beyond health care'.** This strategy recognizes the role of initiatives in legislation, financial policies, taxation and social structures.

Health Education and Health Promotion: the Physiotherapist's Role

A simplistic definition of the role of a health promoter is 'someone who uses all the knowledge and skills available to them to improve the health and well-being of the individuals and communities in which they live and work'. This definition can be adapted and expanded by individuals or professions to reflect their involvement in health promotion.

Physiotherapists, with their educational background in health science and holistic management of health problems, are health professionals with a major role in the treatment and alleviation of health problems. Their commitment to improving the health and well-being of their patients means that they will continue to be integrally involved in health education. Multiple avenues and opportunities will be utilized including schools, workplaces, hospitals and health facilities, community venues, sporting and health clubs, retirement villages, senior citizens' halls, hostels and nursing homes. In addition, physiotherapists are well placed to play a vital role in health promotion, by accepting the challenge identified in Ottawa in 1986 by extending beyond the physiotherapist / patient partnership to address issues pertinent to groups, communities and societies.

References

Bates IJ and Winder AE (1984) *Introduction to Health Education.* Palo Alto: Mayfield Publishing.

Broom DH (1991) *Damned If We Do – Contradictions in Women's Health Care*, p. 2. North Sydney: Allen and Unwin.

Chiarelli P (1987) *Women's Waterworks.* Rushcutters Bay, NSW: Century Magazines.

Chiarelli P and Markwell S (1992) *Let's Get Things Moving.* Rushcutters Bay, NSW: Gore and Osment Publications.

Collins M (ed) (1987) *Women's Health through Lifestages – The Physiotherapist's Contribution.* Sydney: Australian Physiotherapy Association (NSW Branch).

Commonwealth Department of Community Services and Health (1989) *National Women's Health Policy – Advancing Women's Health in Australia.* Canberra: AGPS.

Council of Australian Governments (COAG) Task Force on Health and Community Services (1995) *Health and Community Services: Meeting People's Needs Better. A Discussion Paper.* Canberra: COAG.

Edmonds B (1988) The certificate in health education: a personal perspective. *Physiotherapy Practice* 4: 26–29.

Evans R (1984) Licensure, consumer ignorance and agency. In: Evans, R *Strained Mercy: The Economics of Canadian Health Care*, p. 74. Toronto: Butterworths.

Mitchell L (1987) *Simple Relaxation.* London: John Murray.

Noble E (1978) *Essential Exercises for the Child-Bearing Year.* London: John Murray.

Noble E (1983) *Childbirth with Insight.* Boston: Houghton Mifflin.

Ottawa Charter for Health Promotion (1986) *An International Conference on Health Promotion: The Move Towards a New Public Health.* Ottawa: World Health Organization.

Polden M and Mantle J (1990) *Physiotherapy in Obstetrics and Gynaecology.* Oxford: Butterworth Heinemann.

Polden M and Whiteford W (1992) *The Postnatal Exercise Book.* London: Frances Lincoln.

Richardson B (1994) Health promotion and education. In: Richardson B and Eastlake A (eds) *Physiotherapy in Occupational Health: Management Prevention and Health Promotion in the Workplace.* Oxford: Butterworth Heinemann.

Ritchie JE (1991) From health education to education for health in Australia: a historical perspective. *Health Promotion International* 6: 157–163.

Saltman D (1991) *Women and Health: An Introduction to Issues*, p. 51. Sydney: Harcourt Brace Jovanovich.

Simons J (1987) *Pregnant and in Perfect Shape: Exercising During Pregnancy and After.* Melbourne: Nelson.

Sundin J (1989) *Face to Face with Childbirth: A Comprehensive Active Childbirth Preparation Program.* Sydney: Horwitz Grahame.

Wilder E (ed) (1988) *Obstetric and Gynaecological Physical Therapy.* Clinics in Physical Therapy 20. Edinburgh: Churchill Livingstone.

Williams M and Booth D (1985) *Antenatal Education.* Edinburgh: Churchill Livingstone.

World Health Organization (1978) *Alma-Ata 1978: Primary Health Care. Report of the Proceedings of the Conference held at Alma-Ata, 6–12 September.* Geneva: World Health Organization.

World Health Organization (1981) *Global Strategy for Health for All by the Year 2000.* Geneva: World Health Organization.

World Health Organization (1986) *Intersectoral Action for Health: The Role of Intersectoral Cooperation in National Strategies for Health for All.* Geneva: World Health Organization.

World Health Organization (1987) *Health Promotion in the Working World. Report on a Joint Meeting Organized by the Federal Centre for Health Education (Cologne, 1985).* Copenhagen: World Health Organization.

Part One

Adolescence

2

Puberty and Menarche

HELEN KERR

Neuroendocrinology of Puberty
•
Physical Changes of Puberty
•
Menarche

The transition from childhood to adulthood is called *adolescence*. It includes the physical changes which are part of puberty as well as psychological and social changes. Clarke (1991) defines the psychological and social development that needs to be achieved in adolescence thus.

- To become comfortable with body image.
- To become comfortable with sexual development.
- To make vocational choices.
- To develop abstract thinking.
- To gain independence.
- To form mutually responsible sexual relationships.
- To develop moral attitudes.

The adolescent patient has an undeserved reputation as 'difficult'. Young people appreciate a respectful, non-judgemental and empathic approach from health professionals. Confidentiality is usually a particularly important issue for adolescents working towards independence and autonomy. The young patient should be reassured that the consultation is confidential and she will not be discussed with anyone without her permission and knowledge. An awareness of influences on her life such as home and education environments, peer activities, drugs and sexuality and the prevalence of eating disorders and depression in this age group allows appropriate and sensitive assessment (Bennett, 1988).

Puberty is the term used to describe the biological changes which occur as a child develops and becomes capable of reproduction. In girls this involves, in addition to somatic growth, breast development, enlargement of ovaries, uterus and vagina, the growth of pubic and axillary hair and the establishment of the menstrual cycle. During puberty one of the most obvious events is *menarche*, which means the onset of menstruation. The onset of puberty and its progress are controlled by a part of the base of the brain called the *hypothalamus* and by the adjacent *pituitary gland*.

Neuroendocrinology of Puberty

In the following discussion, the activation of the neuroendocrine pathways of puberty and the physical changes which ensue are reviewed. A young gymnast's case history is used to illustrate some of the factors which may influence development.

The specific mechanisms controlling the time of onset of puberty are complex and still incompletely understood. It is thought that as the central nervous system matures, the restraint of the hypothalamus lessens. Puberty is then heralded by a resurgence of pulsatile, episodic nocturnal secretion of gonadotropin-releasing hormone (GnRH) from the hypothalamus. The hypothalamic–pituitary–ovarian axis, which has been relatively quiescent since early childhood, is thus reactivated (Edmonds, 1989; Rosenfield and Barnes, 1993). Figure 2.1 illustrates the neuroendocrine pathways

Figure 2.1 Neuroendocrine pathways controlling puberty (hypothalamic–pituitary–ovarian and hypothalamic–pituitary–adrenal axes).

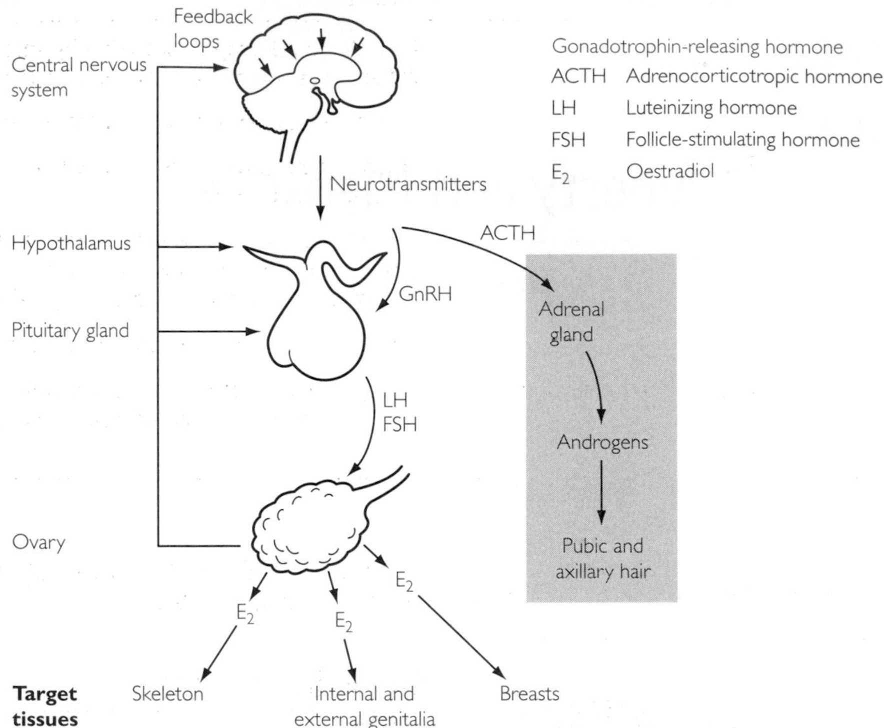

controlling puberty and Table 2.1 summarizes the actions of the principal hormones involved.

Frisch (1990) has hypothesized that a critical weight for height must be achieved to allow pubertal development. She argues that the absolute and relative fat content of the body are important. Adipose tissue is a significant source of extragonadal oestrogen and body weight influences the metabolism of oestrogens to more or less potent forms. Frisch (1990) also postulates that menarche and ovulation are delayed until the body contains enough fat stores to support a pregnancy and lactation. However, these theories have recently been challenged (Stanton et al, 1992). They do not seem to apply to populations whose members have a low average body weight.

Julie-Anne is a 15-year-old elite gymnast. She started gymnastics when she was seven. She trains for 25 hours per week. She has already competed in several international championships and hopes to be selected for the Olympic team. She has not reached menarche. She is 153 cm in height (50th centile for a 12-year-old) and 36 kg in weight (25th centile for a 12-year old). Her skeletal maturity is equivalent to a normal 13-year-old. She has unilateral breast development (breast bud Tanner stage 2). She has no pubic or axillary hair.

Figure 2.2 shows the usual temporal relationship of menarche to the growth spurt of puberty and breast and pubic hair development. From this data Julie-Anne would be expected to have significant breast and pubic hair growth even if she had not reached menarche.

Physical Changes of Puberty

An important aspect of pubertal development is the considerable variability in the age of onset of changes and the time taken to complete these changes. There is also some variation in the order of appearance of the pubertal changes (Wheeler, 1991).

Skeletal growth

Height velocity or skeletal growth increases as an early pubertal event in girls (it is a later pubertal event in boys). A girl grows at 6–11 cm for the year she is growing fastest (peak height velocity). Leg length increases before trunk length and foot length increases before calf and thigh length. Hip width increases relative to shoulder width early in female puberty (Wheeler, 1991). Skeletal maturity, the ossification of the skeleton, can be studied radiographically. Radiographs of the left hand and wrist are compared with standards and expressed as equivalent to normal for a particular chronological age (Greulich and Pyle, 1959).

Table 2.1 Actions of main hormones of female puberty and menstrual cycle

Hormone	Site of origin	Action
Gonadotrophin-releasing hormone	Hypothalamus	Pulsatile gonadotrophin secretion by anterior pituitary gland initiates and controls puberty and menstrual cycle
Follicle-stimulating hormone	Pituitary	Ovarian follicle development leads to oestrogen production
Luteinizing hormone	Pituitary	Androgen and progestogen production by ovary; mid-cycle surge induces ovulation
Oestradiol	Ovary	Growth spurt; epiphyseal fusion; breast and genitalia development; female fat distribution; production of proliferative endometrium. Triggers mid-cycle surge of luteinizing hormone
Progesterone	Ovary	Breast development; production of secretory endometrium
Androgens	Adrenal gland and ovary	Pubic, axillary and other body hair growth; muscle mass increase; skin thickening and increased sebum production by sebaceous glands

Figure 2.2 Pubertal events. (Modified from Llewellyn-Jones (1990) with permission.)

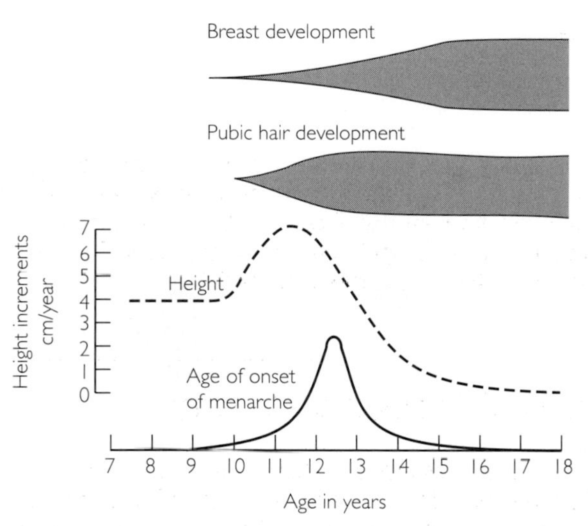

Skeletal maturity is the most valuable investigation in the assessment of delayed and precocious puberty. Menarche usually occurs at a skeletal maturity equivalent to a chronological age of 12.5–14.5 years (Kreipe, 1992).

Changes in body composition

Lean body mass increases during puberty and reaches a peak at menarche in girls. Increase in muscle strength lags behind muscle size by a few months (Wheeler, 1991). Fat mass increases throughout puberty, particularly in the lower trunk and thighs. Lean body mass to fat ratio changes from 5:1 at the onset of puberty to 3:1 at menarche (Kreipe, 1992).

Genitalia changes

EXTERNAL

There is deposition of fat on the mons pubis early in puberty. The labia majora become larger and wrinkled. Young women sometimes fear that their labia are abnormal but there is considerable normal variation in size and shape. The clitoris enlarges slightly.

INTERNAL

The ovaries, uterus, fallopian tubes and vagina increase in size. The vagina develops stratified epithelium. The vaginal secretions become acidic because of colonization by lactobacilli. A physiological vaginal discharge, which may cause concern to the pubertal girl, develops. The endometrium (lining of the uterus) does not thicken significantly until shortly before menarche.

Breast changes

Figure 2.3 illustrates usual breast development during puberty. Uneven breast development is common but sometimes concerns young women. The girl should be reassured that the mature breasts are usually reasonably symmetrical. Investigation such as biopsy of a unilateral breast bud may lead to distortion of the developing breast.

Pubic hair

Figure 2.4 illustrates pubic hair development. Pubic hair development usually follows breast development but 15% of normal girls develop pubic hair before breast enlargement.

Figure 2.3 Breast growth in puberty. Stage 1: prepubertal breast. Stage 2: breast bud, areolar diameter enlarges. Stage 3: further enlargement, smooth contour between breast mound and areola. Stage 4: projection of areola and nipple beyond breast mound. Stage 5: adult contour breast, projection of nipple only. (Reproduced from Gardener and Saunders (1993) with permission.)

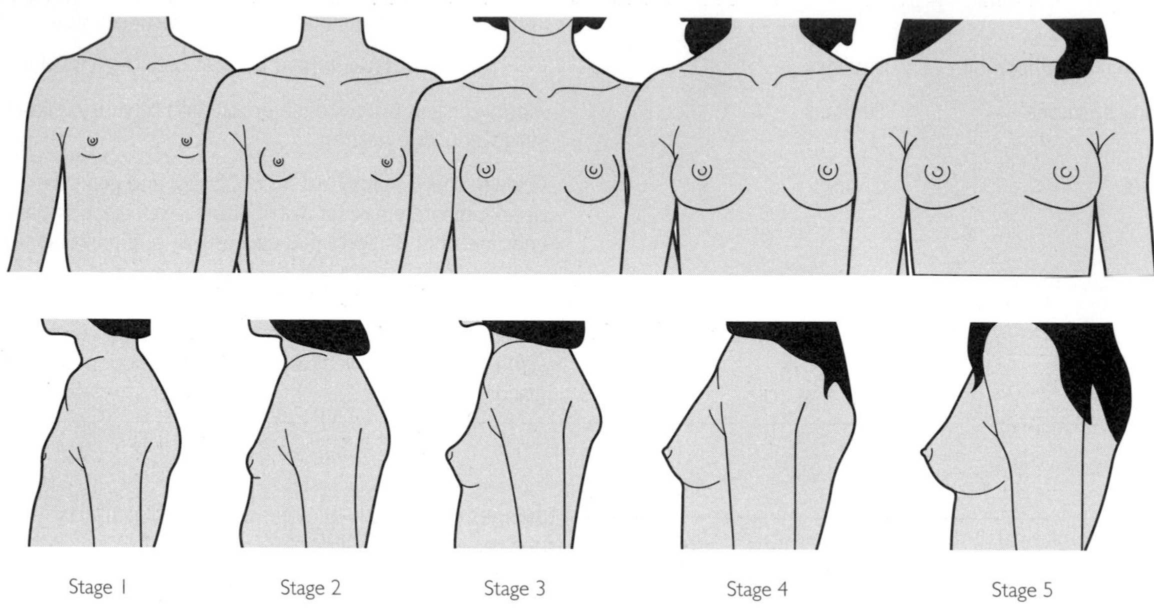

Figure 2.4 Pubic hair development. Stage 1: no pubic hair. Stage 2: sparse growth of long, fine, slightly pigmented hair along labia. Stage 3: hair darker, coarser, curled and spread on to pubes. Stage 4: adult type hair confined to pubes. Stage 5: extension of hair on to medial thighs.

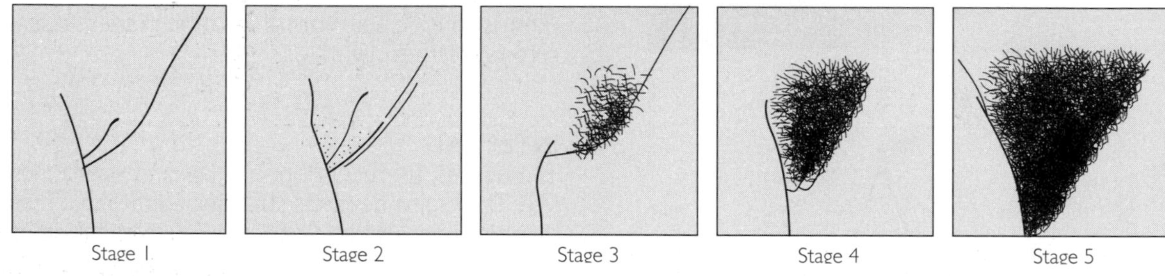

Axillary hair and skin changes

Axillary hair usually develops after pubic hair. The skin thickens and sebaceous and sweat glands begin to function. Increased sebum production almost invariably results in some degree of acne occurring during adolescence.

Menarche

Menarche occurs between 10 and 16 years of age. The average age of menarche in affluent countries is now 12.8; in 1840 it was 16.5. The reasons for this trend are not fully understood but are assumed to be because of improved health and nutrition. There is evidence that the trend to earlier menarche has been levelling off or even reversing in the last 25 years (Rees, 1993). The mythology surrounding menarche and menstruation will be discussed in Chapter 6.

The menstrual cycle

The hormone levels and ovarian follicle and endometrial development during an ovulating cycle are illustrated in Figure 2.5. Initially, the menstrual cycle is usually anovulatory (i.e. ovulation does not occur) and about half the cycles are anovulatory during the first two years following menarche (Rosenfield and Barnes, 1993).

The ovaries contain several hundred thousand immature ova at puberty. During the menstrual cycle, between 10 and 100 ova begin to develop but one dominant follicle emerges. This follicle secretes a hormone, oestradiol, and raises the oestradiol concentration to a critical level, triggering at about mid-cycle a surge of luteinizing hormone from the

Figure 2.5 Hormone levels and ovarian follicle and endometrial development during an ovarian cycle. (From RU486, Ulmann et al. Copyright © 1990 by Scientific American, Inc. All rights reserved.)

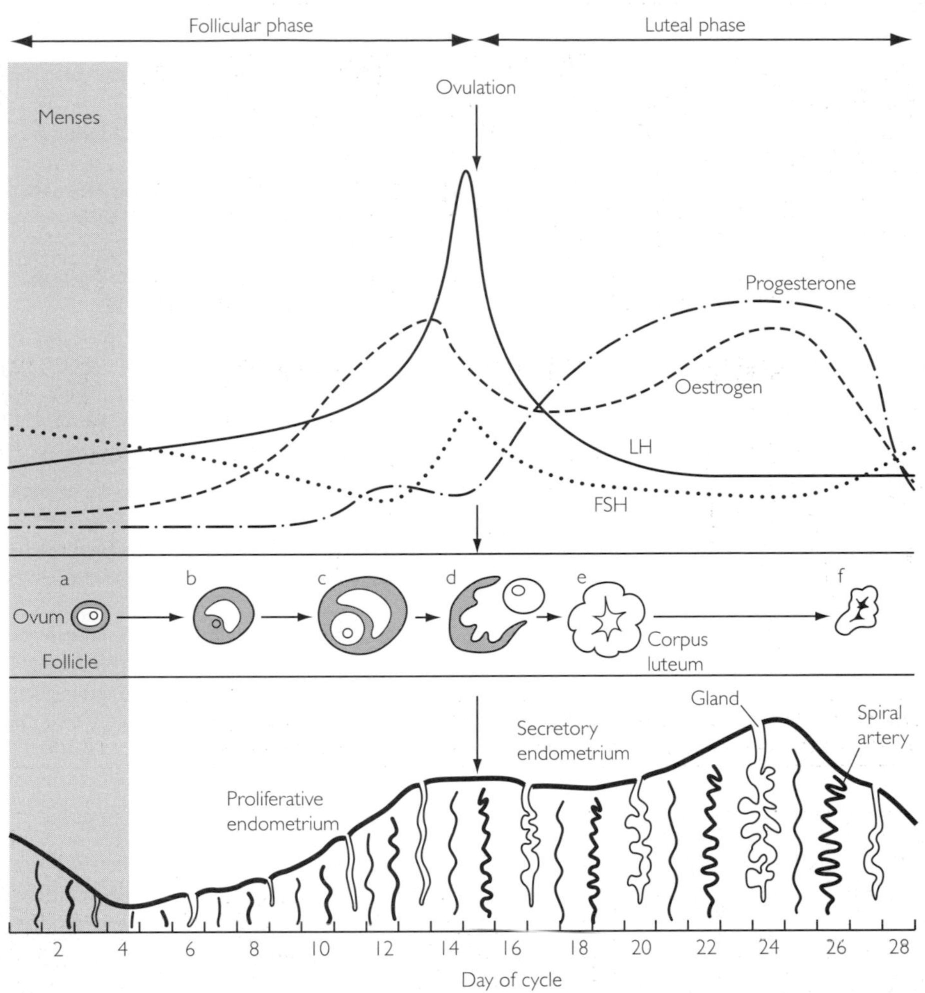

pituitary gland. The peak of luteinizing hormone triggers ovulation in which the ovum is shed from the follicle. (This positive feedback mechanism from ovary to pituitary and hypothalamus indicates female sexual maturity.) Following ovulation, the follicle forms the corpus luteum which secretes progesterone. Progesterone creates a proliferative endometrium in preparation for a possible pregnancy. If pregnancy does not occur, the corpus luteum degenerates, the endometrium is shed and menstruation occurs. There is a wide range of normal cycle lengths in the first years after menarche.

Julie-Anne is an international athlete in an appearance-based sport. Small size is an advantage in gymnastics and thin, early adolescent body shape is favoured. She is significantly under weight and height for her age. She has signs of early puberty. We do not know whether she has begun her pubertal growth spurt. Short stature, pubertal delay and late menarche are common amongst female gymnasts (Rees, 1993) (as Julie-Anne has only very early breast development she is fairly unlikely to reach menarche by age 16). Heavy training schedules combined with dietary restriction to maintain slimness may impede the normal pubertal growth spurt (Theintz et al, 1993).

Restricted diets may be imposed upon the athlete by parents or coach or may be self-imposed. Other studies have shown that intensive training does not affect the age at menarche (Baxter-Jones et al, 1994). It has been postulated that later menarche in gymnasts is, at least in part, due to a genetic predisposition to delayed puberty. However, it is known that intense exercise plays an important role in suppression of the hypothalamic–pituitary–ovarian axis and inadequate calorie intake further delays growth. There is concern that the intensive training regimes and rigid lifestyle endured by some competitive athletes may have long-term adverse psychological, hormonal and musculoskeletal effects, including the possibility of decreased bone density and osteopenia. These areas are further discussed in Chapter 4. There is need for further studies to make it possible to devise safe training regimes, nutrition programmes and appropriate support for young athletes (Mansfield and Emans, 1993).

Summary

It is important to recognize the considerable normal variation in the pubertal process. More research is needed to elucidate the specific mechanisms which trigger puberty. The reasons for the trend to earlier menarche and the recent apparent reversal of this trend also deserve further study, as does the impact of exercise, nutrition and stress on the initiation and progress of puberty.

Dysfunctions which can occur in the menstrual cycle and the physiological and psychological influences on the adolescent will be highlighted in Chapter 6.

References

Baxter-Jones AD, Helms P, Baines-Preece J et al. (1994) Menarche in intensively trained gymnasts, swimmers and tennis players. *Annals of Human Biology* **21**: 407–415.

Bennett DL (1988) Understanding the adolescent patient. *Australian Family Physician* **17**: 345–346.

Clarke S (1991) How to treat the adolescent. *Australian Doctor Weekly*, **7 June**, 111.

Edmonds DK (1989) Menstrual change in adolescence. *Baillière's Clinical Obstetrics and Gynaecology* **3**: 329–339.

Frisch RE (1990) The right weight: body fat, menarche and ovulation. *Baillière's Clinical Obstetrics and Gynaecology* **4**: 419–436.

Gardener K and Saunders J (1993) *Women's Problems in General Practice*, 3rd edn. Oxford: Oxford University Press.

Greulich WW and Pyle SI (1959) *Radiographic Atlas of Skeletal Development of the Hand and Wrist*, 2nd edn. Stanford: Stanford University Press.

Kreipe RE (1992) Normal somatic adolescent growth and development. In: McAnarney ER, Kreipe RE, Orr DP et al (eds) *Textbook of Adolescent Medicine*, pp. 44–67. Philadelphia: W.B. Saunders.

Llewellyn-Jones D (1990) *Fundamentals of Obstetrics and Gynaecology. Vol 2 Gynaecology*, 5th edn, p. 263. London: Faber and Faber.

Mansfield MJ and Emans SJ (1993) Growth in female gymnasts: should training decrease during puberty? *Journal of Pediatrics* **122**: 237–240.

Rees M (1993) Menarche. When and why? *Lancet* **342**: 1375–1376.

Rosenfield RL and Barnes RB (1993) Menstrual disorders in adolescence. *Endocrinology and Metabolism Clinics of North America* **22**: 491–505.

Stanton WR, Kelly JL, Bunyan DA et al (1992) Expected gain in body mass and onset of menarche. *Australian and New Zealand Journal of Obstetrics and Gynaecology* **32**: 338–340.

Theintz GE, Howald H, Weiss U et al (1993) Evidence for a reduction of growth potential in adolescent female gymnasts. *Journal of Pediatrics* **122**: 306–313.

Ulmann A, Teutsch G and Philbert D (1990) RU486. *Scientific American 262*: 21.

Wheeler MD (1991) Physical changes of puberty. *Endocrinology and Metabolism Clinics of North America* **20**: 1–15.

3

Adolescence and the Musculoskeletal System

MELISSA HEWITT-LOCKE

In the 1990s female adolescents are playing a variety of sports that influence the neuromusculoskeletal system. Traditionally girls have been involved in sports such as netball, softball, gymnastics, swimming and athletics. With more sports being available to the public at large, activities that have previously been considered the sporting domain of males, such as cycling, basketball and rugby union, are attracting adolescent girls. The influence of growth in combination with the varied demands of different sports means that there are many orthopaedic conditions that are unique to the growing child / adolescent.

Currently literature predominantly looks at the adolescent group as a whole – males and females. This chapter therefore pertains to both females and males but special consideration has been given to uniquely female conditions.

Orthopaedic Factors

Adolescents achieve approximately half their bone growth in their pubertal years (Parfitt, 1994) with the pubertal time frame being on average five years (Barnes, 1975). Their musculoskeletal system undergoes many changes in a relatively short time. Bones grow at a rapid rate and the musculotendinous units that cross joints have difficulty lengthening at a concomitant rate. A number of injuries appear to be specifically related to the bone growth in adolescence.

Joint biomechanics may be affected during periods of rapid bone growth. An associated change in sensory feedback from the joints and overlying muscles may lead to changes of muscle co-ordination about the joints. It is not uncommon to see the adolescent (female or male) who is 'outgrowing' their body and appears awkward and gangly. As a consequence of this temporary alteration in muscle co-ordination, joint protection may be compromised and injuries may occur.

Increased muscle tension pulling on a bony insertion often results in a traction apophysitis. The patellar and Achilles tendons and hip musculature insertions are the most frequently affected sites.

Rapid alterations in lower limb biomechanics during adolescence also predispose the female to conditions of overuse. Tibial stress syndrome, patellofemoral and heel pain are commonly seen and require physiotherapy involvement. Snapping hip syndrome, whilst not unique to adolescent females, is frequently seen in this group. Girls participating in running and jumping sports are particularly susceptible.

Rapid bone turnover during the teenage years results in a higher incidence of fractures, especially in the physically active subset (Parfitt, 1994). The forearm is most commonly affected. Stress fractures are also seen, with the foot and tibia frequently involved. Growth plate injuries are unique to children and adolescents. Precise diagnosis and correction are required to prevent future disturbances in limb growth. Avulsion fractures are also seen in adolescence and will often occur instead of a ligament sprain.

Disorders linked to growth become more obvious during puberty. An existing idiopathic scoliosis or postural kyphosis may increase in the teenage years or become evident for the first time. Management of these conditions relies on intervention occurring before growth ceases. Physiotherapists are extensively involved with this group and require a good knowledge of the effects of growth on the musculoskeletal system.

Back pain is a serious ailment at all times of life but requires particular attention in adolescence. Sinister causes of the pain must be eliminated and good postural habits and back care formulated.

If a female has specific sports skills, by the time she reaches adolescence she will already be training and competing at a moderate to high level. Whilst wide sports experience is desirable until growth ceases, it is more likely that adolescents participate in one or at the most two sports. Consequently demands are repeatedly made on certain body parts specific to that sport's requirements. Swimming, netball, tennis, athletics (both track and field) and gymnastics are the sports that mostly involve teenage girls. Each has particular areas of risk with respect to injury, both acute and overuse.

In this section, orthopaedic factors that affect the adolescent female will be addressed with particular emphasis on physiotherapy management.

Bone growth

Rapid bone growth occurs during puberty which for females is 9.5–14.5 years of age (Barnes, 1975). Approximately two years after the commencement of puberty, girls achieve their peak height velocity (PHV) (Tanner, 1962). On average PHV is 8 cm per year, with the average age of PHV in girls being just above 12 years of age (Barnes, 1975). Six to twelve months prior to menarche, girls will reach their maximal growth rate and maintain this rate for 2–3 months. Only 5–10% of adult height will be gained after menarche but girls may continue growing linearly up to 19 years of age. In most instances, however, linear growth has ceased by 17 years (Roche and Davila, 1972).

The epiphyseal plates located at either end of the bones allow longitudinal growth and are the site for formation of joint surfaces. Apophyses are also bony growth sites and are where major tendons and ligamentous groups attach. The two areas where bone formation occurs are zones of inherent weakness and are therefore susceptible to injury during the growth phase (Andrish, 1990; Wojtys, 1987). Figure 3.1 illustrates the anatomy of these two zones.

Developing bone is particularly adaptable to different mechanical loads and this ability to 'remodel' itself decreases once maturity is reached. Consequently, physical exercise during childhood and especially puberty has a significant effect on bone growth and development.

Figure 3.1 Bony growth sites in the immature skeleton.

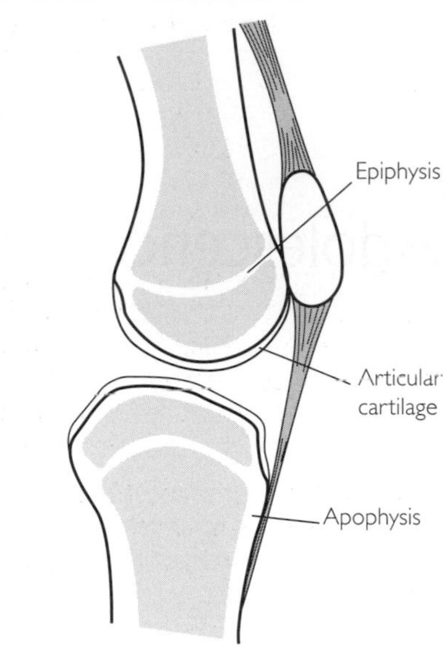

Fractures

In adolescence, an increase in the porosity of the bone cortex occurs as a result of an increase in intracortical bone turnover. This bone turnover makes available adequate amounts of calcium for bone lengthening to occur at the growth plates. It is during this stage of growth that an increased incidence of fractures exists (Parfitt, 1994).

The likelihood of fractures during adolescence is also increased by the height and weight gains, in combination with greater participation in competitive sport, associated with this period. Fractures are primarily due to accidents, contact sports (where high velocities are attained) or as a result of incorrect landing techniques in sports (e.g. a dismount from the uneven bars in gymnastics or a heavy fall after an attempted rebound in basketball).

The radius and ulna are the most commonly fractured bones in the adolescent. This is most likely due to the type of sports played and the incidence of falls associated with them. As growing bone has a good blood supply, healing of fractures usually occurs quickly and with minimal complications. Treatment is via immobilization in a plaster cast unless a rotational or angular deformity with displacement is present. In this instance, open reduction and internal fixation followed by a period of immobilization occurs. A degree of latitude in the healing position is allowed depending on the amount of growth the adolescent has left.

Clavicle fractures are also common in the adolescent and associated with falls. The medial epiphyseal plate closes last of all in the body, at an age range between 18 and 24 years. Table 3.1 demonstrates the mechanism of injury, commonly involved sports and activities, signs/symptoms and the method of treatment associated with clavicular fracture.

Following the period of immobilization, rehabilitation must aim to prevent any stiffness in the glenohumeral joint and

Table 3.1 Clavicle fractures in adolescence

Mechanism of injury	Sports activities	Signs / symptoms	Treatment
Fall on shoulder	Horse riding Basketball Cycling	• Pain on palpation medially (not over sternoclavicular jt) • Localized swelling + / – deformity	• Immobilization with sling / Fig. 8 restraint 7–10 days • Neck / elbow ROM at 7–10 days
Tackling	Football	• Restricted shoulder and neck movement	• Progressive strength exercises

thoracic spine. Weakness of the scapular muscles is often associated with clavicular fractures and if not addressed, will result in long-term scapular and thoracic dysfunction. In adolescent females who sustain shoulder girdle injuries careful attention to the sternum and sternocostal joints is required. Stiffness and associated pain in these joints is common.

The lower leg and ankle are the most commonly fractured sites in the lower limb. Early physiotherapy input is vital to prevent joint stiffness, restore strength and ensure full return to activities of daily living and / or sports participation. Each centre has different protocols for the management of all fractures (stable or unstable). Generally, however, a period of non-weight bearing is followed by partial weight bearing, range gaining, strengthening, co-ordination and balance activities.

Hydrotherapy is an excellent modality for improving joint range, minimizing pain and developing strength. The support of the water can allow otherwise painful movement to occur. Progressions for strengthening can be gradually regained via resistance exercises using weights, elastic exercising equipment or gym facilities. Adolescents enjoy the use of gym equipment for any rehabilitation and good gains in strength can be expected within 6–8 weeks of a specific supervised weights programme being instigated. Body weight exercises are a useful and safe means of strengthening muscle groups.

GROWTH PLATE FRACTURES

The growth plate relies on the fibrous periosteum that inserts into the epiphysis and perichondrium (Fig 3.1) to stabilize it biomechanically and minimize the risk of injury (Andrish, 1990). Ligaments and tendons attach at the perichondrial zone and the tension that these structures receive is transferred to the growth plate. The ligaments that surround the growth plates are 3–5 times stronger than the epiphyseal plate, which results in adolescents sustaining injuries of the growth plate more frequently than the ligamentous damage that occurs in adults (Strizak and Stroberg, 1986).

Due to the influence of ligamentous tension on it, the growth plate is most susceptible to a torsional stress. Pivoting on a fixed foot in netball is a classic example of fracture mechanism. Due to anatomy and biomechanics associated with the injury, growth plate fractures commonly occur at the knee joint. The adolescent who suffers an acute joint injury should be examined for possible epiphyseal / growth plate disruption. Immediate diagnosis is essential to prevent abnormalities of adult limb length, joint function and limb alignment (Anderson, 1991). The signs and symptoms of a growth plate injury are listed in the box. An X-ray will confirm the diagnosis. In the acute growth plate fracture with an undisplaced fragment, the X-ray will appear normal for 10–14 days. After that, there is an obvious periosteal reaction on X-ray (Andrish, 1990).

Signs and symptoms of a growth plate injury

Tense and painful joint

+/– Instability

Tenderness over joint line on palpation

STRESS FRACTURES

Stress fractures are more common in the adolescent female who participates in weight-bearing sports that are endurance in nature or have repetitive high-impact manoeuvres. Ballet dancers, triathletes, basketball players and gymnasts are more likely to sustain stress fractures, with the lumbar spine, navicular and tibia commonly involved.

A 16-year-old triathlete presented complaining of left-sided low back pain and upper posterior thigh pain that had been present for 12 months after falling from her bike during a race. Initially the pain was only present when running and eased with rest. Swimming and cycling were pain free and fitness activities such as skipping were unimpaired.

Training and competing continued and pain became evident when riding her bike and skipping. By wearing a very firmly fitting wetsuit the pain was controlled when skipping and running.

Body weight was low and skinfold measurements were minimal. A bone mineral density (BMD) scan showed reduced BMD at the sites of wrist, lumbar spine and neck of femur. The athlete had been amenorrhoeic for 18 months.

Pain became worse on walking, standing and when moving from sitting to an upright position. On palpation, the fourth and fifth lumbar and first sacral apophyseal joints were tender. Lumbar spine movement was not restricted but positive neural tension was exhibited via a slump and straight leg raise test (Fig. 3.2) (Butler, 1991).

A bone scan demonstrated an unhealed stress fracture of the fifth lumbar vertebrae.

When a stress fracture becomes evident it is usually associated with a sudden increase in activity or a change in the athlete's training surface. With lower limb stress fractures a change in footwear may have occurred. Eating disorders and/or menstrual problems such as amenorrhoea have also been associated with stress fractures in teenage athletes (Highet, 1989). Tables 3.2 and 3.3 present the stages of stress fractures and the appropriate levels of mobility.

Some suggested non-weight-bearing activities while the stress fracture heals could include pool running as well as cycling. Such activities would maintain cardiovascular and muscular fitness. It is often difficult to encourage the adolescent to slow down whilst healing occurs as they do not perceive that the stress fracture is a serious injury.

AVULSION FRACTURES

Bony apophyses are bone growth sites and are therefore susceptible to injury. Major tendon and ligamentous groups attach at these sites, e.g. the tibial tubercle for the patellar tendon. Acute avulsion of an apophyseal centre can occur. The forces that cause an apophyseal avulsion in adolescents usually lead to a musculotendinous or muscle tear in the adult population (Anderson, 1991).

Adolescents sustain avulsion fractures because the involved growth plate has closed but not fused (Meyers, 1988). In the adolescent female the elbow, knee and pelvis are common injury sites and high-velocity activities are often the cause.

Elbow avulsion injuries

Throwing sports such as softball and javelin exert different forces on the elbow at different phases of the throwing action (Andrish, 1990; Meyers, 1988). It is these varying and high-velocity forces that may cause fragmentation of the trochlea, olecranon and/or medial epicondyle in the adolescent involved in throwing sports (Andrish, 1990; Meyers, 1988). Table 3.4 describes the three phases of throwing and the anatomical changes that occur with each action.

Treatment of avulsion fractures about the elbow involves cast immobilization for three weeks. Open reduction and internal fixation are necessary if there is displacement. Some surgeons advocate open fixation and early careful movement (Micheli, 1989). If the radial head is involved in an elbow injury there is an early loss of forearm pronation and supination. If these areas are not quickly targeted, stiffness in these ranges is permanent. In caring for avulsion fractures about the elbow, assessment of paraesthesia in the forearm and hand must be routine as ulnar nerve involvement is not uncommon.

Physiotherapy goals therefore are achievement of full joint range, restoration of strength (via gradual progression) and eventual full return of function prior to sports competition. The elbow joint clinically responds poorly to passive input,

Figure 3.2 Straight-leg raise test to demonstrate the presence of adverse neural tension in the lower limb. Restricted range of motion and a line of pain in the posterior thigh which increases with dorsiflexion of the ankle or head flexion is a positive sign for irritation of the sciatic nerve.

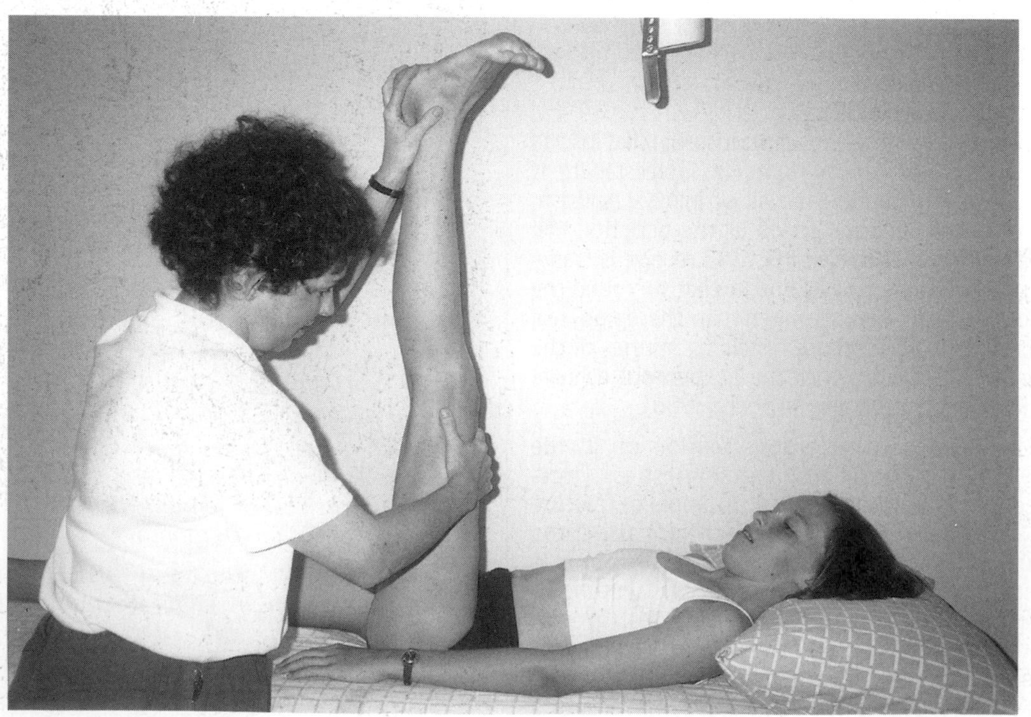

Table 3.2 Signs and symptoms of stress fractures

Initial onset	Dull ache with training/competition	Decreased pain with rest
Progresses to	Sharp persistent pain at start of exercise. Decreased pain as body warms up. Pain at end of exercise session	Pain gradually eases with rest
Finally	Constant ache with superimposed sharp pain with exercise	Does not ease with rest

Table 3.3 Stress fractures and recommended levels of mobility for healing

Initial onset of pain	Rest and non-weight-bearing (NWB) activities
Persistent pain that eases	Partial weight bearing (PWB) on crutches + NWB activities
Constant pain	NWB + air cast/brace for immobilization + NWB activities

therefore range of motion should be achieved via active means. Adolescents often respond well to hydrotherapy activities combined with throwing games, such as one-on-one water polo, which is one approach to restoration of full range of movement.

Tibial tuberosity avulsion fractures

Avulsion fractures of the tibial tuberosity are commonly seen in adolescents between 12 and 16 years of age. This is just before the apophysis fuses with the tibia. There can be two mechanisms of injury: a strong quadriceps contraction when the knee is flexed and the foot fixed or a violent passive flexion of the knee when the quadriceps are contracted maximally. Commonly, these occur in motor vehicle accidents or contact sports such as basketball or rugby for females and football codes for males. The first mechanism is seen as the basketballer goes to 'lay up' but has someone standing on her foot. The second mechanism is seen when the running player is tackled around the shins from front on and the leg is passively flexed. The signs and symptoms of a tibial tuberosity avulsion fracture appear in the box.

Signs and symptoms of tibial tuberosity avulsion fracture

Unable to actively extend knee joint

Severe localized pain over anterior inferior aspect of knee

Localized swelling

Higher patella height compared to unaffected limb (confirmed by lateral X-ray)

If there is no displacement of the tibial tuberosity the patient's leg is immobilized in extension in a cylinder cast or knee immobilizer (one month). Open reduction is necessary in the presence of displaced fragments. The physiotherapist must ensure full return of knee flexion as well as quadriceps and hamstring strength. Eccentric quadriceps control is a vital prerequisite for returning to sport. Exercises may begin by the slowly controlled descent from a stair (Fig. 3.3). Proprioceptive function is commonly

Table 3.4 Phases and forces associated with throwing

Phases	Forces
Wind-up/cocking	Medial distraction and lateral compression of elbow joint. Translational forces across olecranon and humeral joint surfaces (at end of wind-up)
Acceleration	Neutralization of forces
Follow through	Triceps brachii create compression and shearing forces at the radiocarpal joint as forearm pronates to release the ball

Figure 3.3 Eccentric control of the quadriceps muscles using a slow controlled descent from a stair. Care should be taken to ensure that the patient maintains trunk and pelvic stability and that the hip is in neutral rotation or even slightly externally rotated. This will promote appropriate lower limb biomechanics and muscle activation.

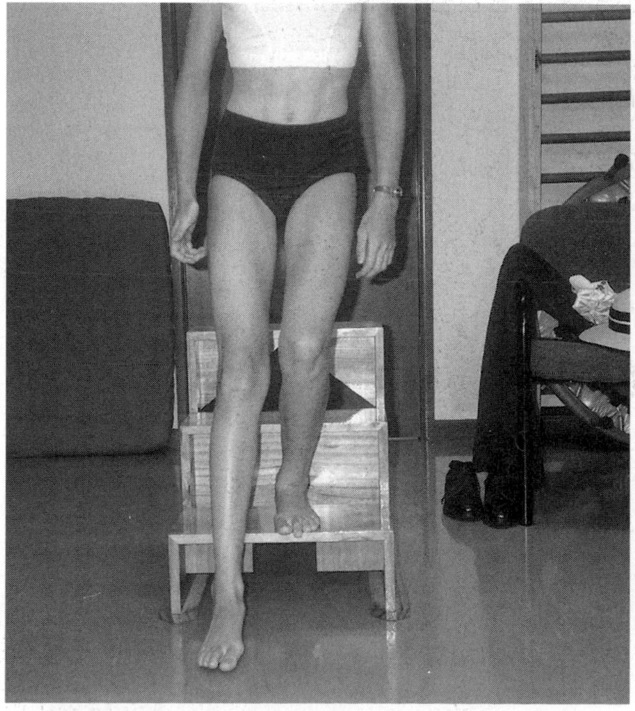

decreased and exercises to improve muscle activity and co-ordination under increasingly difficult situations are indicated (Janda and Vavrova, 1994) (e.g. innovative and challenging use of labile surfaces such as balance boards).

Tightness of the rectus femoris is common in patients presenting with tibial avulsion. It is unclear whether this is a predisposing factor or a result of the avulsion injury. Regardless of whether it is the cause of injury, effective lengthening of the muscle is indicated. The prone position is used initially and then standing can be used for a home programme (Fig. 3.4). Maintenance of posterior pelvic tilt is essential during the technique to ensure maximum distance between the origin and insertion and effective lengthening and to avoid any lordosis associated with anterior pelvic tilt. In addition, assessment and practice of high-level agility skills are necessary to ensure safe return to sport. Such skills might include rapid jumping or hopping in different directions at different speeds (Fig. 3.5).

Tibial spine avulsion

Forceful hyperextension of the knee with tibial rotation or a direct blow to the lower thigh may be responsible for avulsion of the tibial spine in adolescent pre-pubertal children. The tibial eminence is not completely ossified at this age and is weaker than the attached anterior cruciate ligament (ACL) (Smith and Tao, 1995). The adolescent will present with a swollen and painful knee joint as a result of bleeding into the joint.

Outcome for this injury is always positive but knee extension range can be limited. The physiotherapist must attempt to minimize loss of knee extension. As for the other avulsion fractures, treatment is via casting or open reduction and fixation according to the extent of the injury. It is important for physiotherapists to be aware that the ACL can be stretched or partially torn with this injury. Meniscal damage can also occur, as can collateral ligament disruption (Smith and Tao, 1995). It was once believed that ligament damage was rare in the skeletally immature patient because the growth plate was weaker and therefore the site of likely damage. Due to improved arthroscopic techniques and clinical diagnostic tests, ligament and meniscal damage has been demonstrated in adolescents and therefore requires appropriate management.

Anterior superior iliac spine (ASIS) avulsion

Growth plate fusion occurs earlier at the anterior inferior iliac spine (AIIS) than at the anterior superior iliac spine (ASIS), reducing the risk of avulsion of the AIIS (Karlin, 1986). However, sartorius, tensor fascia lata, external and internal oblique abdominal muscles and the inguinal ligament either originate or insert at the ASIS. Avulsion of the ASIS has been cited in association with explosive hip flexor action in sprinters (Karlin, 1986), primarily due to the action of sartorius.

Figure 3.4 Sustained passive stretch to the hip flexors and knee extensors, particularly rectus femoris. Care should be taken to ensure that there is no increase in the anterior pelvic tilt or lumbar lordosis during the technique.

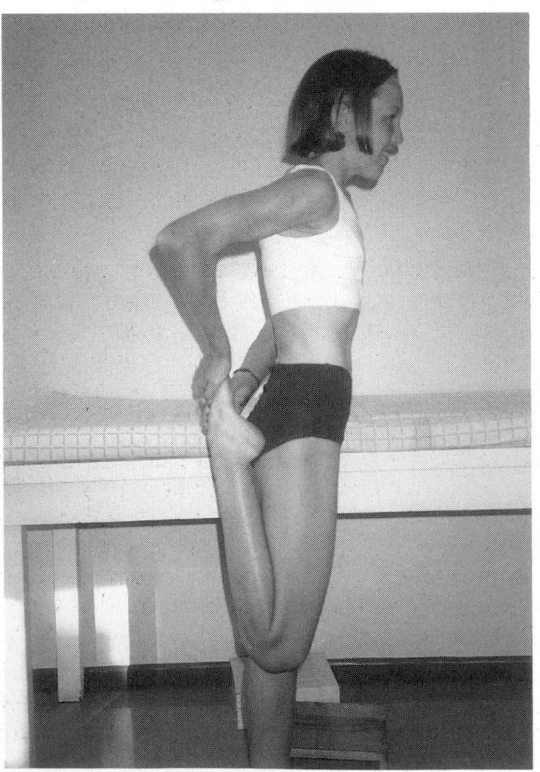

Figure 3.5 Agility exercises combine change in direction of movement at varying speeds and base of support. Bilateral jumping can progress to single-leg hopping.

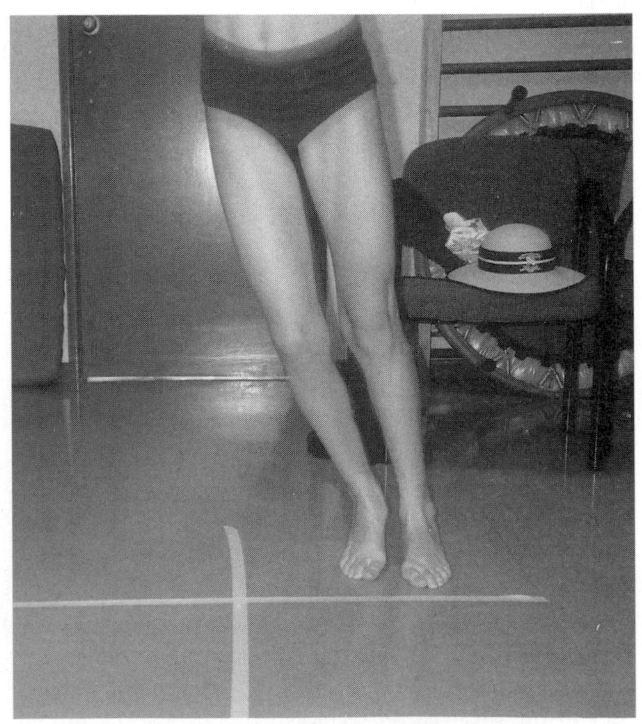

On examination the patient will experience pain on the sit-up manoeuvre, hip flexion, hip abduction and prone knee flexion in combination with hip extension. Initial management includes rest with partial to non-weight-bearing activities limited by pain. Isometric exercises of the hip and trunk and, subsequently, range of motion exercises for these areas are commenced as pain allows. Muscle lengthening regimes are then commenced. Hydrotherapy and pool running are useful interim activities prior to dry land running. Rigorous warm-up is essential prior to competition to minimize the likelihood of injury recurrence or muscle strains. Again, high-level agility skills must be assessed and practised before returning to sport.

TRACTION APOPHYSITIS

Repetitive loading of the apophysis via tensile forces may result in a traction apophysitis in young athletes (Schmidt and Henry, 1989). It is reported that in periods of rapid growth the skeletally immature athlete is more prone to apophysitis due to the pull of tensed muscles on the apophyseal growth sites (Micheli and Fehlandt, 1992). The tibial tubercle and calcaneal apophysis are commonly affected (Micheli and Ireland, 1987). When an adult is exposed to similar traction forces tendonitis is more likely. In all age groups, lower limb alignment with a muscular presentation of tightness of specific biarticular muscles and weakness in antagonist muscle groups clinically appears causal to this presentation. Throwing activities have been cited by Ireland and Hutchinson (1995) as the most likely cause of upper limb apophysitis. The repetitive stresses of throwing irritate the apophysis of the olecranon as the elbow is rapidly extended from a flexed position.

When treating apophysitis it is important to remember that it is a condition linked with growth and often occurs in two areas concurrently (Carter and Aldridge, 1988). The treatment approach to apophysitis is summarized in the box.

Treatment of apophysitis

- Local application of ice/ultrasound (care over growth plate with ultrasound application)
- Pain-free activity
- Supervised stretching programme
- Strengthening programme (eccentric work important in chronic cases) (Stanish, 1995)
- Advice regarding warm-up and cool-down sessions prior to training and competition
- Orthotics to correct biomechanics (lower limb apophysitis)
- A foam heel raise (occasionally used) to provide symptomatic relief (calcaneal apophysitis)

Anatomical factors of females associated with injury

Significant changes in lower limb biomechanics occur during the adolescent growth spurt.

The female pelvis is wider than in males and affects the biomechanics of other lower limb joints, particularly the knee joint. Carbon (1992) considers that this anatomical difference disadvantages the female in weight-bearing sports. Pain or discomfort about the knee are commonly reported during adolescence. Ankle sprains in sports predominantly played by females, such as netball, are common, which may be an artefact of either the increased joint range or the sport-specific environment (surface and rules). Increased ligament laxity around the patella may alter patellar tracking and result in patellofemoral stress (Griffin, 1994).

Increasing levels of circulating oestrogen result in a body shape that is unique to women. Females have narrower shoulders and a greater carrying angle at the elbow and are thus at a mechanical disadvantage in throwing sports compared with males.

Female basal levels of the hormone relaxin are higher than in the adolescent male population, resulting in greater joint flexibility. This is most commonly seen at the shoulders, knees, ankles and patellofemoral joints. Overuse syndromes such as swimmer's shoulder and thrower's (little leaguer's) elbow may occur as a result of poorly stabilized joints undertaking large ranges of motion at high repetitions and forces.

Bones grow faster than associated musculotendinous structures and alterations in flexibility and a propensity for muscular imbalances are reported (Karlin, 1986). These imbalances contribute to alterations in limb alignment (Elliott, 1991). In the lower limb this can result in gait pattern disturbances that may predispose the growing athlete to chronic injury (Strizak and Stroberg, 1986). These problems are more commonly seen in the growing female who is already biomechanically disadvantaged.

Individual teenagers may take variable lengths of time to adjust to these changes in flexibility and associated deficits in motor co-ordination may occur (Wotjys, 1987). The reacquisition of speed, strength and finally skill in their chosen sports can be delayed, with an increased likelihood of acute injury in this period.

Maturational assessment (classified via the attainment of sexual characteristics, e.g. development of genitalia, presence of pubic hair) measures an adolescent's progression towards physical maturity (Caine and Broekhoff, 1987). This assessment is important as a marker of physical ability and potential compared to chronological age. Its usefulness is highlighted when considering injuries caused by loss of flexibility and muscle–tendon imbalances.

Pre- and post-pubertal growth spurts can be reliably predicted via maturational assessment. Biomechanical changes can be monitored during these growth spurts and the physiotherapist can advise the individual, parents and coaches on training programmes and sport participation. Emphasis on stretching activities is warranted. When this does not occur the skeletally immature athlete is at risk of injury.

Training errors involving inadequate warm-up and cool-down sessions, rapid increases in the intensity, frequency and/or duration of sessions and changed footwear or training surface will all contribute to overuse injuries.

> *A 12-year-old cross-country runner showed promise in the sport after only one season. Wanting to perform well in her new sport, she commenced running every afternoon with her father in the off-season. She was also swimming and attended training once or twice per day, averaging 2–5 kilometres per day. Her running routes involved hills and she commenced running three kilometres per day, increasing to five kilometres over the next 10 days.*
>
> *A rapid growth spurt also occurred in this time. Within a month of commencing her running training, she presented with patellofemoral pain bilaterally and bilateral calcaneal apophysitis. Her pain was exacerbated by running and walking up and down hills and stairs and on swimming breast-stroke. She was unable to squat fully without pain.*

Patellofemoral stress syndrome

The epiphyseal growth plates of the knee joint contribute the greatest amount to adult lower limb length and are the fastest growing in the body (Strizak and Stroberg, 1986). It is suggested that rapid changes in the length of these long bones may alter the balance of the quadriceps mechanism. An outcome associated with this change is patellofemoral stress syndrome. The signs and symptoms of patellofemoral stress syndrome are highlighted in Table 3.5.

Rapid growth can result in tightness of the iliotibial band due to the large area of fibrous band. In addition, the vastus medialis appears to be less able to achieve appropriate activation, possibly due to changes in patella alignment or via inhibitory mechanisms. The patella is usually displaced laterally and proximally in these subjects. It is hypothesized that these muscular changes may contribute to patellofemoral stress syndrome (O'Neill et al, 1992; Strizak and Stroberg, 1986). The path that the patella takes as the knee flexes and extends is determined by the bony contours of the patella and the intercondylar notch, the length of the patellofemoral retinaculum and the contraction of the vastus medialis obliquus (Strizak and Stroberg, 1986).

Table 3.5 Signs and symptoms of patellofemoral stress syndrome

Retropatellar pain that affects one or both limbs
Occasional superficial lateral patellar pain
Often exacerbated by a rapid growth spurt
Pain on running, ascending or descending stairs/hills, squatting, jumping
Pain after prolonged sitting
Occasional crepitus on knee flexion and extension.
A softening and fissuring of the articular cartilage of the patella (chondromalacia patella) (Strizak & Stroberg, 1986). This is confirmed via arthroscopy

Lengthening of the iliotibial band and hamstring muscles has been shown to be effective in the treatment of this condition (O'Neill et al, 1992). McConnell (1986) also advocates taping the patella medially to promote improvements of patella tracking during movement. Taping should be used in association with eccentric quadriceps strengthening to reduce pain and restore function. Proprioception and postural balance are often reduced and activities to improve these, such as balance board, mini trampoline balancing and one-legged standing with eyes shut, are beneficial treatment techniques.

Iliotibial band friction syndrome

Iliotibial band (ITB) friction syndrome is thought to be caused by sudden growth in combination with changes in physical activity. Because the female adolescent has a wider pelvis than the adolescent male, ITB friction syndrome is commonly seen in girls who cycle or run. Pain may be felt over the greater trochanter and in some cases a trochanteric bursitis develops (Paletta and Andrish, 1995). Pain may also be experienced over the fibular head, lateral aspect of the knee or along the posterior edge of the ITB. Commonly used treatment techniques are listed in the box.

Treatment techniques for ITB friction syndrome

- Restrict painful activities
- Local application of ice (acute stage)
- Connective tissue massage
- Ultrasound/deep heat therapy
- ITB and hamstring stretches
- Assessment of lower limb biomechanics (modify if required)
- Orthotics (as required)
- Assessment of sporting and training techniques: programmes, surfaces, footwear, equipment
- Maintenance of cardiovascular and local muscular endurance, e.g. via pool running

Snapping hip syndrome

Female adolescents of all sporting persuasions are prone to snapping hip syndrome (Paletta and Andrish, 1995). There are a number of possible causes for this phenomenon. Firstly, ITB syndrome can be a cause, with a snapping sensation and discomfort over the greater trochanter being reported. Hip flexion and extension with internal rotation will reproduce the pain. Secondly, tenosynovitis of the iliopsoas tendon near the lesser trochanter or as it crosses the iliopectineal eminence may also be the cause of snapping hip syndrome. The patient complains of snapping and discomfort in the groin or anterior hip region. Management of presenting signs and symptoms is appropriate and techniques of muscle lengthening and muscle strengthening are likely to be employed. In some instances surgical release of the iliopsoas tendon sheath or iliopsoas lengthening has given positive results (Jacobsen and Allen, 1990).

Swimmer's or thrower's shoulder

Shoulder pain is a common complaint in adolescent swimmers and often occurs as sudden growth spurts alter muscle length and strength and trunk posture. As previously mentioned, adolescent females demonstrate a greater ligament laxity and the shoulder is commonly affected in the active female. The incidence of swimmer's shoulder is said to increase proportionately with ability, with 57% of championship swimmers complaining of shoulder pain (Meyers, 1988). The pain is often associated with impingement of the supraspinatus tendon below the coracoacromial arch (Fig. 3.6). Occasionally the tendon of the long head of biceps brachii is involved (Andrish, 1990). Predisposing sports are swimming, throwing events and racquet sports (Meyers, 1988; Micheli and Fehlandt, 1992; Ryu et al, 1988).

It has been suggested that a more prominent acromion anteriorly and an increase in the amount of inferior angulation of the acromion may be predisposing factors (Neer, 1972). Anterior shoulder instability may cause impingement (Micheli, 1983). Weakened stretched anterior structures allow a traction injury of the rotator cuff tendons to occur and inflammation results.

Figure 3.6 Posterior view of shoulder musculature and anatomy.

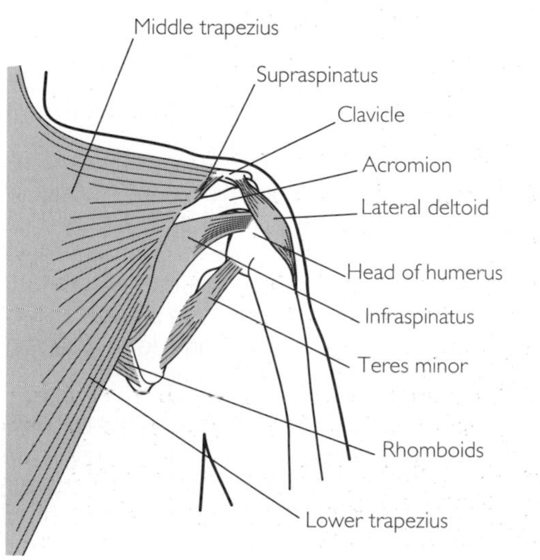

Pre-existing pathology in combination with excessive internal loading of the tendons and capsule may cause swimmer's shoulder (Nirschl, 1986). An associated muscular weakness results. A muscular imbalance about the shoulder joint then causes the humeral head to move superiorly in the glenoid, causing impingement.

Regardless of the cause of swimmer's shoulder, practitioners agree that effective results are achieved via assessment of tight and weak structures and the instigation of appropriate lengthening and subsequently strengthening techniques. Occasionally non-steroidal anti-inflammatory agents are necessary but care with their administration is required. Range of movement exercises and muscle lengthening are commenced within pain limits.

The weak rotator cuff musculature is initially strengthened with the shoulder in less than 90° abduction to prevent impingement pain. Hand weights or elastic exercising equipment may be used through range as inflammation subsides. General shoulder strengthening is also important and as pain subsides and strength improves, exercises above 90° are incorporated into the rehabilitation programme.

Poor biomechanics of the scapula are not uncommon in these patients and weakness is evident in the lower and middle trapezii, rhomboids major and minor. Retraining of scapular rhythm is essential. Lower trapezius strength is particularly important in this group of patients to minimize elevation and upward rotation of the inferior angle of the scapula as the arm is elevated. Scapular retraction and depression exercises often commence in the prone position, progressing to controlled elevation exercises, e.g. abducting the arm slowly and controlling scapular depressions and spinal curvature (Fig. 3.7). As strength improves, exercises can be incorporated into a supervised weight-training programme.

Taping of the scapula is an extremely valuable facilitatory technique as it can provide afferent input to the athlete regarding scapular position. Most common applications of the tape would follow the line of the lower trapezius from the spine of the scapula to the mid-thoracic region (Fig. 3.8). A porous sports tape is commonly used and remains in place for up to three days. Care with skin sensitivity is important and gradual weaning is necessary to allow recruitment of shoulder-stabilizing muscles.

Cervical and thoracic spine pain and stiffness are common in patients who suffer from swimmer's shoulder. Assessment of range of movement, joint pain and stiffness, muscle length and strength as well as neural tension is imperative to prevent recurrence of the symptoms. In the quickly developing female adolescent, self-consciousness about her changing body can cause her to develop a 'round-backed' posture. This results in a narrowing of the sub-acromial arch that can cause impingement with repetitive shoulder elevation. Postural advice is extremely important in this group of girls.

Training regimes and technique must also be assessed as these commonly exacerbate shoulder pain and contribute

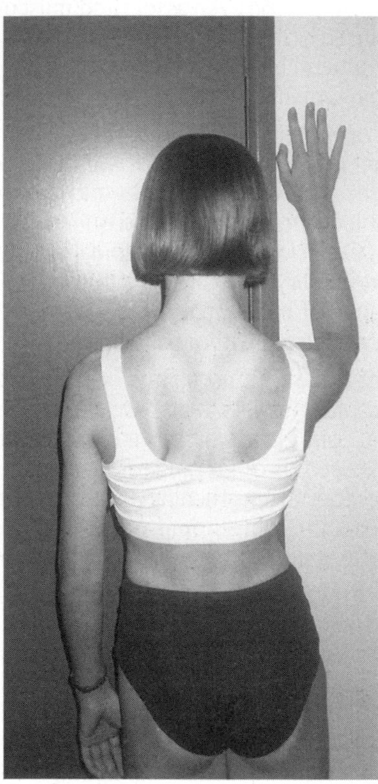

Figure 3.7 Scapular stabilizing muscles can be retrained in function as the arm is elevated. The subject is instructed to stabilize and control scapular and trunk position while slowly elevating the arm. Scapular movement is allowed. The focus is on the time and degree of movement, promoting the stability of the scapula and the coactivity of the serratus anterior and the lower trapezius as upward scapular rotators.

to its tendency to recur. A gradual return to training and competitive levels is required.

Back pain

Persistent back pain should never be ignored in the child or adolescent. Growth is considered to be a major cause of back pain and injuries (Jackson and Cuillo, 1986; Keene and Drummond, 1985; Sward et al., 1990). In periods of rapid growth the hamstrings and lumbar dorsal fascia become tight, causing an alteration in the spine's position. Changes in proprioception from altered afferent feedback may also occur. Rapid changes to joint biomechanics may influence afferent input from the area, thus contributing to alterations in proprioceptive function. In the spinal joints such sensory and motor changes may result in an acute injury during sports activities or lifting.

When bone growth outstrips muscular and ligamentous flexibility recurrent inflammation of the lumbar apophyseal joints and iliac apophysis as well as strains of the extensor musculature can occur (Keene and Drummond, 1985; Sward et al, 1990). Local tenderness is present on palpation and tightness is demonstrated in the hamstrings, lumbar dorsal fascia and hip flexors. Local treatment to relieve joint pain

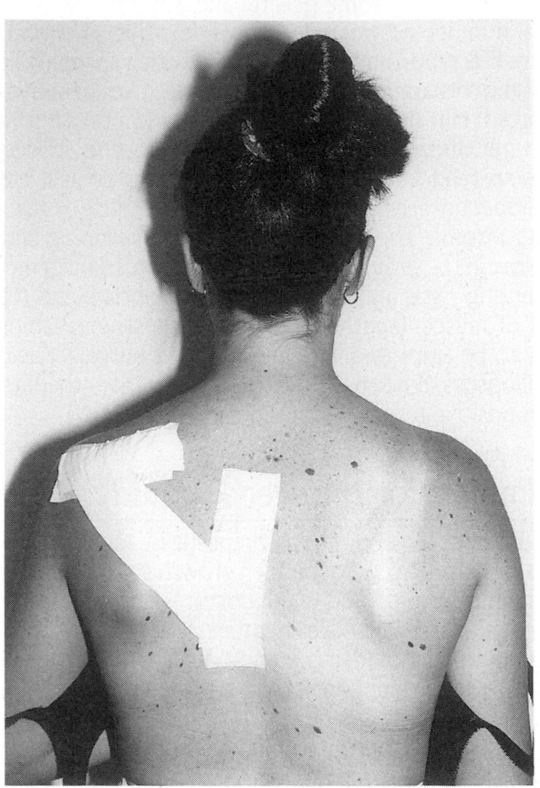

Figure 3.8 Taping of the scapula with rigid strapping tape. The tape should be applied with the scapula in the corrected position and while the subject holds the spine in normal alignment.

and muscular stretches provide good relief. Prophylactic stretching in the growing population will negate the occurrence of lordotic low back pain. Physiotherapists should encourage adolescent patients, especially those who play sport, to carry out a flexibility programme on a daily basis.

The trunk links the upper and lower extremities and in most physical activities one or all limbs are involved in transmitting energy to achieve the requirements of the movement or sporting technique. If the trunk extensors and abdominal muscles are weak, poor support is offered to the spine and an increased tendency towards back injury results. Hamstring and hip flexor length must also be considered. If these muscles are tight the lumbar spine loses its natural lordosis and its ability to transfer forces.

Certain sports predispose the young female athlete to injury. Gymnastics, diving, ballet and skating (both ice and roller) report a high incidence of back injuries and pain (Griffin, 1994). Acute injuries are more common in diving and gymnastics whilst overuse type injuries are common in gymnastics, volleyball, rowing and long-distance running (Goldberg, 1980; Harvey and Tanner, 1991).

In the adolescent most acute back injuries are muscular strains and sprains (Harvey and Tanner, 1991; Jackson and Cuillo, 1986). The mechanism of injury is usually one of lifting and/or twisting. The following case history highlights the signs and symptoms and appropriate treatment regime for adolescents who sustain a back injury of muscular origin.

A 16-year-old gymnast presents with marked tenderness directly over the spinous processes of her first to third lumbar vertebrae with tenderness and spasm of the paraspinal muscles following a training session the day previously that involved back walkovers.

Whilst no pain was felt during training, the girl complained of a 'tired, stiff back' that evening after sitting at her desk and completing homework. On examination, restriction of all movements, but particularly extension and flexion, was evident. Straight-leg raise was reduced to 60° bilaterally with no referred pain but back pain was reproduced with the manoeuvre. Moving from lying to sitting and sitting to standing was painful. Relief was obtained via lying supine and a hot shower.

Treatment included rest and restricted activity within pain limits. Passive physiological intervertebral movements and appropriate electrotherapy were used. As ice irritated the pain, heat was used as an analgesic. Ice is often effective in reducing inflammation. Ranging exercises such as pelvic tilting and supine rotations were instigated within pain limits. Strengthening and stretching exercises were introduced as the pain eased over the next 2–3 days. Treatment was daily for two days and then twice daily for the rest of the week. At this stage activities of daily living were pain free and active movement was full range. Pain was still evident on palpation of the lumbar spine and at the extreme of a straight-leg raise manoeuvre. Gymnastics training was commenced within pain limits at 12 days post-injury. Emphasis on warm-up and stretching programmes, plus a continuation of strengthening work for the abdominal, gluteal and lower back musculature, was reiterated at the final treatment at 17 days.

Sprains and strains respond quickly to effective treatment and the athlete usually returns to sport within two weeks of sustaining the injury. By three weeks the adolescent should have returned to their previous activity levels. If they have persistent back pain it is important that the physiotherapist refers the patient to a medical practitioner to exclude congenital abnormalities or neoplasms.

It is important to note that sedentary adolescents complain more of back pain than their counterparts who engage in unstructured exercise/sport (Salminen et al, 1993). Computer games and television watching may cause posturally related back pain and devotees of these 'sports' require special attention. As girls progress through adolescence the level of activity in organized and recreational sport decreases (Heath et al, 1994). They are therefore more at risk of posturally related back pain than their male counterparts.

Pars interarticularis disorders

Stress fractures of the pars interarticularis (Fig. 3.9), either unilaterally or bilaterally, can occur in young female athletes (Letts et al, 1986). Gymnasts and divers are most commonly affected, with the injury resulting from repetitive lumbar

Figure 3.9 Vertebral anatomy.

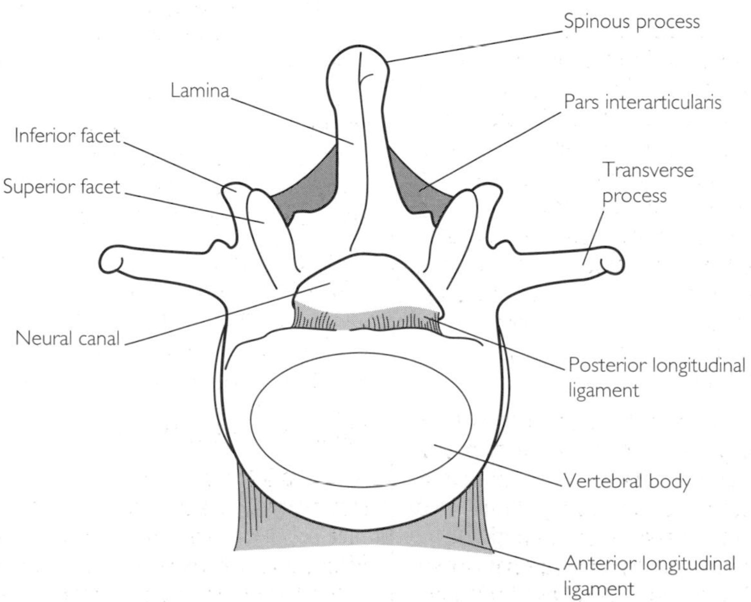

spine flexion and extension. The loading does not need to be great as it is the cyclical behaviour of this movement that creates the stress. It is believed that one side fractures and then, as more load is placed on the opposite pars, an associated microfracture results (Letts et al, 1986). Management is via immobilization, usually in a thoracolumbar spine orthosis.

Back care, posture education and safe lifting techniques are essential components to treatment (Robertson and Lee, 1990). Advice on prevention of injury when playing sport is important. Athletes with unilateral fractures often return to their chosen sports and those with bilateral involvement may also do so with care. The adolescent is advised to avoid contact sports and seek medical attention if a recurrence of symptoms occurs (Letts et al, 1986). If symptoms recur with a chosen sport then the athlete will have to cease that sport or change the activities she performs.

SPONDYLOLYSIS

Spondylolysis is caused by repetitive hyperextension movements of the lumbar spine. The fifth lumbar vertebra is most commonly affected (Letts et al, 1986), with a defect occurring through the pars interarticularis. It may be unilateral, as seen in the throwing sports, such as javelin, judo and diving which involve rotation to one side as the spine is hyperextended. In gymnastics, where back walkovers and dismounts involve pure hyperextension, bilateral defects occur.

The child complains of a chronic ache in the region that is exacerbated by hyperextension and rotation. Extension of the hip also reproduces the pain.

Characteristically, these young athletes have tight hip flexors and hamstrings and weak abdominal muscles. Cessation of the painful activity and rest are required to alleviate the symptoms. Bracing or support with a thoracolumbar spinal orthosis or soft brace is often required and hydrotherapy is useful for pain relief. Strengthening and stretching programmes are commenced as pain settles.

Lumbar facet syndrome

Lumbar facet syndrome can cause acute back pain (Jackson and Cuillo, 1986). As in disorders of the pars interarticularis, it is the result of repetitive hyperextension of the lumbar spine and is seen in sports such as diving and gymnastics. Pain is associated with this condition as the spinal nerves run close to the facet joints and inflammation around these joints results in referred neural pain. Straight-leg raise manoeuvres are always restricted and reproduce pain for this reason. Movement from the forwardly flexed position to neutral reproduces pain. Rest is the initial treatment. Appropriate strengthening of the lumbar stabilizing muscles and stretching of tight musculature is required. Hydrotherapy is extremely beneficial. Occasionally the use of a back support / brace is required to allow pain-free daily activity.

Disc herniations

Whilst intervertebral disc herniations are not common in the adolescent athlete, they have been reported (McKenzie, 1981; Weinert and Rizzo, 1992) and should be considered in the presence of low back or buttock pain +/− leg pain that is difficult to diagnose. The female adolescent who presents with disc herniation is commonly a gymnast. Risk factors are rapid growth spurts and adolescents who are in a high percentile for weight and height (Weinert and Rizzo, 1992). Table 3.6 describes the signs and symptoms and treatment regime for adolescents sustaining discal herniation.

Scoliosis

Idiopathic scoliosis (IS) is the most common spinal deformity in the adolescent female (Fig. 3.10). The spine rotates about its longitudinal axis and deviates laterally (Miyasaki, 1980). Its reported incidence varies between 0.3% and 13.3% depending on the screening protocol implemented (Ebenbichler et al, 1994). The cause of scoliosis is unknown and many hypotheses have been presented. Asymmetry of

Table 3.6 Signs and symptoms and treatment options of disc herniations in adolescents

Signs and symptoms	Treatment options
Decreased forward flexion	Non-steroidal anti-inflammatory drugs
Decreased ipsilateral side flexion	Rest + brace to stabilize region
Flattened lumbar lordosis	Passive extension exercises
+/− Contralateral list	Self-traction
Restricted straight-leg raise	Mechanical traction (prone)
+/− Referred leg pain	Pain-relieving electrotherapy
	Passive physiological intervertebral movements
	Stabilizing exercises, e.g. abdominal hollowing exercises
	Gentle stretching
	Gradual increase in activity and return to sport (within pain limits)
	Surgical intervention a last resort

Figure 3.10 Idiopathic scoliosis. Notice the prominent rib hump on the right in standing. This will be exaggerated in the forward flexed posture.

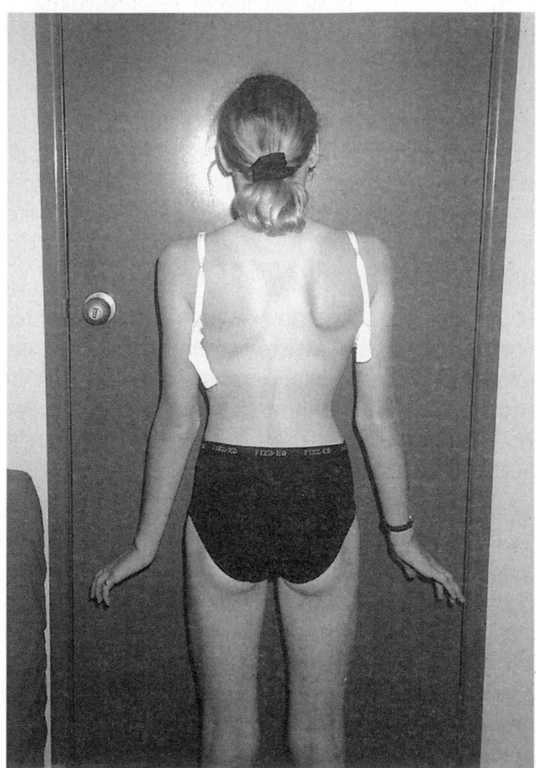

the multifidus muscle group (Kennelly and Stokes, 1993), an increased degree of femoral neck anteversion especially in one limb (Saji et al, 1995), disorders of growth (Goldberg et al, 1993) and disturbances in proprioception +/− generalized joint laxity (Fernandez-Bermejo et al, 1993) have been linked with IS.

It has been shown that girls with IS have a younger age at menarche and an earlier pubertal growth spurt (Goldberg et al, 1993; Hazebroek-Kampschreur et al, 1994). If scoliosis is detected prior to the onset of menarche a better outcome has been seen (Hazebroek-Kampschreur et al, 1994). The type and severity of the curve are also indicative of prognosis (Ebenbichler et al, 1994) and if skeletal maturity has not been reached – as assessed by the development of the ischial apophysis (Risser's sign) – treatment is more likely to be successful (Dhar et al, 1993).

Scoliosis curves can change rapidly and regular monitoring is therefore essential. Management of IS depends on the degree of the presenting curve. Table 3.7 lists the treatment regime of IS according to the extent of the curve.

Physiotherapy input can be invaluable with the compliant patient whose curve is <25°. Postural correction and reinforcement have been shown to be effective with more biologically mature patients, i.e. early onset of menarche (Birbaumer et al, 1994).

Many different braces are used to manage rapidly progressive curves and those between 25° and 45°. Milwaukee (Farady, 1983), Boston (Wynarsky and Schultz, 1989; Ylikoski et al, 1989) and Charleston bending (Price et al, 1990) braces have all been used in the treatment of scoliosis and provide a passive three-point correction of the curve. A brace is worn 23 hours per day to achieve maximum correction whilst some skeletal growth is available (Miyasaki, 1980). As growth slows the brace may be worn for 18 hours per day (Yancey and Micheli, 1994).

Researchers agree that the success of bracing relies on early detection and treatment (Farady, 1983; Focarile et al, 1991; Wynarsky and Schultz, 1989). Results are better if treatment commences before menarche, if a rapid growth spurt occurs before or during treatment (Ylikoski et al, 1989) and if commenced when curves are <30° (Lonstein and Winter, 1994). Bracing has been found to reduce the rib hump associated with IS but the improvement is not substantial enough to improve the cosmetic appearance (Theologis et al, 1993). Once a brace is removed, Montgomery et al (1990) report that IS curves will progress an average of 5.1°. This progression usually occurs within the first two years following cessation of brace wearing.

Routinely, adolescents who require bracing carry out a home exercise programme. Swimming is encouraged as a principal means of fitness, as the buoyancy of the water relieves pressure on the spine. Any non-contact sport, preferably incorporating bilateral arm movements, is encouraged. Specific exercises are taught to improve muscle strength and length but are not designed to correct the

Table 3.7 Management of idiopathic scoliosis according to the degree of curvature

Degree of curvature	Management
<25°	3-monthly review by orthopaedic specialist +/− X-ray, physiotherapy input via exercise and postural correction
Rapidly progressing <25°	Bracing +/− physiotherapy (Ebenbichler et al, 1994)
25–45°	Bracing +/− physiotherapy (Ebenbichler et al, 1994) Lateral electrical surface stimulation (LESS)
>45°	Posterior +/− anterior spinal fusion
Curves unresponsive to conservative treatment Rib humps >15° Curves >60°	Rib resection + spinal fusion (Harvey et al, 1993)

curvature. Improvement in posture is a byproduct of performing the exercise programme. Sensory motor training to encourage appropriate muscular co-ordination of the spine is indicated and should be encouraged. Programmes of progressive exercises for such applications have been developed (Janda and Vavrova, 1994).

After 4–6 weeks of wearing the brace the adolescent attends for an exercise programme. These are initially done out of the brace and are carried out 5–7 times per week. Table 3.8 lists some exercises commonly used. As the adolescent improves, exercises are performed in the brace. More difficult abdominal exercises are introduced. Lateral flexion activities to stretch the trunk are encouraged.

Most adolescents enjoy weight training or aerobics so an exercise programme incorporating these activities assists compliance. Adequate instruction and supervision of these programmes is essential. As muscle length and strength improve the programme must be modified. Physiotherapists are ideally placed to advise on back care, posture and brace wearing and should include these areas in their treatment regime.

Lateral electrical surface stimulation (LESS) has been used in the treatment of adolescent IS since 1977, with many researchers advocating its use. Curve progressions of less than 10° have been reported in up to 65% of patients (Bertrand et al, 1992; Swank et al, 1989).

Researchers report that whilst LESS is an effective means of treating IS curves greater than 30°, there are problems with its application (Bertrand et al, 1992). Physiotherapists using this as a treatment technique must be proficient in the selection of appropriate patients; correct on/off times, intensity of stimulating current and electrode placement are also important. Electrodes are placed at the apex of the curve on the convex side. If positioning is incorrect, the risk of curve progression may be increased. Compliance results are mixed according to various researchers. Skin rashes, sleep disturbances and patient concern regarding correct electrode placement have been reported as negatively affecting compliance (Swank et al, 1989). Others claim that LESS has a better psychological effect on adolescents treated (Bertrand et al, 1992).

If the curve is not held by bracing or LESS, surgery, via rod or segmental instrumentation, is the next mode of treatment. Segmental spinal instrumentation is popular as it affords a three-dimensional correction of the deformity (Bergoin, 1993). Researchers advocate that surgeons ensure that segmental lordosis is maintained in the lumbar spine to allow the spine to withstand the natural ageing process (Bridwell, 1994), as there is evidence to suggest that a loss of spinal length occurs in the skeletally immature girl following spinal fusion (Hsu and Upadhyay, 1994).

Post-operative physiotherapy care aims to prevent respiratory complications and assist in attainment of independent pain-free transfers and mobility. No post-operative immobilization is required unless the scoliosis is particularly severe. Upon discharge, the adolescent often returns for back care advice.

It is important to note that adolescents with IS are more likely to suffer back pain in later life. In a retrospective study where 1476 subjects with IS responded and were compared to a control group, 73% experienced at least one episode of back pain in the previous year compared to 56% in the control group. The IS patients reported more diffuse, constant severe pain and complained more often of limitations in activities of daily living (Mayo et al, 1994). Patients with IS felt that they were not as healthy as their age-related peers, reported more episodes of arthritis and females demonstrated a poorer self-image (Goldberg et al, 1994).

Physiotherapists caring for adolescents with IS play a vital role in back care and postural education. Encouragement of these patients to maintain an active lifestyle and adopt good postural and safe lifting habits is essential. The physiotherapist, in combination with a psychologist, social worker or occupational therapist, may be able to set up exercise classes that positively target body image. As people now live longer, quality of life is precious and prevention plays a major role in physiotherapy care.

Table 3.8 Suggested exercises for conservative treatment of idiopathic scoliosis

Exercise	Aim of treatment
Posterior pelvic tilting	Initiates lower abdominal strength
supine, knees flexed	Stretches back extensors
supine, knees extended	
standing	
Active back extension	Facilitates back strengthening
prone	
push-ups	
Thoracic expansion and extension exercises	Lengthen dorsal thoracic muscles/spine
standing with a deep inspiration	
Straight-leg raise manoeuvres	Lengthen hamstrings/neural structures
Hip extension and abduction activities	Strengthen gluteals
Activities on labile surfaces, balance shoes, wobble boards, gymnastic balls, trampoline	Increase co-ordination of paraspinal muscles and muscles of the pelvis

Kyphosis

Normal values for the thoracic kyphosis are between 20° and 40° of angulation (Sachs et al, 1987). When the curve of the thoracic spine exceeds this, it is described as either a postural kyphosis or Scheuermann's thoracic kyphosis.

Postural kyphosis is a result of tightness in the lumbodorsal fascia, hamstrings and hip flexors. A round-backed posture develops as the adolescent attempts to maintain a centre of balance. Adolescents present with an increased lumbar and cervical lordosis and are unable to extend their thoracic spine when they perform a prone hyperextension manoeuvre. The individual rarely complains of pain but seeks advice because of cosmetic appearance.

Scheuermann's kyphosis (spinal osteochondritis) has a genetic component and is thought to be an autosomal dominant-inherited condition (Baker, 1988). It is not confined only to the thoracic spine and is seen in 20–30% of the population. Incidence is equal in males and females, but males are usually symptomatic, suffering back pain and stiffness. More than three vertebrae must be wedge shaped by more than 5° to classify a curve as a Scheurmann's kyphosis. Vertebral end plate irregularity occurs anteriorly and Schmorl's nodes – herniations of the nucleus pulposus into the vertebral bodies – are present (Baker, 1988).

Researchers report positive results when postural kyphoses with curves <60° are treated via exercise and postural biofeedback (Sachs et al, 1987). If a curve is greater than 70° and progressive, pain and respiratory impairment result. Spinal fusion is the treatment of choice. In a retrospective study Sachs et al (1987) reported a surgical correction initially up to 50% of the measured curve. Two years later, however, a progressive loss of correction was reported.

Treatment of kyphotic curves between 40° and 60° is with a thoracolumbar spinal orthosis. An extension in the form of a breast plate will be added if the curve is high. The brace is worn 18–23 hours per day until growth ceases or the curve reduces to normal values. Exercises are given to improve muscle strength, length and postural control. If the curve is relatively small, exercise alone may be the treatment of choice.

Exercises are directed towards lengthening the lumbodorsal fascia, erector spinae, quadratus lumborum, hamstrings, gluteals, hip flexors and pectoral muscles if found to be tight. Strengthening activities are initiated once flexibility has improved and neck flexors, scapular stabilizing muscles, abdominal groups and gluteals are specifically targeted. Postural setting is a useful way of improving posture. Occasionally taping of the scapulae in a retracted position, with the thoracic spine in slight extension, and the pelvis held in neutral provides proprioceptive and sensory feedback to the adolescent to promote a better posture. Sports underlay is used and can be left in place for up to three days. Care with sensitive skin is essential and gradual weaning from the strapping is important to allow the muscles to reflexly correct the adolescent's flexed posture.

This section has covered common orthopaedic conditions affecting adolescent females. The physiotherapist is in a unique position to treat and educate the teenage girl to minimize the adverse impact of growth on her musculoskeletal system. Appropriate knowledge of the grow ing musculoskeletal system is therefore required by all physiotherapists caring for children and adolescents. It is insufficient to adopt the principles of assessment and treatment used with adults when caring for skeletally immature females.

Hormonal Factors

As well as being a time when significant musculoskeletal changes occur, adolescence is also a time of great hormonal adjustments. Apart from menopause and pregnancy there is no other time in a female's life when such significant hormonal changes take place. Hormonal and orthopaedic factors combine to cause a significant evolution within the young girl's body.

Stages of pubertal development will be discussed in this section. The effect of breast development on posture and pain in the adolescent girl and the effect of menstruation on physical performance will be covered. The impact of increasing levels of the hormone relaxin, which affects ligament laxity and predisposes the female adolescent to joint sprains, will also be discussed.

Tanner's stages of physical development

When treating adolescents, the extent of their physical growth and maturity must be considered. An X-ray of the iliac crest will confirm the potential for bone growth by measuring the amount of ossification at the growth plate (Risser's sign) (Dhar et al, 1993) but clinical observation of development is an effective means of assessing pubertal stages.

Tanner (1962) reports that growth during adolescence is positively correlated with a sequence of changes in the reproductive system. The onset of menses, pubic hair development and breast development follow a pattern. Approximately two years after the commencement of breast development, menses commences. Menstruation occurs when there is a slowing of linear growth. Prior to this slowing, peak height velocity occurs (Barnes, 1975).

Postural implications of breast development

For many girls the attainment of breasts is not without physical complications. In those who have significant breast development, alterations in posture can occur. Many girls are self-conscious about the development of breast tissue. When this is combined with a significant gain in height, they may adopt a round-shouldered posture in an attempt to camouflage their shape.

Pain and stiffness in the thoracic spine can occur and if posture is not corrected the adolescent female can develop a postural kyphosis. The associated compensatory curvatures in cervical and lumbar regions may also lead to neck and low back pain. As previously mentioned, upper limb function may be affected by the biomechanical restrictions of a thoracic kyphosis with overuse injuries of the shoulder as a possible sequelae. A pattern of weakness and tightness may develop in the trunk, shoulder and pelvic girdles. In such a case, a cycle of muscular imbalances and postural problems is created.

Early recognition of postural adaptations to physical changes is an essential role of the physiotherapist. Postural education and training in combination with positive input regarding self-image are warranted. Ideally postural awareness and back care should be practised prior to the pubertal growth spurt. Health and physical education classes in the primary school and early secondary school are the ideal forum for discussion and advice on back care and posture. A programme of active participation in correction of posture is essential to build the necessary individual kinaesthetic awareness of appropriate joint positions.

Many adolescent females who have significant breast development complain of breast pain when undertaking their sporting activities (Griffin, 1994). Running and jumping sports cause most problems. Often all that is required is good sports underwear to provide maximum support.

Recent literature suggests that females participate less in sport as they mature (Heath et al, 1994). One of the reasons for this may be that pubertal girls are self-conscious in displaying their developing body in swimming costumes and sports outfits.

The segregation of sport from the time of pubertal growth (i.e. 11–12 years of age) may not only be appropriate because of the inequality in strength and speed between males and females, but also because it allows the developing girl to gain confidence in her changing physical appearance.

The effect of menstruation on athletic performance

There is no scientific evidence to suggest that menstruation affects athletic performance. Some of the best results in Olympic games have been from women who were menstruating whilst competing (Thomas, 1974). Anecdotally, some females report that they do not perform as well at their chosen sport when they menstruate. Most commonly reported are complaints of abdominal cramps and discomfort, breast tenderness, fluid retention and back pain. Emotionally the athletes complain that they are irritable, depressed and often fatigued. It is worth considering that the risk for injury increases with fatigue.

Athletes have also reported sustaining more musculoskeletal injuries and having impaired co-ordination when menstruating (Mickan, 1993). It must be stressed that these phenomena have not been scientifically proven, but the recognition of impaired performance in individuals during menstruation should not be ignored.

Adolescents should not be dissuaded from exercising because of menstruation. Some young females may not use tampons because of cultural or religious beliefs and obviously swimming is difficult for this group when menstruating. Sympathy is important and they should not be forced to participate. All aspects of life require good hygiene. Reinforcement of cleanliness whilst menstruating is vital and regular changing of sanitary protection should be encouraged, especially when partaking in physical exercise.

The effect of relaxin on ligaments and muscles

In females the onset of puberty comes with an increase in the hormone relaxin which affects the ligaments and muscles (Carbon, 1992). As a result females have more ligamentous laxity than males which, in combination with the aforementioned biomechanical changes seen during growth in the adolescent female, increases their risk of ligamentous injury.

Physiotherapists caring for teenage girls with pre-existing ligament sprains need to be aware of this predisposition to reinjury as a result of increased levels of circulating relaxin. Re-education of body awareness in combination with appropriate strengthening is an integral part of treatment. Janda (personal communication) has noted clinically the marked change in gait patterns in adolescent females as the pelvic stability alters with ligamentous changes. Often, it is at this stage of life that females develop excessive anterior tilt and lateral pelvic shift associated with the stance phase of gait. Such a gait pattern in itself is likely to lead to development of pelvic girdle and trunk muscle imbalance which may be a precursor to later pain syndromes (Bullock-Saxton et al, 1994).

Relaxin also has an effect on muscle tissue. Adolescence is an ideal time to commence education on the role of the pelvic floor and the means of maintaining its function (see Chapters 7 and 8 more information).

The physiotherapist who cares for adolescent females requires a working knowledge of the orthopaedic and hormonal changes that occur during puberty. Conditions that are unique to this group require accurate assessment and precise treatment to prevent any long-term deleterious effects. This section has highlighted the more frequently seen orthopaedic conditions of adolescent females and the impact of hormonal changes on this group.

References

Anderson SJ (1991) Acute knee injuries in young athletes. *The Physician and Sportsmedicine* **19(11)**: 69–76.

Andrish JT (1990) Upper extremity injuries in the skeletally immature athlete. In: Nicholas JA & Hershman EB (eds) *Upper Extremity in Sports Medicine*, pp. 673–688. St Louis: C.V. Mosby.

Baker KG (1988) Scheuermann's disease. A review. *Australian Journal of Physiotherapy* **34(3)**: 165–169.

Barnes HV (1975) Physical growth and development during puberty. *Medical Clinics of North America* **59**: 1305–1317.

Bergoin M (1993) Management of idiopathic scoliosis in children. *Annals of Pediatrics (Paris)* **40(4)**: 259–269.

Bertrand SL, Drvaric DM and Lange N (1992) Electrical stimulation for idiopathic scoliosis. *Clinical Orthopaedics and Related Research* **276**: 176–181.

Birbaumer N, Flor H, Cevey B et al (1994) Behavioral treatment of scoliosis and kyphosis. *Journal of Psychosomatic Research* **38(6)**: 623–628.

Bridwell KH (1994) Surgical treatment of adolescent idiopathic scoliosis: the basics and the controversies. *Spine* **19(9)**: 1095–1100.

Bullock-Saxton JE, Janda V and Bullock MI (1994) Reflex activation of the gluteal muscles in walking. *Spine* **18**: 704–708.

Butler, DS (1991) *Mobilisation of the Nervous System*. Melbourne: Churchill Livingstone.

Caine DJ and Broekhoff J (1987) Maturity assessment: a viable preventive measure against physical and psychological insult to the young athlete? *The Physician and Sportsmedicine* **15**: 67–80.

Carbon RJ (1992) The female athlete. In: Bloomfield J, Fricker PA and Fitch KD (eds) *Textbook of Science and Medicine in Sport*, pp. 467–487. Carlton: Blackwell Scientific Publications.

Carter SR and Aldridge MJ (1988) Stress injury of the distal radial growth plate. *Journal of Bone and Joint Bone Surgery* **70-B(5)**: 834–836.

Dhar S, Dangerfield PH, Dorgan JC et al (1993) Correlation between bone age and Risser's sign in adolescent idiopathic scoliosis. *Spine* **18(1)**: 14–19.

Ebenbichler G, Liederer A and Lack W (1994) Scoliosis and its conservative treatment possibilities. *Wien Med Wochenschr* **144(24)**: 593–604.

Elliott B (1991) *Adolescent Overuse Sporting Injuries: A Biomechanical Review.* Australian Council for Health, Physical Education and Recreation. National Conference Proceedings.

Farady JA (1983) Current principles in the nonoperative management of structural adolescent idiopathic scoliosis. *Physical Therapy* **63(4)**: 512–522.

Fernandez-Bermejo E, Garcia-Jimenez MA, Fernandez-Palomeque C et al (1993) Adolescent idiopathic scoliosis and joint laxity. A study with somatosensory evoked potentials. *Spine* **18(7)**: 918–922.

Focarile FA, Bonaldi A, Giarolo M et al (1991) Effectiveness of nonsurgical treatment for idiopathic scoliosis. Overview of available evidence. *Spine* **16(4)**: 395–401.

Goldberg CJ, Dowling FE and Fogarty EE (1993) Adolescent idiopathic scoliosis – early menarche, normal growth. *Spine* **18(5)**: 529–535.

Goldberg MJ (1980) Gymnastic injuries. *Orthopedic Clinics of North America* **11**: 717–726

Goldberg MS, Mayo NE, Poitras B et al (1994) The Ste-Justine Adolescent Idiopathic Scoliosis Cohort Study. Part II: Perception of health, self and body image, and participation in physical activities. *Spine* **19(14)**: 1562–1572.

Griffin LY (1994) The young female athlete In: Stanitski CL, DeLee JC and Drez Jr D (eds) *Pediatric and Adolescent Sports Medicine*, vol. 3, pp. 16–23. Philadelphia: W.B. Saunders.

Harvey Jr CJ, Betz RR, Clements DH et al (1993) Are there indications for partial rib resection in patients with adolescent idiopathic scoliosis treated with Cotrel-Dubousset instrumentation? *Spine* **18(12)**: 1593–1598.

Harvey J and Tanner S (1991) Low back pain in young athletes: a practical approach. *Sports Medicine* **12(6)**: 394–406.

Hazebroek-Kampschreur AA, Hofman A, van Dijk AP et al (1994) Determinants of trunk abnormalities in adolescence. *International Journal of Epidemiology* **23(6)**: 1242–1247.

Heath GW, Pratt M, Warren CW et al (1994) Physical activity patterns in American high school students. Results from the 1990 Youth Risk Behavior Survey. *Archives of Pediatric and Adolescent Medicine* **148(11)**: 1131–1136.

Highet R (1989) Athletic amenorrhea: an update on aetiology, complications and management. *Sports Medicine (Auckland)* **7(2)**: 82–108.

Hsu LC and Upadhyay SS (1994) Effect of spinal fusion on growth of the spine and lower limbs in girls with adolescent idiopathic scoliosis: a longitudinal study. *Journal of Pediatric Orthopedics* **14(5)**: 564–568.

Ireland ML and Hutchinson MR (1995) Upper extremity injuries in young athletes. *Clinics in Sports Medicine* **14(3)**: 533–569.

Jackson DW and Cuillo JV (1986) Injuries of the spine in the skeletally immature athlete. In: Nicholas JA and Hershman EB (eds) *The Lower Extremity and Spine in Sports Medicine*, pp. 1333–1374. St Louis: C.V. Mosby.

Jacobsen T and Allen WC (1990) Surgical correction of the snapping iliopsoas tendon. *American Journal of Sports Medicine* **18**: 470.

Janda V and Vavrova M (1994) Sensory motor stimulation: a video. Body Control Systems Australia, Brisbane.

Karlin LI (1986) Injuries to the hip and pelvis in the skeletally immature athlete. In: Nicholas JA and Hershman EB (eds) *The Lower Extremity and Spine in Sports Medicine*, pp. 1292–1332. St Louis: C.V. Mosby.

Keene JS and Drummond DS (1985) Mechanical back pain in the athlete. *Comprehensive Therapy* **11**: 7–14.

Kennelly K and Stokes MJ (1993) Pattern of asymmetry of paraspinal muscle size in adolescent idiopathic scoliosis examined by real-time ultrasound imaging. A preliminary study. *Spine* **18(7)**: 913–917.

Letts M, Smallman T, Afanasiev R et al (1986) Fracture of the pars interarticularis in adolescent athletes. A clinical–biomechanical analysis. *Journal of Pediatric Orthopedics* **6**: 40–46.

Lonstein JE and Winter RB (1994) The Milwaukee brace for the treatment of adolescent idiopathic scoliosis. A review of one thousand and twenty patients. *Journal of Bone and Joint Surgery* **76(8)**: 1207–1221.

Mayo NE, Goldberg MS, Poitras B et al (1994) The Ste-Justine Adolescent Idiopathic Scoliosis Cohort Study. Part III: Back pain. *Spine* **19(14)**: 1573–1581.

McConnell J (1986) The management of chondromalacia patellae. A long term solution. *Australian Journal of Physiotherapy* **32(4)**: 215–223.

McKenzie RA (1981) *The Lumbar Spine. Mechanical Diagnosis and Therapy.* Lower Hutt, New Zealand: Spinal Publications.

Meyers JF (1988) Injuries to the shoulder girdle and elbow. In: Sullivan JA and Grana WA (eds) *The Pediatric Athlete*, pp. 143–153. Park Ridges, IL: American Academy of Orthopedic Surgeons.

Micheli LJ (1983) Overuse injuries in children's sports: the growth factor. *Orthopedic Clinics of North America* **14**: 337–360.

Micheli LJ (1989) Elbow pain in a little league pitcher. In: Smith NJ (ed) *Common Problems in Pediatric Sports Medicine*, pp. 233. Chicago: Yearbook Publishers.

Micheli LJ and Fehlandt AF (1992) Overuse injuries to tendons and apophyses in children and adolescents. *Clinics in Sports Medicine* **11(4)**: 713–726.

Micheli LJ and Ireland ML (1987) Prevention and management of calcaneal apophysitis in children: an overuse syndrome. *Journal of Pediatric Orthopedics* **7(1)**: 34–38.

Mickan P (1993) *The Sporting Cycle: The Hormonal Factor and Elite Women Athletes.* Adelaide: Department of Recreation and Sport.

Miyasaki AA (1980) Immediate influence of the thoracic flexion exercise on vertebral position in Milwaukee brace wearers. *Physical Therapy* **60(8)**: 1005–1009.

Montgomery F, Willner S and Appelgren G (1990) Long-term follow-up of patients with adolescent idiopathic scoliosis treated conservatively: an analysis of the clinical value of progression. *Journal of Pediatric Orthopedics* **10(1)**: 48–52.

Neer CS II (1972) Anterior instability for the chronic impingement syndrome in the shoulder: A preliminary report. *Journal of Bone and Joint Surgery* **54(A)**: 41–50.

Nirschl RP (1986) Shoulder tendinitis. In: Pettrone FA (ed) *Symposium on Upper Extremity Injuries in Athletes*, Chapter 28. St Louis: C.V. Mosby.

O'Neill DB, Micheli LJ and Warner JP (1992) Patellofemoral stress: a prospective analysis of exercise treatment in adolescents and adults. *American Journal of Sports Medicine* **20(2)**: 151–155.

Paletta GA and Andrish JT (1995) Injuries about the hip and pelvis in the young athlete. *Clinics in Sports Medicine* **14(3)**: 591–628.

Parfitt AM (1994) The two faces of growth: benefits and risks to bone integrity. *Osteoporosis International* **4**: 382–398.

Price CT, Scott DS, Reed Jr FE et al (1990) Nighttime bracing for adolescent idiopathic scoliosis with the Charleston bending brace. Preliminary Report. *Spine* **15(12)**: 1294–1299.

Robertson HC and Lee VL (1990) Effects of back care lessons on sitting and lifting by primary students. *Australian Journal of Physiotherapy* **36(4)**: 245–248.

Roche AF and Davila GH (1972) Late adolescent growth in stature. *Pediatrics* **50**: 874–880.

Ryu RK, McCormick J, Jobe FW et al (1988). An electromyographic analysis of shoulder function in tennis players. *American Journal of Sports Medicine* **16(5)**: 481–485.

Sachs B, Bradford D, Winter R et al (1987) Scheuermann kyphosis. Follow-up of Milwaukee brace treatment. *Journal of Bone and Joint Surgery* **69-A(1)**: 50–57.

Saji MJ, Upadhyay SS and Leong JC (1995) Increased femoral neck-shaft angles in adolescent idiopathic scoliosis. *Spine* **20(3)**: 303–311.

Salminen JJ, Oksanen A, Maki P et al (1993) Leisure time physical activity in the young. Correlation with low back pain, spinal mobility and trunk muscle strength in 15-year-old school children. *International Journal of Sports Medicine* **14**: 406–410.

Schmidt DR and Henry JH (1989) Stress injuries of the adolescent extensor mechanism. *Clinics in Sports Medicine* **8(2)**: 343–355.

Smith AD and Tao SS (1995) Knee injuries in young athletes. *Clinics in Sports Medicine* **14(3)**: 629–650.

Stanish WD (1995) Lower leg foot and ankle injuries in young athletes. *Clinics in Sports Medicine* **14(3)**: 651–668.

Strizak AM and Stroberg AJ (1986) Knee injuries in the skeletally immature athlete. In: Nicholas JA and Hershman EB (eds) *The Lower Extremity and Spine in Sports Medicine*, pp. 1261–1291. St Louis: C.V. Mosby.

Swank SM, Brown JC, Jennings MV and Conradi C (1989) Lateral electrical surface stimulation in idiopathic scoliosis. Experience in two private practices. *Spine* **14(12)**: 1293–1295.

Sward L, Eriksson B and Peterson L (1990) Anthropometric characteristics, passive hip flexion, and spinal mobility in relation to back pain in athletes. *Spine* **15**: 376–382.

Tanner JM (1962) *Growth at Adolescence*, 2nd edn. Oxford: Blackwell Scientific Publications.

Theologis TN, Jefferson RJ, Simpson AH et al (1993) Quantifying the cosmetic defect of adolescent idiopathic scoliosis. *Spine* **18(7)**: 909–912.

Thomas CL (1974) Special problems of the female athlete. In: Ryan AJ and Allman FL Jr (eds) *Sports Medicine*, pp. 347–373. New York: Academic Press.

Weinert AM and Rizzo TD (1992) Nonoperative management of multilevel lumbar disk herniations in the adolescent athlete. *Mayo Clinic Proceedings* **67**: 137–141.

Wotjys EM (1987) Sports injuries in the immature athlete. *Orthopedic Clinics of North America* **18(4)**: 689–694.

Wynarsky GT and Schultz AB (1989) Trunk muscle activity in braced scoliosis patients. *Spine* **14(12)**: 1283–1286.

Yancey RA and Micheli LJ (1994) Thoracolumbar spine injuries in pediatric sports. In: Stanitski CL, DeLee JC and Drez Jr D (eds) *Pediatric and Adolescent Sports Medicine*, pp. 169–170. Philadelphia: W.B. Saunders.

Ylikoski M, Peltonen J and Poussa M (1989) Biological factors and predictability of bracing in adolescent idiopathic scoliosis. *Journal of Pediatric Orthopedics* **9(6)**: 680–683.

4

Diet and Exercise for the Adolescent

MELISSA HEWITT-LOCKE

Normal Dietary Requirements during the Growth Spurt and Risk Factors
•
The Importance of Appropriate Exercise to the Adolescent Female
•
Exercise: Skeletal Integrity versus Skeletal Damage
•
Exercise, Menstruation and Reproductive Function
•
The Impact of Exercise in Adolescence on Adult Health
•
Psychological Benefits of Exercise

Adolescence is a time of massive growth potential. Apart from early infancy, no other time in life can compare with the physical maturation and sexual development that occurs in adolescence (Bergen-Cico and Short, 1992). Adequate dietary intake of nutrients, vitamins and minerals as well as participation in physical activity assist the adolescent in achieving sexual development, peak height and adequate levels of physical fitness (Bergen-Cico and Short, 1992; Prentice and Bates, 1994).

Patterns of adult behaviour including dieting and concepts of health and wellness are established in late childhood and early adolescence (Bull, 1992; Kelder et al, 1994). The family unit plays a vital role in influencing the teenager with respect to health behaviours and dieting (Rossow and Rise, 1994). It is essential, therefore, that adolescents (and their parents) are informed about a well-balanced diet and develop good eating habits to achieve their full growth potential (Bergen-Cico and Short, 1992; Prentice and Bates, 1994). Health risks of adulthood that are associated with a poor or inadequate diet in the teen years, such as coronary heart disease, arthritis, osteoporosis and some cancers, may then be minimized (Moore et al, 1992; Must et al, 1992; Panico et al, 1987; Withers et al, 1987).

Exercise has been shown to have positive effects on bone modelling (Frost, 1992) and prevention of osteoporosis (De Cree et al, 1991; Welten et al, 1994). It has been argued that too much exercise in the adolescent female can lead to menstrual problems and increase the risk of stress fractures and is often associated with inappropriate dieting behaviours (Highet, 1989). Participation in physical exercise from an early age improves fitness and minimizes the risk of obesity. It has been shown that the overweight adolescent often becomes the obese adult (Brouhard, 1995) and associated with this are the previously mentioned health risks (Must et al, 1992).

In this chapter the importance of a normal diet and appropriate exercise to the adolescent female will be discussed. Physiotherapists are often involved in caring for teenage sporting teams as well as seeing adolescent girls in the clinical setting. It is therefore essential that the practitioner has a working knowledge of appropriate dietary and exercise requirements so that patients may be advised on correct habits. Patients requiring individual assistance should be referred to a dietitian / nutritionist.

Normal Dietary Requirements during the Growth Spurt and Risk Factors

In this section basic nutrition will be discussed, including energy requirements for adolescent females. Special reference to calcium and iron levels will be made. Dietary supplements will also be discussed. The differing dietary requirements of the elite adolescent athlete as opposed to the sedentary adolescent girl will be highlighted.

It is important that dietary information is readily available for young girls. In a longitudinal study of adolescent smoking, physical activity and food choice behaviours, Kelder et al (1994) concluded that there is an 'early consolidation of health behaviour'. The authors of this study believe that because adult health behaviours are set down at an early age, education and intervention should begin prior to 11–12 years of age. Schmalz (1993) found that adolescents involved in at least one sporting activity were unaware of the principles of a good diet as well as the unique caloric and nutritional demands of their chosen sport. This being the case, health professionals in contact with young athletes must reinforce sound dietary advice.

Basic nutrition

No two people have the same energy requirements as individual resting metabolic rates and levels of activity vary. Body size also plays a major part in energy requirements (Grandjean, 1990). It is generally recommended that an adolescent female of 11–15 years of age with a mean weight of 42 kg requires 10 400 kJ per day to ensure complete bone and tissue growth. Girls from 15–18 years of age (mean body weight 55 kg) have a requirement of 9200 kJ per day (Bourke, 1992). It is important that adolescents have a well-balanced diet including varying amounts of foods from the major food groups. The balance of food groups generally advocated appears in Table 4.1.

It is recommended that the sources of energy include:

1. Carbohydrates 50–60%
2. Protein 10–15%
3. Fats 30–35%

The adolescent athlete who trains at a moderate intensity will require 60–70% of their energy intake as carbohydrates. Very few adults, let alone adolescents, know how much food contains the necessary amounts of carbohydrates. Adolescents require precise information on food intake to meet the demands of growth and exercise.

The growing teenager requires 2 g of protein for every kilogram of body weight. Whilst fat is a major source of energy, high-fat diets are not recommended as they increase the risk of obesity, heart disease and some cancers (Grandjean, 1990; Moore et al, 1992).

Calcium requirements

It is well accepted that calcium intake is an important area of nutritional concern for females. Calcium is essential not only for the development of strong bones but also for the attainment of full growth. Calcium also affects the contractility of muscle and the transmission of nerve impulses.

Prentice and Bates (1994), in their study of children and adolescents in Third World countries, concluded that inadequate dietary intakes of calcium may result in linear growth (i.e. peak height) retardation. Zinc and phosphorus are also essential for peak height attainment, as is magnesium for bone development (Bergen-Cico and Short, 1992).

Soroko et al (1994) have shown a positive correlation between lifetime milk consumption and bone mineral density (BMD) in adolescent females and adult women. A positive effect on BMD was seen in both the appendicular skeleton (measured at the mid-radius) and the axial skeleton (spine) in regular milk drinkers. If inadequate amounts of calcium are consumed during the teenage and early adult years, BMD in later life is commonly reduced (see Chapter 32 for further details).

Recommended daily allowances (RDA) of calcium for females

Age	*Milligrams of calcium (mg)*
12–15 years	1000 mg
16–18 years	800 mg
Athletic adolescents	1000–1500 mg (Bourke, 1992)

Table 4.1 The recommended balance of food groups per day

Small amounts	Moderate amounts	Large amounts
Alcohol	Fish	Bread / cereals
Fats / oils	Meat	Legumes
Sugar	Chicken	Potatoes
	Nuts	Rice
	Eggs	Pasta / noodles
	Milk	Fruit / juice
	Cheese	
	Yoghurt	

Adolescent females involved in high-level sport and therefore training on a daily basis benefit from calcium supplementation to their diet. No deleterious effects have been reported and the positive benefits on bone growth and maintenance cannot be ignored.

Table 4.2 lists foods that provide approximately 200 mg of calcium per serving.

Table 4.2 Foods providing 200 mg of calcium

Food	Quantity
Baked beans	2 cups
Hard cheese	25 g
Low fat milk	125 ml
Sardines (with bones)	35 g
Soya milk	140 ml
Tofu	160 g
Yoghurt	125 ml

Adolescent females are often concerned about body image and are loath to eat dairy products because of the associated fat content. Reduced-fat dairy products are a good source of calcium and can be fortified with extra calcium. Lactose-intolerance sufferers can include soya milk in their diet to ensure adequate calcium intake.

Too much protein and salt in a diet will affect calcium retention. Excessive amounts of alcohol, caffeine, unprocessed bran and foods rich in oxalate (such as spinach) will affect the body's capacity to absorb calcium. It is imperative that a patient who requires dietary advice is referred to a nutritionist/dietitian.

Iron requirements

Iron plays an important role in the production of the body's energy. It is an essential component of haemoglobin, which transports oxygen in the blood. Adolescents involved in aerobic activities therefore require adequate amounts of iron in their diet. There are two main forms of dietary iron. Haem iron is easily absorbed in the body whilst non-haem iron requires animal sources of protein and vitamin C to assist absorption. Excessive amounts of caffeine, tannins and fibre in the diet reduce the body's capacity to absorb non-haem iron.

Table 4.3 Recommended daily allowances (RDA) of iron for childhood and adolescents and foods providing 2 mg per serving.

Children	**6–8 mg**
Adolescents	**10–13 mg**
Food	*Quantity*
Lean beef	50 g
Chicken	200 g
Liver	20 g
Spinach	1/2 cup

Table 4.3 indicates the recommended daily allowance of iron for children and adolescents, as well as those foods that provide 2 mg of iron per serving.

Iron-rich foods

Haem iron foods	*Non-haem iron foods*
Red meat	Breakfast cereals
Poultry	Rice
Seafood	Pasta
Liver*	Bread
Kidney*	Vegetables and legumes
	Fruit
	Tofu

*Denotes richest sources of iron

Anaemia occurs when the blood iron levels and the stores of iron in the body (serum ferritin) are reduced. It is more common in females because of iron lost during menstruation. Females are also more likely to restrict their intake of red meat because of the perceived increased fat content of this food. As red meat is an excellent source of iron, these women often have inadequate intakes of iron.

An increase in iron loss may occur when strenuous exercise is performed. Increased sweating and urine output, as well as destruction of blood cells, are the causes. Iron stores also are reduced as a consequence of the growth spurt (Grandjean, 1990). When treating female adolescent athletes, it is important to be aware of the signs of early anaemia, which include impaired athletic performance and fatigue.

Fatigue increases the likelihood of sustaining injury. Physiotherapists can minimize this risk by ensuring that their patients are aware of the association between fatigue, injury and reduced iron stores. Reduced ferritin levels can impair athletic performance, commonly seen in endurance events (Rowland et al, 1987).

This is highlighted by the results of a study by Nelson et al (1994). These researchers found that 20% of a sample of 114 11–14-year-old schoolgirls demonstrated mild anaemia and compromised physical performance during a step test with a slower return to resting heart rate at 1 minute post-testing.

If anaemia is untreated, symptoms worsen. The athlete commonly complains of shortness of breath and dizziness. It is important that athletes are screened pre-season to exclude pre-existing anaemia and also mid-season, especially if training is intense and/or the athlete is complaining of the aforementioned symptoms (Rowland et al, 1987).

Magazanik et al (1990) report that there is a high incidence of serum iron deficiency in female athletes. In their study of young female athletes involved in intensive training, they concluded that their serum ferritin and haematological status improved when daily iron supplements were given in the training period. If iron supplements are used, regulation by a doctor or nutritionist is essential and an iron-rich diet must be enforced.

Dieting

Two-thirds of adolescent girls are unhappy with their weight and body shape (Moore, 1993). Dieting is becoming more frequent in younger age groups. In a study of 9- and 14-year-olds Hill et al (1992) found that girls in both age groups equally expressed unhappiness with their body shape and weight. Their perceived 'ideal' body was slimmer than their existing body shape and that of non-dieters in the group. Half of the sample were 'of average or below average weight index for their age' (Hill et al, 1992).

It is believed that the unavoidable change in body shape at the start of puberty leads to poor self-esteem. This triggers the teenage girl into a dieting behaviour (Koff and Rierdan, 1993). Advertising and reporting in adolescent women's magazines has changed from 1970 to 1990, with a heightened awareness of physical fitness and a concomitant tendency towards leaner, more streamlined models (Guillen and Barr, 1994). The message the media send teenage girls is that a slim svelte body is the norm. To counter the media image, the provision of educational programmes to encourage adolescents to adopt healthy eating habits and exercise is promoted by Emmons (1994). The need for dieting at such an early age is then avoided.

Regular smoking by adolescents to control their body weight and appetite has been reported by Camp et al (1993). In a study of 659 American high school students, 39% of females and 12% of males used smoking to decrease their appetite, with the females also adopting restrained eating patterns. This societal trend is interesting and disturbing. The health risks associated with smoking are great. Education again plays a vital role in preventing adolescents adopting unhealthy practices.

Adolescent females involved in particular sports are more prone to dieting than their non-sporting counterparts, with female athletes reported as being at higher risk of developing eating disorders (Taub and Blinde, 1992). In a study of competitive swimmers aged 9–18 years, Dummer et al (1987) found that 41% attempted to reduce their weight and 17.5% tried to increase their body weight. Of the group, only 16.5% were overweight and 16.6% were underweight. They concluded that the swimmers were encouraged to perform to the best of their ability whilst reducing their percentage body weight. The swimmers reported that most pressure came from parents, friends and to a lesser extent coaches. The concern lies in the fact that even the skeletally immature athletes in this sample were encouraged to diet.

Swimming is usually considered a sport that has fewer problems with dieting. Ballet, gymnastics and athletics are sports that promote a slim body image. Clarkson et al (1985) studied adolescent female ballet dancers and found that their mean percent body fat was 16.4, significantly less than non-athletic controls. More disturbing, however, was an 'average absolute total caloric intake 25% lower than the recommended intake' (Clarkson et al, 1985).

Adolescents participating in high-level sport have increased energy requirements and therefore must be careful to adopt a complete diet. Endurance athletes (e.g. cross-country runners and long-distance swimmers) require more carbohydrate and protein in their diet. Power- and strength-related sports require more protein and a general increase in caloric intake to support muscular development (Grandjean, 1990).

Dietary supplements

A well-balanced diet including a variety of foods from the five food groups ensures that nutrient requirements are met.

The non-sporting adolescent rarely uses dietary supplements but those who play competitive sport and indeed adolescents aspiring to elite sports participation actively seek vitamin/mineral supplements. Sobal and Marquart (1994) administered a questionnaire to 742 adolescent athletes and found that 38% used vitamin/mineral supplements. Reasons for their use included improved athletic performance, treatment of illness and maintenance of healthy growth. Of these athletes, 62% believed that supplement use improved athletic performance.

Research has shown that vitamin and mineral supplementation above the RDA does not improve athletic performance (Grandjean, 1990). Athletes with high-energy diets are usually consuming more than the RDA of vitamins and minerals from their diet alone. Webster and Barr (1995), in a study of adolescent female gymnasts and speed skaters, found that calcium intake was greater in the sports groups than in a control group of normally active adolescents.

Recent research has looked at the benefits of nutritional antioxidants on improved athletic performance. It has been suggested that when antioxidants are ingested, performance is improved in athletes who participate in high-intensity sports that require repeatable efforts (Kanter and Williams, 1995). Sprint swimming and cycling are good examples of these sports. More adolescents are looking at antioxidants as a viable means of improving sports performance. It is important to inform adolescents that whilst antioxidants may have a positive effect on performance, fat-soluble vitamins such as vitamins A, D, E and K can become toxic when ingested in high doses (Grandjean, 1990).

A multivitamin is appropriate when an adolescent must limit their caloric intake for some reason, is unable to eat certain food groups or has poor/unusual dietary preferences (Grandjean, 1990). Often vegetarianism becomes popular with teenage females and these girls may have a diet lacking in vitamins and minerals.

The same arguments about vitamin/mineral supplementation can be used for protein and amino acid supplements. Excessive protein in the diet can result in dehydration and renal and liver disorders (Grandjean, 1990). Recent research suggests that creatine supplementation improves athletic performance in activities that require repeated bouts of high-power exercise (e.g. sprint cyclists and runners). It is also important for athletes who have low dietary concentrations of creatine, such as vegetarians (Greenhaff, 1995).

A healthy diet in adolescence ensures complete bone and tissue development and growth and the appropriate levels of energy to participate in activities of daily life and moderate sporting pursuits. Elite athletes require more kilojoules per day to provide enough energy for their sports participation. If dietary levels of carbohydrates are inadequate fatigue will result (Walberg-Rankin, 1995). This has been demonstrated in aerobic endurance activities that are of medium intensity. Adolescent athletes who are watching their carbohydrate intake because of weight concerns are a target population. It is important to remember that patients are more susceptible to injury when fatigued.

Dieting is a common occurrence in the adolescent female population, with many girls who diet weighing less than their ideal body weight. Education on sound eating and exercise is vital to ensure good health of this population group. Self-esteem is often low in adolescence, with a pubertal change in body shape resulting in dissatisfaction. Hence dieting behaviours are adopted.

Positive reinforcement of personal qualities and participation, rather than physical attributes, is important. Health professionals caring for teenage girls must place emphasis on these factors rather than a slim physique and lean body mass. Athletes involved in sports such as gymnastics and endurance running are extremely susceptible and therefore, extra care must be taken with this subset. Close liaison with a nutritionist or sports physician is important if the practising physiotherapist has concerns about the dietary well-being of a patient.

The Importance of Appropriate Exercise to the Adolescent Female

It has long been established that exercise has positive benefits on the health and well-being of all individuals. In the teenage years regular exercise has been shown to have positive associations with weight control, motor co-ordination, cardiovascular fitness and the development of skeletal integrity and normal muscle tissue (Carbon, 1992). Exercise has also been shown to play an important role in pain management, social development and the psychological well-being of adolescents (Naughton and Carlson, 1995).

Excessive exercise in the form of intensive training, however, can have significant short- and long-term ill effects. Menstrual disturbances including athletic amenorrhoea, stress fractures and growth disturbances, fatigue, overuse injuries and eating disorders have been associated with high levels of exercise (Highet, 1989; Martin and Bailey, 1987; Taub and Blinde, 1992; Theintz et al, 1993). Long-term sequelae may include alterations in fertility, bone density and skeletal integrity.

Debate on the appropriate amount of exercise for adolescent females and its positive and negative effects has many sides. This section will highlight the pros and cons of exercise in the growing female, with special reference to areas of interest for physiotherapy. It is important that health carers, coaches, parents and adolescents themselves consider the benefits of exercise and balance the positive and negative aspects of physical activity.

Appropriate exercise levels in childhood versus puberty

Research shows that athletic ability varies with stages of maturation (Griffin, 1994). Sports involvement up until puberty aims for children to achieve and maintain cardiovascular fitness (Naughton and Carlson, 1995). Pleasure in participating, social interaction and the development of physical skills should be the emphasis of sport in this age group.

It is suggested that up until puberty, sport participation should be non-specific (Griffin, 1994). This allows children to derive enjoyment from a number of sports and minimizes the risk of musculoskeletal stresses of one sport being placed on the physically immature skeleton. Females begin their pubertal development, on average, between 11 and 13 years of age. With puberty a radical change in body shape usually occurs. There is a natural deposition of fat in adolescent females that results in previous sports participation often becoming difficult.

The whip-like 10-year-old gymnast who wins all the competitions may find her chosen sport difficult if she suddenly grows 10 cm in height and physically matures. The adolescent swimmer who physically matures at an earlier age than her peers, however, may suddenly find endurance races easier as an increase in body fat improves buoyancy and reduces the work of her sport.

Playing a number of sports as a child is therefore even more important for females than for males. A broad base of sport skills is ensured and disappointment and a disinclination to continue sports participation if puberty causes an individual's body shape to significantly alter are avoided.

Aerobic power is an indicator of endurance capacity and has been found to improve with training in girls of all ages. It is more marked after the initial growth spurt (peak height velocity – PHV) in boys and girls. The ability to improve aerobic power is at its lowest during the female's growth spurt (Bar-Or, 1988) and this ability reaches a plateau after 14 years of age (Armstrong and Welsman, 1994).

Anaerobic power is an indicator of short burst strength activities. It is significantly lower in childhood, but increases steadily with age. Nindl et al (1994) report that after girls reach 11–12 years of age there is not a marked increase in anaerobic capacity. Bale et al (1992) report that anaerobic power increases linearly throughout adolescence in both males and females up to 18 years. Success in sprint sports and strength-specific weight training is therefore more effective if commenced after puberty.

Exercise capacity of females versus males

In childhood, boys and girls have equal athletic ability and experts agree that up to approximately 11 years of age, coeducational sporting activities are appropriate (Griffin, 1994).

After the pubertal growth spurt, males and females demonstrate significant physical and physiological differences. Teenage girls on average gain less height and weight than their male counterparts. Percentage body fat and muscle mass differ (Griffin, 1994), as demonstrated in Figure 4.1. This results in a lesser ability to generate the power required to propel a greater body weight.

When the above phenomena are combined with the smaller thorax, heart and vital capacity but greater respiratory rate of post-pubertal females, an unequal base exists for post-pubertal male and female athletes to compete. Cardiac output is less because of the smaller heart size and at the same VO_{2max}, females have a higher heart rate. Haemoglobin levels are also lower in the adolescent female. All these factors result in a reduced oxygen-carrying capacity in the female athlete (Van De Loo and Johnson, 1995). At this stage of development it is vital that females are given the opportunity to play sport and be successful in competition. This means that after puberty competitive sport must occur between females and not between the two sexes.

Figure 4.1 Adolescent body fat and muscle mass.

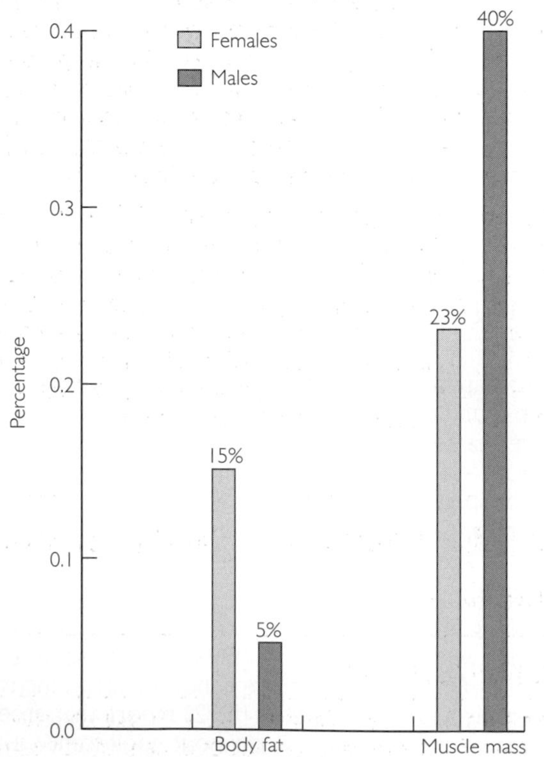

Whilst males have a genetic predisposition to strength, females may require physical activity to attain and maintain strength (Glenmark et al, 1994). This is a further reason why female adolescents should be encouraged to participate in physical activities.

In a study of sport participation in North American high school students, Heath et al (1994) found that 52% of girls did not participate in physical education. Although 43% of boys also did not participate, vigorous activity was more common in boys than girls. As adolescents progressed towards university, sports participation decreased.

Rowland and Freedson (1994) conclude that from the age of six to 16 years there is a 50% decrease in physical activity. The health risks of inactive teenagers when they reach adulthood cannot be ignored. Clinicians agree that a minimum of 20–30 minutes of physical activity 3–5 times per week should be encouraged throughout adolescence and into adult life.

Exercise: Skeletal Integrity versus Skeletal Damage

The effect of exercise on bone growth and stature

As previously mentioned, approximately half of peak adult bone mass is attained during the pubertal growth spurt (Parfitt, 1994). In this time the bone is particularly sensitive to mechanical loading. Adolescence therefore is an important time for weight bearing and physical activity to occur.

Whilst physical exercise is considered vital during the teenage years to achieve high levels of bone density, researchers voice concern regarding too much exercise and its effect on stature and the increased risk of skeletal injuries, especially stress fractures.

The growth and maturity of elite female gymnasts was investigated at the 1987 World Championship Artistic Gymnastics by Claessens et al (1992). A control sample of non-athletic girls aged 13–20 years was also studied. They concluded that gymnasts were significantly shorter and lighter with narrower hips and shoulders. The differences were most apparent after 17 years of age.

A comparison of the growth of female volleyball players and the general population in the 9–13 age range was undertaken by Malina (1994). Volleyball players were significantly taller but near the median for body weight.

The argument on whether stature is affected by early training is heated. Malina (1994) suggests that at elite levels of sport there is a natural selection and those athletes have the physical characteristics required by their sport regardless of sports participation.

In sports where stature is small, the consensus seems to be that heavy training (characterized as more than 18 hours per week) commencing before puberty and continued throughout the teenage years does alter growth rate to an extent that full adult height is not achieved (Theintz et al, 1993).

Gymnastics and ballet are sports where most concern is voiced. The reason for the inhibition of growth is uncertain. Suppression of the hypothalamus–pituitary system (which controls growth) occurs. Exercise in combination with the metabolic effects of dieting are thought to be the cause of this inhibition (Theintz et al, 1993).

An 11-year-old female primary school student is a keen gymnast in the development squad of her sport. She presents to physiotherapy six times over four months with seemingly trivial muscle strains that respond within one treatment. She has been feeling very tired at school and not doing her homework because she is 'just too tired' after training. She has put on a little bit of weight in the last six months and the girls at gymnastics have been teasing her. She is running home from training rather than catching the bus and has taken to missing lunch and not eating meat or desserts if she can feed the dog without Mum seeing.

Her increased levels of activity along with her change in diet have resulted in her being anaemic. Referral to a sports physician and dietitian and a moderate fitness programme are initiated. Her training schedule is discussed with her coach and varied to allow little bouts of activity over a longer training session with more rest days. She is reassured that she will not lose her place in the squad. Her energy levels return to normal over 3–4 months and she ceases having muscular sprains associated with her former fatigue.

Bone mineral density

In the adolescent female osteoporosis refers to inadequate bone formation and early bone loss, resulting in reduced bone mass and an increased susceptibility to fractures. In childhood more bone is laid down than is resorbed. Throughout adolescence the two processes balance each other but bone becomes stronger and thicker.

Physical exercise is essential in adolescence to ensure attainment of peak bone density. A good diet and a regular menstrual cycle also positively affect bone mass. Excessive caffeine and alcohol decrease BMD, as does smoking. Heredity plays a part in the attainment of peak BMD, with small-boned, thin females and those of Asian or Caucasian descent more likely to be affected by osteoporosis.

The relationships between physical activity, dietary calcium, menstrual history and BMD in competitive female college gymnasts was studied by Kirchner et al (1995). Comparison of BMD between this group and anthropometrically matched non-athletes was also investigated. It was found that despite inadequate dietary calcium and a high incidence of menstrual irregularities, the gymnasts had a higher BMD in the axial and appendicular skeleton than the control group.

It is proposed that the mechanical loading that occurs in gymnastics provides a great stimulus for bone mineralization. Although the girls had been training for a long period of time (mean 11.1+/−0.5 years) and had commenced training at a mean age of 6.2+/−0.4 years, the authors argued that physical activity during a time of rapid bone deposition was responsible for the increased BMD in the gymnasts. The hypothesis that females with a genetic predisposition to high BMD may select and be successful at gymnastics is raised.

Many researchers believe that physical exercise is vital because of its positive benefits on BMD (De Cree et al, 1991). The effects of weight-bearing and non-weight-bearing exercise on BMD were examined by McCulloch et al (1992). They compared os calcis BMD in adolescent soccer players and swimmers (males and females). The soccer players had the highest BMD at this site in both sexes. This study supports the belief that weight-bearing exercise is of more benefit in increasing BMD. However, recent clinical work suggests that exercise need not only be weight bearing. Activities that involve large muscle groups, e.g. swimming and cycling, may be as beneficial as weight-bearing activity in improving BMD in the areas that are affected by the muscle groups involved. Research in this area is warranted.

Strength- and power-trained athletes have been shown to have a high bone mineral content (BMC) and BMD (Suominen, 1993). Recent research suggests that in certain strength and power sports, intensive training over many years may increase BMD in specific sites even in the presence of amenorrhoea (see Chapter 6 for information on amenorrhoea). Elite ice skaters have been shown to have increased BMD in the lower skeleton even in the presence of menstrual irregularities (Slemenda and Johnson, 1993).

The effect of weight-bearing activity, daily calcium intake and body weight on the attainment of peak bone mass in males and females from 13 to 27 years of age was examined by Welten et al (1994). They concluded that weight-bearing activity and a normal body weight for age in adolescence and early adult life were essential to achieve the highest peak bone mass possible (in the lumbar spine) by 27 years of age. The debate on exercise and BMD continues.

Exercise, Menstruation and Reproductive Function

Amenorrhoea

There are two types of amenorrhoea. *Primary amenorrhoea* is when the adolescent has not commenced menstruation by 16 years of age. *Secondary amenorrhoea* occurs in the female who has already commenced menses but has 3–6 consecutive months when her periods are absent or has only 3–5 periods per year. This topic is discussed further in Chapter 6.

Since the early 1970s researchers have studied the relationship between physical exercise and amenorrhoea. 'Athletic amenorrhoea' most commonly occurs in sports that are aerobic in nature and require lower body weights and percentage body fats, with athletics, ballet, gymnastics and aerobics being good examples (Highet, 1989).

Whilst intensity of training is linked with amenorrhoea, eating disorders, dieting, psychological and emotional stress and delayed menarche are also important variables to consider (Prior et al, 1992). It is well documented that women who are chronically hypo-oestrogenaemic have accelerated bone loss over time with the most rapid loss (4% per year) occurring just after the cessation of periods (Highet, 1989).

In athletes who suffer amenorrhoea for more than one year, cancellous bone density decreases but cortical bone mass remains the same (Griffin, 1994). This loss of BMD at highly trabecular bone sites (e.g. the navicular) increases the athlete's susceptibility to stress fractures (Martin and Bailey, 1987). Early detection and management of amenorrhoea is therefore essential.

Intensive training before the onset of menstruation is thought to cause amenorrhoea. Amenorrhoeic athletes were compared with athletes with regular menstrual cycles by Baer and Taper (1992). The amenorrhoeic group ran more miles per week, had been training for longer and had commenced training before or at the onset of menses.

The impact of inadequate nutrition on amenorrhoea cannot be ignored. Researchers have shown a positive relationship between a lower caloric intake and amenorrhoea in athletes (Kaiserauer et al, 1989). They maintain that the imbalance between energy intake and output (in terms of exercise intensity) rather than the exercise level itself is more responsible for amenorrhoea.

The good news for athletes is that once the level of training has been reduced or ceased, amenorrhoea rarely continues for more than two months (Stager, 1984). Increased body weight also usually reverses the complaint. Training levels can decrease whilst body weight remains low and menstruation will resume. For the elite athlete who wishes to continue in her sport there is little comfort in these findings. In this group of females oestrogen therapy may be required to prevent the long-term side effect of osteoporosis (Griffin, 1994).

There is no evidence to suggest that an athlete's reproductive function is altered permanently by amenorrhoea (Stager, 1984). Many elite female athletes go on to have a family after episodes of amenorrhoea. The most significant side effect of this condition is the potential loss of bone mineral (as previously mentioned).

It is important to remember that secondary amenorrhoea may not be caused by sports participation. Pregnancy must be excluded in the adolescent athlete as well as emotional stresses, eating disorders and weight loss.

Dysmenorrhoea

Dysmenorrhoea is classified as primary or secondary in nature and describes pain that is experienced during the menstrual cycle. Primary dysmenorrhoea may be uterine or ovarian in nature and it is estimated that it has been experienced by 5–50% of adolescent girls. Secondary dysmenorrhoea is due to pelvic pathology and is outside the scope of this chapter.

Exercise has been associated with a reduction in premenstrual symptoms and pain associated with menstruation (Carbon, 1992). It is believed that the premenstrual symptoms of breast pain, tension and excessive fluid are minimized by exercise.

Reasons that exercising females may suffer less from dysmenorrhoea are:

- reduction of prostaglandins – the uterine pain mediators;
- alterations in central neurotransmitters;
- the release of endorphins that moderate pain;
- an increased resistance to pain that results from fitness training.

In females who suffer from severe dysmenorrhoea, non-steroidal anti-inflammatory drugs are often prescribed. Their antiprostaglandin function reduces period pain. Oral contraception (OCP) may be used to minimize menstrual pain by inhibiting ovulation and thereby lowering prostaglandin levels.

The Impact of Exercise in Adolescence on Adult Health

Obesity in adolescence and childhood has been significantly linked as a risk factor for obesity in adult life (Brouhard, 1995). Traditionally obesity was considered a disorder of food intake, but more evidence supports the importance of energy expenditure in preventing obesity in both the short and long term (King and Tribble, 1991). Obesity not only interferes with physical activity, but also increases the risk of ischaemic heart disease, some cancers and elevated blood pressures (Moore et al, 1992; Must et al, 1992; Withers et al, 1987).

Children of poorer physical fitness demonstrate a significantly higher systolic blood pressure. Increases in physical activity result in lower blood pressures in children and adolescents, with regular physical fitness reducing the risk of coronary artery disease (Panico et al, 1987).

Recent research with females at risk of breast cancer concludes that those who engage in at least 3.8 hours per week of physical exercise from menarche have a reduced risk of breast cancer compared to inactive women (Bernstein et al, 1994). Alteration in ovarian function in response to hormonal changes as a result of exercise is thought to be the cause.

The importance of exercise for long-term health is emphasized. Physiotherapists have a good knowledge base of exercise and fitness. In the area of adolescent health the emphasis should be on prevention of problems. Physiotherapists, in combination with sports scientists and human movement graduates, need to become more involved with general fitness programmes.

Psychological Benefits of Exercise

The psychological benefits of exercise are not exclusive to female adolescents. People regularly engaging in exercise report that they are better able to cope with day-to-day physical and emotional life stresses and have a positive self-image (Griffin, 1994).

The reasons why adolescents persist with exercise were investigated by Douthitt (1994). Overwhelmingly, in the female population studied, reasons included 'perceived global self-worth and perceived physical appearance'.

In a study of pregnant adolescents, Koniak-Griffin (1994) found that an exercising group had a significant increase in self-esteem and a decrease in depressive symptoms compared to controls. Not surprisingly, physical discomforts also diminished. As physiotherapists play a major role in exercise in the child-bearing year, this is important information and highlights the need for involvement in fitness classes with pregnant teenagers.

The importance of good nutrition and exercise in the adolescent years cannot be ignored. Physiotherapists in combination with other health professionals are well equipped to inform young females about appropriate levels of exercise, the importance of playing many sports at a young age and the dangers of an inappropriate diet to present and future health and wellness. The emphasis of our care should be prevention. Health education is vital when working with teenagers.

References

Armstrong N and Welsman JR (1994) Assessment and interpretation of aerobic fitness in children and adolescents. *Exercise Sports Science Review* **22**: 435–476.

Baer JT and Taper LJ (1992) Amenorrheic and eumenorrheic adolescent runners: dietary intake and exercise training status. *Journal of American Diet Association* **92(1)**: 89–91.

Bale P, Mayhew JL, Piper FC et al (1992) Biological and performance variables in relation to age in male and female adolescent athletes. *Journal of Sports Medicine and Physical Fitness* **32**: 142–148.

Bar-Or O (1988) The prepubescent female. In: Shangold MM, Mirkin G (eds) *Women and Exercise: Physiology and Sports Medicine*, pp. 109–19. Philadelphia: F.A. Davis.

Bergen-Cico DK and Short SH (1992) Dietary intakes, energy expenditures, and anthropometric characteristics of adolescent female cross-country runners. *Journal of American Dietary Association* **92(5)**: 611–612.

Bernstein L, Henderson BE, Hanisch R et al (1994) Physical exercise and reduced risk of cancer in young women. *Journal of National Cancer Institute* **86**: 1403–1408.

Bourke L. (1992) Fine tuning – how much and when? In: Bourke L (ed) *The complete guide to food for sports performance*, pp. 27–45. North Sydney: Allen and Unwin.

Brouhard BH (1995) Hypertension in children and adolescents. *Cleve Clinical Journal of Medicine* **62(1)**: 21–28.

Bull NL (1992) Dietary habits, food consumption, and nutrient intake during adolescence. *Journal of Adolescent Health* **13(5)**: 384–388.

Camp DE, Klesges RC and Relyea G (1993) The relationship between body weight concerns and adolescent smoking. *Health Psychology* **12(1)**: 24–32.

Carbon RJ (1992) The female athlete. In: Bloomfield J, Fricker PA, Fitch KD (eds) *Textbook of Science and Medicine in Sport*, pp. 467–487. Melbourne: Blackwell Scientific Publications.

Claessens AL, Malina RM, Lefevre J et al (1992) Growth and menarcheal status of elite female gymnasts. *Medicine Science Sports and Exercise* **24(7)**: 755–763.

Clarkson PM, Freedson PS, Keller B et al (1985) Maximal oxygen uptake, nutritional patterns and body composition of adolescent female ballet dancers. *Research Quarterly Exercise and Sport* **56(2)**: 180–185.

De Cree C, Vermeulen A and Ostyn M (1991) Are high-performance young women athletes doomed to become low-performance old wives? *Journal of Sports Medicine and Physical Fitness* **31**: 108–114.

Douthitt VL (1994) Psychological determinants of adolescent exercise adherence. *Adolescence* **29(115)**: 711–722.

Dummer GM, Rosen LW, Heusner WW et al (1987) Pathogenic weight-control behaviors of young competitive swimmers. *Physician and Sports Medicine* **15**: 75–84.

Emmons L (1994) Predisposing factors differentiating adolescent dieters and non dieters. *Journal of American Dietary Association* **94(7)**: 725–728.

Frost HM (1992) Perspectives: bone's mechanical usage windows. *Bone and Mineral* **19**: 257–271.

Glenmark B, Hedberg G, Kaisjer L et al (1994) Muscle strength from adolescence to adulthood – relationship to muscle fibre types. *European Journal of Applied Physiology* **68(1)**: 9–19.

Grandjean AC (1990) Sports nutrition. In: Mellion MB, Walsh WM and Shelton GL (eds) *The Team Physician's Handbook*, pp. 78–91. Philadelphia: Hanley and Belfus Inc.

Greenhaff PL (1995) Creatine and its application as an ergogenic aid. *International Journal of Sports Nutrition* **5**: S100–S110.

Griffin LY (1994) The young female athlete. In: Stanitski CL, DeLee JC and Drez D (eds) *Pediatric and Adolescent Sports Medicine*, vol. 3, pp. 16–23. Philadelphia: W.B. Saunders.

Guillen EO and Barr SI (1994) Nutrition, dieting and fitness messages in a magazine for adolescent women, 1970–1990. *Journal of Adolescent Health* **15(6)**: 464–472.

Heath GW, Pratt M, Warren CW et al (1994) Physical activity patterns in American high school students. Results from the 1990 Youth Risk Behavior Survey. *Archives of Pediatric and Adolescent Medicine* **148(11)**: 1131–1136.

Highet R (1989) Athletic amenorrhea: an update on aetiology, complications and management. *Sports Medicine (Auckland)* **7(2)**: 82–108.

Hill AJ, Oliver S and Rogers PJ (1992) Eating in the adult world: the rise of dieting in childhood and adolescence. *British Journal of Clinical Psychology* **31(Pt 1)**: 95–105.

Kaiserauer S, Snyder AC, Sleeper M et al (1989) Nutritional, physiological and menstrual status of distance runners. *Medicine Science Sports and Exercise* **21**: 120–125.

Kanter MM and Williams MH (1995) Antioxidants, carnitine, and choline as putative ergogenic aids. *International Journal of Sports Nutrition* **5**: S120–S131.

Kelder SH, Perry CL, Klepp KI et al (1994) Longitudinal tracking of adolescent smoking, physical activity, and food choice behaviors. *American Journal of Public Health* **84(7)**: 1121–1126.

King AC and Tribble DL (1991) The role of exercise in weight regulation in nonathletes. *Sports Medicine* **11(5)**: 331–349.

Kirchner EM, Lewis RD and O'Connor PJ (1995) Bone mineral density and dietary intake of female college gymnasts. *Medicine Science Sports and Exercise* **27(4)**: 543–549.

Koff E and Rierdan J (1993) Advanced pubertal development and eating disturbance in early adolescent girls. *Journal of Adolescent Health* **14(6)**: 433–439.

Koniak-Griffin D (1994) Aerobic exercise, psychological well-being and physical discomforts during adolescent pregnancy. *Research and Nursing Health* **17(4)**: 253–263.

Magazanik A, Weinstein Y, Abarbanel, J et al (1990) Effect of an iron supplement on body iron status and aerobic capacity of young training women. *European Journal of Applied Physiology* **62**: 317–323.

Malina RM (1994) Attained size and growth rate of female volleyball players between 9 and 13 years of age. *Pediatrics Exercise and Science* **6(3)**: 257–266.

Martin AD and Bailey DA (1987) Review: skeletal integrity in amenorrheic athletes. *Australian Journal of Science and Medicine in Sport* **19(2)**: 3–7.

McCulloch RG, Bailey DA, Whalen RL et al (1992) Bone density and bone mineral content of adolescent soccer athletes and competitive swimmers. *Pediatric Exercise Science* **4(4)**: 319–330.

Moore DC (1993) Body image and eating behavior in adolescents. *Journal of American College of Nutrition* **12(5)**: 505–510.

Moore J, Campana J, Lam M et al (1992) Participation in school physical education and selected dietary patterns among high school students – United States, 1991. *Journal of School Health* **62(8)**: 392–394.

Must A, Jacques PF, Dallal GE et al (1992) Long-term morbidity and mortality of overweight adolescents. A follow-up of the Harvard growth study of 1922 to 1935. *New England Journal of Medicine* **327(19)**: 1350–1355.

Naughton G and Carlson J (1995) Physiological aspects of youth sport: developmental or detrimental? *Sport and Health* **13(2)**: 5–7.

Nelson M, Bakaliou F and Trivedi A (1994) Iron-deficiency anaemia and physical performance in adolescent girls from different ethnic backgrounds. *British Journal of Nutrition* **72(3)**: 427–433.

Nindl BC, Mahar MT, Harman EA et al (1994) Lower and upper body anaerobic performance in male and female adolescent athletes. *Medicine Science Sports and Exercise* **27(1)**: 235–241.

Panico S, Celentano E, Krogh V et al (1987) Physical activity and its relationship to blood pressure in school children. *Journal of Chronic Disability* **40**: 925–930.

Parfitt AM (1994) The two faces of growth: benefits and risks to bone integrity. *Osteoporosis International* **4**: 382–398.

Prentice A and Bates CJ (1994) Adequacy of dietary mineral supply for human bone growth and mineralisation. *European Journal of Clinical Nutrition* **48(Suppl 1)**: S161–S176.

Prior JC, Vigna YM and McKay DW (1992) Reproduction of the athletic woman: new understandings of physiology and management. *Sports Medicine (Auckland)* **14(3)**: 190–199.

Rossow I and Rise J (1994) Concordance of parental and adolescent health behaviours. *Society for Science and Medicine* **38(9)**: 1299–1305.

RowlandTW and Freedson PS (1994) Physical activity, fitness, and health in children: a close look. *Pediatrics* **93(4)**: 669–672.

Rowland TW, Black SA and Kelleher JF (1987) Iron deficiency in adolescent endurance athletes. *Journal of Adolescent Health Care* **8**: 322–326.

Schmalz K (1993) Nutritional beliefs and practices of adolescent athletes. *Journal of School Nursing* **9(2)**: 18–22.

Slemenda CW and Johnson CC (1993) High intensity activities in young women: site specific bone mass effects among female figure skaters. *Bone and Mineral* **20**: 125–132.

Sobal J and Marquart LF (1994) Vitamin / mineral supplement use among high school athletes. *Adolescence* **29(116)**: 835–843.

Soroko S, Holbrook TL, Edelstein S et al (1994) Lifetime milk consumption and bone mineral density in older women. *American Journal of Public Health* **84(8)**: 1319–1322.

Stager JM (1984) Reversibility of amenorrhea in athletes. *Sports Medicine (Auckland)* **1(5)**: 765–767.

Suominen H (1993) Bone mineral density and long term exercise: an overview of cross-sectional athlete studies. *Sports Medicine (Auckland)* **16(5)**: 316–330.

Taub DE and Blinde EM (1992) Eating disorders among adolescent female athletes: influence of athletic participation and sport team membership. *Adolescence* **27(108)**: 833–848.

Theintz GE, Howald H, Weiss U et al (1993) Evidence for a reduction of growth potential in adolescent female gymnasts. *Journal of Pediatrics* **122(2)**: 306–313.

Van De Loo DA and Johnson MD (1995) The young female athlete. *Clinics in Sports Medicine* **14(3)**: 687–707.

Walberg-Rankin J (1995) Dietary carbohydrate as an ergogenic aid for prolonged and brief competitions in sport. *International Journal of Sport Nutrition* **5**: S13–S28.

Webster BL and Barr SI (1995) Calcium intakes of adolescent female gymnasts and speed skaters: lack of association with dieting behavior. *International Journal of Sport Nutrition* **5(1)**: 2–12.

Welten DC, Kemper HCG, Post GB et al (1994) Weight-bearing activity during youth is a more important factor for peak bone mass than calcium intake. *Journal of Bone and Mineral Research* **9(7)**: 1089–1096.

Withers RT, Norton KI, Craig NP et al (1987) The relative body fat and anthropometric prediction of body density of South Australian females aged 17–35 years. *European Journal of Applied Physiology* **56**: 181–190.

5

Eating Disorders

HELEN KERR

The eating disorders, anorexia nervosa and bulimia nervosa, usually present in adolescence. There is a vast literature about eating disorders and there are some strongly held opinions about aetiology and management. Some of these views will be discussed. However, it is important to be aware that there are significant deficiencies and inconsistencies in the published research. These are:

- too few large-scale population studies;
- too much reliance on hospital-based data;
- a lack of replication of studies, especially those which seem to indicate significant advances;
- a scarcity of adequately controlled studies.

Only a few of the factors associated with eating disorders can be considered to be adequately understood (Gillberg, 1994).

Agreement on the diagnostic criteria for anorexia nervosa and bulimia nervosa now exists, however, which is the initial step in ensuring some continuity of evaluation (American Psychiatric Association, 1994).

Criteria for Diagnosing Anorexia Nervosa

- Refusal to maintain body weight at or above normal minimum for age and height (e.g. weight loss leading to maintenance of body weight less than 85% of that expected or failure to make expected weight gain during period of growth (usually puberty) leading to body weight less than 85% of that expected).
- Intense fear of gaining weight or becoming fat, even though underweight.
- Disturbance in the way in which the body weight or shape is experienced, undue influence of body weight or shape on self-evaluation or denial of the seriousness of the current low body weight (Fig. 5.1).
- In postmenarcheal females, amenorrhoea, i.e. the absence of at least three consecutive menstrual cycles (women on the oral contraceptive pill will have withdrawal bleeds but are considered to have amenorrhoea for the purposes of diagnosis of anorexia nervosa).

Two anorexia nervosa subtypes are also recognized:

1. restricting type – no regular binge eating or purging behaviour (i.e. self-induced vomiting or misuse of laxatives, diuretics or enemas);
2. binge-eating/purging type – regular binge eating or purging.

Criteria for Diagnosing Bulimia Nervosa

- Recurrent episodes of binge eating. An episode of binge eating is characterized by both of the following:

(a) eating in a discrete period of time an amount of food that is definitely larger than most people would eat during a similar period of time and under similar circumstances;
(b) a sense of lack of control over eating during the episode.

- Recurrent inappropriate compensatory behaviour in order to prevent weight gain, such as self-induced vomiting, misuse of laxatives, diuretics, enemas or other medications, fasting or excessive exercise.
- The binge eating and inappropriate compensatory behaviours both occur on average at least twice a week for three months.
- Self-evaluation is unduly influenced by body shape and weight.
- The disturbance does not occur exclusively during episodes of anorexia nervosa.

Two bulimia nervosa subtypes are also recognized:

1. purging type – regular episodes of self-induced vomiting or misuse of laxatives, diuretics or enemas;
2. non-purging type – regular use of other inappropriate compensatory behaviours such as fasting or excessive exercise.

There are many young women who exhibit disordered eating and some of the features of anorexia nervosa and bulimia nervosa, but do not meet the above criteria.

Prevalence and Epidemiology

There is a consensus view that the prevalence of eating disorders is increasing. The reported rates depend on the diagnostic criteria used. The usually quoted prevalence figure for anorexia nervosa in allegedly high-risk groups of young women is 1% (Crisp et al, 1976). High-risk people are in occupations or situations where pressure is put on them to maintain a very slim physique, e.g. ballet dancers, models, girls from private schools (Freeman and Newton, 1993). However, Garner and Garfinkel (1980) report 3.5% of fashion students and 7.6% of professional ballet students have anorexia nervosa. Prevalence rates for bulimia nervosa of up to 19% have been reported among female college students (Powers, 1994). Eating disorders have until recently been thought to occur mainly in Western-oriented countries and predominantly in young women from higher socioeconomic groups, but there is evidence of an increase in these disorders in the developing world and in women of all socioeconomic groups (Pate et al, 1992).

Eating disorders do occur in males but are much more common in females. Anorexia nervosa typically begins in adolescence with a peak age of onset between 14 and 17. Bulimia nervosa usually presents later in adolescence or young adulthood (Holden, 1989).

Though there is at present debate about the prevalence and epidemiology of eating disorders there is no doubt that anorexia and bulimia nervosa cause considerable disability and distress. There is also a significant mortality from these disorders, both as a direct consequence of the condition and from suicide (Holden, 1989).

In the following discussion the diagnosis, clinical features, suggested aetiology, recommended management and reported prognosis will be reviewed using illustrative case histories. Obesity and a recent advance in understanding its aetiology will be briefly described.

Kate is a 16-year-old ballet dancer. She sees the general practitioner recommended by her ballet school to request 'diet pills'. She weighs 52 kg and is 170 cm tall. She is accompanied by Melissa, her 15-year-old friend who is also a ballet dancer. They tell the doctor that their teacher has advised Kate to lose some weight. She has already lost 2 kg but is finding it difficult to get down to 50 kg (the weight recommended by the teacher). They report that some of the students induce vomiting or take laxatives to control their weight but Kate wants to lose weight 'safely'. Kate has not had a period for two months. She had her menarche at 13 years and has had fairly regular periods until now. She has never had sexual intercourse.

At 52 kg Kate is already underweight for her height. A useful index for assessing healthy weight is the body mass index (BMI). The index is calculated from the formula (wt in kg) ÷ (ht in m)^2. The following categories are usually recognized:

<15	Emaciated
15–20	Underweight
20–25	Normal
25–30	Overweight
30–40	Moderately obese
>40	Severely obese

Kate's BMI would thus be calculated at 52 kg ÷ (1.7 m)^2, which gives her a BMI score of 18 and a classification of underweight.

Kate seems relieved when the doctor says she does not need diet pills and that she is underweight at 52 kg. The general practitioner also says that she understands that ballet dancers are often required to maintain a low weight but that at least Kate should allow herself to regain the 2 kg she has lost. The doctor asks if she can telephone the ballet school's principal to discuss the problem. Initially Kate and Melissa are unsure but when the general practitioner explains that she need not reveal their names but that she would say only that she is concerned that inappropriate advice may be being given to students, they agree. When telephoned, the principal expresses dismay at the situation and organizes a joint meeting with the general practitioner, the physiotherapist used by the school, a dietitian, the ballet teachers and some student representatives to discuss appropriate nutrition, training programmes and minimum weight recommendations for students.

Kate is underweight and has missed a period. She does not, however, meet the diagnostic criteria for anorexia nervosa.

Is Kate at increased risk of developing disordered eating?

Social dieting seems to merge into the spectrum of disordered eating and eating disorders (Holden, 1989). Young women in appearance-based occupations seem to be at increased risk of developing anorexia nervosa (Garner and Garfinkel, 1980). The personality traits which make a good ballet dancer – hard working, perfectionist, ambitious – may also predispose to anorexia nervosa.

Educational intervention will presumably help to prevent the development of eating disorders. The provision of information to patients about the detrimental physical effects of eating disorders early in the condition is a useful management strategy (Freeman and Newton, 1993). It is postulated that intervention before the development of the disorder will be more effective, but further evaluation of such programmes is necessary.

Figure 5.1 Distortion of body image.

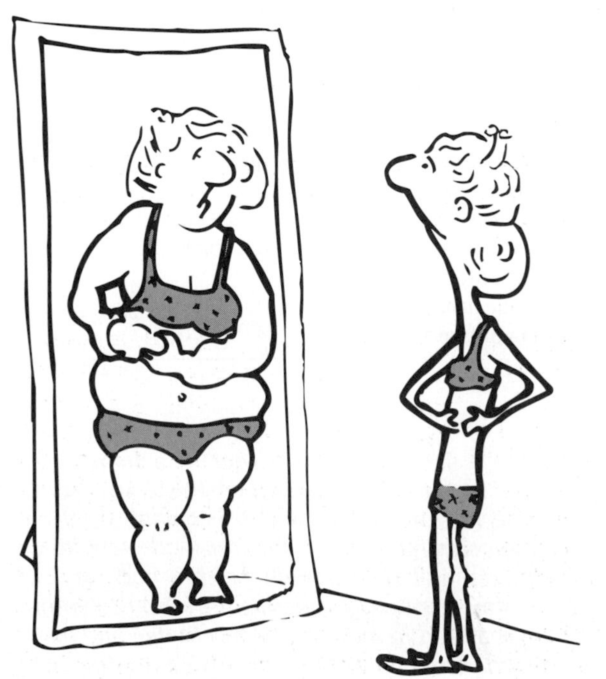

Gillian is 17 and a very highly achieving university student. She attends the student health service because the principal of her residential college has requested her to do so. Gillian's friends had spoken to the principal because they were concerned about her weight loss, how little she was eating and her overexercising. Gillian denies that there is any problem and says she feels perfectly well. On direct questioning she reports that she eats muesli and skim milk for breakfast, salad for lunch and meat and vegetables for dinner, in similar quantities to other students. She says she sometimes eats ice cream and cake. She seems distant, perhaps a little supercilious, but polite and seemingly co-operative. On further questioning Gillian says she has been hospitalized in the past because of her low weight. She agrees to the student health service doctor obtaining a copy of her past medical records and reluctantly agrees to be weighed and measured. She weighs 42 kg and is 163 cm in height (third centile for weight, 50th centile for height for a 17-year-old; BMI 15.8). She is on the contraceptive pill for 'period control'. She is not sexually active.

Gillian's reluctance to admit that there is a problem is a common feature of anorexia nervosa. Her friends and the college principal are much more worried than she seems to be. Young women who lose weight because of physical illness are usually very concerned, feel unwell and seek medical help. Gillian reports a fairly restricted diet. Most anorexia nervosa sufferers are preoccupied with food and are reasonably well informed about nutrition though they often hold distorted opinions about adequate diets. The diet of an anorexia nervosa patient is reported, on average, to contain one-sixth of the energy, one-sixth of the carbohydrate, one-third of the protein and one-ninth of the fat of a normal woman's diet (Abraham and Llewellyn-Jones, 1987).

When William Gull first named anorexia nervosa in 1874 (the condition was first described by Richard Morton in 1689) he reported his patient as having 'want of appetite'. In fact, most sufferers are very hungry but resist eating because of their obsession about weight gain and body shape. Gillian is not outwardly acknowledging that she has a problem. A usual characteristic of anorexia nervosa patients is a tendency to deceive or manipulate those who are trying to make her alter her behaviour. Gillian is terrified of gaining weight and fears losing control of her food intake. She already feels coerced by those who are trying to help her. The commonest problem in the management of eating disorders is that the patient and the health professionals and/or family become embroiled in a battle for control. Most patients with eating disorders are obsessed with self-control. The attempted imposition of outside control is doomed to failure. Co-operation, collaboration and the building of an open, trusting therapeutic relationship seems to be the way forward (Anon, 1995).

Gillian's medical records (from the general practitioner who looked after her at boarding school) reveal that she began to lose weight shortly after menarche. Her periods started when she was 12. She had four or five periods in the first year and then they stopped. After six months amenorrhoea her mother took her to see a general practitioner. She was started on the oral contraceptive pill to 'regularize' her periods. Gillian's parents then moved overseas and she went to boarding school. During Gillian's second term at school the staff became concerned about her weight loss and social isolation (she had made friends initially but seemed now to be a 'loner'). She was referred to the school general practitioner but despite his intervention she continued to lose weight and was admitted to hospital. She was 14, 163 cm in height and 36 kg in weight (between the 75th and 90th centile for height, at the third centile for weight; BMI 13.5) (Fig. 5.2). The hospital records reported that Gillian complained of cold hands and feet and difficulty with concentration on her school work. She expressed concern about the work she was missing and her impending examinations. She was emaciated and dehydrated, had dry skin and lanugo hair on her face, neck and forearms. Her heart rate was 50 per minute, systolic blood pressure was 80 mmHg, diastolic blood pressure 40 mmHg and temperature 36°C. Dental examination showed loss of dental enamel. She had a low serum potassium and electrocardiographic abnormalities consistent with this.

A re-feeding programme had resulted in reasonable weight gain (though she was found to be hiding food rather than eating it early in the treatment) but she had reached a plateau at 45 kg (BMI 17).

She had individual psychotherapy and her mother and she (her mother had returned from overseas when Gillian was admitted to hospital) had a few sessions of family therapy. She was discharged from hospital after three months. She had sat her school examinations in hospital and had done very well.

Shortly afterwards Gillian's family moved to another city where her father, who is an army officer, had been posted. Gillian went to live with her parents and brother who was at university in this city. She went to a day school.

Tables 5.1 and 5.2 summarize the typical physical and psychological features of anorexia nervosa, many of which are exhibited by Gillian. The physical effects are largely adaptive measures by the semistarved body to conserve energy. The psychological features seem to both precede and be a result of the eating disorder (Freeman and Newton, 1993; Nussbaum, 1992; Powers, 1994).

Figure 5.2 Typical anorexic appearance. (Reproduced from Abraham and Llewellyn-Jones (1987) with permission of Oxford University Press.)

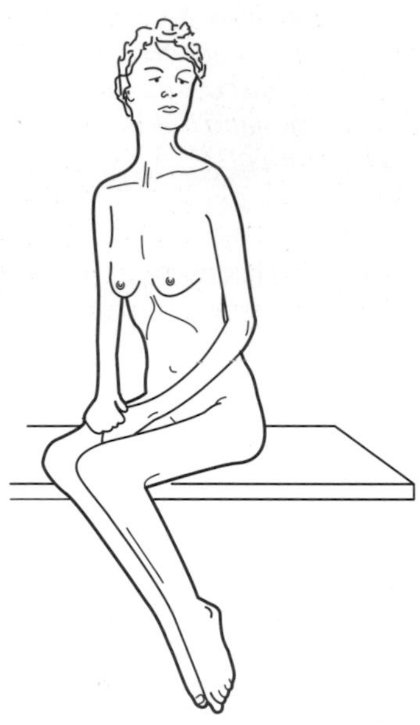

Table 5.1 Common physical features of anorexia nervosa patients

- Severe weight loss with loss of subcutaneous fat and muscle bulk
- Reduced metabolic rate with decreased heart rate, blood pressure and temperature
- Reduced or arrested growth rate if not fully grown
- Decreased gastrointestinal function leading to bloating and constipation
- Decreased renal function with reduced ability to concentrate urine
- Osteopenia and possible osteoporosis
- Impaired cardiac function mainly due to electrolyte disturbance
- Depressed hypothalamic–pituitary–ovarian axis leading to amenorrhoea, pre-pubertal hormone levels and failure to progress through puberty if pre-pubertal or pubertal
- Possible cerebral atrophy
- Dry cracked skin and lanugo hair growth (soft downy hair on face, neck, arms and back)
- Dental problems with erosion of dental enamel due to gastric acid in the mouth from self-induced vomiting
- Dizziness, tiredness
- Cold, blue hands and feet
- Swelling of face and ankles

Sophie, a 19-year-old manager in a hamburger store, started to diet at school when she was about 17. She was then 59 kg and 160 cm tall (BMI 23) and says she 'hated being fat'. A friend had taken a photograph of her, though Sophie had tried to avoid being photographed. She reports: 'Something snapped in me'. She began to diet and exercise and reduced her weight to 46 kg over the next three months. She remembers then going into the student refectory at her college and being unable to resist the iced buns. She began to binge and vomit. Since then her weight has fluctuated between 50 kg and 55 kg. She says she wants to stop bingeing, that she is 'so sick of this' and that she has 'wasted enough time on it'. She lives with her parents but thinks they are unaware of her problem. She has recently confided in her boyfriend and was frightened that he would reject her but he has been concerned and sympathetic and urged her to get help.

Table 5.2 Common psychological features of anorexia nervosa patients

- Distorted body image
- Food preoccupation
- Poor self-esteem with overwhelming sense of ineffectiveness
- Obsessional, perfectionist, overachieving
- Higher than average prevalence of history of sexual abuse
- Depressed, anxious, emotionally labile, social withdrawal
- Strong-willed and controlling but also 'good' and compliant
- Uncommunicative, secretive, distrustful
- Other self-destructive behaviour (e.g. suicide attempts, self-cutting, drug abuse)

Bulimia nervosa is a recently defined disorder compared with anorexia nervosa (Russell, 1979) but there is considerable overlap between the two conditions. Sophie shows some typical bulimic features. She binges in secret, she spends a significant amount of money on food which she hoards for binges. Abraham and Llewellyn-Jones (1987) report quantities of food 3–30 times that which would normally be consumed in one day being eaten during a binge. Sophie shows the typical bulimic cycle. Her weight fluctuates but is within the normal range. Some bulimia nervosa sufferers are underweight, others overweight. Recurrent vomiting may cause swelling of the face (due to parotid gland enlargement), hoarseness of the voice and dental problems. Knuckles may show calluses or ulceration because of repeatedly sticking the fingers down the throat to induce vomiting.

Bulimic patients may exhibit many of the features shown in Table 5.1. They may also share with anorexic patients the psychological characteristics listed in Table 5.2. The bulimic girl is likely to be more socially integrated than her anorexic sister. She is likely to be less rigidly controlled (in some respects the bulimic patient is a 'failed' anorexia nervosa sufferer) and may be more likely to engage in other self-harming behaviour like substance abuse.

Aetiology of Eating Disorders

Why do young women develop these self-destructive and distressing disorders?

The consensus view seems to be that there are probably many causes and that there is a complex interplay of each or some of these causes in an individual patient (Nussbaum, 1992).

SOCIOCULTURAL FACTORS

The desire to be thin seems to be a prerequisite for the development of an eating disorder. Dawn French, the rotund British comedienne, calls the glamorization of today's pencil-thin models a 'massive tyranny. 47% of women in the UK are size 16 or over but are nowhere to be seen' (Brown, 1994).

Adolescent girls become increasingly dissatisfied with their bodies as they grow up. Overperception of body size is found amongst teenage girls in many countries (Abraham and Llewellyn-Jones, 1987). Model agencies are prescriptive about the acceptable female body – young women have the 'ideal' of the extremely slim, androgynous woman presented to them by Western-style media. The magazine image of the beautiful woman is becoming more tubular, less curvaceous, taller and lighter (Guillen and Barr, 1994). It is therefore not surprising that some adolescent women find it difficult to accept the normal rounding of their bodies as they mature.

GENETIC, FAMILY, PERSONALITY AND BIOLOGICAL FACTORS

Studies of twins have shown anorexia nervosa occurs more frequently in monozygotic compared with dizygotic twins (Holland et al, 1984), suggesting a genetic component. Family patterns such as failure to deal with conflict, superficial patterns of communication and inadequate boundaries between individuals have been implicated as significant aetiological factors. The role of sexual abuse in the development of eating disorders is not clear. Poor self-image and problems with overcontrol of emotions are common personality traits in sufferers but it is not evident whether these are a cause or a result of the eating disorder. There is also the possibility of a primary hypothalamic abnormality in anorexic and bulimic patients (Lask and Bryant-Waugh, 1993).

Management of Eating Disorders

As there is no consensus view with regard to the cause, it is not surprising that there are many suggested management strategies for eating disorders. Early recognition and assessment of anorexic and bulimic behaviour allows intervention before the young woman is seriously ill and demoralized.

Management should address physical, psychological and family aspects. A collaborative approach with the patient seems likely to be more successful but there are adherents of a more authoritarian regime. Hospitalization is essential if the patient has severe signs of starvation, dehydration or electrolyte imbalance or is severely depressed and at risk of suicide. Individual and family psychotherapy are usually employed. Cognitive behavioural therapy is often advocated, especially for the bulimic patient, with strategies like diary keeping to help identify triggers for binge behaviour.

Medication is probably of little benefit in anorexia nervosa unless there is coexisting depression. In bulimia nervosa antidepressant medication, especially serotonin reuptake inhibitors like fluoxetine, may be of value. There is a shortage of designated treatment centres even in the affluent world and there is a need for improved hospital facilities and better training for community-based health professionals (Lask and Bryant-Waugh, 1993).

Prognosis of Eating Disorders

Studies of the prognosis of eating disorders reveal a prolonged illness course over several years. About half of the patients with anorexia nervosa become well though years after apparent recovery many women still report reverting to anorexic behaviour if stressed. About a quarter of patients show significant improvement and the remaining quarter remain chronically ill (Lask and Bryant-Waugh, 1993). The prognosis in bulimia nervosa is probably more hopeful, with at least two-thirds making a full recovery, at least in the short term (Holden, 1989).

Obesity

In some cultures, for example in Tonga, the obese are considered particularly beautiful but in Western-orientated societies this is no longer so. Obese people endure derogatory comments and pejorative associations are made – 'fat and unfit', 'fat and lazy', 'fat and stupid', 'fat and ugly'. Young women seem to be more vulnerable to these negative attitudes than young men. Enormous amounts of time and money are spent attempting to lose weight. Dieting is a multibillion dollar industry but only 2% of adult dieters lose weight long term (Freeman and Newton, 1993). Adolescent dieters may fare a little better. There is now doubt that mild obesity (BMI 25–30) contributes to ill health though moderate and severe obesity do increase morbidity and mortality. There is even evidence that mildly overweight women have a lower mortality rate than women of normal weight (Freeman and Newton, 1993).

Recently there has been renewed interest in a genetic cause for obesity and the detailed description of an 'obesity gene' in mice (Zhang et al, 1994). This gene is believed to have a human counterpart and may provide further evidence for the 'set point' theory of the aetiology of obesity. This theory postulates that an individual has a predetermined body mass and if food intake or physical activity is changed the metabolic rate alters to defend this body mass.

This biological theory of obesity does not mean that the obese adolescent should not be encouraged to lose weight but that pharmacological treatment may be more useful than has hitherto been thought. Unsuccessful treatment strategies demoralize and victimize patients. Realistic goals should be agreed upon by patient and health professional, concentrating on gradual changes towards more healthy eating and a more active lifestyle.

The damaging cycle of diet–weight gain–diet should be explained and discouraged. Skinfold measurements and waist measurements may be a more useful assessment of progress than weight as they can show loss of fat even when weight is unchanged.

Summary

Anorexia nervosa, bulimia nervosa and obesity are not yet adequately understood. There are now agreed diagnostic criteria for these disorders and this will lead to improved interpretation of data. Education of young people, parents and health professionals seems to be desirable, as does the collaborative approach to management. Rigorous assessment of outcomes is necessary. Designated clinics need to be further developed.

References

Abraham S and Llewellyn-Jones D (1987) *Eating Disorders: The Facts*, 2nd edn. Oxford: Oxford University Press.

American Psychiatric Association (1994) *Diagnostic and Statistical Manual of Mental Disorders*, 4th edn, pp. 544–550. Washington DC: American Psychiatric Association.

Anonymous (1995) Personal view. Which option would you take? *British Medical Journal* **311**: 635–636.

Brown J (1994) Time out with Dawn French. Big is beautiful. *New Weekly* **November 21**: 34–35.

Crisp AH, Palmer RL and Kalucy RS (1976) How common is anorexia nervosa? A prevalence study. *British Journal of Psychiatry* **128**: 549.

Freeman C and Newton R (1993) Eating disorders. In: McPherson A (ed) *Women's Problems in General Practice*, 3rd edn, pp. 424–447. Oxford: Oxford University Press.

Garner DM and Garfinkel PE (1980) Sociocultural factors in the development of anorexia nervosa. *Psychological Medicine* **10**: 647–656.

Gillberg C (1994) Whither research in anorexia and bulimia nervosa. *British Journal of Hospital Medicine* **51**: 209–215.

Guillen EO and Barr SI (1994) Nutrition, dieting and fitness messages in a magazine for adolescent women, 1970–1990. *Journal of Adolescent Health* **11**: 464–472.

Holden NL (1989) Eating disorders. *Baillière's Clinical Obstetrics and Gynaecology* **3**: 705–727.

Holland AJ, Hall A, Murray R et al (1984) Anorexia nervosa: a study of 34 twin pairs and one set of triplets. *British Journal of Psychiatry* **145**: 414–419.

Lask B and Bryant-Waugh R (1993) Editorial: eating disorders. *British Journal of Hospital Medicine* **49**: 531–533.

Nussbaum MP (1992) Nutritional conditions. In: McAnarney ER, Kreipe RE, Orr DP et al (eds) *Textbook of Adolescent Medicine*, pp. 536–553. Philadelphia: W.B. Saunders.

Pate JE, Pumariega AJ, Hester C et al (1992) Cross-cultural patterns in eating disorders: a review. *Academic Child and Adolescent Psychiatry* **31**: 802–809.

Powers PS (1994) Eating disorders. In: Sanfilippo JS (ed) *Pediatric and Adolescent Gynecology*, pp. 397–416. Philadelphia: W.B. Saunders.

Russell GFM (1979) Bulimia nervosa. An ominous variant of anorexia nervosa. *Psychological Medicine* **9**: 429–448.

Zhang Y, Proenca R, Maffei M et al (1994) Positional cloning of the mouse obese gene and its human homologue. *Nature* **372**: 425–432.

6

Menstrual and Perimenstrual Problems: Impact on the Adolescent

HELEN KERR

Historical and Societal Perspective
•
Dysmenorrhoea (Painful Periods)
•
Premenstrual Syndrome
•
Menorrhagia (Heavy Periods)
•
Amenorrhoea and Oligomenorrhoea (Absent and Infrequent Periods)

Historical and Societal Perspective

Menstruation more than any other bodily function has, throughout history, been encumbered with a conflicting and complex mythology. Ancient people had no idea why women bled and so menstruating women and menstrual blood were, and still sometimes are, regarded with fear and awe.

> Oh! menstruating woman, thou art a fiend from which all nature should be closely screened. (Ancient rhyme quoted by Walker, 1983)

In some 'primitive' societies, a girl was subject to a period of seclusion at menarche. This was usually followed by celebration and feasting to acknowledge her new status. Islamic and Judaeo-Christian teachings are full of references to the menstruating woman as unclean, polluting and shameful. Some orthodox followers of these religions still observe rituals which reflect these views.

It is not surprising that studies of young contemporary women reveal ambivalent attitudes about menarche and menstruation (Abraham et al, 1985; Snowden and Christian, 1983).

In some cultures, predominantly in Middle Eastern, Asian and North African countries, girls may marry at menarche, regardless of their age. Such early marriage contributes significantly to obstetric, gynaecological and neonatal problems.

In Western-style societies, menarche is often a covert event for which girls are ill prepared and they may be frightened or ashamed (Abraham et al, 1985).

Emily's menarcheal story

I only found out about periods a few months before mine began. I was 10. It was embarrassing when my friends first began talking about periods and I didn't know what they were. My friends didn't really explain very well and I didn't want to ask too many questions and make myself look even more stupid. So I really didn't know what to expect. For a while, every time I went to the toilet I was scared that there would be blood between my legs. Then one day there was. I didn't know how to tell Mum. I thought maybe she'd be angry. She wasn't angry but she wasn't too happy either. She sighed and said 'Oh well, it happens to us all'. She gave me some pads and that was about it.

Young people learn from the behaviour patterns of their families, peers, school and the wider community. Within the family, health behaviours and attitudes are modelled.

Cumming et al (1994) reviewed sexuality education and sources of information about menstruation and found young people's knowledge to be inadequate despite the availability of some excellent educational material. He emphasized the need to use the 'teachable moment' and to create an 'askable atmosphere'. Parents, health professionals and educators need to feel comfortable discussing sexual development issues. Health education programmes developed in co-operation with young people and using peer educators are more effective than programmes devised and imposed by adult educators (Jay et al, 1984). Young people's existing relevant beliefs and attitudes about the subject need to be known before appropriate education can be planned (Adler et al 1990). People are more likely to absorb information and change their attitudes if they believe the educator is similar to them in lifestyle and understands their issues. This is particularly true for young people who sometimes feel unable to identify with or trust adults (Sloane and Zimmer, 1993).

Some young women fare better than Emily.

Debbie's menarcheal story

When I was about 10 or 11 Mum explained to me all about periods. In fact, I didn't get mine until I was 15. I felt like a bit of a freak because all my girlfriends had started their periods a long time ago. But Mum assured me that I was still perfectly normal and that soon they would come. She was right. Even though I was desperate to start menstruating it was still a shock to see the blood. When Mum came home from work I told her and we both started to cry. She hugged me and explained that she was crying because she was going to miss the little girl that I had been. My Mum was a bit of an old hippie and she got the idea to have a special dinner where I would be presented as a woman. I wasn't too sure, but she was only going to ask her sister and my Dad (Mum and Dad are amicably separated). The next night I had to get all dressed up and then Mum took me into the lounge where Dad and Aunty Clare were and she said, 'This is our daughter and our niece. She is now a woman and I would like us to spend this evening remembering the beautiful little girl that she was and she can tell us all about the incredible woman that she is going to be'. Dad and Aunty clapped. Even though I was glad none of my friends could see this, it was really nice. After we had dinner, Mum and Dad and Aunty Clare all gave a little speech saying what they thought was special about me. I'm really glad that the milestone of menarche was observed in such a special way for me.

Debbie's mother seems to have devised a positive and joyful acknowledgement of her daughter's menarche.

A girl's expectations of her menstrual cycles are determined by social, educational and family influences (Brooks-Gunn and Ruble, 1982). The role model her mother provides is an important part of these influences.

Dysmenorrhoea (Painful Periods)

Until the last two or three decades, women who complained of dysmenorrhoea and other menstrual symptoms were often regarded as neurotic. There is now considerable evidence that the pain of primary dysmenorrhoea (primary or spasmodic dysmenorrhoea occurs in the absence of recognizable pelvic disease) is caused by uterine hypercontractility mediated by prostaglandins and other similar substances.

Jenny is 16 and attends her general practitioner's surgery in obvious distress complaining of acute abdominal pain. Her period has just started. Jenny's menarche occurred when she was 12. She does not remember the first two periods being painful but since then she has had variable discomfort with most periods, which occur about every 29 days. The pain usually starts with the onset of bleeding. She has crampy lower abdominal and back pain which sometimes radiates to her anterior thighs. Occasionally she has missed school because of the pain but usually she takes a couple of paracetamol and lies down with a hot water bottle on her abdomen and within an hour or so can function again. Today's pain is the worst she has ever experienced. She is crying, rolling around on the examination couch and is clearly frightened. She says she has vomited once and passed loose stools twice since the onset of severe pain two hours ago. She also complains of a headache. She reports that she has not missed any periods and that this period has occurred 'on time'.

It is important to establish that a girl with vaginal bleeding and abdominal pain is not pregnant. A spontaneous abortion or an ectopic (extrauterine) pregnancy should be considered. Jenny is not pregnant. The pain, its distribution and its association with normal menstruation is typical of primary dysmenorrhoea. She has had similar but not so severe symptoms in the past.

Dysmenorrhoea may manifest as low lumbar and/or anterior thigh pain (referred uterine pain) without abdominal pain. A woman may therefore present directly to a physiotherapist assuming the pain is due to mechanical joint dysfunction. It is important for the physiotherapist to ask whether lumbar or thigh pain is temporally related to menstruation.

Prevalence of dysmenorrhoea

Dysmenorrhoea in adolescent girls is extremely common. About 90% of high school students complain of painful periods and about one-third of these will be severely affected. Dysmenorrhoea is the leading cause of school absenteeism in adolescent girls (Wilson et al, 1989).

Jenny is examined and reassured that her pain is not an indication of a serious disorder. The mechanism of pain in dysmenorrhoea and the use of medication is explained. She takes two naproxen sodium tablets (a prostaglandin-inhibiting agent) and within 30 minutes is much more comfortable and relieved. Jenny is sexually active and using condoms. She says she prefers not to use the combined oral contraceptive pill.

Many girls are unaware of the cause of dysmenorrhoea and that effective therapy is available (Wilson et al, 1989).

Aetiology of dysmenorrhoea

Dysmenorrhoea is caused by excessive synthesis of prostaglandins and probably also of leukotrienes and vasopressin. These substances cause uterine hypercontractility and ischaemic pain. Intrauterine pressure measurements of up to 400 mmHg have been measured during the spasms of dysmenorrhoea (Fraser, 1992).

Treatment of dysmenorrhoea

Seventy to ninety percent of adolescent patients with severe dysmenorrhoea respond well to prostaglandin-inhibiting drugs. The combined oral contraceptive pill relieves the symptoms of most of those patients not helped or only partially relieved by antiprostaglandin medication (Rosenfeld and Barnes, 1993). Many sexually active young women choose this method of contraception and enjoy the non-contraceptive benefit of pain-free periods. The combination of contraceptive pill and prostaglandin-inhibiting drug is safe and effective.

Non-drug management, including acupuncture, hypnosis, behaviour modification therapy and osteopathy, may be helpful.

Although dysmenorrhoea has a known physical cause, as with any painful condition education, reassurance and stress reduction measures help the sufferer to cope better.

Secondary dysmenorrhoea

If dysmenorrhoea in an adolescent woman does not respond to a combination of an antiprostaglandin agent and a combined oral contraceptive pill, she may have an underlying pelvic disorder. Endometriosis, a common but incompletely understood disease, may cause dysmenorrhoea. In endometriosis, extrauterine endometrial tissue thickens and is shed with the hormonal cycle and can cause severe dysmenorrhoea, dyspareunia (painful intercourse) and infertility. Laparoscopy is required to make a definitive diagnosis.

Pelvic infection, usually caused by sexually transmitted disease, may also lead to refractory dysmenorrhoea.

Premenstrual Syndrome

Premenstrual syndrome (PMS), previously called premenstrual tension (PMT), is characterized by a cluster of physical and psychological symptoms which occur in the luteal phase of the menstrual cycle and disappear within a few days of the onset of menstruation. The cause is unknown. Earlier research concentrated on older women but adolescent women report similar rates of premenstrual symptoms (Wilson et al, 1989). In some women, a single symptom predominates but more than 150 symptoms have been described in premenstrual syndrome, none of which is specific to the syndrome. It is therefore not surprising that a debate continues about whether the syndrome is a true entity. There is concern amongst some that acknowledgment of a menstrually related disorder with psychological symptoms like anger and irritability will stigmatize women. There is also concern that descriptions of the syndrome focus on negative symptoms and ignore the positive mood and energy changes which some women report in the premenstrual phase (Reid, 1991). While the debate continues, many women are aware of emotional or physical changes occurring in association with the menstrual cycle.

Definition of premenstrual syndrome

Sampson (1989) has subdivided the many definitions of premenstrual syndrome into the general population's definition, the scientific research definition and the clinician's definition. This seems useful to highlight the importance of knowing exactly what is being discussed.

THE GENERAL POPULATION'S DEFINITION

A recent Australian advertisement for an over-the-counter PMT remedy asserts 'PMT is believed to affect almost all women from time to time, and to be a chronic monthly burden for as many as 40% . . .' The same advertisement claims that sufferers have included '. . . Maria Callas and Joan Crawford, Sylvia Plath, Elizabeth the First and poor old Queen Victoria' and continues, 'So, if you suffer PMT, you are in good company'.

Michelle is 18. She lives at home with her father. Her mother, who has bipolar disorder (manic depression), is at present in hospital. Michelle presents saying she has PMT and her father has advised her to seek treatment. She says she gets irrationally angry with her father. This tendency is not worse premenstrually. As she talks it becomes evident that she is angry with her father. She reports that he repeatedly tells her that she is stupid and will never amount to anything. She begins to cry as she relates this and says she feels guilty because he has always given her everything she wants. She is working as a child carer during the day and studying at night to try to gain university entrance requirements to study early childhood education.

Michelle is suffering from emotional abuse, not premenstrual syndrome. There is a tendency for imprecise and all-inclusive 'definitions' of premenstrual syndrome to be used to avoid confronting other issues.

THE SCIENTIFIC RESEARCH DEFINITION

The American Psychiatric Association's *Diagnostic and Statistical Manual of Mental Disorders* (American Psychiatric Association, 1994) currently refers to premenstrual syndrome as premenstrual dysphoric disorder. The criteria for diagnosis are detailed in Table 6.1. Using these strict criteria, the prevalence of premenstrual syndrome in women in their reproductive years is 3–8% (Steiner et al, 1995).

The establishment of precise diagnostic criteria allows critical evaluation of premenstrual syndrome. However, there is concern among many that defining the disorder as a mental health problem will restrict research into possible physical causes.

THE CLINICIAN'S DEFINITION

Lee-Lin is a 20-year-old post-graduate student. She requests information about oral contraception. She also says that she has noticed marked mood changes, bloating of her abdomen, uncomfortable fullness in the breasts and headaches in the few days before her period starts. She becomes irritable with her family and boyfriend, feels hopeless and is easily moved to tears. She recognizes that her anger is over trivial matters and her 'desperate' feelings are 'not reasonable' but feels powerless to control her behaviour or her thoughts. She has a heavy academic workload and says she does not work effectively in the premenstrual week. Within two days of her period starting she feels a 'completely different person'. Her usual confidence and equanimity are restored.

She decides to use the combined oral contraceptive pill for contraception and asks if this is likely to affect her premenstrual symptoms. She starts on a low dose monophasic pill and three months later reports a marked alleviation of her premenstrual symptoms. She is delighted.

Table 6.1 Research criteria for premenstrual dysphoric disorder (APA, 1994)

A. In most menstrual cycles during the past year, five (or more) of the following symptoms were present for most of the time during the last week of the luteal phase, began to remit within a few days after the onset of the follicular phase and were absent in the week post-menses, with at least one of the symptoms being either (1), (2), (3) or (4).

1. Markedly depressed mood, feelings of hopelessness or self-deprecating thoughts
2. Marked anxiety, tension, feelings of being 'keyed up' or 'on edge'
3. Marked affective lability (e.g. feeling suddenly sad or tearful or increased sensitivity to rejection)
4. Persistent and marked anger or irritability or increased interpersonal conflicts
5. Decreased interest in usual activities (e.g. work, school, friends, hobbies)
6. Subjective sense of difficulty in concentrating
7. Lethargy, easy fatiguability or marked lack of energy
8. Marked change in appetite, overeating or specific food cravings
9. Hypersomnia or insomnia
10. A subjective sense of being overwhelmed or out of control
11. Other physical symptoms, such as breast tenderness or swelling, headaches, joint or muscle pain, a sensation of 'bloating', weight gain

B. The disturbance markedly interferes with work or school or with usual social activities and relationship with others (e.g. avoidance of social activities, decreased productivity and efficiency at work or school).

C. The disturbance is not merely an exacerbation of the symptoms of another disorder, such as major depressive disorder, panic disorder, dysthymic disorder or a personality disorder (although it may be superimposed on any of these disorders).

D. Criteria A, B and C must be confirmed by prospective daily ratings during at least two consecutive symptomatic cycles. (The diagnosis may be made provisionally prior to this confirmation.)

Does Lee-Lin have premenstrual syndrome? This has not been established by prospective charting of her symptoms as required by the American Psychiatric Association (1994) diagnostic criteria, but Lee-Lin requested oral contraception and now finds her symptoms largely resolved. She has been advised that the 'pill' may help with her premenstrual symptoms. Is the improvement due to the placebo effect?

The health professional's definition of premenstrual syndrome should not be as all-embracing as the advertiser's nor as restrictive and exclusive as the researcher's definition. Women should, if possible, complete a menstrual diary for at least two cycles prior to treatment. This prospective charting may reveal symptoms unrelated in time to the menstrual cycle, symptoms throughout the cycle but with a premenstrual exacerbation (perimenstrual distress) or premenstrual syndrome with absence of symptoms postmenses (Sampson, 1989).

Aetiology of premenstrual syndrome

The cause of premenstrual syndrome is unknown but is probably complex and multifactorial. No consistently abnormal patterns of hormones, nutritional deficiencies or predictable coexisting psychiatric disorders have been found. Premenstrual syndrome does seem to be a 'Western' disorder, unlike dysmenorrhoea and menstrual mood changes which occur in societies throughout the world (Sampson, 1989). Recently, serotonin abnormalities have been implicated in the aetiology and it has been suggested that the syndrome is a form of atypical depression (Steiner et al, 1995).

Management of premenstrual syndrome

As many causes have been postulated for premenstrual syndrome, it is inevitable that many treatments have also been suggested. Defining the woman's symptom complex as accurately as possible and considering relevant gynaecological, contraceptive and psychosocial factors is essential. This comprehensive assessment is not only necessary to devise a rational management plan, but women report that having the problem acknowledged and taken seriously is itself helpful. The menstrual chart helps to define the problem and can also prompt useful self-help strategies, for example not scheduling avoidable stressful activities in the premenstrual time.

Information and education about menstruation and menstrual cycle problems can reduce anxiety and distress. Self-help education material is available but much of it is biased and promotes particular treatments based on unsubstantiated opinions about aetiology. A broad but discerning approach encompassing healthy lifestyle changes, improved stress management and specific symptom relief measures helps the majority of women with premenstrual syndrome.

Regular exercisers have fewer premenstrual symptoms than non-exercisers (Aganoff and Boyle, 1994). It has been suggested that this benefit is related to endorphin production. Manipulative therapy has been advocated in premenstrual syndrome as it is postulated that endorphins are released during spinal manipulation.

Specific treatments

The potential side effects of specific remedies must be considered, as must possible toxicity in pregnancy.

PYRIDOXINE (VITAMIN B6) AND EVENING PRIMROSE OIL (GAMMA-LINOLENIC ACID)

Many women report benefits from pyridoxine, evening primrose oil and preparations containing both substances. Pyridoxine is a co-factor in the metabolism of the neurotransmitters dopamine, noradrenaline and serotonin. Gamma-linolenic acid is a precursor of prostaglandin E and an intermediary in the production of essential fatty acids. Deficiencies of pyridoxine and gamma-linolenic acid have been postulated in premenstrual syndrome.

There are no consistent findings in the literature about the efficacy of these substances. Pyridoxine may cause gastrointestinal side effects and there may be a risk of producing neuropathy with larger doses. Nausea, softening of the stools and headaches are side effects reported with evening primrose oil.

PROSTAGLANDIN INHIBITORS

Antiprostaglandin medication may be helpful in controlling mood and physical symptoms but may also cause gastrointestinal side effects.

ENDOCRINE TREATMENTS

Combined oral contraceptives, oestrogens, progesterone and progestogens, bromocriptine, danazol (an androgen) and gonadotropin-releasing hormone agonists have been used with reported benefit in individual women but with no reproducible proven benefit in studies.

DIURETICS

Spironolactone, the aldosterone antagonist diuretic, may be useful.

SEROTONIN REUPTAKE INHIBITORS

Fluoxetine and other serotonin reuptake inhibitors have been shown recently to be more effective than placebo in the treatment of premenstrual syndrome (Steiner et al, 1995).

Summary

Premenstrual syndrome is a nebulous cyclic disorder of unknown cause affecting women throughout their reproductive lives. It causes significant disability to a minority and lesser problems to a majority of women. Further research into the causes of premenstrual syndrome is necessary, as is scientific assessment of the many suggested treatments.

Menorrhagia (Heavy Periods)

About 30% of adolescent women complain of heavy periods. Average menstrual blood loss is 40 ml per cycle while menorrhagia is menstrual blood loss of more than 80 ml each cycle. Self-estimation of blood loss is very unreliable. The research method for assessment of menstrual blood loss is the conversion of the blood in pads or tampons to alkaline haematin which can then be quantified colorimetrically.

Bleeding disorders are present in about 20% of adolescents with menorrhagia. Heavy or irregular bleeding may be caused by anovulatory cycles. This may occur in adolescence because of immaturity of the feedback mechanisms to the hypothalamus and pituitary, resulting in lack of ovulation and lack of formation of the corpus luteum. Oestrogen, unopposed by progesterone, leads to endometrial overgrowth and subsequent heavy bleeding. Antiprostaglandins and/or the oral contraceptive pill will decrease blood loss by about 50% (Rosenfeld and Barnes, 1993).

Amenorrhoea and Oligomenorrhoea (Absent and Infrequent Periods)

Pregnancy must always be considered in the adolescent who complains of amenorrhoea, even if she has never had a period. In primary amenorrhoea (never menstruated), pubertal development should be assessed. Chromosomal abnormalities such as Turner syndrome (chromosome pattern 45XO or 45XO/46XX) lead to delayed puberty and short stature but are usually recognized earlier in childhood. Delayed puberty and menarche are much more likely to be physiological (no underlying pathology) or due to excessive exercise and/or anorexia nervosa.

Polycystic ovarian syndrome is a common cause of secondary amenorrhoea or oligomenorrhoea in adolescent women. About 90% of women with oligomenorrhoea and 30% with amenorrhoea may have this condition. Hirsutism (excessive hairiness), acne and obesity may be associated.

Menstrual irregularities may be caused by any factor or disease process which interferes with the hypothalamic–pituitary–ovarian axis, the endometrium and the outflow of blood from the uterus.

Summary

Menstrual cycle problems can impair the quality of many young women's lives. Although much more needs to be discovered about the aetiology and treatment of these conditions, better education about menarche, menstruation and the remedies available if there are problems could alleviate much distress.

ACKNOWLEDGEMENTS

My thanks go to Ruth Ratcliffe for menarcheal stories.

References

Abraham S, Fraser I, Gebski V et al (1985) Menstruation, menstrual protection and menstrual cycle problems. *Medical Journal of Australia* **142**: 247–251.

Adler NE, Kegeles SM, Irwin CE et al (1990) An assessment of decision processes. *Journal of Pediatrics* **116**: 463–469.

Aganoff JA and Boyle GJ (1994) Aerobic exercise, mood states and menstrual cycle symptoms. *Journal of Psychosomatic Research* **38**: 183–191.

American Psychiatric Association (1994) *Diagnostic and Statistical Manual of Mental Disorders*, 4th edn, pp. 715–718. Washington DC: APA.

Brooks-Gunn J and Ruble DN (1982) The development of menstrual-related beliefs and behaviors during early adolescence. *Child Development* **53**: 1567–1577.

Cumming DC, Cumming CE and Kieran DK (1994) Menstrual mythology and sources of information about menstruation. *American Journal of Obstetrics and Gynecology* **164**: 472–476.

Fraser IS (1992) Prostaglandins, prostaglandin inhibitors and their roles in gynaecological disorders. *Baillière's Clinical Obstetrics and Gynaecology* **6**: 829–857.

Jay MS, DuRant RH, Shoffilt T et al (1984) Effect of peer counsellors on adolescent compliance in use of oral contraceptives. *Pediatrics* **73**: 126–130.

Reid RL (1991) Premenstrual syndrome. *New England Journal of Medicine* **324**: 1208–1210.

Rosenfeld RL and Barnes RB (1993) Menstrual disorders in adolescence. *Endocrinology and Metabolism Clinics of North America* **22**: 491–505.

Sampson GA (1989) Premenstrual syndrome. *Baillière's Clinical Obstetrics and Gynaecology* **3**: 687–704.

Sloane BC and Zimmer CG (1993) The power of peer education. *Journal of American College Health* **41**: 241–245.

Snowden R and Christian B (1983) Patterns and perception of menstruation: a cross cultural study. In: Dennerstein L and Senarclens M (eds) *The Young Woman: Psychosomatic Aspects of Obstetrics and Gynaecology*, pp. 47–54. International Congress Series 618. Amsterdam: Excerpta Medica.

Steiner M, Steinberg S, Stewart D et al (1995) Fluoxetine in the treatment of premenstrual dysphoria. *New England Journal of Medicine* **332**: 1531–1534.

Walker BG (1983) *The Woman's Encyclopedia of Myths and Secrets*, p. 643. New York: Harper Collins.

Wilson CA, Keye C and Keye WR (1989) A survey of adolescent dysmenorrhoea and premenstrual symptom frequency. *Journal of Adolescent Health Care* **10**: 317–322.

7

The Pelvic Floor and its Related Organs

RUTH SAPSFORD

The pelvic floor muscles (PFM) and the function of organs associated with these muscles form an important aspect of work for physiotherapists involved in women's health. The functional disorders of that area of the body are frequently the sequelae of the hormonal and reproductive process. Certainly the high incidence of urinary incontinence in the middle decades and the defaecation difficulties peri- and post-menopausally are related to parturition. They can also occur unrelated to vaginal deliveries.

However, problems occur at all ages, so it seems relevant to introduce pelvic floor (PF) anatomy and normal pelvic organ function at this stage. Problems experienced by adolescent girls will be described in the next chapter, but for details of management of the various conditions refer to Chapter 30.

While anatomy – the structure – doesn't change, it has been realized that descriptions of anatomy from aged and embalmed cadavers do not truly reflect the relationships between organs and muscles that occur in living subjects. Consequently, there are now many reports of physiological, ultrasound, magnetic resonance imaging and electromyographic studies which provide a truer picture of the PF and its associated organ function. Whilst the basic description of muscles is taken from traditional anatomy sources (*Gray's Anatomy*, 1995; Netter, 1989) there is some variation in nomenclature regarding parts of the PFM amongst current researchers (DeLancey, 1994a). Clarification of the full role of PFM will come from further research into the function of the PF and its relation with other trunk muscles, rather than from that related to isolated organ function. A knowledge of the present understanding of this anatomy is essential for physiotherapists treating pelvic organ dysfunction.

Superficial Pelvic Floor Muscles

The PF is considered by some writers to consist of the pelvic organs outside the peritoneum, the endopelvic fascia, the deep and superficial muscle layers and their intervening fibrous diaphragms. The muscular diaphragm which supports the pelvic contents and helps prevent their prolapse through the bony pelvic outlet consists of the superficial muscle groups of both the urogenital and anal triangles and the deep group, which is termed the levator ani. Fascia invests these muscles and forms the connection between organs, muscles and the pelvic walls.

External anal sphincter (EAS)

This is a true sphincter muscle and is frequently described in three parts – subcutaneous, superficial and deep – though separate parts have not always been demonstrated at dissection (Ayoub, 1979). The *subcutaneous* segment has circular fibres which insert into the skin and cause skin puckering as they contract. The *superficial* section has fibres which encircle the anus and attach posteriorly to the tip of the coccyx and anteriorly to the perineal body. The *deep* part is a true sphincter and the fibres of puborectalis are incorporated into it.

ACTION

The EAS assists in maintaining anal closure at rest, being responsible for up to 30% of this pressure (Lestar et al, 1989). It maintains a low level of activity in sleep (Floyd and Walls, 1953). It contracts strongly when there are increases in intra-abdominal pressure (IAP) and with voluntary effort.

Superficial perineal muscles

The *ischiocavernosus* arises from the ischial tuberosity and inserts into the side and undersurface of the crus of the clitoris. The *bulbospongiosus* arises from the perineal body and, encircling the vagina and urethra, inserts across the body of the clitoris. These two muscles act upon the clitoris and are probably involved in the female sexual response (DeLancey, 1994b). The bulbospongiosus closes the vaginal orifice.

The *transversus perinei superficialis* arises from the ischial tuberosity and inserts into the *perineal body*, which is a fibromuscular structure set in the mid-point of the perineum, between the anus and the vagina. It acts as the hub of the superficial muscle complex and its stability contributes to the efficient functioning of those muscles as well as providing support for the anal canal (Fig. 7.1). Fibres from the levator ani also attach to it. Stretch and tearing of fibromuscular tissues are not uncommon during childbirth and often compromise perineal body stability.

The *striated urogenital sphincter* muscle is now considered to consist of three parts (Oelrich, 1983). The lower two segments take the place of the deep transverse perinei in the male.

1. The *sphincter urethrae* surrounds the urethra in its mid-region. The circularly directed fibres tend to be deficient posteriorly in the adult and the muscle inserts into fibrous tissue. This has been called the rhabdosphincter.
2. The *compressor urethrae* is continuous above with the urethral sphincter. It arises from the ischiopubic rami, travels forward and medially to arch across the anterior surface of the urethra.
3. The *sphincter urethrovaginalis* blends with the compressor urethrae above and arises from the anterior side of the urethra. It passes posteriorly along the urethra and vagina to insert posterior to the vagina into the opposite muscle and perineal body.

The three muscles act to compress, retract and elongate the urethra. The lower two are probably responsible for voluntary interruption of micturition. In nulliparae, an average time of 1.96 seconds is needed to stop the flow of urine in mid-stream but in multiparae it takes longer, a mean of 4.4 seconds (Sampselle and DeLancey, 1992).

Deep Pelvic Floor Muscle Group

Levator ani

Three muscles are usually classified as the levator ani and it is important to understand them separately as they can function in different ways. If you consider that the human

Figure 7.1 Muscles of the female urogenital and anal triangles.

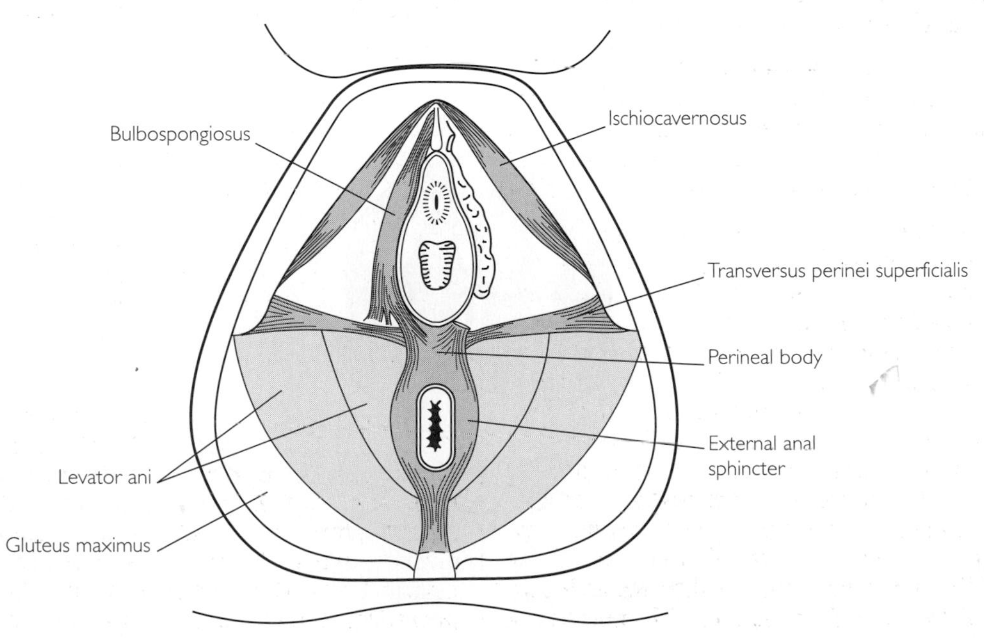

levator ani has evolved from the tailed animal species you will understand how the different functions have arisen. In dogs, the pubococcygeus pulls the tail between the legs, while the iliococcygeus and ischiococcygeus wag the tail from side to side (Figs 7.2 and 7.3).

The *puborectalis* arises from the posterior surface of the pubic bone in conjunction with the pubococcygeus and, passing backwards alongside the urethra, vagina and the rectum, it inserts into the muscle from the other side. It forms a U-shaped sling around the anorectal junction, where it is incorporated into the deep anal sphincter. It is inferior to the levator plate. It pulls the anorectal junction anteriorly, thus assisting in anal closure. Puborectalis and the external anal sphincter are considered to act as one unit.

The *pubococcygeus* arises from the posterior surface of the pubic bone and the fascia over the obturator internus and passes backwards with the puborectalis, contributing varying slips to the vagina, perineal body and the rectum. It joins with the muscle of the other side posterior to the anus to form the anococcygeal ligament and through this inserts into the anterior surface of the coccyx. It tends to pull the coccyx forward, elevates all the pelvic organs and compresses the rectum and vagina.

Figure 7.2 Levator ani – perineal aspect.

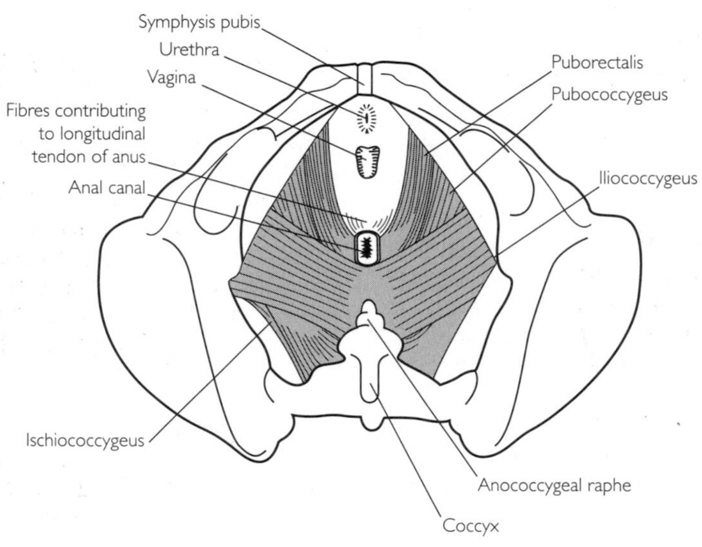

Figure 7.3 Levator ani – pelvic aspect.

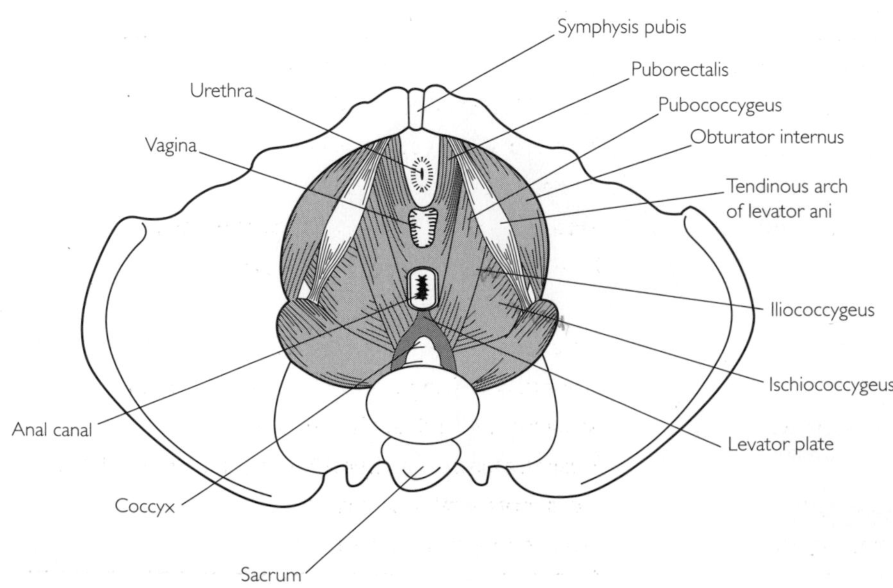

The *iliococcygeus* arises from the fascia over the obturator internus and the ischial spine and passes posteromedially to join the muscle of the other side, posterior to the anus and inferior to the pubococcygeus. It inserts into the fibrous anococcygeal raphe and the lateral margins of the lower surface of the coccyx. It tends to pull the coccyx from side to side and elevates the rectum which lies on the levator plate. The *levator plate* is the term applied to the combined layers of pubococcygei and iliococcygei that unite posterior to the anorectal junction and insert into the coccyx. In the anterior part of the pelvic floor the opening between the two pubococcygei is often termed the *levator hiatus*.

The *ischiococcygeus* can be considered as part of the levator ani or as a separate muscle. It arises from the ischial spine and the sacrospinous ligament and inserts into the lateral margins of the upper coccyx and lower sacrum. It exhibits marked individual variation. It provides support for pelvic contents and contributes to sacroiliac joint stability.

Overall the levator ani is almost horizontal in the sagittal plane, with a slight downward bow. It is gutter shaped in the coronal view.

There have been differences of opinion regarding the innervation of the periurethral sphincters and the PF for a long time. It would seem that there is considerable individual variation in the nerve supply and some of the muscles probably receive innervation via both the pelvic surface, from direct branches of sacral nerve roots, and the perineal surface from branches of the pudendal nerve. Table 7.1 details the motor nerve supply of the perineal and pelvic floor muscles. Motor and sensory branches may travel in different nerves. Recent work has been carried out on male cadavers and it is unknown whether there are gender variations.

Action of the Pelvic Floor Muscles

A better understanding of PF function has been achieved by means of modern investigation techniques. However, a study of levator myography (Berglas and Rubin, 1953) was the first to show the true relationships of organs to muscles (Fig. 7.4). The levator plate, rectum and vagina were defined by barium and their positions at rest and on straining were recorded.

It is easier to understand the mechanics of a combined PFM contraction by studying Figure 7.5, which is based on these X-ray studies. During a pelvic floor contraction the anorectal junction, the vagina and urethra are pulled anteriorly; all the organs are lifted forwards and in a cephalad direction and the rectum and vagina are compressed.

Magnetic resonance imaging (MRI)

A recent study (Christensen et al, 1995) demonstrated that with a submaximal sustained contraction (one and a half minutes were required for MRI), the PF moved the bladder and urethra upwards, lifting the posterior bladder wall a mean of 7 mm. Anterosuperior movement was observed in all organs. Fast scanning MRI (2–10 seconds) demonstrated increased obliquity of the levator plate on straining in normal subjects (Goodrich et al, 1993). This confirmed the earlier findings of Berglas and Rubin (1953).

Ultrasound

Perineal ultrasound studies have measured the lift of the bladder neck during voluntary maximal PFM contraction at

Table 7.1 Nerve supply to the muscles of the pelvic floor

Muscle	Nerve supply	
External anal sphincter	Inferior haemorrhoidal branch of pudendal N	S2
Ischiocavernosus	Perineal branch of pudendal N	S2
Bulbospongiosus	Perineal branch of pudendal N	S2
Transversus perinei sup.	Perineal branch of pudendal N	S2
Urogenital sphincter	Sensory – dorsal N clitoris, branch of pudendal N	S3
	Motor – perineal branch of pudendal N	S3
	– pelvic sacral roots	S2, 3
Puborectalis	Sacral roots – pelvic suface – ipsilateral	S3
	Proximal branch of pudendal N – perineal surface	
Pubococcygeus	Sacral roots – pelvic surface – ipsilateral	S3, 4
	Proximal branch of pudendal N – perineal/asymmetrical	
Iliococcygeus	Sacral roots – pelvic surface	S3, 4
Ischiococcygeus	Sacral roots – pelvic surface	S3, 4

(Percy et al, 1981; Jeunemann et al, 1988; Zvara et al, 1994; Narayan et al, 1995)

Figure 7.4 X-ray of a nulliparous female in relaxed standing. The rectum (R) and vagina (V), outlined with barium, are positioned over a slightly oblique levator plate (Lp). X marks the anterior margin of the levator plate. On straining, the levator plate becomes more oblique and the organs are pressed against it. (Reproduced from Berglas and Rubin (1953) with permission of *Surgery, Gynecology and Obstetrics.*)

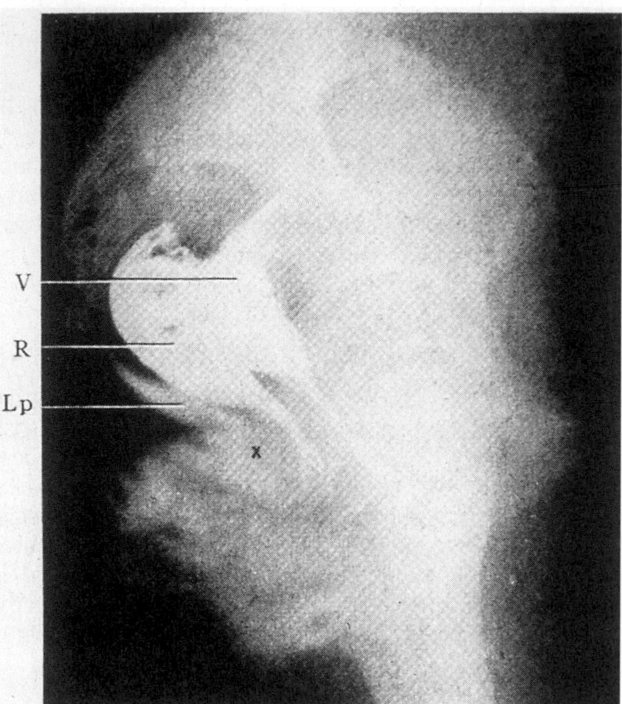

Figure 7.5 Drawing of a normal vaginal axis of the living showing an almost horizontal upper vagina and rectum lying upon and parallel to the levator plate. The latter is formed by fusion of pubococcygei muscles posterior to the rectum. (Copyright Dr DH Nichols. Reproduced from Nichols and Randall (1989) with permission of Williams and Wilkins and the authors.)

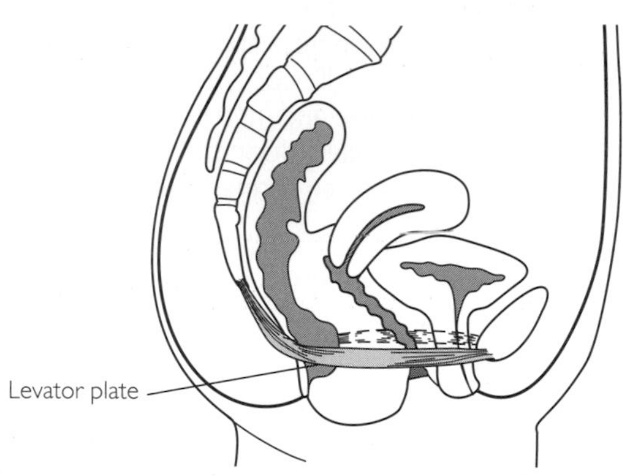

8.5 mm in normal subjects (Wise et al, 1992). PFM thickness varied from 7.9 to 10.9 mm in normals at rest, with a mean increase of 2.2 mm on contraction (Klarskov et al, 1991).

Electromyography (EMG)

Many kinesiological EMG studies have been carried out and record muscle activity at rest and during various activities. Pubococcygeal activity has been recorded by fine-wire EMG with the subject at rest in the supine position (Deindl et al, 1993). In normal continent nulliparous females during voluntary PF holds, activity can be sustained over a long period – up to 647 seconds with an empty bladder and 600 seconds with a full one – but there is marked individual variation (Deindl et al, 1993). Using vaginal surface electrodes, EMG of pubococcygeus was compared with baseline readings in supine. A strong posterior pelvic tilt in supine generated EMG activity of baseline × 2, standing generated baseline × 5 and resisted hip adduction generated baseline × 10 activity (Santiesteban, 1988).

Associated activity

There is increasing evidence of an interaction between the pelvic floor and the abdominal wall, but the extent of this interaction, and the mechanisms which effect it, are not understood at present. PFM maximal contractions performed by well-trained subjects without any visible movement of the rest of the body produced EMG activity in the rectus abdominis (Bo et al, 1990). However, a recent fine-wire EMG study by Sapsford et al (1997a) demonstrated that activity occurred in all the abdominal muscles during a maximal PFM contraction. It occurred principally in transversus abdominis and the obliques, with least activity in rectus abdominis. The position of the lumbar spine affected the activity, with a significant increase in external oblique (EO) EMG activity in subjects in a posterior pelvic tilt position.

A concentric needle electrode inserted into the periurethral levator ani recorded pelvic floor activity associated with hip and trunk movements – hip adduction, gluteal contraction, posterior pelvic tilt and sit ups (Bo and Stien, 1994). Fine-wire EMG receptors inserted into pubococcygeus recorded activity in that muscle during a variety of isometric abdominal exercises such as 'hollowing' (TrA) and 'bracing' (TrA and EO) (Sapsford et al 1997b).

Histology

Stabilizing and supporting muscles exhibit tonic muscle activity and have a high proportion of slow-twitch muscle fibres. PFM are support muscles and different studies, detailed in Table 7.2, confirm high numbers of slow-twitch (type 1) fibres.

Muscle spindles have been found in all muscles. Oestrogen receptors have not been identified in striated muscle cells of the female pubococcygeus, but some have been isolated from the connective tissue of the levator ani (Bernstein et al, 1995).

Table 7.2 Distribution of fibre types in pelvic floor muscles

Muscle	Type I fibres
Pubococcygeus – anterior (Gilpin et al, 1989)	67%
– posterior	76%
Puborectalis (Swash, 1992)	75%
Periurethral levator ani (Gosling et al, 1981)	95%
External anal sphincter (Swash, 1992)	78%

Connective Tissue Supports of Pelvic Organs

The endopelvic fascia, fibromuscular tissue containing abundant smooth muscle fibres, surrounds the pelvic organs and, attaching to the pelvic side walls, suspends the organs. This fascia is thickened in several areas to form 'ligaments' which do not have the structure of true ligaments.

The rectum is attached along the lines of the sacral foraminae to the curve of the sacrum. The parametrium is that section of the fascia attached to the uterus and is made up of the cardinal and uterosacral ligaments which support the uterus. It continues down the vagina as the paracolpium (attached to the vagina), the upper part supporting the upper vagina over the rectum and levator plate and the lower part holding the lower vagina between the bladder and the rectum. Pubocervical fascia supports the bladder and consists of the covering of the anterior vaginal wall and its attachment to the pelvic side walls. Rectovaginal fascia, which attaches the posterior vaginal wall to the pelvic side walls, prevents the rectum from protruding forwards. Suburethral fascia attaches to the arcus tendineus fascia pelvis and the medial border of the levator ani (DeLancey, 1994a). The lower vagina is fused to the levator muscle, perineal body, urethra and perineal membrane. Pubourethral ligaments, from the mid-region of the urethra, attach to the pubic bones and contribute to urethral support.

Tearing and stretching of the endopelvic fascia result in loss of support for the organs. Ageing and genetic factors may compound the original problem. Together they contribute to organ prolapse (see Chapters 27 and 28).

The Role of the Pelvic Floor Muscles in the Female

There is still much to be discovered about how these muscles function in normal subjects in daily living. Due to their inaccessibility, testing is difficult and until recently physiotherapists have tended to consider that the PF was only of concern to therapists working in the region of women's health. Muscle function research has generally been the province of therapists working in musculoskeletal and sports physiotherapy areas. Now there is an awareness of the coactivated function of the PF with limb and trunk muscles in many activities (Bo and Stien, 1994; Markwell and Sapsford, 1995; Sapsford et al, 1996; Sapsford et al 1997b; Voss et al, 1985). Activation of the PF can facilitate contraction of other muscle groups, e.g. abdominal, and vice versa.

The role of the pelvic floor

- Supports the pelvic organs
- Integral to increases in intra-abdominal pressure
- Maintains the anorectal angle, contributing to faecal continence
- Provides rectal support during defaecation
- Reinforces urethral closure during increases of intra-abdominal pressure
- Has an inhibitory effect on bladder activity
- Assists in 'unloading' the spine
- Assists in pelvispinal stability
- Contributes to sexual arousal and performance

Pelvic organ support

The muscles provide constant support of the organ load in the upright position. Fascia envelops the muscles and, with the ligaments, attaches organs to the side walls of the pelvis, but these connections are not strong enough to provide continuous support (Nichols and Randall, 1989). The ligaments attached to the organs, like those around any joint, limit the extent of movement under pressure. If called upon to provide the sole support, they gradually lengthen.

Relationship to intra-abdominal pressure

The contraction of the PF has been noted with increased IAP. Constantinou and Govan (1982) have reported a periurethral contraction preceding the increase in IAP by 250 milliseconds in normal nulliparous subjects. This early activation of the pelvic floor appears to correlate with early activation of the deep abdominal muscles in specific activities (Hodges and Richardson, 1996). Research is in progress to identify the nature of the contributions of the PF muscles to the generation of IAP.

Maintaining the anorectal angle

The junction between the rectum and the anus is approximately 90° at rest (Bartram and Mahieu, 1992). This angle is decreased when the external anal sphincter and the puborectalis contract to defer imminent defaecation in an inappropriate situation (see Fig. 7.12).

Rectal support during defaecation

When the IAP is increased to initiate or sustain defaecation, rectal support is provided by the underlying muscles of the levator plate. Pubococcygeal activity has been recorded by EMG during defaecation in normal subjects (Lubowski et al, 1992). Other muscles of the levator plate also contribute.

Urethral closure

A strong sudden PFM contraction reinforces urethral closure during voluntary interruption of micturition (Vereecken and Verduyn, 1970). During the increased IAP of an effort activity, the PF contraction lifts the bladder neck higher into the abdominal pressure zone, where transmitted abdominal pressure reinforces proximal urethral closure and prevents any urine escaping (see Fig. 7.9).

Bladder inhibition

The normal resting muscle tone of the pubococcygeus tends to inhibit the sacral micturition centre in spinal cord segments S2, 3 and 4 (Mahony et al, 1977). This inhibition defers detrusor activation, resulting in larger bladder volumes with less frequent voiding.

'Unloading' the spine

The load of the upper body in the erect position would be entirely transmitted by the vertebral column if the IAP was zero. The static pressure created by a rigid abdominal cylinder can act to support the upper part of the body and therefore 'unload' the spine. This involves abdominal, dorsal, diaphragmatic and PF muscles (Grillner et al, 1978). Recent studies indicate that the coactivation of all these muscles is an essential prerequisite for developing appropriate IAP, thus supporting the spine (Hodges, personal communication).

Pelvispinal stability

The ischiococcygeus arises from the sacrospinous ligament and ischial spine and inserts into the lower part of the sacrum. Thus, strength in this muscle contributes to the stability of the sacrum, by providing a counternutation force (posterior shift of the base of the sacrum).

Sexual function

The superficial perineal muscles which insert around the crus and the body of the clitoris affect the vascular status of those organs, inhibiting venous return, and probably contribute to sexual response (DeLancey, 1994b). In discussion of PF strength, it has been stated that achievement of orgasm is significantly related to maximum PF squeeze pressure (Dougherty et al, 1986). However, not all authors agree on this.

Pelvic Floor Muscle Strength

The normal pelvic floor muscle, like all striated muscle, develops its strength from the demands placed upon it. Gordon and Logue (1985) found that subjects participating in regular fitness activities had stronger PFM, as measured by vaginal squeeze pressure, than those leading more sedentary lives. This applied whether they were parous or not. Specific PFM exercises were not practised regularly by most of those undertaking other fitness activities. The same response, of increased strength with increased physical activity, may not occur, however, in cases of significant pelvic floor pathology.

The Pelvic Organs

Urinary bladder

The bladder is a smooth muscle hollow viscus in which urine is stored. It is the only smooth muscle organ under voluntary control. Its shape varies with its degree of fullness, being collapsed within the lesser pelvis immediately posterior to the pubic bone when empty and rising into the abdomen, to a maximum of 5 cm above the pubic symphysis, when full. It is attached by ligaments and fascia to the side walls of the pelvis. Its triangular base is directed posteroinferiorly and is closely related to the anterior vaginal wall.

The very extensible transitional epithelium is attached to the smooth muscle (detrusor) walls. The three muscle layers of the detrusor are not distinct and this interlacing arrangement allows the extensibility required for filling with a minimal increase of pressure. The triangular base, the trigone, has thicker muscle and smoother mucosa and does not allow distension. The apex of the triangle is the lowest part and the urethra exits the bladder at this point through the neck of the bladder (Fig. 7.6). The urethra lies within the substance of the bladder walls for a short distance. The two ureters enter the bladder at the base of the trigone, traversing the muscle wall obliquely, thus ensuring closure and preventing reflux during bladder contraction when voiding.

In women without any PF laxity, the urethrovesical junction should be at the level of or above the superior margin of the pubic symphysis at rest in supine (Blaivas and Olsson, 1988) (Fig. 7.7).

URINE PRODUCTION

The kidneys control blood concentration and volume by removing surplus water and solute; they help regulate blood pH and remove toxic wastes. Of the 180 litres of blood filtered each day, approximately 1% of filtrate goes into

Figure 7.6 Simplified structure of the bladder and urethra with their efferent nerve supplies. α = alpha-adrenergic sympathetic nerve endings; β = beta-adrenergic sympathetic nerve endings; —— somatic efferent nerves; ---- parasympathetic nerves; ······ sympathetic nerves.

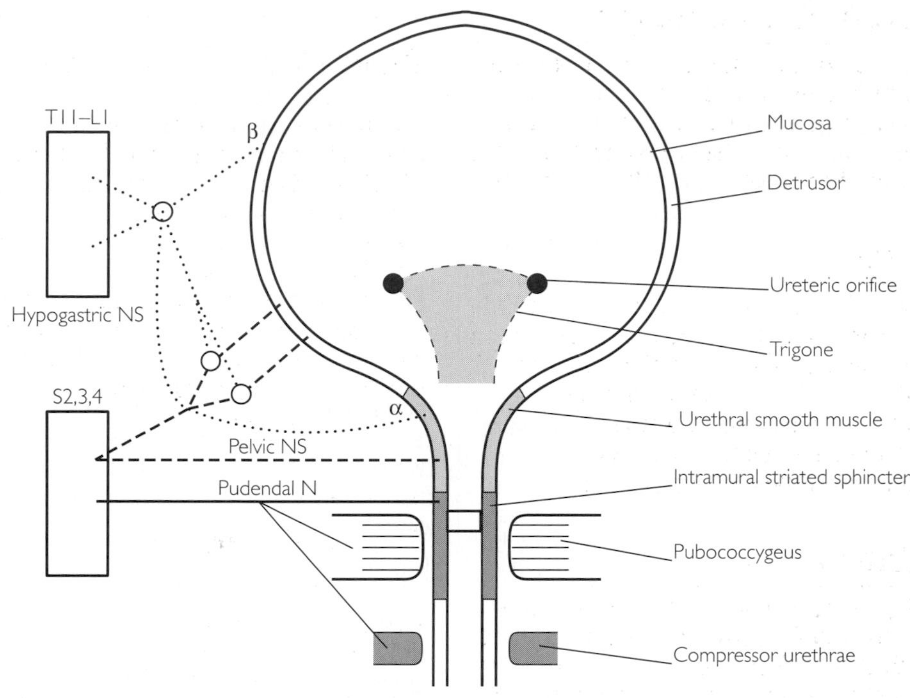

Figure 7.7 X-ray illustrating the position of the bladder base in relation to the symphysis pubis. Residual urine is in the bladder. Note the intrauterine contraceptive device (Lippes loop). (X-ray courtesy of Sue Markwell.)

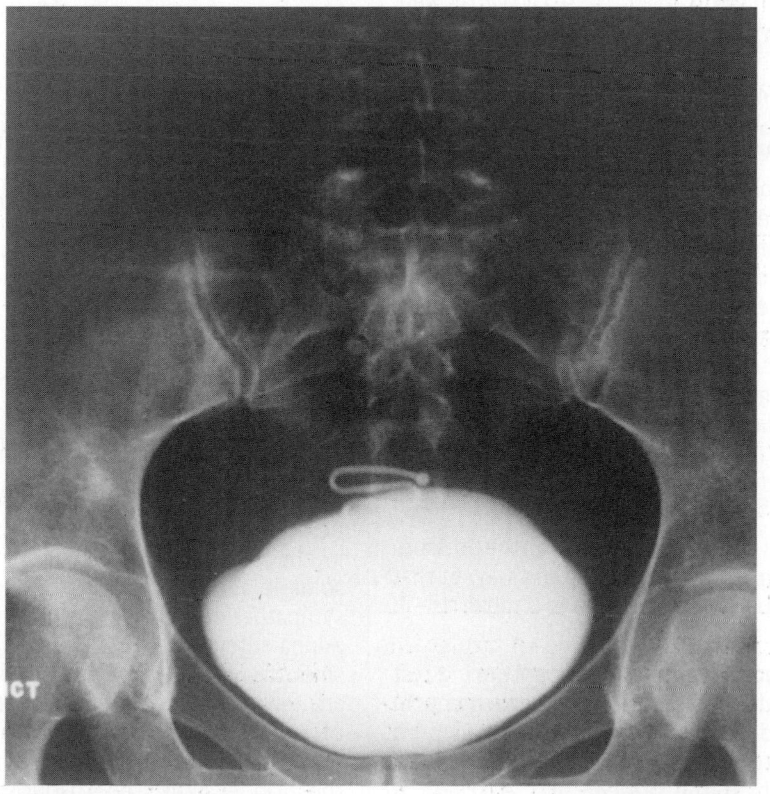

the urine, representing 1–2 litres of urine a day. On a normal diet, a minimum of about 500 ml of urine per day is needed to excrete urinary solutes, mainly urea and electrolytes. Antidiuretic hormone (ADH) controls the rate at which water is lost by controlling the permeability of the renal collecting ducts to water. Night urine production decreases under the effect of ADH.

The volume of urine produced and hence the rate of bladder filling is dependent on fluid intake, ambient temperature, intake of alcohol and other drugs and psychological state. Coffee, tea and alcohol are diuretics. Nervousness can cause increased amounts of urine as cerebral impulses increase blood pressure and renal filtration (Tortora and Anagnostakos, 1987).

BLADDER FUNCTION

Urine is continually entering the bladder, but the pressure remains low, usually <10 cmH_2O. The development of bladder capacity continues until adolescence. Approximate capacity for different ages is calculated at 30 ml per year, plus an extra two years, so that a 14-year-old could be expected to have a capacity of around 450–480 ml. The first sensation of filling generally occurs at 40% of cystometric bladder capacity (the bladder capacity during filling via catheter during cystometry) and the desire to void at 70–75% of capacity (Wyndaele, 1990).

In healthy females with a median age of 40 years, day frequency of voiding was 5.7 times (Boedker et al, 1989). A desire to void normally occurred at 380 ml, with a feeling of extreme fullness at 500 ml. In this series 22% of the women got up once at night to void. These capacities were measured by frequency/volume charts and there was no correlation with age. In other series the functional bladder capacity is smaller. A bladder capacity of 600 ml is considered the upper limit of normal in urodynamic studies, but there is no absolute maximum bladder capacity.

Bladder function with physiological filling varies from that recorded during catheter filling at cystometry. Assessment of normal filling and emptying responses has been made possible by the use of computer technology in ambulatory monitoring. In females, voided volumes were lower (340 ml), voiding pressures higher (60 cmH_2O) and urine flow rates were higher (28 ml sec^{-1}) during continuous ambulatory monitoring than those obtained in conventional urodynamic studies (Robertson et al, 1994).

BLADDER FILLING

As the bladder fills from 0 ml to 350–400 ml, the pressure rises from 0 to 5–10 cmH_2O in early filling and stays at that level until almost at capacity, when there is a rapid rise in pressure.

There is minimal tonic activity in the levator ani during rest in a supine position, with increases during movement. In standing there is a gradual increase in electrical activity in the urethral sphincter, to reinforce closure, and the levator ani, to support weight, as the bladder fills. A cough is accompanied by intense EMG activity in the striated muscles (Vereecken and Verduyn, 1970).

Late in the filling process there are periodic acute increases in bladder pressure (micturition waves) as the detrusor contracts in response to bladder wall stretch. The contraction subsides after a while and the conscious feeling of fullness fades. The urethra remains closed and its closure can be reinforced voluntarily by the contraction of the surrounding striated muscle. This compresses the urethra and elongates it, pulling the bladder neck in a cephalad direction.

The urethra

This is a multilayered tube, 6 mm in diameter, extending from the bladder neck 3–4 cm to the external urethral meatus on the perineum. Its proximal portion (15%) (DeLancey, 1994b) is within the bladder wall. It passes between the two sides of the levator ani but has no direct attachment to these muscles. It lies against the anterior vaginal wall and the lower two-thirds are inseparable from it.

The urethral epithelium is oestrogen sensitive. The submucosa is highly vascular and the resultant sponginess of the urethral wall contributes to urethral closure. This vascularity is also dependent on oestrogen. Elastic fibres in the connective tissue exert continuous tension and contribute to the static closure with little expenditure of energy. The viscoelastic closing mechanism is an important factor in prevention of urinary leakage (Lose et al, 1989). The smooth muscle is continuous with the bladder, yet distinct from it. The circular layer is poorly developed, but the longitudinal layer has more substance and probably functions to shorten the urethra during micturition (DeLancey, 1994b).

The striated intramural sphincter, sometimes called the *rhabdosphincter*, surrounds the urethra in its middle third. It is thicker anteriorly and is composed of slow-twitch fibres of small size, without any muscle spindles (Gosling et al, 1981), though a later study disputes this. In the lower third of the urethra, in the region between 60% and 80% of its length, the closing pressure is enhanced by the periurethral sphincter musculature (Fig. 7.8).

BLADDER AND URETHRAL INNERVATION

Afferent fibres from the bladder mucosa, detrusor muscle, urethral mucosa and smooth muscle, intramural striated sphincter, the levator ani and compressor urethrae travel via either the pelvic nerves or the pudendal nerves to the sacral cord (S2, 3, 4) and so to higher levels in the cord and to the brain. Efferent nerves are both somatic and autonomic (see Fig. 7.6). Cholinergic (parasympathetic) activity results in detrusor contraction. Alpha-adrenergic (sympathetic) activity contributes to smooth muscle closure in the proximal urethra. There are few beta-adrenergic sympathetic fibres in the dome of the bladder. Other sympathetic input may be mediated through the parasympathetic ganglia close to the bladder wall. The rhabdosphincter is supplied from

Figure 7.8 Approximate spatial relationships of muscles along the length of the female urethra, illustrated in percentages of the length, from proximal to distal.

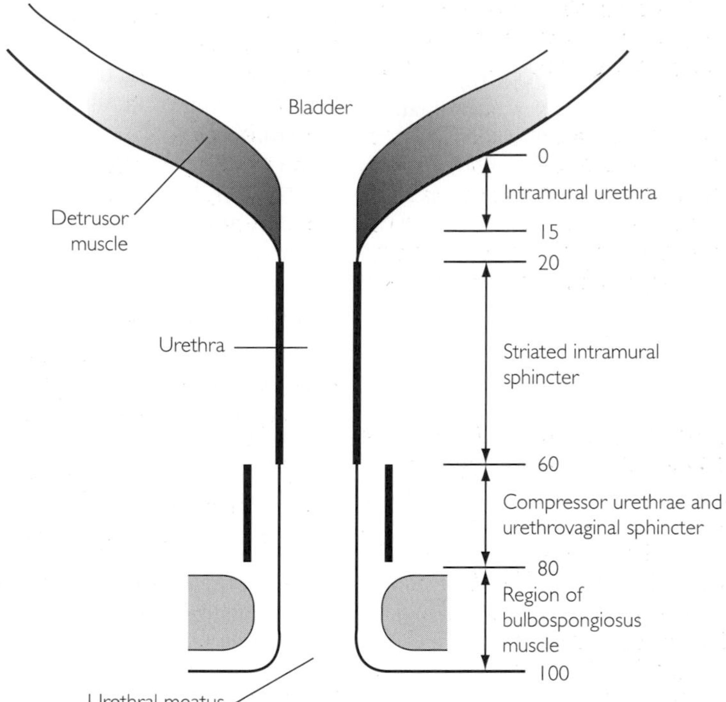

the pudendal nerve. In the male a second innervation has been identified from direct sacral branches on the pelvic surface (Zvara et al, 1994) and this parallels the previously reported nerve supply, via the pelvic nerves, in the female (Gosling, 1979) (see Table 7.1 for other striated muscle innervation).

Urethrovesical innervation is a complex mechanism and it is now well documented that there are non-adrenergic non-cholinergic (NANC) nerve receptors in the detrusor muscle. This has implications when considering the effect of medications on modification of detrusor behaviour.

URETHRAL FUNCTION

The urethra must stay closed and water-tight except when emptying. Maximal pressure is recorded in the region between 20% and 60% of the urethral length (Oelrich, 1983) (see Fig. 7.8). This area of generated pressure is greater than bladder pressure and is called the *functional urethral length*. In normal women (mean age of 46 years) the functional length is approximately 3 cm. Maximal urethral closing pressure (MUCP) varies with age, being approximately 75 cmH_2O during the 20s and falling to about 30 cmH_2O in women over 60 years (Hilton and Stanton, 1983). In a normal urethra the bladder neck can be seen to close within 0.25 seconds in a stop test during voiding (Gosling, 1979). This necessarily precedes cessation of urine flow.

The urethral closing pressure is measured during urodynamic studies as the difference between the intravesical pressure and the intraurethral pressure at the level of the sphincter. Rises of abdominal pressure are transmitted to the proximal urethra where they augment the sphincter and effectively maintain urethral closing pressure (Fig. 7.9). The closing pressure with effort, as in sneeze, cough, lift, etc., is reinforced by periurethral and levator ani muscle activity and the transmitted IAP. Studies show that pressure is greatest in the lower urethra in the region of the compressor urethrae muscle, precedes the rise in IAP and can be double the abdominal pressure (Constantinou and Govan, 1982).

Micturition

Micturition is an integrated striated and smooth muscle process. The sequence of activities in the process of voiding is as follows.

THE PROCESS OF MICTURITION

- The person sits or squats.
- The pelvic floor and periurethral sphincter muscles relax.
- The bladder neck descends.
- The diaphragm and the abdominal wall contract, minimally.
- The trigone contracts, opening the posterior bladder neck, and occludes the ureteric orifices.
- The bladder neck funnels and urine enters.
- There is a cessation of EMG activity in the urethral sphincter, the pelvic floor and the external anal sphincter (Vereecken and Verduyn, 1970). This electrical silence begins before the increase in bladder pressure.

Figure 7.9 Illustrating the relationship between increases in intra-abdominal pressure and intravesical and intraurethral pressures. The continent state of an anatomically normal patient is represented. An increase in intra-abdominal pressure is noted by the large arrow being applied directly to the bladder. Increases applied to the proximal urethra are indicated by the smaller arrows. The lower limit of the physiologic 'body cavity', or usual position of the pelvic diaphragm, is indicated by the dotted line. (Copyright Dr DH Nichols. Reproduced from Nichols and Randall (1989) with permission of Williams and Wilkins and the authors.)

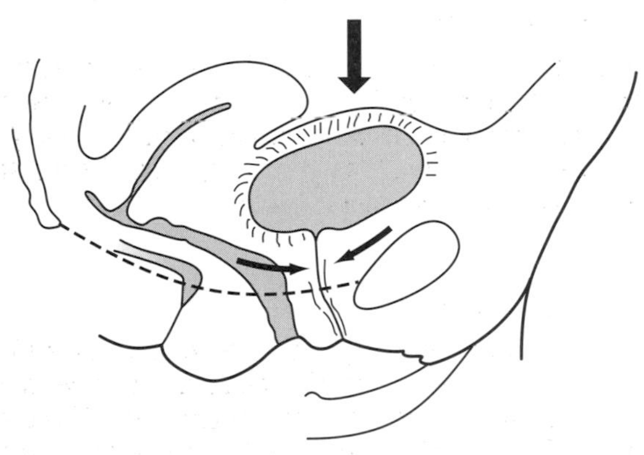

- The detrusor contracts and the urethra is pulled open, becoming shorter and wider. There is an increase of intravesical pressure. The posterior urethrovesical angle is lost.
- Urine flows until the bladder is empty, to a residue of virtually 0 ml. The rate of flow varies with the volume. (Peak flow rate on continuous monitoring was 23–28 ml sec^{-1} and maximum pressures reached 60–100 cmH_2O (Robertson et al, 1994).)
- The detrusor then relaxes, the urethral closing pressure is reinstated and the pelvic floor regains its low level of activity.
- The trigone resumes its normal tone.

If, however, the woman does not sit on the toilet seat but crouches above it (84.8% of women never sit on public toilet seats), the flow of urine is slower and the bladder may not empty completely, leaving a residue, measured by ultrasound, three times that recorded after seated voiding (Moore and Richmond, 1989). One explanation of this is that the urethra and pelvic floor do not relax completely in the crouching position when the glutei are functioning (Bo and Stein, 1994).

NEUROLOGICAL CONTROL OF BLADDER AND URETHRAL FUNCTION

Neurological control of continence and micturition involves extensive connections in both the peripheral and central nervous systems. Somatic sensory and motor neurones, sympathetic and parasympathetic neurones, the sacral micturition centre, ascending and descending spinal tracts and several centres within the brain (medulla, pons, cerebellum, frontal lobes, the sensory and motor cortex) all contribute to efficient function.

In infants bladder emptying is a reflex controlled, via the sacral micturition reflex centre (S2,3,4), by cerebral centres. All infant voiding triggered some sleep changes – either waking, limb or facial movements, change from quiet sleep to REM sleep or heart and respiratory rate changes. There was more marked awakening in older children (Yeung, 1995). Gradually function is modified by higher centres. By the time the child is five years old full control has generally developed.

In the mature subject there is conscious awareness of bladder fullness and sometimes of pelvic floor muscle activity. The ability to facilitate or inhibit the integrated pelvic floor/detrusor action required to empty the bladder is the basis of urinary continence. Micturition is generally initiated by conscious decision, at an appropriate time and place, and does not require a full bladder. Cortical centres stimulate the pontine micturition centre to initiate detrusor contraction via spinal tracts and the parasympathetic pathways and at the same time inhibit sympathetic bladder storage activity and urethral and pelvic floor closing activity. A simple way to remember the basic detrusor control is 'sympathetic stores and parasympathetic pours'.

The storage and voiding processes are controlled by a series of reflexes that contribute to urine storage, deferment of voiding, initiation of micturition, sustained detrusor contraction and sphincter relaxation to completion of voiding, interruption of voiding and resumed storage (Mahony et al, 1977).

Urinary continence

Continence is the ability to store and retain urine, with conscious control over the time and place of emptying. Physical disability which limits access to toilets can place severe restrictions on continence. Inability to locate a toilet or physical restraints to access (e.g. being confined in a broken down elevator) can cause any person to be incontinent under such circumstances. What are the physiological factors that contribute to urinary continence?

- A compliant and stable detrusor which allows bladder filling to a normal volume of 300–400 ml without any intermittent or sustained increases of pressure (not above 10 cmH_2O) during the filling.
- A bladder neck and proximal urethra that remain closed and do not allow egress of urine during the storage phase.
- An adequate and stable urethral closing pressure. It must be greater than the pressure of the bladder and the urine it contains and must not fluctuate spontaneously or under provocation.
- During increases of IAP, that pressure must be transmitted to the proximal urethra to counteract the abdominal pressure exerted on the bladder.
- Good neurological control of all the storage and voiding processes.

The uterus and vagina

The vagina is a fibromuscular tubal structure between the urethrovesical and the anorectal systems. It is a potential space and at rest the anterior and posterior walls are in contact. The epithelium is stratified squamous and in its well-oestrogenized state, the thickened walls form transverse folds called rugae, which are particularly noticeable on the anterior vaginal wall. The walls are thin when oestrogen levels are low before puberty and after the menopause. From the posterior wall of the vaginal introitus (entrance) to the posterior vaginal fornix it is 7–8 cm in length. The vagina rests on the rectum over the levator plate and is supported by the endopelvic fascia. It passes between the pubococcygeus and may get muscle slips from it. Lower down, it is surrounded by the urethrovaginal sphincter and the bulbospongiosus is in contact on each side. The urethra and bladder approximate the anterior wall and the rectovaginal septum and the perineal body the posterior wall.

The vagina functions as an organ for coitus, a repository for seminal fluid, a menstrual passage and a childbirth passage. During sexual arousal the inner two-thirds lengthen and widen. The outer third becomes grossly engorged, thus reducing the lumen, to form the orgasmic platform. These changes revert rapidly following orgasm, but take much longer to resolve if orgasm does not occur.

Details of uterine structure and function are covered in the section on the physiology of pregnancy in Chapter 10.

The rectum

The rectum is the lowest part of the gastrointestinal (GI) tract and is continuous above with the sigmoid colon and below with the anal canal. It begins at the level of S3 in the mid-line, lies in the sacrococcygeal curve, rests on the levator plate and ends in front of the tip of the coccyx at the anorectal flexure. It is covered by peritoneum in its upper two-thirds and this is reflected from the rectum onto the posterior vaginal wall, forming the base of the rectouterine pouch (pouch of Douglas). It is about 12 cm in length and its distal end is dilated to form the rectal ampulla. Its walls are composed of two layers of smooth muscle – inner circular and outer longitudinal. At its distal end the circular muscle layer thickens to form the internal anal sphincter and the longitudinal layer is augmented by slips from the pubococcygei.

INNERVATION

The rectal mucosa has abundant non-myelinated nerves supplied via the presacral and middle rectal plexuses. The sympathetic supply is a continuation of the hypogastric plexus (T7–12, L1–2) travelling with the inferior mesenteric artery. The parasympathetic supply is from the visceral branches of S2, 3 and 4 travelling in the pelvic splanchnic (nervi erigentes) nerves.

Much of the control of the activities of the GI tract is carried out at a local level by the enteric nervous system without input from the autonomic system. Non-adrenergic non-cholinergic (NANC) nerve endings are frequently found in this intrinsic system (Fig. 7.10).

RECTAL FUNCTION

The rectum is normally empty, with a resting pressure of 2–5 cmH_2O, and its role is that of a temporary storage container until a suitable time presents for emptying. The ease with which the contents are emptied is dependent on many factors, one of which is appropriate consistency. Consistency of rectal contents varies with fluid and solid intake, but is also affected by GI motility. A simple explanation of intestinal motility is contained in Table 7.3.

GI transit times in normal subjects are prolonged in the second and third trimesters of pregnancy and in the luteal phase of the menstrual cycle. Progesterone is the probable cause of this delay. Coffee has profound effects on the GI system in some people (both male and female). It can increase rectosigmoid motility within four minutes of ingestion, with the effects lasting 30 minutes. Hot water does not have the same effect. Susceptible subjects have a desire to defaecate within 20 minutes of drinking coffee (Brown et al, 1990).

Rectal motor activity tends to propel contents in a retrograde direction, away from the anus towards the lower pressure area of the sigmoid colon. This activity ceases after meals, allowing the gastrocolic reflex to initiate rectal filling and defaecation. Retrograde motor activity is greater at night (Rao and Welcher, 1994) and its purpose may be to

Figure 7.10 The enteric nervous system, which plays a large part in control of gastrointestinal function, has a sensory submucosal plexus (Meissner's) and a motor intermuscular plexus (Auerbach's).

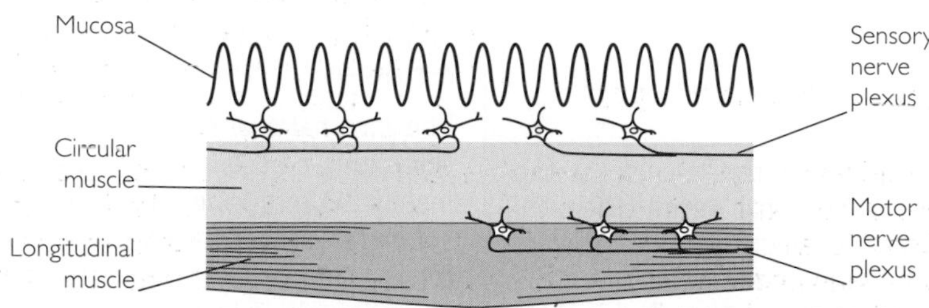

Table 7.3 Gastrointestinal function, motility and timing in normal subjects. The direction of movement of contents is indicated by arrows

Area	Action	Movement	Transit time
Mouth/pharynx/ oesophagus	Forward propulsion	Integrated smooth/striated muscle action	Liquids – 1 second Solids – 4–8 seconds
Stomach	Food break down	Mixing waves ⟲	Empties in 2–6 hours
Small intestine	Digestion	Segmentation ← → Peristalsis →	Empties 0.5–1 litre in 3–5 hours
Large intestine	Water and electrolyte absorption	Segmenting ← → Retrograde ← Giant propagating waves ⟶	Colon transit times: female 50 hours (max) male 35 hours (max)
Rectum	Container	Retrograde ← Peristalsis is rare in normals during defaecation	Empties in 11–20 seconds

Figure 7.11 The anal canal. In the upper canal the mucosa and underlying muscle are ridged into 6–10 vertical folds, which end distally in the anal valves half way down the canal. The submucosal tissue is very vascular, with a venous plexus called the haemorrhoidal plexus in the region of the anal valves. Three muscles contribute to the anal sphincter mechanism – the smooth muscle internal sphincter, striated muscle external sphincter and the combined smooth and striated conjoined longitudinal tendon of the anus.

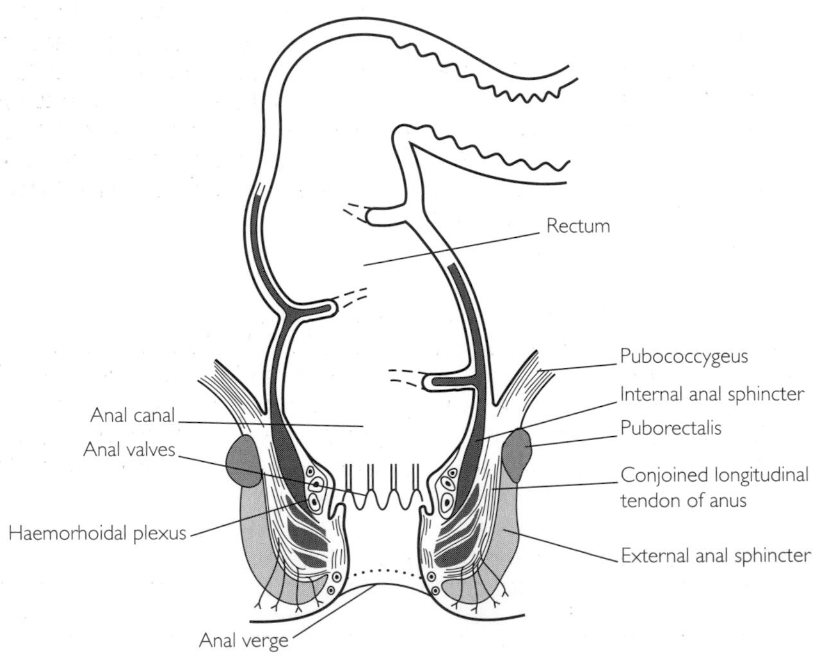

prevent contents reaching the anal region and so prevent nocturnal defaecation.

The anal canal

This begins at the level of the tip of the coccyx, at the anorectal flexure, and ends at the anal verge (the anal skin), which at rest in normal subjects in side lying is approximately 2 cm above the level of the ischial tuberosities (Womack et al, 1986). The length of the canal is 2.5–4.5 cm (longer in males) and it is an anteroposterior slit with its lateral walls in apposition. Its length increases with voluntary contraction of the external anal sphincter and puborectalis and decreases when the rectum is full (Fig. 7.11).

The *internal anal sphincter* consists of smooth muscle, a thickening of the circular muscle of the GI tract, approximately 30 mm long and 2–3 mm thick. The *external anal sphincter*, concentrically placed outside the internal sphincter, is a circular layer of striated muscle which incorporates the puborectalis in its deepest part. Between the two muscle layers, the longitudinal smooth muscle of the rectum is joined by slips from the medial borders of the pubococcygei forming the *conjoined longitudinal tendon of the anus*. This splits to be inserted into both the internal and external sphincters (see Fig. 7.11).

INNERVATION

The anal mucosa is sensitive to pain, temperature, touch, pressure and friction extending from above the anal valves to the hairy skin interface (Cherry and Rothenberger, 1988). Sensory fibres travel in the inferior haemorrhoidal nerves to S2, 3 and 4.

The motor supply is as follows.

- Sympathetic via hypogastric nerves: alpha-adrenergic contracts the internal sphincter, beta-adrenergic possibly relaxes it.
- Parasympathetic via the pelvic nerves: role inconclusive.
- Enteric nervous system – intramural: control of the rectoanal inhibitory reflex.
- Somatic via inferior haemorrhoidal branch of pudendal nerve: contracts the external sphincter.

ANAL SPHINCTER ACTIVITY

A basal resting pressure, highest 1–2 cm from the anal verge, keeps the anal sphincter closed. The internal sphincter is generally considered to provide 85% of this pressure. More recently, 70% of the closure has been attributed to it (Lestar et al, 1989). Intermittent internal sphincter relaxation occurs, unrelated to rectal filling, 3–5 times an hour, thus allowing anal sampling of rectal contents and discrimination between them.

Maximal squeeze pressure from the voluntary external sphincter contraction is greatest in the distal part of the canal and decreases proximally. It is generally twice as high as the resting pressure but can only be sustained for a short time, less than one minute. Rises in IAP are accompanied by increases in external sphincter pressure. Maximal cough-generated external sphincter pressure is greater than maximal voluntary squeeze pressure (Meagher et al, 1993).

There is great variation in normal values for resting and squeeze pressures, depending on equipment used and the age and sex of the subjects (Table 7.4). The effect of vaginal delivery on these values can be significant (see Chapter 23).

RECTAL FILLING

Giant propagating waves, triggered by food intake (gastrocolic reflex) and on waking, propel intestinal contents from the transverse colon to the rectum. Rectal filling creates different sensations – awareness, need to defaecate and discomfort (Table 7.5). These are probably pressure activated (Broens et al, 1994), but for some time it was considered that perception of these sensations was through stretch receptors in the pelvic floor muscles and their associated connective tissue.

As the rectum fills, the anal resting pressure fluctuates. This pressure decrease allows the anal mucosa to 'sample' the rectal contents, whether gas, liquid or solid. Gas can be expelled without passing solid contents. Rapid intermittent rectal filling leads to a sustained drop in internal sphincter pressure. This is called the rectoanal inhibitory reflex (RAIR) and precedes defaecation. The reflex is mediated through the myenteric plexus. Spontaneous increases in striated anal sphincter activity occur to maintain anal closure until the rectum can be emptied. This response to a drop in internal sphincter pressure also occurs in sleep (Orkin and Tissaw, 1994). If defaecation is deferred the rectum accommodates, the sensation fades and the sphincter pressure is gradually restored.

Defaecation

Defaecation, like swallowing and micturition, is a visceral and somatic process, involving diaphragmatic, abdominal, pelvic floor and colonic activity. It occurs between three times a day and three times a week in 94% of the population

Table 7.4 Normal anal pressures, mean values (Akervall et al 1990)

	Male	Female	Ageing effect
Maximal resting IAS	80.6 cmH_2O	76.2 cmH_2O	↓ 0.5% per year
Maximal squeeze EAS	327 cmH_2O	199 cmH_2O	↓ 1% per year

Table 7.5 Rectal sensations and approximate volume values taken as norms

Sensory threshold volume (STV)	Lowest distension-producing sensation	<30 ml
Defaecation threshold volume (DTV)	Threshold causing desire to defaecate	80–120 ml
Maximal tolerable volume (MTV)	Maximal distension causing great discomfort/pain	180–240 ml

These volumes are usually calculated using an air-filled balloon. There is marked variation even in normals

(Drossman et al, 1982). It proceeds through the following steps.

- Peristalsis propels contents into the rectum.
- Initial awareness of filling occurs – sensory threshold volume.
- Intermittent distension activates the rectoanal inhibitory reflex.
- Anal canal sampling of rectal contents occurs.
- With further filling the inhibitory reflex is sustained and the desire to defaecate is perceived – defaecation threshold volume.
- Puborectalis and external anal sphincter maintain anal closure until it is convenient to empty.
- At an acceptable time and place the subject sits or squats. Squatting widens the anorectal angle and lengthens the external anal aperture (Tagart, 1966).
- The pelvic floor relaxes.
- With increased IAP (obliques, transversus and diaphragm) the pelvic floor descends 1–2 cm and puborectalis and external anal sphincter release.
- The anorectal angle widens (to about 135°) and the anal canal funnels and shortens.
- As defaecation proceeds the increased IAP compresses the rectum against the actively supporting levator plate (Lubowski et al, 1992).
- Rectal emptying continues until complete, either with sustained IAP or with colonic peristalsis (peristaltic rectal contraction is rare in normals during defaecation).
- A 'closing reflex', a sharp burst of EMG activity, occurs in puborectalis, external anal sphincter and the PF at the end of defaecation, restoring normal position and pressure gradients.

Figure 7.12 The anorectal angle at rest, contracted and during defaecation. At rest anal closure is maintained predominantly by the internal anal sphincter. When defaecation is deferred puborectalis and the anal sphincter are contracted, the anus is lengthened and the anorectal angle decreased. During defaecation, the anorectal angle increases and the anal canal funnels and is shortened.

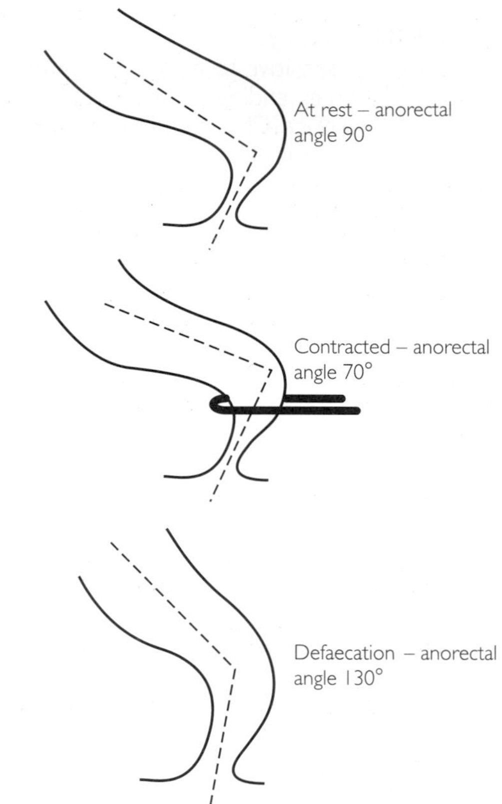

Faecal continence

As well as being able to empty the rectum effectively, each person needs to have absolute control over all actions associated with this. Continence has been defined as 'the ability to perceive, retain and evacuate rectal contents at a suitable time and place' (Kuijpers, 1990).

What maintains continence?

- *Anal canal high pressure zone.* Anal pressure is always greater than rectal pressure other than during defaecation. It increases with increases in IAP and is greater in the distal canal.
- *Anorectal angle.* Puborectalis contraction narrows the anorectal angle and lengthens the anal canal.
- *Rectal compliance and capacity.* Slow or intermittent filling allows time for rectal muscle accommodation, but inflammation and scarring can limit this.
- *Rectal sensation.* The sensory threshold volume varies, but awareness of rectal filling is a prerequisite for external sphincter response to internal sphincter relaxation.
- *Rectoanal inhibitory reflex.* The minimal volume to decrease internal sphincter pressure (10–30 ml) is termed the rectoanal inhibitory reflex threshold. External sphincter pressure increases simultaneously. Regular internal sphincter relaxation allows anal sampling of rectal contents.
- *Stool volume and consistency.* A large volume of liquid contents can overcome any continence mechanism.
- *Colorectal motility.* Rectal pressure is usually greater than sigmoid colon pressure and retrograde contractions tend to keep the rectum empty. Rapid propulsion of colonic contents may not allow time for rectal accommodation.

This description of the anatomy and function of the pelvic organs and pelvic floor muscles provides the student with a background understanding before treating patients with problems. Dysfunction associated with the pelvic floor and organs is dealt with in the age-relevant sections of this book – Chapters 8, 23, 28 and 29.

References

Akervall S, Nordgren S, Fasth S et al (1990) The effects of age, gender and parity on rectoanal functions in adults. *Scandanavian Journal of Gastroenterology* **25**: 1247–1256.

Ayoub SF (1979) Anatomy of the external anal sphincter in man. *Acta Anatomica* **105**: 25–36.

Bartram CI and Mahieu PHG (1992) Evacuation proctography and anal endosonography. In: Henry MM and Swash M (eds) *Coloproctology and the Pelvic Floor*, 2nd edn, p. 149. Oxford: Butterworth Heinemann Ltd.

Berglas B and Rubin IC (1953) Study of the supportive structures of the uterus by levator myography. *Surgery, Gynecology and Obstetrics* **97**: 677–692.

Bernstein I, Balslev E, Bodker A et al (1995) Estrogen receptors in the human levator ani muscles. *Neurourology and Urodynamics* **14**: 520–521.

Blaivas JG and Olsson CA (1988) Stress incontinence: classification and surgical approach. *Journal of Urology* **139**: 727–731.

Bo K and Stien R (1994) Needle EMG registration of striated urethral wall and pelvic floor muscle activity patterns during cough, valsalva, abdominal, hip adductor and gluteal muscle contractions in nulliparous healthy females. *Neurourology and Urodynamics* **13**: 35–41.

Bo K, Kvarstein B, Hagen R et al (1990) Pelvic floor muscle exercise for the treatment of female stress incontinence. 2. Validity of vaginal pressure measurements of pelvic floor muscle strength and the necessity of supplementary methods for control of correct contraction. *Neurourology and Urodynamics* **9**: 479–487.

Boedker A, Lendorf A, H-Neilsen A et al (1989) Micturition pattern assessed by the frequency/volume chart in healthy population of men and women. *Neurourology and Urodynamics* **8**: 421–422.

Broens PMA, Penninckx FM, Lestar B et al (1994) The trigger for rectal filling sensation. *International Journal of Colorectal Diseases* **9**: 1–4.

Brown SR, Cann PA and Read NW (1990) Effect of coffee on distal colon function. *Gut* **31**: 450–453.

Cherry DA and Rothenberger DA (1988) Pelvic floor physiology. *Surgical Clinics of North America* **68**: 1217–1230.

Christensen LL, Djurhuus JC and Constantinou CE (1995) Imaging of pelvic floor contractions using MRI. *Neurourology and Urodynamics* **14**: 209–216.

Constantinou CE and Govan DE (1982) Spatial distribution and timing of transmitted and reflexly generated urethral pressures in healthy women. *Journal of Urology* **127**: 964–969.

Deindl FM, Vodusek DB, Hesse U et al (1993) Activity patterns of pubococcygeal muscles in nulliparous continent women. *British Journal of Urology* **72**: 46–51.

DeLancey JOL (1994a) The anatomy of the pelvic floor. *Current Opinion in Obstetrics and Gynecology* **6**: 313–316.

DeLancey JOL (1994b) Functional anatomy of the pelvic floor and urinary continence mechanism. In: Schussler B, Laycock J, Norton P and Stanton S (eds) *Pelvic Floor Reeducation*, p. 9–21. London: Springer-Verlag.

Dougherty MC, Abrams R and McKey PL. (1986) An instrument to assess the dynamic characteristics of the circumvaginal musculature. *Nursing Research* **35**: 202–206.

Drossman DA, Sandler RS, McKee DC et al (1982) Bowel patterns among subjects not seeking health care. *Gastroenterology* **83**: 529–534.

Floyd WF and Walls EW (1953) Electromyography of the sphincter ani externus in humans. *Journal of Physiology* **122**: 599–604.

Gilpin SA, Gosling JA, Smith ARB et al (1989) The pathogenesis of genitourinary prolapse and stress incontinence of urine. A histological and histochemical study. *British Journal of Obstetrics and Gynaecology* **96**: 15–23.

Goodrich MA, Webb MJ, King BF et al (1993) Magnetic resonance imaging of pelvic floor relaxation: dynamic analysis and evaluation of patients before and after surgical repair. *Obstetrics and Gynecology* **82**: 883–891.

Gordon H and Logue M (1985) Perineal muscle function after childbirth. *Lancet* **2**: 123–125.

Gosling JA (1979) The structure of the bladder and urethra in relation to function. *Urologic Clinics of North America* **6**: 31–38.

Gosling JA, Dixon JS, Critchley HOD et al (1981) A comparative study of the human external sphincter and periurethral levator ani muscles. *British Journal of Urology* **53**: 35–41.

Gray's Anatomy (1995) 38th edn, p. 831–835. Edinburgh: Churchill Livingstone.

Grillner S, Nilsson J and Thortensson A (1978) Intra-abdominal pressure changes during natural movements in man. *Acta Physiologica Scandanavica* **103**: 275–283.

Hilton P and Stanton SL (1983) Urethral pressure measurement by microtransducer: the results in symptom free women and in those with genuine stress incontinence. *British Journal of Obstetrics and Gynaecology* **90**: 919–933.

Hodges PW and Richardson CA (1996) Inefficient muscular stabilisation of the lumbar spine associated with low back pain. *Spine* **22**: 2640–2650.

Jeunemann K-P, Lue TF, Schmidt RA et al (1988) Clinical significance of sacral and pudendal anatomy. *Journal of Urology* **139**: 74–80.

Kelleher CJ, Cardozo LD, Wise BG et al (1992) The impact of urinary incontinence on sexual function. *Neurourology and Urodynamics* **11**: 359–360.

Klarskov P, Bernstein I, Juul N et al (1991) Pelvic floor muscle thickness measured by perineal ultrasonography. *Neurourology and Urodynamics* **10**: 388–389.

Kuijpers JHC (1990) Anatomy and physiology of the mechanism of continence. *Netherlands Journal of Medicine* **37**: S2–5.

Lestar B, Penninckx F and Kerremans R (1989) The composition of anal basal pressure. An in vivo or in vitro study in man. *International Journal of Colorectal Diseases* **4**: 118–122.

Lose G, Colstrup H and Thind P (1989) Urethral elastance in healthy and stress incontinent women. *Neurourology and Urodynamics* **8**: 370–372.

Lubowski DZ, King DW and Finlay IG (1992) Electromyography of the pubococcygeus muscles in patients with obstructed defaecation. *International Journal of Colorectal Diseases* **7**: 184–187.

Mahony DT, Laferte RO and Blais DJ (1977) Integral storage and voiding reflexes. *Urology* **9**: 95–106.

Markwell SJ and Sapsford RR (1995) Physiotherapy management of obstructed defaecation. *Australian Journal of Physiotherapy* **41**: 279–283.

Meagher AP, Lubowski DZ and King DW (1993) The cough response of the anal sphincter. *International Journal of Colorectal Diseases* **8**: 217–219.

Moore KH and Richmond D (1989) Crouching over the toilet seat: prevalence, and effect on micturition. *Neurourology and Urodynamics* **8**: 422–424.

Narayan P, Konety B, Aslam K et al (1995) Neuroanatomy of the external urethral sphincter: implications for urinary continence preservation during radical prostate surgery. *Journal of Urology* **153**: 337–341.

Netter FH (1989) *Atlas of Human Anatomy.* USA: Ciba-Geigy.

Nichols DH and Randall CL (1989) *Vaginal Surgery*, 3rd edn, p. 463. Baltimore: Williams and Wilkins.

Oelrich TM (1983) The striated urogenital sphincter in the female. *Anatomical Record* **205**: 223–232.

Orkin BA and Tissaw M (1994) The rectoanal inhibitory reflex: the contractile component and sleep stages. *Gastroenterology* **107**: 1247.

Percy JP, Neill ME, Swash M et al (1981) Electrophysiological study of motor nerve supply of pelvic floor. *Lancet* **1**: 16–17.

Rao SSC and Welcher K (1994) Periodic rectal motor activity in humans – the nocturnal gatekeeper? *Gastroenterology* **107**: 1233.

Robertson AS, Griffiths CJ, Ramsden PD et al (1994) Bladder function in healthy volunteers: ambulatory monitoring and conventional urodynamic studies. *British Journal of Urology* **73**: 242–249.

Sampselle CM and DeLancey JOL (1992) The urine stream interruption test and pelvic muscle function. *Nursing Research* 41: 73–77.

Santiesteban AJ (1988) Electromyographic and dynamometric characteristics of female pelvic floor musculature. *Physical Therapy* **68**: 344–351.

Sapsford RR, Markwell SJ and Richardson CA (1996) Abdominal muscles and the anal sphincter: their interaction during defaecation. Proceedings of the Australian Physiotherapy Association National Congress, Brisbane, pp. 103–104.

Sapsford RR, Hodges PW and Richardson CA (1997a) Activation of the abdominal muscles is a normal response to contraction of the pelvic floor muscles. *Conference Abstract. International Continence Society, Yokohama*, 117.

Sapsford RR, Hodges PW and Richardson CA et al (1997b) Activation of pubococcygeus during a variety of isometric abdominal exercises. *Conference Abstract. International Continence Society, Yokohama*, 115.

Swash M (1992) Histopathology of the pelvic floor muscles in pelvic floor disorders. In: Henry MM and Swash M (eds) *Coloproctology and the Pelvic Floor*, 2nd edn, p. 175. Oxford. Butterworth Heinemann Ltd.

Tagart REB (1966) The anal canal and rectum: their varying relationship and its effect on anal continence. *Diseases of Colon and Rectum* **9**: 449–452.

Tortora GJ and Anagnostakos NP (1987) *Principles of Anatomy and Physiology*, 5th edn. New York: Harper and Row.

Vereecken RL and Verduyn H (1970) The electrical activity of the paraurethral and perineal muscles in normal and pathological conditions. *British Journal of Urology* **42**: 457–463.

Voss DE, Ionta MK and Myers BJ (1985) *Proprioceptive Neuromuscular Facilitation*, 3rd edn, p. 326. Philadelphia: Harper and Row.

Wise BG, Khullar V and Cardozo LD (1992) Bladder neck movement during pelvic floor contraction and intravaginal electrical stimulation in women with and without genuine stress incontinence. *Neurourology and Urodynamics* **11**: 309–311.

Womack NR, Morrison JFB and Williams NS (1986) The role of pelvic floor denervation in the aetiology of idiopathic faecal incontinence. *British Journal of Surgery* **73**: 404–407.

Wyndaele JJ (1990) Studies on the different clinical sensations during bladder filling. *Neurourology and Urodynamics* **9**: 353–354.

Yeung CK (1995) The normal infant bladder. *Scandanavian Journal of Urology and Nephrology* (Suppl 173): 19–23.

Zvara P, Carrier S, Kour N-W et al (1994) The detailed neuroanatomy of the human striated urethral sphincter. *British Journal of Urology* **74**: 182–187.

8

Urinary Dysfunction in Adolescence

RUTH SAPSFORD

Urethrovesical Dysfunction

Physiotherapists who work in the area of women's health need to be aware that aspects of pelvic floor dysfunction that relate to urethrovesical and anorectal systems can occur in adolescents. Definitions, descriptions, signs, symptoms, assessment and management (medical and physiotherapeutic) of all pelvic floor functional problems are contained in Chapters 28, 29 and 30. Overlap across age groups occurs constantly, so the age group divisions in this book are arbitrary.

Urethrovesical Dysfunction

In a normal bladder there is little increase in pressure during filling, until capacity is approached. The bladder is said to be 'stable', hence a 'stable detrusor'. With an overactive detrusor there are spontaneous or provoked involuntary contractions which the person cannot suppress. This may be termed bladder instability and can occur during filling when the person is trying to inhibit micturition. There can be an urge to void followed by urine loss or spontaneous loss without warning. Detrusor overactivity and instability occur in all age groups and are one cause of urinary incontinence.

Incontinence is an involuntary loss of urine which is a social or hygienic problem and is objectively demonstrable (Abrams et al, 1988). It is a symptom. There are different types of incontinence and physiotherapy is not appropriate in all of them. But not all bladder dysfunction results in incontinence.

Adolescence is defined as the period between childhood and maturity, extending from 12 to 21 years in females (*Shorter Oxford English Dictionary*). A recent survey in the UK looked at urinary symptoms in 665 11–12-year-old girls (Swithinbank et al, 1994). Follow-up surveys are planned for four years later. Urinary urgency occurred in 12.2%, bed wetting in 3.5%, with occasional day-time wetting in 16.6%. Laughing was the most common cause of urine loss. There was some resistance to participation in the survey from school staff, parents and children. It seems urinary incontinence is still a taboo subject and was considered too sensitive to be discussed in school.

This section on adolescents lists relevant problems with a brief management outline. Detailed descriptions of management are included in Chapter 30.

Urinary tract infection

Before any treatment for incontinence is undertaken, urinary tract infection (UTI) must be eliminated. The most common infection, in 95% of cases, is the bacteria *Escherichia coli*, found in normal rectal flora. Sufferers present with frequent and urgent voiding and with burning or discomfort on voiding. They may also have a fever. Treatment is by antibacterial agents. Young schoolgirls have about a 2%

incidence of UTI and usually outgrow the susceptibility around puberty. However, when they become sexually active UTI becomes common again. Infection can precipitate urge incontinence and nocturnal enuresis. Physiotherapists are not involved in management of infection, but must be aware of the part it plays in incontinence and the need for adequate treatment.

Nocturnal enuresis

Enuresis means an involuntary loss of urine. If there is loss during sleep it is termed nocturnal enuresis (Abrams et al, 1988). Nocturnal enuresis is familial, with a fivefold risk if the mother was a sufferer and a sevenfold risk if the father was a sufferer. Primary nocturnal enuresis can persist into adolescence. In this case the subject has never been dry at night for a minimum of six months. Secondary nocturnal enuresis recurs after the subject has been dry at night for at least six months and it frequently has a psychological background. The depth of sleep amongst sufferers is not a factor in this condition, as enuretic episodes occur in all stages of sleep. Controls and those who suffer from bed wetting were found to have similar sleep patterns.

PATHOGENESIS

1. Small functional bladder capacity (there is usually normal capacity under anaesthesia).
2. Nocturnal polyuria (excessive nocturnal urine production).
3. Detrusor overactivity, often associated with day-time frequency, urgency and urine loss.
4. Lack of normal arousal from sleep in response to bladder filling.

However, it seems that a combination of these factors can occur and the rate of bladder filling may be a contributing factor, as enuretic episodes often occur in the earlier hours of the night.

A bladder capacity of around 200–250 ml is needed to enable a child to sleep through the night with a dry bed, if urine production is normal (Troup and Hodgson, 1971). Children with small functional bladder capacities will experience day frequency too. This small capacity may be triggered by a low level of detrusor overactivity. Management aims to increase day-time bladder capacity by a bladder training programme and benefits for the night should follow. Care must be taken that bladder capacities are kept within reasonable levels (see Chapter 30). Increased vesical pressures can contribute to upper urinary tract damage, due to reflux of urine, and a combination of large bladder volumes and high urethral sphincter pressures to prevent urine loss may result in problems.

If nocturnal urine production is large then a normal capacity bladder will be inadequate. In these children there may be insufficient night-time production of antidiuretic hormone (ADH), resulting in large volumes of dilute urine. Management can be either by learning to wake at night to a full bladder, using an enuresis alarm to assist in this, or by the replacement of antidiuretic hormone, using desmopressin. This is administered at bed-time either orally or via a nasal spray and the drug is absorbed through the mucosa. It is also available in tablet-form. This treatment may not be available in all countries. Relapse rates are quite high when hormonal treatment is withdrawn (see Chapter 30 for further treatment details).

Overactive detrusor function causes the bladder to contract inappropriately, resulting in incontinence. It can occur both day and night. An adolescent with this problem may void frequently during the day in response to urgency. Volumes are usually smaller than normal. However, the person is not woken at night. Management includes urge control techniques and bladder training to increase day-time capacity. Hopefully, the improved control will carry over into the night. Medication which quietens detrusor activity is frequently used (see Chapter 30).

Electroencephalographic studies combined with bladder pressure measurements (cystometrograms) showed that a certain number of bed wetters did not get the normal arousal from sleep in response to bladder stretch with filling (Azuma et al, 1990). Management consists of monitoring for five consecutive nights and waking the person when the EEG patterns change. Cures have been reported in 25% and improvement in 53% of cases (Terasaki et al, 1990).

Tracy, a slightly built, shy 16-year-old girl, presented for treatment for nocturnal enuresis. She wet the bed nightly and had been dry for a period of 3–4 months when she was quite young. Medical investigation when she was younger, including IVP, showed no abnormalities. A trial of imipramine led to an allergic response. An enuresis alarm had been tried when younger, but it was very disruptive of sleep for the family and so was discontinued. Tracy was not an active person, preferrring to listen to music with friends rather than play sport.

Her frequency/volume chart showed three voids a day, each of around 250–300 ml. She had no urgency and was able to defer voiding easily during the day. Despite it being summer, her daily fluid intake was reportedly approximately 1000 ml. Her voided volume at night was 600–700 ml. This was ascertained by weighing her bedding and night attire both dry and wet. It was difficult to confirm accuracy of these figures.

She was encouraged to increase her fluid intake and defer voiding to increase day-time bladder capacity. It was decided to trial an enuresis alarm during the summer school holidays. A body worn personal alarm was used. After two weeks Tracy was waking on her own to the alarm and only the pantyliner was wet. She passed a large volume of urine into the toilet on waking. Three weeks later Tracy reported that she sometimes woke before the alarm and she had increased her fluid intake. She had also taken the plastic sheeting off her bed.

After another three weeks Tracy reported that she had been dry for two weeks, sometimes waking at night to void and sometimes sleeping right through the night. She had discontinued use of the alarm. It was suggested that she continue with her increased fluid intake.

Genuine stress incontinence (GSI)

This is usually regarded as a problem related to pregnancy and parturition. However, there are a number of papers confirming its occurrence in nulliparous females. Genuine stress incontinence (GSI) is an involuntary loss of urine occurring when, in the absence of a detrusor contraction, the intravesical pressure exceeds the maximum urethral pressure (Abrams et al, 1988). Urine loss occurs during increased intra-abdominal pressure with sneezing, coughing, running , jumping, etc. Loss is small, usually a spot loss, occurring simultaneously with the increase in IAP.

Nulliparous university students reported a 26% incidence of GSI (Bo et al, 1989), while in another series 28% of nulliparous university sporting women reported urine loss while participating in their sport (Nygaard et al, 1994). For some of these, the problem had commenced during high school, especially with high-impact activities. In more detailed clinical investigations of nullipara, poor urethral closing pressures during coughing were demonstrated in the majority of sufferers and more than half of them had weak pelvic floors (Bo et al, 1994). A number also had hypermobile joints. Elite gymnasts reported urine loss during tumbling, trampolining, jumping and landing. Those with longer training hours were susceptible to loss (Warren, 1993). These were probably the more advanced students undertaking the more difficult manoeuvres.

Dysfunctional voiding

One form of this problem is an inco-ordination of voiding which can occur in young girls. The detrusor muscle contracts but the urethral sphincter fails to relax. One explanation of its cause relates to the development of normal urinary control. Infants have a reflex voiding process and as control develops there is a time when continence is perhaps due to urethral sphincter and periurethral muscle contraction rather than detrusor suppression. This pattern may partially persist in some children. Inco-ordinate voiding may also be related to painful voiding, incontinence, embarrassment, stress, sexual abuse or straining at defaecation. The position adopted on the toilet may also be a factor.

There may be:

- premature interruption of urine flow and incomplete voiding;
- an inco-ordination of sphincter and detrusor, sometimes dribbling small amounts and at others having a reasonable flow;
- marked day frequency, small voids and perhaps nocturnal enuresis;
- a large increase in bladder pressure to force the sphincter to release or force urine past it.

Some of these problems can persist into adolescence. Physiotherapists can contribute to the management by teaching relaxed sitting with foot support for voiding, relaxation of the PF and sphincter and encouraging adequate time for the voiding. Voiding in a squatting position can be helpful. The process of outlet release, similar to that used in defaecation retraining, can be helpful (see Chapter 30).

Giggle incontinence

There is a sudden involuntary partial or complete emptying of the bladder. It occurs without warning during or after a bout of giggling or hysterical laughter. It often begins around 5–7 years and tends to resolve by 12 years, though urgency and leakage can continue into adult life (Glahn, 1979). It possibly results from detrusor instability triggered by the repeated or sustained increase in intra-abdominal pressure and generally occurs during the latter half of the bladder-filling phase. In one study, on testing, detrusor function and bladder pressures were normal and it was impossible to measure these during laughter (Cisternino and Passerini-Glazel, 1995). While it is stated that girls eventually grow out of it, giggle incontinence can cause severe embarrassment and the sufferer is often ridiculed by her peers. Sufferers are encouraged to use urge control techniques during laughter to inhibit detrusor activity (see Chapter 30). Pelvic floor exercises may be helpful. In some cases medication to quieten the detrusor is prescribed.

Urgency and urge incontinence

Urge incontinence is an involuntary loss of urine associated with a strong desire to void (Abrams et al, 1988). Urgency may be associated with two types of dysfunction. Hypersensitivity results in sensory urgency. This often occurs with UTI when the bladder mucosa is irritated. There is a frequent desire to void but urine loss is uncommon. Overactive detrusor function results in motor urgency and is more likely to result in loss. This loss is usually of greater volume than with stress incontinence and can often result in wet underwear and wet legs. Day-time loss may result from detrusor instability triggered by increases in intra-abdominal pressure or with impact. In this case the sufferer is dry at night when she is at rest. Management consists of urge control techniques and, if appropriate, bladder training and pelvic floor re-education (see Chapter 30).

While the conditions listed in this section occur in adolescence, they can continue into adult life. Intervention at this stage, with improvement of the condition, will have a positive effect on self-esteem as well as giving a sense of being in control.

References

Abrams P, Blaivas JG, Stanton SL and Andersen JT (1988) The standardisation of terminology of lower urinary tract function. *Scandanavian Journal of Urology and Nephrology* **114**: 5–19.

Azuma Y, Terasaki T and Watanabe H (1990) A new classification of enuresis founded on overnight simultaneous monitoring of electroencephalography and cystometry. *Neurourology and Urodynamics* **9**: 446.

Bo K, Hagen R, Kvarstein B et al (1989) Female stress urinary incontinence and participation in different sport and social activities. *Scandanavian Journal of Sports Sciences* **11**: 117–121.

Bo K, Stien R, Kulseng-Hanssen S et al (1994) Clinical and urodynamic assessment of nulliparous young women with and without stress incontinence symptoms: a case control study. *Obstetrics and Gynecology* **84**: 1028–1032.

Cisternino A and Passerini-Glazel G (1995) Bladder dysfunction in children. *Scandanavian Journal of Urology and Nephrology* (Suppl) **173**: 25–29.

Glahn BE (1979) Giggle incontinence (enuresis risoria). A study and an aetiological hypothesis. *British Journal of Urology* **51**: 363–366.

Nygaard IE, Thompson FL, Svengalis SL et al (1994) Urinary incontinence in elite nulliparous athletes. *Obstetrics and Gynecology* **84**: 183–187.

Swithinbank LV, Carr JC and Abrams PH (1994) Longitudinal study of urinary symptoms in children. *Scandanavian Journal of Urology and Nephrology* (Suppl) **163**: 67–73.

Terasaki T, Azuma Y and Watanabe H (1990) Development and result of therapeutic machine of enuresis based on overnight simultaneous monitoring of electroencephalography and cystometry. *Neurourology and Urodynamics* **9**: 449–450.

Troup CW and Hodgson NB (1971) Nocturnal functional bladder capacity in enuretic children. *Journal of Urology* **105**: 129–132.

Warren B (1993) A qualitative investigation into the prevalence of stress urinary incontinence in a population of elite, nulliparous, female gymnasts randomly selected from throughout Australia. *Newsletter of the Curtin University of Technology.* **1**: 14–15.

9

Sexual Function and Common Sexual Issues

JANE HOWARD

Sexuality is a very important part of women's lives. Women who have problems with sexuality often have difficulty in finding a health professional in whom to confide. An understanding of female sexuality and some common sexual issues will enable the physiotherapist to respond to women's sexual health concerns in an effective manner. When physiotherapists become comfortable discussing sexual issues and have knowledge about them, they may facilitate healthy and adaptive attitudes to relationships between young people and help them access information about safe sex and contraception. In particular, it is necesssary to have some knowledge, an accepting attitude and some skills to treat women for their pelvic floor dysfunction. It is advisable to keep up to date with knowledge and to have a referral network for difficult cases.

This chapter begins with the physiology of sexual desire and the female sexual response. Common sexual problems are then described. Sexual issues for women with illness or disability and adolescent women are followed by a short section on sexual abuse. Contraceptive methods are briefly discussed and the chapter finishes with an overview of sexually transmitted infection.

Sexuality is a complex interaction of biological, psychological and social factors which develop over a lifetime. It encompasses all things pertaining to being male or female. The social aspects involve culture, family, peer influences and expectations, whereas biological involvement includes innate characteristics such as gender, hormones, health, anatomy and physiology. Psychological factors revolve around feelings, experiences and personal meanings.

Female Sexual Desire

Sexual desire may take the form of erotic fantasy, sexual attraction to another person or desire for sexual activity. Sexual desire is probably shaped by social, cultural and psychological factors and is dependent on the functioning of the limbic system of the brain, the higher centres of the brain and hormones, particularly testosterone.

Female Sexual Response

Sexual response may be divided into four stages:

1. arousal
2. plateau
3. orgasm
4. resolution

Arousal

An intact nervous system is necessary for sexual arousal. The parasympathetic nervous system is responsible for arousal via sacral nerve roots 2, 3 and 4 although the sympathetic nervous system is probably involved in orgasm. Skin sensation in the genital area is important for arousal. Sexual arousal occurs in waves and there are general bodily changes and genital changes which occur at the time.

GENERAL BODILY CHANGES

There is general vasocongestion and muscle tone is increased. The heart and respiratory rates increase whilst the blood pressure rises. Feelings of excitement occur. There may be a flush on the skin of the chest and neck, together with increased sweating.

GENITAL CHANGES

There is a marked increase in blood flow to the genitals. The clitoris enlarges with blood and retracts under the clitoral hood whilst the corpora cavernosa (two erectile structures around the vaginal opening) become engorged with blood. The labia minora increase in size. The pelvic muscles also become congested and the lower vaginal wall becomes swollen and oedematous, whilst the upper vagina balloons out. The uterus is also congested and rises up out of the pelvis. Lubrication occurs by serum from the blood passing through the vaginal wall into the vagina (transudation). A few drops of fluid may be secreted from Bartholin's glands.

Plateau

This is the time of maximal arousal. The breasts become enlarged and the nipples become erect. The pupil of the eye may become dilated and salivation may occur.

Orgasm

During orgasm the pelvic floor muscles contract in a rhythmic fashion every 0.8 seconds, expelling blood and fluid which has accumulated in the tissues during arousal. The muscles contract 5–15 times and the earliest contractions are the most pleasurable. Spasms of other muscle groups such as the abdominal muscles, thighs and buttocks may also occur in orgasm. Loss of small quantities of urine is common in orgasm.

Orgasm may be associated with an altered state of consciousness. Some women are able to orgasm more than once if sexual stimulation is continued. Some women are never able to reach high levels of sexual arousal and do not orgasm, whilst others orgasm occasionally (Fig. 9.1). Women often think that it is not essential to orgasm every time they have sex, whereas their partners are much more likely to view orgasm as essential.

Resolution

There is a rapid return to normal after orgasm and many women have a subjective feeling of calm. During resolution, blood from the genitals returns to the general circulation and all the changes associated with arousal disappear. If orgasm does not occur then resolution takes longer.

Figure 9.1 Varieties of normal female sexual response, detailing arousal, plateau, orgasm and resolution phases.

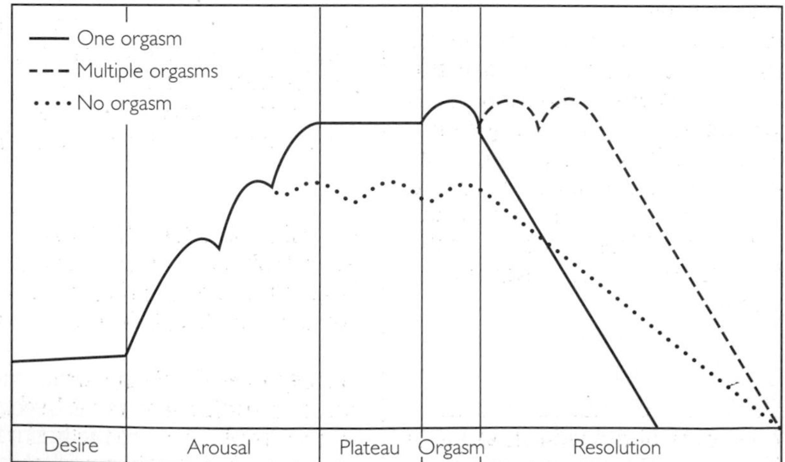

Female Sexual Dysfunction

Sexual dysfunction in women is very common. Michael et al (1994) reported that one woman in five stated that sex did not give them pleasure. Some studies have shown that a percentage of women never actually experience sexual desire, although they may be able to respond sexually when in a sexual situation.

The main female sexual dysfunctions are:

- lack of libido;
- failure of arousal;
- vaginismus;
- failure to orgasm;
- dyspareunia.

Lack of libido

A lack of interest in sex is a common sexual problem for women at all ages. It is particularly prevalent in women who have suffered sexual abuse, women who are depressed, in the late stages of pregnancy and post-partum and also in post-menopausal women. Social, psychological and physical factors are involved to varying degrees.

Failure of sexual arousal

This may occur along with lack of libido. However, there may be no problems with libido although there is a lack of arousal. Often the failure to become aroused is due to the woman never really having an opportunity to discover what is stimulating for her. This situation is very common in women whose partners have premature ejaculation when there is little time for arousal. The problem may also occur as a result of damage to the pelvic autonomic nervous system which is responsible for sexual arousal.

Vaginismus

This is a condition where the muscles at the vaginal outlet go into spasm on any attempt to penetrate the vagina with a penis, a tampon or a finger. Spasm of the adductor muscles of the thighs may also reflexly occur on attempted penetration. Any pressure on the pubococcygeus muscle when it is in spasm is perceived as painful (see Chapter 7). Vaginismus usually occurs in women who lack knowledge about the anatomy and physiology of the vagina and who are also anxious about intercourse. Occasionally it may result from sexual abuse, a painful vaginal infection or a painful examination, e.g. a Pap smear. Figure 9.2 illustrates the process of taking a Pap smear.

Failure to orgasm

Hite (1977) reported that only one-third of women were able to orgasm during sexual intercourse whereas two-thirds are able to orgasm with stimulation of the clitoris. Some women are able to get highly aroused but do not orgasm, whereas others fail to orgasm because they do not get very aroused. Treatment is aimed at increasing knowledge about sexual arousal and genital anatomy and encouraging self-stimulation. Attention is paid to improving focus in sexual arousal, because women commonly allow their minds to wander away from sexual thoughts in sexual activity. Teaching acceptance of body shape and self-assertiveness are also important.

Figure 9.2 The process of taking a Pap (Papanicolaou) smear. Columnar and squamous epithelium are scraped from the cervix using an Ayres spatula.

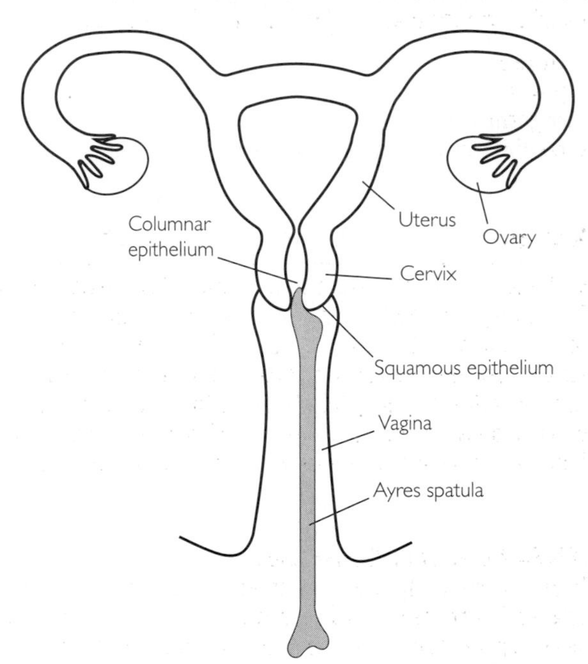

Dyspareunia

Dyspareunia means that sexual intercourse is painful. This pain may be categorized into superficial pain, which occurs on initial penetration, or deep dyspareunia which occurs on deep penetration. There are a large number of causes for painful sexual intercourse and most of them are physical. Therefore it is always important to refer the woman for a general medical and genital examination.

CAUSES OF DYSPAREUNIA

Vaginal infections Recurrent *Candida albicans* causes soreness of the vagina and may result in vaginal fissures. These are particularly painful on urination.

Sexually transmissible infections Herpes genitalis tends to cause episodic dyspareunia lasting a week or two at a time. Human papilloma virus (HPV) may cause long-term dyspareunia when it affects the skin in the lower vagina and vulva. *Gonorrhoea* and *Chlamydia* cause cervicitis and this may result in deep dyspareunia.

Chronic dermatitis Skin conditions are common in the vulval region and often give rise to inflammation of the vulva and dyspareunia.

Laser treatment Laser treatment to the vagina and vulva for HPV infection causes scarring of the skin tissue and lack of elasticity.

Hymenal remnants The hymen usually disappears in foetal life, but occasionally there are strands of tissue across the opening or an arc of hymenal remnant on one side. In both cases penetration will result in pain.

Uterine fibroids Benign uterine wall tumours are common in women in their 30s and 40s and may feel uncomfortable in intercourse.

Endometriosis In this condition endometrial cells occur outside the uterus and then undergo hormonal changes with the menstrual cycle. Bleeding at the time of the period causes scarring in local tissue. Endometriosis causes severe dyspareunia and dysmenorrhoea.

Ovarian cysts Painful intercourse, with the pain located on the side of the cyst, is common.

Constipation A full rectum may protrude into the posterior vaginal wall, deforming its shape and capacity.

Cystitis Bladder infections and urethritis may cause discomfort during intercourse.

Episiotomy Sexual intercourse may be avoided post-partum due to episiotomy pain. Post-partum superficial dyspareunia occurred in 60% of women in one survey. One-fifth of them had not resumed intercourse three months post-delivery (Hay-Smith and Mantle, 1996). See Chapter 19 for early management of episiotomies.

Radiotherapy Treatment of cervical cancer may involve radiotherapy to the vagina which may result in scarring and fibrosis, causing dyspareunia.

Other Problems

Vaginal flatus is a common problem for women. Release of air trapped in the vagina may occur in sexual activity and make embarrassing noises. If this happens occasionally it is normal. In some women who have pelvic floor damage after childbirth vaginal flatus may occur at any time (see Chapter 28).

Sexuality and Disability

Any medical condition or disability can have an effect on sexuality. These effects may be psychological, physical or both.

Changes in appearance or behaviour are likely to have an effect on self-esteem and body image and may lead to avoidance of social and sexual contact. Women with lifelong disabilities are often overprotected, have little education about sex and personal relationships and limited opportunity to meet suitable partners. For these women hormonal control of fertility, to prevent pregnancy, should be tried before resorting to hysterectomy. Many women with disabilities suffer sexual exploitation and those with an intellectual disability may not understand the meaning of sex.

Conditions which affect the blood and nerve supply to the genitals, such as diabetes, multiple sclerosis, spinal cord injury and spina bifida, are likely to affect sexual arousal. Autonomic nervous system damage may compromise both arousal and orgasm. Upper motor neurone damage, e.g. cerebral palsy, may result in hip adductor spasms and difficulty in positioning for penetration.

Catheters and ostomy bags create aesthetic and physical problems.

Sexual Issues for Adolescent Women

> Sexuality is a complex and confusing aspect of life . . . adolescence is a critical period in the upsurge of sex drives, the development of sexual values and the initiation of sexual behaviour (Moore and Rosenthal, 1993)

Sexual orientation

Sexual development occurs in stages. Bancroft and Machover Reinish (1990) described three principal strands of sexual development: gender identity, sexual response and capacity for intimate dyadic relationships. These strands begin to develop in foetal life, but integrate in adolescence. Sexual orientation is simply the sexual interest in another person. This may involve sexual fantasy, attraction to another person or sexual activity with another person. Heterosexuals are sexually interested in a person of the opposite sex; homosexuals are drawn to a person of the same sex. Homosexual women are called lesbians. Bisexual people are interested in both sexes and asexual people do not have any sexual interest at all. Trans-sexuals are those who think they belong in a body of the opposite sex and wish to change sex. Trans-sexuality is a rare condition in women.

Most modern industrial societies polarize sexual orientation into heterosexuality or homosexuality. However, in recent times there seems to be more tolerance of homosexuality and bisexuality but homophobia, the irrational fear of homosexual behaviour, is still evident in public attitudes.

The process of self-identification as a lesbian and the disclosure of that identity to others is known as 'coming out'. Michael et al (1994) report that only 3.5% women ever experience a homosexual attraction and less than 1% of women have sexual activity with another woman.

Sexual behaviour in female adolescence

Present society defines sexual roles for women less clearly than in the past. Puberty occurs at an earlier age and marriage is often delayed. Single motherhood is more socially acceptable than ever before and effective contraception and safe abortion services allow women to choose when to have children. Adolescent sexuality has gained more acceptance in recent decades.

MASTURBATION

Erotic fantasy and masturbation are not well researched, as these behaviours are considered to be very private. In the past, Western culture considered masturbation to be generally harmful and addictive, but it is now considered to be normal behaviour. Katchadourian (1990) reports that young girls begin to masturbate at an average age of 12 years, two years earlier than boys, and have a lower rate of masturbation.

Self-stimulation is a way to learn about sexual arousal. There are no known ill effects of masturbation and a partner is not required. Erotic fantasy helps in the development of sexual orientation and sexual identity.

SEXUAL BEHAVIOUR WITH A PARTNER

Most young women move from holding hands with a partner to kissing and petting, progressing to sexual intercourse over a period of time. Sexual behaviour with a partner may begin around the age of 13 years. Boys tend to want more sexual intimacy than girls and sometimes unwanted sexual activity occurs.

AGE AT FIRST SEXUAL INTERCOURSE

A trend towards sexual experience at a younger age has occurred in the last two decades. Sixty percent of 17-year-olds reported being non-virgins and 80% of adolescents reported their first episode of sexual intercourse between the ages of 14 and 19 years (Goldman and Goldman, 1988). Adolescents appear to be more sexually adventurous than in the past and may engage in oral and anal sex more often.

SEXUAL RELATIONSHIPS

Adolescent relationships fall into two main categories: serial monogamy and sexual adventuring. Serial monogamy relates to sequential relationships with one partner at a time. Sexual adventuring is sexual activity with a number of sexual partners. Casual sexual activity and risky sexual behaviour is less common amongst girls than boys. Early engagement in sexual activity and risky sexual behaviour is often associated with drinking, smoking, truancy and delinquency. These teenage problems may have common origins in breakdown of family relationships, abuse and poor self-esteem.

ADOLESCENT PROSTITUTION

This is a serious problem which has increased since the 1970s. Young girls enter prostitution as a way of surviving abuse, lack of education, substance abuse, crime and family stress.

Sexual Abuse

Sexual abuse is an issue for women of all ages. There is a continuum of sexual abuse from sexual suggestions to violent rape.

Sexual assault

The incidence of sexual assault is thought to be much higher than reported. Govey (1991) found that 52% of female university students reported that they had experienced some form of sexual victimization. Rape or attempted rape was reported by 25%. Roberts (1992) found that one-third of 14-year-old boys believed it was reasonable to rape a girl if she led him on.

Child sexual abuse

Goldman and Goldman (1988) report that 28% of Australian girls experience some form of sexual abuse, by an older person, during childhood. More than 90% of such incidents are perpetrated by men. The abuse may range from leering and touching to intercourse with violence. Girls respond to abuse with shock, fear and revulsion. The long-term effects of sexual abuse are:

- depression;
- poor self-esteem;
- substance abuse;
- sexual dysfunction;
- failure to form relationships;
- lack of trust in men;
- bowel dysfunction.

Responding to a woman who discloses sexual abuse

There are several important ways to respond to a woman who discloses sexual abuse.

- Believe her – it is not your job to validate her story.

- Tell her you are sorry that this happened.
- Tell her it is not her fault.
- Tell her sexual abuse is common and she is not alone.
- Suggest she seek professional help – have readily available telephone numbers of 'care after sexual assault' services, psychologists, rape crisis counsellors and family planning centres.
- Refrain from asking for details about the abuse.

Contraception

Fertility control is an issue for all women of child-bearing age. Contraception has become highly developed in the last three decades and a number of different methods are generally available. Throughout a woman's reproductive years her methods of fertility control may change. With the advent of the HIV epidemic, the condom has become extremely significant, in that it is the only contraceptive method providing protection against sexually transmitted infections. Research continues into new methods of contraception.

Hormonal contraception

COMBINED ORAL CONTRACEPTIVE PILL

The pill contains two hormones, oestrogen and progestogen, which are taken daily for 21 days followed by a seven-day break. During this break the woman will have a period. Over the years hormone dosages have been lowered and side effects minimized. With correct usage the pregnancy rate is one per 100 women taking the pill each year. In practice, user failure rate increases the pregnancy rate to eight per 100 women per year.

Serious side effects of strokes, thrombosis or heart attacks are now very low, but smokers are at higher risk. The combined pill is not recommended for smokers over 35, but is safe for non-smokers up to the age of 50, provided they are without the risk factors of obesity, diabetes, heart disease and hypertension.

The oral contraceptive pill has been shown to protect against cancer of the endometrium and cancer of the ovary. In young women who take the pill for five years before their first pregnancy, there may be an increased risk of breast cancer at a young age, but breast cancer in young women is rare. Risk of cancer of the cervix is higher in pill users, but it may be related to human papilloma virus (HPV) infection, early onset of intercourse, multiple partners and smoking.

EMERGENCY CONTRACEPTION

There are two successful methods of preventing pregnancy after sexual intercourse:

1. a high dosage of oral contraceptive within 72 hours (2% pregnancy rate);
2. insertion of a copper-bearing intrauterine contraceptive device (IUCD) within five days (nil pregnancy rate).

General practitioners, family planning clinics and sexual health clinics are all able to provide emergency contraception, but many women are unaware of its availability.

PROGESTOGEN-ONLY PILL

This pill is useful for women who are lactating and those who are unable to take oestrogen. It is often used in smokers over the age of 35. It has to be taken within three hours of the same time every day and has a failure rate of two pregnancies per 100 women each year.

DEPO MEDROXY PROGESTERONE ACETATE (DMPA)

This progesterone is given by injection three-monthly. The pregnancy rate is less than one per 100 users. Periods may cease and there is a delay of up to six months in return of fertility after cessation of use. It can be used during lactation without affecting milk supply.

HORMONAL IMPLANTS

Slow release of progestogen from Silastic rods inserted under the skin can provide effective contraception for five years. Availability is limited at present.

Intrauterine contraceptive device (IUCD)

These are an important alternative for women who have side effects on hormones. Two devices are readily available and can be worn for 5–8 years, with pregnancy rates of one per 100 users per year. The method is inappropriate for those at risk of sexually transmitted infections, as any infection is more likely to spread to the fallopian tubes and cause infertility.

Barrier methods

DIAPHRAGM

This is inserted into the vagina by the woman prior to intercourse and removed six hours later. It is used in conjunction with a spermicide. Failure rates are quoted as 3–5 pregnancies per 100 users per year, but may be higher.

CONDOM

The condom has a 2% failure rate and provides protection against sexually transmissible diseases. Occasionally women or their partners are allergic to latex or the lubricant and so are unable to use this method. Careful use is important.

SPERMICIDES

These are various creams, foams and pessaries which are placed in the vagina before intercourse to kill spermatozoa and prevent conception. Spermicide alone has a high failure rate. Diaphragms are used with spermicides and condom use may be combined with a spermicide.

Periodic abstinence

By observing the nature of vaginal mucus at different times in the menstrual cycle and taking her body temperature every day, a woman can learn to detect when she ovulates each month. By avoiding sexual intercourse at the fertile time she can avoid pregnancy. In practice this method has a high failure rate and it is recommended that women who want to use this method should seek professional advice first (see Chapter 10).

Permanent methods

FEMALE STERILIZATION

This procedure, in which clips or rings occlude the fallopian tubes, is done laparoscopically under a general anaesthetic. It is an effective permanent procedure, with a 50% chance of successful reversal.

VASECTOMY

Male sterilization involves an operation under local anaesthetic to sever the vasa deferentia. The risks of the procedure are minimal and there appear to be no long-term effects apart from sterility.

New methods

- Vaginal rings, impregnated with hormones, function in a similar way to the oral contraceptive pill.
- Female vinyl condoms, a once-only device, have a high failure rate.
- Hormone (progestogen)-releasing IUCDs are available in some countries.
- Vaccines to prevent pregnancy are being researched.
- RU486 is a post-coital contraceptive. Optimal dosages are still being determined.
- Regular testosterone injections for three months in men will prevent sperm production and cause temporary infertility. Further investigation of this method is in progress.

Abortion

Termination of pregnancy is usually performed in the first trimester of pregnancy and only occasionally in the second trimester. It is performed legally for medical, psychological or social reasons. Termination of pregnancy is a straightforward medical procedure with few short-term or long-term complications. Approximately 80 000 women in Australia have a termination of pregnancy each year and fertile women of all ages are represented in the abortion figures. Suction curettage is the procedure most often used, with either a local or a general anaesthetic.

All contraceptive methods have a failure rate and women are usually very clear about whether they wish to continue with a pregnancy. Abortion services are very important to women's mental and physical health. In countries where there are no legal abortion services thousands of women die each year from the complications of illegal abortion.

RU486

RU486 is known as the abortion pill and has been the subject of great controversy in recent times. This drug is used in combination with prostaglandins to cause an abortion in early pregnancy. Surgery is usually avoided and the woman can attend a clinic as an outpatient. This drug is not yet available in all countries.

Teenage Pregnancy

The number of teenagers giving birth in Australia has decreased from 28.1 per 1000 in 1980 to 21.9 per 1000 in 1992 (Australian Bureau of Statistics, 1980, 1992). The majority of them are aged 18 and 19 years, with numbers decreasing in the under-16s. In 1981, 58.9% of the teenagers giving birth were unmarried and this figure rose to 82.5% in 1990. The teenage birthrate in the Australian Aboriginal population is much higher than in the general population.

Countries which are accepting of adolescent sexuality, teach their children about it and provide contraceptive services have a lower rate of teenage pregnancy than countries who try to prohibit teenage sexuality and teach abstinence.

Sexually Transmitted Infections

Young people aged 15–19 years have the highest incidence of sexually transmitted infection (STI) and those aged 20–24 years the second highest. People with multiple sexual partners have a higher risk than those with one long-term partner.

The most important STIs in the Western world are caused by bacteria, spirochaetes, viruses or parasites (see Table 9.1).

Transmission

Methods of transmission of STIs include:

- sexual intercourse, e.g. gonorrhoea, chlamydia;
- broken skin contact with an infectious lesion, e.g. herpes, human papilloma virus;
- mother to infant during pregnancy via the placenta in blood, e.g. hepatitis B, HIV, syphilis, or during childbirth, e.g. herpes, chlamydia;

Table 9.1 The most common sexually transmitted infections

Causative agents	Types of infection
Bacteria	Chlamydia, gonorrhoea donovanosis, chancroid, lymphogranuloma venereum (mainly occur in central and northern Australia)
Spirochaetes	Syphilis
Viruses	Human immunodeficiency virus (HIV), herpes types 1 & 2, hepatitis B, hepatitis C, human papilloma virus (HPV), molluscum contagiosum
Parasites	Pediculosis pubis, scabies

- sharing injecting equipment – hepatitis C, hepatitis B, HIV;
- needlestick injury – hepatitis C, hepatitis B, HIV;
- organ donation – hepatitis C, hepatitis B, HIV;
- artificial insemination – hepatitis C, hepatitis B, HIV;
- breast feeding, e.g. HIV.

Workplace safety guidelines to protect healthcare workers from infections

Health workers must protect their own safety by following protocols, a sample of which is listed below. Each workplace will have its own protocols.

- Hand washing before and after examining each patient.
- Wearing gloves on both hands when likely to contact body fluids.
- Do not resheath needles.
- Dispose of sharps immediately after use in a rigid-walled sharps container.
- Safe disposal of body fluid-contaminated wastes.
- Autoclaving equipment at the specified temperature.
- Clear protocols for staff.

Management of sexually transmitted infections

TESTING

Testing is available for anyone who feels that they may be at risk of infection or who has symptoms such as a vaginal discharge, genital sores or lumps or painful sexual intercourse. The tests which are used to diagnose STI include throat, endocervical, vaginal and anal swabs. Blood tests are used to diagnose HIV, hepatitis B , hepatitis C and syphilis. Many medical practitioners obtain written consent from the client prior to an HIV test. Careful pre-test counselling to explain the significance of testing for HIV is essential. The test for hepatitis C is not yet perfectly reliable, so its use tends to be limited.

TREATMENT

Antibiotic therapy is curative for chlamydia, gonorrhoea, syphilis and donovanosis. The parasitic infections are easily cured with lotions. There is no cure for viral infections but there is a treatment to alleviate herpes and several therapies to alleviate HIV. Genital warts can be treated by various paints, diathermy, cryotherapy or laser vaporization.

CONTACT TRACING

It is important to counsel the person about the nature of the infection and encourage testing and treatment of the partner or partners. Encouraging safe sexual behaviour is essential. Occasionally a professional contact tracer is asked to contact partners.

FOLLOW-UP TESTING

It is usual to repeat the testing after treatment to assess the response to treatment.

Long-term consequences of STI

PELVIC INFLAMMATORY DISEASE (PID)

Gonorrhoea, chlamydia and other infections can cause PID, which is an infection of the fallopian tubes. Resultant scarring can give rise to infertility, pelvic pain, dyspareunia or rectal pain.

SYPHILIS

Syphilis can cause lesions in many parts of the body, giving rise to neurological, joint, heart and skin problems.

HIV

This virus causes a progressive loss of immunity to infection. Opportunistic infections develop in the lungs, bowel, vagina and mouth. The late stage of the infection is known as acquired immune deficiency syndrome (AIDS) and occurs 8–10 years after initial infection. At the late stage of HIV infection, opportunistic infections in the lungs, bowel and nervous system, along with cancers, overwhelm the person.

The virus initially affected the male homosexual community but has also spread to partners of bisexual men and into the heterosexual community. Babies of infected mothers, IV drug users, recipients of blood products (prior to understanding its method of transmission), health-care workers (needlestick injuries, etc.) and sex workers have also been infected. At this time the male homosexual community has the highest infection rate. Currently there is no cure, so prevention involves the use of condoms in all new or casual sexual relationships. The infection can be spread by both males and females. Health-care workers must take universal precautions.

HEPATITIS B

In Australia, 5% of the caucasian population carry markers for previous hepatitis B infection and 0.1–0.3% are carriers and remain infectious. In Australian Aboriginal and Torres Strait Islanders and also in south east Asian populations, 60–90% have markers of infection and up to 30% are carriers. Chronic liver disease and liver cancer may result from previous hepatitis B infection.

HEPATITIS C

Half of those infected with this virus become chronic virus carriers. Twenty to thirty percent of people infected with hepatitis C progress to cirrhosis of the liver in 20 years and of these, a proportion will develop cancer (NH&MRC, 1994).

HUMAN PAPILLOMA VIRUS

This virus causes the development of genital warts, with the whole genital tract being involved, often subclinically. Warty growth is usually on the exterior and infectivity is greatest soon after the development of the lesion. With a good immune system lesions disappear after a few months. Treatment of persistent lesions is with cautery, laser, cryotherapy and certain topical creams.

Certain HPV subtypes are associated with pre-invasive and invasive cancer of the cervix and lower genital tract. This can occur within two years. The outcome from HPV infection depends on the effectiveness of the body's immune system to control the virus. Advice regarding immunity and factors which affect it should be given to all women with HPV. Cervical smear screening – a Pap smear – is recommended for all women who are or who have been sexually active.

HERPES VIRUS

Herpes simplex is an extremely common infection which may occur around the mouth or genitals and occasionally elsewhere. Herpes is manifest in short attacks of mild to severe discomfort. Vulvovaginal burning, itching and hyperaesthesia can occur in the active phase, accompanied by erythema, blisters and shallow ulcers. The vagina and/or cervix can be affected, with a watery discharge being the main symptom. Attacks recur at intervals, with around half the sufferers developing immunity after one or two attacks. Treatment is with acyclovir and its long-term use is effective in controlling most recurrences. During vaginal delivery the baby is at risk if active infection is present.

Prevention of sexually transmitted infections

SAFE SEX

Condoms should be used carefully every time intercourse occurs unless both partners have had no other sexual partners or both have been recently tested for STI and plan to have no other partners. Testing is recommended before stopping the use of condoms in a steady relationship. The more sexual partners a person has, the higher the risk of STI.

VACCINATION

Hepatitis B vaccination is available in three doses given over a six-month period. Vaccination is recommended for particular groups with a higher risk of infection (see box). It is likely that the vaccine will be recommended for everyone in the near future.

Groups for whom hepatitis B vaccination is recommended

Injecting drug users

Health workers

People in institutions

Those with multiple sexual partners

Indigenous Australians

Sexual partners of hepatitis B carriers

Infants of mothers who are hepatitis B carriers

Those who have been sexually assaulted

SAFE NEEDLE PRACTICES

New needles and syringes should be used on each occasion. The Australian National Council on AIDS has announced recommended guidelines for cleaning needles and syringes. However, using new equipment on each occasion is the safest way to prevent infection and cleaning needles and syringes is not recommended.

SAFE TATTOOING AND ACUPUNCTURE

Before having a tattoo or acupuncture, it is important to check that the operator autoclaves the needles prior to use.

This chapter provides a basic introduction to sexual function and common sexual issues for young women, to help physiotherapists in their work with these women. Sexual dysfunction is common and problems with contraception and sexually transmitted infections are very common.

References

Albion St AIDS Centre (1994) *The AIDS Manual*, 3rd edn. Sydney: MacLennon and Petty.

Australian Bureau of Statistics (1980, 1992) *Births Australia*. Catalogue no. 3301.0.

Bancroft J and Machover Reinish J (1990) *Adolescence and Puberty*, New York: Oxford University Press.

Goldman J and Goldman R (1988) *Show Me Yours. Understanding Children's Sexuality.* Ringwood, Victoria, Australia: Penguin.

Govey N (1991) Sexual victimisation prevalence among New Zealand university students. *Journal of Counselling and Clinical Psychology* **59**: 464–466.

Hay-Smith J and Mantle J (1996) Surveys of the experience and perceptions of post-natal superficial dyspareunia of post-natal women, general practitioners and physiotherapists. *Physiotherapy* **82**: 91–97.

Hite S (1977) *The Hite Report*. Sydney: Paul Hamlyn.

Katchadourian H (1990) Sexuality. In: Feldman SS and Elliot GR (eds) *At the Threshold: The Developing Adolescent*. Cambridge, MA: Harvard University Press.

Michael RT, Gannon JH and Lauman EO (1994) *Sex in America: A Definitive Survey*. Boston: Little, Brown.

Moore S and Rosenthal D (1993) *Sexuality in Adolescence*. London: Routledge.

National Health and Medical Research Council of Australia (1994) *Hepatitis C*. Canberra: Commonwealth of Australia.

Roberts G (1992) 'Rape OK if led on' say third of boys. *The Age*, Melbourne. 5/9/92, p. 6.

Further Reading

Bass E and Davis L (1993) *Beginning to Heal: a First Guide for Survivors of Child Sexual Abuse*. London: Cedar.

Boston Women's Health Collective (1992) *The New Our Bodies Ourselves. A Book by and for Women. Updated and Expanded for the 1990s*. New York: Touchstone.

Cooke K (1993) *The Modern Girl's Guide to Safe Sex*, 2nd edn. Ringwood, Victoria, Australia: McPhee Gribble.

Guillebaud J (1993) *Contraception. Your Questions Answered*, 2nd edn. Edinburgh: Churchill Livingstone.

Haseltine F, Cole S and Gray D (1993) *Reproductive Issues for Persons with Physical Disabilities*. Baltimore: Paul H. Brookes.

Kitzinger S (1985) *Women's Experience of Sex*. London: Penguin.

McClosky J (1992) *Your Sexual Health*. Kewdale, Western Australia: Elephas.

Montgomery B and Morris L (1992) *Successful Sex: How to Make your Sex Life more Enjoyable and Solve Common Problems*, 2nd edn. Melbourne: Viking O'Neill.

National Health and Medical Research Council of Australia (1992) *Handbook on Sexually Transmitted Diseases*, 3rd edn. Canberra: Commonwealth of Australia.

Part Two

The Child-bearing Year

10

Overview of Pregnancy and the Puerperium

KATE COPELAND

Conception
•
Anatomy of the Female Reproductive System
•
Pregnancy Trimesters and Tests
•
Role of Physiotherapy in Pregnancy
•
Complications of Pregnancy
•
Labour
•
Puerperium
•
Lactation

The child-bearing year (CBY) is a term that has been used by physiotherapists and others for many decades. Noble (1976, p. 1) defined it as the time 'from conception through post-partum adjustment'. Pregnancy itself is often divided into 'trimesters', each equating to approximately three months. A simplistic view of the CBY can be seen as **four** trimesters – nine months of pregnancy plus the first three months after the birth of the baby. Detailed information about the role of the physiotherapist with respect to women's health during the CBY is outlined in the chapters that follow.

Effective clinical practice for physiotherapists is based on a sound knowledge and understanding of anatomy and physiology and of the social and psychological aspects of each stage of the CBY.

This chapter provides an introduction and review of:

- the menstrual cycle;
- female anatomy;
- pregnancy tests;
- the role of the physiotherapist;
- complications which may occur during pregnancy;
- stages of labour;
- physiology of labour;
- the puerperium (after the baby is born);
- lactation.

Provision of advice, education, health promotion, treatment, support and liaison are some of the aspects of physiotherapy interaction with women during pregnancy, birth and the early days with a new baby.

The aims of obstetric physiotherapy have been summarized by Marshall (1981) as follows.

1. To promote good health, poise and a sense of well-being during pregnancy and encourage preventive medicine.
2. To give women the opportunity to discuss their fears and expectations in a relaxed and sympathetic atmosphere and to acquire positive and accurate information about pregnancy and labour.
3. To offer instruction in skills to conserve energy, raise pain tolerance levels and maintain control during labour.
4. To alleviate the stresses and strains of pregnancy.
5. To rehabilitate women during the puerperium to full physical activity and mental well-being.

Marshall and Walsh (1994) further commented that obstetric physiotherapists 'have to consider the special needs of each individual mother and address the multi-faceted nature of the individual in terms of her physical activities, her comforts, her psychological and emotional maturity and development, her spiritual aspirations, expectations and desires'. They comment that an obstetric physiotherapist, by working in close harmony with both the prospective mother and other members of the health team, can play a truly unique role in enhancing the quality and dignity of giving birth and in the longer term mothering and parenting.

Physiotherapists may come into contact with pregnant women in a multitude of ways.

- At educational sessions provided by hospital clinics, community health centres or local communities.
- By referral from GPs, hospital doctors or specialists for treatment of a particular physical problem.
- By patient self-referral for information, advice or treatment.
- At pregnancy exercise classes, including 'pregnastics' and 'aquarobics'.
- At a sports injury clinic.
- At a session organized by a specific group, such as young parents programme (teenage pregnancy).
- Management of a pre-existing illness, injury or disability, including rheumatoid arthritis, spinal injury, etc.

Regardless of whether you are working within a general hospital, in a specialist physiotherapy practice, in manipulative or sports physiotherapy or in a community setting, a knowledge and understanding of the effects and implications of pregnancy and the puerperium is essential. It must be remembered by all physiotherapists that women comprise approximately 50% of the total population and that all women from teenagers to those in their 50s are within their reproductive years. The reproductive period usually continues until the supply of ova runs out, but with advances in scientific techniques such as the use of artificial hormone stimulation and zygote implantation, pregnancies have been reported in women nearing 60 years of age.

Physiotherapy within a team of health providers is another important aspect in the CBY. The members of the team may vary depending on the location, both geographic and social, and may include obstetricians, gynaecologists, paediatricians, general practitioners, midwives, nurses, social workers, dietitians and others.

Conception

In the human, conception takes place around the time of ovulation, approximately day 10–16 in the menstrual cycle (see Chapter 11). Around 200 million sperm in 4 ml of seminal fluid are deposited in the upper vagina during sexual intercourse. The sperm swim up through the uterus to the outer third of the fallopian tubes, where fertilization takes place.

If fertilized, the egg continues along the fallopian tube towards the uterine cavity and initiates the production of hormones to prevent menstruation. The fertilized ovum implants onto the wall of the uterus and creates the area which then develops into the placenta.

Associated with the menstrual cycle are identifiable changes in vaginal secretions. These changes are the basis for the Billings method of birth control (Billings and Westmore, 1980; Billings et al, 1989) which allows women and their partners to gain knowledge of their fertility based on the appearance of the vaginal mucus. Dependent on the needs of the individual, this knowledge may be used to increase the chances of pregnancy or to avoid fertile times.

Figure 10.1 Flow chart of conceptual process from fertilization to foetus.

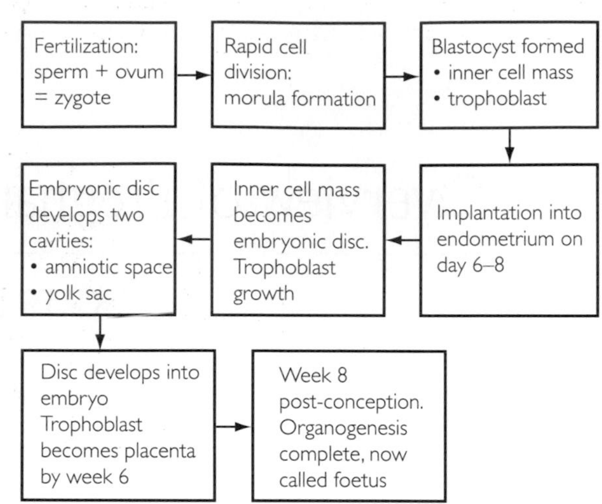

Anatomy of the Female Reproductive System

Knowledge of external and internal female genitalia is important for the clinical physiotherapist. It is also important for women generally to have an understanding about their own bodies, appearance and function and changes which occur. The first edition of the Boston Women's Health Book Collective (1973) *Our Bodies, Ourselves* provided information to women as consumers of health care, including the suggestion that women should take a mirror and look at their own genitalia (Fig. 10.2).

In the non-pregnant woman, the *uterus* is an 8 cm long, hollow, thick-walled muscular organ, lying behind the bladder and in front of the rectum. It is sometimes described as being shaped like an upside-down pear. Consisting of the fundus, the body, the isthmus and the cervix, the uterus is bent forward and tilted to overhang the bladder from behind and above (Fig. 10.3). The isthmus develops into the lower segment of the uterus during pregnancy. The neck of the uterus is the *cervix* which is the lower constricted part of the uterus. It projects down into the vaginal vault, with the vaginal walls surrounding the cervix. The lowest point of the cervix is called the *external os.*

The *vagina* is a 10 cm long canal which proceeds from the cervix to the perineum. Its walls are involuted into folds called rugae which are capable of expanding considerably to allow the passage of the baby during childbirth.

The *ovaries* lie at the back of the peritoneum, hanging by a mesentery called the mesovarium. Each ovary is covered by a layer of cells known as the germinal layer. At ovulation the ovum erupts through the ovary into the peritoneal cavity. It

Figure 10.2 Female external genitalia. Mons veneris = (mons pubis) fatty tissue overlaying the junction of the two pubic bones (symphysis pubis); labia majora = (major lips) hair-covered skinfolds; labia minora = (minor lips) smaller and more delicate; clitoris = homologue of the male penis; vestibule = area enclosed by labia minora; urethral meatus (external urinary orifice); Vaginal orifice = opens onto lower part of the vestibule; Bartholin's ducts = open into the vestibule at its posterolateral aspect; perineum = area outlined by the vaginal fourchette anteriorly and the anus posteriorly.

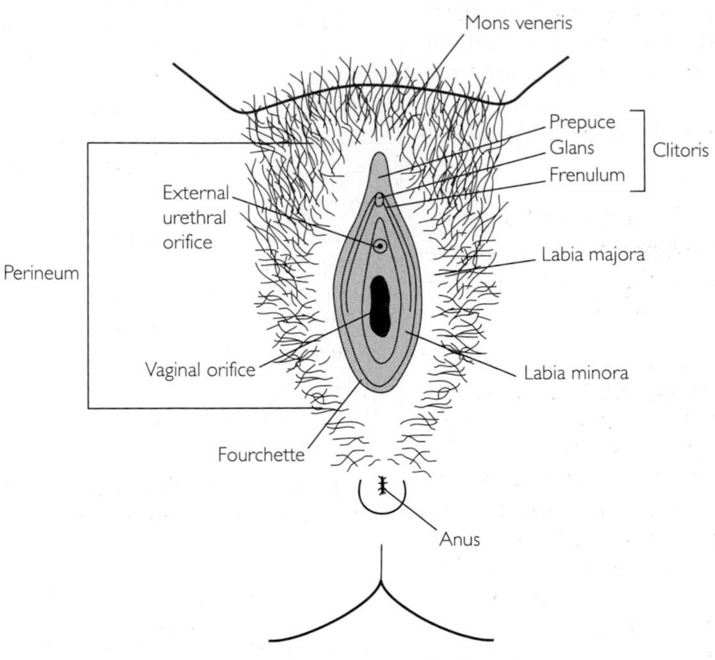

Figure 10.3 Median section through the female pelvis.

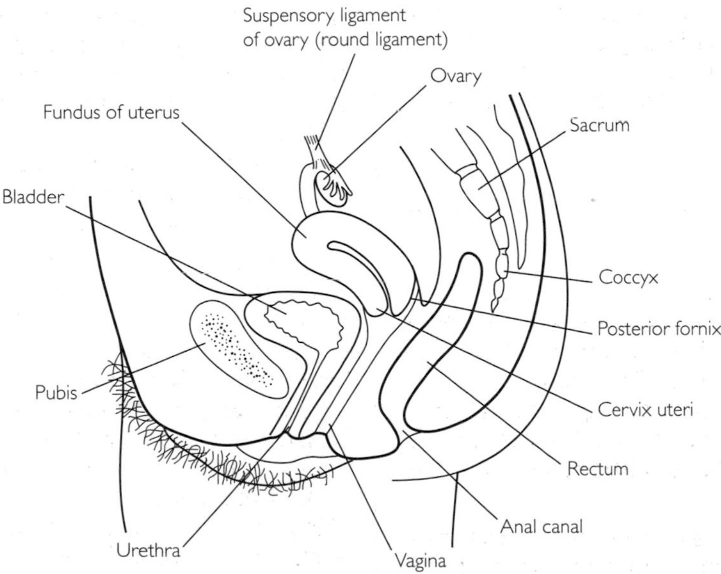

is then gathered by the fimbriae into the fallopian tube. The *fallopian tubes* lie in the upper part of a transverse fold of the peritoneum called the broad ligament.

Also part of the female reproductive system are the *breasts*. Changes begin early in pregnancy and continue through to the birth of the baby and afterwards (see Chapter 11 and section on lactation, p. 106).

Skeletal supports

The birth canal is comprised of fibromuscular and bony structures – the bony pelvis, the brim, the pelvic cavity and the outlet.

The *bony pelvis* consists of four bones – the two innominates (each made up of the pubis, ischium and ilium), the sacrum and the coccyx. These bones are joined by strong ligaments at the sacroiliac joints and pubic symphysis and loosely connected at the sacrococcygeal joint. The sacrum curves backwards and downwards, making the superior border quite prominent – the sacral promontory. The pelvic aspect of the sacrum is concave, contributing to some of the curve of the birth canal when combined with the coccyx. Together they measure a curve of 11–13 cm in length. Anteriorly the canal consists of the symphysis pubis, approximately 4–5 cm long.

The *brim* of the pelvis is described by the sacral promontory, the wings of the sacrum, the iliopectineal lines and the superior aspect of the pubic bones. Four characteristic brim outlines have been described (Fig. 10.6):

Figure 10.4 Sectional diagram showing ovaries, uterus and fallopian tubes.

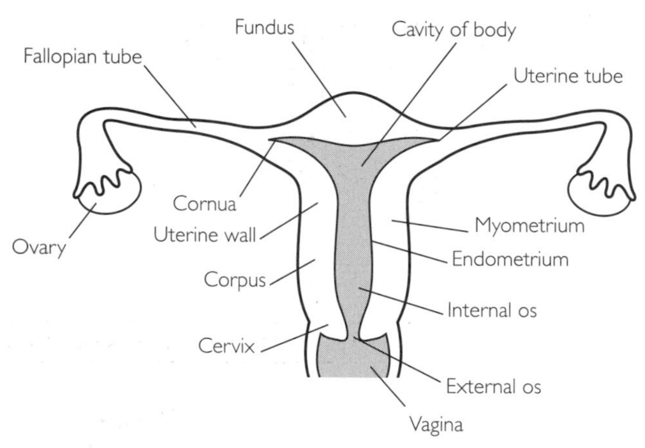

1. the gynaecoid, which is the most common shape and is almost round;
2. the android or male, which is heart shaped;
3. the anthropoid, which is more oval with its longest axis anteroposteriorly;
4. the platypelloid, which is longer transversely.

The differences in these pelvic shapes determine to a large degree the way in which the baby passes through the birth canal (Fig. 10.7).

The *pelvic cavity* is bounded by the curve of the sacrum posteriorly, the pubic bones anteriorly and the innominates laterally. The lower part of the cavity is also known as the plane of least dimensions. The ischial spines are located about mid-way in the birth canal and are used as a reference point for the descent of the baby during labour. With the ischial spines being 0, the position of the baby's head is described as being up to 5 cm above (−5 to −1) or below (+1 to + 5) the ischial spines (see Fig. 10.8).

The *pelvic outlet* is outlined by the ischial tuberosities, the subpubic arch, the coccyx and the sacrotuberous ligaments (see Fig. 10.9).

During pregnancy, the ligamentous connections of the bony pelvis are loosened by the effects of relaxin and problems of pain and instability of the pelvic girdle are relatively common. Refer to Chapter 14 for information on assessment and management of these problems.

Preconception health issues

It has been stated that all women intending pregnancy should be in optimal physical condition (Fisher, 1989). Although some individuals and groups are strongly in favour of preconceptual care and advice, there is limited

Figure 10.5 Female bony pelvis detailing pelvic inlet diameters.

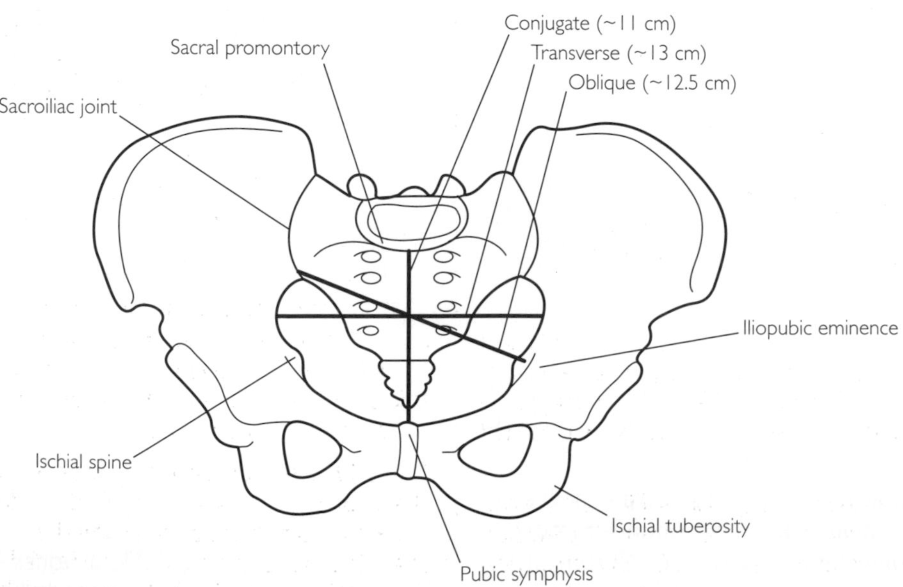

Figure 10.6 Variation in shape of the pelvic brim. A Gynaecoid, almost round: 55% of women. B Android, heart shaped due to projecting sacral promontory and narrow fore-pelvis: 20% of women. C Anthropoid, oval and, like the android pelvis, tends to have mid-pelvic narrowing: 20% of women. D Platypelloid, transversely oval, usually a shallow pelvis with capacious outlet: 5% of women. (Reproduced from Beischer and Mackay (1986) with permission of NA Beischer.)

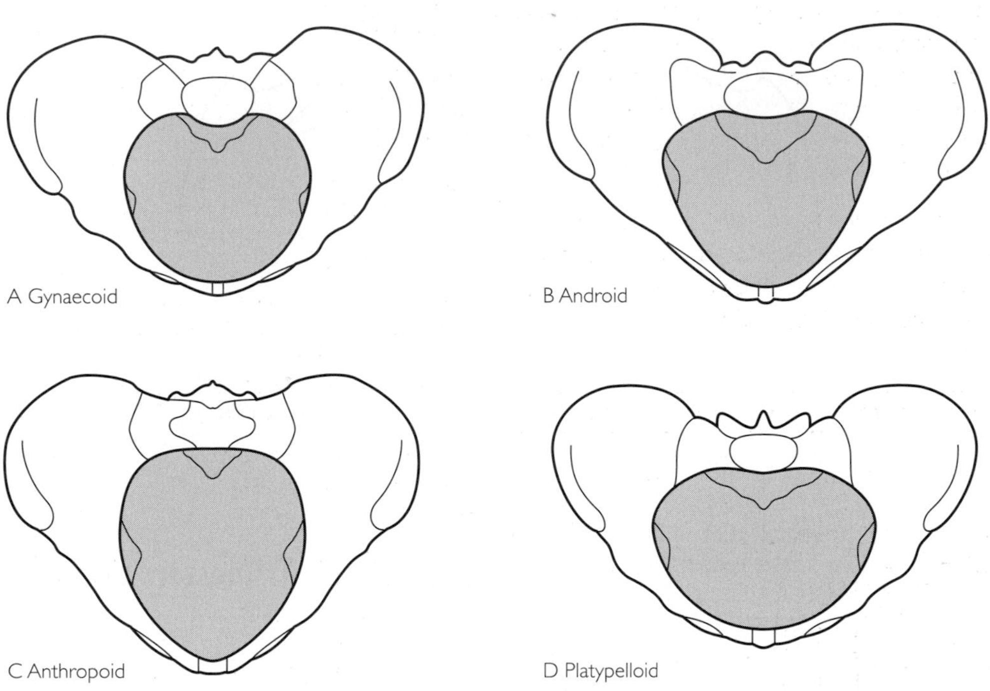

Figure 10.7 The birth canal.

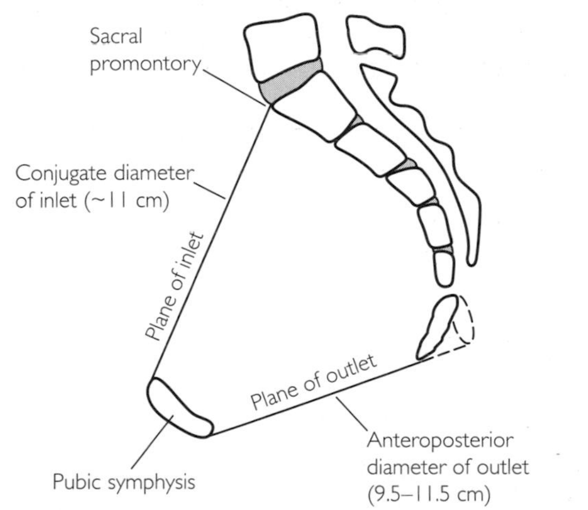

Figure 10.8 The descent of the fetal head in relation to the ischial spines.

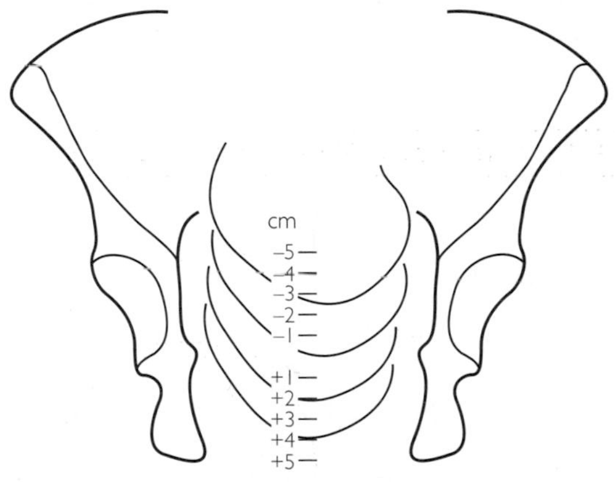

empirical evidence as yet to support their stance. Enkin et al (1989) state that 'on the basis of present knowledge its (pre-pregnancy advice) beneficial effects are likely to be extremely modest and it cannot automatically be regarded as harmless'.

An opportunity for pre-pregnancy counselling, advice and testing is offered by a negative pregnancy test. The medical practitioner and the woman can use this time to review medication and the use of non-prescribed drugs, to check rubella status and discuss immunization if appropriate, to check for possible pregnancy risk factors which require evaluation and management, to discuss the use of vitamin and other diet supplementation and the need for caution during exercise programmes.

The evidence that cigarette smoking may have harmful effects on the foetus is strong. Clear evidence links maternal smoking and reduced birth weight (Burton et al, 1989; Cliver et al, 1992; Cnattingius, 1992; Luke, 1994; MacArthur and Knox, 1988; Olsen, 1992; Roquer et al, 1995).

Figure 10.9 The female pelvic outlet.

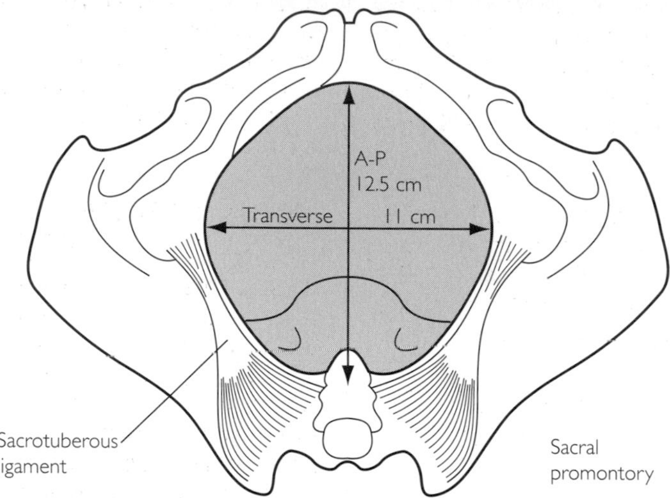

Several components of pre-natal diet influence foetal growth, including vitamin A, folate, calcium and iron. Low maternal and newborn levels of vitamin A are strongly associated with intrauterine growth retardation (Luke, 1994). It is known, however, that fat-soluble vitamins such as A and D can cause metabolic changes and supplementation should not be undertaken except with medical or pharmaceutical advice and supervision.

Niebyl (1995) recommends that women who have previously had an infant with a neural tube defect should supplement their diet with 4 mg folic acid each day from at least four weeks before conception and throughout the first three months of pregnancy and that all women capable of becoming pregnant should consume 0.4 mg folic acid each day. Although the cause of neural tube defects is often unknown, possible causes include genetic influences, nutritional deficiency or drugs. A decrease in folate intake has been associated with an increased risk of such defects (Mills et al, 1992; Rush, 1994; Yates et al, 1987). Recent studies support the concept that folic acid supplements will decrease both the recurrent risk and first occurrence of neural tube defects (Center for Disease Control, 1991; MRC, 1991). Bower and Stanley (1989), in an Australian case-control study in the first six weeks of pregnancy, found there was a clear dose-related association with free folate intake and the risk of neural tube defects.

A recent study has found that daily zinc supplementation in women with relatively low plasma zinc concentrations is associated with greater infant birth weights and head circumferences (Goldenberg et al, 1995).

Pregnancy Trimesters and Tests

First trimester

Many women are unaware of their pregnancy for the first 4–6 weeks. Despite this, growth and development of the foetus proceeds at a phenomenal rate. The first three months of pregnancy include a period of adjustment to the fact of having a baby and to the physical changes beginning in the body.

Simons (1987) noted that:

> The effects of these physiological changes have long been underrated, not by the medical profession but by women themselves. How many of us in our pregnancies acknowledge and accept the fact that we are more vulnerable to injury, more susceptible to strain and need to accommodate the changes that pregnancy brings?

MORNING SICKNESS

Nausea and vomiting are the most frequent, the most characteristic and perhaps the most troublesome symptoms of early pregnancy. In a recent study from an urban practice in the United Kingdom, of 363 women from mixed socioeconomic backgrounds 28% experienced nausea and an additional 52% had both nausea and vomiting (Gadsby et al, 1993). The aetiology of nausea in pregnancy is still unknown and the variety of treatments that have been recommended reflect the multitude of theories as to the underlying cause (Enkin et al, 1995).

Prior to the 1980s, thalidomide was frequently prescribed for the relief of pregnancy-related nausea and vomiting. It was not until a causal relationship was established between babies born with missing or deformed limbs and the mother's use of thalidomide that it was removed from sale. After this, the most widely used drug prescribed for the treatment of nausea and vomiting in pregnancy was Debendox. Since its removal from the market (as a direct result of litigation against the manufacturers) there has been an increased use of alternative medication for treating nausea and vomiting, although concerns about potentially harmful effects on the foetus have limited the use of medication.

Non-pharmacological management of nausea and vomiting
Kahn (1988) noted that transcutaneous electrical nerve stimulation (TENS) was being used to reduce morning sickness discomfort. Success was achieved using a high rate of 120 Hz with a medium pulse width of 150 microseconds stimulating the traditional 'hoku' position (the web space between thumb and forefinger). Interestingly, it was noted that this technique did not seem to work if used on the left arm.

De Aloysio and Penacchioni (1992) demonstrated that the use of bands that apply pressure to the Neiguan acupressure point on the wrist between the flexor carpi radialis and the palmaris longus muscles is effective in reducing nausea and vomiting of pregnancy in 60% of patients.

Evans et al (1993) investigated the use of sensory afferent stimulation (SAS) delivering a continuous current of up to 20 mA to the wrist for treating pregnancy-induced nausea and vomiting. Despite a small sample size, 87% of the study subjects recorded improvement in symptoms with the SAS unit. Of the 13 subjects who reported no change in symptoms while using the placebo device, 11 had improvement with the SAS unit. Conversely, although 10 patients reported improvement with the placebo unit, only one (10%) failed to improve with the SAS unit also. Their results suggest that sensory afferent stimulation is beneficial in reducing nausea and vomiting during the periods of stimulation.

McMillan (1994) combined stimulation of the acupuncture point with transcutaneous electrical stimulation (TCES) to control sickness in patients following orthopaedic surgery. It should be noted that TCES is a term used interchangeably with TENS and transcutaneous nerve stimulation (TCNS).

A prospective trial comparing acupressure bands, sensory afferent stimulation and TENS for control of nausea of pregnancy would be most interesting.

Nausea and vomiting of intense severity is termed *hyperemesis gravidarum* and may require hospital management, including the use of intravenous therapy (Bashiri et al, 1995). If extremely prolonged, hyperemesis gravidarum should promote consideration of thyrotoxicosis (Ladwig et al, 1995). Mothers with high carbohydrate intake in early pregnancy tended to have smaller placentas and lower birthweight babies (Godfrey et al, 1996). Morning sickness may be an advantage in these cases. Prednisolone has been shown to be an effective treatment for severe hyperemesis gravidarum, where other measures have failed (Nelson-Perry, 1995).

OTHER COMMONS SIGNS OF EARLY PREGNANCY
Other common signs and symptoms of early pregnancy include breast changes, urinary frequency, vaginal discharge and tiredness/sleepiness (see Fig. 10.10 and Table 10.1 for more details). These are primarily due to the physiological changes occurring during early pregnancy and are explained in more detail in Chapter 11.

Second trimester

The second three months are usually more comfortable for women. Changes which may occur at this time include development of stretch marks, production of colostrum (precursor to milk production from the breasts), problems with heartburn, indigestion and constipation, potential for urinary infections, varicose veins and backache. The mother also becomes aware of foetal movements. Once again, these changes are primarily due to the physiological changes occurring and are explained in more detail in Chapter 11. Table 10.2 outlines changes in the second trimester.

With respect to heartburn or indigestion, antacids are often used by women for relief. One concern which has been highlighted is the potential adverse effects of antacids containing aluminium, which are often used by women for relief (Kirschbaum and Schoolwerth, 1989; Monteagudo et al, 1989; Winship 1992, 1993). Effects include interference with iron absorption and specifically the potential for metabolic alkalosis and fluid overload in both the foetus and the mother (Baron et al, 1993). Antacids can be prescribed for relief of persistent heartburn after the first trimester, but should be reserved for the most troublesome symptoms. The use of simple remedies should be offered, although formal evidence of their efficacy is not available. Clinical experience suggests the usefulness of measures such as:

- use of small frequent meals;
- exclusion of foods that exacerbate symptoms such as fatty food, chocolate, alcohol, tea and coffee, and cigarettes;
- squatting to pick things up rather than bending over;
- not going to bed for at least 2–3 hours after eating;
- propping up the bed head to help keep acid from entering the oesophagus.

Third trimester

The third three months of pregnancy is a time of marked growth for the baby and therefore expansion of the mother's abdomen. Changes which may be noted at this time include breathlessness, problems with heartburn, urinary frequency, cramps, muscle and nerve twinges, charged emotions including anticipation and anxiety, and Braxton Hicks contractions.

In the last months of pregnancy, many women notice that the uterus goes through periods of hardening and tightening. These contractions, which are usually painless, are called Braxton Hicks contractions and are believed to play a part in increasing circulation to the uterus and the baby. Towards

Figure 10.10 Details of foetal organ development.

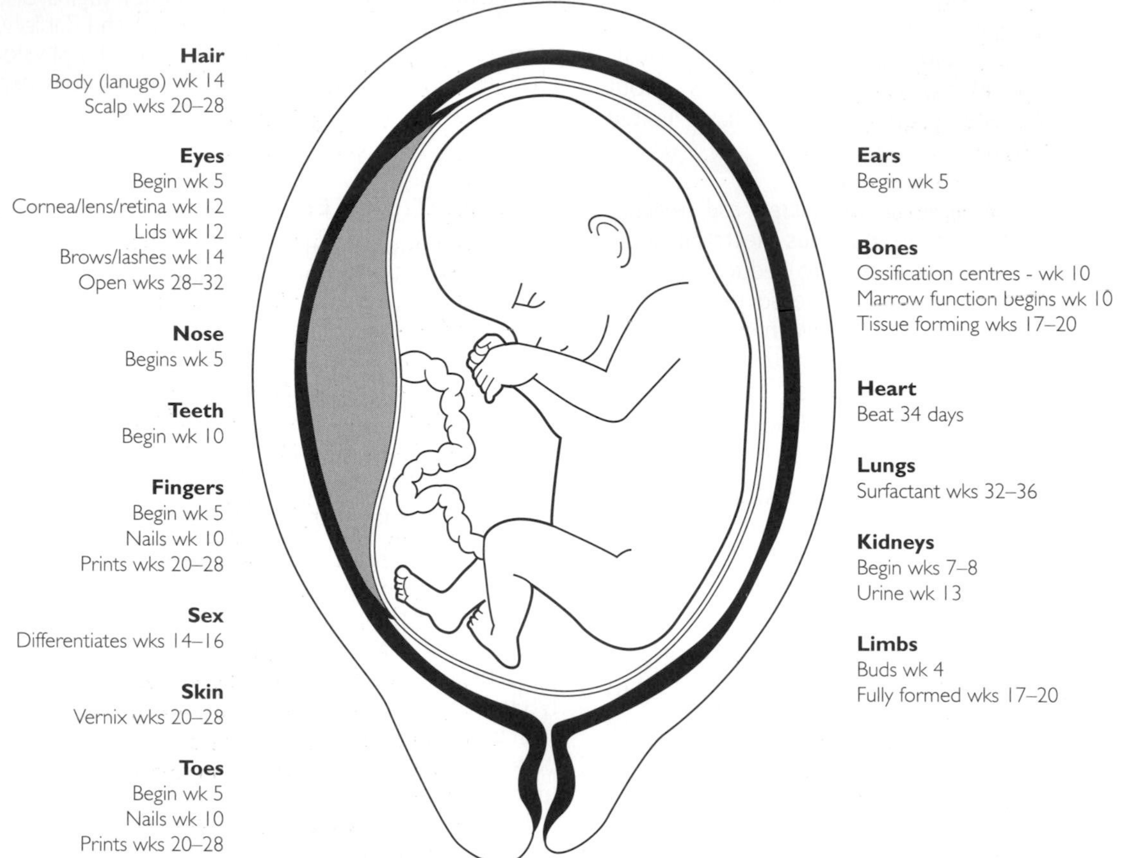

the end of the pregnancy, they may increase in frequency and intensity and may be mistaken for labour contractions. Some women find that being physically active triggers these contractions and a change in activity (such as lying down) will often stop them. This differentiates them from 'true' labour pains which are not responsive to changes in activity levels. Braxton Hicks contractions are sometimes referred to as 'false' labour when they occur close to term. Changes during the third trimester are outlined in Table 10.3.

In the last few weeks of pregnancy, women may be aware of 'lightening', which describes the sensation felt when the baby's head settles into the pelvis and takes some of the pressure away from the diaphragm and ribs. An understanding of the physiological changes occurring at this time is required and can be found in Chapter 11.

Discomforts of pregnancy

Nearly all women experience some degree of discomfort and/or pain during pregnancy. A lot of these problems can be minimized with simple self-help techniques. A summary of the more common discomforts and ways to alleviate them are contained in Table 10.4.

It is important to bear in mind the difference between minor discomforts and symptoms of a more serious nature requiring referral to the woman's medical adviser. As physiotherapists we are frequently asked about these discomforts and we can provide assistance in many instances (see Chapters 14, 16 and 24).

Pregnancy tests and investigations

A variety of tests and investigations is available for use during pregnancy to monitor the health and well-being of mother and baby. A list of these is given in the Appendix at the end of this chapter.

Role of Physiotherapy in Pregnancy

There are a number of ways in which a physiotherapist can provide valuable input and assistance in the course of pregnancy. They are listed here and will be covered in the sections which follow.

Table 10.1 Changes in mother and foetus during the first trimester of pregnancy

Mother	Foetus
0–6 weeks • Unaware of conception till first period missed at 4–5 weeks • May be asymptomatic • Blood/urine tests positive. 95% accurate five days post-conception; 100% accurate 10 days post-conception	• Conception day 10–16 days into cycle. Gametes join to form zygote • Zygote → morula (1–3 days) → blastocyst (4–6 days) → embryo • Implants into uterine wall day 6–8 • Week 2 – Inner cell mass flattens and forms embryonic disc. Primitive uteroplacental circulation and amniotic and yolk sac cavities. • Week 3 – Chorionic sac, villi developed on surface. Villi become vascular. Major development of hearing and nervous systems • Week 4 – Musculoskeletal and nervous development. Arm and leg buds. Adopting C-shaped curve • Week 5 – Embryo and body stalk enveloped in amnion.
Week 7–13 • Amenorrhoea – spotting may occur at time period due • Morning sickness – affects more than 60% of women to some degree • Urinary frequency – effects of progesterone and uterus pressing on bladder • Breasts begin to enlarge due to alveoli development. Pigmentation increases at nipple and areola • Increased vaginal secretions • Fatigue	• Week 7–8 – Rectal/urinary separation. Foetal endocrine glands begin to function. Facial clefts closed • Week 10 – Now called a foetus. Primitive nervous system function at reflex level • Week 12 – Foetus is 10 cm long and weighs 30 g • Week 13 – All organs formed

- Education aimed at prevention of musculoskeletal strains (Chapters 14, 15, 16, 21).
- Provision of information and advice on management or minimization of common physical discomforts of pregnancy (Chapters 15, 16 and 24).
- Optimal physical fitness and preparation for the changes which occur during pregnancy and after the baby is born (Chapter 16).
- Assessment and treatment of musculoskeletal disorders (Chapters 14 and 24).
- Physical coping skills for labour (Chapter 18).
- Education (with other health professionals) on promotion of health and healthy lifestyles, both for the present and the future (Chapters 15, 16 and 19).
- Creating an awareness of the physical changes which will be experienced after the baby is born (Chapter 19).
- Provision of information and advice about ergonomic aspects of life with a new baby or young child (Chapters 20 and 21).

Complications of Pregnancy

It has been estimated that about 50% of women have a normal pregnancy, with a normal delivery after a spontaneous onset of labour (Beischer et al, 1989). Complications can vary markedly in both incidence and severity.

Reasons for antenatal hospital admission

The more common reasons for hospital admission among antenatal women are listed in the box.

- Cervical incompetence
- Hypertension
- Antepartum haemorrhage (major bleeding during pregnancy)

Table 10.2 Changes in mother and foetus during the second trimester of pregnancy

Mother	Foetus
Week 14–16	
• Uterus has emerged from pelvis to enter abdominal cavity • Palpable above pubic bones • Backache may develop • Excess oil produced in skin → acne • Increased perspiration	• Yolk sac disappears – all foetal nourishment from placenta • Weight 120 g • Length 20 cm
Week 17–20	
• Foetal movements felt by mother • Increased blood volume • Weight gain • Waist thickens • Pigmentation changes continue	• Foetus sleeping 20 hours per day • Alternating rest and activity periods • Heart beat 140–150 beats per minute • Finger / toe nails nearly to end of digits • Body elongates • Rapid growth of torso and legs • Weight 360 g • Height 25 cm
Week 20–28	
• Indigestion • Constipation • Varicose veins • Increased awareness of foetal movement • Braxton Hicks contractions occasionally felt • Chloasma (facial pigmentation)	• Reacts to outside stimuli – sound, movement • Lanugo covers body • Liquor 1.2 l • Weight 400–600 g • Length 30–35 cm

- Placental abruption (separation of the normally implanted placenta)
- Placenta praevia (placenta is situated partly or wholly in the lower uterine segment of the uterus)
- Intrauterine growth retardation
- Multiple pregnancy (e.g. triplets, quadruplets)
- Pre-eclampsia / eclampsia (pre-eclampsia is the condition which precedes eclampsia, a convulsive state which is now rare. Pre-eclampsia is quite common, with recognized clinical features, but the basic cause is not yet determined)

Hypertensive disorders in some form occur in about one-quarter of all pregnancies. Pre-eclampsia, a pregnancy-induced hypertension, commonly occurs in the last trimester, with signs of oedema of hands and face, hypertension and proteinuria. Infrequently, this can lead to eclampsia when fitting occurs before, during or after labour. Management is by bed rest. Chronic hypertension occurs before 20 weeks of pregnancy or pre-dates pregnancy. Pre-eclampsia can be superimposed on this. Antihypertensive agents, as well as bed rest, may be necessary in both cases.

Antepartum haemorrhage is caused most commonly by placenta praevia, in which the placenta is implanted low on the uterine wall or over the internal os. Bleeding generally occurs in the third trimester as the lower uterine segment develops and thins. Depending on foetal status, uterine activity and the extent of the blood loss, management by hospitalization aims to increase foetal maturity. In severe bleeding, immediate caesarean section is indicated. Antepartum haemorrhage from placental abruption is generally managed by immediate delivery.

Pre-term labour (between 20 and 37 weeks) *and premature rupture of membranes* (which exposes the foetus to infection) are managed whenever possible to prolong the pregnancy and increase foetal maturity. These can both require prolonged hospitalization.

Multiple pregnancies have increased in incidence since fertility drugs and IVF procedures came into use. Pregnancies with two, three or more babies result in prematurity and bed rest in hospital, especially with more than two babies, is aimed at increasing foetal maturity.

The perinatal mortality rate is lowest in the 25–29-year age group (11.7 per 1000 births) and highest when the mother is 40 years or more (27.8 per 1000 births) (Beischer and Mackay, 1986).

Associated medical and surgical complications

Women who suffer from medical disorders frequently find that the condition changes in response to the pregnancy. Close medical monitoring is necessary. In cardiac disease

Table 10.3 Changes in mother and foetus during the third trimester of pregnancy

Mother	Foetus
Week 29–32	
• Mood swings increase • Varicose veins • Haemorrhoids • Lower limb oedema • Pubic symphysis and SIJ pain • Round ligament pain	• Fat deposits increasing. Scalp hair well defined • Taste and smell developed • Foetal organs begin to function • Foetus now begins to metabolize nutrients, drugs for itself • Weight 1.2 kg • Length 35–40 cm
Week 32–36	
• Frequency of urination • Braxton Hicks contractions more uncomfortable • Breathlessness • Sleeping difficulties • Indigestion • Constipation • Diastasis of rectus abdominis may occur	• Continues to deposit subcutaneous fat • Foetus settles into birth position – usually cephalic • May be breech • Weight 2.4–2.7 kg • Length 40–45 cm
Week 36–40	
• Urinary frequency • Breathlessness • Sleeping difficulties • Pressure in pelvis after baby 'drops' • Navel may evert • Haemorrhoids, varicose veins may worsen • Lower limb oedema increases • Fatigue • 'Sick of being pregnant' • 'Show' in the days or hours preceding labour	• Lanugo disappears – may have small amount at birth • Finger, toe nails firm and extend past tips • Vernix coating decreased, mainly in skin creases – groin, knees, neck, elbows • Weight 3.3 kg (2.5–4.5 kg) • Length 45–55 cm

pregnancy can create severe maternal problems and in diabetes both mother and foetus can be affected.

Disorders which may be aggravated by pregnancy

Renal disease, diabetes mellitus, psychiatric disorder, asthma, essential hypertension, venous thrombosis, epilepsy, cardiac disease, tumours, acute appendicitis, acute cholecystitis, splenectomy

Pregnancy disorders – maternal and foetal

- Foetal maldevelopment (chromosomal disorders, e.g. Down syndrome; neural tube defects, e.g. spina bifida, anencephaly)
- Abortion (miscarriage) – spontaneous, therapeutic, septic
- Ectopic pregnancy (implantation of the foetus occurs outside the uterine cavity, usually in the fallopian tube)
- Hydatidiform mole (developmental abnormality of the trophoblast or placenta)
- Choriocarcinoma (malignant tumour of the trophoblast; approximately half originate in a hydatidiform mole)
- Polyhydramnios (excess amniotic fluid for the gestational period)
- Oligohydramnios (amniotic fluid less than 200 ml). May occur with placental failure or foetal malformation. May lead to positional abnormalities, e.g. talipes
- Blood group incompatibility (different blood group factors between the mother and the foetus). Transfer of cells through the placenta may lead to the mother developing antibodies. After delivery anti-D gammaglobulin administration provides protection for future pregnancies
- Foetoplacental dysfunction
- Foetal positioning – breech, transverse, oblique

Table 10.4 Common discomforts of pregnancy

Discomfort	Cause	Self-help
Urinary frequency	Pressure of uterus on bladder, increased bladder filling. UTI	Empty bladder often. Pelvic floor exercise to support extra weight of uterus. Seek medical advice if infection present
Constipation	Slowing of bowel activity due to: increase in progesterone levels; decrease in activity levels; inadequate fluid intake; ingestion of increased iron	Increase soluble fibre and fluid intake. Increase activity levels – exercise, walking. Change iron supplement (seek medical advice). Regular toilet habits
Haemorrhoids	Constipation. Increased uterine weight pressing on bowel / pelvic veins	Increase fibre and fluids. Analgesia – seek medical advice. Ice packs. Pad for support. Defaecation retraining
Nausea / vomiting	Increase in oestrogen levels → metabolic changes Increase in progesterone → slower emptying of stomach → nausea. Cardiac sphincter relaxation	Small frequent meals. Eat before rising (dry toast, crackers). Avoid greasy and rich food. Usually self-limiting 6–16 weeks
Heartburn	Pressure of uterus on stomach. Progesterone in early pregnancy causes slower emptying, causes increase in reflux. Cardiac sphincter more relaxed due to progesterone	Light frequent meals. Sleep in semirecumbent position. Restrict intake prior to retiring. Ingest milk. Antacid preparations (seek medical advice). Avoid fatty foods, coffee and smoking
Fainting	Vasodilation in early pregnancy. Uterine pressure on inferior vena cava in late pregnancy	Avoid overheating, crowds. Do not stand or rise from lying too quickly. Avoid prolonged standing. Lie down at first indication of feeling faint. Avoid supine lying
Varicose veins	Increase in progesterone and oestrogen. Increase blood volume. Pressure of uterus on pelvic veins	Support hosiery. Avoid prolonged standing. Walk rather than stand. Elevate feet when lying. Rest frequently with feet elevated
Vulval varicosities	As above	Sanitary pad for support. Avoid prolonged standing, squatting. Avoid constipation, straining.
Oedema in lower limbs	Progesterone and gravity cause venous engorgement	Avoid prolonged standing. Walk rather than stand. Rest with feet elevated

Table 10.4 continued

Discomfort	Cause	Self-help
Backache	Relaxin causes looser ligaments → joint laxity, increase in thoracic and lumbar curves. Softening of ligaments	Postural awareness. Ergonomic advice. Lumbosacral support belt. Stability exercises. Strengthening exercises. Rest.
Tender breasts	Oestrogen and progesterone cause an increase in growth	Firm bra for support. Warmth. Physiotherapy treatment for associated thoracic pain
Muscle cramps	Ischaemia, pressure of uterus on nerves. Possibly phosphates in milk	Calf stretches during day. Support stockings. Medical advice re calcium source. Massage. Avoid maximum plantar flexion motion. When women feel cramp beginning, stretches into dorsiflexion, massage
Carpal tunnel syndrome	Swelling in hand/wrist compresses median and ulnar nerves	Working/resting splints. Contrast bathing to increase circulation and decrease oedema. Physiotherapy treatment. Ice, elevation when resting. Muscle pump exercises
Insomnia	Increase in discomfort as pregnancy progresses. Vivid dreams. Anxiety	Relaxation techniques. Rest if cannot sleep. Physiotherapy advice re sleeping positions. Visualization and stress management techniques

Table 10.5 Complications of pregnancy

- Ectopic pregnancy
- Hydatidiform mole
- Choriocarcinoma
- Abortion
- Premature rupture of membranes
- Abruptio placentae
- Placenta praevia
- Polyhydramnios
- Hyperemesis gravidarum
- Haemolytic disease
- Deliveries between 20–28 weeks gestation
- Pre-eclampsia
- Threatened abortion
- Infection of the genital tract
- Maternal obesity
- Contracted pelvis
- Ante-partum haemorrhage
- Multiple pregnancy
- Incompetent cervix
- Prolonged pregnancy (>42 weeks)
- Post-partum haemorrhage
- Prolonged labour
- Hepatitis
- Jaundice
- Eclampsia
- Rupture of uterus
- Stillbirth

Table 10.5 provides a more extensive list of disorders of pregnancy.

The practising physiotherapist needs an understanding of the potential complications which can occur during pregnancy and an awareness of the magnitude and severity of each. This knowledge enables the physiotherapist to modify their treatment plans for maximum benefit.

For additional information, refer to Llewellyn-Jones (1994) or Beischer et al (1989).

Labour

Labour is the term applied to the maternal process culminating in the birth of a baby. There are some well-recognized signs which indicate that labour is imminent (pre-labour signs) and these include:

- lightening, where the baby's head engages into the pelvis. As described earlier, this is often more marked with a first pregnancy and may happen 2–4 weeks before labour begins. With second and subsequent babies, it may not happen until labour begins;
- Braxton Hicks contractions, previously described. These tend to occur more frequently towards the end of pregnancy;
- increased mucous discharge from the vagina;
- weight loss of around 1 kg in the week before labour begins;
- nesting behaviours – spurts of energy, sudden cleaning/painting/sewing/decorating;
- increased pelvic pressure;
- slight diarrhoea or wind in the bowel.

Signs of labour

- Regular contractions felt in the abdomen or groin, low in the back or in the legs. The uterus can be felt hardening at the same time. Contractions tend to become longer, stronger and closer together. These contrast with Braxton Hicks contractions which may come in sets but do not progress in this way.
- A 'show' of mucous discharge from the vagina, which may be stained with blood.
- Rupture of the membranes – the 'bag of waters' which surrounds the baby leaks or breaks. This is less common; only about 10% of labours begin with the waters leaking.
- Some women experience constant minor backache, with bouts of stronger back pain, during labour.

Stages of labour

FIRST STAGE

Usually described as being from the onset of regular contractions to full dilation of the cervix. Initially the cervix softens, shortens and begins to dilate. As contractions become longer, stronger and closer together, dilation of the cervix continues. When fully dilated the cervix has stretched open to a diameter of 10 cm. At the same time the baby moves deep down into the pelvis. When the uterine muscle fibres contract, they do not relax to their original length but to the shortened position.

SECOND STAGE

The second stage of labour is the time from full dilation of the cervix until the birth of the baby. Some midwives do not consider that second stage begins until the urge to push is felt.

Many women find the urge to push irresistible, but some experience very little desire to push. As second stage progresses, the baby moves along the birth canal. The contractions are usually stronger, but may occur less frequently (see Chapter 17).

THIRD STAGE

The third stage of labour is from the birth of the baby until delivery of the placenta (or afterbirth). Once the baby is born, the cord is clamped and cut. The uterus continues to contract and this causes the placenta to disengage from the uterine wall. In Australia, the administration of intramuscular syntometrine or ergometrine at the time of delivery of the baby's shoulders is used to contract the uterus strongly and decrease the potential for post-partum haemorrhage. This action also tends to reduce the length of the third stage of labour (Chapter 17).

Once delivered, the placenta and membranes are examined to ensure that they are complete. At this time, the perineum is examined to check for any tear or graze. If an episiotomy has been performed, this will be repaired.

For some women, the placenta does not separate spontaneously. Gentle manoeuvres such as cord traction may be attempted. If these are unsuccessful, then manual removal of the placenta under anaesthetic is indicated.

Mechanics of labour

When the foetus reaches full growth at 40 weeks (38–42 week normal range), the pregnancy is said to be at term. In most pregnancies the head of the baby is the presenting part (cephalic or vertex presentation). In 4% of pregnancies, the baby is breech or bottom first, with legs crossed or extended or even foot first (footling breech). A very few mothers have a baby in transverse lie, with the baby lying across the uterus, which will necessitate caesarean delivery (Llewellyn-Jones, 1994).

CARDINAL MOVEMENTS

The position of the baby is described with respect to the baby's head in relation to the pelvis. When labour commences, the head of the foetus is usually left or right occiput transverse (LOT or ROT) or may be partly anterior (LOA or ROA) (Fig. 10.11)

Rotation and descent of the baby through the pelvis are described as the cardinal movements. These are described in detail in the caption to Figure 10.12. The sequence of cardinal movements is: engagement, descent, flexion, internal rotation, extension, external restitution of the head, expulsion.

The position of the mother in labour can assist the process of descent. By being upright in the first stage of labour, the abdominal wall is able to relax and gravity can assist the uterus to fall forward, directing the head into the pelvic inlet and applying pressure to the cervix (Liu, 1989). In second stage, squatting increases the pelvic diameter, with a 1 cm increase in transverse and 0.5–2 cm increase in antero-posterior diameters (Roberts, 1980).

For further reading see Chapters 17 and 18.

Figure 10.11 Positions of the foetal occiput during descent in second stage of labour.

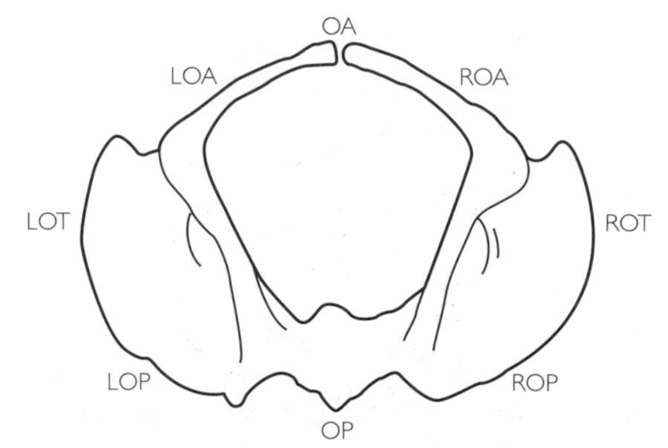

Figure 10.12 (Caption appears at foot of p. 105)

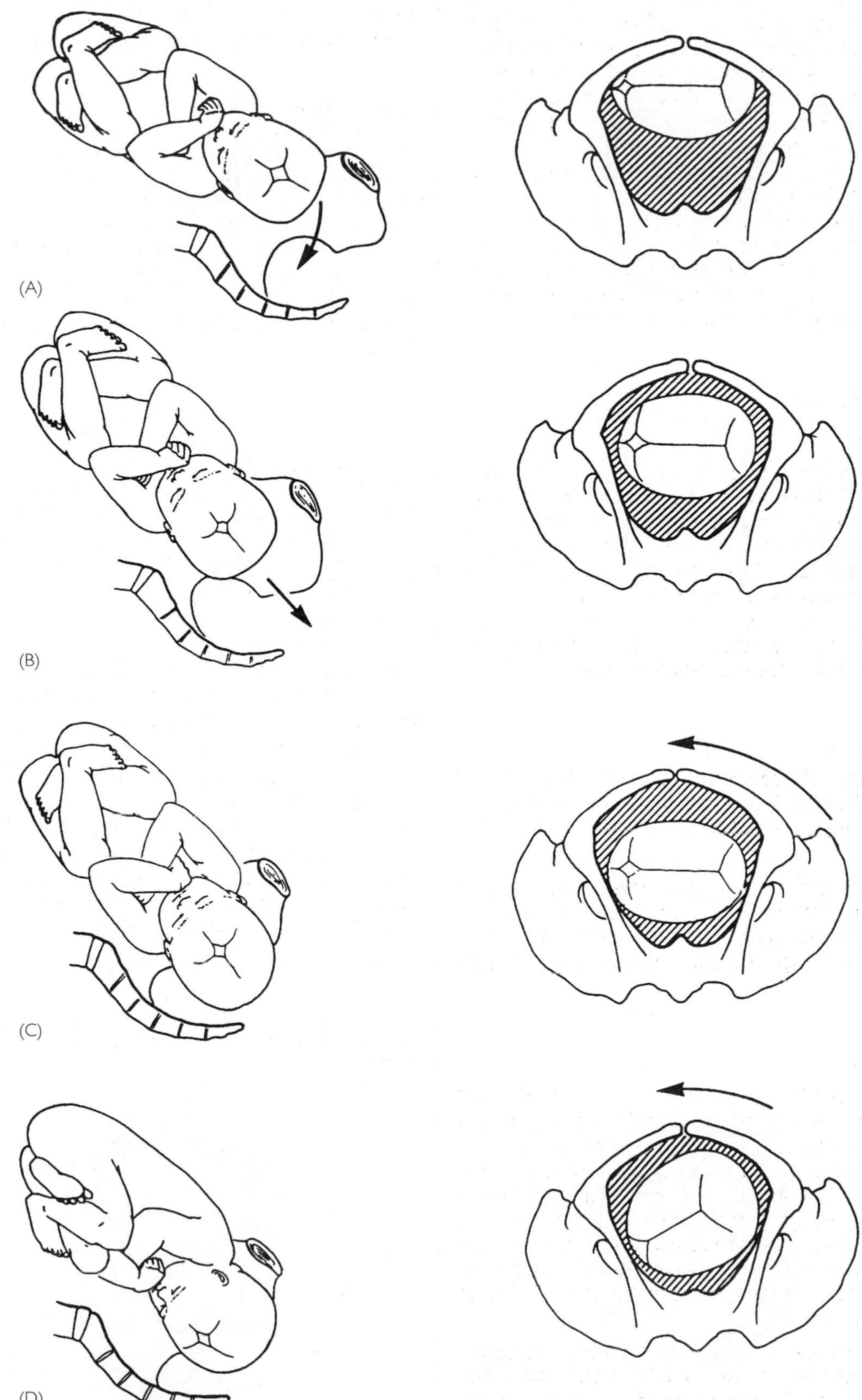

Figure 10.12 (Caption opposite)

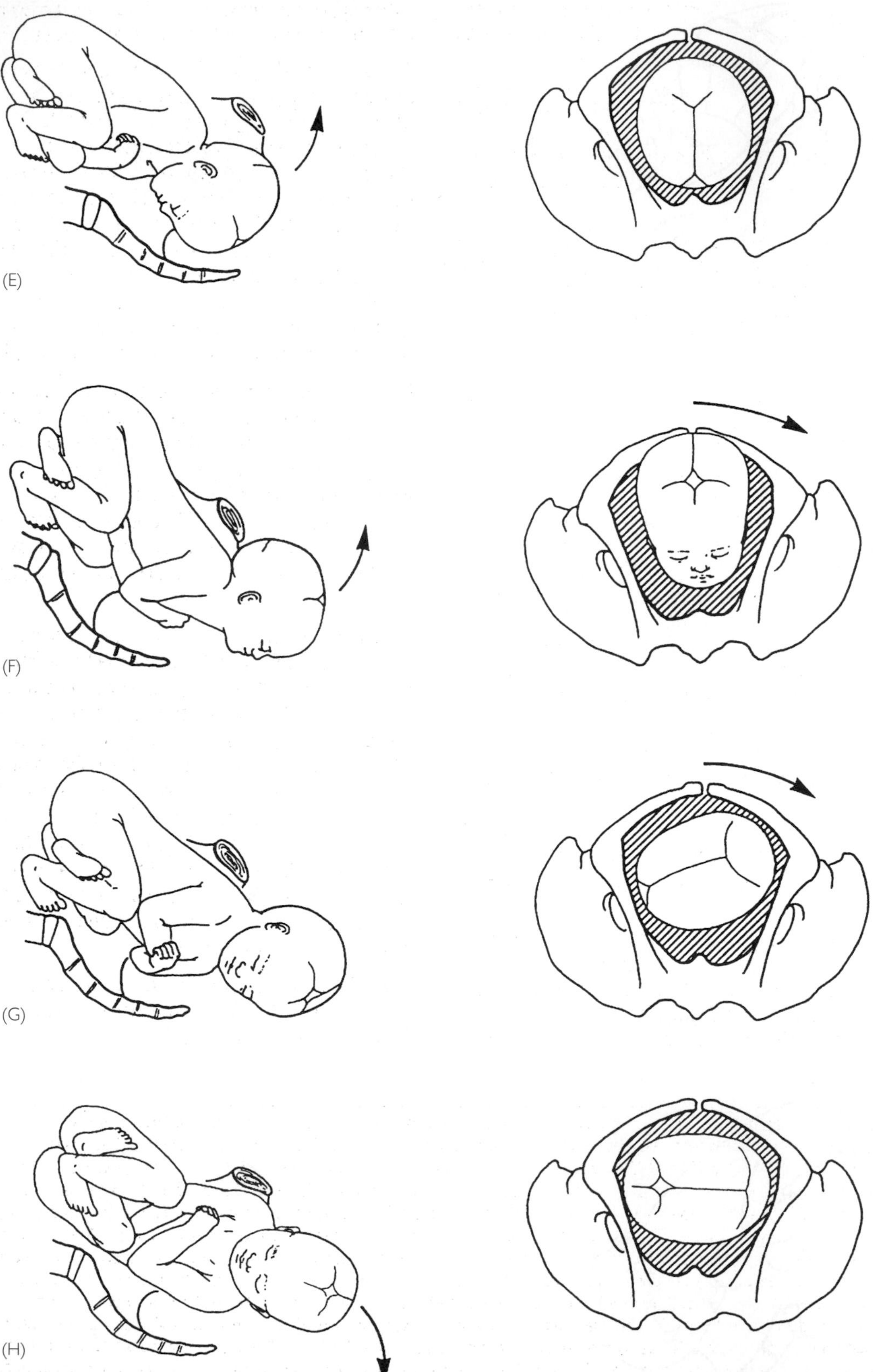

HOW LONG IS LABOUR?

Unfortunately it is impossible to know how long labour will take. Women who have had several children often comment that each labour is very different from the others. In general, giving birth to the first baby takes longer than giving birth to subsequent children. In first labours, the cervix effaces (flattens and shortens) before dilation begins. In subsequent labours, effacement and dilation occur concurrently (Beischer and Mackay, 1986). It is thought this may contribute to the shortened time for first stage in subsequent labours.

The average length of the first stage of labour with a first baby is from 12 to 14 hours, with second stage from 1/2 to two hours. Third stage of labour is approximately 1/2 hour. The total range therefore is between two and 36 hours.

Puerperium

By convention, the puerperium lasts for six weeks from the birth of the baby. During this time the physiological changes which occurred during pregnancy revert to the non-pregnant state. However, many changes take longer than six weeks. Physiotherapists are particularly interested in changes occurring during the first three months after the delivery, the so-called fourth trimester of the CBY, though a number of musculoskeletal conditions require much longer than this to return to normal.

The endocrinological changes which occurred during pregnancy revert rapidly. Hours after the birth of the baby and the delivery of the placenta, the levels of maternal hormones HPL and HCG fall rapidly and are undetectable in serum by two and 10 days respectively. Similarly, oestrogen and progesterone levels also fall rapidly, reaching non-pregnant levels by seven days after birth.

The cardiovascular system reverts to the non-pregnant state over two weeks. After the first 24 hours, the blood and plasma volumes begin to return to the non-pregnant state. For 10 days, the raised coagulation factors persist but are balanced by a rise in fibrinolytic activity.

The perineum may have been damaged during birth, either by an episiotomy or by a tear. The damage is repaired by suturing, but oedema of the tissues may have occurred and will persist for some days (refer to Chapter 19).

The uterus undergoes the most marked changes. After the delivery of the placenta, the uterus is approximately the size of a 20-week pregnancy and weighs 1000 g. It rapidly becomes smaller and by the end of the first week it weighs about 500 g and is tucked back into the pelvis. By six weeks post-partum it again approximates its pre-pregnant size and weight (50 g). Most women continue to bleed from the vagina for between two and six weeks after the birth as the uterine lining completely sheds. If the bleeding becomes significantly heavier than a period, offensive or accompanied by pain or fever, this may indicate an underlying infection and medical advice and treatment should be sought.

If the woman is not breast feeding, her periods are likely to return 6–8 weeks after the birth. If she continues to breast feed, they may take anything from two or three months to two years or even longer. Contraception may be needed as early as three weeks after the birth. A woman who is fully breast feeding is extremely unlikely to conceive within six weeks of delivery. However, as ovulation may occur before the first period, contraception will be required after this time.

A barrier method (condoms or diaphram) or a progesterone-only pill (sometimes termed the 'mini-pill') can be used while breast feeding. A contraceptive pill containing oestrogen will decrease the breast milk. In addition, during pregnancy there are changes in the clotting factors which increase the risk of thromboembolic complications. The oestrogen-containing contraceptive pill is therefore not recommended for any woman under four weeks post-partum. For women who have previously used the 'Billings method' for contraception, a warning that cervical mucus is affected during breast feeding and that additional methods are required should be given during their hospital stay.

For additional information on post-partum physiological changes, refer to Llewellyn-Jones (1994), de Swiet (1991) or Beischer and Mackay (1986).

Figure 10.12 Cardinal movements of the foetus during second stage of labour. The mechanism of delivery from the left occipitolateral position (LOT). This is an explanation of the steps or movements the foetus undergoes to negotiate the birth canal. Each step is illustrated by paired diagrams of the pelvis viewed laterally and of the head as palpated from below during vaginal examination. **A.** The head enters the pelvic brim with the posterior parietal bone presenting. Both fontanelles are shown at the same station as would be the case if flexion was incomplete. **B.** Lateral flexion of the head on the neck enables the head to descend and engagement has occurred. The head is now synclitic. **C.** Further lateral flexion allows descent of the head past the pubic symphysis; 90° internal (anterior) rotation of the occiput is required. **D.** The occiput has rotated 45° towards the front. The shoulders have rotated with the head which is not always the case. The sagittal suture lies in the right oblique diameter of the pelvis. **E.** Internal (anterior) rotation of the occiput is complete. Further descent has occurred. The sagittal suture lies in the anteroposterior diameter of the outlet. The head now begins to extend. **F.** Birth of the head is due to extension with the pubic symphysis acting as fulcrum; 45° restitution will now occur. **G.** Restitution of the head is due to the twist on the neck (due to internal rotation) being undone. Had the shoulders not rotated 45° with the head (see D, above), restitution would have been through 90°; 45° external rotation will now occur. **H.** External rotation of the head is due to internal (anterior) rotation of the shoulders. This movement does not occur if internal rotation of the head is unaccompanied by movement of the trunk as the shoulders are already in the anteroposterior diameter of the pelvis. Traction on the head directed posteriorly releases the anterior shoulder from beneath the pubic symphysis. (Reproduced from Beischer and Mackay (1986) with permission of NA Beischer.)

Lactation

It has been said by Ebrahim (1991) that 'For the first time mother there are three essentials for successful lactation: provision of information, building-up confidence and dealing efficiently with problems as they arise'. As physiotherapists, we can assist our obstetric patients with the first two requirements and refer appropriately for the third, if we have an understanding of the process and factors involved in lactation.

Physiology of the breast

The breast is made up of 15–20 lobes embedded in fat and fibrous tissue radiating from the nipple. These lobes drain towards the nipple through the excretory lactiferous ducts. Behind the nipple, they expand to form the lactiferous sinus. These lobes are separated by septa, through which blood vessels, nerves and lymphatics flow. The basic secretory or milk-producing units of the lobes are alveoli, small sacs off the alveolar ducts. Surrounding the alveoli are basket cells which are contractile and are responsible for ejection of the milk from the alveoli to the ducts.

From puberty to onset of first pregnancy, the breast has well-defined lobes but scanty alveoli development. The hormonal changes that occur early in the first pregnancy prompt a spectacular phase of growth and proliferation. Early in pregnancy, there is hyperplasia of ductor and secretory elements. Later in pregnancy, there is hyperplasia of alveoli and secretion begins. There is a decrease of supporting tissue, fat and fibrous connecting tissue (see Fig. 11.4).

Within 48 hours of birth, the alveolar epithelium changes and continuously increases its secretory activity. The alveoli become distended with milk and the contraction of 'basket' cells propels the milk into the ducts, lactiferous ducts and sinuses.

Lactational performance is related, physiologically, to endocrine, nutritional and psychological factors in the mother.

Endocrine factors associated with lactation

The process of getting milk to the baby from the breast has three stages:

1. Prolactin is secreted from the anterior pituitary glands and stimulates milk production in the alveoli.
2. When the baby suckles at the nipple, sensory receptors in the hypothalamus stimulate the post-pituitary to secrete oxytocin. Oxytocin stimulates the myoepithelial cells surrounding the alveoli to contract and force the milk along the ducts to the sinuses under the areola. This is called the 'let-down' or 'milk ejection' reflex. Milk may drip or spurt from the nipple when let-down occurs, whether or not the baby is attached. Let-down can be stimulated by the sight or sound of a baby (not necessarily one's own), as well as the baby's suckling. Oxytocin is also responsible for stimulation of uterine contractions in early post-partum. Many women, particularly multiparae, complain of painful uterine cramping and increased uterine blood flow during breast feeding in the first few days after the birth.
3. At the start of a feed, the baby suckles in a shallow rapid 'suck, suck' pattern. After let-down occurs, the sucking changes to a deeper 'suck, swallow' pattern. The continued stimulation at the nipple sends further messages to the hypothalamus and the cycle continues. In simple terms, the more the baby suckles, the more milk the mother makes. Supply = Demand (Phillips, 1991).

Nutritional factors associated with lactation

Breast milk is a living substance which constantly changes to meet the changing requirements of the baby. Colostrum (first milk) is formed as early as the 12th week of pregnancy and after the birth is available to the baby for the first 2–3 days. Colostrum, which is rich in protein (8.5%), contains immunoglobulins, fat-soluble vitamins and minerals and has a low lactose and fat content, thus providing all the baby's nutritional requirements. As the milk 'comes in', there is a period of transition where the baby receives a mixture of mature milk and colostrum. In this time, the fat content and calories increase and the protein decreases to around 1%.

Mature breast milk, which is produced from this time on, is bluish-white in appearance. It contains 88.3% water, 1% protein, 3.5% fats which are polyunsaturated, 7% carbo-

Figure 10.13 Positioning the baby for breast feeding. Milk ejection reflex: the baby suckles (a) and sensory impulses are transmitted to the spinal cord (b) then to the hypothalamus (c), there causing prolactin (d) and oxytocin (e) secretion simultaneously. Within 30–60 seconds milk begins to flow.

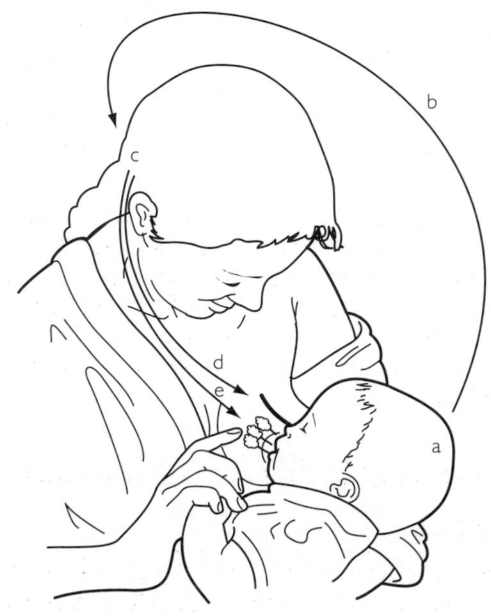

hydrate and 0.2% minerals. Sodium and calcium levels are stable in the milk, while iron levels are low but extremely bioavailable. The energy content of breast milk is 294 kJ 100 ml^{-1}. Over any 24-hour period, the proportion of water in breast milk alters to accommodate the baby's needs. In hot climates, the water content increases to prevent dehydration (Ebrahim, 1991; Minchin, 1985).

Psychological factors associated with lactation

The success or failure of breast feeding can depend on psychological factors. Mothers need to be encouraged and supported in their efforts to breast feed. Negative comments and attitudes, however unintentional, can be devastating for a new mother beginning to breast feed.

The emphasis on the health benefits of breast feeding should not be at the expense of the more social benefits. For some women, the information regarding decreased cost, father's ability to bottle feed expressed breast milk and easier night feeding may be the contributing factors in their decision to breast feed, rather than the perceived health benefit to the infant (Losch et al, 1995).

Minchin (1985) stated that:

> There are three essentials for successful lactation:
>
> 1. the parturient mother in whom physiologic mechanisms have caused the breasts to form milk;
> 2. the infant with his in-born reflexes which enable him to obtain milk, and
> 3. the immediate attendant of the mother, who can help to create the correct environment and act as a catalyst so that the physiologic processes in the mother and the baby can come together and operate in harmony.

Minchin states that the early days after the birth of the baby are crucial. Physiologically most mothers are able to secrete milk but success in lactation requires much more. It has been said that successful breast feeding is a learned skill, not an inherent one. Because of this, attention to details such as the correct way of holding the baby, the position of the mother during feeding, the protractility of the nipples, the baby's reactions and response to the feeding situation and so on are all important.

Primary contact for breast-feeding women is with the midwife. In the community setting, organizations such as Nursing Mothers Association of Australia and the La Leche League (UK, USA and NZ) provide an invaluable counselling role. In both settings, the physiotherapist working in women's health can provide valuable expertise and assistance.

Role of physiotherapy with lactating women

Physiotherapists require a knowledge and understanding of breast feeding. Their special clinical skills of teaching relaxation, posture correction and positioning can be of great benefit to the new mother.

RELAXATION

Relaxation techniques learned in ante-natal classes can be applied selectively whilst breast feeding to facilitate the let-down reflex, increase the mother's physical comfort and her emotional satisfaction with the process. A number of women will benefit from relaxation training post-partum. Reciprocal relaxation is particularly useful (Mitchell, 1988). Relaxation cassette tapes may be useful for both mother and baby at feed times, but warnings should be given against falling asleep if very relaxed.

POSTURE

The physiotherapist's knowledge of anatomy, combined with their understanding of the effects of body positioning, enables them to assist the mother into positions which support her back and avoid awkward postures. In sitting, a mother needs low back support; a pillow to support the baby and prevent tension in the mother's back, shoulders and neck; a foot stool to increase hip flexion, help maintain lumbar lordosis and maintain the baby's position; and often a special cushion that allows sitting without painful perineal pressure (see Chapter 19).

When lying, comfortable positioning is assisted by the use of pillows behind the back, between the knees and carefully positioned under the head ensuring that the shoulders are not elevated. With care, this can be a particularly comfortable position for women following delivery by caesarean section.

POSITION OF BABY

To enable effective attachment at the breast and to reduce the possibility of nipple damage, the baby needs to be positioned at breast height. Usually a pillow or two is required on the mother's lap to achieve this. A simple reminder is 'Chest to chest and chin to breast' (Nursing Mothers Association of Australia, 1993). The midwife will teach the mother to breast feed, but the physiotherapist's attention to posture and relaxation can make the task easier.

Benefits of breast feeding

The Australian National Health and Medical Research Council (NH&MRC, 1993) states:

> The promotion of breast feeding is a public health message. Support and encouragement at all levels of the community is essential to maintain and improve the rates and duration of breast feeding in Australian women, particularly those who are disadvantaged in any way. The inclusion of breast feeding in the dietary guidelines is aimed at contributing to the health of all Australians from birth.

The contribution breast feeding can make to the health of the population has been supported by research into the benefits, short- and long-term, of breast feeding. Some of the trials to date have looked at disease immunity, intelligence and otitis media.

Dewey et al (1995) found that breast-fed infants who fed for at least 12 months, when matched for variables to formula-fed infants, had a 50% reduction in diarrhoeal illness and 19% fewer episodes of otitis media, with reduced duration of episodes.

Pisacane et al (1994) suggest that breast feeding has a strong protective effect against acute lower respiratory infection. However, there does not seem to be any protection against pertussis type illness. In a longitudinal study from birth to nine years, Lanting et al (1994) found, after adjusting for variables, '. . a small advantageous effect of breast feeding on neurological status at nine years of age'. It is suggested that the longer chain polyunsaturated fatty acids in breast milk may have a role since they are vital for brain development.

Prospective and epidemiological studies have demonstrated the relationship between exclusive breast feeding for at least four months and a decrease in Crohn's disease, childhood cancers and childhood onset diabetes mellitus (Lawrence, 1995). Prospective studies have also shown a decrease in infant onset asthma, infantile eczema and rhinitis in the first two years of life in infants breast fed exclusively for at least six months and protected from other known family allergens, such as smoking.

Other studies which find protective effects against necrotizing enterocolitis (Buescher, 1994) and urinary tract infection (Wold and Hansen, 1994) add to the ever-increasing research establishing the importance of breast feeding in maintaining infant well-being.

Another area of research emerging in recent years is re-establishing the role of breast feeding as a contraceptive. Short (1994), Kennedy and Visness (1992) and Short et al (1991) all found reliable contraceptive protection in breast-feeding women. Kennedy and Visness found that pregnancy rates for breast-feeding mothers were 3% at six months if they remained amenorrhoeic. This rate of protection is similar to that of usual contraceptive methods used in the first year of parenthood.

Breast feeding alone is not a contraceptive long term. Once menses resumes, other methods of contraception are required. Women do become pregnant when breast feeding, as many can attest.

Problems can occur at any stage of lactation. Breast engorgement usually occurs in the first few days following birth. A blocked lactiferous duct can occur at any stage but is often precipitated by a physical cause such as tight bra or pressure. Mastitis, an inflammatory/infective process, tends to occur in the early post-partum period (first four weeks). Physiotherapy management has been used for these conditions (see Chapter 24).

Formula feeding

There are times when lactation does not succeed, despite the mother's and midwife's best efforts. Mothers who then formula feed their infants require sensitive support and encouragement. Principles such as those discussed for position of the mother and baby still apply and every effort should be made to make the mother as comfortable as possible, physically and emotionally. Relaxation can be invaluable for the mother at this time, as she may be very upset when feeding has not gone as anticipated.

Working and breast feeding

Working and breast feeding are not mutually exclusive. Many women choose to combine a career outside the home with breast feeding their baby. Facilities for expressing and storing breast milk or having the baby brought to the workplace for feeds are recent initiatives. All mothers working outside the home deserve full support from family and the workplace, regardless of their choice of feeding methods.

WHO/UNICEF Breastfeeding in the 1990s

In July 1990, WHO/UNICEF produced and adopted a policy document on infant feeding in the 1990s. The document, the Innocenti Declaration, states in part:

> As a global goal for optimal maternal and child health and nutrition, all women should be enabled to practise exclusive breast feeding and all infants should be fed exclusively on breast milk from birth to four to six months of age. Thereafter, children should continue to be breast fed, while receiving appropriate and adequate complementary foods, for up to two years of age or beyond.

In its document *Healthy People 2000* (Dept of Health and Human Services, 1990), the declared aim of the Australian government is to have 80% of infants breast fed at three months of age by the year 2000.

As health professionals promoting primary health care, physiotherapists can play an active role in helping mothers achieve the goals set by WHO/UNICEF (1990) and national governments.

References

Baron TH, Ramirez B and Richter JE (1993) Gastrointestinal motility disorders during pregnancy. *American College of Physicians* **118**(5): 366–375.

Bashiri A, Neumann L, Maymon E and Katz M (1995) Hyperemesis gravidarum: epidemiologic features, complications and outcome. *European Journal of Obstetrics and Gynecology and Reproductive Biology* **63**: 135–138.

Beischer NA and Mackay EV (1986) *Obstetrics and the Newborn: An Illustrated Textbook*, 2nd edn. Sydney: W.B. Saunders.

Beischer NA, Mackay EV and Purcal NK (1989) *Care of the Pregnant Woman and Her Baby*, 2nd edn. Sydney: W.B. Saunders / Baillière Tindall.

Billings E and Westmore A (1980) *The Billings Method: Controlling Fertility without Drugs or Devices*. Richmond, Victoria, Australia: A. O'Donovan.

Billings EL, Billings JL and Catarinich M (1989) *Billings Atlas of the Ovulation Method: the Mucus Patterns of Fertility and Infertility*. Melbourne: Ovulation Method Research and Reference Centre of Australia.

Boston Women's Health Book Collective (1973) *Our Bodies, Ourselves: A Book By and For Women*. New York: Simon and Schuster.

Bower C and Stanley FJ (1989) Dietary folate as a risk factor for neural tube defects: evidence from a case-control study in Western Australia. *Medical Journal of Australia* **150**: 613.

Buescher ES (1994) Host defense mechanisms of human milk and their relations to enteric infections and necrotizing enterocolitis. *Clinical Perinatology* **21**: 247–262.

Burton GJ, Palmer ME and Dalton KJ (1989) Morphometric differences between the placental vasculature of non-smokers, smokers and ex-smokers. *British Journal of Obstetrics and Gynaecology* **96**: 907–915.

Center for Disease Control (1991) Use of folic acid for prevention of spina bifida and other neural tube defects 1983–1991. *Mortality and Morbidity Weekly Reports* **40**: 513.

Cliver SP, Goldenberg RL, Cutter GR et al (1992) The relationships among psychosocial profile, maternal size, and smoking in predicting fetal growth retardation. *Obstetrics and Gynecology* **80**(2): 262–267.

Cnattingius S (1992) Smoking during pregnancy. Pregnancy risks and sociodemographic characteristics among pregnant smokers. *International Journal of Technology Assessment in Health Care* **8(Suppl 1)**: 91–95.

De Aloysio D and Penacchioni P (1992) Morning sickness control in early pregnancy by Neiguan point pressure. *Obstetrics and Gynecology* **80**: 852–854.

Department of Health and Human Services (1990) *Healthy People 2000*. National Health Promotion and Disease Prevention Objectives. Conference Edition Sept 1990. in NH&MRC, Dietary Guidelines for Australians 1993.

De Swiet M (1991) The Cardiovascular System. In Hytten F and Chamberlain G (eds) *Clinical Physiology in Obstetrics*, 2nd edn, pp. 3–38. Oxford: Blackwell Scientific Publications.

Dewey KG, Heinig MJ and Nommsen-Rivers LA (1995) Differences in morbidity between breastfed and formula fed infants. *Journal of Pediatrics* **126**: 696–701.

Ebrahim GJ (1991) *Breastfeeding: The Biological Option*, 2nd edn, p. v, pp. 49–87. London: Macmillan Press.

Enkin M, Keirse MJNC and Chalmers I (1989) *A Guide to Effective Care in Pregnancy and Childbirth*. Oxford: Oxford University Press.

Enkin M, Keirse MJNC, Renfrew M and Neilson J (1995) *A Guide to Effective Care in Pregnancy and Childbirth*. 2nd edn. Oxford: Oxford University Press.

Evans AT, Samuels SN, Marshall C and Bertolucci LE (1993) Suppression of pregnancy-induced nausea and vomiting with sensory afferent stimulation. *Journal of Reproductive Medicine* **38**: 603–606.

Fisher M (ed) (1989) *Guide to Clinical Preventive Services: A Report of the US Preventive Services Task Force*. Baltimore: Williams and Wilkins.

Gadsby R, Barnie-Adshead AM and Jagger C (1993) A prospective study of nausea and vomiting during pregnancy. *British Journal of General Practice* **43**: 245–248.

Godfrey K, Robinson S, Barker C et al (1996) Maternal nutrition in early and late pregnancy in relation to placental and fetal growth. *British Medical Journal* **312**: 410–414.

Goldenberg RL, Tsunenobu T, Neggers Y et al (1995) The effect of zinc supplementation on pregnancy outcome. *Journal of the American Medical Association* **274**(6): 463–468.

Kahn J (1988) Electrical modalities in obstetrics and gynecology. In: Wilder E (ed) (1988) *Obstetric and Gynecologic Physical Therapy*, pp. 113–129. New York: Churchill Livingstone.

Kennedy KI and Visness CM (1992) Contraceptive efficacy of lactational amenorrhoea. *Lancet* **339**: 227–230.

Kirschbaum BB and Schoolwerth AC (1989) Acute aluminium toxicity associated with oral citrate and aluminium-containing antacids. *American Journal of the Medical Sciences* **297**(1): 9–11.

Ladwig P, Coles R, Fischer E and Spurrett B (1995) Thyrotoxicosis in pregnancy presenting as pancytopenia. *Australian and New Zealand Journal of Obstetrics and Gynaecology* **35**: 457–460.

Lanting CI, Fidler V, Huisman M et al (1994) Neurological differences between 9 year old children fed breastmilk or formula milk as babies. *Lancet* **344**: 1319–1322.

Lawrence R (1995) The clinician's role in teaching proper infant feeding techniques. *Journal of Paediatrics* **126**: S112-S117.

Lewis TLT and Chamberlain GVP (eds) (1995) *Gynaecology by Ten Teachers*, 16th edn. London: Edward Arnold.

Liu YC (1989) Cited in: Blackburn ST and Loper DL (1992) *Maternal, Fetal and Neonatal Physiology: A Clinical Perspective*, pp. 109–135. Philadelphia: W.B. Saunders.

Llewellyn-Jones D (1994) *Fundamentals of Obstetrics and Gynaecology*, 6th edn. Sydney: C.V. Mosby.

Losch M, Dungy CI, Russell D and Dusdieker LB (1995) Impact of attitudes on maternal decisions regarding infant feeding. *Journal of Paediatrics* **126**: 507–514.

Luke B (1994) Nutritional influences on fetal growth. *Clinical Obstetrics and Gynecology* **37**(3): 538–549.

MacArthur C and Knox EG (1988) Smoking in pregnancy – effects of stopping at different stages. *British Journal of Obstetrics and Gynaecology* **95**: 551–555.

Marshall K (1981) Pain relief in labour: the role of the physiotherapist. *Physiotherapy* **67**(1): 8–11.

Marshall K and Walsh DM (1994) Health of mother and child: striking the balance. *Physiotherapy* **80**(11): 767–768.

McMillan CM (1994) Transcutaneous electrical stimulation of Neiguan anti-emetic acupuncture point in controlling sickness following opioid analgesia in major orthopaedic surgery. *Physiotherapy* **80**(1): 5–9.

Mills JL, Tuomilechto J, Yu KF et al (1992) Maternal vitamin levels during pregnancies producing infants with neural tube defects. *Journal of Pediatrics* **120**: 863.

Minchin M (1985) *Breastfeeding Matters: What We Need to Know about Infant Feeding*. Sydney: Alma Publications / George Allen and Unwin.

Mitchell L (1988) Simple Relaxation: *The Mitchell Method of Physiological Relaxation for Easing Tension*, 2nd edn. London: John Murray.

Monteagudo FSE, Cassidy MJD and Folb PI (1989) Recent developments in aluminium toxicity. *Medical Toxicology* **4**: 1–16.

MRC Vitamin Study Research Group (1991) Prevention of neural tube defects: results of the Medical Research Council Vitamin Study. *Lancet* **338**: 131.

NH&MRC (1993) *Dietary Guidelines for Australians*, pp. 1–110. Canberra: Australian Government Publishing Service.

Nelson-Perry C (1995) 27th British Obstetrics and Gynaecology Conference, Dublin.

Niebyl JR (1995) Folic acid supplementation to prevent birth defects. *Contemporary Obstetrics and Gynecology* **40**(6): 43–50.

Noble E (1976) *Essential Exercises for the Childbearing Year. A Guide to Health and Comfort Before and After the Birth of Your Baby.* London: John Murray.

Nursing Mothers Association of Australia (1993) *Hospital Resources Booklet*. Nunawading: Nursing Mothers Association of Australia.

Olsen J (1992) Cigarette smoking in pregnancy and fetal growth. Does the type of tobacco play a role? *International Journal of Epidemiology* **21**(2): 279–284.

Phillips V (1991) *Successful Breastfeeding*, 2nd edn. Nunawading: Nursing Mothers Association of Australia.

Pisacane A, Graziano L, Zona G et al (1994). Breastfeeding and acute lower respiratory infection. *Acta Paediatrica* **83**: 714–718.

Roberts J (1980) Cited in: Blackburn ST and Loper DL (1992) *Maternal, Fetal and Neonatal Physiology: A Clinical Perspective*, pp. 109–135. Philadelphia: W.B. Saunders.

Roquer JM, Figueras J, Botet F and Jimenez R (1995) Influence on fetal growth of exposure to tobacco smoke during pregnancy. *Acta Paediatrica* **84** (2): 118–121.

Rush D (1994) Periconceptual folate and neural tube defect. *American Journal of Clinical Nutrition* **59** (Suppl): 511.

Short RV (1994) What the breast does for the baby, and what the baby does for the breast. *Australian and New Zealand Journal of Obstetrics and Gynaecology* **34**: 262–264.

Short RV, Lewis PR, Renfree MB and Shaw G (1991) Contraceptive effects of extended lactational amenorrhoea: beyond the Bellagio Consensus. *Lancet* **337**: 715–717.

Simons J (1987) *Pregnant and in Perfect Shape – Exercising During Pregnancy and After.* Melbourne: Nelson Publishers.

WHO/UNICEF (1990) The Innocenti Declaration. Cited in: *Hospital Resources Booklet* (1993) p. 4. Nunawading: Nursing Mothers Association of Australia.

Winship KA (1992) Toxicity of aluminium. *Adverse Drug Reactions and Toxicological Review* **11**(2): 126–141.

Winship KA (1993) Toxicity of aluminium. *Adverse Drug Reactions and Toxicological Review* **12**(3): 183–184.

Wold AE and Hansen LA (1994) Defence factors in human milk. *Current Opinions in Gastroenterology* **10**: 652–658.

Yates JRW, Ferguson-Smith MA, Shenkin A et al (1987) Is disordered folate metabolism the basis for the genetic predisposition to neural tube defects? *Clinical Genetics* **31**: 279.

Further Reading

Beischer NA, Mackay EV and Purcal NK (1989) *Care of the Pregnant Woman and Her Baby*, 2nd edn. Sydney: W.B. Saunders/Baillière Tindall.

Chalmers I, Enkin M and Keirse MJNC (1989) *Effective Care in Pregnancy and Childbirth. Volume 1: Pregnancy.* Oxford: Oxford University Press.

Chalmers I, Enkin M and Keirse MJNC (1989) *Effective Care in Pregnancy and Childbirth Volume 2: Childbirth.* Oxford: Oxford University Press.

Hytten F and Chamberlain G (eds) (1991) *Clinical Physiology in Obstetrics*, 2nd edn. Oxford: Blackwell Scientific Publications.

Llewellyn-Jones D (1994) *Fundamentals of Obstetrics and Gynaecology*, 6th edn. Sydney: C.V. Mosby.

Queenan JT (ed) (1994) *The Management of High Risk Pregnancy*, 3rd edn. Boston: Blackwell Scientific Publications.

Appendix

Pregnancy Tests and Investigations

Urine tests

- Pregnancy test – the diagnostic tests depend on the detection of a hormone, human chorionic gonadotropin (HCG) in the urine. The level of HCG reaches its highest point in normal pregnancy between eight and 12 weeks. Abnormally high levels occur with multiple pregnancy and with hydatidiform mole and choriocarcinoma (Lewis and Chamberlain, 1995). HCG is found in its most concentrated form in the first urine passed in the early morning. The tests are highly reliable but a false-negative test may occur if the test is performed too early (before six weeks from the last menstrual period) or too late (after 16 weeks from the last menstrual period) in the pregnancy.
- Routine testing – on each ante-natal visit to the doctor or clinic the urine is examined to exclude the presence of sugar, protein and ketones, which may indicate potential problems with the pregnancy.
- Mid-stream urine test is an examination of urine to exclude presence of asymptomatic bacteriuria. A proportion of women in early pregnancy have significant bacteriuria and require antibiotics to prevent development of further problems.

Routine blood tests

- Haemoglobin estimation, used to detect anaemia.
- Blood group and rhesus factor, to ensure access to cross-matched blood in the event of haemorrhage during pregnancy, labour or the puerperium. Also used to identify rhesus incompatability between mother and infant blood types.
- Serological tests for syphilis or other venereal infection (VDRL), to allow identification and adequate treatment of mother and baby.
- Rubella antibodies are tested to ascertain if the woman is immune or susceptible. If she is susceptible and rubella is contracted in early pregnancy, this can result in foetal abnormalities (deafness, cataract, heart defects). If the woman is susceptible, vaccination is usually offered after the birth of the baby.

Specific blood tests

- Haemoglobin electrophoresis to detect conditions such as sickle cell disease and thalassaemia in negroid or Mediterranean women.
- Serum alpha-fetoproteins to detect open neural tube defects such as spina bifida or anencephaly.
- Hepatitis (A, B, C) screening to detect presence of hepatitis and avoid infection of health-care workers during blood taking or delivery.
- HIV/AIDS screening to detect presence of HIV/AIDS and avoid infection of health-care workers during blood taking or delivery.
- Glucose tolerance test to measure the woman's ability to stabilize blood sugar levels after ingestion of glucose. A random finding of glucose in the urine is common in pregnancy (see Chapter 11). This test may be used to exclude diabetes mellitus in pregnancy where there is a close family history of diabetes, marked obesity, any history of a previous baby weighing over 4.5 kg or unexplained stillbirth. The test begins with a fasting blood sugar and urine specimen. The woman takes glucose by mouth, then blood and urine samples are collected at half-hourly intervals for two hours.

Ultrasound

Diagnostic ultrasound is commonly used in obstetrics for the identification of early pregnancy, accurate pregnancy dating, assessment of foetal growth, early diagnosis of multiple pregnancy, estimation of foetal health, diagnosis of certain congenital abnormalities, localization of the placental site and as an adjunct to other tests such as amniocentesis.

X-rays

Since the availability of ultrasound, the use of X-rays during pregnancy has reduced to almost nil, because of the potential radiation hazard to the baby.

Amniocentesis

Amniotic fluid is withdrawn from the uterus for analysis. Indications for use include detection of some foetal abnormalities such as Down syndrome and open neural tube defects, identification of sex in sex-linked disorders such as haemophilia and Duchenne muscular dystrophy and identification of biochemical disorders. This procedure is usually performed at 16–18 weeks of pregnancy. Risks of complications, in the order of 1–2%, include abortion, preterm labour and limb deformities. Results usually take 3–4 weeks, which means the pregnancy is well advanced before the results are known.

Chorionic villus sampling

This test is also used for foetal abnormality, usually between nine and 12 weeks of pregnancy. Guided by ultrasound, a small tissue sample is taken from the edge of the placenta (the chorion) and tested to exclude abnormalities such as Down syndrome, spina bifida, sex-linked disease or chromosomal abnormalities. Risks of complications such as miscarriage, in the order of 2–5%, have to be balanced against the fact that testing is conducted earlier in the pregnancy and that results are available within three days.

Oestriol tests

Assessment of the amounts of oestriol or human placental lactogen (HPL) gives an indication of the functioning of the placenta. For oestriol tests, blood tests are conducted three times over five days to determine if the oestriol level is stable or falling. For the HPL test, blood samples on two consecutive days are assessed and give a faster result. However, they are rarely used now as they have been superseded by ultrasound.

Foetal movement recording (kick chart)

One sign of a healthy baby is vigorous movement. The pregnant woman may be asked to record the time it takes for the foetus to move 10 times (any time from a few minutes to 12 hours). Low movement counts indicate a need for closer foetal monitoring.

Antenatal cardiotocography (CTG)

Foetal heart rate traces can be recorded using a cardiotocograph. A normal trace shows a foetal heart rate of between 100–160 beats per minute. Abnormalities may give warning that the foetus is in jeopardy and should be delivered. Indications include low movement count, evidence of placental insufficiency, antenatal bleeding, following amniocentesis or in cases of multiple pregnancy.

11

Pregnancy and the Puerperium: Physiological Changes

ROBYN SHARPE

Cardiovascular System
•
Respiratory System
•
Immune System
•
Digestive System
•
Weight Gain in Pregnancy
•
Urinary System
•
Skin
•
Breasts
•
Endocrine System
•
Musculoskeletal Changes Associated with Pregnancy
•
Reproductive System
•
Nervous System
•
Puerperium

The woman who understands the changes occurring in her body during pregnancy will be able to co-operate more fully with her health-care team, gain more benefit from their care and participate in her own management. Physiotherapists dealing with these women must be aware of the multitude of endocrine and physiological changes which are involved in the formation of an optimal foetal environment.

Cardiovascular System

The cardiovascular system undergoes great changes during pregnancy. Overall, there is an increase in cardiac output, increased oxygen consumption, decreased peripheral resistance and a rapid throbbing pulse. Some of these changes, such as breathlessness, a racing heart and warm hands, will be noticed by the pregnant woman and the physiotherapist treating her and may require modification of any treatment being given.

Cardiac output

Changes in cardiac output (stroke volume × heart rate) include:

- 40% increase in the first trimester, persisting throughout pregnancy;
- stroke volume increasing by 30%;
- heart rate increasing by 15 beats per minute.

The increased output is directed to the uterus, kidneys and, it is thought, the gastrointestinal tract. Blood flow in the uterus increases during pregnancy to approximately 500 ml min^{-1} at term (Beischer and Mackay, 1986; de Swiet, 1991; Robson et al, 1987).

Blood pressure

There is little change in arterial blood pressure or systolic pressure during pregnancy. Diastolic pressure decreases slightly in mid-pregnancy, returning to normal levels in late pregnancy. Normal values for blood pressure in pregnancy are less than 140/90. Pregnancy-induced hypertension (PIH) is diagnosed when systolic pressure increases by more than 30 mmHg or diastolic increases by more than 15 mmHg (Blackburn and Loper, 1992). Ferguson et al (1994) have developed normalcy curves for blood pressure in pregnancy which allow for variation throughout the duration of the pregnancy.

Supine hypotension

When the pregnant woman lies supine the cardiac output is decreased because of uterine compression of the inferior vena cava. This is known as supine hypotension (Fig. 11.1). Arterial blood pressure is lower than in the sitting position and symptoms can range from minimal central cardiovascular alteration to severe syncopal shock. Moving the woman into a side-lying position usually gives symptomatic relief (Kinsella and Lohmann, 1994). This is an important consideration for the physiotherapist treating pregnant women. Treatment positions may need to be modified to avoid unnecessary discomfort for the patient.

Venous blood pressure

There is little alteration of venous blood pressure during pregnancy. It may rise in the lower limbs due to hydrostatic and mechanical pressures in the pelvis. When standing, this rise may result in lower limb oedema, varicosities and distension in the veins. Central venous pressure is usually unaltered but may decrease in late pregnancy when the woman is supine (de Swiet, 1991; Gaudin et al, 1989).

Peripheral resistance

A 20% decrease occurs as a result of a basically unaltered blood pressure and an increased cardiac output. Blood flow increases, especially to the hands and feet, causing sensations of warmth and a partial immunity to cold.

Figure 11.1 Postural (supine) hypotension syndrome. Transverse section of the abdomen in late pregnancy illustrating that the pressure of the uterus and contents is most likely to compress the inferior vena cava when the patient is on her back. Cardiac output increases 10% when the patient turns to the right lateral position and 20% when turning to the left lateral position, the preferred position for rest in pregnancy. (Reproduced from Beischer and Mackay (1986) with permission of NA Beischer.)

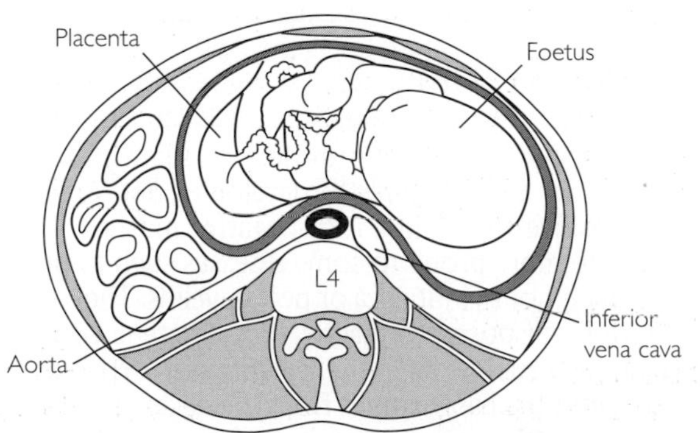

Peripheral vasodilatation

It is thought that this occurs because progesterone reduces the effects of angiotensin in the blood, making the pregnant woman more reliant on sympathetic nervous control to maintain tone in the blood vessels. Women with Raynaud's disease may experience relief from this painful condition during pregnancy because of the vasodilatation occurring. Nasal mucous membranes are congested, which may result in epistaxis (nose bleed), palmar erythema, vascular spiders and haemangioma may occur on the skin (de Swiet, 1991; Beischer et al, 1989).

Blood volume

Plasma volume increases by 50% while red cell mass increases by 20–30%, resulting in a total blood volume increase of 40%, from 4.0 litres to 5.5 litres. The effective haemodilution is known as *physiological anaemia*. The blood is able to circulate more freely and promotes better heat exchange from the dilated blood vessels in the skin. The increase in blood volume allows the woman to withstand the average blood loss at delivery of 500 ml without adverse effects (Beischer and Mackay, 1986).

Heart

The elevated diaphragm in pregnancy raises and rotates the heart so that the apex is more lateral and higher than usual. This may cause a false impression of enlargement. Electrocardiograph (ECG) changes may occur which mimic ischaemic heart disease. There is an increased tendency to supraventricular tachycardia, atrial or ventricular systoles and rhythm disturbances (Gaudin et al, 1989).

Myocardial contractility

This increases throughout pregnancy due to lengthening of the muscle fibres, causing mild ventricular hypertrophy. Increased blood volume and venous return results in an increased diameter of the left atrium.

Cardiovascular changes at delivery and puerperium

Blood pressure and cardiac output both increase during labour. Initially, after delivery, the cardiac output increases. It then decreases shortly after and returns to normal levels by two weeks post-partum. It is during these two weeks that the majority of cardiovascular parameters change the most. Only mild ventricular hypertrophy remains by five months after the birth (Duvekot and Peeters, 1994).

Plasma volume gradually decreases following delivery, mainly by diuresis (urination), and the red cell mass is slowly reduced so that blood volume is restored to pre-pregnant levels (Letsky, 1991). Blood loss at parturition is greatest in the first hour. Only 80 ml of blood is passed in the lochia in the next 72 hours. A healthy woman may lose up to 1000 ml at delivery without incurring a significant decrease in haemoglobin. If the woman has had an episiotomy, tear or uterine atony, the blood loss may be greater. During the six weeks post-partum, the haematological system returns to pre-pregnant status (Llewellyn-Jones, 1994).

Folate deficiency, if untreated during the pregnancy, may become clinically significant after delivery, especially in lactating women. Megaloblastic anaemia is a result of continuing folate deficiency (Letsky, 1991).

Respiratory System

The respiratory system is not as stressed as the cardiovascular system by pregnancy. Pregnant women frequently notice shortness of breath, due in part to increased congestion in lung capillaries, as well as increased respiratory centre sensitivity.

Patients with respiratory disease tend not to deteriorate as much as those with cardiac problems. Various studies have shown asthma to improve, worsen or remain unchanged during pregnancy. Fortunately, severe asthma is rare during labour and delivery (Blackburn and Loper, 1992; de Swiet, 1991). Other studies have shown that steroid-dependent asthmatic women have an increased risk of pre-term and low birth-weight babies (Clark, 1993; Kelly et al, 1995; Perlow et al, 1992). Reducing known risks (smoking, recreational drugs, dust and other triggers) during pregnancy helps to lesson the impact of asthma on the pregnant woman (Greenberger, 1992).

Information on gas exchange, particularly oxygen consumption, remains contradictory. However, it appears that there is an increase in basal oxygen consumption of 30–40 ml min^{-1}. This increase in oxygen consumption, combined with a 40% increase in minute ventilation, causes hyperventilation in pregnancy, especially when the increased effectiveness of breathing by the diaphragm is taken into account.

Functionally, the pregnant woman at rest tends to increase her ventilation by breathing more deeply. Alveolar ventilation is increased by up to 50%, despite dilated bronchioles, increasing the physiological dead space. During pregnancy the subcostal angle increases from 68° in early pregnancy to 103° in late pregnancy (Fig. 11.2)

During pregnancy breathing is more diaphragmatic than costal, with the diaphragm rising by 4 cm and the chest diameter increasing by 2 cm. There is also greater travel of the diaphragm during inspiration (Mobius, 1961; Thomson and Cohen, 1938). Table 11.1 illustrates a summary of changes in the respiratory system.

Figure 11.2 The rib cage in pregnancy (black) and non-pregnant (stippled), showing the increased subcostal angle, the increased transverse diameter and the raised diaphragm.

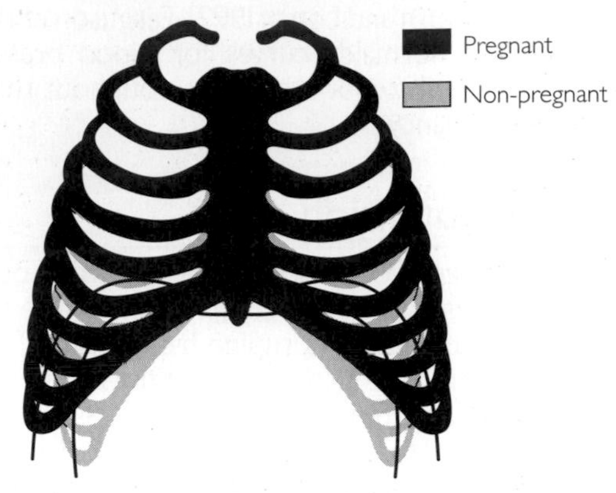

Table 11.1 Respiratory changes in pregnancy (from Blackburn and Loper, 1992; de Swiet, 1991)

Parameter	Non-pregnant state	Pregnant state
Vital capacity	3200 ml	3200 ml
Tidal volume	450 ml	600 ml
Residual volume	1000 ml	800 ml
Inspiratory capacity	2500 ml	2650 ml
Expiratory reserve	700 ml	550 ml
Functional residual capacity	1700 ml	1350 ml
Total lung volume	4200 ml	4000 ml
P_{O_2}	85 mmHg	92 mmHg
P_{CO_2}	35 mmHg	30 mmHg
pH	7.4	7.4
Oxygen consumption		Increased by 20%
CO_2 tension		Decreased
Diaphragm		Raised by 40 mm
Chest diameter		Increased by 20 mm
Respiratory rate		Unchanged
Subcostal angle	68°	103°

Immune System

In pregnancy, the immune system is slightly depressed generally but is still capable of developing antibodies from an Rh-positive foetus in an Rh-negative mother. Pregnant women are more prone to some diseases such as pneumococcal pneumonia, influenza or poliomyelitis. They may also be more predisposed to reactivation of latent viruses, e.g. cytomegalovirus (CMV) or herpes (Stirrat, 1991). Protection of the foetus probably comes from the decidua and trophoblast and not the uterus as a whole (Stirrat, 1991).

The baby is protected against transplacental and post-natal infections by passive antibodies from six weeks of pregnancy to nine months of age. As a foetus, the baby receives immunoglobulin-G (IgG) by placental transfer, gaining passive immunity. Of the four immunoglobulins produced by the mother, IgG is the only one which crosses the placenta (Stirrat, 1991). Active transfer continues from six weeks to 22 weeks at a slow, steady rate. Around 22 weeks there is a rapid increase so that by 26 weeks gestation, maternal and foetal concentrations of IgG are equal. Maternal IgG is maintained in the baby's circulation until it disappears around nine months post-partum (Beischer et al, 1989).

Digestive System

'Morning sickness', nausea and/or vomiting occur most commonly in early pregnancy but may occur throughout pregnancy for some women. The term 'morning' is inaccurate as the nausea may occur at any time of day or night or, indeed, all day. Excessive vomiting in pregnancy (hyperemesis gravidarum) affects a small percentage of women and may necessitate hospital admission in the first trimester. It is thought that human chorionic gonadotropin (HCG), which rises in early pregnancy, may trigger nausea. Odours and certain foods are other causes of nausea in some women. Appetite increases in early pregnancy and may persist throughout the pregnancy. The upward pressure of the uterus on the stomach reduces the capacity for large amounts of food in late pregnancy, which may be compensated for by snacking more frequently on smaller amounts of food.

Occasionally pregnant women report abnormal cravings for substances such as coal or chalk (*pica*). More common are cravings for foods which are salted and spiced rather than sweet. This was thought to be due to a dulling of taste sense during pregnancy but a trial comparing pregnant and non-pregnant women found that all taste thresholds were raised in pregnancy, i.e. sweet, sour, salt and bitter. Increased thirst is also noted throughout pregnancy. The effects of pregnancy on the alimentary canal are listed in Table 11.2.

Weight Gain in Pregnancy

Weight gain in the first 20 weeks of pregnancy is small (0–2 kg). It then increases to 1.0 kg per month to 30 weeks, further increasing to 1.0 kg per fortnight between 30 and 40 weeks (Beischer et al, 1989), (Fig. 11.3). Some women gain much less (<5 kg) and others much more (>20 kg). The Institute of Medicine (1990) conducted a National (US) Natality Survey which indicated that the continuing rise in maternal weight gain over the past 30 years has corresponded with an increase in mean foetal weight. This has resulted in new guidelines for maternal weight gain, dependent on the pre-pregnant weight and body mass index (BMI) of the mother, as outlined in the box below.

Table 11.2 Effect of pregnancy on alimentary canal (from Baron et al, 1993)

Anatomy	Effect
Mouth	Gingival oedema → tendency to gum bleed Teeth – no demineralization. Increase in cavities, particularly 5–7 months. Saliva – 1–2 l day^{-1} secreted. No increase in normal amount. May appear to be more due to difficulty swallowing saliva
Oesophagus	Decreased competence of lower oesophageal sphincter → heartburn Decreased sphincter response to hormonal and physiological stimuli Decreased sphincter response to increased abdominal pressure
Stomach	Decreased gastric secretions. Decreased motility → slower emptying times. Progesterone → decreased tone → nausea
Small intestine	Increased functional efficiency. Increased transit time → increased absorption time
Large intestine	Progesterone → increased relaxation of smooth muscle → constipation Increased water absorption in colon → constipation
Gall bladder	Increased bile concentration → increased risk of gall stone formation Size of gall bladder increases progressively over pregnancy

BMI <19.8	30–40 lb (13.5–18 kg)
BMI > 19.8–26.0	25–35 lb (12.0–16 kg)
BMI >26.0	15–20 lb (6.5–9 kg)

As physiotherapists, we can help reduce the mother's anxiety about her weight gain during pregnancy by being aware that many researchers regard weighing the mother as 'an ante-natal ritual', whose influence on clinical management is questionable (Abrams, 1994; Cogswell et al, 1995; Ekblad and Grenman, 1992; Hytten, 1990; Luke, 1994; May and Mahlmeister 1994).

Maternal weight gain or loss is a poor indication of foetal well-being and is affected by variations in weighing methods and equipment (Hytten, 1990).

Growth of the foetus is a complex issue. The major influences are the uterine environment and the mother. Nutritional deprivation in the first trimester may have adverse effects on the placental structure. The strongest link with foetal growth appears to be the pre-pregnancy weight of the mother, when compared with weight gain in pregnancy.

Figure 11.3 Distribution of weight gain in pregnancy.

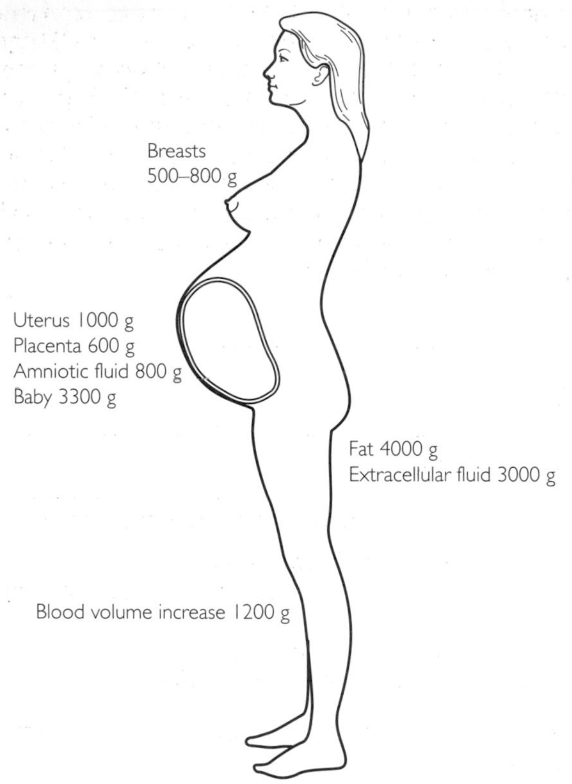

The higher the pre-pregnancy weight, the less is the effect of pregnant weight gain. Weight gains of less than 5 kg may be associated with a risk of intrauterine growth retardation (IUGR) (Spinillo et al, 1994). In a study looking at average and overweight women and the link with high birth-weight babies, Cogswell et al (1995) found that overweight women (BMI >29.0) who gained more than 35 lb (16 kg) had an increased risk of a high birth-weight infant (>4000 g). Weight gain and energy intake need to be tailored to the individual. Ideals of weight gain cannot be determined purely from research. Major maternity hospitals usually have a dietetics department to whom patients can be referred, particularly if they are worried about their weight gain in pregnancy.

Alcohol

The National Health and Medical Research Council (NH&MRC) Dietary Guidelines for Australians (1993) recommend no alcohol intake during pregnancy and refraining from alcohol during lactation. If alcohol is drunk, it should be after the infant has fed. It is now widely recognized that excessive alcohol intake, defined as more than two standard drinks/day or binge drinking, may be linked to foetal alcohol syndrome. Physiotherapists need to have current information about these recommendations as questions on nutrition, alcohol and smoking are frequently asked in ante-natal education and exercise classes.

Lactation

During lactation, adequate nutrition is important for both maternal and infant well-being. Todd and Parnell (1994) undertook a study of 73 breast-feeding women over a period of 12 months. They found the energy intake to be lower than required, at 8411 kJ when the Australian Recommended Nutritional Intake (RNI) is 10 500 kJ. All the women maintained lactation, although their calcium and zinc intake was regarded as inadequate. After the birth of their baby, many women are reluctant to lose weight for fear of interfering with lactation. In a study by Dusdieker et al (1994), 22 breast-feeding women embarked on a supervised weight reduction programme. After 10 weeks, the mean weight loss was 4.8 kg. Milk production was not adversely affected and the quality and quantity of milk remained satisfactory. The infants all achieved expected weight gain for age when weights were compared before and after the 10-week period.

Calcium

Calcium is important not only for maternal well-being (prevention of osteoporosis in later years), but also for bone deposition in the infant. By term, the foetal skeleton contains 30 g of calcium, which the foetus will take from maternal calcium stores, i.e. bone, if maternal calcium intake is less than adequate. The recommended daily intake for pregnant and lactating women is 1200 mg per day (Repke, 1994a). For US, UK and Australian women, the principal source of calcium is dairy foods but 75% of women of childbearing age do not receive the RNI of calcium per day. In women for whom dietary intake of calcium is not possible, calcium supplementation may be necessary. Care is required with supplementation when other supplements are being taken. Magnesium, zinc and iron may inhibit calcium absorption and should be given separately to decrease competition for absorption in the gastrointestinal tract (Repke, 1994a).

A recent study has shown that lactating women lose significantly more bone during the first six months postpartum compared to non-lactating women. After weaning, the lactating women gained significantly more bone than did non-lactating women. The study concluded that lactation may not result in net bone loss (Kalkwarf and Specker, 1995).

Birth weight and gestational length may be increased with supplementary calcium and magnesium during pregnancy (Luke, 1994) and high levels of calcium supplementation (2 g elemental calcium or 5 g calcium carbonate) per day appear to reduce PIH and the risk of pre-eclampsia (Repke, 1994b).

Folate

It is now well recognized that folate deficiency in early pregnancy is related to neural tube defects such as spina bifida, anencephaly and encephalocoele. At the time of neural tube development (around 3–4 weeks post-conception), most women are unaware of the pregnancy. Folate intake therefore needs to be adequate before conception.

Folate deficiency is one of the most common vitamin deficiencies. The recommended intake is 0.36 mg day^{-1} to prevent neural tube defects. Very large quantities of fruit, vegetables, cereals and juices are required to meet this intake solely from the diet so supplementation is suggested for all women planning to conceive. The other benefits of folate supplementation in women may include reducing the risks of some cancers and vascular disease (Mason, 1994). The NH&MRC (1993) advised the National Food Authority to recommend folate fortification of several cereal-based foods, juices and yeast extracts. This was approved in 1995 as a recommendation but is not mandatory. There have been concerns about vitamin B_{12} neuropathy associated with folate fortification (Metz, 1995). However, the levels of folate required to produce this (>1 mg day^{-1}) are much greater than the level of fortification recommended (0.36 mg day^{-1}) (Rush, 1994). It is recommended that clients at risk of having infants with neural tube defects be referred to their medical adviser (see Chapter 10).

Metabolism

Average daily energy requirements in pregnancy necessitate an intake, depending on activity, of 8500–10 000 kJ. Increased demand for protein, calcium and iron in pregnancy can be met with a normal balanced diet. Supplemental vitamins may be prescribed for some women who cannot achieve this.

The Dietary Guidelines for Australians (NH&MRC, 1993) provide useful information to help avoid undue weight gain in pregnancy. The balance of food types should be similar to that of non-pregnant females (see Chapter 4).

Most nutrients are carried in the blood at lower concentrations than the non-pregnant state. Hytten (1991) suggests this general decrease in levels of nutrients results in an increased transfer to the foetus instead of maternal tissues. The placenta appears to be more efficient than the maternal tissues at taking up nutrients from maternal blood at the lower levels of concentration. Thus the balance is favourable to the foetus rather than the mother. The mother alters her physiological and biochemical environment to provide optimal conditions for the foetus.

Urinary System

Progesterone, with its effects on smooth muscle generally in pregnancy, causes dilatation of the renal pelves and ureters. The ureters also elongate to accommodate the increasing size of the uterus. Later in pregnancy, the uterus compresses the ureters at the pelvic brim, causing a slowing of urine flow. Combined with an increase in urine output, this predisposes the pregnant woman to frequency, which can occur quite early in pregnancy and, for some, urinary tract infections. Blood volume to the kidneys is increased and there is an increase of 40% in renal blood flow glomeru filtration rate. This may result in changes in tubular reabsorption, with substances such as sugar, folic acid and water-soluble vitamins being excreted in maternal urine (Sturgiss et al, 1994). Diabetes can occur in pregnant women, some of whom are already predisposed to it genetically. Sugar levels return to normal after delivery in most women (gestational diabetics) but may remain elevated and become established diabetes. Stress and urge incontinence are commonly reported in pregnancy. The causes are many and complex and a thorough assessment is required to improve continence (see Chapters 23 and 28).

Skin

Pigmentation

Pigmentation changes occurring in pregnancy include:

- darkening of the areola on the breasts;
- linea nigra (vertical brown stripe down abdominal midline);
- increase in colouring on the vulva;
- chloasma (increased facial pigmentation).

These changes in pigmentation usually resolve gradually after delivery.

Striae gravidarum (stretch marks)

Striae gravidarum (stretch marks) occur on the abdomen, breasts, thighs and buttocks of most women to varying degrees. It is thought they are caused by changes in the elastic fibres and collagen in the dermis. The dermis ruptures and overstretches the epidermis, causing scarring. The marks are permanent, but change from blue / red wide marks to smaller silvery lines over time. Some women are more genetically susceptible than others. Massage, creams, oils and lotions will not prevent or remove the scars, but may help decrease the tight dry feelings of stretched skin. Undue weight gain may increase the stretch marks. Very marked striae may indicate impending pre-eclampsia (Beischer et al, 1989).

Sayer et al (1990) found women with stress incontinence and prolapsed bladder neck had a significantly greater incidence of abdominal striae. There was also an association with hypermobile joints. These findings are of interest to the physiotherapist treating obstetric patients.

Hair loss

After the birth of her baby, the mother may notice increased hair loss and worry that she is going bald. This perception occurs because during pregnancy there is a marked reduction in normal hair loss, as a result of an increased growth phase of the hair follicles. Hair growth and loss usually return to pre-pregnancy rates by 20 weeks ton and Lewes, 1982; Wong and Ellis,

Breasts

In early pregnancy many women experience tenderness and fullness in the breasts as they begin enlarging under the influence of the hormones relaxin, progesterone and oestrogen. Pigmentation changes include darkening of the areola and nipple. From around 12 weeks of pregnancy, the breasts begin to make the first milk (colostrum). Some women will leak or be able to express this fluid during pregnancy.

Montgomery's tubercles develop from enlarging sebaceous glands around the areola and secrete sebum as lubrication to keep the nipple and areola supple (Fig. 11.4). Breast weight increases in pregnancy by approximately 500–800 g. The blood supply to the breast also increases, with veins becoming visible, along with stretch marks in some women. Breast size is unrelated to capacity for milk production. The proportion of glandular versus fat tissue is more relevant to the capability to produce milk.

Nutritionally, mothers require an extra 2000 kJ per day to fulfil the demands of breast feeding. Mature milk production commences 24–96 hours post-partum. Stimulation of the nipple by frequent feeding in the first 24 hours causes an earlier changeover from colostrum to mature milk by stimulating prolactin production. Colostrum is rich in protein and antibodies and assists in providing immunity, particularly to gastroenteritis, in the baby (Beischer et al, 1989; Ebrahim, 1991).

Figure 11.4 The lactating breast.

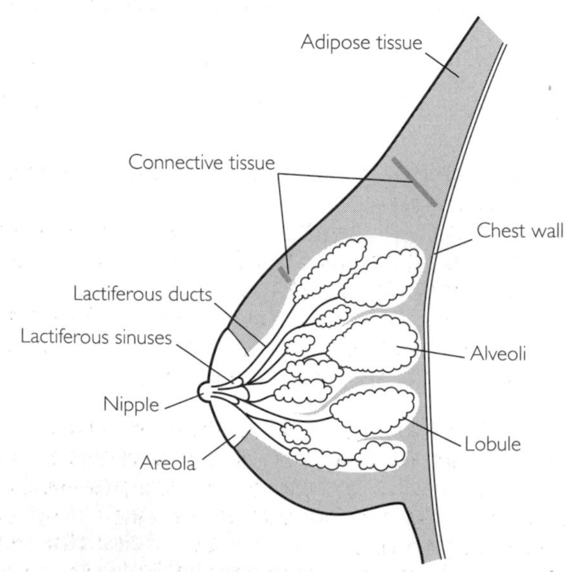

Endocrine System

During pregnancy, many organs of the body secrete hormones which affect the expectant mother. The effects of each of these hormones are outlined in Table 11.3.

Musculoskeletal Changes Associated with Pregnancy

Relaxin, progesterones, oestrogen and cortisols cause a generalized increase in joint laxity and range. These effects seem to be greater in multigravidae than in primigravidae. It takes 3–6 months for the body to return to the pre-pregnant state. Posture is adapted during pregnancy to compensate for the increasing abdominal size. Thoracic and lumbar curves increase, as does strain on joints. As a result, back pain is a common symptom in pregnancy, affecting more than 50% of pregnant women.

Other symptoms commonly seen by physiotherapists include carpal tunnel problems, caused by oedema in arms and hands compressing the distal segments of the median and ulnar nerves. This generally occurs later in pregnancy but has been noted around 16 weeks in some women. The muscles of the abdominal wall adapt to increasing foetal growth with stretching of the muscle fibres, widening and at times splitting of the linea alba and softening of the aponeurosis and fibrous sheaths. Diastasis of the recti muscles requires care in exercise and may necessitate external support. The maternal centre of gravity shifts posteriorly to accommodate the increase in abdominal size (Fig. 11.5). This in turn reduces stability and may result in the 'waddling gait' associated with pregnancy (Bullock et al, 1987; Romen et al, 1991). Musculoskeletal changes and physiotherapy treatment are discussed in Chapter 14.

Cramp

Many women experience painful muscle cramps during pregnancy, particularly in the lower limbs. The cause of these cramps has been variously reported as impaired venous blood flow due to increased pelvic pressure from the foetus, vasodilatation and changes in phosphate and calcium metabolism (Page and Page, 1953). Calcium may need to be given in supplemental form to alleviate this possible cause of cramp. Deep venous thrombosis (DVT) is a rare source of painful legs in pregnancy (<1%) (Lee et al, 1990). If a patient complains of painful legs, a careful and detailed assessment by the physiotherapist should be made. If the therapist suspects a DVT, the patient should be referred immediately to her doctor. Regular calf stretches during the day, warmth and support hosiery can all help to alleviate the painful problem of cramp. The patient is also advised to massage the affected part after the cramp releases and to encourage active release, to reduce post-cramp

Table 11.3 Hormones – action and pregnancy changes

Hormones	Action
Anterior pituitary	
Follicle-stimulating hormone (FSH)	Ovarian development, follicle development, follicle to ovum release, corpus luteum production
Luteinizing hormone (LH)	Corpus luteum growth, follicle release
Prolactin	General growth, lipid metabolism and blood product growth During pregnancy – uterine growth and activity, breast development, milk synthesis
Human placental lactogen (HPL)	Mobilizes free fatty acids During pregnancy – foetal growth via carbohydrate metabolism
Human growth hormone (HGH)	Growth of skeleton, connective tissue, muscle and organs During pregnancy – foetal growth
Adrenocorticotrophic hormone (ACTH)	Production of corticosteroids, regulates metabolism of fat, protein and carbohydrate, controls body fluid mineral concentration During pregnancy – foetal production of CTH
Posterior pituitary	
Oxytocin	Pregnancy – uterine activity, labour Puerperium – milk ejection reflex
Vasopressin (ADH)	Antidiuretic hormone – fluid resorption from renal tubules During pregnancy – possible role in fluid resorption from foetal lungs (Cummings et al, 1995)
Ovary	
Progesterone	Cyclical endometrial glycogen storage, breast alveolar stimulation During pregnancy – relaxes smooth muscle tone, breast development, increases body temperature, decreases arterial and alveoli $P\text{CO}_2$
Oestrogen	Puberty changes, cyclical endometrial, myometrial and breast duct stimulation. During pregnancy – myometrial fibre enlargement
Relaxin	During pregnancy – uteroplacental circulation (Jauniaux et al, 1994), uterine growth, possible foetal growth, relaxes ligaments, modifies collagen–mucopolysaccharide relationship of cervix and pelvic joints (Klopper, 1991)
Placenta	
Human chorionic gonadotropin (HCG)	During pregnancy – maintains corpus luteum function, regulates placental oestrogen, possible suppression of maternal immune reaction to foetus (Llewellyn-Jones, 1994)
Thyroid	
Triiodo-thyronine T3	Controls metabolic rate During pregnancy – mild hyperthyroidism, increase of metabolic rate, cardiac output, pulse rate. Affects heat tolerance. Six weeks post-partum returns to pre-pregnancy values (Burrows et al, 1994)

soreness. She should be encouraged to avoid leg stretches into plantar flexion in bed. If the women senses a cramp developing she can prevent it by actively stretching the muscles involved.

Reproductive System

Uterus

In the non-pregnant woman the uterus is approximately the size of a pear, weighs around 60 g and can hold 6 ml. By 40 weeks of pregnancy the uterus weighs 1000 g and can hold 5000 ml.

The myometrium of the uterus has three muscle layers (Fig. 11.6).

- The inner circular layer pulls open the lower segment and cervix in labour.
- The middle oblique layer is involved in the expulsive contractions of labour and in clamping off bleeding vessels after placental delivery.
- The outer longitudinal layer thickens to form a strong upper segment which pushes the foetus down into the more passive lower segment in labour.

The perimetrium is part of the peritoneum. It is able to allow unrestricted uterine growth owing to its extension into the pouch of Douglas posteriorly and the uterovesical pouch anteriorly. The endometrium is the inner lining of the uterus. In pregnancy it is called the decidua (Bennett and Brown, 1993; Blackburn and Loper, 1992; Gaudin et al, 1989).

Figure 11.5 Biomechanical changes in pregnancy.

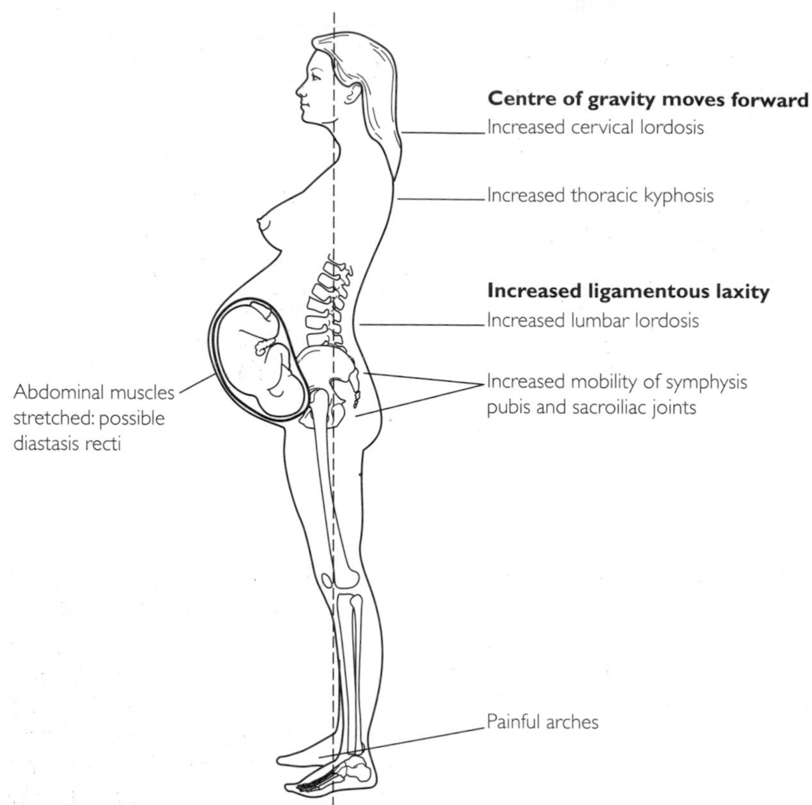

Figure 11.6 The muscle layers of the uterus.

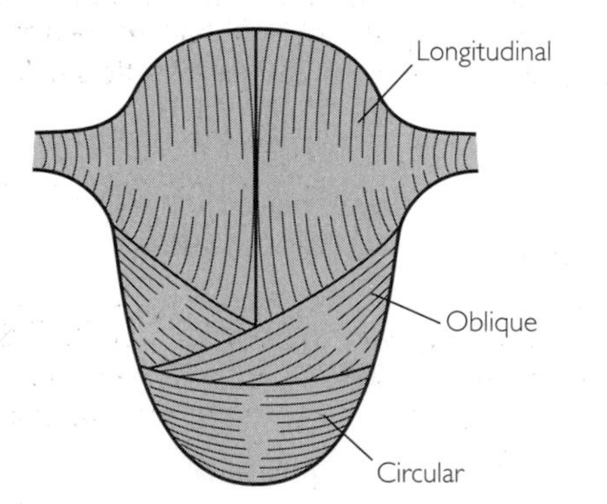

Foetal movements are felt by the primigravida at around 18–20 weeks and 14–16 weeks in the multigravida. At 14–16 weeks the foetal heart can be heard using a Sonic-aid and by 24–26 weeks with a stethoscope.

The contractile protein actomyosin is responsible for most of the increase in muscle fibres. Later in pregnancy the fibres also stretch, causing thinning of the uterine wall, especially in the lower segment.

For the first 12 weeks, the uterus remains a pelvic organ. It then grows out into the abdominal cavity and can be palpated above the pubic bone. By 20 weeks it is at umbilical height and reaches the xiphisternum by 36 weeks in the primigravida and 40 weeks in the multigravida (Fig. 11.7).

The uterus contracts throughout pregnancy from approximately eight weeks on but the contractions may not be noticed by the mother until 28 weeks or so. As pregnancy progresses the contractions become stronger under the influence of prostaglandins being released from the decidua. These contractions, also called Braxton Hicks, are painless for most women but may be distressing for others. They have a role in the formation of the lower uterine segment in later pregnancy, as they draw the isthmus up to form this segment. The sensitivity of the uterus to oxytocin increases in pregnancy by up to 100 times (Beischer et al, 1989).

Some interesting findings about oxytocin and its changing level in the maternal bloodstream over 24 hours indicate that plasma oxytocin levels are significantly higher around midnight in the pregnant woman at 37–39 weeks gestation (Fuchs et al, 1992). In the light of this and similar findings, it has been suggested that a more chronotherapeutic approach to inducing labour may reduce the required dosage of oxytocin or prostaglandin (Honnebier and Nathanielsz, 1994).

Cervix

The cervix enlarges because of increasing vascularity and softens under the influence of oestrogen and progesterone

Figure 11.7 Fundal height in primiparous and multiparous pregnancies.

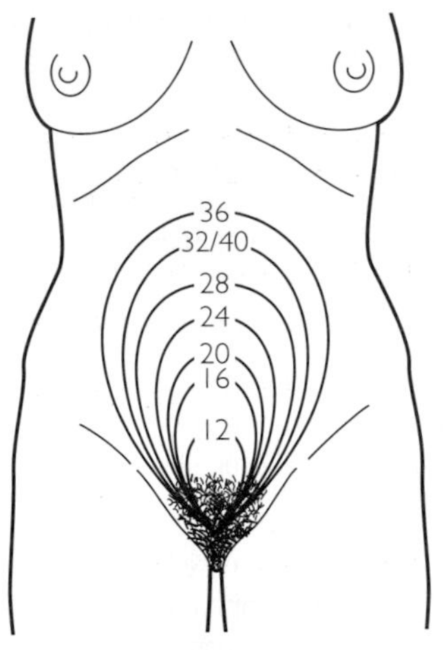

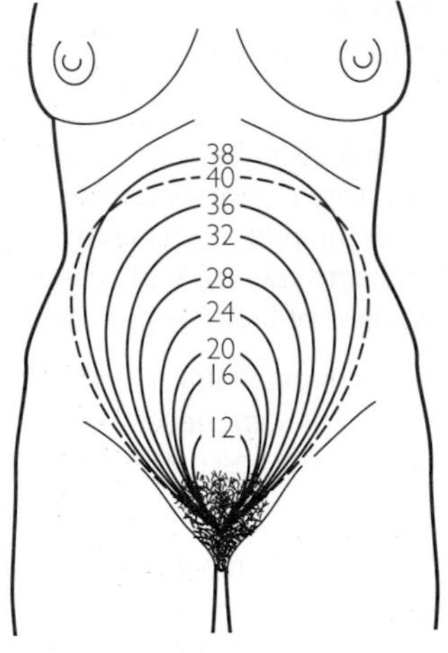

as pregnancy progresses. The colour changes early on from pink to violet, due to the effects of progesterone. Ripening of the cervix occurs due to the effect of prostaglandin and relaxin as labour becomes imminent. As pregnancy continues, a thick mucous plug, the *operculum*, forms in the cervical canal. It comes away at the onset of labour – the 'show'.

Vagina

The vagina changes in colour and firmness, similar to the cervix. Glycogen increases in the squamous cells and thus predisposes toward monilial infection (thrush). The muscle layer of the vagina thickens and the connective tissue surrounding the vagina allows it to become more elastic. These changes make it possible for the vagina to dilate during the second stage of labour to allow the passage of the foetus.

Nervous System

As previously mentioned, fluid retention can compress nerves passing through narrow canals. One example is compression in the carpal tunnel, causing pain, numbness and weakness in the hand. It was thought that women's cognitive ability decreased in pregnancy but Schneider (1988) showed no deterioration in mental ability from the pre-pregnant state to late pregnancy, on a series of intelligence tests. However, anxiety, increased mood lability, vivid nightmares and insomnia are all well documented in pregnancy. The exact aetiology of these changes is not known, but is thought to be hormonal.

Visual changes

In pregnancy, tear volume is decreased, with an associated alteration in the trilaminar tear film. Raised oestrogen and progesterone levels in pregnancy reduce secretion of mucin by the goblet cells of the conjunctival surface.

The cornea also changes in pregnancy. It contains 70% water and as such is affected by an increase in extracellular fluid. Oedema may result. Corneal sensitivity is reduced in pregnancy, resulting in minor irritations becoming major before they are noticed by the woman. There is also a change in the curvature of the cornea, related to raised oestrogen levels (Farrall, 1974).

All of these changes have been noted to cause difficulties for pregnant women who wear contact lenses. Sometimes problems occur post-partum as well. It is suggested that in women who develop symptoms, contact lenses should be worn less often and not overnight (Imafidon, 1992).

Puerperium

Physiological changes in the puerperium include a return to pre-pregnancy levels of most body systems and a change in the action of others – for example, lactation in the breast.

Endocrine changes take some time to occur, with relaxin effects being maintained for 12 weeks despite a cessation of production by four days post-partum. This has implications for the musculoskeletal system, in restricting the intensity of exercise during this time and ensuring that principles of good posture and back care are considered.

The cardiovascular system returns to normal within two weeks, with blood volume returning to the pre-pregnant level. A lot of fluid is passed as urine in the first few days post-partum to achieve this reduction (Beischer et al, 1989).

Skin changes gradually return to the pre-pregnant state. It may take many weeks for chloasma and the linea nigra to fade.

Table 11.4 Changes in some systems associated with pregnancy

Cardiovascular	Cardiac output increases by 40%; slight decrease in BP mid-pregnancy then increasing to normal Supine hypotension in late pregnancy. Peripheral vasodilatation – warm extremities Limb oedema
Respiratory	Tidal volume increases by 40%; vital capacity increases slightly. Inspiratory capacity increases by 300 ml; subcostal angle increases by 35° O_2 consumption increases by 20%; respiratory rate unchanged Diaphragm rises by 4 cm; chest diameter increases by 2 cm Shortness of breath – hyperventilatory effort from respiratory centre sensitivity
Immune system	Baby receives immunity from mother via placental transfer of IgG Mother has some general depression of maternal immunity so does not reject foetus. Slightly predisposed to reactivating latent viruses and some illnesses, e.g. influenza, pneumococcal pneumonia
Digestive system	Nausea in early months – morning, noon and night. Increase in appetite Weight gain 10–14 kg. Heartburn (decreasing lower oesophageal sphincter competence) Slower emptying of stomach; slower mobility and absorption rates in small intestine Constipation due to decrease in motility in large intestine and increased water reabsorption Gall bladder increase in bile concentration → increased risk of gall stones
Urinary system	Frequency in early and late pregnancy → tubular reabsorption changes → increase in sugar excretion
Skin	Increase in pigmentation of areola, face, abdomen, linea nigra Striae gravidarum (stretch marks) Increased oiliness because of increased sebum production
Breasts	Increase in size by 500–800 g. Colostrum may leak from 12 weeks on Veins more prominent because of increase in blood supply. Stretch marks may occur
Endocrine	See Table 11.3
Musculoskeletal	Joint laxity and stretching. Muscle stretching. Postural changes due to increased spinal curvature
Reproductive	Uterine growth. Breast enlargement. Cervix softens and changes colour. Vagina is more susceptible to thrush
Neurological	Increased mood lability. No decrease in intellectual performance. More prone to compression of distal nerves because of increase in fluid (e.g. carpal tunnel)

The digestive system alters after birth. Breast-feeding mothers often maintain an increased appetite in order to provide the extra energy required for lactation.

The respiratory system returns to normal soon after delivery. Oxygen saturation has been measured at 98% the day after delivery, whereas in labour it has been as low as 87% (de Swiet, 1991).

The changes in pregnancy are summarized in Table 11.4.

Knowledge of the changes which occur during pregnancy and the puerperium and their resultant problems is essential for physiotherapists working with women in the child-bearing year. While this text provides a brief outline of these changes, readers are encouraged to refer to the recommended reading for further information.

References

Abrams B (1994) Weight gain and energy intake during pregnancy. *Clinical Obstetrics and Gynaecology* **37**: 515–527.

Baron TH, Ramirez B and Richter JE (1993) Gastrointestinal motility disorders during pregnancy. *Annals of Internal Medicine* **118**: 366–375.

Beischer N and Mackay E (1986) *Obstetrics and the New Born, 2nd edn*. Sydney: W.B. Saunders/Baillière Tindall.

Beischer N, Mackay E and Purcal N (1989) *Care of the Pregnant Woman and Her Baby*, 2nd edn. Sydney: W.B. Saunders/Baillière Tindall.

Bennett VR and Brown LK (eds) (1993) *Myles Textbook for Midwives*, 12th edn, pp. 13–64. London: Churchill Livingstone.

Blackburn ST and Loper DL (1992) *Maternal, Fetal and Neonatal Physiology: A Clinical Perspective*. Philadelphia: W.B. Saunders.

Bullock JE, Jull GA and Bullock MI (1987) The relationship of low back pain to post-ural changes during pregnancy. *Australian Journal of Physiotherapy* **33**: 10–17.

Burrows G, Fisher D and Larsen PR (1994) Maternal and fetal thyroid function. *New England Journal of Medicine* **331**: 1072–1077.

Clark SL and the National Asthma Education Program Working Group (1993) Asthma in pregnancy. *Obstetrics and Gynecology* **82**: 1036–1040.

Cogswell ME, Serdula MK, Hungerford DW and Yip R (1995) Gestational weight gain among average weight and overweight women – What is excessive? *American Journal of Obstetrics and Gynecology* **172**: 705–712.

Cummings JL, Carlton DP, Poulain FR et al (1995) Vasopressin effects on liquid lung volume in fetal sheep. *Paediatric Research* **38**: 30–35.

de Swiet M (1991) The cardiovascular system, in Hytten F and Chamberlain G (eds) *Clinical Physiology in Obstetrics*, 2nd edn, pp. 3–38. Oxford: Blackwell Scientific Publications.

Dusdieker LB, Hemingway DL and Stumbo PH (1994) Is milk production impaired by dieting during lactation? *American Journal of Clinical Nutrition* **59**: 833–840.

Duvekot JJ and Peeters LL (1994) Maternal cardiovascular haemodynamic adaptation to pregnancy. *Obstetrics and Gynaecological Survey* **49**: S1–14.

Ebrahim GJ (1991) *Breastfeeding: The Biological Option*, 2nd edn, pp. 49–87. London: Macmillan.

Ekblad U and Grenman S (1992) Obese women and women with excess weightgain in pregnancy. *International Journal of Gynaecology and Obstetrics* **39**: 277–283.

Farrall HP (1974) A study of the effects of orally administered female hormones on the volume and composition of lacrimal fluid related to the toleration of corneal contact lenses. Cited in Imafidon CO (1992) Contact lenses in pregnancy. *British Journal of Obstetrics and Gynaecology* **99**: 865–868.

Ferguson JH, Neubauer BL and Shaar CJ (1994) Ambulatory blood pressure monitoring during pregnancy. Establishment of standards of normalcy. *American Journal of Hypertension* **7**: 838–843.

Fuchs AR, Behrens O and Liu H (1992) Cited in Honnebier MBOM and Nathanielsz PW (1994) Primate parturition and the role of the circadian system. *European Journal of Obstetrics and Gynaecology and Reproductive Biology* **55**: 200.

Gaudin AJ, Jones KC, Cotanche JG et al (1989) *Human Anatomy and Physiology*, pp. 733–749. Florida: Harcourt Brace Jovanovich.

Greenberger PA (1992) Asthma in pregnancy. *Clinics in Chest Medicine* **13**: 597–605.

Honnebier MBOM and Nathanielsz PW (1994) Primate parturition and the role of the circadian system. *European Journal of Obstetrics and Gynaecology and Reproductive Biology* **55**: 193–203.

Hytten F (1990) Is it important or even useful to measure weight gain in pregnancy? *Midwifery* **6**: 28–32.

Hytten FE (1991) Nutrition, in Hytten F and Chamberlain G (eds) *Clinical Physiology in Obstetrics*, 2nd edn, pp. 150–172. Oxford: Blackwell Scientific Publications.

Imafidon CO (1992) Contact lenses in pregnancy. *British Journal of Obstetrics and Gynaecology* **99**: 865–868.

Institute of Medicine (IOM) (1990) *Nutrition during Pregnancy, Weight Gain and Nutrient Supplements. Report of the Subcommittee on Nutritional Status and Weight Gain during Pregnancy, Subcommittee on Dietary Intake and Nutrient Supplements during Pregnancy, Subcommittee on Dietary Intake and Nutritional Status during Pregnancy and Lactation.* Food and Nutrition Board. Washington, DC: National Academy Press.

Jauniaux E, Johnson MR, Jurkovic D et al (1994) The role of relaxin in the development of the uteroplacental circulation in early pregnancy. *Obstetrics and Gynaecology* **84**: 338–342.

Kalkwarf HJ and Specker BL (1995) Bone mineral loss during lactation and recovery after weaning. *Obstetrics and Gynecology* **86**: 27–32.

Kelly YJ, Brabin BJ, Milligan P et al (1995) Maternal asthma, premature birth, and the risk of respiratory morbidity in schoolchildren in Merseyside. *Thorax* **50**: 525–530.

Kinsella SM and Lohmann G (1994) Supine hypotensive syndrome. *Obstetrics and Gynaecology* **84**: 774–788.

Klopper A (1991) The hypothalamus and pituitary gland, in Hytten F and Chamberlain G (eds) *Clinical Physiology in Obstetrics*, 2nd edn, p. 382. Oxford: Blackwell Scientific Publications.

Lee RV, McCombs LE and Mezzadri FC (1990) Pregnant legs, painful legs: the obstetricians' dilemma. *Obstetrics and Gynaecological Survey* **45**: 290–298.

Letsky E (1991) The haematological system, in Hytten F and Chamberlain G (eds) *Clinical Physiology in Obstetrics*, 2nd edn, pp. 39–45. Oxford: Blackwell Scientific Publications.

Llewellyn-Jones D (1994) *Fundamentals of Obstetrics and Gynaecology*, 6th edn, pp. 29–33. London: C.V. Mosby.

Luke B (1994) Nutritional influences on foetal growth. *Clinical Obstetrics and Gynaecology* **37**: 538–549.

Mason JB (1994) Folate and colonic carcinogenesis: searching for a mechanistic understanding. *Journal of Nutritional Biochemistry* **5**: 170–175.

May KA and Mahlmeister LR (1994) *Maternal and Neonatal Nursing*, 3rd edn, pp. 282–283, 403–410. Philadelphia: JB Lippincott.

Metz J (1995) Folate, B12 and neural tube defects. *Medical Journal of Australia* **163**: 231–232.

Mobius WV (1961) Cited by de Swiet M (1991) The respiratory system, in Hytten F and Chamberlain G (eds) *Clinical Physiology in Obstetrics*, 2nd edn, pp. 83–100. Oxford: Blackwell Scientific Publications.

NH&MRC Dietary Guidelines for Australians (1993) Canberra: Australian Government Publishing Service.

Page EW and Page EP (1953) Cited in Lee RV, McCombs LE and Mezzadri FC (1990) Pregnant legs, painful legs: the obstetricians' dilemma. *Obstetrics and Gynaecological Survey* **45**: 290–298.

Perlow JH, Montgomery D, Morgan MA et al (1992) Severity of asthma and perinatal outcome. *American Journal of Obstetrics and Gynecology* **167**: 963–967.

Repke JT (1994a) Calcium homeostasis in pregnancy. *Clinical Obstetrics and Gynaecology* **37**: 59–65.

Repke JT (1994b) Calcium and vitamin D. *Clinical Obstetrics and Gynaecology* **37**: 550–557.

Robson SC, Dunlop W, Moore W and Hunter S (1987) Cited by de Swiet M (1991) The cardiovascular system, in Hytten F and Chamberlain G (eds) *Clinical Physiology in Obstetrics*, 2nd edn, pp. 3–38. Oxford: Blackwell Scientific Publications.

Romen Y, Masaki DI and Mittelmark RA (1991) Physiological and endocrine adjustments to pregnancy in Mittelmark RA, Wiswell RA and Drinkwater BL (eds) *Exercise in Pregnancy*, 2nd edn, pp. 9–29. Baltimore: Williams and Wilkins.

Rush D (1994) Periconceptual folate and neural tube defect. *American Journal of Clinical Nutrition* **59**: 511S–515S.

Sayer TR, Dixon JS, Hosker GL and Warrell DW (1990) A study of paraurethral connective tissue in women with stress incontinence of urine. *Neurourology and Urodynamics* **9**: 319–320.

Schneider Z (1988) Thinking and learning in pregnancy. PhD thesis. Melbourne: Faculty of Education, Monash University.

Spinillo A, Capuzzo E, Piazzi G et al (1994) Maternal high risk factors and severity of growth deficit in small for gestational age infants. *Early Human Development* **38**: 35–43.

Stirrat G (1991) The immune system in Hytten F and Chamberlain G (eds) *Clinical Physiology in Obstetrics*, 2nd edn, pp. 101–109. Oxford: Blackwell Scientific Publications.

Sturgiss SN, Dunlop W and Davison JM (1994) Renal haemodynamics and tubular function in human pregnancy. *Clinical Obstetrics and Gynaecology* **8**: 209–234.

Thomson KJ and Cohen ME (1938) Cited by de Swiet M (1991) The respiratory system, in Hytten F and Chamberlain G (eds) *Clinical Physiology in Obstetrics*, 2nd edn, pp. 83–100. Oxford: Blackwell Scientific Publications.

Todd JM and Parnell WR (1994) Nutrient intakes of women who are breastfeeding. *European Journal of Clinical Nutrition* **48**: 567–574.

Winton GB and Lewes CW (1982) Cited in Blackburn ST and Loper DL (1992) *Maternal, Fetal and Neonatal Physiology: A Clinical Perspective.* Philadelphia: W.B. Saunders.

Wong RC and Ellis CN (1984) Cited in Blackburn ST and Loper DL (1992) *Maternal, Fetal and Neonatal Physiology: A Clinical Perspective.* Philadelphia: W.B. Saunders.

Recommended reading

PHYSIOLOGY

Gaudin HJ, Jones KC, Cotanche JG et al (1989) *Human Anatomy and Physiology.* Florida: Harcourt Brace Jovanovich.

Hytten F and Chamberlain G (eds) (1991) *Clinical Physiology in Obstetrics*, 2nd edn. Oxford: Blackwell Scientific Publications.

PREGNANCY

Beischer NA, Mackay EV and Purcal NK (1989) *Care of the Pregnant Woman and Her Baby*, 2nd edn. Sydney: WB Saunders/Baillière Tindall.

LACTATION

Ebrahim GJ (1991) *Breastfeeding, the Biological Option*, 2nd edn. London: Macmillan.

Minchin M (1985) *Breastfeeding Matters: What We Need to Know about Infant Feeding*. Sydney: Alma Publications/George Allen and Unwin.

CONCEPTION

Hytten F and Chamberlain G (eds) (1991) *Clinical Physiology in Obstetrics*, 2nd edn. Oxford: Blackwell Scientific Publications.

12

The Psychological and Emotional Aspects of Child Bearing

KAREN COOMBES AND RACHEL DARKEN

Pregnancy and giving birth are special and unique events and a multitude of human experience exists, so that relying on a single impression to describe the act of giving birth and the lead-up to it would be inaccurate and unrealistic. From conception to the labour and delivery and often for a period afterwards, a woman will be bombarded by a barrage of emotions, often differing between two individual women, between two different pregnancies in the same woman and depending on the stage in the continuum of events. Aspects and sensations of pregnancy and birth that are enjoyable for some women may be disliked or even distressful for others. This variation exists just as the physiological pattern of labour and delivery is unpredictable and highly individual.

Certainly racial, cultural and ethnic background have a definite influence on a woman's psychological status during these times. Indeed, distinct nationalities will have their own unique customs and common emotional scenarios at particular phases of pregnancy and birth. It is accepted that these obvious differences exist in a multicultural society together with certain similarities across the human race as a whole. Nevertheless, the journey from conception to birth is likely to bring with it problems, challenges, excitement and happiness for the woman, her partner and her family.

Physiotherapists have a large educational role during the ante-natal and post-natal periods and in maintaining a holistic service it is vital to enquire not only about a woman's physical condition but also her psychological status. An understanding of the variations of normal that can exist on the emotional plane throughout the birthing process and afterwards aids in identifying women who may be at risk of developing problems post-natally, those actually experiencing post-natal problems and obtaining the early intervention of professional expertise to assist them. Sufficient knowledge can also help physiotherapists recognize states of mind that will naturally pass without posing a threat to the woman's mental health.

Emotional and Psychological Changes Through the Ante-natal Period

The news of a pregnancy, whether it be a joyous or daunting occasion for a couple, will bring with it in the nine months to follow multiple tests of inner strength and flexibility as well as relationship stability. Major physical changes are occurring continually within the mother-to-be as the pregnancy advances, requiring the woman and her family to adapt accordingly through emotional and psychological channels. The family unit will be growing alongside the growing baby, both in number as well as in knowledge and wisdom about the birthing process.

Each trimester of pregnancy can generally be related to one of three psychological states – acknowledgement, consolidation and preparation – in response to the progression from conception to the actual commencement of labour. A woman's mechanisms of coping throughout each stage are dependent upon such variables as her physical condition, social and family support networks, the reaction evoked in the woman by her pregnancy and the significance she attaches to it.

A special meaning or definition is attributed to a pregnancy by each woman, her partner and her family, and emotional responses throughout the pregnancy are dictated by these. The high degree of individuality between pregnancies in different families or between different pregnancies within the same family indicates that the significance attached to a pregnancy may be quite variable between people and between pregnancies in the same woman.

Creation of a new life for some couples is an overt expression of the love they feel for one another or simply a natural progression of their special bond. Yet other couples conceive in order to repair a failing marriage or hold the relationship together by establishing a common interest for the pair (Kitzinger, 1977). If during childhood a woman felt isolated or unloved or in fact feels lonely in her adult life, her own pregnancy may engender hopes of obtaining the love she was denied or of filling the emptiness. Pregnancy may give a woman with low self-esteem a sense of achievement, particularly if she feels most aspects of her life have been insignificant or unsuccessful (Kitzinger, 1977).

There may be negativity associated with falling pregnant if the woman views the growing baby as a foreign entity invading her body. If the conception occurs later in life the woman may feel embarrassed and attempt to hide the fact, yet society today accepts women child bearing into their forties (Kitzinger, 1977).

Upon confirmation that she is pregnant and throughout the first trimester, major hormonal and physiological changes within the woman become coupled with psychological acknowledgement of the growing baby inside her. During this phase she will firstly undergo the realization that she is pregnant and subsequently begin to link meaning and definition to the idea depending on her circumstances. A totally new and different role is imminent for the woman, particularly if it is her first pregnancy. She will either deliberately or automatically attune to her inbuilt impressions and memories of her own childhood upbringing, basing her parenting skills and strategies on those of her parents (Kitzinger, 1977).

The woman will be mentally coming to terms with her new status and lability during the early ante-natal period may manifest itself as moments of happiness and sadness in close succession. Such highs and lows form part of a normal process in the adjustment to pregnancy. The pregnancy itself may cause feelings of indifference, with periods of ecstasy and excitement about the situation interspersed with the intrusion of misery and dread. Guilt may then prevail in the latter case, with the woman feeling as though she is rejecting her baby despite the fact that these feelings may be beyond her control.

Emotions may overflow into other areas of life or relationships if there is a lack of understanding as to what is being experienced by the woman. In particular, confusion and bewilderment at the woman's behaviour may consume her partner, which in turn may threaten the relationship, a situation that was non-existent prior to the pregnancy (Kitzinger, 1977). Hormonal changes, apart from contributing psychologically, can elicit physical repercussions associated with being pregnant. Unfortunately, these added stresses arise at a time when the commencement of pregnancy is concealed from the outside world and when fatigue created by the hormonal and physiological adjustments is setting in. Consequently, the mother-to-be may not be receiving the additional assistance that would be beneficial even at this early stage to assist in alleviating her physical and psychological load (Kitzinger, 1977).

Sweet (1988) suggests an emotional shift from the fourth to the sixth month of pregnancy from 'being pregnant' to 'expecting a baby'. During this consolidation phase there is a settling of emotional turmoil as acceptance of the pregnancy has occurred and the body has become accustomed to the altered hormonal and physical conditions. Awareness of the pregnancy by others is heightened as the enlarged female dimensions become noticeable and the baby's activity can be felt, thus precipitating the enhanced care and support that may have been forgotten during the first trimester (Kitzinger, 1977). The mother-to-be is now the centre point of the pregnancy. She tends to adopt increasing responsibility for another human being, often reflected in a shift towards a healthier lifestyle. The cessation of such 'bad' habits as smoking and excessive alcohol intake occurs to prevent adverse effects on her baby.

The couple's relationship may alter, with attention predominantly on the mother-to-be causing possible separation between them. This is often because the father feels like an intruder on his partner's time or is feeling isolated from her due to her often heavy schedule. The mother-to-be is also likely to become more attentive to her baby as the pregnancy continues, possibly causing her partner to feel neglected, however unintentionally.

This is probably also partially attributable to the increasing relevance of female relationships throughout the second trimester, where there is strong identification between the mother-to-be and all other women who have also moved through the childbirth experience (Kitzinger, 1977). These bonds are bound to elicit sentiments of empathy, of having been through similar circumstances. The sharing of emotions associated with labour and delivery and the giving of advice, education and reassurance concerning the impending events all greatly help to ease a woman's fears and anxieties about what lies ahead.

Nevertheless, in the quest to maintain the closeness of the relationship throughout the onslaught of seemingly maternal issues, the parents should participate in birth preparations as a couple and identify with their partner's feelings through the ups and downs of pregnancy. Open communication will also facilitate the resolution of any conflict to create a harmonious relationship into which a child will soon be born.

Preparation consumes the final three months of pregnancy where there tends to be mixed feelings regarding the impending labour and delivery. As the time of birth draws nearer the mother-to-be may become impatient, wishing it would all be over or she may alternatively become quite anxious and fearful of the unknown (Kitzinger, 1986). In particular, she may be concerned about not living up to expectations during the labour or fulfilling her role as a mother (Kitzinger, 1977). She may wonder if she will remember all she has learnt through her ante-natal classes, self-education and discussion with other women.

As the preparatory phase implies, the woman may become very busy getting ready for the new addition to the family or she may adopt a deep sense of calm and serenity, waiting for nature to take its course. Her self-image is greatly affected by the notion that her once familiar dimensions have been transformed into an alien body and continue to change regularly. Towards the end of the nine months the woman may begin to feel like a used vessel existing solely to incubate her growing baby (Kitzinger, 1977).

The sheer burden of the extra weight she must carry means an increase in physical lethargy, necessitating numerous short rest periods throughout the day, also compounded by the possibility of interrupted sleep due to her more pronounced shape later in the pregnancy. The woman may feel physically unattractive to her partner and correspondingly experience a decline in her libido, though there are some women who become quite sexual during pregnancy. Concentration levels for complicated mental tasks may decrease and the woman may daydream frequently, though disturbing fantasies about herself and the baby may come to the fore.

In today's society a woman who is expecting a baby will most often leave her career or occupation, albeit temporarily. She may opt to give up her job completely to raise her child and may then fall victim to a minor identity crisis, especially if she has had major involvement in work duties and high ambitions for progression. There may be concomitant social drawbacks such as emotional isolation with the change to the usual daily environment and absence of colleagues and friends, not to mention the possibility of financial hardship on the family with the loss of one income. Jimenez and Newton (1982), however, related reported job commitment to emotions in the third trimester of pregnancy and six weeks post-partum in 120 primiparae. It was discovered that women who adapt well to work also adapt well to child bearing and women who scored high in job commitment had more favourable psychological and emotional experiences in the first pregnancy and post-partum period on some measures.

Where a woman experiences periods of absence from work as a result of falling pregnant successively, a more common scenario today in contrast to leaving a career altogether, her responses may be similar though not as marked, more short-lived and more prevalent in the initial phases of giving up work for each pregnancy. Alternatively, some mothers-to-be may jump at the opportunity of adopting the role of home maker, particularly if their occupation or career is dissatisfying and they are seeking to add another dimension to their lives.

Apart from teaching women the basic physical aspects of childbirth, ante-natal classes offer social contact for mothers-to-be and facilitate the sharing of emotions and group problem solving. Physiotherapists can mediate this conversation, offer their ideas on what to expect emotionally at this time, give reassurance and support and provide solutions based on their knowledge, but must also know their limitations and when to refer on to other avenues of treatment.

Emotional and Psychological Aspects of Childbirth

For the expectant mother, pregnancy seems to last for such a long time that she may become preoccupied with her status, viewing the pregnancy as a way of life and often somewhat oblivious to the impending arrival of new life. The challenge of labour will evoke responses and feelings in a woman that are largely dependent on the type of delivery she has, the attitude of her attendants, her personality and the relationship she has with her partner (Corkill, 1996). Active involvement of the mother and support from her partner during birth produce more positive physical and psychological outcomes (Henneborn and Cogan, 1975).

A number of conflicting emotions may arise at different phases of labour or indeed in close succession during one particular stage. Kitzinger (1987) describes excitement, doubt, hope, fear, anxiety, joy, anger, weariness, irritation, disbelief, satisfaction and peace. Certainly at the 'breaking of the waters' a woman could feel sick, anxious, frightened and excited all at once, due respectively to the physical phenomenon itself, the possible ambivalence of the hospital setting, the daunting nature of the time to come and the anticipation of another human being entering the room.

Labour and delivery are more often than not considered to be painful events, yet for women with a strong sense of self the experience can be one of creative growth and maturation (Price, 1988). Relaxation and sheer pleasure can prevail when the woman observes that her strategies for the management of labour, studied so meticulously ante-natally, are successful in smoothly guiding her through the turbulent uterine contractions. It is common for the woman to be consumed by the movements occurring in her body, often being unaware of others around her and losing sense of time (Beels, 1978).

Where the labour advances to the expulsive stage, the woman may experience a second wind of increased energy and alertness. With the emergence of the baby's head a sensuous enjoyable feeling may overcome her, together with the fascination at viewing the reality of a child, nine months in the making. The woman may find it quite natural, empowering and satisfying to accommodate to her body's physical task through emotional sounds and comforting movements, losing her inhibitions and rebelling against conservative ideas during childbirth (Beels, 1978). Following the bringing of a child into the world, the mother may be overwhelmed and feel disbelief that the baby, particularly size-wise, has emerged from inside her. She may be surprised that she was able to lose her inhibitions without being worried or self-conscious about doing so, dispelling her preconceptions from the ante-natal period (Kitzinger, 1987).

Alternatively, the birth may not be seen as positively by other women. It may be deemed an ordeal to be endured due to the invasiveness of the situation, loss of bodily control and self-consciousness that it involves. Embarrassment and weakening may then ensue. It can be seen as humiliating and conjure feelings of helplessness and vulnerability, particularly if there has been any previous history of physical or sexual abuse (Corkill, 1996) or the woman has experienced a traumatic labour and delivery in the past. If the woman is lacking in emotional support she may feel isolated in her plight and disorientated without reassurance in a strange environment. She may wonder how much more her anatomy can endure and become angry at the baby for putting her through such a trauma, though this is usually short-lived (Kitzinger, 1987). The woman may feel quite self-centred throughout this intense time, forgetting the equally traumatic experience of the newborn.

If her progress is not as favourable as expected it can be quite tiring and depressing with seemingly little return for maximum effort. If the labour is felt to have gone on for too long the woman may become irritable, particularly towards her partner (Beels, 1978), whom she may not realize is enduring the same emotions though obviously to a much lesser extent. In either the enjoyable or more difficult case the mother-to-be will appreciate the strength and support displayed by her partner, regardless of whether this is overtly expressed by her. Frustration may ensue at being instructed to push when the woman feels she is already at her limit and the numerous different commands by those present can seem like harassment despite the best intentions (Beels, 1978). The emergence of the baby's head can be a painful, overwhelming, bursting sensation.

Throughout the birthing process, the use of technological equipment for monitoring the vital signs of the baby may provoke anxiety in the mother that something is wrong, even though she may be sure in her own mind that all is well (Kitzinger, 1987). It may be disappointing to have other assistive intervention when difficulties arise if the woman had planned on managing the birth independently. It is often easy to lose sight of the reason for labour, that is, to give birth to new life, and instead focus on the gruelling nature of the task, forgetting the light at the end of the tunnel.

These two quite different scenarios illustrate the extremes of pleasure and pain that a labour and delivery can bring. Yet the individuality of each birth can mean that both positive and negative features are present during its course and this is usually the case. The woman's self-esteem and self-image are deeply influenced by her perceived success or failure at child bearing (Corkill, 1996). Having a caesarean section has a profound psychological impact on a woman. There is often a shattering of confidence, guilt and anxiety at the inability to perform the most natural womanly function of having a baby and it can be hurtful for these mothers to learn of complication-free vaginal deliveries (Kitzinger, 1987).

However, childbirth is not a pass or fail examination of womanhood or indeed motherhood. A normal birth is impossible to describe or achieve as there is really no such thing. Mothers should rejoice at the uniqueness of their birthing process, whether it be totally favourable or fraught with difficulty, and bear in mind that the importance lies in the outcome of a new baby arriving into the world.

If physiotherapists are aware of the diversity of human emotions during labour and delivery, they can offer a thorough selection of educational opportunities for women to gain maximum satisfaction from these events. Obviously teaching coping mechanisms is important to alleviate fear and apprehension but techniques of empowerment can be encouraged, including active participation in the birthing process and decreasing inhibition in preference to conservative strategies. Providing the woman with choices to facilitate these enables her to be self-determining during childbirth, rather than passively obeying instructions.

Emotional and Psychological Changes Associated with the Post-natal Period

There appears to be a series of emotions that may affect a new mother after she has given birth. These generally indicate the ease with which the woman is adjusting to motherhood and span from harmless in nature to quite dangerous with respect to her own and her child's well-being.

Normal emotional and psychological changes in the post-natal period

Following such a climactic process as pregnancy and giving birth, the hopes, preparations and excitement that had been escalating since the initial notification of the pregnancy turn to a feeling of being let down after the nine month wait is all over (Kitzinger, 1977). The majority of the new mother's life had been focused on the labour and delivery and when this state no longer exists an empty feeling can remain, despite the fact that she will immediately have her hands full caring for her newborn.

Approximately 40–60% of new mothers will experience some depression post-partum similar to premenstrual tension (BCFPND, 1996a) and this is quite normal bearing in mind the substantial immediate change to the woman's lifestyle. This can be attributed, more specifically, to the notion that the mother is living in a transitional state. She hovers between grieving over the loss of her past identity and idealized image of her baby to being preoccupied with the newborn, paranoid about its health and protective of the baby where hospital staff are concerned (Kitzinger, 1977). This mild transient depressive state has been termed the 'baby blues' and is not considered to be a mental illness. It has been associated with a difficult labour, a hospital rather than a home birth, the birth of a premature baby and a new mother who experiences violent mood swings (Kitzinger, 1977). Grieving will also be a prime issue in the cases where a baby is born ill, has a disability or is stillborn and these add complexity to the emotional issues associated with the birth alone.

The onset of the post-partum blues occurs on the third or fourth day following delivery and it can continue for up to a few weeks with obvious signs and symptoms being tearfulness, fatigue, irritability, labile mood, insomnia, anxiety and hostility towards her partner (BCFPND, 1996a). Apart from the mourning process associated with leaving her 'old' self in the past and overexaggerating the needs of her child, the mother may exhibit mannerisms associated with the trials of caring for a newborn, including analysing or lacking confidence in her mothering skills and feeling guilty for becoming emotional when the baby cries or behaves temperamentally (Kitzinger, 1977). Normally the new mother will become accustomed to the different demands being placed upon her and become more comfortable with her mothering role.

Abnormal emotional and psychological changes in the post-natal period

When there is adverse feeling almost all of the time after giving birth, despite having a well-behaved baby, the mother is moving further along the distress scale. If the gradual successful adaptation to the new lifestyle that most women experience does not occur then post-natal depression (PND) is imminent and this occurs in 15–20% of new mothers (BCFPND, 1996a). Instead there may be an incongruence between the mother's ideal life and reality, often precipitated by obsessional striving to live up to too high expectations. This superwoman syndrome, where the mother attempts to successfully juggle several aspects of her life in conjunction with the new baby (Auchincloss, personal communication), leads to dejection when plans fail to come to fruition.

Post-partum depression can be a direct extension of the baby blues with respect to the symptoms experienced, though more severe and persistent. The symptoms of this distressful phenomenon may, however, develop a few weeks or months post-partum when the blues have long ago subsided (Sved-Williams, 1995). The Brisbane Centre for Postnatal Disorders (BCFPND) defines an average onset of within six weeks post-childbirth and a duration of two weeks to one year. Ongoing PND may exist where subsequent pregnancies occur (BCFPND, 1996a).

It appears that symptoms of PND are the same as those that are prevalent at other lifestyle stages (O'Hara et al, 1990), except the frequency of specific traits such as high anxiety, irritability (Boyce and Stubbs, 1994), fear, panic attacks and obsessional thoughts about the baby are higher in PND (Buist, 1995). More generally, though, the woman may display overt signs to observers or complain of a variety of problems. These include:

- crying a lot or crying about small upsets;
- hating herself;
- hating her baby because she feels he/she is inconvenient and unpredictable;
- denial of her baby's existence;
- being afraid of harming her baby;
- sleeping poorly despite her baby being asleep;
- being terrified of being alone;
- not feeling any sex drive (libido);
- feeling she cannot cope with anything, e.g. housework;
- appetite disturbance;
- agitation or retardation;
- poor memory and poor concentration;
- feelings of inadequacy;
- guilt feelings over performance as a mother;
- insomnia;
- fatigue;
- complaints of ill health;
- mood swings;
- social withdrawal;
- despondency;
- tension in relationships, especially with her partner (Sved-Williams, 1995; BCFPND, 1996a).

There appears to be inconclusive evidence as to a single cause of PND and prevailing views reflect a multifactorial approach contributing to its development. Biological, gynaecological, obstetric, psychopathological, cognitive-behavioural, sociocultural and psychosocial factors are thought to be involved (Chen, 1995).

Specifically, causes of PND include hormonal changes at the end of pregnancy affecting women whose brain chemistry is vulnerable, particularly a dramatic decrease in oestrogen and progesterone (Buist, 1995); an irritable baby who sleeps very little; a mother's general lack of self-confidence; lack of support from significant others; the mother having had a difficult upbringing herself; being a perfectionist; past history of depression for any reason; physical problems following childbirth; and having a premature baby or one that is suffering with particular health problems (Sved-Williams, 1995). This list is by no means exhaustive.

Buist (1995) believes that some women are at particular risk of the disorder. These risk factors include a past history or family history of depression, past history of premenstrual tension, past history of abuse as a child, obsessional personality and problems with a partner or marital difficulties. Other contributors to a more likely incidence of PND have been early discharge post-delivery (especially in the first 24 hours afterwards) (Boyce, personal communication), lack of support (Dennerstein et al, 1989), obstetric interventions during childbirth (Astbury et al, 1994), being a young mother (Chapman, 1995), a history of infertility or being a mature mother, with the latter being due to unreal expectations of herself whilst leading a multifaceted life.

It is imperative that physiotherapists are aware of the signs and symptoms associated with PND as often these health professionals have ongoing contact with new mothers as they strive to regain physical attributes, improve fitness, form sound ergonomic habits while caring for their new baby, manage stress, achieve relaxation and manage any specific pathological conditions arising from giving birth.

Screening for PND should be performed by any health professional as a regular part of post-partum care because the disorder is common and after childbirth is a period in which women have substantial dealings with the medical profession. It is often difficult to detect PND due to the similarities between the characteristic symptoms suffered and those of the normal post-partum scene (Quayle, 1995). The Edinburgh Postnatal Depression Scale (EPDS) is a 10-item questionnaire widely used in many countries to assist in the screening process approximately 6–8 weeks post-partum (Cox et al, 1987).

Often women feel ashamed of admitting the existence of difficulties in the post-natal period, particularly if they have always coped well with life problems in the past and have never sought any personal or professional assistance or they have expectations of perfection surrounding the care of their newborn baby and own personal well-being. Recognizing that she is experiencing the effects of a condition and accepting that a course of action is necessary are the first steps a woman takes in the resolution of PND (Sved-Williams, 1995).

With assistance, women with PND should experience some improvement in approximately six weeks (Quayle, 1995), so early identification is extremely valuable in preventing the unnecessary continuation of problems. Physiotherapists may often detect the existence of PND through their communication and observation skills with new mothers. They may also assist in the woman's realization of her individual problems post-partum, enforcing their seriousness, reassuring her that shame is not warranted and offering advice as to the appropriate opportunities for professional help.

It may be that with the support of an understanding partner or family, a woman is able to remedy her situation. Certain lifestyle changes may assist, including having time away from her baby if it is happy and healthy, participating in regular exercise, spending time by herself and with her partner, as well as being involved in adult conversation (Auchincloss, personal communication). These may help the woman feel a more complete person rather than solely existing as a mother. She obtains a break from any stresses that exist and can take pleasure in some activities from her previous days, whilst being assured that her baby is safe and being cared for.

If a woman feels isolated or embarrassed about her inability to cope independently, however, she may opt for professional advice immediately in preference to consulting loved ones (Sved-Williams, 1995). Certainly today's society maintains the belief that a new mother should be successful in the simultaneous management of her home life, family, marriage, busy career and social commitments, not to mention caring for an often temperamental new baby. In response to society's pressures, the mother may not wish to worry or burden those around her and is also able to keep the situation private.

It is crucial that physiotherapists and other health professionals treating this client group recognize and acknowledge the existence of post-natal depression. It also helps to hasten the process of obtaining assistance for new mothers with PND if service providers having early and / or ongoing contact with them have access to information about the condition.

Physiotherapists could liaise with community and family health service nurses, general practitioners or community health centres to acquire this knowledge and there are a number of books on the subject for both health professionals and new mothers (Sved-Williams, 1995). However, if problems persist despite education it is appropriate to refer the client for more specialized assistance.

Professional assistance can take the form of medication, stress management, discussion about the current situation and marital intervention (Chapman, 1995). PND needs to be managed in terms of the family unit, including the partner and the baby (Buist, 1995), as all can suffer the effects and in fact there is potential for long-term consequences on the cognitive development of the infant (Murray, 1992).

Cognitive behaviour therapy programmes are available in some areas and focus on the role transition from career woman to mother and the accompanying sense of loss, coping with increased workloads, stress and conflict resolution strategies, assertion skills, support network advice, myths of motherhood and aspects of PND development (BCFPND, 1996b). Round-the-clock services exist in a number of areas. Contact the social work department for a list of resource / support centres. GPs may refer the new mother with PND to a psychiatrist (Sved-Williams, 1995).

Support groups are also available where women have the opportunity to take charge and self-manage their situations and this may be an option for those concerned with not overburdening their families and friends or those who have high expectations of themselves. A listening approach to PND treatment empowers women to make individual decisions.

The Brisbane Centre for Post-natal Disorders is an example of a centre which promotes such services as inpatient and outpatient treatment for the mother and her child, a PND clinic, fathers' group, ante-natal education, consultation liaison service, telephone counselling and health professional education.

Special support organizations may offer telephone counselling by women who have previously suffered from PND and can therefore empathize, as well as liaison with a number of professionals. Courses and group contact may be available. It is recommended that the woman consult her GP before contacting a support organization simply to ensure the prescription of medications, if necessary, and to establish that no health risks to the woman and her child are apparent (Sved-Williams, 1995). It is also advised that before embarking on another pregnancy the woman should wait till her child is two years of age and she has ceased medication for at least a year, due to the high risk of relapse in subsequent pregnancies (Buist, 1995).

Inpatient treatment is indicated in the case of moderate to severe symptoms of PND with inadequate community or family support, worsening illness or failure to respond to outpatient treatment or a suicidal or infanticidal mother (Buist, 1995). Along the continuum of post-natal disorders, the most severe in nature is when a woman exhibits post-partum psychosis and this in fact constitutes a psychiatric emergency. The onset of this condition, on average within the first two weeks (Sved-Williams, 1995), has been shown to be associated with increased sensitivity of dopamine receptors in the hypothalamus, which may be triggered by the sharp fall in circulating oestrogen concentrations (Wieck et al, 1991).

Post-partum psychosis occurs in 1–2 women per 1000 deliveries (BCFPND, 1996a), particularly in women with bipolar mood disorder and in those with a history of previous mental illness (Kitzinger, 1977). They may either be manic or depressed. Signs and symptoms of mania include irritability, euphoria, confusion, hyperactivity, poor judgement, inability to adequately care for themselves or their baby and feeling little need for sleep. Depression, as a subcategory of post-partum psychosis, is more pronounced than in PND with the mother exhibiting volatile behaviour and experiencing command hallucinations and delusions that her baby is impaired or even dead. She may feel perplexity, guilt concerning her lack of love for her child or overconcern for the baby's health or safety (BCFPND, 1996a). With the risk of infanticide and suicide inherent in post-partum psychosis, the need increases for physiotherapists to identify the warning signs and refer the woman to the appropriate professional agencies for help, as with the occurrence of PND.

Physiotherapists have an ongoing contribution to make to the physical and psychological domains of women's health along the path from pregnancy to the post-partum period, in order to provide this client group with total care. Physiotherapy education sessions need to focus on varied techniques to benefit women with different schools of thought and individual personalities and be flexible enough to allow discussion on emotional issues as well as physical facts. An awareness of normal and abnormal psychological parameters is paramount, as is the judgement to realize when referral elsewhere is warranted for the mother's safety and that of her baby.

References

Astbury J, Brown S, Lumley J and Small R (1994) Birth events, birth experiences and social differences in post-natal depression. *Australian Journal of Public Health* **18**: 176–184.

BCFPND (Brisbane Centre for Post-natal Disorders) (1996a) Post partum affective disorders. Statistical newsletter.

BCFPND (Brisbane Centre for Post-natal Disorders) (1996b) Effects of post-natal disorders on children. Newsletter No 2, January.

Beels C (1978) *The Childbirth Book*, pp. 117–179. London: Turnstone Books.

Boyce PM and Stubbs JM (1994) The importance of postnatal depression. *Medical Journal of Australia* **161**: 471–472.

Buist A (1995) Postnatal depression. *Medical Observer Continuing Medical Education* **June**: 1–2.

Chapman M (1995) Conference report on post-natal disorders. *Australian Doctor* **22nd September**: 41–42.

Chen CH (1995) Etiology of post-partum depression – a review. *Kao-Hsiung-I-Hsueh-Ko-Hsueh-Tsa-Chih* **11**(1): 1–7.

Corkill A (1996) Effects of the birth of a first baby on a couple's sexual relationship. *British Journal of Midwifery* **4**(2): 70–73.

Cox JL, Holden JM and Sagovsky R (1987) Detection of post-natal depression, development of the 10 item postnatal depression scale. *British Journal of Psychiatry* **150**: 782–786.

Dennerstein L, Lehert P and Riphagen F (1989) Postpartum depression – risk factors. *Journal of Psychosomatic Obstetrics and Gynaecology* **10** (Suppl): 53–65.

Henneborn WJ and Cogan R (1975) The effect of husband participation on reported pain and probability of medication during labor and birth. *Journal of Psychosomatic Research* **19**: 215–222.

Jimenez MH and Newton N (1982) Job orientation and adjustment to pregnancy and early motherhood. *Birth* **9**(3): 157–163.

Kitzinger S (1977) *Education and Counselling for Childbirth*, pp. 89–111, 265–270. London: Baillière Tindall.

Kitzinger S (1986) *Pregnancy and Childbirth*, pp. 188–190. London: Doubleday Australia Pty Ltd.

Kitzinger S (1987) *Giving Birth – How It Really Feels*. London: Victor Gollancz Ltd.

Murray L (1992) The impact of postnatal depression on infant development. *Journal of Psychology and Psychiatry* **33**: 543–561.

O'Hara MW, Zekoski EM, Philipps LH and Wright EJ (1990) Controlled prospective study of postpartum mood disorders: comparison of childbearing and nonchildbearing women. *Journal of Abnormal Psychology* **99**: 3–15.

Price J (1988) *Motherhood – What It Does to Your Mind*. London: Pandora.

Quayle S (1995) Therapy update. *Australian Doctor – Continuing Medical Education* **9th June**: 67–68.

Sved-Williams A (1995) Postpartum depression and the baby blues. *BLISS Newsletter* 7: 1–8.

Sweet BR (1982) *Mayes' Midwifery: A Textbook for Midwives*, 11th edn. London: Baillière Tindall.

Wieck A, Kumar R, Hirst AD et al (1991) Increased sensitivity of dopamine receptors and recurrence of affective psychosis after childbirth. *British Medical Journal* **303**(6803): 613–616.

13

Perinatal Sexuality

JANE HOWARD

Effect of Pregnancy on Sexuality and Sexual Behaviour
•
Effect of Lactation on Sexuality

Perinatal sexual experience varies for different women. There are many factors which influence the psychological and physical changes in sexuality in pregnancy and the puerperium, including:

- personal and cultural beliefs;
- nature of the sexual relationship;
- health and mood;
- medical restrictions;
- belief in myths: sex in pregnancy is taboo; pregnant women are unclean; intercourse will harm the woman/ foetus;
- health of the baby;
- episiotomy;
- fatigue.

Effect of Pregnancy on Sexuality and Sexual Behaviour

Many studies have shown a declining libido and sexual enjoyment for women as pregnancy progresses (Barclay et al, 1994; Masters and Johnson, 1966; Solberg et al, 1973). In early pregnancy this has been attributed to tiredness, nausea and sore breasts. In later pregnancy it has been attributed to increasing girth causing a negative effect on body image and also difficulty in finding a comfortable position. There is also a fear of harming the baby. It has been suggested that dyspareunia and apareunia are common in the last trimester, with many women ceasing intercourse because of physical discomfort (Reamy et al, 1982; Solberg et al, 1973). The response of the partner to the pregnancy and the changing body image may be positive or negative.

The effect of sexual intercourse on the foetus is an area of controversy. Some research has shown an increase in foetal distress in the babies of women who were still having sexual intercourse prior to labour. Other research finds no increase. Some women avoid intercourse in late pregnancy in case they harm the foetus.

Post-partum sexuality

Much confusion exists about the actual time to resume sexual intercourse after childbirth and so unsubstantiated advice is often given by health professionals. Studies have shown that women vary in their return to sexual activity. There may be a diminished desire and decreased frequency of intercourse for up to two years (Bing and Colman, 1977). Masters and Johnson (1966) showed that a group of lactating women resumed intercourse within 2–3 weeks of delivery and reported higher levels of sexual tension than prior to their pregnancy. For others, the enormous burden of caring for a new baby causes tension, anxiety and tiredness and the extra workload decreased sexual desire.

Post-natal depression affects about one in 10 women and is often undiagnosed for long periods of time. Symptoms of fatigue, loss of libido, hostility and confusion are common. Post-partum, men are likely to feel excluded from the emotional attachment of the mother with her baby and this may also affect the sexual relationship.

Bleeding from the placental site on the uterine wall ceases at 2–4 weeks post-partum and episiotomies may be healed by this time, so that intercourse can occur any time after two weeks post-partum, when the couple are ready. However, it has been reported by Abraham et al (1990) that one in five women takes more than two months to achieve comfortable intercourse. In a recent survey, 60% of the respondents experienced post-natal superficial dyspareunia (Hay-Smith and Mantle, 1996).

Effect of Lactation on Sexuality

High levels of prolactin hormone in lactating women cause low sexual desire. Low oestrogen levels in lactating women may cause the vaginal skin to be thin and atrophic and lack of lubrication causes dyspareunia. Breasts may be sore in lactation and let-down may occur in sexual arousal, causing embarrassment or making a mess to be cleaned up later. Some women are sexually stimulated by breast feeding and if they reach orgasm in this manner they may feel guilt.

In general terms, women are likely to have decreas desire and sexual activity as pregnancy progresse partner's reaction to pregnancy may affect sexual acti Post-partum there is a major change in the woman's life an sexuality is likely to be affected in a negative way. The extra work involved in caring for a new baby, lack of sleep, anxiety and depression may all affect women's sexuality.

References

Abraham S, Child A, Ferry J et al (1990) Recovery after childbirth: a preliminary prospective study. *Medical Journal of Australia* **152**: 9–12.

Barclay L, McDonald P and Loughlin J (1994) Sexuality and pregnancy: an interview study. *Australian and New Zealand Journal of Obstetrics and Gynaecology* **34**: 1–7.

Bing E and Colman L (1977) Cited in Fogel C and Lauver D (1990) *Sexual Health Promotion.* London: Harcourt Brace Jovanovich.

Hay-Smith J and Mantle J (1996) Surveys of the experience and perceptions of post-natal superficial dyspareunia of post-natal women, general practitioners and physiotherapists. *Physiotherapy* **82**: 91–97.

Masters W and Johnson V (1966) *Human Sexual Response.* Boston: Little Brown.

Reamy R, White S, Darvell W et al (1982) Sexuality and pregnancy: a prospective study. *Journal of Reproductive Medicine* **27**: 321–327.

Solberg D, Butler J and Wagner N (1973) Sexual behaviour in pregnancy. *New England Journal of Medicine* **288**: 1098.

Further reading

Kitzinger S (1985) *Women's Experience of Sex.* London: Penguin.

14

Musculoskeletal Changes Associated with the Perinatal Period

JOANNE BULLOCK-SAXTON

The extraordinarily rapid physiological and physical changes which occur during the ante-natal and post-natal period require significant musculoskeletal adaptation. These changes may be implicated in the development of pain syndromes which may need to be controlled or relieved by physiotherapy intervention. In addition, latent problems of a musculoskeletal nature existing prior to pregnancy may be exacerbated due to the pregnancy itself or the woman may sustain a musculoskeletal injury unrelated to the pregnancy. In each case, physiotherapy management may be required.

Chapters 10 and 11 have described many of the physiological changes associated with pregnancy, including the increase of hormonal concentrations, the release of relaxin (MacLennan, 1983), the changes in blood volume and respiratory rate (Chapter 11), as well as the development and growth of the foetus (Chapter 10). Each of these may directly or indirectly affect the musculoskeletal system. Foetal growth alone is responsible for one of the most obvious musculoskeletal changes associated with pregnancy, which is the expansion of the abdomen.

While there are many musculoskeletal disorders potentially influenced by pregnancy, there are some which are particularly common and require specific focus. Posture, development of spinal or pelvic pain and the lengthening of abdominal and pelvic floor muscles are common to most pregnant women. The relationships between pregnancy and these features, as well as relevant physiotherapy interventions, are the focus of this section. The pelvic floor dysfunctions associated with the puerperium are thoroughly discussed in Chapter 23 and will not be addressed here, although clearly, they do fall within the scope of musculoskeletal disorders.

Neuromuscular and Articular Relationships

To understand the influence of pregnancy on the musculoskeletal system, it is important to recognize the interactions which occur with any imposed change. The musculoskeletal system is composed of three subsystems: the muscular, articular and neural systems. Janda (1978) has asserted that it is impossible to have damage or change in any one system without its being reflected in each of the other two systems. Current research has provided justification for this proposal. However, in their attempt to relieve pain and discomfort, clinicians may inadvertently neglect to consider the 'wider' view of presenting symptoms. Such an omission is often reflected in recurrence of the patient's symptoms some time later. By considering each of the three associated subsystems, the clinician can evaluate the patient's pain or dysfunction in a global manner.

One of the most significant changes to the musculoskeletal system early in pregnancy is in the degree of passive restraint offered by the collagenous tissues surrounding the articulations. Hainline (1994) explains that oestrogen causes proliferation of connective tissue and that relaxin acts to provide vascularization and softening of this connective tissue. It is not surprising, therefore, that increases in joint laxity can be measured in multiple joints during pregnancy (Calguneri et al, 1982). The most notable biomechanical effects of the influence of these hormones is in the symphysis pubis where the width has been reported to increase from 0.5 mm to 12 mm and where vertical displacement of the symphysis may result. Such a change in the passive restraint of any joint is bound to have significant influences on the afferent input to the spinal cord and higher cortical centres. Certainly studies of the proprioceptive acuity of subjects with hypermobile joints indicate that they have a lesser sensitivity than subjects with normal joint mobility (Hall et al, 1995; Mallik et al, 1994). Prospective research into the effect of pregnancy hormones on joint proprioceptive acuity could help to explain many of the clinically observed changes in gait and balance which appear to take place prior to any major changes occurring in uterine size. Studies of the long-term effects of such alterations in ligament and capsular laxity could contribute much to our understanding of joint degeneration.

While the muscle spindle is undoubtedly the primary organ responsible for proprioceptive sense, the role of the joints should not be discounted. On the basis of their research, Johannsson et al (1991) have developed a convincing argument for the importance of the influence of articular mechanoreceptor reflexes on the preprogramming of muscle stiffness via the gamma motor neurone loop, i.e. via regulation of the muscle spindle tension. Extrapolation of this information for the pregnant woman suggests not only that joint movement is less restricted by ligaments and capsule but also that muscle stiffness may be reduced, leading to a decrease in muscle responsiveness to perturbations. This may be one reason for clinical reports of a sense of decreased balance during pregnancy.

Many research studies have provided an insight into the characteristic muscle responses associated with changes in joint afferent information. While these studies have not focused upon pregnancy, their findings have some relevance when the implications of musculoskeletal disorders are being considered. It is therefore of value to review such findings in the broad context of muscle response to articular changes. In early animal studies, Ekholm et al (1960) investigated the response to various articular stimuli of the decerebrate and, in some cases, the spinalized cat. They found that increasing the articular pressure, as well as pinching the articular capsule, led to quadriceps (i.e. extensor) inhibition, while pinching the knee capsule elicited a response from the knee flexors (biceps femoris). Two decades later, Stokes and Young (1984) studied human muscles and considered that joint injury can inhibit the activity of muscles, leading to weakness and wasting. They measured the rectified integrated EMG of both quadriceps muscles of patients who had had a meniscetomy by arthroscopy and recorded large decreases (80%) in quadriceps (i.e. extensor) activation on the side of surgery. Inhibition persisted for up to 15 days post-operatively (30–40%), despite the lack of pain at this time. A possible mechanism for this inhibition might be the stimulation of those joint afferents in the capsule which are receptive to pressure caused by joint effusion. Indeed, in 1965, De Andrade et al (1965) revealed that in normal human subjects and those with pathology, infusion of saline into the knee joint was responsible for decreased activation of the quadriceps. Results of recent studies by Iles et al (1990) have indicated that as the volume of effusion is increased, the amplitude of H-reflex is decreased and that even apparently *imperceptible volumes* of saline could inhibit quadriceps activation. In these studies, the inhibition of the joint extensors following changes in the afferent stimulation from the joints has been highlighted.

These muscular responses are not only localized to the area of injury. Freeman and Wyke (1966) contributed much to the understanding of the activity of many muscles of the lower limb and the importance of afferent information from the joint for normal regulation of muscle activity. Although it is difficult to extrapolate results from animal studies to human behaviour, Wyke's (1967) observations must be noted. He observed that in the cat, an injury of the capsule and/or ligaments influences muscle activity not only in muscles which cross the injured joint, but also in those which are remote from it. Wyke stressed the fact that 'Interruption of the flow of impulses from the mechanoreceptors in a joint capsule into the central nervous system should result in clinically evident disturbances of perception of joint position and movement and of the reflexes concerned with posture and gait'. Wyke also argued that the articular sensory information was vital to normal postural reflexes. Thus, the arthrokinetic reflex might be considered as a triggering factor which would initiate a whole chain of adaptation reactions, eventually resulting in a changed movement pattern. The possibility that sensory deficits associated with localized injury in one part of the body influence muscle function in another and may ultimately lead to pain has considerable implications for the physiotherapist, influencing both the preventive and therapeutic approaches to patient care.

The inter-relationships between articular, muscular and neural system are now being considered more broadly by researchers from a variety of fields. Such progress will assist in the eventual understanding of human responses to injury and the development of effective treatment protocols. For instance, Coderre and Melzack (1987) described an augmented pain sensitivity in a much wider central nervous distribution than might be expected following injury. These authors were investigating responses to pain stimuli and noted a decrease in the threshold for stimulation in the dorsal horn neurones which influenced the response of efferent pathways to further sensory stimuli. Woolf (1983) has reported similar central nervous adaptations to altered afferent input and recorded these on the contralateral limb. Grubb et al (1993) have recently reported changes in spinal neurone receptive fields ipsilaterally, contralaterally and at different segmental levels in rats with chronic inflammation of the ankle joint, where afferent information has been distorted by injury. Such research portrays the potential global effect of an injury or a change in afferent information not only on the ipsilateral spinal cord connections, but also with contralateral, ascending and descending neurones. As the neural pathways influence the afferent and efferent pathways in each of these spinal cord areas, the effect of a single injury, potentially, can be magnified and reflected throughout sites of the body.

The relevance of these studies to the physiotherapist dealing with musculoskeletal disorders is that they highlight the need to recognize the pattern of changes in the muscular and neural systems as a result of changes in the afferent information to the joint. These changes are not only local but also extend throughout the body. It is clear that treatment for musculoskeletal disorders must address all components of the system and must reflect a broad perspective of the body. An example is given below.

A pregnant woman (18 weeks) presents to your clinic complaining of low back pain which is worse at the end of the day and has been bothering her for the last three weeks. She suffered a very brief incident of back pain one year ago, which settled within a few days of rest. Her occupation as a physical education teacher at a secondary school involves being on her feet frequently throughout the day. The subjective examination reveals to you that the pain is worse on the days that she goes for a (3 km) jog and is relieved primarily by bed rest and heat. Her previous medical history is insignificant, although when you enquire about previous lower limb injuries she mentions that she had a severe ankle sprain four years ago. She thinks her ankle sprain was on the right-hand side. She is not on any medications, suffers from no neurological symptoms and is generally healthy.

On observation of the patient's posture, it is clear that her right forefoot demonstrates more pronation, her femur is more internally rotated on the right and the pelvis is anteriorly tilted and rotated around the transverse axis in a counter-clockwise direction. The muscles of the gluteal region on the right appear to be weaker and there is an increased activity of the lumbar erector spinae (more predominant on the left). During gait, the patient has a shorter stance phase on the right, limited by decreased right hip extension. Adequate relative hip extension on the right side for the toe off phase is generated by hyperextension of the lumbar spine. Active movement tests demonstrate a reproduction of the patient's type and area of pain by extension of the spine and by a posterior anterior directed pressure on the L5 and L4 vertebral levels. Neither of these spinal levels is assessed as stiff during palpation. The gluteals on the right-hand side are weak on muscle testing.

Local treatment to the spinal level provides immediate relief of symptoms which lasts no longer than a few days. Treatment directed at normalizing the lower limb muscle length, strengthening the gluteals, providing an insole to correct the forefoot pronation and increasing the speed of activation of the abdominals and gluteals via conscious activation and then proprioceptive training to stabilize the lumbar spine and pelvis during gait proves to have an effect on eliminating the pain over the long term.

Such a case illustrates the interactivity of different body parts. It is quite likely that the original ankle sprain was sufficient to instigate subtle changes in the recruitment and activation of the pelvic muscles (Bullock-Saxton, 1991, 1994). Over time, these changes, as well as the injury itself, may have caused changes in the posture and thus biomechanics of the lower limb and, subsequently, the pelvis. Decreased activation of the muscles and poor joint biomechanics may then have been exacerbated in the pregnancy due to changes in joint laxity. At this stage, the subclinical adaptations were exaggerated and pain was a result. Treatment of the local site (L4 and L5) only was not effective, as this was merely the site where musculoskeletal changes of other body parts were reflected, i.e. the symptom and not the cause. The cause in this case was multifactorial and required a similar therapeutic approach. The relevance to clinical practice is that assessment and treatment must encompass a review of all three subsystems.

The Influence of Pregnancy on Posture

Postural adaptations appear to be a natural consequence of pregnancy. Of concern to physiotherapists is the nature and degree of any individual's postural adaptations to the constantly changing forces upon them, as well as the possible maintenance of new postures in the post-natal period. The physiotherapist must place emphasis on directing and training women to ensure that their newly assumed posture does not overstress any one body segment since the outcome of this could be fatigue, microtrauma and pain.

The most obvious physical features in pregnancy influencing the woman's posture are the alterations in body mass and the consequent changes in the centre of gravity. Apart from the growth of the foetus, which at term weighs approximately 3.5 kg, the woman's body mass increases because of growth of the uterus, placenta and membranes and the increased volume of amniotic fluid and circulating blood (O'Connor, 1969). Danforth (1967) estimates that part of the approximate 9 kg total increase is due to an increase in breast size, added fat and, in particular, retention of fluid provoked by the level of oestrogens (Hainline, 1994; O'Connor, 1969).

Because of the implications for musculoskeletal changes and subsequent pain, it is important to consider the nature of any postural adaptation in some detail. It is also important to review these postural responses both during and after pregnancy and to consider the role physiotherapy may play in ensuring the alignment of the body minimizes joint stress and the development of pain.

Normal posture

Descriptions of the correct upright position vary in their emphasis. A lot of attention was paid to postural definitions by mid-20th century authors and their ideas are still relevant today. Segmental alignment, pelvic inclination, carriage of the head and neck, the distribution of the weight on the feet, the curves of the spine, abdominal protuberance, chest position and centre of gravity are all mentioned by various authors (Massey, 1943). Definitions may be categorized as descriptive or anatomical.

From a descriptive point of view, Basmajian (1965) has proposed that in a limited sense, posture could be considered to be the upright, well-balanced stance of the human subject in a 'normal' position. In the same vein, Calliet (1981) claims that static spinal configuration can be considered 'good posture' if it is effortless, non-fatiguing and painless when the individual remains erect for reasonable periods. Kendall et al (1993) remind us that an evaluation of postural faults necessitates a standard by which individual postures may be judged. They quote the Posture Committee of the American Academy of Orthopedic Surgeons' concept of good posture as being that state of muscular and skeletal balance which protects the supporting structures of the body against injury or progressive deformity irrespective of the attitude in which they are working. Under such conditions, muscles function most efficiently and optimum positions are provided for thoracic and abdominal organs.

Anatomically, the definition of normal posture is described in terms of the relationships of the body and its parts to the line of gravity (Massey, 1943). For example, Basmajian (1965) has stated that to maintain equilibrium in a standing posture with the least expenditure of internal energy, a vertical line dropped from the centre of gravity should fall downward through an inert supporting column of bones. Kendall et al (1952) referred to this as the vertical intersection line of two planes of reference (frontal and sagittal), each of which hypothetically divides the body into two sections of equal weight. This line is analogous to the gravity line. In the idealized normal erect posture, the line of gravity passes through the mastoid processes, a point just in front of the shoulder joints, the hip joints (or just behind), and just in front of the knee and ankle joints. According to Hollinshead (1976), its relationship with the spine is that it passes through C7 and T1, in front of most of the thoracic region, but again through the vertebral bodies at about the thoracolumbar junction. In the lumbar region it passes close to the centre of L4. When so situated, the least energy expenditure is required of the back musculature (Floyd and Silver, 1950; Portnoy and Morin, 1956). Hollinshead (1976) maintains that if one of the spinal curves is exaggerated so as to throw the line of gravity too far from its usual position, it can be restored without additional musculature strain only by altering a curve in the opposite direction. Some evidence of this was supplied by Cureton and Wickens (1935), who found a low but significant inverse relationship between kyphosis and the gravity line of the body.

It is clear that the 'ideal' posture, so described here, is not really the 'normal' posture. Individual and ethnic variations abound and it is these variations, as well as the degree of their difference from 'ideal', which appear to change with the progression of the pregnancy.

Postural changes associated with pregnancy

A review of the literature on the determination of the exact nature of the postural changes associated with pregnancy offers a somewhat confusing picture. While there is general consensus in the literature that changes occur, there are differing opinions as to what form these changes take. Many of the initial comments about postural changes during pregnancy were based on clinical observation and it was not until the late 1970s and 1980s that a series of objective measurements were performed on women during their pregnancy to determine the exact nature of the postural changes. Unfortunately, even with objective measurements, there is still confusion as to the nature of the adaptation. Hummel (1987) has tried to classify the nature of the centre of gravity change and the various options that may be associated with this. He reports a tendency to an increased anterior displacement of the line of gravity in pregnant females. However, this is not significantly different from normal individuals. Hummel suggests that the natural tendency to anterior displacement may be counterbalanced by a number of options such as increased activation of the gastrocnemius and soleus muscles, an active posterior displacement of the body (which would require increased muscular effort), extension of the hip joint or posterior displacement of the upper trunk. It is clear that the mechanisms that may be used to achieve an active posterior displacement of the body may include increase of the lumbosacral angle, an increase of the lumbar curvature or a displacement of the pelvis anteriorly with a simultaneous displacement of the shoulders posteriorly, which may be reflected in greater degrees of thoracic kyphosis. Table 14.1 details the various adaptations listed by authors interested in this topic.

The general consensus is that there is an exaggeration of the lumbar curvature and possibly the thoracic curvature, although the description of the means by which these changes occur differs. Some argue that there is an increase in the lumbosacral angle due to posterior displacement of the upper trunk and an anterior shift of the pelvis (extending the hip). Others suggest an active increase in lumbar lordosis to compensate for the abdominal enlargement.

Table 14.1 Proposed postural adaptations during pregnancy

Postural change	Reference
Increased lumbar lordosis	Sands, 1958; Spankus, 1965; Bullock et al, 1987; Hummell, 1987; Bullock-Saxton, 1991; Dumas et al, 1995a
Anteriorly displaced sacrum	Sands, 1958; Spankus, 1965
Posterior displacement of the trunk, thus increasing the lumbar lordosis	Rhodes, 1958; Danforth, 1967; Nwuga, 1982; Hummell, 1987
Bending forward over enlarging uterus	Cyriax, 1965
Extension of the hip joint	Hummell, 1987
Flattening of the lumbar spine	Snijders et al, 1976
Increased thoracic kyphosis	Bullock-Saxton, 1991; Hummell, 1987

In contrast to the predicted increase in lumbar lordosis during pregnancy, Snijders et al's (1976) study of the posture of pregnant women found that a straightening of the lumbar spine occurred in their Dutch subjects. A recent study by Dumas et al (1995) from Canada assessed posture in 65 women during pregnancy and the effect of participating in an exercise programme during pregnancy. Two groups were formed with one receiving the exercise intervention and the other no intervention (controls). Measurements of lordosis and kyphosis were calculated from a lateral photograph of the subject with markers placed on various spinous processes from T1 to L5. Four assessments were made, three during the pregnancy and one post-partum. Results revealed that in the control group the lordosis steadily increased over the pregnancy and was maintained in the post-partum period. However, in the exercise group the lordosis increased to the second trimester, decreased in the third trimester and increased again at the post-partum period. On the other hand, little change in the kyphosis curvature was found over the entire period of pregnancy.

The changes identified by Dumas et al (1995a) seem to agree with those reported by Bullock-Saxton (1991) who found an increase in lordosis during pregnancy (Bullock et al, 1987) and a maintenance of that lordosis post pregnancy (Bullock-Saxton, 1991). In contrast, however, Bullock-Saxton (1991) found that the kyphosis also changed during pregnancy. Hummel (1987) also reported an increase in the sagittal profile of the lumbar spine and the thoracic spine after the 30th week of pregnancy. However, Hummel was careful to explain that while in some subjects the curves increased markedly, in others they did not, while in some subjects flattening of curves appeared to occur. Other authors studying the effect of pregnancy on the lumbar curve (Östgaard et al, 1993) have found no significant change in depth of lumbar curve during pregnancy. Differences in research findings throughout the world may represent differences in measurement technique, time of assessment during the pregnancy, ethnic differences in initial posture type as well as the initial pre-pregnancy postures of the women to be tested.

Another fascinating result of Dumas et al's (1995a) study is the effect of parity on lordosis in the last eight weeks of pregnancy. Those women who had borne more than one child prior to the current pregnancy showed a marked increase in the degree of lordosis, particularly at the third trimester. By the post-partum period, the lordosis had slightly decreased but was still significantly greater than in women who had no previous children. Dumas et al (1995a) suggested that this could reflect a difference in the daily functional activities between the two groups, where women with other children may be involved in carrying them and may also have a higher housework load. Such a daily routine could cause fatigue and so prevent the women from maintaining lumbar stability.

It is clear that while the general trend in the literature suggests an exaggeration in the spinal curves during pregnancy, it is essential that each woman be assessed individually. It is the opinion of the author that the nature of the spinal curve changes occurring during pregnancy are related to the woman's prior pregnancy curvature. For instance, a pre-pregnancy posture that incorporated some degree of anterior pelvic shift, hip extension and posterior translation of the upper trunk would be likely to be exaggerated during pregnancy.

To date, no study has attempted to classify the women's posture in the early stages of pregnancy and monitor the nature of adaptations in relation to this classification. Such a prospective study would be somewhat time consuming, but well worth while for an understanding of pregnancy-induced postural adaptations.

Kendall et al (1993) have defined certain posture types in comparison to the so-called 'ideal posture' , e.g. flat back; kypholordosis or sway back. In posture observation, the clinician usually makes a judgement regarding the postural type of the client. Landmarks such as pelvic inclination, the position of the line of gravity and the depth and extent of lumbar and thoracic curvatures provide the clinical cues to allow a classification. Table 14.2 identifies the differences in alignment, quality of curvature and relationship with the line of gravity, all of which are considered in the classification process. Such classification forms the basis upon which physiotherapists assess qualitative aspects of posture and joint control during movement. With this in mind, it seems reasonable to argue that many of the objective studies to date have identified and measured spinal posture in a rather gross fashion, considering many spinal segments all together. Posture studies need to address issues associated with other important features such as initial posture classification, the sites of maximum curvature depth and transition between curves, joint stiffness and control and document these progressively through pregnancy. Figures 14.1–14.3 highlight the differences in characteristic postures between pregnant women (Figs 14.1a and 14.2a), as well as the differences in posture presentation when two pregnant women fall within the same category (Figs 14.2a and 14.3a). Figure 14.1a illustrates a woman 14 weeks pregnant whose

Table 14.2 Body positions influencing the judgement of postural type

Body part	Ideal	Kypholordosis	Sway back	Flat back
Head	Neutral position log: through external auditory meatus	Forward log: slightly posterior to the external auditory meatus	Forward log: through the occipital bone	Forward log: through occipital bone
Cervical spine	Slightly convex anteriorly log: through the dens/odontoid process of the axis, through the bodies of the cervical vertebrae	Hyperextended log: only passes through some of the upper cervical vertebral bodies	Slightly hyperextended log: passes through lower cervical vertebral bodies only or not at all	Slightly extended log: passes through lower cervical vertebral bodies only or not at all
Scapulae	Flat against back	Abducted and/or protracted	May be normal	May be normal
Thoracic spine	Gentle convex curve	Increased flexion	Increased flexion extending into the upper lumbar vertebrae	Increased flexion in upper thoracic spine, lower thoracic has little or no convex curvature
Lumbar spine	Gentle concave curve log: through the bodies of the lumbar vertebrae	Hyperextended log: posterior to the vertebral bodies	Fairly flat spine, possibly with a very short concave curve at L5–S1 log: may not pass through lumbar vertebrae at all	Flexed log: through the vertebral bodies
Pelvis	ASIS and PSIS on same horizontal plane log: through the sacral promontory	Anterior tilt (ASIS rotated inferiorly, PSIS rotated superiorly)	Posterior tilt (ASIS rotated superiorly, PSIS rotated inferiorly) or neutral position	Pelvis posterior tilt (ASIS rotated superiorly, PSIS rotated inferiorly)
Hip joints	Neutral flexion and extension log: slightly posterior to the centre of the hip joint	Flexed log: slightly posterior to the centre of the hip joint	Hyperextended log: posterior to the hip joint	Extended log: posterior to the hip joints
Knee joints	Neutral flexion and extension log: slightly anterior to the centre of the knee joint	Slightly hyperextended log: anterior to the centre of the knee joint	Hyperextended log: through centre of the knee	Extended log: slightly anterior to the centre of the knee
Ankle joints	Neutral log: slightly anterior to the lateral malleolus, through the calcaneocuboid joint	Slight plantar flexion due to the slight knee hyperextension log: anterior to the lateral malleolus, anterior to the calcaneocuboid joint	Neutral tendency for plantar flexion due to knee position is compensated by anterior shift of the pelvis and hyperextension of the hips	Slight plantar flexion log: slightly anterior to the lateral malleolus, through the calcaneocuboid joint

log: line of gravity

posture would be classified as sway back. Figure 14.1b illustrates the same woman at 36 weeks gestation, when the sway-back posture has slightly exaggerated. Figure 14.2a illustrates a woman whose posture in the early part of her pregnancy would be classified as lordotic, the characteristics of which have been exaggerated towards term (Fig. 14.2b). Figures 14.3a and 14.3b illustrate a similar result in another individual. It is clear from these illustrations that there is a large individual variation in the presentation and degree of postural changes assumed. The fact that the initial postural deviations are exaggerated during pregnancy can be explained by considering that tissue resistance is less in the direction of the natural habitual posture.

Post-natal Posture

Because the mass of the extruded abdomen and the hormonal changes during pregnancy are considered to

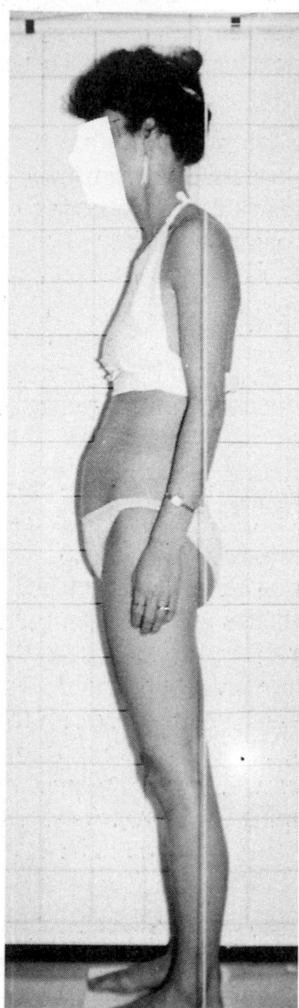

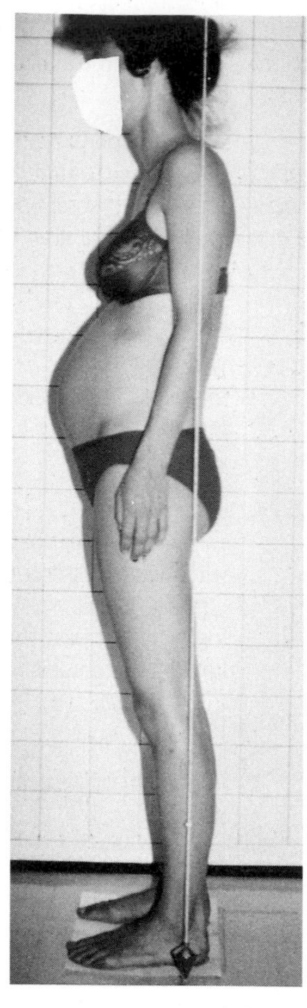

Figure 14.1 (a) Sway-backed posture of a woman at 14 weeks gestation. (b) Sway-backed posture of the same woman has maintained its characteristics by 36 weeks gestation.

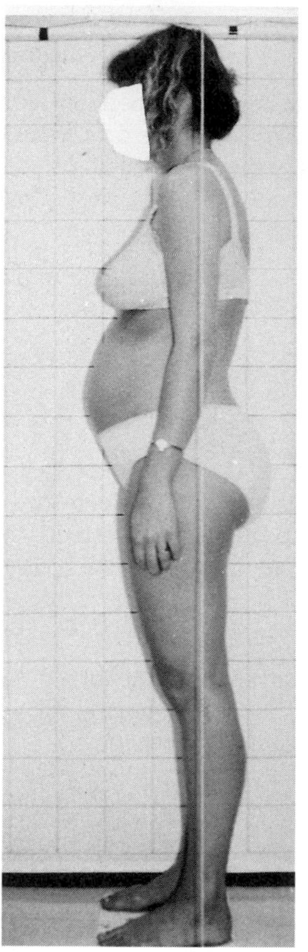

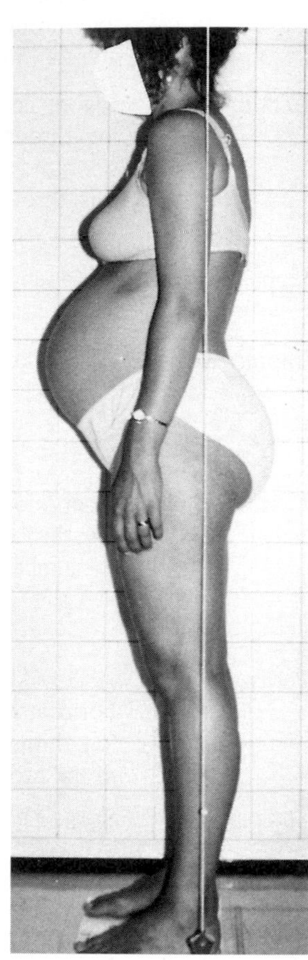

Figure 14.2 (a) A woman with a lordotic posture observed at 16 weeks gestation. (b) The same woman has an increase in the lordosis and also in the kyphosis at 38 weeks gestation. Note that the transition between the kyphosis and lordosis occurs rather abruptly at approximately the L3 level.

be influential in altering spinal curvatures, it is often assumed that following the birth of the baby, the posture will return to that of the 'pre-pregnant' state. Noting the postural changes found to occur in pregnancy from the 14th week and onwards during the ante-natal period (Bullock et al, 1987), Bullock-Saxton (1991) carried out a study to try to identify the so-called 'original' posture by assessing women in the post-natal period. The result of this study (Bullock-Saxton, 1991) was unexpected, but has since been confirmed by Dumas et al (1995a). It was found that the posture in the post-natal period was not significantly different from that measured at the late stages of pregnancy, the increase in postural curves measured during the pregnancy being maintained even three months post-natally. Figure 14.4 illustrates the posture of a woman in the early part of her pregnancy, at term and three months post-natally.

Such a result suggests that the women have subconsciously altered their body perception for stance and, without intervention, have maintained this posture of exaggerated curvatures. As the postural curves are greater than in the early part of the pregnancy, the possibility for decreased control of the spine, higher loads and greater shearing forces at the spine seems augmented. Subsequent pain may well develop as the mother takes on new tasks associated with the care of the newborn. Obviously, physiotherapy intervention for postural retraining in the post-natal period may be of considerable value.

Physiotherapy treatment options

One of the most valuable components of treatment offered to any pregnant woman is to explain the importance of posture to the quality of her movement during daily activities. It is movement and its dysfunction which are usually associated with the development of pain. The posture from which the movement is initiated and performed plays an essential role in ensuring optimal joint biomechanics. The ante-natal class setting is an obvious arena in which to address this issue.

Figure 14.5 illustrates the application of postural education in four-point kneeling, in sitting and in standing using a mirror. The treatment aims to increase the ability of the trunk muscles to coactivate and support the spine in as

Figure 14.3 (a) At 15 weeks, this woman demonstrates a lordotic posture with a convex curve which appears to extend into the mid-thoracic region and the degree of lordosis appears to be less exaggerated than that of the woman in Fig. 14.2. (b) Progression of postural curves occurs in the same direction as Fig. 14.3a only with some slight exaggeration of their degree.

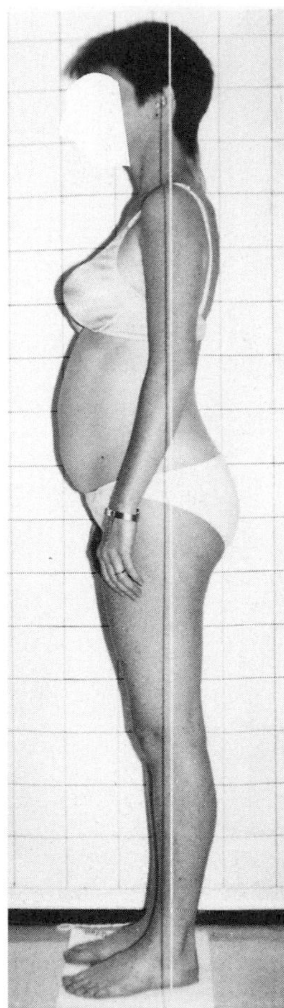
a

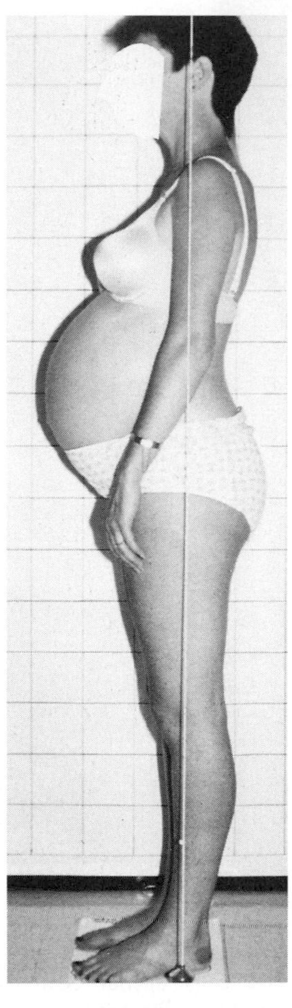
b

close to a neutral position as possible. Such an achievement would ensure that the spine was supported and that the distribution of pressures over the spinal joints and pelvis was as even as possible. In each of these postures, the therapist reminds the woman to focus on the alignment of three main spinal areas, i.e. the pelvis, the thoracolumbar junction and the head (Hamilton, personal communication). Initial alignment of these three areas appears to assist in the appropriate alignment of the lumbar and thoracic spine, as well as the shoulder girdle and lower limbs. Control of spinal posture is often easiest to initiate in four-point kneeling, as in this position lower limb alignment and its effect on the pelvis can be eliminated. It is also a pleasant position for the woman as the pregnancy progresses, serving to reduce the pressure of the growing foetus. However, the four-point kneeling position does require some degree of shoulder girdle stability. From this position, the woman can easily move the pelvis and can identify a neutral pelvic tilt, neutral lumbar, thoracic and cervical curvatures. She can also position the head and eventually elongate the entire spine by an active effort to increase the distance between the top of the head and the sacrum (without altering the neutral curvatures achieved). Such a specific posture requires a large degree of co-contraction of the trunk and shoulder girdle muscles and helps to train them for activities of daily living. Once the correct alignment has been achieved, a posture rod can be placed on the woman's spine and the contact on bony points used as a form of pressure feedback. Such a device can be useful for home exercise.

When close to neutral pelvic and spinal posture has been achieved, attention can be paid to sitting posture. This is done most easily when the height of the stool is such that the hips are at approximately 60° of flexion, as it throws the weight more directly onto the ischial tuberosities. However, chairs of different heights may also be used. Figure 14.5b illustrates a relaxed spinal posture in sitting in a woman of 37 weeks gestation. Activities of the upper limbs are encouraged during this posture, with concentration on control of the spinal curvatures.

Achieving alignment in standing where the joints are close to a neutral position is desirable to encourage balanced muscular control (Janda and Vavrova, 1994). This may be taught initially with frequent feedback, through use of a mirror and verbal encouragement. The therapist can use a number of facilitatory handling techniques to achieve the appropriate joint posture control. Visualization, verbal feedback, tactile facilitation (such as light pressure cues on the top of the head, the pelvis, the thoracolumbar junction and also the inferior angle of the scapula), sweep tapping of specific muscles and adhesive taping as a proprioceptive stimulus are just a few approaches that can assist in facilitating active joint alignment.

Once the woman understands how to hold her body posture as close to neutral as possible, the muscular control can be challenged by decreasing the base of support as well as by offering unstable surfaces as a basis for maintaining balance. Such techniques help to make maintaining postural control more automatic in nature. An essential component of treatment is to ensure that the appropriate muscle activity is at a subconscious level, otherwise the effects will not be maintained (Janda and Vavrova, 1994). Many approaches may be used to enhance active control of postural stability. For example, in four point kneeling, the base of support may be decreased by raising one limb (Fig. 14.6) and then oblique upper and lower limbs while endeavouring to maintain postural stability. A further challenge may be introduced by the addition of an unstable surface (such as an exercise ball, rocking or wobble board) under one of the supporting body parts. Such an approach used for sitting posture control is illustrated in Figure 14.7. Figure 14.7a illustrates use of a self-inflating tube (Torso, South Australia) which has unidirectional instability and Figure 14.7b an exercise ball. Both of these devices facilitate endurance of muscular contraction. Therapy would concentrate on appropriately controlled slow then rapid upper and lower limb movements to integrate the control into the appropriate motor plan (Janda and Vavrova, 1994).

Standing posture control can be challenged by the use of unstable surfaces such as wobble boards or balance shoes

Figure 14.4 (a) Posture of a primigravida at 14 weeks. (b) Posture at 36 weeks gestation. (c) Posture at 12 weeks post-natal. Note that the quality and depth of the spinal curvatures at this stage emulate that of the late pregnancy observation.

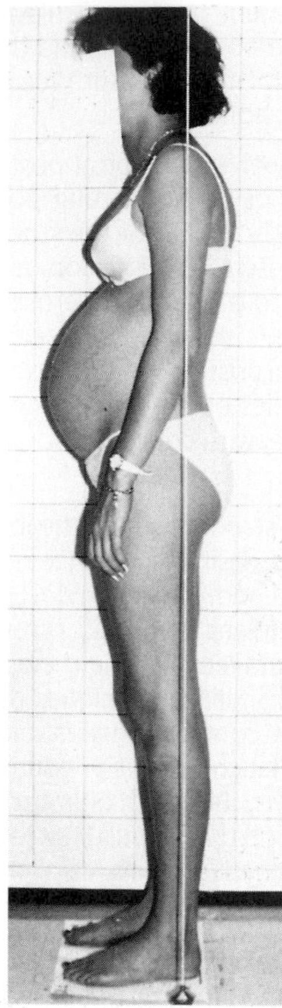
a

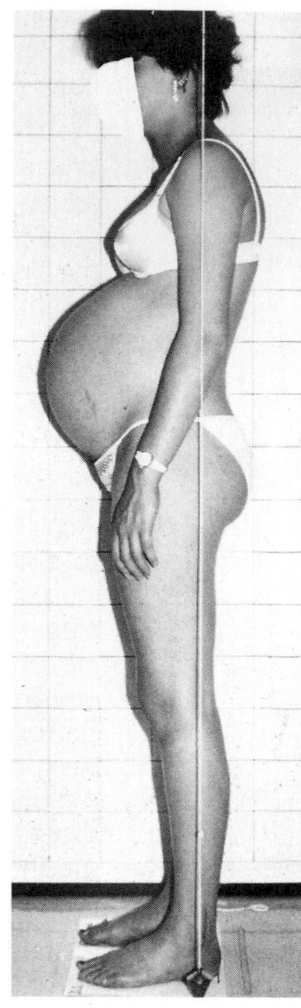
b

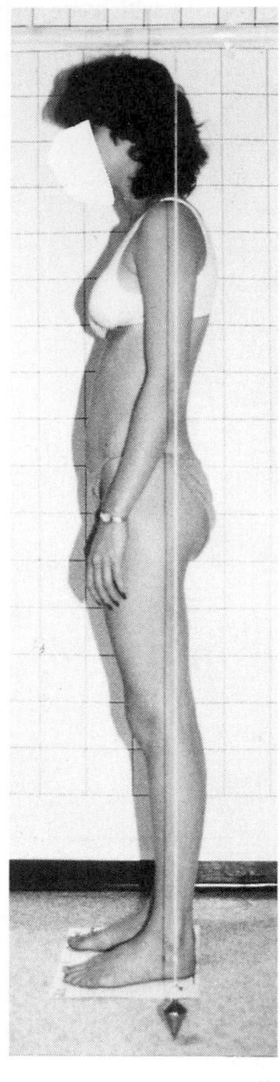
c

(Bullock-Saxton et al, 1993) (Fig. 14.8a). The latter consist of a cork sandal with a moulded sole and a rubber hemisphere attached to the undersole. Wearing these sandals, the woman takes short quick steps while balancing on the supporting hemisphere (controlled by hip and knee flexion) and maintaining pelvic control (hip hitching is a common error). To gain the desired effect, the sandal must not touch the floor, the toes should stay in contact with the sandal and large steps should not be attempted. Research studies have shown that this improves activation of the trunk musculature and the shoes are therefore recommended for postural retraining as well as following lower limb injuries. Such co-ordination training should be performed frequently for short periods of no more than two minutes per session, each day. An added advantage of wearing these shoes is the overall effect on improvement of balance in standing (Bullock-Saxton, unpublished data). Figure 14.8c illustrates the use of a wobble board for the control of standing posture in the post-natal period.

Once the woman can control her pelvic and spinal posture, it is helpful to provide training in appropriate reaching and lifting methods. This is particularly important in the post-natal period where the frequency of lifting is increased due to the woman's care of the infant. Safety in lifting requires not only spinal control, but also lower limb muscular strength. Progressive exercises controlling the spine and lower limb can be prescribed. The woman must be aware of the importance of maintaining spinal control through muscular contraction and of controlling the lower limb alignment. Figures 14.9a and b illustrate the progression from initial weight shift training to controlling a lunge, a component of some lifting manoeuvres.

Jane enrolled for her first ante-natal class when she was 24 weeks pregnant. Part of the class education was about the effect of the pregnancy on her posture. She vaguely remembered that in primary school the teachers had talked about posture, but she had not taken much notice. She had rather a slim build and had always been able to hyper-extend her knees and elbows and used to do tricks with her thumbs which made her friends exclaim with distaste. The physiotherapist incorporated an assessment of posture and trunk control during upper and lower limb movement for the group during the tea break, after she had described the possible changes associated with pregnancy. The

Figure 14.5 (a) Four-point kneeling is an excellent position for training postural awareness and the co-activation of trunk muscles. The knees are positioned directly under the hips and the hands directly under the shoulders, with some elbow flexion. A pillow under the ankle ensures that the ankles are not forced into plantar flexion. The physiotherapist pays particular attention to facilitating the active holding of neutral curves of the spinal column. This may be achieved by light pressure cues at lumbar, thoracolumbar and neck areas and verbal feedback. Asking the woman to consider elongation of the spine is also helpful for facilitation of trunk muscle activity. At the end of the treatment session, the woman should be able to achieve this neutral posture by herself. (b) The neutral spine posture with slight elongation of the spine ('Elevate the top of your head toward the ceiling') is practised in the sitting posture. (c) Training the neutral spine posture in standing with the use of visual feedback (mirror) and light touch facilitation to the pelvis, thoracolumbar region and head. Often this posture is easier to achieve with slight flexion of the hips and knees. The hips should also be in neutral or slightly externally rotated so that the projection of an imaginary line through the centre of the thigh falls over the second toe of the foot. Pay attention to the alignment of the scapula also and ensure that correction of scapula position occurs independent of changes in thoracic spine curvature.

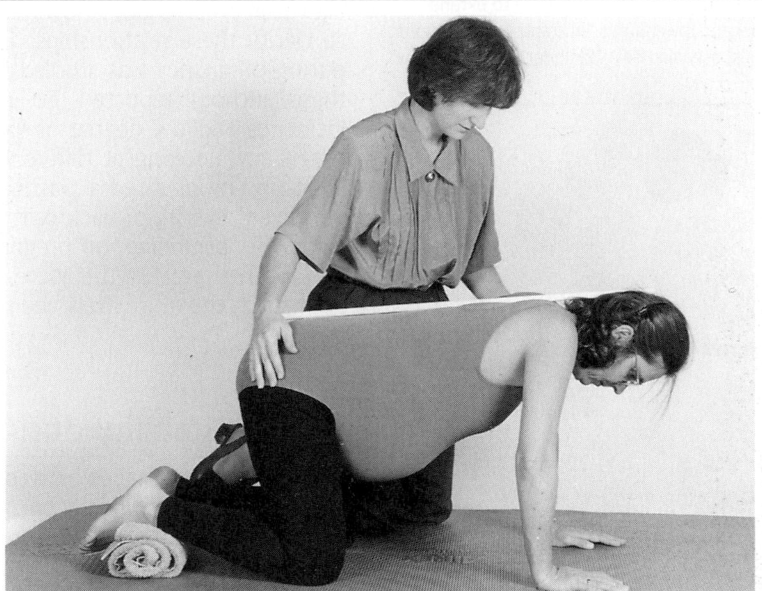

a

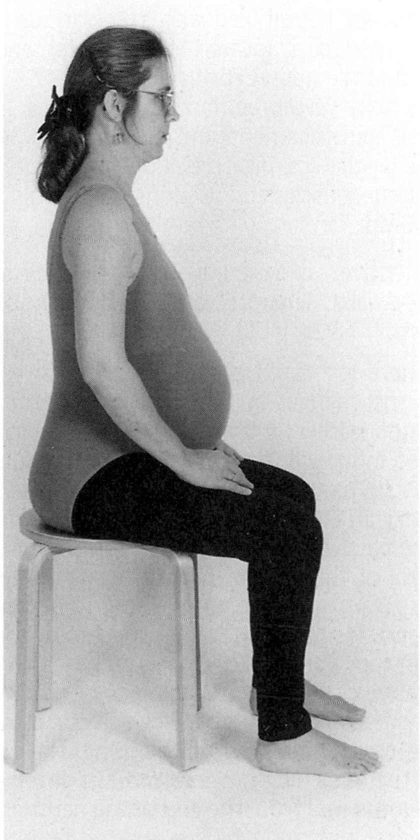

b

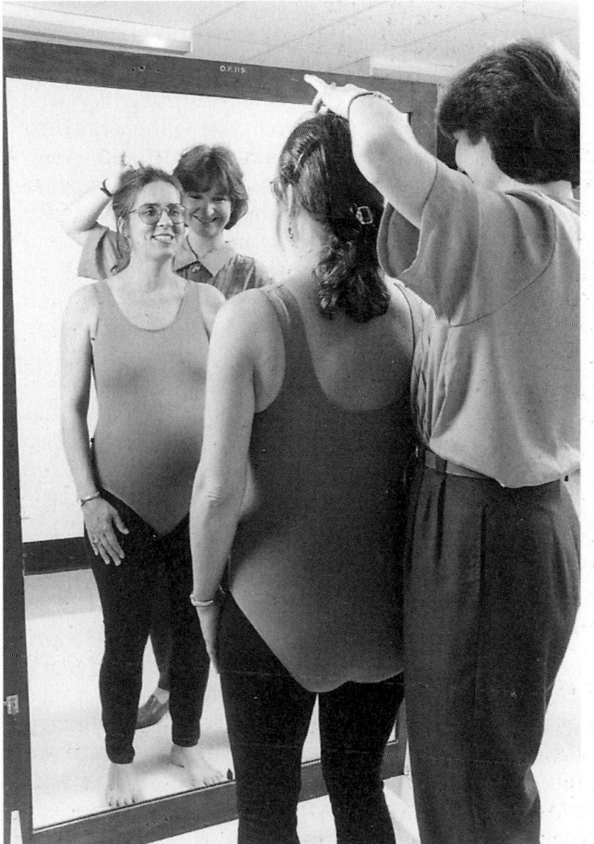

c

Figure 14.6 Progression of difficulty for the control of trunk posture is to decrease the base of support (i.e. increasing the load demands on the system) or to add unstable surfaces or perturbations to the system (challenging the co-ordination of appropriate muscular activation). This figure illustrates the raising of the left upper limb while holding neutral posture. The posture rod is used as a form of pressure feedback for the woman, who is aware of the points of her spine in contact with the cylindrical bar (the posture rod should be of reasonable mass). If, during the exercise, there is a loss of ability to control the spine, the rod will no longer contact the same points on the spine or it will roll away from the centre of the back. Other options for decreasing base of support are to extend a lower limb or to lift oblique upper and lower limbs. Unstable bases (rocking or wobble boards or exercise balls) may also be used under the supporting surfaces.

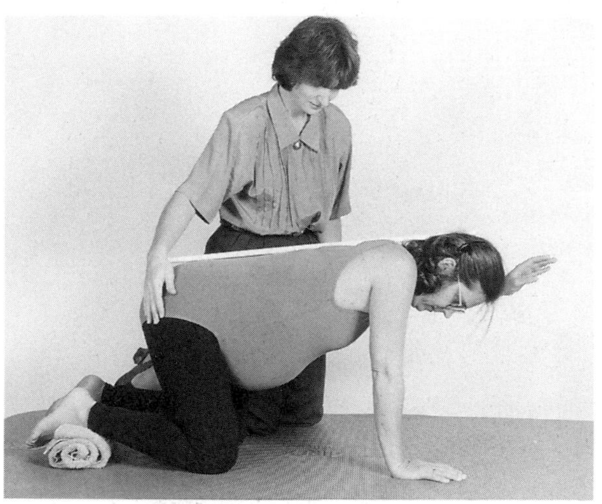

physiotherapist had said to Jane that it was important that she learn to control her posture which was already of a kypholordotic type. Jane was first taught to control her pelvic alignment in four-point kneeling and asked to practise this with a posture rod provided by the physiotherapist. She was also asked to try to adapt the same spinal posture in sitting and standing and this was checked before she left. Jane watched the mirror as she adjusted her posture and saw that she looked taller. When she tried to control her spine with movement, she noticed that she felt more stable. It seemed reasonable to her to work at improving the strength of her postural muscles. At subsequent visits, the physiotherapist added different exercises which were fun to do while Jane was working. By the time that Jane had her baby girl she was aware of her posture and although her whole body felt unusual after the baby was born, she was able to consider the three main areas of the pelvis, upper low back and head. She found that raising her head toward the ceiling but not poking out her chin seemed to help place the rest of her body into balance. She did notice that although she sometimes forgot about her posture, it was usually in the back of her mind and she liked the graceful appearance and sense of control of movement that it gave her.

Posture and Pain

Evidence from experimental studies shows that posture does alter during pregnancy. It has also been shown that low back pain is a common complaint during pregnancy. It could be assumed therefore that these two factors may be related. A review of the literature suggests that a relationship does exist between some aspects of posture and low back pain presentation. However, more research is required to clarify these relationships. The incidence of back pain during pregnancy was studied by Bullock et al (1987) and these authors reported no relationship between pain incidence and the degree of lordosis or kyphosis during pregnancy. Looking at different parameters, Dumas et al (1995b) demonstrated a positive correlation between the perceived severity of back pain and the change in lordosis from the beginning of pregnancy to the post-partum period. The greater the increase in lordosis during the pregnancy, the more likely the person was to suffer severe back pain.

Spinal instability during pregnancy

The possible relationship between posture, muscle function changes and back pain may be explained by Panjabi's (1992a, 1992b) hypothesis of spinal stability and instability in which he proposed that spinal stability is dependent on the co-ordinated interaction of three subsystems:

1. *control subsystem:* neural feedback from various force and motion transducers, located in ligaments, tendons and muscles, and the neural control centres;
2. *passive subsystem:* vertebrae, facet articulations, intervertebral discs, spinal ligaments and joint capsules, as well as the passive mechanical properties of the muscle;
3. *active subsystem:* muscles and tendons surrounding the vertebral column.

'These passive, active, and neural control subsystems, although conceptually separate, are functionally interdependent' (Panjabi, 1992a, p. 384).

In pregnancy, there is a rapid change in the passive subsystem, due to the changes in the circulating hormones. For reasons stated earlier in this chapter, such changes undoubtedly also influence the active and control subsystems. Panjabi (1992b) has proposed that a possible cause for instability is either an increase in the range of motion not restrained by the passive subsystem (the neutral zone) or a decreased control of this area by the active subsystem. In either situation, a portion of the normal range of motion is not controlled and this may lead to increased shear forces, microtrauma and pain. Panjabi (1992b) has defined that part of the normal range of motion with minimal internal resistance to movement as the neutral zone, which corresponds closely with the neutral position of the joint. The elastic zone comprises the remaining range of motion of the joint and is the range measured from the end of the neutral zone to the physiological limit and which is resisted by internal

Figure 14.7 Progressions of posture demands in sitting are to use an unstable base. A unidirectional self-inflating tube (Torso, Adelaide) can be used to challenge stability in the anteroposterior direction and also the lateral direction. Such a device is easily transportable and can be used readily in work situations. (b) Therapeutic exercise balls provide a multidirectional unstable base of support (wobble boards may also be used). In addition, the compressibility of the ball can provide extra proprioceptive stimulation due to joint compression achieved by gently bouncing down into the ball, while maintaining a neutral posture.

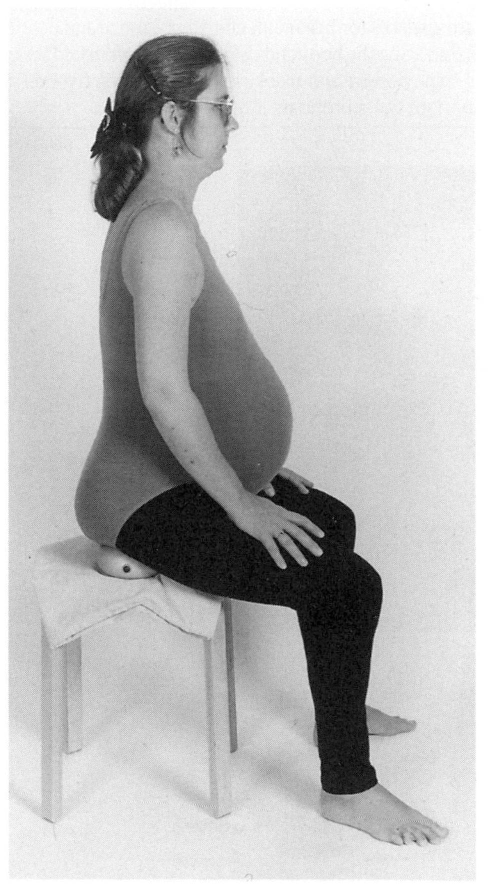

a

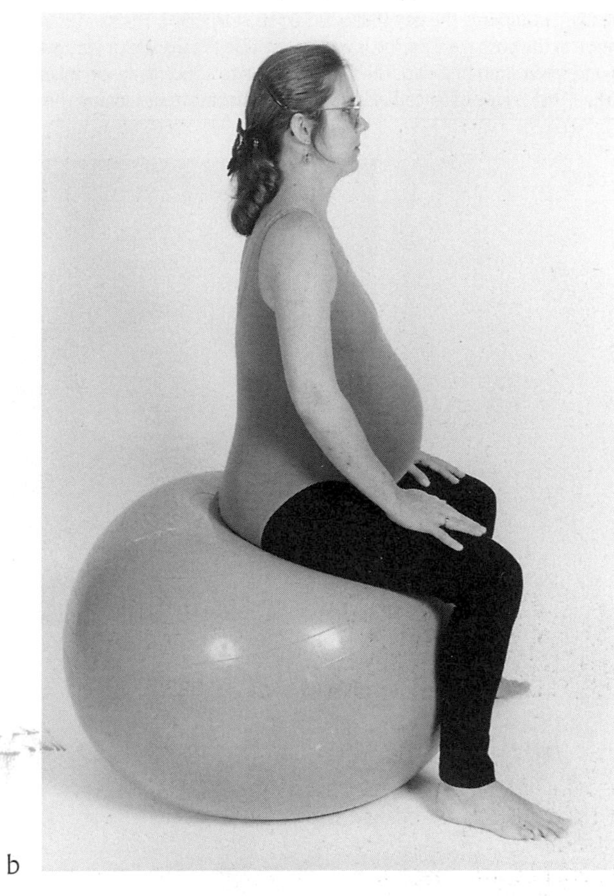

b

passive restraints. Panjabi (1992b) argues that spinal instability is apparent when there is a relatively large neutral zone in proportion to the total range of motion. He also asserts that the presence of pain is magnified by increases in spinal instability (Panjabi, 1992b). While this theory has not been applied to the pregnant population, it is a feasible extrapolation of these propositions. It could explain the very early onset of low back pain (though often not severe) in pregnancy, even prior to the ascent of the foetus into the abdominal region. It must be remembered that ligamentous changes occur very early in the pregnancy (Hainline, 1994) and could be responsible for alterations in spinal stability.

Spinal stability and the abdominal musculature

It is apparent that spinal stability may be affected by pregnancy due to changes in ligamentous restraint. A further potential influence of pregnancy on spinal stability could be through the lengthening of the abdominal muscles and the consequential change in their ability to generate tension (Gilleard, 1992). As it is clear that spinal stability may be a factor to consider in the development of low back pain in pregnant women, it is important to review research investigating the relationship between spinal stability and abdominal muscle activation.

The results of recent research have provided a convincing argument for the importance of the transversus abdominis in the stability of the lumbar spine (Hodges and Richardson, 1996, 1997; Richardson and Jull, 1994, 1995; Richardson et al, 1990, 1992). Cresswell et al (1992) identified the contribution of the transversus abdominis to generation of intra-abdominal pressure. The role of the deeply placed transversus abdominis as a potential stabilizer of the spine was proposed by Richardson and Jull (1994, 1995), who considered that it was able to increase the anterior stability and contribute to the posterior stability of the lumbar spine via its attachment to the thoracolumbar fascia. Hodges and Richardson (1997a) showed that in normal individuals, the transversus abdominis was activated prior to all other abdominal muscles, irrespective of the direction of movement being generated. This landmark

Figure 14.8 (a) Balance sandals have a dense but slightly compressible hemisphere placed in the centre of the base of the shoe (Body Control Systems Australia, Brisbane). They provide an unstable base of support during walking activities and as such increase the afferent information from the lower limb. Janda and Vavrova (1994) recommend their use for postural education, as well as balance and proprioceptive rehabilitation. (b) Training in the use of the balance sandals requires specific attention to reinforcement of appropriate movement patterns. The woman should keep her feet in contact with the sandals at all times via activation of the lumbricals of the feet. The sandal should make contact on the floor only through the hemisphere. Small rapid steps are taken with controlled flexion and extension at the hip and knee. The pelvis and spine should be held in neutral posture and the trunk elongated. There should be no hip hitching during gait due to overactivity of the quadratus lumborum. The woman can wear the shoes for short periods of time (two minutes maximum), frequently throughout the day (Bullock-Saxton et al, 1993). The sandals are best worn on hard surfaces for maximum effect. (c) Balance and posture re-education in the post-natal period is warranted. Use of a wobble or rocking board is helpful in displacing the body and demanding co-ordinated activation of trunk and lower limb muscles. The woman needs to concentrate on maintaining the neutral spine posture and trunk elongation during the exercise. Increasing the degree of knee flexion will also assist in strengthening the quadriceps, so important for appropriate lifting techniques.

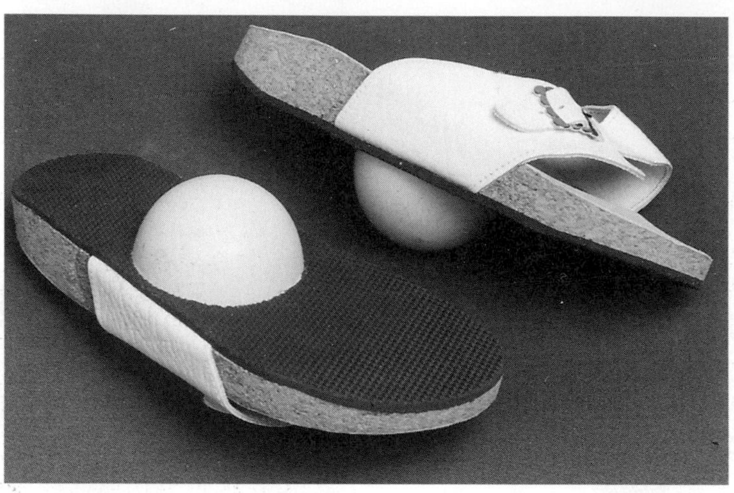

a

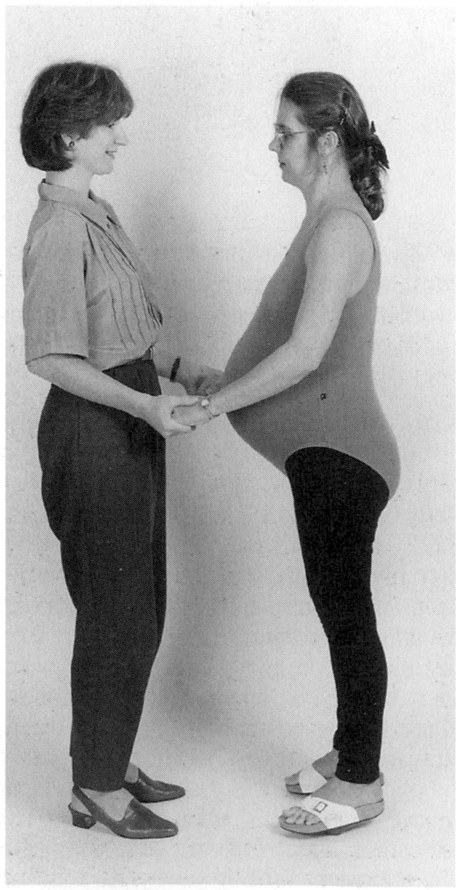

b

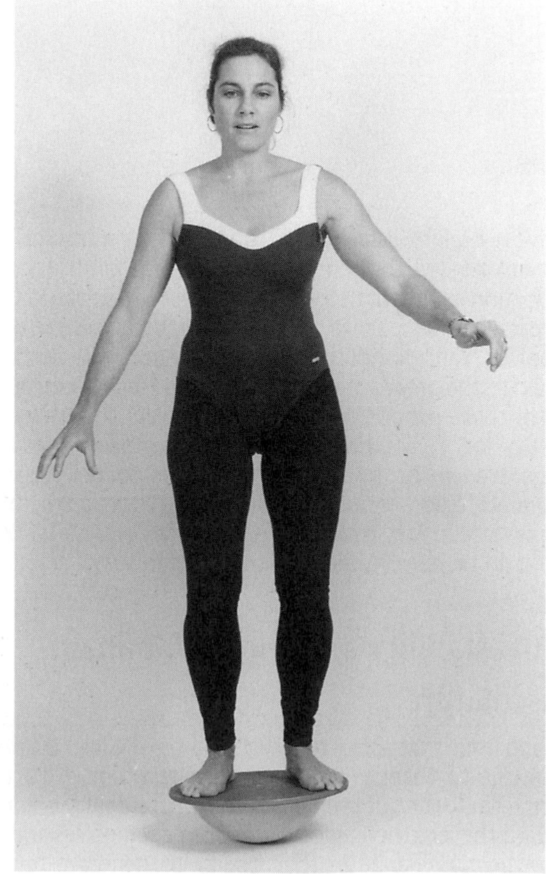

c

Figure 14.9 (a) Initial weight shift training can concentrate on spinal posture while increasing the loads on the lower limbs. Also pay attention to the control of femoral rotation (aviod internal rotation of the femur). (b) Exercising the lower limbs to support weight in a controlled manner is essential to achieving appropriate lifting behaviour. The spine can be maintained in neutral and the woman concentrates on spinal stability while she lunges forward onto the front leg.

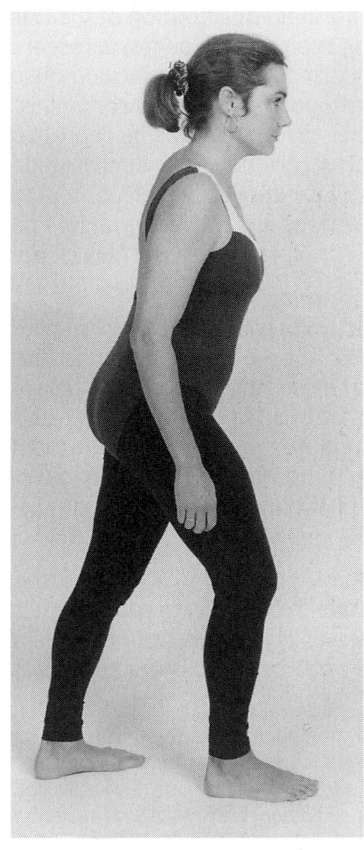

a

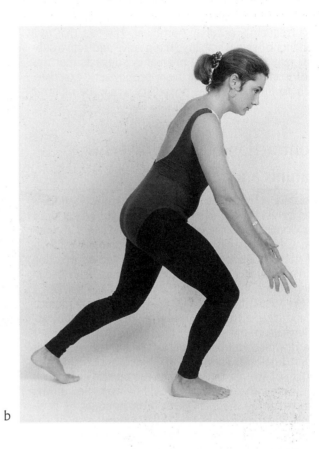

b

research used fine-wire EMG to investigate the relative recruitment of anterior and posterior trunk muscles as well as upper and lower limb muscles in a variety of motions causing rotations of the lumbar spine. Following the collation of this normative data, Hodges and Richardson (1997b) demonstrated that in patients with chronic low back pain, the activation of the transversus abdominis was significantly delayed. It no longer acted in anticipation of a movement, but rather responded to the movement. Their subsequent research has found that training the low back pain subjects to activate the transversus abdominis has led to a decrease in recurrence of symptoms.

The role of the multifidus as a potential spinal stabilizer was proposed by Bergmark (1989), who considered that the direction of the segmental fibres of this muscle as well as their lever arm was insufficient to generate significant torque for motion. Hides et al (1994) demonstrated with real-time diagnostic ultrasound that in low back pain patients the cross-sectional area of the multifidus was significantly decreased on the side of pain. Hides et al (1996) illustrated that specific exercises to restore activation of the multifidus led to a decrease in the incidence of subsequent back pain episodes.

These research findings appear to support the need to train specific activation of the transversus abdominis and multifidus to improve spinal stability in low back pain subjects (Richardson and Jull, 1995) and suggest that once this is achieved, movements requiring controlled activation of all muscles of the trunk should be introduced into the rehabilitation programme. In this way, the focus of treatment has turned from reporting the number of abdominal curls that can be performed by a patient to confirming the ability to maintain stability of the pelvis during functional activities. In Jull's view (personal communication), clinical observations suggest that this is probably due to the fact that overemphasis on the activity of multijoint muscles such as the rectus abdominis and the obliques inhibits the activation of the transversus abdominis.

The research reported above highlights the point that the emphasis in early rehabilitation should be on the isolated activation of the multifidus and transversus abdominis so that the establishment of a motor plan incorporating their appropriate and early activation may be encouraged. This may be achieved by the co-contraction of the multifidus, transversus abdominis and the pelvic floor (Richardson and Jull, 1995). The inter-relationship between the pelvic floor and the abdominal muscles is currently under further investigation and is described in Chapter 23. Richardson and Jull (1995) provide a detailed description of the coactivation of the transversus abdominis and multifidus and the reader is encouraged to review their paper on this topic. It appears relevant to consider the application of these exercises for the pregnant and post-natal woman, for whom low back pain is a frequently occurring problem. The fact that two components of spinal stability (the passive and active subsystems) may be affected by pregnancy suggests that this group of women may benefit from prophylactic exercises. Research to investigate this possibility would be of great value.

Co-contraction of the transversus abdominis and multifidus

The isolated activation of the transversus abdominis is achieved by asking the subject to slowly and gently draw in the abdominal muscles, particularly in the lower abdominal area. Often, there is a simultaneous isometric contraction of the multifidus posteriorly and this co-contraction assists in maintaining the neutral spine posture described in an earlier section of this chapter (Richardson and Jull, 1995). Figure 14.10 illustrates the sagittal view of the abdomen before and after a transversus and multifidus co-contraction. Richardson and Jull (1995) consider that the easiest posture in which to learn the activity of these muscles is four-point kneeling. They feel that this position provides some form of stretch facilitation to the muscle group. It is easy to imagine that this effect would be magnified during pregnancy. During pregnancy, the woman could be positioned as illustrated in Figure 14.5a, without use of the posture rod. Post-natally, particularly until the vaginal and uterine wall have healed (approximately six weeks post-partum), a modification of four-point kneeling can be adopted (Fig. 14.11) to avoid the remote possibility of air embolus. It is often helpful for the physiotherapist to facilitate the activation of the muscle by placing her hand on the lower abdomen. The instruction for the contraction is best given thus: 'Breathe in, breathe out, now slowly draw your abdomen away from my hand, now resume breathing'.

Figure 14.10 (a) Sagittal view of the relaxed abdomen. (b) Sagittal view of abdomen after transversus abdominis and multifidus co-contraction.

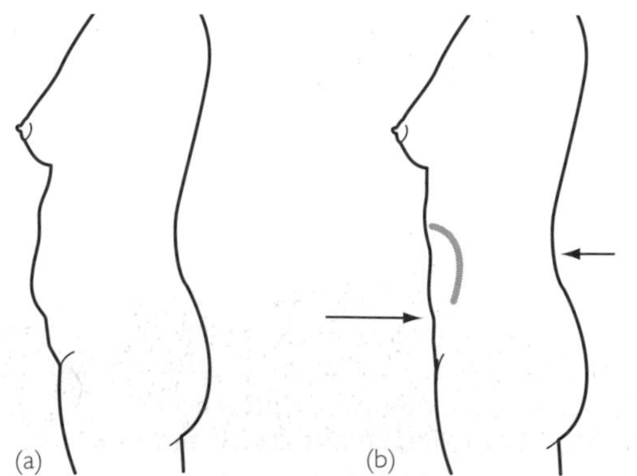

Performing the contraction after the outbreath avoids the possibility of the woman using an incorrect technique of negative pressure during inspiration, as well as capitalizing on the decreased threshold of activation of the transversus abdominis following expiration (Hodges, personal communication). Other incorrect techniques include the overactivation of the external oblique or rectus abdominis. In such circumstances, either the rib cage will be depressed during the activation (external oblique) or the lumbar spine will flex (rectus abdominis). Use of EMG biofeedback to inhibit action of external oblique and/or rectus abdominis during the early isolated training of transversus abdominis is recommended.

Richardson and Jull (1995) have suggested that the co-contraction of the pelvic floor is also helpful in facilitating the correct activation of these muscles. Sapsford (personal communication) feels that it is important that the pelvic floor muscles are drawn upwards slowly and not by a rapid closure of the sphincters. A full bladder has also been found to be an inhibitory factor in facilitation of these muscle groups (Hodges, personal communication).

The specific facilitation provided by the physiotherapist is an essential component of achieving appropriate contraction of the transversus abdominis. It is essential that the patient does not try too hard and overactivate inappropri-

Figure 14.11 In the early post-natal period, transversus abdominis activation can be taught in a modification of four-point kneeling, where the upper trunk is elevated and neutral spine posture maintained. The four-point posture (and its modification) seems to provide a stretch facilitation to the abdominal wall, which assists in the achievement of the appropriate contraction. The therapist can assist by placing her hand on the lower abdominal wall or by deep pressure to the transversus abdominis just medial and inferior to the ASIS. The woman should gently breathe in, then breathe out and slowly draw the abdomen toward her spine and away from the therapist's hand. No movement of the spine or depression of the rib cage should occur during the activity. All contractions should be slow. Once the contraction has been achieved, breathing should resume and the contraction held for up to 10 seconds. Co-contraction of multifidus and/or the pelvic floor can assist in achieving the transversus abdominis activation (Richardson and Jull, 1995). This training can be progressed to prone lying see Richardson and Jull (1995).

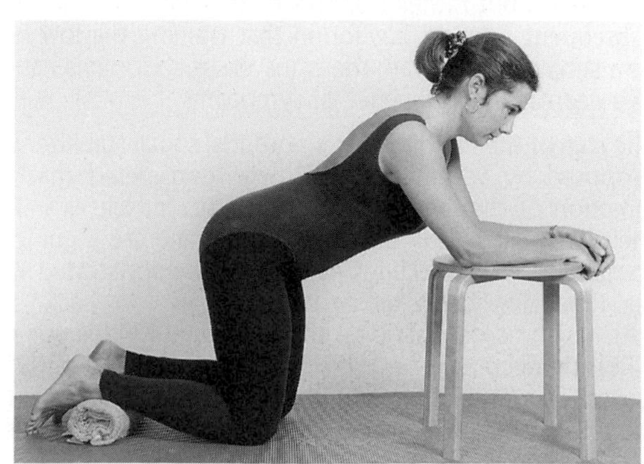

ate synergists. Verbal cues, facilitatory handling, specific positioning as well as relevant co-activation patterns are techniques the physiotherapist will need to employ to achieve results.

The activity to encourage multifidus muscle action is an isometric holding of a small proportion of maximum voluntary contraction (MVC) (approximately 30% MVC; Richardson, personal communication). Some women have difficulty in activating the muscle in this way and it may help them to imagine that they are tightening a string between their sacrum and their occiput without moving their spine. Placement of the physiotherapist's hands on these two areas and provision of a light pressure cue can also be helpful. It is essential that the muscle contractions are performed slowly to try to augment the recruitment of the tonic motor units (Richardson and Jull, 1995).

Once the woman is able to perform appropriate co-contraction of the transversus and multifidus, holding for an arbitrary 10 seconds, and to repeat it 10 times, it is important that the function of these muscles is integrated with the other trunk musculature to provide stability (Richardson and Jull, 1995). The premise is that with specific training, the early activation of the transversus abdominis will be facilitated and so the muscle will assist in supporting the lumbar spine during activities. With the woman concentrating on spinal and pelvic stability, an early exercise for integration is to increase the load on the muscles. This can be achieved in sitting or standing with the spine in the neutral posture, flexing or extending slightly at the hips only and maintaining the erect and neutral posture (Fig. 14.12). To develop rotary stability, higher loads can be added to the pelvis with the woman in supine and the patient controlling the pelvic motion while actively allowing the flexed hip to abduct (Fig. 14.13a) or by slowly extending the flexed hip and knee (Fig. 14.13b). The physiotherapist could be quite imaginative in selecting exercises that encourage integrated control of the pelvis and spine. Bridging and lunging are two useful positions. It is essential that the woman concentrates on stability. Richardson and Jull (personal communication) consider that once integration has been achieved, it is essential for the physiotherapist to continue to monitor the isolated activation of the deep muscles (transversus abdominis and multifidus).

Figure 14.12 An early integration of transversus abdominis activity with all other abdominal muscles can be to increase the load on the trunk via backward inclination. The woman should maintain the neutral posture and extend at the hips. Placing the thumb on the ASIS and the first finger on the ribs can give some feedback on the maintenance of spinal alignment.

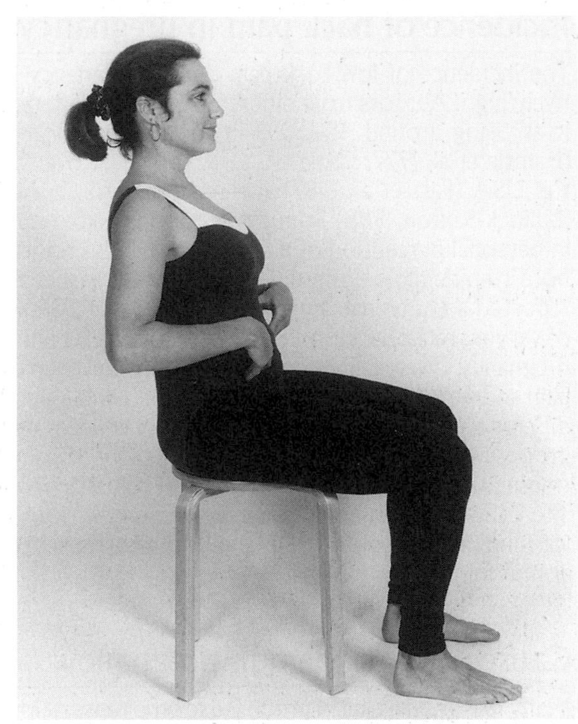

Figure 14.13 (a) During integration of abdominal muscle activity, concentration is placed on maintaining pelvic stability. The woman can monitor her pelvic movement by placing her hands on the ASIS. Use of a pressure biofeedback device (Chattanooga, Brisbane) (Richardson and Jull, 1995) can also assist in providing information on control of trunk rotation. By slowly allowing one leg to fall outwards from flexion into abduction, a rotation force is generated on the pelvis which the co-activation of the abdominal muscles must resist to maintain pelvic stability. (b) Maintaining pelvic stability in anterior and posterior tilt can be achieved by adding limb loads of flexion and extension of the limb with and without (a progression) support on the heel. Once again, the woman must ensure that the pelvis maintains stability and does not change its alignment during the performance of the exercise.

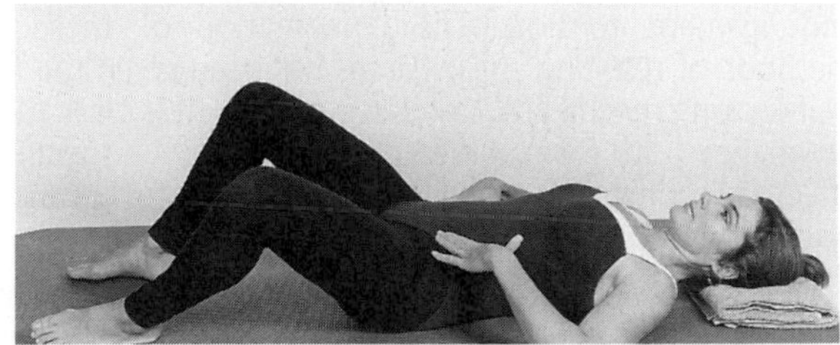

a

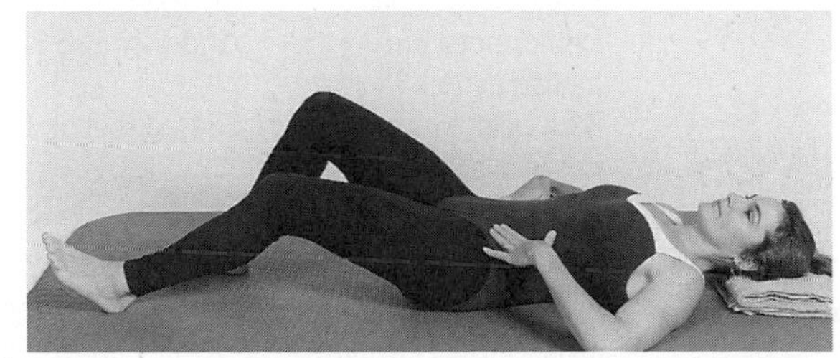

b

Spinal Pain during Pregnancy and Post-partum

Incidence of back pain in pregnancy

The incidence of low back pain during pregnancy is relatively high. Authors from different countries have reported it as being around 48–50% in the UK and Scandinavia (Mantle et al, 1977; Östgaard et al, 1991), just over 56% in the USA (Fast et al, 1987) and near to 70% in Australia (Bullock-Saxton, 1988). Ethnicity is considered to be a factor in personal perception of pain and as such is important to note in epidemiological studies. For example, Fast et al (1987) reported a study involving a questionnaire of 200 women of varying racial background in relation to back pain during pregnancy. Overall, 56% of the patients complained of back pain and 44% complained of no pain. There was a significant difference in the ethnic distribution between the two groups where Caucasians complained of back pain more frequently and Hispanics complained of pain less frequently. The other two ethnic groups represented (African-American and Asian) demonstrated similar proportions of people complaining of back pain.

Causes of back pain in pregnancy

Many reasons have been proposed for the cause of low back pain during pregnancy. Rungee (1993) provides an excellent review of this topic covering epidemiology, aetiology, prophylaxis, evaluation and treatment. While directed at orthopaedic surgeons, his review of the literature is of great relevance to physiotherapy and highlights the diversity of causes associated with this problem. Indeed, Östgaard et al (1993) have commented on the mulifactorial nature of low back pain during pregnancy and the wide variety of variables associated with either the incidence or the severity of this musculoskeletal condition, as Table 14.3 illustrates. It is clear that physiotherapy assessment needs to encompass a thorough review of history and the factors influencing pain behaviour and it should also determine objective signs so that symptoms may be related to mechanical causes.

Table 14.3 Factors related to the development of low back pain and sacroiliac pain during pregnancy

Symptom	Proposed causative factor	Reference
Low back pain	Weight gain during pregnancy	Östgaard et al, 1991
	Rapid postural changes	Rungee, 1993
	Vascular effects	Rungee, 1993
	Previous back pain experienced during menstruation	Östgaard and Andersson, 1992
	Back pain in previous pregnancies	Östgaard et al, 1991
	Repetitive lifting/ bending	Östgaard and Andersson, 1992
Sacroiliac pain	Pelvic insufficiency due to hormonal changes	Östgaard et al, 1991

Much of the literature does not clearly distinguish the differences in origin of pain, labelling all pregnancy-induced symptoms as emanating from the 'low back'. In a large Scandinavian survey of 855 pregnant women, Östgaard et al (1991) asked women at each visit to illustrate the area of their back pain on a body chart as well as to indicate its severity on a visual analogue scale. Forty-nine percent of women complained of having suffered some back pain during their pregnancy and 36% of that particular sample stated that they had significant pain. From the pain drawings of the back pain group, it appeared that there were three major regions associated with this pain:

1. pain above the lumbar region only;
2. pain in the lumbar region with or without radiation to one or both legs;
3. pain over the sacroiliac area sometimes with radiation to the side.

Pain in the symphysis pubis was apparent in all groups.

Östgaard et al (1991) found no correlation between the incidence of back pain and the weight gained during pregnancy. For this reason, they considered that the incidence of back pain could be explained only by the biomechanical overloading associated with pregnancy.

The possible means by which changes in the quality of the ligamentous and capsular restraints may affect spinal stability and result in pain have been discussed. In addition, it must be remembered that pelvic stability changes significantly during the course of pregnancy. Softening of pelvic ligaments and the pubic symphysis are responsible for altered biomechanics, increased shear and pain (Hainline, 1994; Östgaard et al, 1991). Reports of recent research by Vleeming et al (1990a, 1990b) have described the components of stability for the sacroiliac joint. These anatomists and bioengineers describe the sacroiliac joint as a friction joint, which is based on the principles of two sources of force generation. The first, termed form closure, refers to a stable situation with closely fitting joint surfaces, where no extra forces are needed to maintain the state of the system. While the sacroiliac joints would have a significant amount of form closure, if this were the only stability mechanism it would make mobility impossible. The second mechanism of force generation is termed force closure, which is generated by the compression offered by relevant muscle contraction and ligament tension. The combination of these two methods of resisting shear forces has been given the term 'self-locking mechanism' by these authors. It is clear that in pregnancy both form and force closure may be specifically affected, leading to less ability to resist shear forces and the possibility of pain.

Relaxin plays a significant role in the laxity of the symphysis pubis as well as the collagenous ligamentous structures of the pelvis (MacLennan, 1983; MacLennan et al, 1986). The result is the widening of pubic symphysis and sacroiliac joints, affecting the degree to which the sacroiliac joints are firmly opposed. Vleeming et al (1990b) identify four muscles which can affect the force closure, these being erector spinae, gluteus maximus, latissimus dorsi and biceps femoris. While pregnancy may not directly affect these muscles, many postures may predispose to different activity levels prior to pregnancy. The increasing demands for force closure generated by the ligamentous laxity may tip the balance for subjects starting with poor muscle function.

While there is still much to be discovered about factors associated with pregnancy-induced spinal and pelvic pain, it appears that some areas and their causes can be broadly identified. Rungee (1993) feels that there is strong evidence to support the view that the most severe backache is usually associated with sacroiliac dysfunction resulting from the change in level of relaxin in the early part of the pregnancy. Low back pain may also develop due to mechanical changes associated with rapid postural changes as the foetus grows. As reported earlier, Dumas et al (1995b), in correlating severity of pain with change in lordosis from early pregnancy to post-partum, demonstrated by use of a pain diary that the greater the increase in lordosis during pregnancy, the more likely was the person to suffer severe back pain. This was qualified by the statement that the correlation only explained 9–13% of the variance, although it was rather significant. In addition, these researchers correlated knee joint laxity scores with severity of pain as documented in a pain diary and found that at the end of pregnancy, those women with a large increase in laxity compared to post-partum laxity measures were likely to have the most severe back pain. Again they made these statements hesitantly due to the level of r, where r equals nearly 27% of the explanation.

Radicular symptoms are thought to be most probably due to mechanical pressure of ligaments, spinal structures or nerve roots and also possibly to the effect of 'lightening', an event occurring in the final four weeks of pregnancy. This is due to the descent of the foetus into the pelvic cavity, so relieving the pressure on the diaphragm and upper abdominal cavity and making breathing easier for the pregnant woman.

Recent literature appears to be identifying a pain related to the 'history of time and weight-bearing experienced in the posterior pelvis, deep in the gluteal area'. For example, Östgaard et al (1995) report that the patients' pain drawings illustrate a well-defined area of stabbing pain in the buttocks distal and lateral to the L5–S1 area, with or without radiation to the posterior thigh, but not into the foot. The pain is reproduced or exacerbated by a posterior pelvic pain provocation test. Associated with this are pain-free movements in the hips and spine, no nerve root syndrome and a typical pain caused by turning in bed. Östgaard et al (1995) explain that the mechanical cause of posterior pelvic pain is not clear at this stage, although there is suggestion that it may be related to the sacroiliac joint. They feel that it is essential to differentiate between standard low back pain per se and posterior pelvic pain and they feel that there is a correlation between a positive response to the posterior pelvic pain provocation test and the incidence of posterior pelvic pain.

The pain provocation test is carried out with the patient lying supine and the tested leg flexed at hip and knee with the hip at 90° flexion. The therapist applies a light longitudinal compression down the length of the femur while stabilizing the other side of the pelvis with the second hand. Compression is provided by movement of the therapist's body over the leg. Östgaard et al (1995) recommend the use of only a light compression through the femur to try to elicit the pain. The test is positive when the patient reports a familiar well-localized pain deep in the gluteal area. Östgaard et al (1995) also prefer the term 'posterior pelvic pain' since there is no specific evidence of the anatomical location of the pain. The important feature differentiating between standard low back pain and posterior pelvic pain seems to be that posterior pelvic pain often becomes worse during back muscle training, which may be a treatment offered to low back patients. These authors emphasize that doing the provocation test alone is insufficient for an examination of the presenting pain and that it is important to do a thorough clinical examination of the lumbar spine to ascertain other possible mechanical reasons for pain.

Rungee (1993) suggests that a herniated nucleus pulposus, tumours and infection are all possible causes of low back pain during pregnancy, although they are rare. Symptoms may range from mild to severe. To make a diagnosis of herniated nucleus pulposus, one would expect to find the appropriate clinical findings of weakness, dermatomal sensory paraesthesia and possibly diminished reflexes. Bowel and bladder incontinence may be difficult to differentiate in the pregnant patient due to symptoms associated with these organs in pregnancy. In the area of prophylaxis, Rungee (1993) draws on the literature and suggests that instruction in lifting techniques and overhead working mechanics to avoid lumbar strain should be given.

Treatment approaches to low back pain during pregnancy

It is clear that when a woman presents to the physiotherapist during the ante-natal period with low back pain, the standard subjective and objective assessments for spinal pain are necessary. While the mechanical features associated with pregnancy may be the cause, this cannot be a presumption and other factors must be considered (Rungee, 1993).

Maitland (1991) outlines an important conceptual approach to the assessment of musculoskeletal disorders. He reminds the clinician that during the subjective examination, the patient should be listened to with an open mind, so that known theory may be integrated with the clinical picture presented. He warns against the use of suggestive words for the source of pain, so as to avoid decision-making bias. The importance of not only determining the site of the pain but also understanding the pain behaviour in detail enables the clinician to appreciate the significance of the symptoms and responses of the patient.

Maitland (1991) considers that joint or muscular examination aims to identify the source of the disorder and also the pain. Careful movement of the joint in normal physiological planes as well as accessory planes is recommended. Such movements of the spine are illustrated by Maitland (1986). The essential component in assessment is the identification of a 'particular movement, activity or function that will reproduce symptoms' (Maitland, 1991, p. 5) for identification of cause. Differentiation tests and accurate recording of movement range and pain are essential components of the clinician's approach to diagnosis. The period of gestation will obviously influence the type of tests performed during an objective examination of a pregnant woman. As the abdomen enlarges, physiological movements of the spine will be limited. This factor will also influence the positioning for examination of accessory movements of the spine. Figure 14.14 illustrates the preferable posture for lumbar spine examination later in pregnancy. This position may also be used for treatment. Note that the abdomen and the upper leg are supported.

Depending on the presentation of the patient, the available treatment options may be wide and varied. In Maitland's (1991) opinion, 'So long as patients present with different symptoms and signs, there will have to be changes in the techniques to free the patients of their symptoms' (p. 6).

In the case of pregnancy, much spinal pain and particularly pelvic pain may be associated with excessive mobility. Local treatment to any inflamed joint would be recommended, bearing in mind any contraindications to electrotherapy in the ante-natal period. In addition, corsets of various forms may be useful in providing an increase in stability. If this is the case, then once fitted, the relief is usually apparent. However, if fitting a woman with a brace it is important that a variety of styles be tried, as often there is an individual difference in response to corsets designed to perform similar tasks (Livingstone, personal communication). Figure 14.15 illustrates corsets for lumbar spine, SIJ and pubic symphysis dysfunction.

Each treatment session can be divided into three components (Maitland, 1991): examination of the patient (to determine the effect of the disorder on the patient and on movements of her affected joint areas), treatment techniques and evaluation (to determine the effectiveness of a technique). The latter evaluation should be applied throughout treatment and at its completion (Maitland, 1991).

Mary, a 32-year-old bank clerk of 28 weeks gestation G_1P_1, presented to the ante-natal physiotherapist Jane with moderate low back pain centrally located between L3 and L5 and radiating equally on both sides about 4–5 cm from the centre of the spine. Occasionally when the pain was more severe, there was some radiation into both upper buttock areas. In nature, the pain was like a deep ache and it tended to occur toward the end of the day, especially if Mary had been attending the teller section and standing on her feet for longer than an hour at a time. She did not feel that any particular movements of the spine exacerbated her symptoms, although she was careful to try to bend her knees more when lifting and she was aware that her movements were getting more restricted. The pain was relieved when she lay on her side, with heat from the bath and with massage from her husband. There was usually no pain when she awoke in the morning. The episodes of pain during the day have been increasing in frequency during the week, going from approximately twice a week a month ago to nearly every day now. She had no previous history of any spinal or hip pain and is

Figure 14.14 Lumbar spine assessment during late pregnancy can be performed in side lying with support to the abdomen and lower limbs with pillows.

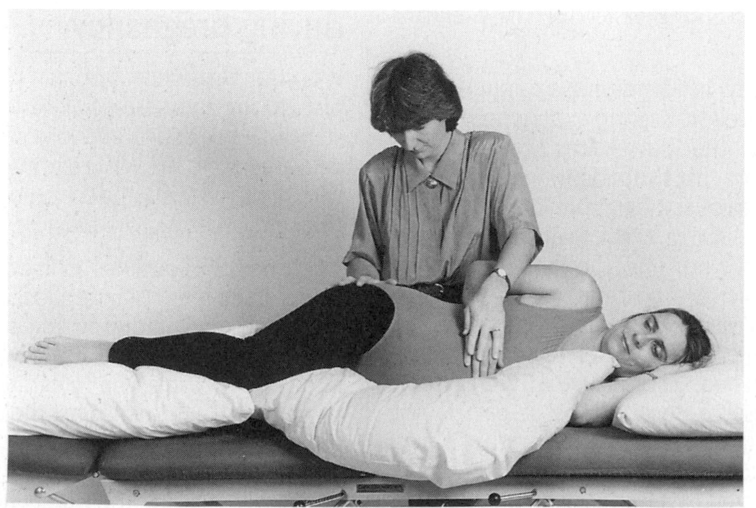

Figure 14.15 (a) A neoprene corset for the lumbar spine. Two straps can be tensioned around the lumbar segments to provide extra support. (b) The corset is now orientated with the straps around the sacroiliac joints (SIJ) in order to increase SIJ stability. (c) A narrow belt which can be used for providing support to the SIJ and the pubic symphysis. It is helpful to place the quick-release buckle toward the front to allow the woman to easily decrease the tension when she sits.

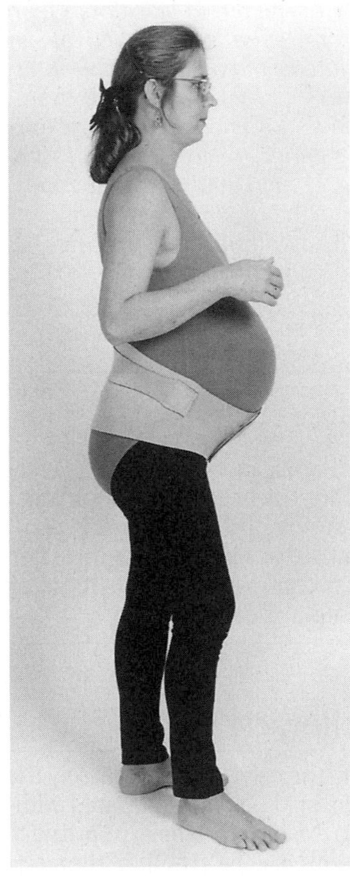
a

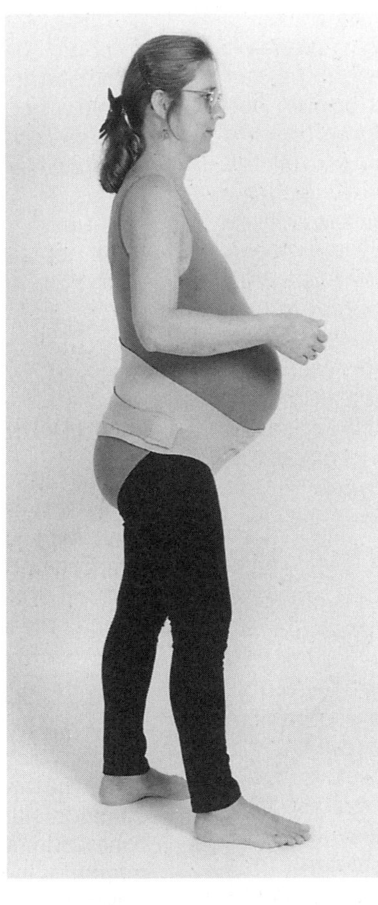
b

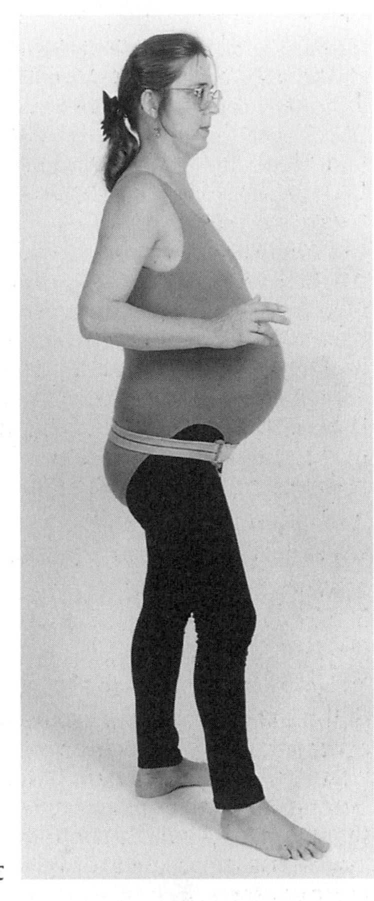
c

taking no medications for any other complaint. She is well and her obstetrician is pleased with the progress of the pregnancy.

Objectively, forward flexion of the spine (range of motion: second finger touching the superior border of the patella) produced minor pain in the area of discomfort. Other movements were not painful, although the full range of motion in lateral flexion was limited due to the abdomen. On palpation, the erector spinae muscles were very tight and deep palpation was uncomfortable.* Assessment of rotation of the lumbar segments revealed a slight restriction in physiological range and an increased resistance to movement, particularly at L3–4.* Active extension of the lumbar spine, performed in side lying and resisted by pressure applied to the sacrum, also caused some discomfort in the area of pain.*

Jane initiated treatment with gentle passive rotation of the lumbar segments in side lying (see Fig. 14.14). Reassessment of the points marked (that is, those activities which reproduced her symptoms) revealed an improvement in the range of motion of the L3–4 segment and an improvement in the quality of end feel. The muscle tightness of the lumbar erector spinae was slightly less and forward flexion did not reproduce pain until the second finger reached below the patella. From these responses, the physiotherapist felt that the pain was primarily associated with muscle fatigue of the lumbar erector spinae and multifidus as well as poor spinal stability and that this was also affecting the quality of the joint movement in the mid-lumbar levels. Gentle mobilization appeared to have decreased some of the local muscle spasm, but Jane felt that it would provide temporary relief only. The treatment was performed once more and then reassessed. All signs had improved, but not completely resolved. So that Mary could manage her pain at home, she was taught to control her spinal posture in four-point kneeling and to activate the transversus abdominis and multifidus (see p. 148). Jane also fitted Mary with a neoprene back support for use particularly on those days when she was working at the teller desk and on her feet.*

They spent some time finding the brace that was comfortable and were able to cut away some excess neoprene just near the anterior hip to allow Mary to sit comfortably.

Mary returned for a reassessment two weeks later. She had been conscientiously performing her home programme and the episodes of pain had become less intense, only of a mild nature and now occurred only when she stood for the full day. Jane progressed the exercises for postural control, adding the more challenging activities of increasing load and additional limb movement. Jane also discussed the modification of exercises in the post-natal period and took the opportunity to revise with Mary her lifting techniques and to discuss suitable heights of the baby bath and baby change table. Mary found that the combination of back support and active muscle activity to maintain spinal stability controlled her episodes of pain for the remainder of her pregnancy.

Georgia was 28 years old and 36 weeks pregnant with her second child. She had been experiencing a sharp stabbing pain in the buttocks for the past two weeks that was elicited by rolling over in bed, walking up and down stairs and fast walking. No apparent incident was associated with the onset of her symptoms. The pain was quite severe and was sharp only for the moment that the exacerbating movement was being performed, after which there was a sense of a deep ache which lasted only for a few minutes. If she did not perform the movements that caused pain, she had no discomfort. While she felt that she did not have too long to wait for the birth of her second child, the pain was interfering with her normal movements and the care of her 18-month-old baby boy. She had not had any problems of this nature during her first pregnancy, but during the birth of her son, Jason, she had considerable pain in the same area and he had been an occipito–posterior presentation (OP) and her second stage labour had been quite long. However, after Jason's birth she was not aware of any back discomfort. She is healthy with no other medical complications.

The nature of Georgia's pain is suggestive of a joint dysfunction and the movements that are exacerbating her pain would be those that generate shear, particularly around the sacroiliac joint and pubic symphysis. The presentation of the symptoms toward the later stage of her pregnancy may indicate that the laxity of the pelvis in combination with the weight of the foetus have led to the failure of the SIJ to maintain form or force closure. A suggested approach would be to provide some external stability from a SIJ or pubic symphysis strap (Fig. 14.15b, 14.15c). If this treatment is to be useful in Georgia's case, this strap should relieve the intensity in each of the exacerbating movements. Such a response would support the diagnosis of instability of the SIJ. In addition, Georgia could benefit from exercises to activate and strengthen the gluteus maximus, as this muscle often becomes weak or hypotonic in SIJ dysfunction (Janda, 1986) and it is considered an important component in generated form/force closure of the SIJ (Vleeming et al, 1990b). Georgia can be trained to activate the gluteus maximus of the stance leg and the contralateral latissimus dorsi to help to provide stability during gait.

Warning

While passive physiological and accessory movement of the joints are useful treatment techniques for pain relief and joint stiffness during the child-bearing year, it is important to recognize that high-velocity thrust manipulation of the joints is contraindicated due to the alteration in the ligamentous and capsular laxity.

Pain from the thoracic spine

While the low back and the pelvis are undoubtedly the most common sites of pain in the spine associated with pregnancy, others may also exist. For example, pain, tingling and numbness in the forearms may be a result of thoracic outlet syndrome or pain in the thoracic spine during respiration may exist and be exacerbated during pregnancy. Bookhout and Boissonnault (1988) state that expansion of the rib cage occurs as a result of pregnancy where the transverse diameter of the chest increases and the diaphragm becomes elevated. It is interesting to note that the subcostal angle increases prior to the exertion of mechanical pressure on the ribs by the growing foetus. They suggest that the neurovascular bundle over the first rib may become stretched during this elevation. The increasing chest circumference may also be responsible for any mechanical aggravation of the costovertebral joints in the thoracic spine, which can be particularly painful in the evening when the patient lies on her side (Bookhout and Boissonnault, 1988).

Bookhout and Boissonnault (1988) describe thoracic outlet syndrome as a common presentation during pregnancy. However, they give no indication of the frequency of its occurrence. The term 'thoracic outlet syndrome' suggests that there is compromise of the brachial plexus, subclavian artery and the subclavian vein, with symptoms from this compromise radiating to the upper extremity. It is common during pregnancy probably because of the elevation of the first rib associated with changed breathing patterns as the foetus increases in size. Such rib elevation may be due to increased activity of the anterior and middle scalene

Figure 14.16 (a) During pregnancy, examination of the thoracic spine (usually performed in prone lying) can be performed in supported sitting over the adjustable plinth. (b) Thoracic spine examination can be performed in sitting in later pregnancy with the physiotherapist supporting the upper trunk and generating rotational movements of the intervertebral segments. (c) Mobilization of the thoracic spine can be actively achieved in side lying and using elevation and protraction of the arm with the woman maintaining eye contact with the hand. In initial training the physiotherapist can stabilize the thoracic segment below by a transverse pressure on the spinous process and encourage localized thoracic spine movement. Holding onto a ball appears to assist in the control and localization of the exercise (Livingstone, personal communication). (d) Use of a self-inflating tube (Torso, Adelaide) placed under the spine can assist in self-mobilization of local stiffness. The tube can be placed with its upper margin on the segment below and the woman can slowly and gently extend over the tube. Of course, the woman must be advised not to remain in the supine position for long. (e) A posture brace can be used to assist in training thoracic spine posture.

a

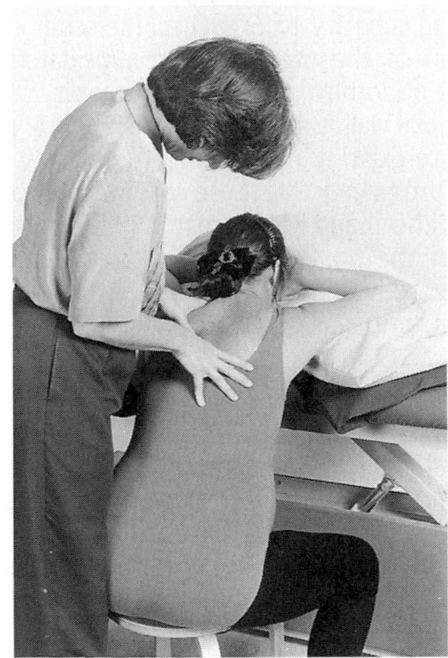

c

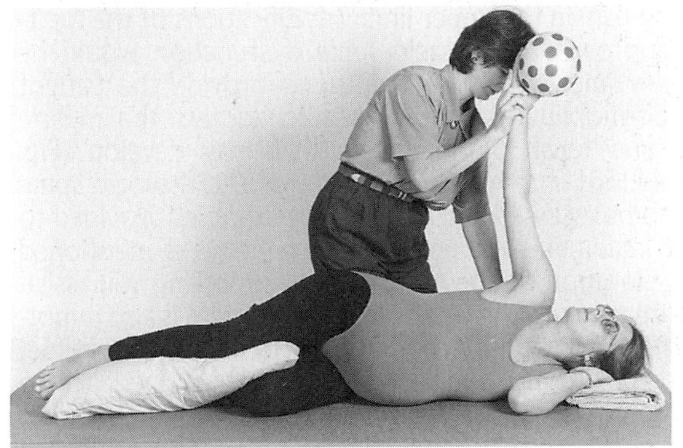

d

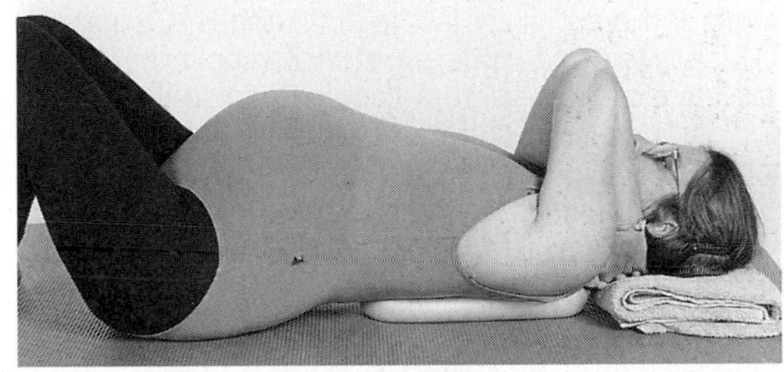

b

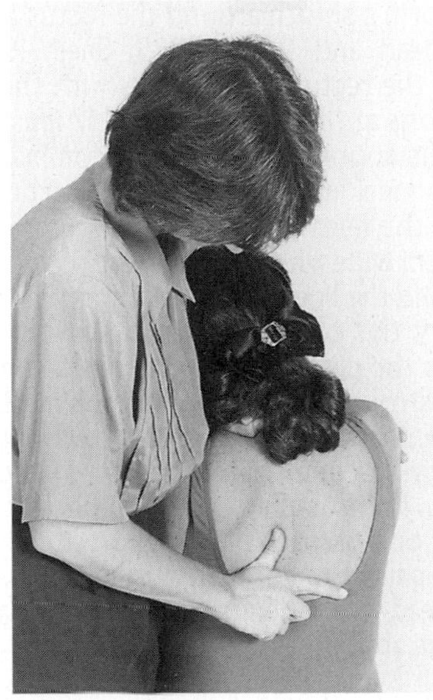

e

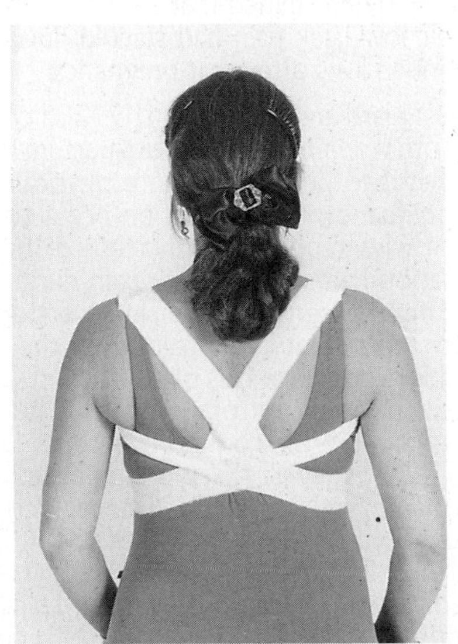

muscles. Compromise would therefore occur by either an increase in the tensile stress of the structures or a decrease in the available space for their movement between the first rib and the clavicle.

It would be natural to assume that anyone with thoracic outlet syndrome requires examination not only of the neck but also of the clavicle, glenohumeral joint, sternoclavicular and acromionoclavicular joints as well as examination of the thoracic spine (Fig. 14.16a, 14.16b). In addition, the upper limb tension test described by Butler (1991) is a necessary component of the examination of someone presenting with radiating pain in the upper limb. Modifications of the treatment approach to thoracic spine dysfunction would be necessary and it is often helpful to provide the patient with self-mobilization techniques to address the muscle spasm and local joint stiffness that may develop (Fig. 14.16c, 14.16d). Further, the posture of the thoracic spine needs to be assessed and appropriate exercises provided to help to maintain alignment of this region. As mentioned earlier, elevation of the head toward the ceiling will assist. Concentration on the position of the scapulae is also important. The use of taping (see Chapter 3) or a brace (Fig. 14.16e) can also be a useful source of proprioceptive feedback to train appropriate thoracic posture.

Post-partum pain

While the majority of spinal and pelvic pain experienced during pregnancy appears to subside within six months post-partum and most likely in the first month (Östgaard et al, 1993), Östgaard and Andersson (1992) report the long-term prevalence of post-partum back pain in some cases, with 7% of women who suffered back pain during pregnancy stating that they still had severe back pain 18 months later. These women need to be identified early in their pregnancy for appropriate management. Östgaard and Andersson (1992) also found that long periods of back pain during pregnancy were associated with a slow regression of back pain after pregnancy. It is interesting to note that in an epidemiological survey of 1746 women in Sweden, Svensson et al (1990) determined that 10% of women considered that their low back pain had started during pregnancy and continued long after that pregnancy.

According to Östgaard and Andersson (1992), a characteristic associated with women suffering post-partum low back pain was that they had performed more physically heavy work prior to pregnancy, the correlation being strong. In addition, women who reported an increase of back pain during menstruation had suffered back pain during earlier pregnancies and multi-pregnant women in general appeared more at risk for persistent back pain after the current pregnancy. Of this group, previous back pain and sick leave because of their back pain from physically heavy and monotonous work were all common factors. Östgaard and Andersson (1992) suggest that the significant amount of lifting performed by mothers of small babies (particularly multiparas) could contribute to the development of back pain (see Chapter 21 for further details). Hayes et al (1987) have determined that the force on the lumbar spine generated during lifting of children can be 2000 N, a considerable load to withstand.

Influence of Pregnancy on the Muscular System

The most marked influence of pregnancy on the muscular system is in the required lengthening of the abdominal wall. The uterus expands and increases in weight more than 20 times exclusive of its contents (Sherwood, 1993). In the non-pregnant state, the uterus weighs approximately 60 g and its capacity is about 6 ml. At term, the weight has increased to 1 kg and the capacity to 5000 ml (Beischer et al, 1989). The expansion of the uterus is accommodated by gross changes in the abdominal wall anatomy, that is, the anatomy of the abdominal wall is markedly influenced by pregnancy. In addition, pre-existing muscle imbalances may be exacerbated during pregnancy and these require appropriate management (Bookhout and Boissonnault, 1988). Some muscles, particularly of the posterior spine and lower limbs, may increase their activity during pregnancy to compensate for changes in centre of gravity.

Anatomy of the abdominal wall

The abdominal wall is bounded superiorly by the infrasternal angle and inferiorly by the iliac crest, inguinal sulcus and pubic sulcus (Kahle et al, 1992). On each side of the mid-line, between the rib cage and the symphysis pubis, lies the rectus abdominis muscle (Hollinshead and Rosse, 1985). The outer, inner and innermost muscle layers of the antero-lateral wall are formed by the external oblique, internal oblique and transversus abdominis muscles respectively. The aponeuroses of the external obliques, internal obliques and transversus abdominis muscles meet in a mid-line raphe where the intertwining of their tendon fibres forms the collagenous linea alba. Before the aponeuroses meet in the linea alba, they form a sheath around the rectus abdominis muscle (Hollinshead and Rosse, 1985; Snell, 1986). The anterior layer of the rectus sheath fuses with the external oblique aponeurosis at this level. Figure 14.17 illustrates the relationship of the aponeurosis of the abdominal muscles. All of the abdominal muscles have an insertion in the median plane to the linea alba. Above the umbilicus, this structure is 1–2 cm wide while below it, the recti muscles lie closer together and the linea alba is narrower (Platzer, 1986). During pregnancy, this connective tissue structure is likely to 'loosen' due to the circulating hormones. There is good evidence that oestrogens may alter the polymerization of acid mucopolysaccharides and thereby have a profound effect on the physicochemical properties of the ground substances which, for example, act as the adhesive between fibres in collagenous tissue (Hytten and Leitch, 1964). In addition to an expanding abdomen during pregnancy, this 'loosening' may lead to a widening of the linea alba, termed 'diastasis of rectus abdominis'.

Diastasis of rectus abdominis

Diastasis recti occurs commonly in pregnancy and incidence rates of 67% (Boissonnlaut and Blaschak, 1988) and 100%

Figure 14.17 Cross-sections of rectus abdominis and its sheath. (1) Above the arcuate line the aponeurosis of the internal oblique (b) divides. Its anterior lamina fuses with the aponeurosis of the external oblique (a) to form the ventral layer of the rectus sheath. Its posterior lamina fuses with the aponeurosis of the transversus abdominis (c) to form the dorsal layer of the rectus sheath. (2) Below the arcuate line the aponeuroses of all three muscles fuse to form the ventral layer of the rectus sheath and the transversalis fascia forms the dorsal layer. (Reproduced with permission from Kendall and McCreary, 1983.)

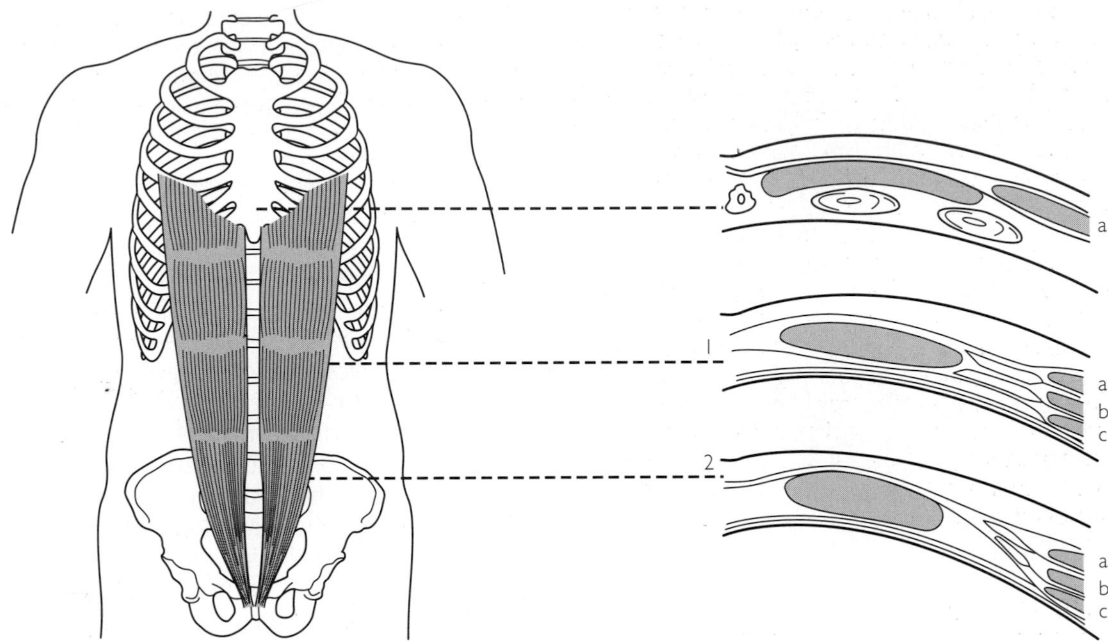

(Bursch, 1987; Hannaford and Tozer, 1985) have been reported. The incidence of different degrees of diastasis, however, does not appear in the literature. Thornton and Thornton (1993) report a case of a divarication of the recti muscles measured at 23 cm, which is clearly a gross separation. Some factors have been considered to have a strong causal relationship with the degree of diastasis (Hannaford and Tozer, 1985; Noble, 1988; Polden and Mantle, 1990) and these include weight gain during pregnancy, age, baby's birth weight, the para status of the mother, connective tissue insufficiency and the level of exercise of the mother. The presence of diastasis recti can be palpated as a hollow or trough between the superficial rectus abdominis muscles. The existence of a separation of the abdominal muscles was documented as early as 1858, when Gray described the recti muscles as 'diverging from one another in their ascent, becoming of considerable breadth after great distension of the abdomen from pregnancy. . .'

The presence of diastasis recti indicates a number of changes to the integrity of the abdominal wall. For example, the viability of the lumbosacral fascia, which provides a circumferential support to the lumbar spine (Miller and Medeiros, 1987) and incorporates the central attachments of the internal oblique and transversus abdominis, may be weakened. The absence of a stable insertion for all abdominal muscles may influence the inter-relationship between attachment and muscle fibre direction. Changes to the angle of insertion of a muscle influences the muscle's line of action (Warwick and Williams, 1973) and subsequently the muscle's functional capabilities. However, currently, there is a paucity of information on the effect of known musculoskeletal adaptations during pregnancy on gross structural changes of specific abdominal muscles.

If such changes do occur, then they would have implications for the way in which the abdominal muscles were activated and for their ability to stabilize the pelvis during activity and under load. Gilleard (1992) found that functional ability of abdominal muscles decreased during and after pregnancy, as reflected in a decreased ability to stabilize the pelvis. Such inadequacies could lead to muscle imbalances, inefficiency in movement, changes in posture and the development of low back pain.

Boissonnault and Kotarinos (1988) suggest that the pyramidalis muscle has its origin anterior to the pubis symphysis. As this is not present in all individuals, it may be a cause for diastasis recti of large proportions. This is because the functional activity of the pyramidalis muscle is to provide tension and reinforcement of the linea alba.

Boissonnault and Kotarinos (1988) suggest that pregnancy hormones are commonly implicated in the softening of connective tissue believed to occur throughout the body. Moore (1983) points out that connective tissues become less supportive as the levels of hormones increase during pregnancy and suggests that these hormones may contribute to loosening of the abdominal fascia. MacLennan's (1983) review of the literature suggests that relaxin appears to affect only those sites which have specific markers for the hormone. To date these have been found in the cervix, myometrium, decidua and breast connective tissue. Another important point is that relaxin has a varying

Figure 14.18 The abdomen of a woman three days post-natally. She demonstrates a ridging of the rectus abdominis during trunk curl and on palpation the diastasis measured 35 mm.

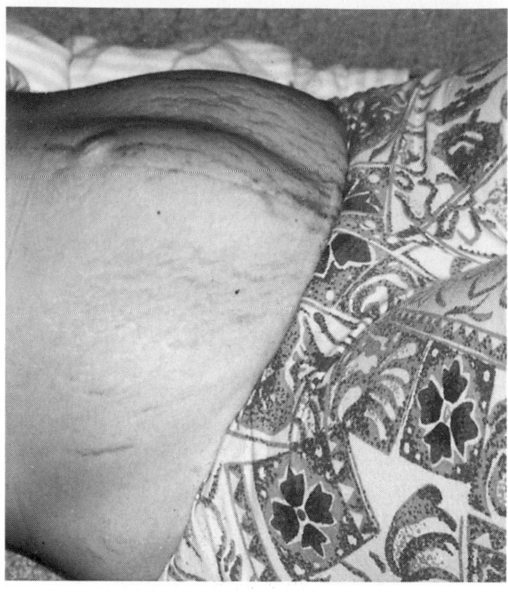

concentration level in the blood during pregnancy, whereas the levels of progesterone and oestrogen tend to increase throughout the pregnancy.

Boissonnault and Kotarinos (1988) suggest that an increase in the size of the diastasis may be due to a combination of the effects of hormonal changes on the linea alba and the mechanical stresses to the abdominal wall. These authors point out that the functional loss associated with diastasis would influence the ability of the abdominal muscles to contract effectively. Figure 14.18 illustrates the abdomen of a post-natal woman with a palpable diastasis of 35 mm just above the umbilicus and a bulging rectus abdominis on contraction. The increase in ligamentous laxity of peripheral joints has been correlated with the size of the abdominal sagittal diameter by Östgaard et al (1993). These findings are interesting for the possible correlation between the development of diastasis (associated with a large abdomen) and the degree of peripheral laxity that may exist.

Management of diastasis of rectus abdominis would be associated with the functional deficits existing in the abdominal musculature. Noble (1988) has suggested that if there is a wide diastasis during active exercise of trunk curl, patients should actively draw the sides of the abdomen closer together with their hands. This may be indicated if there is either a complete or an incomplete tear of the linea alba. However, if there is only a minor degree of diastasis then this activity would be overzealous. In terms of function, it is important that the abdominal obliques and transversus are able to contract well and to be able to increase the intra-abdominal pressure when necessary for lifting and for other functions of bearing down. The relevance of a trunk curl exercise to activities of daily living would have to be questioned. Primarily it is considered that the general function of the abdominals is to provide stability of the spine. This is normally performed through isometric co-contraction and any abdominal exercise regime should emphasize endurance-holding capacity rather than only dynamic concentric contractions aiming to increase strength. Such an exercise programme may consist of promotion of transversus abdominis activation with co-contraction of the pelvic floor which could be taught in modified four-point kneeling (Fig. 14.11) and progressed to upright postures, as described earlier.

In addition to the improvement of muscle activation in the abdominal region, the use of an abdominal corset has been advocated by Thornton and Thornton (1993). Such a device can act as a support for the abdominal wall in the case of gross divarication of the rectus abdominis muscles during pregnancy and patients report a sense of stability in this area on its use. Clinical opinion suggests that a firm support around the waist can act as a reminder to activate the muscles. Rather than a tendency to relax while using a corset, the firm pressure usually generates an increased tension. Consider the situation of abdominal muscle activity when a woman is dressed in loose-fitting flowing clothes, compared to a tight-fitting dress. In loose clothing, the abdominals can easily be relaxed, whereas the opposite appears true for the tight-fitting clothing (Livingstone, personal communication).

A woman at term for her second pregnancy had a rectus divarication measuring 23 cm at the umbilicus. The patient had found symptomatic relief of lumbar pain during pregnancy from the wearing of an abdominal corset. The patient also stated that the corset proved to be useful in the second stage of labour when it was applied after active pushing which had caused the uterus to prolapse through the divarication. (Such a situation created a biomechanical disadvantage and may have prolonged the second stage of labour due to abdominal insufficiency.) The woman was managed post-natally for this gross divarication with the use of Tubigrip around the abdomen for three weeks and a graduated exercise programme. Six months after delivery, the divarication measured 1.5 cm at the umbilicus (Thornton and Thornton, 1993).

A number of corsets are available for post-natal abdominal support. Some clinicians also advocate the use of support girdles in the initial stages post-partum (Livingstone, personal communication). Abdominal supports offer some stimulation for active contraction of the abdominals, particularly if the patient is advised to draw her abdomen away from the support offered by the corset. Figure 14.19 illustrates one abdominal corset and the use of elastic bandages for abdominal support.

Figure 14.19 (a) A broad elastic bandage can be used to provide abdominal support particularly during pregnancy when the abdomen is increasing in size. (b) Abdominal corsets can be used to provide extra support during the post-natal period. The woman can be advised on maintaining appropriate spinal alignment while she periodically draws her abdomen away from the support. In such an application, the support can provide the required stability as well as acting as a pressure biofeedback for facilitation of muscle activation.

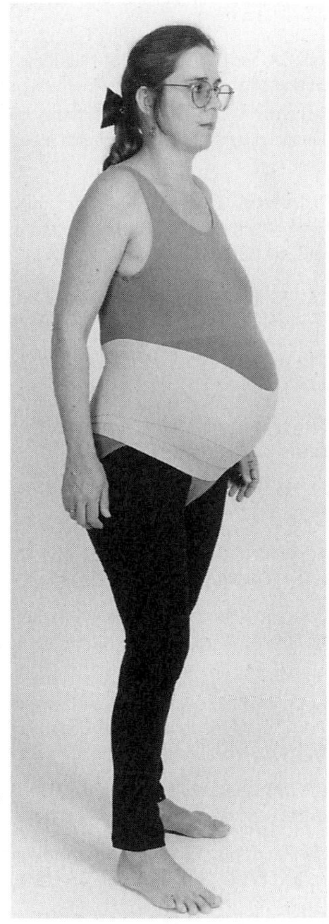

a

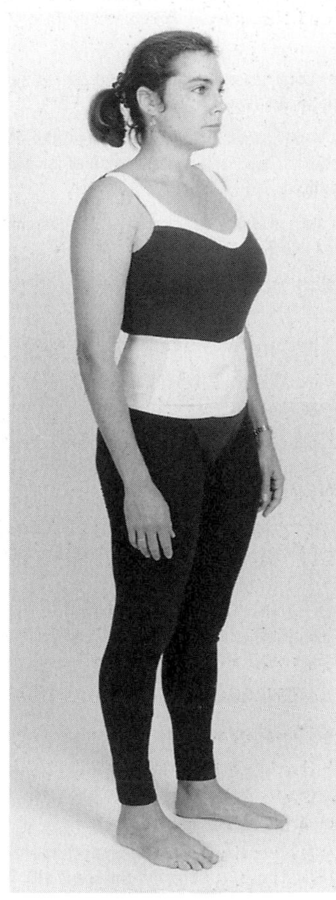

b

Summary

In the child-bearing year the female body illustrates its wonderful capacity to adapt and nurture the growth of the foetus and infant. It is an amazing process of nature. When considering the large musculoskeletal changes that occur in accommodating this function, it is not surprising that some parts of the system suffer dysfunction. Physiotherapy is in a unique situation to offer services to help the woman adapt to her pregnancy and the physical demands of child-care. The physiotherapist's thorough knowledge of anatomy and understanding of the musculoskeletal system, coupled with an appreciation of the particular differences with which a woman in her child-bearing year presents, ensures an active role for physiotherapists in education and management of this period of a woman's life.

References

Basmajian JV (1965). Man's posture. *Archives of Physical Medicine and Rehabilitation* **46**: 25–35.

Beischer N, Mackay E and Purcal N (1989) *Care of the Pregnant Woman and Her Baby*, 2nd edn. London: W.B. Saunders.

Bergmark A (1989) Stability of the lumbar spine. A study in mechanical engineering. *Acta Orthopaedica Scandinavica* **230**(60): 20–24.

Boissonnault J and Blaschak M (1988) Incidence of diastasis recti abdominis during the childbearing year. *Physical Therapy* **68**: 1082–1086.

Boissonnault JS and Kotarinos RK (1988) Diastasis recti. In: Wilder E (ed) *Obstetric and Gynaecologic Physical Therapy, Clinics in Physical Therapy*, Vol. 20, pp. 63–82. New York: Churchill Livingstone.

Bookhout MM and Boissonnault WG (1988) Physical therapy management of musculoskeletal disorders during pregnancy. In: Wilder E (ed) *Obstetric and Gynaecologic Physical Therapy, Clinics in Physical Therapy*, Vol. 20, pp. 17–62. New York: Churchill Livingstone.

Bullock JE, Jull GA and Bullock MI (1987) The relationship of low back pain to postural changes during pregnancy. *Australian Journal of Physiotherapy* **33**(1): 10–17.

Bullock-Saxton JE (1988) Back pain during pregnancy: a retrospective questionnaire. Australian Physiotherapy Association National Conference, Canberra, pp. 84–91.

Bullock-Saxton JE (1991) Changes in posture measured in standing associated with pregnancy and the early post-natal period. *Physiotherapy Theory and Practice* **7**(2): 103–109.

Bullock-Saxton JE (1994) Local sensation changes and altered hip muscle function following repetitive ankle sprain. *Physical Therapy* **74**: 17–31.

Bullock-Saxton JE, Janda V and Bullock MI (1993) Reflex activation of gluteal muscles in walking with balance shoes: an approach to restoration of function for chronic low back pain patients. *Spine* **18**(6): 704–708.

Bursch G (1987) Interrater reliability of diastasis recti abdominis measurement. *Physical Therapy* **67**: 1077–1079.

Butler DS (1991) *Mobilisation of the Nervous System.* Melbourne: Churchill Livingstone.

Calliet R (1981) *Low Back Pain Syndrome*, 3rd edn. Philadelphia: F.A. Davis.

Calguneri M, Bird HA and Wright B (1982) Changes in joint laxity occuring in pregnancy. *Annals of Rheumatic Diseases* **41**: 126–128.

Coderre, TJ and Melzack R (1987) Cutaneous hyperalgesia: contributions of the peripheral and central nervous systems to the increase in pain sensitivity after injury. *Brain Research* **404**: 95–106.

Cresswell AG, Grundstrom A and Thorstensson A (1992) Observations on intra-abdominal pressure and patterns of abdominal intra-muscular activity in man. *Acta Physiologica Scandinavica* **144**: 409–418.

Cureton TK and Wickens JS (1935) The centre of gravity of the human body in the antero-posterior plane and its relation to posture, physical fitness and athletic ability. *Research Quarterly Supplement*, **6**: 93–106.

Cyriax J (1965) *Textbook of Orthopaedic Medicine.* Cassell, London.

Danforth D (1967) Pregnancy and labour. *American Journal of Physical Medicine* **46**: 653–658.

De Andrade JR, Grant C and Dixon A (1965) Joint distension and reflex inhibition in the knee. *Journal of Bone and Joint Surgery* **47A**: 313–322.

Dumas GA, Reid JG, Wolfe LA et al (1995a) Exercise, posture and back pain during pregnancy. Part I. Exercise and posture. *Clinical Biomechanics* **10**: 98–103.

Dumas GA, Reid JG, Wolfe LA et al (1995b) Exercise, posture and back pain during pregnancy. Part II. Exercise and back pain. *Clinical Biomechanics* **10**: 104–109.

Ekholm J, Eklund G and Skøglund S (1960) On the reflex effect from the knee joint of the cat. *Acta Physiologica Scandinavica* **50**: 167–174.

Fast A, Shapiro D, Ducommun EJ et al (1987) Low back pain in pregnancy. *Spine* **12**: 368–371.

Floyd WF and Silver PHS (1950) Electromyographic study of patterns of abdominal activity of the anterior abdominal wall muscles in man. *Journal of Anatomy* **84**: 132–145.

Freeman MAR and Wyke B (1966) Articular contributions to limb muscle reflexes. *British Journal of Surgery* **53**: 61–68.

Gilleard WL (1992) The structure and function of the abdominal muscles during pregnancy and the immediate post-birth period. MSc thesis, University of Wollongong, Australia.

Gray H (1858) *Gray's Anatomy: The Classic First Edition* (reprinted 1991). The Promotional Reprint Company, Great Britain.

Grubb BD, Stiller RU and Schaible HG (1993) Dynamic changes in the receptive field properties of spinal cord neurons with ankle input in rats with chronic unilateral inflammation in the ankle region. *Experimental Brain Research* **92**: 441–452.

Hainline B (1994) Low back pain in pregnancy. In: Devinsky O, Feldmann E and Hainline B (eds). *Neurological Complications of Pregnancy*, pp. 65–76. New York: Raven Press.

Hall MG, Ferrel WR, Sturrock RD et al (1995) The effect of the hypermobility syndrome on knee joint proprioception. *British Journal of Rheumatology* **34**: 121–125.

Hannaford R and Tozer J (1985) An investigation of the incidence, degree, and possible predisposing factors of rectus diastasis in the immediate post-partum period. *Journal of National Obstetrics and Gynaecological Special Group of the Australian Physiotherapy Association* **4**: 29–32.

Hayes WC, Nachemson AL and White AA (1987) Forces in the lumbar spine. In: Camins MB and O'Leary PF (eds) *The Lumbar Spine*, pp. 1–21. New York: Raven Press.

Hides JA, Stokes MJ, Saide M et al (1994) Evidence of lumber multifidus muscle wasting ipsilateral to symptoms in patients with acute/subacute low back pain. *Spine* **19**(2): 165–172.

Hides JA, Richardson CA and Jull GA (1996) Multifidus muscle recovery is not automatic after resolution of acute, first episode low back pain. *Spine* **21**: 2763–2769.

Hodges PW and Richardson CA (1997) Feedforward contraction of transversus abdominis is not influenced by the direction of arm movement. *Experimental Brain Research* (in press).

Hodges PW and Richardson CA (1996) Inefficient muscular stabilisation of the lumbar spine associated with low back pain: a motor control evaluation of transversus abdominis. *Spine.* (in press).

Hollinshead WH (1976) *Functional Anatomy of the Limbs and Back: a Textbook for Students of the Locomotor Apparatus*, 4th edn. Philadelphia: W.B. Saunders.

Hollinshead W and Rosse T (1985) *Textbook of Anatomy.* 4th edn. Philadelphia: Harper and Rowe.

Hummell P (1987) Changes in posture during pregnancy. PhD thesis, Vrije Universiteit de Amsterdam, Academisch Pragshrift.

Hytten F and Leitch I (1964) *The Physiology of Human Pregnancy.* Oxford: Blackwell Scientific Publications.

Iles JF, Stokes M and Young A (1990) Reflex actions of knee joint afferents during contractions of the human quadriceps. *Clinical Physiology* **10**: 489–500.

Janda V (1978) Muscles, central nervous motor regulation and back problems. In: Korr IM (ed) *Neurobiologic Mechanisms in Manipulative Therapy*, pp. 27–41. New York: Plenum Press.

Janda V (1986) Muscle weakness and inhibition (pseudoparesis) in back pain syndromes. In: Grieve GP (ed) *Modern Manual Therapy of the Vertebral Column*, pp. 197–201. Edinburgh: Churchill Livingstone.

Janda V and Vavrova M (1994) *Sensory Motor Stimulation: A Video*, presented by J.E. Bullock-Saxton. Brisbane: Body Control Systems Australia.

Johansson H, Sjölander P and Sojka P (1991) A sensory role for the cruciate ligaments. *Clinical Orthopaedics and Related Research* **268**: 161–178.

Kahle W, Leonhardt H and Platzer W (1992) *Colour Atlas and Textbook of Human Anatomy*, 4th edn. Stuttgart: Georg Thieme.

Kendall HO, Kendall FP and Boynton DA (1952) *Posture and Pain*, p. 204. Malabar, Florida: Malabar Publishing.

Kendall FP and McCreary EK (1983) *Muscles Testing and Function*, 3rd edn. Baltimore: Williams and Wilkins.

Kendall FP, McCreary EK and Provance PG (1993) *Muscles Testing and Function*, 4th edn, p. 451. Baltimore: Williams and Wilkins.

MacLennan AH (1983) The role of relaxin in human reproduction. *Clinical Reproduction and Fertility* **2**: 77–95.

MacLennan AH, Nicholson R and Green RC (1986) Serum relaxin in pregnancy. *Lancet* **2**: 241–245.

Maitland GD (1986) *Vertebral Manipulation*, 4th edn. London: Butterworth.

Maitland GD (1991) *Peripheral Manipulation*, 3rd edn. Oxford: Butterworth Heinmann.

Mallik AK, Ferrell WR, McDonald AG et al (1994) Impaired proprioceptive acuity at the proximal interphalangeal joint in patients with the hypermobility syndrome. *British Journal of Rheumatology* **33**: 631–637.

Mantle MJ, Greenwood RM and Currey HLF (1977) Backache in pregnancy. *Rheumatology and Rehabilitation* **16**: 95–101.

Massey WW (1943) A critical study of objective methods for measuring anterior posterior posture with a simplified technique. *Research Quarterly* **14**: 3–25.

Miller M and Medeiros J (1987) Recruitment of internal oblique and transversus abdominis muscles during the eccentric phase of the curl-up exercise. *Physical Therapy* **67**: 1213–1217.

Moore M (1983) *Realities in Childbearing*. Philadelphia: W.B. Saunders.

Noble E (1988) *Essential Exercises for the Childbearing Year*, 3rd edn. Boston: Houghton Mifflin.

Nwuga VCB (1982) Pregnancy and back pain among upper class Nigerian women. *Australian Journal of Physiotherapy* **28**: 8–11.

O'Connor DT (1969) Some thoughts on the mechanical anatomy of the female pelvis. *Australian Journal of Physiotherapy* **XV**(1): 7–14.

Östgaard HC (1995) Back and posterior pelvic pain in relation to pregnancy. In: Vleeming A, Mooney V, Dorman T and Snijders C (eds). The integrated function of the lumbar spine and sacroiliac joint. *Second Interdisciplinary World Congress on Low Back Pain*, San Diego, pp. 185–188.

Östgaard HC and Andersson GBJ (1992) Postpartum low back pain. *Spine* **17**(1): 53–55.

Östgaard HC, Andersson GBJ, and Karlsson K (1991) Prevalence of back pain in pregnancy. *Spine* **16**: 549–552.

Östgaard HC, Andersson GBJ, Schultz AB et al (1993) Influence of some mechanical factors on low back pain. *Spine* **18**(1): 61–65.

Panjabi M (1992a) The stabilizing system of the spine. Part I Function, dysfunction, adaptation and enhancement. *Journal of Spinal Disorders* **5**: 383–389.

Panjabi M. (1992b) The stabilizing system of the spine. Part II Neutral zone and instability hypothesis. *Journal of Spinal Disorders* **5**(4): 390–397.

Platzer W (1986) Locomotor system, vol. 1. In: Kahle W, Leonhardt H and Platzer W (eds) *Colour Atlas and Textbook of Human Anatomy* in 3 volumes. New York: Georg Thieme.

Polden M and Mantle J (1990) *Physiotherapy in Obstetrics and Gynaecology*. Oxford: Butterworth Heinemann.

Portnoy H and Morin F (1956) Electromyographic studies of the postural muscles in various positions and movements. *American Journal of Physiology* **186**: 122–126.

Rhodes P (1958) Orthopaedic conditions associated with childbearing. *Practitioner* **181**: 305–312.

Richardson CA and Jull GA (1994) Concepts of rehabilitation for spinal stability. In: Boyling JD and Palastanga N (eds) *Grieve's Modern Manual Therapy of the Vertebral Column*, 2nd edn, pp. 705–720. Edinburgh: Churchill Livingstone.

Richardson CA and Jull GA (1995) Muscle control – pain control. What exercises would you prescribe? *Manual Therapy* **1**: 2–10.

Richardson CA, Toppenberg R and Jull GA (1990) An initial evaluation of eight abdominal exercises for their ability to provide stabilisation for the lumbar spine. *Australian Journal of Physiotherapy* **36**(1): 6–11.

Richardson CA, Jull GA, Toppenberg R et al (1992) Techniques for active lumbar stabilisation for spinal protection: a pilot study. *Australian Journal of Physiotherapy* **38**(2): 105–112.

Rungee MJL (1993) Low back pain during pregnancy. *Orthopedics* **16**: 1339–1344.

Sands RX (1958) Backache of pregnancy, a method of treatment. *Obstetrics and Gynaecology* **12**: 670 – 676.

Sherwood R (1993) *Human Physiology: From Cells to Systems*. Minneapolis: St Paul West.

Snell R (1986) *Clinical Anatomy for Medical Students*. Little Brown and Co.

Snijders GJ, Snijder JD and Hoest HT (1976) Change in form of the spine as a consequence of pregnancy. *Digest of the 11th International Conference on Medical and Biological Engineering*, Ottawa, Canada, pp. 670–671.

Spankus JD (1953) Lumbosacral junction; roentgenographic comparison of patients with and without backaches. *Journal of the American Medical Association* **152**: 1610–1613.

Spankus JD (1965) The cause and treatment of low back pain during pregnancy. *Winsonsin Medical Journal* **64**: 303–304.

Stokes M and Young A (1984) The contribution of reflex inhibition to arthrogenous muscle weakness. *Clinical Science* **67**: 7–14.

Svensson H, Andersson GBJ, Hagstad A et al (1990) The relationship of low back pain to pregnancy and gynaecologic factors. *Spine* **15**: 371–374.

Thornton SI and Thornton SJ (1993) Management of gross divarication of the recti abdominis in pregnancy and labour. *Physiotherapy* **79**: 457–458.

Vleeming A, Stoeckart R and Snijders CJ (1990a) Relation between form and function in the sacroiliac joint. Part I Clinical anatomical aspects. *Spine* **15**(2): 130–132.

Vleeming A, Volkers ACW, Snijders CJ et al (1990b) Relation between form and function in the sacroiliac joint. Part II Biomechanical aspects. *Spine* **15**(2): 133–136.

Warwick R and Williams P (eds) (1973) *Gray's Anatomy*, 35th edn. Harlow: Longman.

Woolf, CJ (1983) Evidence for a central component of post-injury pain hypersensitivity. *Nature* **306**: 686–688.

Wyke B (1967) The neurology of joints. *Annals of the Royal College of Surgeons of England* **41**: 25–50.

15

Ante-natal Education

LURLENE LIVINGSTONE, RUTH SAPSFORD AND SUE MARKWELL

Lifestyles that prevail in the 1990s mean that women ante-natally have different needs from previous generations. These women work full time, often until term, many keep fit at the gym and are too tired to cope with evening ante-natal classes. All are aware that pain relief is available, so preparation for labour does not merit the same emphasis as it did for their mothers.

There are many professional women becoming first-time mothers in their 30s and even 40s, who have unrealistic ideas of the demands of a new baby and how they will cope, with little or no family support. So the emphasis of ante-natal education provided by the physiotherapist must change to meet these women's needs. Parenting skills and how to cope with the physical demands of mothering may be more important than how to cope with a labour, in which epidural analgesia is readily available to relieve pain. There are other groups in the community, often disadvantaged, who have special educational needs.

The physiotherapist's input to classes will depend on the setting within which she works. However, for the 'new educator', the experience of observing classes conducted by other physiotherapists is invaluable. Time spent in the labour ward sitting through labours provides an understanding of the infinite variations that can occur. Educators must not base their teaching on their own labour experiences as it is impossible for these to be truly representative. Background knowledge of the child-bearing year and small group teaching principles needs the addition of practical examples to enable effective class taking.

The Setting – Team Approach or Sole Educator?

Physiotherapists can provide ante-natal education in:

1. large obstetric hospitals where other input is provided by some or all of the following: midwives, dietitians, lactation consultants and medical personnel. Clients may be high or low risk and have access to a large range of services;
2. a community setting where a team education structure has been established;
3. a community setting, where the physiotherapist is a sole practitioner but has access to hospitals for labour ward visits by arrangement or can refer clients to other services;
4. a rural setting where the physiotherapist may work in isolation. Her clientele may give birth in a distant centre.

A team may consist of some or all of the following professionals who provide the input outlined.

- *Midwife* – conception, foetal development, routine ante-natal care, healthy pregnancy habits, support services available, emotional changes, complications of pregnancy.

Labour – signs of onset, process of first, second and third stages of labour, delivery methods, episiotomy, role of support persons.
- *Physiotherapist* – physical changes in pregnancy and puerperium, preventive practices, ergonomics, safe exercise guidelines, specific exercises for stability and strengthening, physical management of pregnancy discomforts, musculoskeletal problem management, relaxation, breathing, positioning, coping skills for labour, massage. Postnatal review, joint stability, muscle strengthening, fitness programmes, baby handling and baby massage, specific treatment modalities.
- *Dietitian* – nutrition in pregnancy and for life.
- *Anaesthetist* – pain management in labour.
- *Lactation consultant* – preparation for and process of breast feeding.
- *Child health nurse* – feeding, parenting and health issues.

Seldom are all of these professionals available. Roles are amalgamated and videos and literature etc. used to cover gaps in a programme. Those working in isolation will need to further their education to enable them to provide 'well-rounded' classes. In some areas, liaison between different professional bodies has enabled the development of guidelines for ante-natal education. Professional roles have been defined to give mothers ante-natal education that provides the optimum benefits and utilizes the skills of the educators (APA, 1989).

Figure 15.1 The professional team involved in ante-natal education.

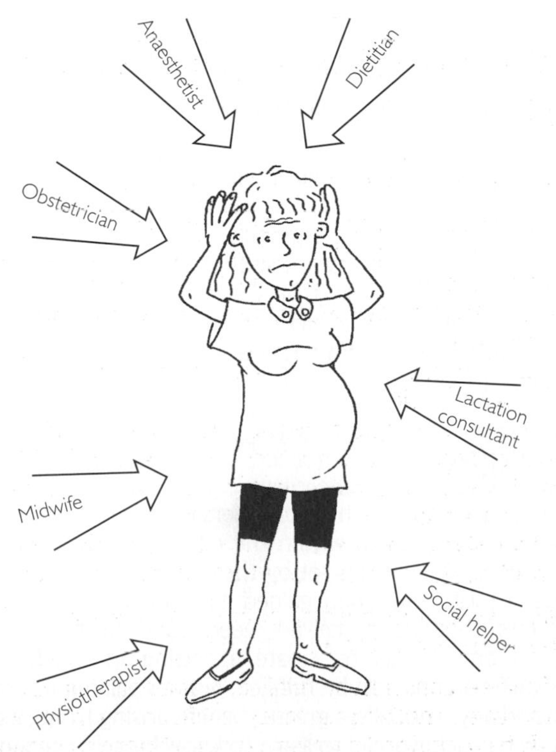

Necessary Knowledg[e] and Resources

Whatever the setting in w[...] therapist must have the following [...] effective classes.

Awareness of the mother's / couple's needs and attitudes

Ideally the physiotherapist should have contact or an interview, either in person or by phone, with each class participant prior to classes. The purpose is to learn about the person / couple, establish a relationship and gain information. Will she attend alone or with a partner? Has she any previous experience or problems? What are her attitudes to and expectations of classes and labour? Are there any relevant cultural factors? What is her work situation?

> Prior attitudes and social relations can affect the way women prepare for and experience birth. Women who feel positive about themselves should view most of their experiences positively, including the experience of giving birth. They feel more in control of their lives and worry less about childbirth (Norr et al, 1977, p. 264).

Some women don't know what they need from classes. Others, usually after a previous experience, have very specific needs and may only require revision of practical aspects. It is almost impossible to provide an appropriate level of information for all the class participants within one group. Perhaps the best approach is for the educator to state at the beginning that she assumes a certain level of knowledge and to pitch the content above a basic level, while avoiding extremes.

The physiotherapist must make each person feel at ease within the class and so enable them to participate fully and gain as much as possible from it. During practical segments, emphasize the self-help strategies for single participants and the help of partners amongst couples.

A father's response to the pregnancy and classes should be considered too. Many fathers, 22.5% in one study, particularly first-time fathers and those less well educated, experience physical symptoms during their wife's pregnancy (Lamb and Lipkin, 1982). This is termed the couvade syndrome, in which the man takes on part of the pregnancy. This is evident in different cultures too. The symptoms include loss of appetite, nausea, vomiting, abdominal pain and toothache. As well as physical symptoms, the educator must be aware of the father's mental attitudes too. A recent survey of fathers' attitudes found that first-time fathers are confused by their changing role and relationship with their partner and the baby and are overwhelmed by the fear that they will not fulfil the role expected of them. They felt that services focused on their partner's labour and the birth of the child and neglected their greatest concerns, that is, their

…entity, their relationships and their future role as …arclay et al, 1996). Perhaps there is a need for a class … to expectant fathers' needs.

Develop small group teaching skills

An ante-natal group can be run in several ways, but group numbers should be small enough to allow the educator and couples/women to get to know each other. The group structure caters for members who have common goals; it should give a sense of belonging, an opportunity to interact and encourage full participation in all group processes. Lecture style and authoritarian presentation prevent the group from functioning in this desired way.

A physiotherapist/teacher must have enthusiasm for the topic and an ability to give the group the required balance of instruction, practice, discussion and participation. Controlling and directing discussion is a skill that improves with practice. The group leader can use questions, elicit opinions or ask for an expression of feelings on a topic to stimulate discussion. When a group functions in an optimum way all members feel comfortable in the situation. In one study, men stated that they often endured and did not enjoy ante-natal education. They often resented the way in which information was presented (Barclay et al, 1996). This statement should make all educators evaluate the way they conduct their classes and modify the process accordingly.

Classes in which members feel at ease can offer peer support to cope with problems and can progress later into young mothers' groups which share the cares and joys of parenting. Life-long friendships can develop.

Provide a suitable venue, equipment and teaching aids to maximize the class experience

All manner of teaching aids are available including models of the pelvis, foetus and uterus and charts, posters, slides, videos and photos. It is not possible to list them here. Before purchasing any, however, it would be a good idea to contact physiotherapists involved in women's health within your own area, for information on sources and suitable material. Remember that your hands are useful teaching aids too. An abundance of material is available from Childbirth Graphics, 1210 Culver Road, Rochester, New York.

Some basic principles apply to the use of aids within the class.

- Keep content simple and clear.
- Make sure material is relevant and stimulating. Use colour for emphasis.
- Aids must be large enough and positioned for the whole group to see.
- Make sure you are thoroughly familiar with all material you intend using.
- Have aids readily at hand for teaching and available for viewing after the class.
- Handle 'living' aids gently, e.g. baby, uterus.
- Do not overuse.
- Review material frequently and update.

The venue should be large enough for the intended group. It should be relatively quiet, well ventilated and heated if appropriate, have easy access to drinking water and a toilet, have enough mats for each mother/couple, be well sign-posted and all linen, equipment and surfaces should be clean. In some classes women are required to bring their own pillows.

Sound theoretical basis

Have a good background knowledge of the processes of pregnancy, parturition and the puerperium (see Chapters 10 and 11). However, the more extensive the reading, the greater knowledge and understanding the educator will have to take to the class. See the recommended reading lists attached to many of the chapters.

Familiarity with the birthing environments which class participants will attend

Whether hospital, birth centre or home is to be the birth place, the educator must be familiar with each and with the facilities available – types of beds and chairs, bath, spa, shower, bean bag, toilet proximity, nitrous oxide (N_2O_2) availability, foetal monitoring, etc. Some centres provide continuity of care where the same small select team of midwives provide care throughout pregnancy and then in labour for 'non-risk' parturients. This has resulted in greater maternal satisfaction for this group, in comparison with mixed medical and normal midwifery labour care, with fewer adverse maternal and neonatal outcomes (Rowley et al, 1995).

The educator must be familiar with the routine conduct of labour within each setting. Policies on ambulation, positions allowed during labour, especially second stage must be known. Are the labour ward staff familiar with the physiotherapist's teaching, so that they can reinforce it? Are music, videotaping the birth and the presence of family and friends allowed? Who applies TENS? Is an anaesthetist available if required?

Flexibility

Have a flexible approach which caters for differing situations and facilitates growth within the educational setting. The atmosphere of a class is set by the educator. Having established a relationship and gained an understanding of the women's/couples' perceived needs and attitudes, the physiotherapist has to create a setting in which each woman's potential can be fulfilled. Besides gaining information and physical skills, a greater benefit arising from classes can be for each woman to learn to know herself. The way in which a teacher listens to, responds to and directs each woman will help her towards this.

A teacher must:

- draw out a woman's capacity to develop an awareness of and response to her own body;
- help build confidence in the woman's own ability to bear a child and to be a good mother;
- help the woman to confront her fears and doubts and work through these to be ready to be a parent.

Ante-natal Class Aims

1. To educate mothers/couples about the physical and emotional changes of pregnancy, labour and the puerperium.
2. To explain the importance of ante-natal care for a healthy and comfortable pregnancy.
3. To prepare the mother/couple to cope with the process of labour to achieve a dignified and satisfying birth.
4. To provide a forum for discussion and exchange of ideas.
5. To improve the confidence of mothers/couples in their ability to cope with all the changes during the child-bearing year and to encourage a sense of responsibility for self and family throughout life.

Figure 15.2 Poor seating arrangements for ante-natal classes.

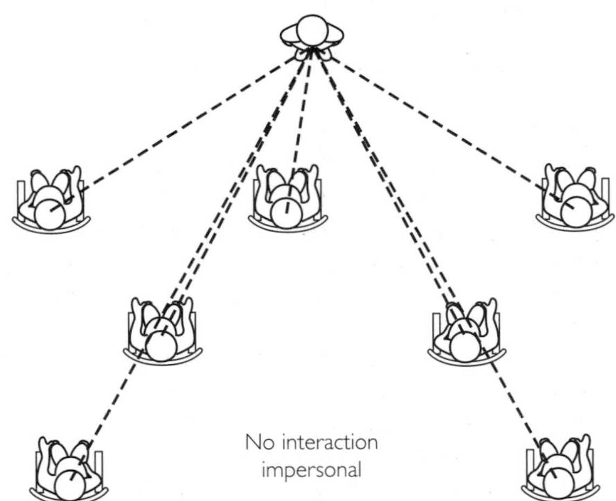

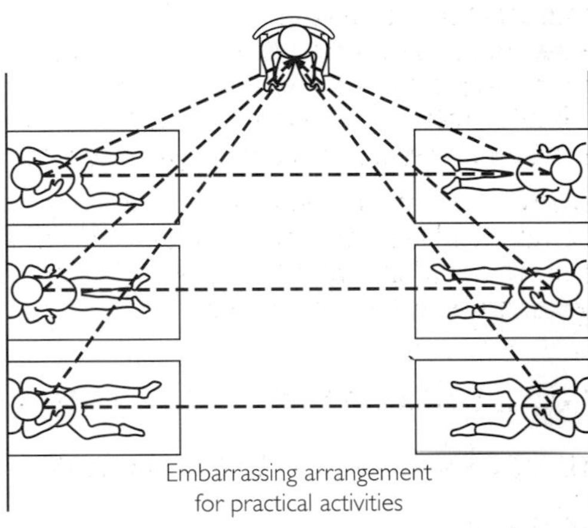

Figure 15.3 Good seating arrangements for ante-natal classes. Group arrangement which allows eye contact, easy visualization of aids, back support and avoids embarrassment is the ideal.

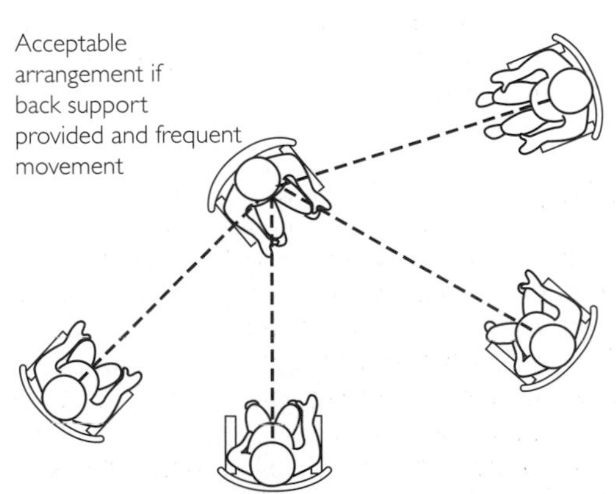

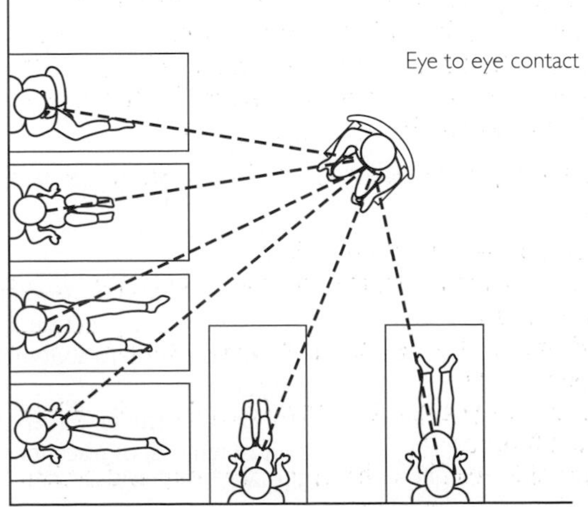

Ante-natal Class Format

The first ante-natal class is, without doubt, the most important. The physiotherapist, as a teacher/facilitator, must establish an atmosphere where mothers/couples feel at ease, can express attitudes and expectations and are able to learn skills to cope with pregnancy, labour and a new baby.

Use of name tags and memorizing and using names individualizes each person. Participation by partners in small tasks – arranging chairs and pillows, writing names, organizing drinks – can break the ice. Allow time for shy persons to adapt. Loose discreet clothing contributes to comfort. Some homely furnishings and 'baby' items and appropriate background music help set the atmosphere.

It is preferable to limit class numbers. Seven to ten women/couples are ideal so that educator–group interaction can occur.

Class participants generally sit on or lie on floor mats. Back support, discreet positioning to avoid embarrassment (see Fig. 15.2), frequent opportunities to move and extra pillows (wedge pillows are useful) provide physical and psychological ease. Arrange mats to allow group interaction and good eye contact (see Fig. 15.3).

In each class information is provided, discussion and questions encouraged and techniques and exercises practised. Motivation is generally high, but enthusiasm, attention span, fatigue, self-consciousness and embarrassment determine behaviour. The physiotherapist must observe and respond to these behaviours and direct the group accord-

Table 15.1 Outline of antenatal class content

Stage of pregnancy	Information	Practical
14–20 weeks	Pregnancy – physiology and psychology, emotional lability, needs of fathers Coping with minor discomforts Warning signs Fetal development Nutrition Postural awareness Back care Ergonomics – workplace, home, nursery (Chapter 21) Relaxation Fitness, safe exercising Referral for specific problems Equipment and furniture (Chapter 20)	Stability/strengthening of muscles – abdominals, pelvic floor, quadriceps, shoulder retractors Postural awareness Use of squatting, cross-leg sitting Defaecation dynamics Relaxation + breath awareness, use in sleep, ADL
28–34 weeks	Onset of labour – true/false When to come to hospital 1st stage of labour – latent/acceleration	Positions for 1st stage – walk, stand, forward lean, chair, high side lie, bean bag
1st stage	Early coping – distraction Induction Routine nursing care/monitoring Types of labour – OA, OP, breech Coping mechanisms – early, distraction; later – position, heat wet/dry, relaxation, breath awareness, massage TENS, N_2O_2, epidural, pethidine, etc. Positioning for epidural Pain and types of pain relief Problems	Relaxation Massage – effleurage, counterirritant TENS N_2O_2 Role play – pain pinch, massage, relaxation
2nd stage	2nd stage of labour Pushing, positions Pain Delivery – position, crowning, episiotomy, tear, head delivery, suction, cord check, syntocinon, baby to abdomen 3rd stage Problems – vacuum, forceps, CS, manual removal of placenta Sutures	Positions – supported squatting, high sitting, high side lie, propped supine Correct pushing technique Breathing Role play – pushing position and technique

ingly, instituting frequent breaks, reviewing information, using short practice sessions, giving brief individual attention and at times providing tactile input for variation. Encouraging the shy, subduing the overexuberant and restoring focus after distraction are all important to the success of the class.

How many classes and how long for each? There are many options. One hour, two hours or even weekend intensive courses can be considered. Give due consideration to attention span as pregnant women become restless easily. What time of day? Each educator will need to know her clientele base, their work routines and means of access to the centre to decide on the most suitable timing.

Class content and sequence

Rather than outlining a strict class structure, it is suggested that classes be in two groups. The early group provides for pregnancy, the later group for labour and the puerperium.

EARLY PREGNANCY CLASSES

Between 14–20 weeks of pregnancy, 2–3 classes should be planned. The content material listed in Table 15.1 assumes that the physiotherapist is the sole educator so adapt this if you are part of a team.

Be aware that nursery equipment and furniture are always changing, and regulations governing safety standards vary between countries and states. It is the responsibility of the physiotherapist taking the classes to know where to direct parents to access appropriate safety information in regard to equipment, furniture and the home. In some places physiotherapy groups have compiled comprehensive guidelines for selection of furniture (e.g. prams, strollers, car seats and much more) with reference to Standards Association regulations.

LATER LABOUR CLASSES

Commencing around 28 weeks, 3–4 classes will be needed to cover labour and the puerperium and these should be completed by 34 weeks. These classes cover the process of labour and how to cope with it. A good way to structure the presentation is to respond to the mother's questions:

- What is happening?
- What will I feel?
- What can I do?
- What can my support person do?
- What can anyone do?

The information and the practice are interwoven throughout the classes.

Early post-natal issues

Ideally, these should be included in the ante-natal class content. Topics should include pain in the perineum and breasts, breast feeding, rooming in, caring and bathing, fatigue, sleep problems, restricting visitors, bladder control, defaecation, post-natal 'blues', importance of exercise, stability and strengthening, help at home and contraception.

Figure 15.4 What can anybody do?

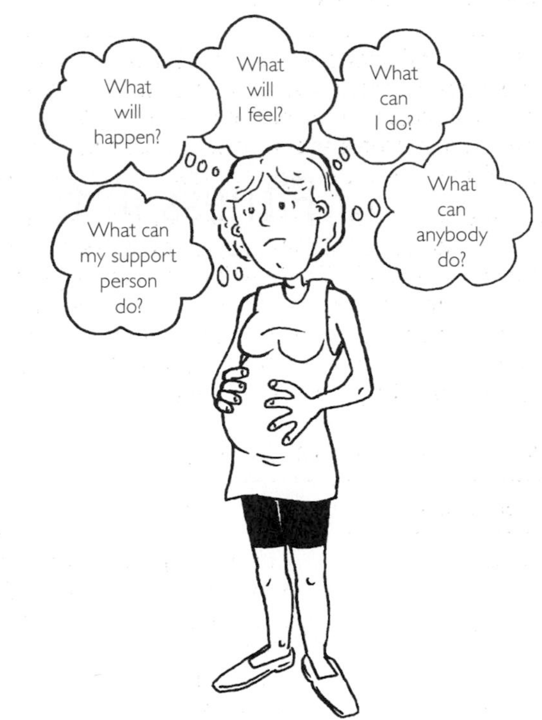

A labour ward visit may be conducted by the physiotherapist or the hospital staff. This familiarizes women/couples with the surroundings and some of the processes. The physiotherapist can use this visit as a realistic practice session for her class members.

Good teaching requires evaluation of one's own efforts, listening to the feedback from participants and adaptation to changing practices, social structures and women's needs.

References

Australian Physiotherapy Association (WA) and Midwives Association of Western Australia (1989) *An Education Programme for the Child-bearing Year*, 2nd edn. Perth, Western Australia: Combined Antenatal Education Committee.

Barclay L, Donovan J and Genovese A (1996) Men's experiences during their partner's first pregnancy. *Australian Journal of Advanced Nursing* **13**: 12–24.

Lamb GS and Lipkin M (1982) Somatic symptoms of expectant fathers. *American Journal of Maternal Child Nursing* **7**: 110–115.

Norr K, Block C, Charles A et al (1977) Explaining pain and enjoyment in childbirth. *Journal of Health and Social Behaviour* **18**: 260–275.

Rowley MJ, Hensley MJ, Brinsmead MW et al (1995) Continuity of care by a midwife team versus routine care during pregnancy and birth: a randomised trial. *Medical Journal of Australia* **163**: 289–293.

Further reading

Kitzinger S (1977) *Education and Counselling for Childbirth*. London: Baillière Tindall.

Williams M and Booth D (1974) *Antenatal Education*, 1st edn. Edinburgh: Churchill Livingstone.

16

Fitness in the Child-bearing Year

KATRINA HORSLEY

This chapter discusses the physiotherapy approach to fitness in the child-bearing year. Although the focus is on pregnancy, exercise in the post-natal period will also be addressed.

Pregnancy is a time of great change and growth – for some an exciting challenging state. For others it may be a time of stress, emotional change and lifestyle reassessment. All of these factors should be considered by the physiotherapist when designing exercise programmes and advising on physical activity during pregnancy and the post-natal period. Therefore, the concept of 'fitness' in pregnancy must encompass emotional, social and psychological aspects in addition to physical fitness.

The Oxford dictionary defines 'fit' as 'to be in harmony with; in suitable condition; to be the right size and shape'. These are all relevant to fitness for the pregnant woman.

Motivation to Exercise

It is important to establish the reason for a woman wishing to exercise during pregnancy. This is appropriate whether she wishes to join a class specifically for pregnancy, continue to play sport, undertake an individual exercise regime or learn a few key exercises in preparation for labour.

Historically, guidelines for exercise during pregnancy were based on social factors and society's attitude towards women (O'Neill et al, 1990). This in turn has influenced women's desire to exercise during pregnancy.

As early as the third century BC, Aristotle attributed difficult childbirth to a sedentary lifestyle. The Romans advocated avoidance of exercise in the first trimester, moderate activity in the second trimester and less activity in the third. The approach to exercise in pregnancy in Victorian England was very conservative (O'Neill et al, 1990).

Today, the increased emphasis on fitness, which developed through the 1980s, is influencing the pregnant woman's attitude to exercise. Furthermore, society's view of the ideal physique will influence some women's perceptions of their changing body shape and body image (Jackson, 1993).

As a consequence of the focus on body shape some women may use exercise as a means to limit weight gain during pregnancy. Physiotherapists need to be aware of normal pregnancy weight gains and refer the woman to a dietitian if indicated. The use of exercise to promote weight loss should be discouraged in pregnancy (Artal and Buckenmeyer, 1995).

The physiotherapist must recognize the differing needs of a fit woman who wishes to continue to exercise safely during pregnancy and those of a woman who has embarked on a 'get fit' campaign in the belief that it will assist her to cope with the physical demands of pregnancy and labour. Therefore, assessment should not only include physical aspects and history but consider psychological influences.

Figure 16.1 Pregnancy is a time of physical and emotional change.

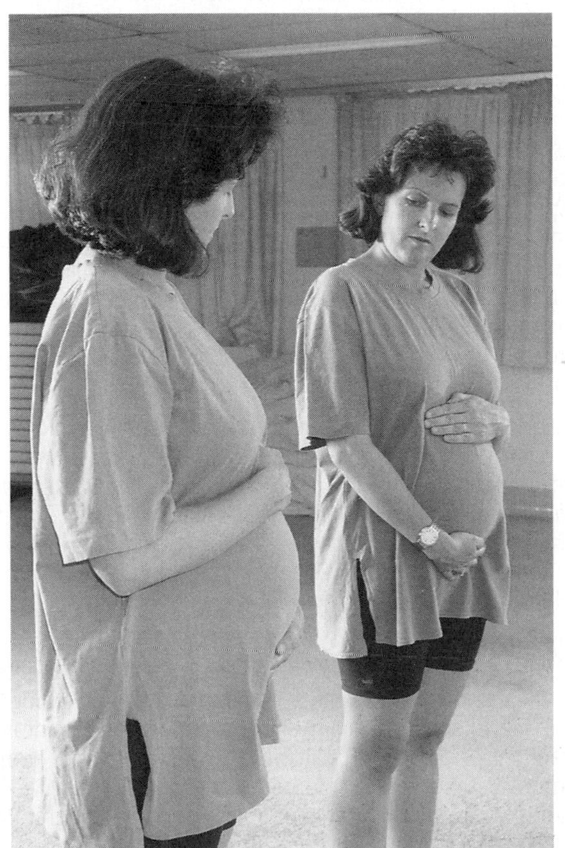

Many authors have noted that pregnancy is an optimum time to establish healthy lifestyle changes, with respect to smoking, exercise, nutrition and weight control, due to women's intrinsic motivation to learn and to maximize the health of their babies (Artal and Buckenmeyer, 1995; Clissold et al, 1991; Freda et al, 1993; Spedding, 1993).

In the promotion of a healthy lifestyle in the child-bearing year, physiotherapists can reinforce the value of exercise and back care as part of the multidisciplinary team involved in ante-natal care. Additionally, many of the aspects of physiotherapy ante-natal education, such as stress management and relaxation, provide the basis for life-long skills. Physiotherapists have unique expertise and skills to offer the pregnant woman who wishes to exercise safely in the child-bearing year. Specifically these include the ability to:

- understand the physiological and biomechanical changes in pregnancy and their influence on exercise;
- assess muscle strength, muscle length and posture;
- analyse movement;
- design exercise programmes;
- reinforce the principles of ante-natal education (such as relaxation, breath awareness and back care);
- manage concurrent musculoskeletal problems associated with the child-bearing year.

Physiotherapists are involved in advising the pregnant woman on exercise prescription in four ways:

1. teaching specific exercise as part of an ante-natal class;
2. conducting specially designed exercise classes for pregnancy;
3. advising on the continuation of sport and physical activity;
4. prescribing exercise as a component of treatment for musculoskeletal conditions.

In summary, factors which influence exercise prescription in pregnancy are women's motivation to exercise, previous experience or activity, current fitness level, health and gestation. Clapp (1994) states that exercise regimes in pregnancy can be flexible and individualized, provided that both the exercise and pregnancy are monitored. Due to our skills and expertise in caring for the child-bearing woman, physiotherapists can offer a holistic approach to the design of exercise in pregnancy and advise on fitness in the child-bearing year.

Safety of Exercise in Pregnancy

If physiotherapists are to encourage women to exercise, the possible benefits and dangers to the woman and the foetus must be considered. Many women are no longer content to be told to go for a stroll or a swim or to use commonsense in their exercise prescription.

Women will ask questions such as:

- Can I still play sport?
- What are the safe limits of exercise?
- Will being fit help my labour?
- What exercises should be avoided?

The physiotherapist must be able to answer these questions based on scientific rationale. The biomechanical and physiological changes of pregnancy in the design and modification of movement must be considered.

The value of exercise in pregnancy is controversial as both benefits and risks have been hypothesized (Hatch et al, 1993). Empirical evidence is difficult to compare due to the great variety in methodologies of studies. Obviously ethical considerations restrict the types of studies which involve pregnant women.

Risks: what does the literature say?

Despite the difficulties in interpreting research, a brief review of current literature is presented to discuss aspects of safety during pregnancy, under the following headings:

1. pregnancy and neonatal outcome;
2. effects of exercise on maternal physiology;
3. effects of exercise on the foetus and placenta;
4. thermoregulation.

PREGNANCY AND NEONATAL OUTCOME

Many women are under the misapprehension that being physically fit will guarantee an easy labour and delivery. It is important that we can present the findings of research in this area.

Rose et al (1991) conducted a study from 1984 to 1988 in which 21 342 women self-rated their physical activity during the second trimester of pregnancy. They found that there was no significant difference in the rates of low birth weight or foetal or neonatal death. Nevertheless, the validity of self-rating could affect the results of this study despite the large sample size.

A study which examined the course of labour after endurance exercise during pregnancy was designed to test the hypothesis that the continuation of regular running or aerobics during the latter half of pregnancy would have a negative effect on the course and outcome of labour. However, the study found that exercisers had a lower incidence of abdominal and vaginal operative delivery and that active labour was shorter for spontaneous vaginal deliveries. The incidence of pre-term labour was similar in the test and control groups, but labour began significantly earlier in the exercise group. Furthermore, signs of foetal stress were less frequent in the exercise group, but neonatal birth weight was reduced. The author concluded that for fit women, regular aerobics or running has a beneficial effect on the course and outcome of labour (Clapp, 1990).

This conclusion was supported by a retrospective survey of 44 women, which found that maternal exercise was associated with a significant decrease in the duration of second stage of labour and reduction in the incidence of obstetric complications (Botkin and Driscoll, 1991). No other obstetric or neonatal outcome differences were found.

Consistent findings between studies suggest that all women decrease activity as pregnancy progresses. Exercisers tend to weigh less, gain less weight and deliver smaller babies than non-exercisers (Sady and Carpenter, 1989).

In summary, some studies indicate that regular exercise is positively correlated with obstetric outcome. Nevertheless, this evidence is not conclusive and comparison between studies is difficult. Artal Mittlemark et al (1991a) summarize that the inability to draw an association between published studies and complications resulting from maternal exercise relates to major design flaws, e.g. lack of randomization, small sample size, lack of appropriate analysis and failure to consider pre-pregnancy fitness levels in evaluating results.

Therefore it is not possible to draw a scientific conclusion that maternal exercise is harmful or beneficial to the outcome of pregnancy from either the maternal or neonatal perspective.

EFFECTS OF EXERCISE ON MATERNAL PHYSIOLOGY

The physiology of pregnancy has been discussed in Chapter 11. This particular section will concentrate on the relationship between the physiology of pregnancy and exercise. Changes in the maternal physiology during pregnancy affect the physiological responses to exercise (Sady and Carpenter, 1989). For further information on physiology the reader is referred to the article by Sady and Carpenter (1989).

Research indicates that a woman who has been physically active prior to pregnancy can maintain enhanced cardiorespiratory responses to acute exercise, if aerobic exercise is continued throughout pregnancy (Pivarnik et al, 1993). During pregnancy cardiac output during submaximal exercise increases above values in non-pregnant women for the same workload. Changes in submaximal VO_2 during pregnancy relate to the type of exercise, increasing more in weight-bearing exercise (Sady and Carpenter, 1989).

A study which was designed to look at the effects of chronic exercise on blood volume expansion during pregnancy concluded that physically active women possessed significantly greater blood volumes than their sedentary counterparts. It also supported the proposal that there was no significant effect on pregnancy outcome in relation to activity (Pivarnik et al, 1994).

Appropriately prescribed endurance exercise programmes for women are associated with the same salutary effects as for men and these benefits can be attained at moderate levels of exercise if long-term compliance is maintained (Franklin et al, 1990). However, the pregnant woman demonstrates significant loss in cardiovascular reserve during gestation, which limits her ability to perform strenuous activity (Wallace and Wisewell, 1991).

Additionally, as the plasma volume increases earlier than the red cell volume a haemodilutional anaemia causes a decline in the oxygen-carrying capacity of the pregnant woman. This must be considered, as exercise increases the demand for oxygen which may further embarrass the capacity in the very obese or anaemic pregnant woman (Sady and Carpenter, 1989).

Most authors recommend modification of exercise programmes during pregnancy, in order for exercise to be safe for the mother and foetus. Physiological response to exercise is related to the gestation of the woman and many precautions relate more to the second and third trimesters (Wisewell, 1991).

EFFECTS OF EXERCISE ON THE FOETUS/PLACENTA

Potential risks to the foetus as a result of maternal exercise are documented as including hyperthermia, abnormal heart rate changes and hypoxia (Jarski and Trippett, 1990). Factors including changes in uteroplacental flow, increased uterine contractions and reduced maternal glucose levels have also been identified as potentially affecting the foetus (Bell and O'Neill, 1994). Potential risks to the foetus related to maternal exercise are summarized in the box.

Potential risks to the foetus from maternal exercise

- Hyperthermia
- Hypoxia
- Abnormal heart rate
- Decreased uteroplacental flow
- Increased uterine contractions
- Reduced maternal glucose levels
- Disruption of maternal endocrine haemostasis
- Poor growth

The major haemodynamic response to exercise is redistribution of blood flow away from the splanchnic organs towards exercising muscles. This has led authors to suggest that blood may be directed away from the foetus to active muscle groups during exercise (Artal and Buckenmeyer, 1995).

Research has shown that the flow of blood in the main uterine artery may decrease during intense exercise. However, animal studies indicate that at least 50% of uterine blood flow would need to be redistributed before the foetus would be negatively affected (Wilkening and Meschia, 1983). A study which found that the foetal heart rate increased significantly during exercise found that no changes occurred in the systolic/diastolic ratio of the velocity of foetal umbilical artery flow (Erkkola et al, 1992). Nevertheless, in this study women were exercising at 70%, 80% and then 92% of the calculated maximum heart rate (which is above the recommended level for pregnancy). It is possible that the augmented cardiac output in pregnancy prevents the compromise of blood flow to the uterus and foetus (Sady and Carpenter, 1989).

Several studies have found that the foetal heart rate increases during and after sustained maternal exercise. It appears that the increase is related to gestational age and the duration, intensity and type of exercise (Clapp et al, 1993). Despite the foetal heart rate increasing or remaining the same with submaximal exertion, a few studies have shown occasional foetal bradycardia with vigorous maternal exercise (Artal Mittlemark et al, 1991a; Bung et al, 1991). This could be related to brief periods of hypoxia (Artal Mittlemark et al, 1991a).

In another study, a cohort of over 800 ante-natal women were recruited to examine the relationship between foetal growth and maternal exercise in each trimester. In fit low-risk women exercise was positively associated with growth (Hatch et al, 1993). With heavier exercise, in those whose energy expenditure was about 2000 kcal per week, larger birth-weight increments were measured.

In contrast, a study designed to test the hypothesis that continuation of running and/or aerobics programme during late pregnancy at or above 50% of preconceptual levels limits foetal growth was conducted by Clapp and Capeless (1990). They studied 77 well-conditioned exercisers and 55 matched controls. Significant reductions in birth weight were seen in the offspring of the exercise group. The authors' conclusion was that continuation of a regular aerobic or running programme at or above a minimal training level, during late pregnancy, results in an asymmetric pattern of growth restriction which primarily impacts on neonatal fat mass.

Research suggests that numerous physiological mechanisms act to increase foetal tolerance to the circulatory and respiratory challenges of moderate maternal exercise (Franklin et al, 1990). Nevertheless, it appears that the effect of exercise on the foetus requires further investigation as the conclusions of studies are inconsistent.

THERMOREGULATION IN PREGNANCY

The possibility of exposing the foetus to hyperthermia has been considered by many studies. These have indicated that maternal hyperthermia is potentially teratogenic, being most hazardous in the first trimester. Abnormalities such as central nervous system conditions (e.g. spina bifida, anencephaly) have been indicated. Much of this research is based on animal models, but exercise in humans can result in core temperatures above the recommended level for pregnancy. Studies suggest that a possible maternal threshold for human teratogenesis is 39.2°C (Artal and Buckenmeyer, 1995).

There is little human evidence that pregnant women exercise to a level of exertion which causes significant hyperthermia, but this conclusion is mostly based in the non-athletic population where exercise is not of high intensity or long duration. In the non-pregnant female strenuous exercise for longer than 30–60 minutes can increase the core temperature to 39°C (Artal Mittlemark et al, 1991b) which is potentially harmful to the foetus. Due to the risks, pregnant women are advised to avoid self-inflicted conditions which may result in core temperatures above 38.9°C (McMurray and Katz, 1990). This advice should also apply to the preconceptual woman attempting to conceive (RACOG, 1994). Women partaking in higher levels of exercise could monitor their rectal temperature to provide some indication of the increase in their core temperature.

Research findings support the hypothesis that the magnitude of exercise-associated thermal stress for the embryo and foetus is markedly reduced by maternal physiological adaptations to pregnancy (Clapp, 1991). These adaptations begin in early pregnancy and include changes in resting temperature, thermal mass, sweating threshold and venous capacitance.

Evidence regarding the risk of overheating in saunas or spas is inconclusive. Nevertheless, Artal and Buckenmeyer (1995) advise avoiding spa temperatures greater that 38.5°C. The situation of entering a spa or sauna after exercise, as may arise in gyms, is considered particularly dangerous in pregnancy. The Royal Australian College of Obstetricians and Gynaecologists (RACOG) recommend that water temperature in pools should not exceed 28–30°C (RACOG, 1994).

McMurray and Katz (1990) argue that water-based exercise may be safer in pregnancy as it provides for greater heat loss. This proposal has been supported by a study which showed that exercise in water at 70% of VO_{2max} was well tolerated and offered several physiological advantages for the pregnant woman when compared to land-based exercise (Katz et al, 1990). The advantages included lower foetal heart rates and lower maternal heart rates and systolic blood pressure.

In a later study comparing the thermoregulation of pregnant women during aerobic exercise on land and in water, results suggested that thermal balance for both media was maintained when women exercised at 70% maximal heart rate for 20 minutes. The conclusion was that for normal fit pregnant women who participate in a moderate exercise programme, heat stress is not a major concern (McMurray et al, 1993).

Summary statement

There is a significant body of knowledge to support the hypothesis that aerobic exercise in normal pregnancy is safe for mother and foetus if modified and of moderate intensity and duration (Artal, 1992; Clapp, 1994; Huch and Erkkola, 1990; Wallace and Engstrom, 1987; Warren, 1991; Wolfe and Mottola, 1993). The data suggest that the clear difference between theoretic concern and observed outcome is best explained by the hypothesis that the physiologic adaptations to exercise and to pregnancy are complementary and foeto-protective (Clapp, 1994). Further research on the chronic effects of specific exercise programmes would contribute to knowledge regarding safe exercise regimes for pregnancy.

Guidelines for Exercise in Pregnancy

In 1985, the American College of Obstetricians and Gynecologists (ACOG) developed safety guidelines for exercising in the child-bearing year. There has been discussion about the conservative nature of these guidelines. In particular, some authors suggested that the ACOG guidelines were too stringent for aerobically fit low-risk ante-natal women (Hatch et al, 1993).

For example, an article by Zeanah and Schlosser (1993), which considered adherence to the ACOG guidelines, indicated that women who had exercised regularly before conceiving, with normal uncomplicated pregnancies, did not adversely affect their pregnancy outcome by exercising in excess of the guidelines. Nevertheless, the study was a retrospective survey of 173 women who exercised during their pregnancy and was not experimental in design.

The variables considered in the study were maternal weight gain, neonatal birth weight, caesarean section rate and gestational age of the newborn. The survey indicated no significant difference in outcomes amongst women who exercised with heart rates above 150 beats per minute for duration longer than 40 minutes when compared to the conforming group (n = 87), except for caesarean rate. The authors proposed that the longer duration (over 40 minutes) and moderate intensity groups had significantly fewer caesarean deliveries than the group which adhered to the guidelines.

Although heart rate is not an ideal measure of exercise intensity it is convenient and practical (Sady and Carpenter, 1989). In general it is recommended that target heart rates in pregnancy and the post-natal period are set at 25–30% lower than the appropriate pre-pregnancy rate. Variations in the available recommendations exist (see Table 16.1).

It is important to remember that both the intensity and duration of exercise will affect core temperature. Sady and Carpenter (1989) report that foetal bradycardia was not recorded at exercise of 180 beats per minute but most authors do not recommend exercise at this intensity due to the risk of hyperthermia. It is proposed that aerobic capacity can be improved safely by a pregnancy exercise programme of moderate physical activity for 30 minutes three times weekly (Mullinax and Dale, 1986).

The ACOG revised the guidelines for exercise in the child-bearing year in February 1994 to provide a more liberal approach. Pivarnik (1994) argues that the increased latitude provided by the guidelines creates increased responsibility for both the pregnant woman and her doctor. Similarly the physiotherapist is responsible for reinforcing the need for the pregnant woman to communicate with her medical practitioner about her exercise regime.

Table 16.1 Variation in guidelines for exercise

ACOG, 1994	Exercise three times a week Modify intensity according to maternal symptoms Stop exercising if fatigued
RACOG, 1994	Decrease exercise intensity by 25–30% Limit strenuous exercise to 15–20 minutes Peak heart rate 140 b/min
ACSM, 1991	15 minute at peak heart rate of 140 b/min 30–45 minute total exercise Athletes exercise less than 75% maximum heart rate

In 1994, the RACOG also developed a pamphlet entitled 'Exercise and Pregnancy', incorporating general guidelines for exercising in the child-bearing year.

These documents provide women and also health professionals involved in advising women on the safety of exercise in the child-bearing year with accepted guidelines to follow. Awareness of these documents is increasingly important in a time of greater medicolegal ramifications of providing professional advice. Physiotherapists should read these and similar documents carefully as they could be used as accepted standards on guidelines to exercise in pregnancy. It is also important to maintain current knowledge of available guidelines as research may result in modification of recommendations. A summary of the guidelines (1996) is provided in the box.

Guidelines for exercise in pregnancy

Consult with medical caregiver before commencing exercise.

Gradually increase exercise if previously sedentary.

Exercise regularly – 3×/week.

Maximum heart rate should not exceed 140–150 b min^{-1} or a limit set in consultation with doctor.

Moderate exercise should not exceed 20 minutes.

Avoid overheating and exercising in hot conditions.

Maintain adequate fluid intake to avoid dehydration.

Do not exercise with a febrile illness.

Ensure adequate warm-up and cool-down periods.

Avoid exercising in supine after the end of the fourth month.

Avoid contact sports after 16 weeks gestation.

Avoid ballistic bounces with stretches and do not stretch to extreme ranges of movement.

Low-impact exercise is preferable.

Full flexion or hyperextension of joints should be avoided.

Activity involving Valsalva manoeuvres should be avoided.

Increase calorie intake to account for exercise needs.

Contraindications to Exercise in Pregnancy

From previous discussion it is apparent that both pregnancy and exercise place increased demands on the cardiovascular and respiratory systems.

Some absolute and relative contraindications to exercise in pregnancy are contained in the box. In some cases medical approval to exercise may be provided dependent on the individual woman's history and presentation. In all cases exercise should not be commenced before medical consultation.

Contraindications to exercise in pregnancy

Diseases of the cardiovascular, respiratory or renal systems

Diabetes

Thyroid disease

History of miscarriage, premature labour, cervical incompetence

Vaginal bleeding or fluid loss

Hypertension

ple pregnancies
bnormal placental function or position
Sudden pain
Decreased foetal movements
Anaemia/blood disorders
Breech presentation in the third trimester

Benefits of Exercise in Pregnancy

As discussed, we need to be aware of the risks and guidelines to safe exercise in pregnancy, but what about the benefits? If physiotherapists are to *promote* exercise in pregnancy we need to understand the benefits of participating in an exercise programme. It is estimated that approximately 10% of Australian women participate in vigorous exercise (Australian Bureau of Statistics, 1992). The proportion of women who exercise during pregnancy is unknown, but some women view pregnancy as a time to adopt an exercise programme (Bell and O'Neill, 1994).

The general benefits of regular aerobic exercise, such as weight control, reduction in coronary artery disease, decreased physical discomforts and positive mental benefits including reduction in anxiety and depression, and modulation of stress levels are documented as having a place in the management of pregnancy (Koniak-Griffin, 1994; Mersy, 1991). These health benefits can be derived from mild and moderate levels of exercise in non-pregnant adults (American College of Sports Medicine, 1991).

Recent studies support the view that in pregnancy, moderate fitness conditioning can augment metabolic and cardiopulmonary capacities without altering foetal development or pregnancy outcome (Wolfe and Mottola, 1993).

A study which examined the relationship between aerobic exercise, maternal self-esteem and physical discomforts during pregnancy found that women who exercised had statistically significant higher self-esteem and lower physical discomfort scores (Wallace et al, 1986). The authors of this study acknowledge that the lack of random assignment to groups may have resulted in selection bias.

The research on the relationship between exercise and labour or outcome of delivery is still not conclusive. There is not sufficient evidence to state categorically that fitness decreases the length of labour, improves obstetric outcome in terms of assisted delivery, use of pharmacological pain relief or other variables or has a major impact on neonatal outcome in either a positive or negative way. Nevertheless, exercise can offer women many other positive benefits that physiotherapists can market in relation to participation in classes. It is important to note that guaranteeing an easier labour should not be listed as a potential benefit.

Some of the less tangible and less quantifiable benefits of exercise in pregnancy, including the social support of group interaction, are probably the most important to the pregnant woman. Artal and Buckenmeyer (1995) summarize the literature on benefits of pregnancy by stating that 'An association between potential health benefits and fitness in pregnancy is yet to be proven; however none doubt that maintaining an active lifestyle improves the quality of life' (p. 63).

The potential benefits of exercise in pregnancy are summarized in the box.

Potential benefits of exercise in pregnancy

Maintains cardiovascular fitness
Improves posture
Decreases physical problems or minor complaints of pregnancy, e.g. backache
Strengthens specific muscles in preparation for pregnancy and labour
Maintains muscle length and flexibility
Assists in maintenance of healthy weight range
Increases body awareness and control
Improves co-ordination, balance and rhythm
Improves breath awareness and control
Improves circulation
Reinforces principles of relaxation
Improves physical well-being and therefore decreases fatigue
Reduces stress and anxiety
Increases endurance and stamina
Provides social interaction
Assists post-natal recovery

Exercise Classes for Pregnancy

There are many advantages in conducting specific exercise classes for pregnancy. Specialized classes can be designed to meet the needs of pregnant women and this objective cannot be achieved in a class provided for the general public.

Benefits of specialized classes include:

- familiarization with a hospital, if classes are conducted where a woman is delivering;
- reinforcement of the principles of physiotherapy antenatal education (e.g. relaxation, breath awareness, back care);
- ability to modify exercises for each woman's individual problems (e.g. carpal tunnel syndrome);
- ability to design exercises which strengthen or stretch

muscle groups affected by the biomechanical changes in pregnancy;
- strengthening of muscle groups to assist ergonomic principles;
- inclusion of pelvic floor exercises and avoidance of strain on the pelvic floor;
- ability to carefully monitor women and adapt exercises accordingly;
- development of camaraderie between women;
- establishment of a network of friends for support during pregnancy and in the post-natal period;
- medical assistance readily accessible.

Pre-class assessment

From a safety perspective all women attending a pregnancy exercise class should inform their medical practitioner of their participation. This is important if a condition developing during the pregnancy requires the modification or cessation of exercise (Artal, 1992). Examples of such changes could be hypertension or the diagnosis of multiple pregnancies.

Attention to determining the following details should form part of the physiotherapy assessment:

- history – obstetric (gestation, previous complications such as threatened premature labour or miscarriages);
- medical condition and any concurrent medical problems;
- current and previous level of activity;
- musculoskeletal problems;
- abdominal strength and presence of a diastasis of the rectus abdominis;
- posture;
- attendance at ante-natal classes;
- doctor's permission to exercise (preferably in writing).

This information should be documented on each woman's assessment sheet where a record of pulse rates and frequency of attendance can be recorded.

Some pregnancy exercise classes encourage women to undergo a detailed individual assessment prior to participation in a class. It is also possible to build assessment into the class structure by encouraging new participants to attend the class early. Time also needs to be allocated at the end of the class to allow the opportunity to answer questions and to provide individual advice.

In line with the increasing emphasis on encouraging women to take responsibility for their health during pregnancy (Pivarnik, 1994), women should be provided with guidelines for safety of exercise in pregnancy. They should also be informed of potential risks (Artal, 1992). Encourage women to listen to their own bodies and not to 'push' themselves during pregnancy.

Women should be encouraged to report any pain with particular exercises and to be aware of the danger signs during exercise. Teaching women how to monitor their own pulse helps them to maintain their heart rate within accepted guidelines.

Features of a pregnancy exercise class

Classes designed for pregnancy differ from normal gym classes in many ways. Some of these differences include:

- small groups (up to 10 is ideal);
- well-ventilated / air-conditioned room;
- low-impact movements;
- slow music with a strong beat;
- carpeted supportive floor;
- mirrors for visual feedback;

Figure 16.2 Assessment of abdominal muscles.

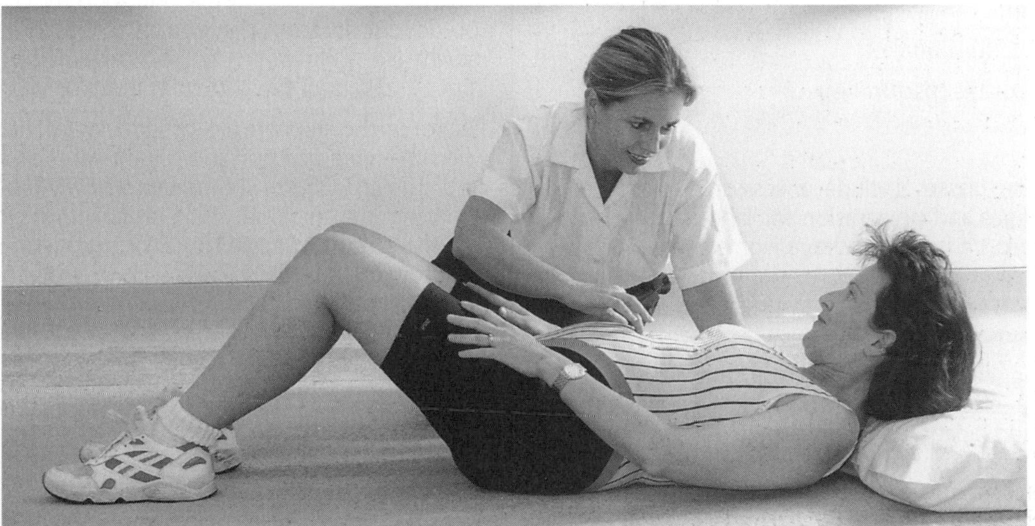

- participants should wear comfortable loose clothing, supportive shoes and bra;
- water available;
- emergency equipment available.

Structure of a pregnancy exercise class

Exercise classes for pregnancy can have quite different approaches and thus cater for different women's needs. Some classes can be similar to a modified low-impact aerobics class with a component of cardiovascular work. Other classes may focus more on slow controlled movements and stretches, incorporating relaxation and breath awareness.

Regardless of the emphasis, an ante-natal exercise class should incorporate ergonomic principles of back care in moving and changing positions, gentle stretches for muscle groups at risk of shortening, practice of relaxation and breath awareness and utilize movements which increase body awareness and control.

An example of one class format is provided in the box.

Class structure

Encourage fluid intake.

Introduction – emphasize safety and correct posture.

Monitor resting pulse.

Warm-up – 10 minutes.

Modified cardiovascular component – 20 minutes.

Monitor pulse and water break.

Gentle cool-down.

Specific strengthening, stability, toning and balance work.

Stretches.

Relaxation.

Encourage fluid intake.

Question or discussion time.

Some exercise classes include a session on aspects of physical changes and preparation for labour in each class. Another approach is to encourage women to attend ante-natal classes and then to reinforce the principles taught in the classes in an experiential way, through movement, in the pregnancy exercise class.

Incorporating co-ordination work in the cardiovascular section of a class promotes body awareness and co-ordination and adaptation of balance to the changing body shape and centre of gravity of pregnancy. It is not uncommon for the physiotherapist to observe women with very poor body awareness, rhythm and co-ordination slowly develop a more 'in tune' control of their bodies and sense of their physical being.

Specific features of the phases of an ante-natal exercise class will be covered in more detail.

INTRODUCTION TO THE CLASS

At the beginning of the class the physiotherapist should introduce herself, outline the structure of the class and general guidelines for exercise. Safety aspects should be reiterated regarding levels of exertion and risk of overheating. Revise the warning signs for exercise and ask women to report *any* unusual symptoms including tachycardia, shortness of breath, dizziness, faintness or vaginal fluid loss.

Warning signs and symptoms

- Tachycardia
- Palpitations
- Shortness of breath
- Dizziness
- Faintness
- Vaginal fluid loss
- Pain

It is important for women to know these signs and symptoms if they will be exercising without supervision at home. If any occur they are to stop exercising and contact their doctor. It is useful to reinforce these messages with written and pictorial posters. However, the most effective way to reinforce correct postures and movement patterns is by role modelling and demonstration.

Remind women that the class comprises individuals of different gestations and that each woman should exercise at her own pace. Encourage her to be responsible for her own body and report any discomfort. If the co-ordination is too difficult instruct the woman to keep her lower limbs moving (to maintain the active muscle pump) and rest her upper limbs, until the pattern is more comfortable.

Reinforce the importance of drawing in her abdominals when changing position and of general posture during the class. The instruction should be to slowly draw the umbilicus towards the spine. Even in pregnancy most women can perform this movement to gain contraction of the transversus abdominis which will assist in protecting the spine (Richardson and Jull, 1995a). Women should be encouraged to breathe normally during any abdominal contractions and not to hold their breath.

WARM-UP

The purpose of a warm-up period in any exercise class is to prepare the body for exercise. Gentle exercise will increase the circulation to all major muscle groups and enhance neural and connective tissue function (Brukner and Kahn, 1994). This theoretically decreases the likelihood of injury.

The increased cardiac output of pregnancy is required to meet the nutritional needs of the foetus and increased renal blood flow (Chapter 11). There is also increased oxygen consumption during pregnancy due to the increased load of the placenta, uterus, breasts, respiratory work and augmented cardiac load (Romem et al, 1991). The increased blood volume leads to a 40% augmentation of cardiac output from the 14th week of pregnancy. To decrease the work of the heart there is also an associated decreased vascular resistance causing venous dilation.

What implications does this have for the physiotherapist conducting an ante-natal exercise class? Adequate warm-up and cool-down periods are even more important in pregnancy due to the changes in blood volume and vascular compliance. Stroke volume declines in the third trimester of pregnancy as the result of diminished venous return due to enhanced venous compliance and intra-abdominal pressure. These changes cause pooling of blood in the lower limbs and pelvis (Morton et al, 1985).

A study of maternal haemodynamics found that in the third trimester, standing was associated with a decrease of more than 15% of cardiac output when compared to the lateral supine position (Katz, 1991). Maintaining a strong muscle pump by activity in the calves will reduce the risk of venous pooling and decreased cardiac stroke volume. This is the rationale for maintaining lower limb movement during the class until the cardiac output has returned to the pre-exercise level.

It has been proposed by some physiotherapists that long-legged exercise tights could assist venous return, but there is no objective research to support this hypothesis. Nevertheless, there is some value in discouraging women from wearing constrictive clothing which may impede blood flow.

Cessation of upper limb activity does not have such a dramatic effect on blood flow and should be the choice if women feel that they are overexerting themselves or are unable to co-ordinate a pattern of movement.

MODIFIED CARDIOVASCULAR SECTION

The aim of this section of the class is to increase heart rate and respiratory rate for a cardiovascular workout. Rather than improving fitness levels, the aim during pregnancy should be to maintain previous fitness levels.

Incorporation of co-ordination work in this section can be of benefit to women in adapting movement to an altering centre of gravity and body shape. However, movement patterns should avoid sudden changes of direction, jumping or jarring motions or high-level balance work (Artal and Buckenmeyer, 1995; Sundin, 1987).

Sequences of low-impact upper and lower limb movement are easier for the woman who has not previously attempted aerobics or aerobic dance. In this way movements can be added progressively to a pattern, building on the complexity of movement. It is not the aim of pregnancy exercise classes to create difficult movement patterns and the physiotherapist should be ready to adapt routines if class members are finding the movements complicated. This may occur particularly with new class members who could be discouraged from attending if the class is too difficult and feelings of clumsiness are reinforced. The physiotherapist should be sensitive to the individual's needs and subtly adapt the class without intimidating participants.

At the conclusion of the cardiovascular section women should take their pulse whilst keeping their lower limbs moving. They can then gauge whether they need to modify their activity level in the next class to stay within the recommended guidelines for heart rate of 140–150 beats minute^{-1}. The pulse rate may actually increase if the lower limbs are not kept moving gently during this monitoring. This can be explained by simple physiology. The cardiac output has been increased during exercise to a level needed to sustain the activity. Remember that:

$$\text{Cardiac output} = \text{stroke volume} \times \text{heart rate}$$

Logically, the heart rate could increase if the stroke volume decreases (as a result of the pooling of blood in the calves) in order to maintain the required cardiac output associated with exercise (Morton et al, 1985).

BREAK

During the break to measure heart rate by monitoring the carotid pulse, women should be encouraged to drink water to maintain adequate levels of hydration. Liberal consumption of liquids before, during and after exercise helps to prevent hyperthermia and dehydration (Artal and Buckenmeyer, 1995). Lower limb activity should be gradually decreased during this period.

COOL-DOWN

As discussed, it is important that women sustain activity in the lower limbs during a cool-down period. This allows the cardiac output and heart rate to return to normal gradually and prevents impediment to circulation through pooling in the lower limbs. The pulse rate should be measured again, to see if the heart rate is gradually returning to a resting level.

STRENGTHENING, STABILITY AND TONING EXERCISES

In this part of the class music should be more gentle to encourage mental and physical relaxation. Exercises incorporate strengthening for muscle groups which become weakened and stretched due to the anatomical adaptations of pregnancy. Classes can incorporate strengthening work for the abdominals, back extensors, gluteals, rhomboids, lower trapezius, hip external rotators, quadriceps and pelvic floor.

Figure 16.3 Monitoring heart rate is advisable.

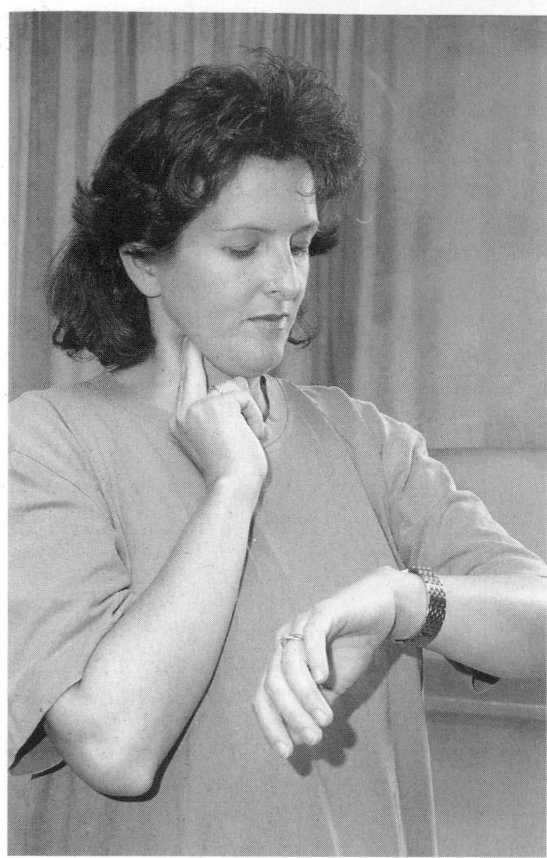

Increasing the strength of groups of muscles such as the quadriceps and the gluteals will assist women in the activities of daily living, such as lifting. Many active labour positions for the first and second stages can be assisted by strengthening of these specific muscle groups. For example, if a woman is standing and draping on her partner, strengthening her rhomboids and quadriceps will assist the stability of her position and decrease the strain on the support person.

Strengthening of the shoulder girdle, biceps and triceps also assists in post-natal activities, including lifting a child and coping with increased laundry. Triceps strengthening also assists bed mobility if operative intervention is required, although this should not be focused on in an ante-natal situation unless a woman is having an elective caesarean.

Small hand weights (0.5–1 kg) are useful in upper limb strengthening exercises, but movement patterns should be monitored closely to ensure smooth controlled movements. Weights should not be used by women with symptoms of carpal tunnel syndrome, such as pain, swelling, paraesthesia or numbness.

Exercise classes provide an ideal opportunity to reinforce ergonomic principles which have been discussed in antenatal classes (see Chapters 15 and 21). This is by demonstration of movement patterns utilizing a 'drawing in' of the abdominals, avoidance of combined flexion and rotation of the spine and in strategies of moving to the floor, such as through kneeling. These principles can be related to improved comfort during pregnancy and activities of caring for a baby, to increase their relevance to the pregnant or post-natal woman.

In this section of the class movement which increases body awareness is also emphasized through slow gentle patterns and movements. Exercises such as pelvic rocking on all fours or in standing can be practised as pain-relieving techniques for labour.

Pelvic floor exercises can be practised and the importance of these exercises reinforced. Slow relaxed breathing should be incorporated to rhythmically co-ordinate with movement, such as inhaling whilst stretching up and exhaling during a curling pattern of movement.

LENGTHENING OF TIGHT SOFT-TISSUE STRUCTURES

The importance of muscle lengthening and gentle stretching after exercise is increased in pregnancy. It is also an opportune time to gently lengthen muscle groups which may have become shortened in adaptation to pregnancy (e.g. hip flexors, piriformis, pectorals and calves). Again, exercises for muscle lengthening can be co-ordinated with breath awareness to reinforce the relationship between exhaling and 'letting go' of muscle tension. Some physiotherapists emphasize the role of the release of tension for labour through such lengthening exercises (Sundin, 1989).

The definitive function of the hormone relaxin, produced by the ovaries, is still unclear. However, it appears that its main functions are relaxation of ligaments and softening and stretching of fibrocartilage by collagenolytic activity, in preparation for labour (Romem et al, 1991). The generalized effects of relaxin on collagen throughout the body have implications for the design of safe lengthening techniques. It is not uncommon to read that the ability to stretch further in pregnancy offers an opportunity to gain extra mobility in stretches. This does not acknowledge the greater risk of overstretching soft tissues in pregnancy and the potential damage that may be caused.

Books written by authors with an incomplete understanding of the combined biomechanical and hormonal influences during pregnancy may promote programmes that risk overstretching soft tissues.

> It is wise to be judicious in your reading and critically evaluate the exercise component of general pregnancy books.

One example of dangerous exercises is partnered stretches, where a support person is assisting the woman to stretch. This decreases the control of the pregnant woman to stretch safely. In a pregnancy exercise class women must be encouraged to lengthen muscles slowly and not to push into the extreme ranges of movement. Ballistic bouncing should also be discouraged.

Figure 16.4 A gentle stretch for the hip flexors. The body weight is moved forward and held over the forward leg, stretching and holding the left hip in extension. The pelvis and lumbar spine should be maintained in a neutral position.

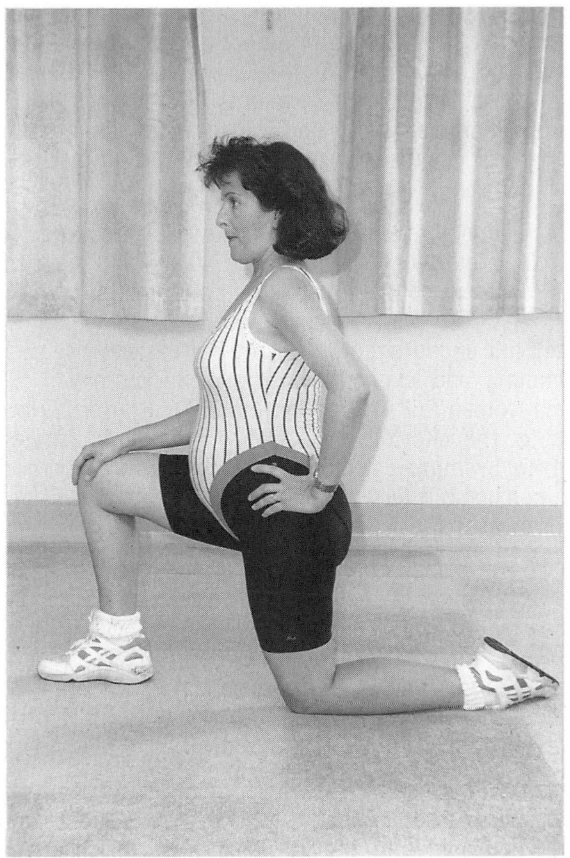

RELAXATION

This is the section of the class that participants report to be the most enjoyable. In an experiential way the principles of relaxation taught in an ante-natal class can be reinforced. Different physiotherapists will have different approaches to teaching relaxation, which can be practised in a variety of positions, such as fully supported in side lying with pillows or supported sitting in a chair or against a wall. Various approaches to relaxation can be incorporated in a class, such as reciprocal relaxation, focusing on breath control, visualization or a combination of all of these methods (see Chapter 18 for more details on relaxation).

CLASS CONCLUSION

At the end of the class, participants will frequently want to discuss aspects of exercise relevant to them as an individual. This may include the need to modify an exercise due to discomfort, sport in pregnancy, return to activity in the post-natal period, etc. Time should be allocated to addressing individual concerns. Again, this reinforces the dual role of the classes as an educative medium.

Kate was a 36-year-old primiparous woman who attended a major teaching hospital for her ante-natal care. She had recently moved to a new city with her partner. The move had caused feelings of apprehension about becoming a new parent without her family and friends close by.

Her first contact with the physiotherapy department was when she and her partner attended ante-natal education classes, which were run in conjunction with the midwives. It was here that she heard about the pregnancy exercise classes at the hospital. Before she became pregnant Kate had kept fit by jogging, but was no longer doing any regular exercise.

Figure 16.5 The right piriformis is stretched as the body weight is lowered towards the right. Stretch of piriformis occurs with hip flexion, adduction and external rotation.

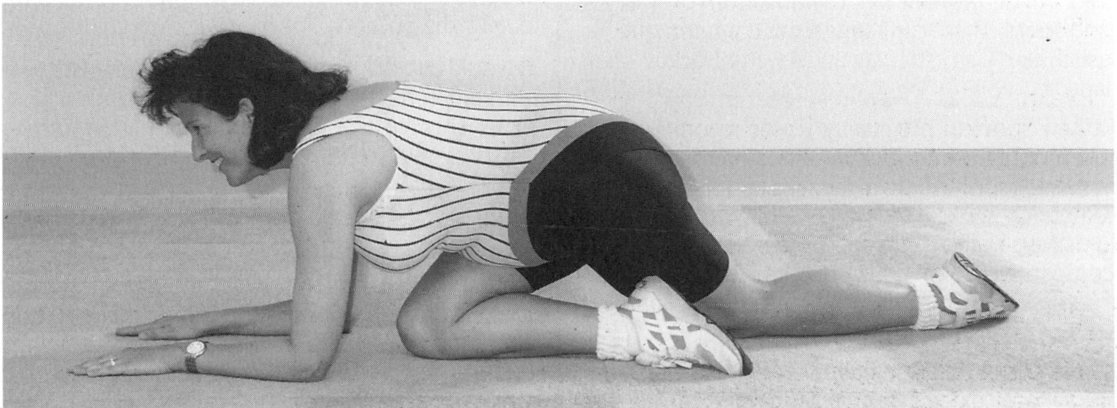

At 20 weeks gestation Kate started to attend the weekly evening pregnancy exercise class. She found that her balance had changed and that she felt unco-ordinated. The physiotherapist reassured her that it was normal to feel a little more clumsy with changes in body shape but that she would improve with practice.

Within a short time Kate had become friendly with other 'regulars' of the class and her body awareness had also improved. She realized that the class was assisting her to practise much of what she had learnt in the ante-natal classes, such as relaxation, back care and breath awareness. The other women in the class had tips on the best places to buy furniture for the baby and Kate felt reassured that her concerns about parenthood were not unusual.

On two mornings a week Kate was getting up early to go for a walk in the cool of the day. She had convinced her partner that he could also benefit from some regular exercise.

At about 33 weeks Kate was experiencing some back pain when rolling over in bed and going up and down stairs. The physiotherapist from the class showed her how to modify her exercise programme and made an appointment for her to be individually assessed and treated. Her back pain decreased, but she still had some discomfort at the end of the day.

When Kate started maternity leave she was able to attend day classes and exercise more regularly. By now the hospital was feeling very familiar to Kate and she would drop in to the midwifery advisory staff to talk about her concerns, such as breast feeding. Her mother was planning to visit after the baby was born, to give her a hand for the first few weeks.

Sport in Pregnancy

Apart from designing exercise programmes physiotherapists should advise women on continuation of various activities and sport. These can range from common queries to the unusual, like: 'Can I still play underwater hockey when I'm pregnant?'.

Learning a new sport in pregnancy is not recommended. Interpretation of guidelines for exercise in pregnancy indicates sports which should be avoided. These include contact sports like netball, hockey, etc. where a blow to the abdomen could risk the health of the foetus. Tennis can be played in a non-competitive manner, but squash places the woman at risk of overheating due to its intensity and confined space.

Scuba diving is contraindicated due to pressure changes and the risks of variable oxygen supply and hypercapnia (Sady and Carpenter, 1989). Horse riding and skiing are dangerous because of the risk of falling and damaging the foetus. Additionally, sports which require agility, balance and strength such as skiing, horse riding and gymnastics can expose the pregnant woman to injury.

This could occur for several reasons. Firstly, as pregnancy progresses the enlarging uterus, breasts and postural changes alter the woman's centre of gravity and affect balance. Secondly, decreased mobility of the joints of the ankles and wrists affects the ability to grip and quickly change direction. This stiffness of the wrists and ankles occurs as a result of water retention in the ground substance of the connective tissue, despite the generalized increased relaxation of ligaments (Romem et al, 1991). Thirdly, increased laxity and joint mobility in pregnancy may predispose the woman to injury of the joints (Botticelli et al, 1991).

More generalized rhythmical exercise involving large muscle groups is recommended (Sady and Carpenter, 1989). Most authors support the continuation of walking or jogging at pre-pregnancy levels (with medical clearance), but encourage non-weight-bearing exercise such as swimming and cycling (Artal and Buckenmeyer, 1995). Some women find mobile cycling difficult after 20 weeks due to the altering centre of gravity and changes in balance. Swimming decreases the likelihood of orthopaedic injury and offers the benefits of buoyancy and gentle resistance of the water.

If a woman wishes to continue to attend a normal gym it is desirable to provide her with advice on the type of classes and activities which are safe. 'New Body' or low-impact classes are safer, but are frequently still too fast and require sudden changes of direction. Step classes are not recommended due to the risk of falling and the potential of aggravating the symphysis pubis joint.

Circuit classes need to be slowed down and the pregnant woman is advised to exercise at her own pace and not at the speed determined by the class or instructor. Weight training should be limited to light weights (2–5 kg) or low resistance on machines to avoid the use of Valsalva manoeuvres. Valsalva manoeuvres can result in decreased venous return to the heart, increased arterial pressure and increased cardiac work. The general emphasis should be on low weights and repetitions. Free weights are not recommended due to the potential for injury if they are dropped.

It would be advantageous for physiotherapists to be familiar with different classes available in gyms and to have personal experience of the level of co-ordination and movement patterns involved.

Tai chi and yoga are often recommended for pregnant women as an adjunct to other forms of exercise (Sundin, 1989). The combination of breath awareness, movement, mental control and stretching should be ideal for pregnancy to increase body awareness. Nevertheless, it is wise to check women's individual programmes as they may not be designed for pregnancy and include undesirable movements and stretches.

Swimming, cycling and aerobic walking have not been associated with reported problems (Jarski and Trippett, 1990). Nevertheless, modification of activity during pregnancy is supported in the literature. Contradictions to exercise include conditions which limit cardiorespiratory reserves (Jarski and Trippett, 1990).

If a woman has been a regular exerciser preconceptually and has a normal pregnancy, she can be encouraged to continue her exercise regime in a moderated form.

The pregnant athlete

This chapter has not discussed exercise advice or prescription for the pregnant athlete attempting to maintain or improve performance. In reconciling the personal goals of childbirth and athletic performance, the major concern is that of risk to the foetus (Artal and Buckenmeyer, 1995).

Readers are referred to the American College of Sports Medicine (ACSM) guidelines which provide position standards on the quality and quantity of physical training and the Hale and Artal Mittlemark (1991) reference for further information.

Exercise and the Common Discomforts of Pregnancy

The physiotherapy management of problems associated with physical changes in pregnancy has been discussed in Chapters 11 and 14.

This section will briefly outline the relationship between some of the minor complaints in pregnancy and the modification of exercises in a class. The term 'minor complaints' is quite misleading as often these are the conditions which cause significant distress to the pregnant woman.

Round ligament pain

The round ligaments are two fibromuscular cords which extend from the uterus to the labia majora. Together with the uterosacral ligament, they act to support the uterus in the correct axis in the pelvis. During pregnancy the round ligaments become hypertrophied and more vascular to accommodate the increasing weight of the uterus.

Round ligament pain is a sharp stitch-like pain in the lower abdomen, often lasting up to 20 minutes and caused by sudden uncontrolled movements of the pelvis, such as rolling over, or changing posture, e.g. moving from sitting to standing. Non-pregnant women may experience this pain when getting up quickly from a chair. Some pregnant women also report that brisk walking causes bilateral pain.

The importance of slow controlled movements with drawing in of the abdominals will assist in prevention of round ligament pain. Therefore correct posture and control of movement must be emphasized throughout the class. Support by a sacroiliac (or trochanter) belt can be useful. If a woman experiences severe pain, sustained posterior pelvic tilting is often pain relieving.

Back pain

The biomechanical changes related to pregnancy and the causes and treatment of back pain have been discussed in Chapter 14. This section of the chapter will only discuss general advice on exercise in relation to back pain.

Simons (1987) believes that exercise classes can incorporate movements designed to create a strong and supple spine. In particular, movements which mobilize and strengthen the thoracic spine assist in preventing stiffness associated with increased thoracic kyphosis.

The finding of the study by Bullock et al (1987) that thoracic kyphosis increases as significantly as lordosis indicates that physiotherapists could devote more attention to this area in treatment and exercise programmes. These exercises can be continued in the post-natal period where enlarged breasts can accentuate poor posture.

Additionally, back care can be reinforced in all movement patterns and in changes of position and role modelling by the physiotherapist's demonstration is vital.

Figure 16.6 The thoracic spine is held in extension and then rotated from side to side.

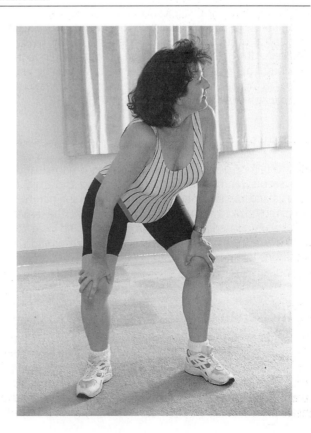

Symphysis pubis pain

'Symphysitis' results from an irritation caused by motion of the symphysis pubis associated with ligamentous laxity (Karzel and Friedman, 1991). Class participants with symphysis pubis pain should avoid unilateral lower limb movements which create a torsional force on the pelvis or a shearing force on the symphysis pubis. Positions which aggravate pain should be avoided. Some women with severe pain find side lying uncomfortable due to unilateral compression of the pelvis. In general, bilateral movements are less painful for these women. For example, if an exercise was aiming to increase hip extensor strength unilateral hip extension on all fours would aggravate symphysis pubis pain. An alternative exercise of bridging (in a controlled, slow pattern) would assist in gluteal strengthening whilst involving a bilateral pattern of movement (see Chapter 19 for further details).

Anterior rib pain

Anterior rib pain may occur from the 34th week of pregnancy, when the fundal height is at a maximum, due to the stretching of the abdominal insertion on the lower ribs. Women should avoid stretching exercises which increase this pain.

Carpal tunnel syndrome

The symptoms of carpal tunnel syndrome can be exacerbated by weight bearing on an outstretched hand, as in four-point kneeling. One suggestion to avoid pain is to advise women to bear the weight on clenched hands with the wrist in neutral to avoid combined extension of the wrist and fingers. Alternatively, the position of forearm support can be used. This is usually preferable to all fours on hands and knees as women are less likely to adopt an overextended lumbar spine in this position.

Oesophageal reflux

Heartburn or oesophageal reflux occurs predominantly in the second and third trimesters, due to the expanding uterus and placenta and relaxation of the sphincters, and is characterized by a burning pain in the chest. The sensation can be aggravated by recumbent positions and in any position where the head is down, such as on forearms and knees. Positions will need to be modified for sufferers of gastro-oesophageal reflux.

Other changes

It is important to be aware of other changes during pregnancy which may occur in an exercise class. These include headaches, fainting and nose bleeds. Remember that micturition is often more frequent in pregnancy and participants may need to leave the class. Facilities should be nearby.

Position for Exercises

Some implications for position have been raised in the above section.

By far the most important guideline relating to position is discussed in the guidelines from both the American and the Australian Colleges of Obstetricians and Gynaecologists where the avoidance of supine lying after the fourth month of pregnancy is recommended. However, there is disagreement about the gestation when supine exercise should be avoided. Early research indicates that physiological changes do not occur until 35–36 weeks gestation (O'Neill and Champion, 1989). In contrast Artal and Buckenmeyer (1995) state that supine exercise should not be performed under any circumstances.

At rest, cardiac output is lower in the supine than in the lateral position (Bell and O'Neill, 1994). The supine position causes symptomatic reduction in cardiac output in about 5% of pregnant women (Kerr, cited by Artal and Buckenmeyer, 1995). This phenomenon is usually referred to as 'supine hypotension' or the 'aortocaval compression syndrome'. It is explained by the gravid uterus compressing the inferior vena cava and reducing the return of venous flow to the heart. The resultant decrease in cardiac output is considered to be potentially dangerous to the foetus and can interfere with uterine circulation. It has also been implicated as a cause of placental abruption (Artal and Buckenmeyer, 1995).

If women are to use a modified supine position for exercise, it should be for dynamic and not static exercise so that the woman is not resting in supine for long periods (e.g. slow controlled bridging). The supine position can be modified by resting on the forearms and using semirecumbent positions. Changing the position to side lying between the use of these modified positions is also warranted.

Nevertheless, the implications in cases of uteroplacental insufficiency or abnormal placental function increase the danger of modified supine positions. Women should be aware of the overt symptoms of supine hypotension (nausea, dizziness) and strategies to adopt if these occur. Firstly, they should be advised to roll onto their side and report symptoms to the physiotherapist. Medical assistance should be sought if symptoms do not subside quickly.

The prone position is not used in ante-natal exercise classes due to feelings of discomfort as the foetus grows.

Exercises in Ante-natal Education Classes

As discussed, pregnancy is a time when women are responsive to lifestyle advice and health education messages. The role of women as health educators in families also means that they can influence the health of their family members. At child-bearing age women are particularly exposed to trauma and receptive to health education, which may prevent later problems, such as incontinence.

Education on women's health issues should ideally commence in schools and be reinforced during ante-natal and post-natal classes and further classes in the community (McIntosh, 1989). For example, early education on the role and function of the pelvic floor could assist in the prevention of some forms of urinary dysfunction. Currently, by the time many women, who are unaware of the role and function of the pelvic floor, attend ante-natal classes, hormonal and anatomical changes are already affecting pelvic organ and pelvic floor muscle function.

Ante-natal class courses differ in length and content. Classes are sometimes conducted in conjunction with other health professionals. Nevertheless, the exercise component taught by physiotherapists needs to be limited to the essential information for pregnancy and the post-natal period. In this way a few important exercises can be taught and reinforced in each class. This is preferable to teaching too many exercises which may be performed poorly at home without supervision. Ideally, more women would attend a pregnancy exercise class where the range of exercises can be more comprehensive and integrated with principles of ante-natal education.

Specific Exercises for Pregnancy

What are the essential exercises to teach in ante-natal classes?

Traditionally most classes have included awareness of the function and changes of the pelvic floor and abdominal muscles. In addition, pelvic rocking and hip adductor stretches have been included. The rationale of teaching the latter two exercises requires examination.

Pelvic floor exercises

The role of pelvic floor exercises has been discussed in Chapter 7. Refer to this chapter for a detailed description of the anatomy of the pelvic floor.

In an ante-natal class, the value of teaching pelvic floor exercises is two fold. The first objective is to provide women with a good understanding of the function of the pelvic floor and its vital role in continence (urinary and faecal), structural support of the pelvic organs and sexual satisfaction for both partners.

The second is to create an awareness of the muscle group so that women increase their control over the pelvic floor and their ability to relax it during the second stage of labour. Nevertheless, Artal and Buckenmeyer (1995) state that the rationale of teaching pelvic floor exercises to avoid tears or episiotomies in labour has never been supported by scientific evidence. There is anecdotal evidence that elite athletes have rigid, inextensible pelvic floors which prolong the second stage of labour. Thus, it could be hypothesized that awareness and the ability to relax the pelvic floor could play a role in the second stage of labour.

Discussing generalized exercises for the pelvic floor differs from exercise prescription for women with symptoms of pelvic floor dysfunction. In cases of dysfunction, individual assessment and medical review are essential to diagnose the cause of the problem and to provide appropriate treatment. Ante-natal classes can provide women with an awareness of the symptoms of poor urinary or faecal control and encourage them to seek the assistance of a physiotherapist. Physiotherapists need to educate women, and health professionals, about the differing roles of exercise in prevention and management of urinary problems and the highly specialized nature of muscle assessment and re-education.

Education on the role of the pelvic floor should begin in the early stages of pregnancy. 'Early Bird' classes for women in their first trimester are the ideal time for education in pregnancy.

Physiotherapists can reinforce the need to commence pelvic floor exercises as early as possible in the post-natal period, which may be before a physiotherapist visits. Women's fears of damaging perineal stitches by exercising can be dispelled and the role of exercise in healing promoted. Providing management strategies for perineal pain will also facilitate the ability to perform early pelvic floor exercises (see Chapter 19).

Regimes which contribute to the prevention of pelvic floor problems can be provided in a class situation. This could include the role of specific exercises, diet, bladder habits, defaecation position and pattern and the role of general exercise in assisting pelvic floor strength.

Some guidelines for urine control include:

- drink adequate fluids;
- avoid constipation and straining;
- perform pelvic floor exercises regularly throughout the day;
- regular general exercise helps;
- maintain a healthy weight range;
- avoid going to the toilet 'just in case';
- seek early help for symptoms;
- avoid smoking which can cause chronic coughing;
- pelvic floor support for effort activities.

Classes aim to provide women with a generalized pelvic floor exercise programme and strategies to progress the programme to improve muscle strength and endurance. In some texts general pelvic floor exercises will be referred to as 'Kegel' exercises.

Quick, strong holds and repetitions of pelvic floor contractions assist in re-education of the fast-twitch muscle fibres which normally work reflexly during activities such as sneezing or coughing. During pregnancy women may experience stress incontinence during coughing or sneezing as a result of combined hormonal and anatomical changes. Teaching women strategies of contracting their pelvic floor muscles when they are about to cough, lift or increase their intra-abdominal pressure may assist in preventing urine loss.

Women also need to be taught the role of the slow-twitch muscle fibres in the supportive function of the pelvic floor. Therefore, teach women to contract the pelvic floor, drawing 'up and into the pelvis', and to maintain a 6–10-second hold, if possible. Women should gradually increase both the length of the contraction and the number of repetitions as their strength and endurance increase. Exercise prescription should start at an achievable level and be slowly progressed.

Physiotherapists use different analogies to explain how to perform a pelvic floor contraction. This is reasonable for initial awareness, but the importance of the exercise should not be minimized by confusing images. Discourage women from repetitive cessation of the flow of micturition as an exercise (as described in some books) as this will not effectively strengthen muscles and could contribute to the retention of urine.

Pelvic tilting

Teaching pelvic tilting is of value to pregnant women as part of a range of pain-relieving techniques for labour. Pelvic rolling combines rocking in a circular motion and uses kinaesthetic input to relieve pain. It can be used in various labour positions and practised during ante-natal classes in combination with other physical techniques, like massage.

The rationale of teaching all women to posterior pelvic tilt to improve their posture assumes that all women adopt an anterior pelvic tilt during pregnancy. This may not be the case. Research on postural changes in pregnancy is difficult as roentgenographic measurement in pregnancy is contra-indicated and other forms of measurement may not be reliable (Gilleard and Brown, 1994). Women should be individually assessed before teaching them to improve their posture by posterior pelvic tilting in standing. Similarly, posterior pelvic tilting is not the panacea to cure back pain, which requires individual assessment, appropriate intervention and exercise prescription (see Chapter 14).

Lengthening of the hip adductor muscles

Lengthening of the hip adductors has been taught in various ways. Physiotherapists have normally encouraged contract–relax techniques as opposed to bilateral stretches in a cross-leg sitting position by pushing the knees to the floor. Overzealous stretches, which are encouraged in some texts, risks damaging the symphysis pubis due to the increased connective tissue laxity associated with pregnancy.

As always, physiotherapists must question the value of the exercise to the pregnant woman. If a woman has very tight adductors, she may find the use of stirrups during delivery overstretches her adductors. However, stirrups are being used less as active birth positions become increasingly adopted. It is an essential component of practice to assess the length of muscles prior to prescribing a lengthening exercise which may not be necessary.

Women who have very tight adductors who wish to squat in labour may benefit from gentle stretches. However, modified squatting positions can be comfortably adopted by a greater segment of the population than full squats, which require a combination of muscle lengths. It is not recommended that women practise full squats as a form of 'training' for labour due to the strain of full flexion on the knees and impediment to lower limb circulation. Varicosities of the vulva and haemorrhoids could also be aggravated.

The best way to stretch the adductors is by unilateral slow stretching, utilizing a contract–relax pattern.

The abdominal muscles

The abdominal muscle group comprises the rectus abdominis, internal and external obliques and the transversus abdominis. There are differing opinions about the objectives of strengthening the abdominal muscles during pregnancy. Physiotherapists have been interested in the function of the abdominal muscle group during pregnancy due to its role in posture, trunk stability and in the active expulsion of the baby in the second stage of labour.

Physiotherapists need to incorporate new knowledge into current practice. The traditional focus on the rectus abdominis needs to be considered in light of the role of the abdominals as a group and the objectives of abdominal strengthening.

Historically, ante-natal classes have focused on concentric exercises for the rectus abdominis by the encouragement of modified 'sit-ups' or 'mini-curls'. As the rectus lengthens during pregnancy with the growth of the foetus, the mechanical advantage of the muscle decreases. Therefore, it has not been considered practical to attempt strengthening exercises in late gestation.

Gilleard's (1992) study showed that as pregnancy progressed the gross structure of the rectus abdominis altered, the ability to stabilize the pelvis decreased and abdominal muscle activation patterns and inter-relationships altered. This was related to the increased length of the rectus abdominis and changes in the angle of insertion of the muscle.

Research on the function of the abdominals in non-pregnant subjects indicates that the internal and external obliques and the transversus abdominis are the prime muscles in providing trunk stability (Richardson et al, 1990; Richardson and Jull, 1995a; APA, 1995). More recent studies by Richardson and Jull (1995b) further isolate the stability role to transversus abdominis and the internal obliques. However, conclusions need to be drawn in recognition of the differing biomechanical factors in the pregnant and post-natal woman.

Nevertheless, it can be argued that the internal obliques and transversus should be the groups targeted during ante-natal class exercise prescription for two reasons. Firstly, the rectus is stretched and mechanically disadvantaged. Secondly:

> Functionally, the abdominal muscle activity that is perhaps more important, especially when considering the loaded upright posture, is the ability of the abdominal muscle group to co-contract isometrically, promoting stability in the lumbopelvic region (Wohlfahrt et al, 1993).

Stability is of prime importance during pregnancy and in the post-natal period due to the increased load of the foetus on the spine, postural changes and the deceased strength of the rectus abdominis.

Therefore the rationale of concentric trunk flexion is questionable, as promotion of the stabilizing role should be a prime consideration when designing a programme to improve the strength and endurance of the abdominal muscle group (Wohlfahrt et al, 1993). Additionally, dynamic exercise does not correlate with improvement in isometric strength (Fleck and Schutt, cited by Wohlfahrt et al, 1993).

Clinical experience suggests that a very useful exercise in the ante-natal period is the transversus abdominis exercise performed on all fours (knees and forearms). In this position the woman can relax her abdomen and is then instructed to lift the baby up towards the spine. The weight of the abdomen provides stretch facilitation for the transversus abdominis and the baby provides additional resistance (see Chapter 14).

Pelvic floor contractions can be performed at the same time as they are a synergistic group. This position should not be adopted in the early post-natal period due to a theoretical risk of air entering the placental site and causing an air embolus. Bridging poses a similar risk and should be avoided until the lochia flow has ceased.

Gilleard (1992) found that post-natally the abdominal muscle inter-relationships had returned to early pregnancy levels by eight weeks post-birth. However, ability to stabilize the pelvis remained low at eight weeks post-birth. A later study proposed that the functional decrement of the rectus muscle post-natally related to an altered biomechanical environment consequent to structural adaptations (Gilleard and Brown, 1994).

Although the serum concentrations of relaxin produced by the corpus luteum of pregnancy decline to normal within 3–7 days post-partum, the anatomic effects may persist for up to 12 weeks (Artal Mittlemark et al, 1991b). However, clinicians find that postural changes and muscle weakness may be present up to 12 months post-natally.

Diastasis of the rectus abdominis

A further complicating factor in appropriate exercise prescription for strengthening the abdominals during pregnancy is the occurrence of a diastasis of the rectus abdominis. The bellies of the rectus abdominis frequently separate at the linea alba during pregnancy as a result of combined hormonal and anatomical changes.

Noble (1976), in her early book *Essential Exercises in the Child-bearing Year*, postulated that obesity, multiple pregnancy, a large foetus or excessive amniotic fluid were predisposing factors in the occurrence of a diastasis. However, a study by Hannaford and Tozer (1985) found no significant relationship between the width of a diastasis and these variables. Noble also indicated that hormonal influences, stretching and sudden exertion further challenged the integrity of the rectus muscle. She believed that a diastasis is normally detected post-natally or in late pregnancy.

Clinically, a diastasis is a frequent finding in post-natal assessment, but in examining women ante-natally a diastasis can often be detected in the second trimester. This finding is supported by a small study of six primigravid women between 14 weeks gestation and eight weeks post-delivery (Gilleard and Brown, 1992). The study found significant changes in the angles of insertion of the rectus abdominis and in the separation of the muscle at and below the umbilicus by 30 weeks gestation.

Ante-natally some women will display a mid-line bulge when concentrically contracting the rectus abdominis, whilst in other women the muscle bellies will tend to separate. There is no substantiated explanation for this difference. The

Figure 16.7 Exercising the transversus abdominis. The back is flat or has a slight lordosis and the abdomen is lax. The lower abdomen is raised towards the spine and held firmly. The pelvis must not move.

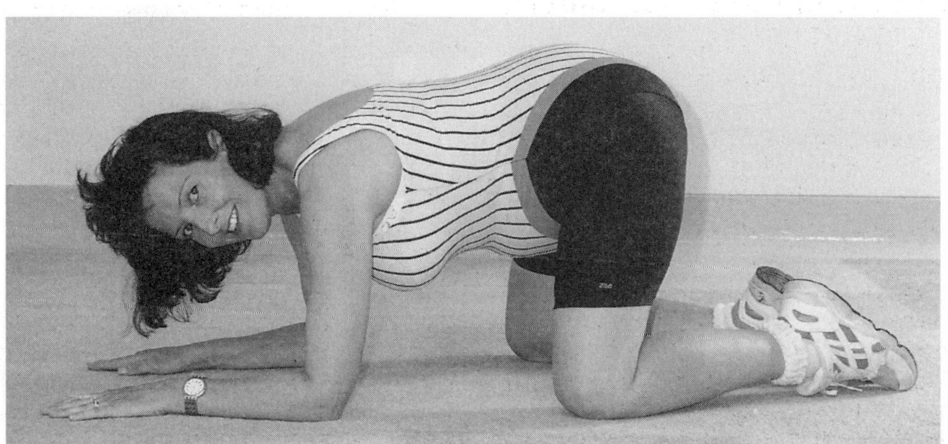

rationale for teaching women to support the abdomen centrally with their hands is not based on scientific evidence. Teaching women to roll to their side to sit up from lying, rather than flexing their trunk, would appear logical in avoiding strain on the rectus abdominis and protecting the back.

In post-natal assessment women have traditionally been instructed to avoid concentric oblique work, such as diagonal sit-ups, for fear of increasing the diastasis. An article by Callinan-Moore (1993, p. 19) states that 'Exercises involving the use of the obliques and transversus should be avoided or closely monitored' in late pregnancy and post-natally. A recent study reported by Ellson and Bullock-Saxton (1995) studied the degree of diastasis with real-time ultrasound scanning and indicated that the non-resisted abdominal curl with rotation did not significantly increase the diastasis from its resting width. Further research is warranted in this area.

The clinician is advised to follow these procedures. Firstly, monitor the effect of diagonal abdominal contractions on diastasis width by palpating the muscles and prescribe exercises accordingly. Secondly, place more emphasis in exercise prescription on restoring strength of the postural endurance fibres of the internal oblique and transversus abdominis muscles activated primarily in their maintenance of pelvic and lumbar stability, rather than in an active (isotonic contraction) role (such as a trunk curl with or without rotation) (see Chapters 14 and 19 for further details).

This can be achieved by low levels of abdominal muscle contractions, which focus on the maintaining of pelvic and lumbar stability during lower limb movements. These exercises are adaptions of those described by Wohlfahrt et al (1993). In crook lying, the pelvis and lower trunk are kept stable by abdominal contraction as the lower limb is slowly moved. One leg remains flexed whilst the other is slowly moved into extension. If the woman is very weak the heel can remain on the bed. A progression is to slowly lift and lower one extended leg off the bed to 30° whilst maintaining pelvic stability. Ante-natally, these exercises can be performed in a semirecumbent position. An airbag device can be used to provide the woman with feedback about her maintenance of lumbar and pelvic stability during the exercises. Such a device is called a pressure biofeedback (Richardson and Jull, 1995b) and has proved to be a useful clinical tool to aid progress of muscle re-education. The same device may be helpful in retraining abdominal muscle activity in cases of gross diastasis in the post-natal period.

The effects of a diastasis on post-natal function are unclear, but the integrity of the abdominal group and thus function are presumably altered. During the immediate post-birth period, separation of the rectus abdominis was shown to be resolving by week four post-natal, but was not complete by week eight (Gilleard and Brown, 1994).

There is still insufficient research to be dogmatic about protocols concerning the influence of diastasis of the rectus abdominis. Therefore we should assess women individually and prescribe exercises appropriate to their muscle strength and function.

In summary, the importance of the active stabilizing of the trunk by the internal obliques and transversus abdominis has contributed to a changing emphasis on these muscle groups in pregnancy exercise classes and the post-natal period. Physiotherapists working in women's health need to maintain an understanding of current research and challenge the rationale of current practice in light of these findings. Furthermore, the function of the abdominal muscles in pregnancy and the implications for exercise prescription is an area in need of further research.

Post-natal Exercise

Individual post-natal exercise prescription is discussed in Chapter 19. This section will cover general exercise in the post-natal period.

Figure 16.8 Trunk stability is maintained by abdominal contraction, while lower limb movement is carried out. The woman should focus on pelvic stability during slow controlled leg movements.

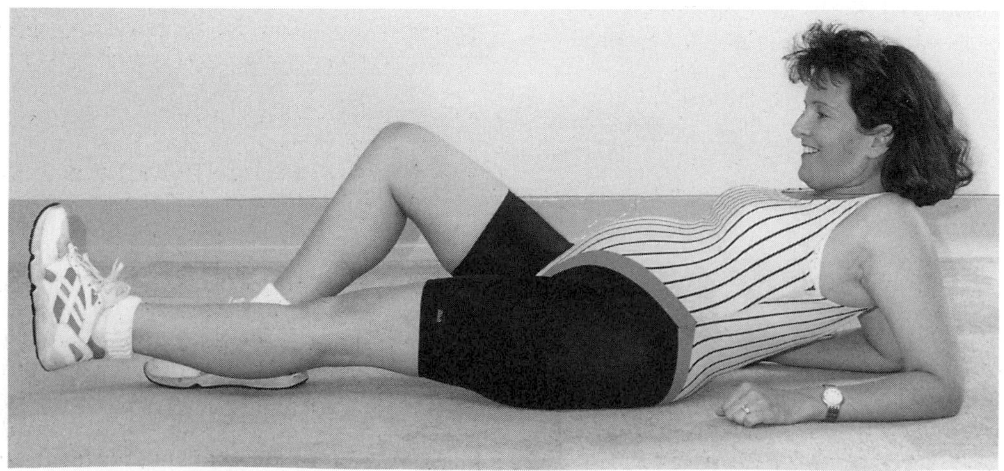

In advising women on the continuation of exercise in the post-natal period, the persistent musculoskeletal and cardiovascular changes need to be considered. The cardiovascular and haemodynamic changes persist for approximately four weeks post-delivery and remain a significant factor during post-partum exercise (Artal Mittlemark et al, 1991a). The musculoskeletal changes persist for a minimum of three months before returning to normal, although some authors have suggested that changes may persist for up to a year.

On average women who do not breast feed gain about 7 kilograms when their weight stabilizes post-partum (Artal Mittlemark et al, 1991a). Therefore exercise in the post-natal period can contribute to weight control in conjunction with healthy eating.

It is also more difficult for women to exercise with the new demands of caring for a baby. This is one of the reasons why specialized classes with child-caring facilities facilitate post-natal exercise. Some women may also form an exercise group, for example swimming, to share the babysitting whilst others are exercising.

Post-natal classes

Whilst in hospital women should be given the opportunity to attend a post-natal class. The structure of the class can be a modification of the ante-natal class outlined above. The class would be shorter in duration and consist of a warm-up period, simple low-impact movements, gentle stretches, posture correction, specific strengthening exercises and relaxation. The class can be attended by most women on the second day after a normal delivery and the fifth day after a caesarean section. Exercises and movement patterns should be modified for women with pain.

However, a group post-natal class should not replace individual assessment and exercise prescription. Individual assessment is needed to tailor post-natal exercises to each woman's presentation and muscle strength, muscle length, pain and posture (see Chapter 19).

The class provides women with a break from the post-natal ward and allows them to focus, if briefly, on their own health and recovery. It should be a chance to reinforce post-natal exercises and include stretches and relaxation to music. Helpful stretches include those for the upper trapezius and pectorals as women are often stiff and tight in this area. This is probably partially related to breast-feeding postures. It is also an ideal opportunity to reinforce ergonomic principles associated with caring for a baby.

Mother and baby classes

Conducting classes for 'mother and baby' performs at least three major functions.

Firstly, it facilitates social interaction for new mothers and gives the opportunity to meet women in a similar situation. If they attended ante-natal classes it will provide an opportunity to strengthen previous friendships. Exchanging experiences about the new role of motherhood, its difficulties and uncertainties is important in reinforcing the normality of their concerns.

Secondly, it provides women with the opportunity to exercise safely until they are able to return to previous levels of activity and generally available classes in the community.

Some classes actively involve the baby in the exercises, which provides an opportunity for women to interact with their baby. If the class does not include 'mother and baby exercises' it is important that women feel free to bring their child to the class so that they are available to feed and comfort their baby as necessary. This may ultimately impose an age restriction on the babies in the class, as the more mobile ones need to be considered from a safety perspective. The role of the class should be to fill the gap between ante-natal classes and other opportunities to exercise in the community.

The third advantage of conducting mother and baby classes is to expose women to the other areas where physiotherapy can assist them. The physiotherapist will be able to assist in the detection and treatment of ongoing post-natal problems like incontinence or back pain. Development of rapport between the therapist and women decreases their reluctance to seek advice on sensitive issues.

Physiotherapists can also provide education about normal baby development and the facilitation of development through everyday handling, play and touch (refer to Chapter 20 for further information).

Physiotherapists can advise on ergonomic problems which women may be experiencing and on the choice of baby equipment (such as slings for carrying). Although many women will have been exposed to this information in ante-natal classes, women's focus in the ante-natal period is often strongly on labour. In the post-natal period the information on ergonomics is more relevant and applicable and therefore better absorbed. Women may also be experiencing back pain caused by poor ergonomics in activities such as feeding, bathing and carrying. Refer to Chapters 19 and 21 for further details.

Conducting classes where mother and baby exercise together has several advantages. These include:

- bonding of mother and baby;
- reinforces ergonomic principles when lifting the baby;
- provides movement experiences for the baby, incorporating gentle vestibular input and head-righting reactions;
- uses the baby as a weight to increase resistance.

The post-natal class can follow a similar format to the exercise ante-natal class. Although the foetus is no longer at risk, the persisting physiologic changes associated with pregnancy dictate a conservative approach to post-natal exercise. The positions of all fours and bridging are contraindicated whilst the woman is still bleeding due to the risk of an air embolus entering the placental site.

Figure 16.9 Strengthening the mother's abdominals and providing vestibular stimulation for the baby. (Reproduced with permission of *The Sunday Mail*, Brisbane.)

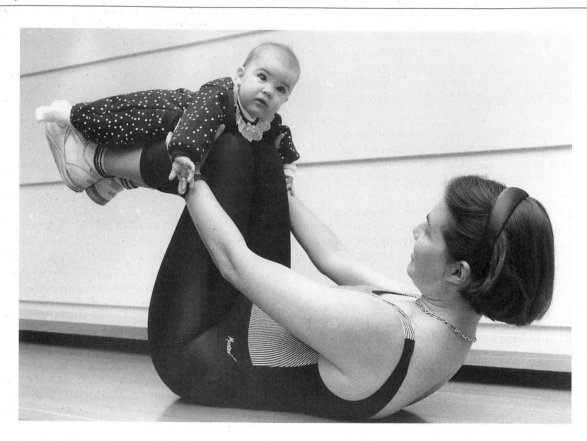

When Kate delivered a baby girl, Emma, she was visited by several of the women from the pregnancy exercise class. The physiotherapist from the class also came to say hello and to encourage her to come to the post-natal class the next day. The ward physiotherapist assessed Kate and provided her with a specific exercise programme.

Kate experienced some back pain after the labour, but responded to a short period of treatment. The physiotherapist reinforced ways to care for her back whilst looking after Emma. Kate was keen to feel as fit as possible when she went home.

On day two post-natal, Kate went to the post-natal exercise class. This gave her the chance to focus on her own health. She realized that she was quite stiff around the neck and shoulders from feeding in a poor position and the stretches and relaxation helped. The physiotherapist revised the principles of good posture for feeding.

The mother and baby class which Kate attended after she went home gave her a chance to catch up with her friends from the classes and to find out what they had called their babies. The class also demonstrated ways of handling babies to stimulate normal development. Although Kate had heard it before, it all made more sense now that she could relate it to the things Emma was doing.

Emma enjoyed the mother and baby exercises they went to, which meant that Kate could be strengthening her abdominal muscles whilst stimulating Emma's development. Kate also tried different carrying slings with Emma. The physiotherapist helped Kate to find the one that offered the most support for her back.

Some of the women from the class decided to form a swimming group so that they could share babysitting whilst exercising.

Apart from improved muscle strength and fitness, Kate realized that the friendship and support she gained from the classes was invaluable. Some of the women from the group still meet regularly for social gatherings and to share experiences about the joys and difficulties of parenthood.

Kate attended the exercise classes for her second pregnancy two years later.

Post-natal Effects of Exercise

A randomized study of the effects of aerobic exercise by lactating women on breast milk volume and composition (n=33) concluded that aerobic exercise performed 4–5 times a week and commenced 6–8 weeks post-partum had no adverse effects on lactation (Dewey et al, 1994). Although a relatively small sample, the study also found that participating in an exercise programme of supervised aerobics at 60–70% of the heart rate reserve for 45 minutes a day, five times a week for 12 weeks, significantly improved the cardiovascular fitness of the post-natal women.

An earlier study had indicated that maximal exercise resulted in a significant increase in lactic acid concentration in breast milk that may be high enough to affect the taste and thus the acceptance of the milk by the infant (Wallace et al, 1992).

These results conflict with a study of vigorously exercising (n=8) and sedentary (n=8) women, whose infants were 9–24 weeks old and exclusively breast fed (Lovelady et al, 1990). This study concluded that there were no differences in milk content, but that exercising women tended to have higher milk volumes.

Dewey and McCrory (1994), in a review of the literature on dieting and physical activity in pregnancy and lactation, conclude that the available data indicate that moderate aerobic exercise is safe and beneficial for most women, if appropriate guidelines are followed. This supports the proposal that moderate aerobic exercise is the most appropriate for the child-bearing year.

How to Get an Exercise Class Started

Frequently physiotherapists and students express concern about the practicalities of establishing exercise classes for the child bearing year. Certainly the theory acts as an essential basis, but then where do we go from there?

As discussed, physiotherapists may offer different styles of class – some more aerobically orientated, others focusing more on body awareness, specific strengthening and breath awareness.

It is useful to look at a range of videos, read different books and attend a variety of low-impact classes offered by gyms. Perhaps consider undertaking an aerobics instructor's course.

These activities will help the physiotherapist to develop an awareness of different styles of exercise classes. It is also important to critically analyse the speed, position and pattern of exercises in order to develop a personal choice of movement as a physiotherapist conducting a specialized class. For some, participation in other classes will also develop personal body awareness and co-ordination.

Then it is a matter of practice. In designing or evaluating exercises, ask yourself 'What is the benefit of this exercise to the pregnant/post-natal woman?'. Try any movement that you will be teaching. Ask yourself 'What does it feel like?'. Jane Simons' (1987) book and video *Pregnant and In Perfect Shape* are helpful in developing these skills.

A last word of advice is not to underestimate the unique combination of skills that you are developing as physiotherapy students or as practising physiotherapists. Your problem-solving skills and analytical approach are assets that will assist you in many walks of life.

Promoting Exercise in the Child-bearing Year – The Physiotherapist's Contribution

The best way to encourage exercise in the child-bearing year is by promoting its benefits to the well-being of the pregnant and post-natal woman. Although there is some indication that fit women have shorter labours, there is insufficient evidence to state this categorically. Therefore an easier labour should never be promoted as a benefit of exercise in pregnancy.

Physiotherapists can certainly market other benefits received from attending their classes, including increased body awareness, group camaraderie and expert advice on the common complaints of pregnancy and subsequent movement modification.

Another way to 'market' the service offered by physiotherapists is to differentiate it from other services. Physiotherapists offer a holistic service and can demonstrate that their exercise classes are specifically designed to meet the needs of women in the child-bearing year.

Conclusion

Physiotherapists have skills and expertise to offer the pregnant woman who wishes to exercise safely in the child-bearing year. In assisting women to make informed choices regarding exercise, physiotherapists need to consider scientific evidence and to keep abreast of current research. This should lead to a critical evaluation of traditional practices and enable the physiotherapist to respond to a more informed consumer.

In discussing specific exercise, this chapter has not been prescriptive, as current knowledge on muscle function and exercise design is changing rapidly. Further research on the relationship between muscle function and the biomechanical changes in pregnancy would assist physiotherapists in designing exercises for the child-bearing year.

Recommendations for exercise designed for the general pregnant population may not be appropriate for individual women. Programmes will differ for the previously aerobically fit pregnant woman and the sedentary, unfit or very overweight woman. Medical conditions and the status of the woman's pregnancy will also have implications for the safety of exercise.

This chapter has provided an overview on which to base clinical experience. When working with pregnant women, it must be remembered that the ultimate goal of pregnancy is a healthy mother and a healthy baby.

References

American College of Obstetricians and Gynecologists (1985) *Exercise During Pregnancy and The Postnatal Period. ACOG Home Exercise Program.* Washington DC: ACOG.

American College of Obstetricians and Gynecologists (1994) Exercise during pregnancy and the postpartum period. Technical Bulletin 189. *International Journal of Gynaecology and Obstetrics* **45**(1): 65–70.

American College of Sports Medicine (1991) *Guidelines for Exercise Testing and Prescription.* Philadelphia: Lea and Febiger.

Artal R (1992) Exercise and pregnancy. *Clinics in Sports Medicine* **11**(2): 363–377.

Artal R and Buckenmeyer PJ (1995) Exercise during pregnancy and postpartum. *Contemporary Obstetrics/Gynecology* **40**(5): 62–90.

Artal Mittlemark R, Dorey FJ and Kirschbaum TH (1991a) Effect of maternal exercise on pregnancy outcome. In: Artal Mittlemark R, Wisewell RA and Drinkwater B (eds) *Exercise in Pregnancy,* 2nd edn, pp. 225–237. Baltimore: Williams and Wilkins.

Artal Mittelmark R, Wisewell A, Drinkwater B and St John-Repovich WE (1991b) Exercise guidelines for pregnancy. In: Artal Mittlemark R, Wisewell RA and Drinkwater B (eds) *Exercise in Pregnancy,* 2nd edn, pp. 299–312. Baltimore: Williams and Wilkins.

Australian Bureau of Statistics (1992) *1989–90 National Survey, Exercise, Australia.* Catalogue No. 4383.0. Canberra: ABS.

Australian Journal of Physiotherapy (1995) *The Lumbar Spine – Stabilisation Training and the Lumbar Motion Segment.* Monograph No 1. Melbourne: Australian Physiotherapy Association.

Bell R and O'Neill M (1994) Exercise and pregnancy: a review. *Birth* **21**(2): 85–95.

Botkin C and Driscoll CE (1991) Maternal exercise: newborn effects. *Family Practice Research Journal* **11**(4): 387–393.

Botticelli TM, Eddy LJ and Larson MA (1991) Lateral instability of the knee joint during pregnancy. Reviewed in *Physical Therapy* **71**(6) (Suppl): 568.

Brukner P and Khan K (1994) *Clinical Sports Medicine.* Australia: McGraw-Hill.

Bullock JE, Jull GA and Bullock MI (1987) The relationship of low back pain to postural changes during pregnancy. *Australian Journal of Physiotherapy* **33**: 10–17.

Bung P, Huch R and Huch A (1991) Maternal and foetal heart rate patterns: a pregnant athlete during training and laboratory exercise tests; a case report. *European Journal of Obstetrics, Gynaecology and Reproductive Biology* **39**(1): 58–62.

Callinan-Moore K (1993) Managing diastasis recti. Australian Physiotherapy Association: *Journal of the National Women's Health Group* **12**(1): 15–19.

Clapp JF (1990) The course of labour after endurance exercise during pregnancy. *American Journal of Obstetrics and Gynecology* **163**(6): 1799–1805.

Clapp JF (1991) The changing thermal response to endurance exercise during pregnancy. *American Journal of Obstetrics and Gynecology* **165**(6): 1684–1689.

Clapp JF (1994) A clinical approach to exercise in pregnancy. *Clinics in Sports Medicine* **13**(2): 443–458.

Clapp JF and Capeless EL (1990) Neonatal morphometrics after endurance exercise during pregnancy. *American Journal of Obstetrics and Gynecology* **163**(6): 1805–1811.

Clapp JF, Little KD and Capeless EL (1993) Fetal heart rate response to sustained recreational exercise. *American Journal of Obstetrics and Gynecology* **168**(1): 198–206.

Clissold TL, Hopkins WG and Seddon RJ (1991) Lifestyle behaviours during pregnancy. *New Zealand Medical Journal* **104**(908): 111–112.

Dewey KG and McCrory MA (1994) Effects of dieting and physical activity on pregnancy and lactation. *American Journal of Clinical Nutrition* **59**(2): 446S–452S.

Dewey KG, Lovelady CA, Nommsen-Rivers LA, McCrory MA and Lonnerdal B (1994) A randomised study of the effects of aerobic exercise by lactating women on breast-milk volume and composition. *New England Journal of Medicine* **330**(7): 449–453.

Ellson D and Bullock-Saxton JE (1995) The effect of abdominal muscle contraction on diastasis recti in post-natal women, determined by diagnostic ultrasound. *Proceedings WCPT Congress,* Washington, p. 1202. Alexandria: APTA.

Erkkola RU, Pirhonen JP and Kivijarvi AK (1992) Flow velocity waveforms in uterine and umbilical arteries during submaximal bicycle exercise in normal pregnancy. *Obstetrics and Gynecology* **79**(4): 611–615.

Franklin BA, Bonzheim K, Wetherbee S, Gordon S and Timmis GC (1990) Exercise and fitness. *Obstetrics and Gynecology Clinics of North America* **17**(4): 817–835.

Freda MC, Anderson HF, Damus K and Merkatz IR (1993) What pregnant women want to know: a comparison of client provider perceptions. *Journal of Obstetrics, Gynaecology and Neonatal Nursing* **22**(3): 237–243.

Gilleard W (1992) The structure and function of the abdominal muscles during pregnancy and the immediate post-birth period. Thesis abstract. Australia: University of Wollongong.

Gilleard WL and Brown JM (1992) Structural changes to the rectus abdominis during pregnancy and immediate post-pregnancy. *Journal of Biomechanics* **25**(7): 728.

Gilleard W and Brown JM (1994) Structure and function of the abdominal muscles during pregnancy and the immediate post-birth period. In: Shiavi R and Wolf S (eds) *Conference Proceedings: Tenth Congress of the International Society of Electrophysiology and Kinesiology.* June 21–24. Charlston, South Carolina, USA.

Hale RW and Artal Mittlemark R (1991) Pregnancy in the elite and professional athlete – a stepwise clinical approach. In: Artal Mittlemark R, Wisewell RA and Drinkwater B (eds) *Exercise in Pregnancy,* 2nd edn, pp. 231–237. Baltimore: Williams and Wilkins.

Hannaford R and Tozer J (1985) An investigation of the incidence and possible predisposing factors of rectus diastasis in the immediate post partum period. *Journal of the National Obstetrical and Gynaecological Special Group, Australian Physiotherapy Association* 4: 29–32.

Hatch MC, Shu XO, McLean DE et al (1993) Maternal exercise during pregnancy, physical fitness, and foetal growth. *American Journal of Epidemiology* **137**(10): 1105–1114.

Huch R and Erkkola R (1990) Pregnancy and exercise – exercise and pregnancy. A short review. *British Journal of Obstetrics and Gynaecology* **97**: 208–214.

Jackson S (1993) Breaking the barriers: women and exercise. *Sports-Medicine News* **August**: 3–4.

Jarski RW and Trippett DL (1990) The risks and benefits of exercise during pregnancy. *Journal of Family Practice* **30**(2): 185–189.

Karzel RP and Friedman MJ (1991) Orthopaedic injuries in pregnancy. In: Artal Mittlemark R, Wisewell RA and Drinkwater B (eds) *Exercise in Pregnancy,* 2nd edn, pp. 123–132. Baltimore: Williams and Wilkins.

Katz VL (1991) Physiological changes during normal pregnancy. *Current Opinions in Obstetrics and Gynecology* **3**(6): 750–758.

Katz VL, McMurray R, Goodwin WE and Cefalo RC (1990) Non-weightbearing exercise during pregnancy on land and during immersion: a comparative study. *American Journal of Perinatology* **7**(3): 281–284.

Koniak-Griffin D (1994) Aerobic exercise, psychological well-being and physical discomforts during adolescent pregnancy. *Research in Nursing and Health* **17**(4): 253–263.

Lovelady CA, Lonnerdal B and Dewey KG (1990) Lactation performance of exercising women. *American Journal of Clinical Nutrition* **52**(1): 103–109.

McIntosh JM (1989) Women – the captive audience. *Physiotherapy* **75**(1): 10–13.

McMurray RG and Katz VL (1990) Thermoregulation in pregnancy. Implications for exercise. *Sports Medicine* **10**(3): 146–158.

McMurray RG, Katz VL, Meyer-Goodwin WE and Cefalo RC (1993) Thermoregulation of pregnant women during aerobic exercise on land and in the water. *American Journal of Perinatology* **10**(2): 178–182.

Mersy DJ (1991) Health benefits of aerobic exercise. *Postgraduate Medicine* **90**(1): 103–107, 110–112.

Morton MJ, Paul MS and Metcalfe J (1985) Exercise during pregnancy. *Medical Clinics of North America* **69**(1): 97–108.

Mullinax KM and Dale E (1986) Some considerations of exercise during pregnancy. *Clinics in Sports Medicine* **5**(3): 559–570.

Noble E (1976) *Essential Exercises in the Childbearing Year.* London: John Murray.

O'Neill M and Champion L (1989) Exercise during pregnancy. What every fitness leader should know. *Journal of the National Womens' Health Group* **8**(2): 9–11.

O'Neill M, Shnier A, Cooper K, Hunyor S and Boyce ES (1990) Historical perspective of exercise during pregnancy. Australian Physiotherapy Association: *Journal of the National Women's Health Group* **9**(2): 7–9.

Pivarnik JM (1994) Maternal exercise during pregnancy *Sports Medicine* **18**(4): 215–217.

Pivarnik JM, Ayres NA, Mauer MB et al (1993) Effects of maternal aerobic fitness on cardiorespiratory responses to exercise. *Medicine and Science in Sport and Exercise* **25**(9): 993–998.

Pivarnik JM, Mauer MB, Ayres NA et al (1994) Effects of chronic exercise on blood volume expansion and hematological indices during pregnancy. *Obstetrics and Gynecology* **83**(2): 265–269.

Richardson CA and Jull GA (1995a) Muscle control – pain control. What exercises would you prescribe? *Manual Therapy* **1**: 2–10.

Richardson CA and Jull GA (1995b) An historical perspective on the development of clinical techniques to evaluate and treat the active stabilizing system of the lumbar spine. *Australian Journal of Physiotherapy,* Monograph **1**: 5–13.

Richardson CA, Toppenberg R and Jull G (1990) An initial evaluation of eight abdominal exercises for their ability to provide stabilisation for the lumbar spine. *Australian Journal of Physiotherapy* **36**(1): 6–11.

Romem Y, Masaki DI and Artal Mittlemark R (1991) Physiological and endocrine adjustments to pregnancy. In: Artal Mittlemark R, Wisewell RA and Drinkwater B (eds) *Exercise in Pregnancy,* 2nd edn, pp. 9–30. Baltimore: Williams and Wilkins.

Rose NC, Haddow JE, Palomaki GE and Knight GJ (1991) Self rated activity level during the second trimester and pregnancy outcome. *Obstetrics and Gynecology* **78**(6): 1078–1080.

Royal Australian College of Obstetricians and Gynaecologists (1994) *Exercise and Pregnancy.* (ACN005474733.) 254 Albert St, East Melbourne 3002.

Sady S and Carpenter M (1989) Aerobic exercise during pregnancy: special considerations. *Sports Medicine* **7**: 357–375.

Simons J (1987) *Pregnant and in Perfect Shape. Exercising during Pregnancy and After.* Melbourne: Nelson.

Spedding S (1993) Pregnancy, exercise and sport – the medical, legal and social issues. *Sport Health* **11**(2): 29–32.

Sundin J (1987) Exercise during pregnancy. In: Collins M (ed) *Women's Health Through Lifestages – the Physiotherapist's Contribution,* pp. 28–45. Australia: Australian Physiotherapy Association (NSW Branch).

Sundin J (1989) *Face to Face with Childbirth. A Comprehensive Active Childbirth Program,* p. 220. Sydney: Horwitz Grahame.

Wallace AM and Engstrom JL (1987) The effects of aerobic exercise on the pregnant woman, foetus and pregnancy outcome: a review. *Journal of Nurse Midwifery* **32**: 277–290.

Wallace AM, Boyer DB, Dan A and Holm K (1986) Aerobic exercise, maternal self esteem, and physical discomforts during pregnancy. *Journal of Nurse Midwifery* **31**(6): 255–262.

Wallace JP and Wisewell RA (1991) Maternal cardiovascular responses to exercise during pregnancy. In: Artal Mittlemark R, Wisewell RA and Drinkwater B (eds) *Exercise in Pregnancy,* 2nd edn, pp. 195–206. Baltimore: Williams and Wilkins.

Wallace JP, Inbar G and Ernsthausen K (1992) Infant acceptance of post-exercise breast milk. *Paediatrics* **89**(6): 1245–1247.

Warren MP (1991) Exercise in women. Effects on reproductive system and pregnancy. *Clinics in Sports Medicine* **10**(1): 131–139.

Wilkening RB and Meschia G (1983) Foetal oxygen uptake, oxygenation and acid based balance as a function of uterine blood flow. *American Journal of Physiology* **244**: H749.

Wisewell RA (1991) Exercise physiology. In: Artal Mittlemark R, Wisewell RA and Drinkwater B (eds) *Exercise in Pregnancy,* 2nd edn, pp. 141–156. Baltimore: Williams and Wilkins.

Wohlfahrt D, Jull G and Richardson C (1993) The relationship between the dynamic and static function of abdominal muscles. *Australian Journal of Physiotherapy* **39**(1): 9–13.

Wolfe LA and Mottola MF (1993) Aerobic exercise in pregnancy: an update. *Canadian Journal of Applied Physiology* **18**(2): 119–147

Zeanah M and Schlosser SP (1993) Adherence to the ACOG guidelines on exercise during pregnancy: effect on pregnancy outcome. *Journal of Obstetric, Gynecological and Neonatal Nursing* **22**(4): 329–335.

17

Physiology of Labour

LURLENE LIVINGSTONE

What Causes the Spontaneous Onset of Labour?
•
Signs that Indicate that Labour is Imminent
•
Induction of Labour
•
The Stages of Labour
•
Disorders and Complications of Labour

It is important for the physiotherapist to have a sound background knowledge of the physiology of labour so that she can answer any questions accurately and be able to direct any enquiries to the appropriate sources. However, complex discussions on physiology during ante-natal classes are unnecessary and time consuming. The physiotherapist's aim is to help the woman understand what is happening to her body so that she is able to work in harmony with it, supported by her partner and those attending her. The information delivered to the couple should be accurate and realistic otherwise there may be a great feeling of disappointment about the experience of childbirth if labour, delivery and the outcome vary from the preconceived norm.

Labour is defined as the process in which the foetus, placenta and secundines are expelled from the uterus via the birth canal after a minimum period of 20 weeks (Beischer and Mackay, 1986).

During labour the uterus, a hollow muscular structure, has the ability to contract and relax, progressively causing the descent of the foetus, the effacing (shortening and thinning) and dilation of the cervix and finally the passive movement of the foetus through the birth canal. Throughout the procedure the contractions increase in intensity, duration and frequency. It is usually difficult to determine the exact time of the onset of labour, as there is development and regression of spontaneous uterine contractility throughout pregnancy, gradually progressing into labour. Cervical dilation and effacement may also be present before labour. It is currently accepted clinically that labour has started when the cervical dilation progresses beyond 2 cm; however, some women in labour experience intense painful sensa-

Table 17.1 Physiological changes in mother and foetus during labour

Maternal respiratory	↑ in ventilation ↓ PCO_2, 22 mmHg at end first stage
Maternal cardiovascular	↑ 10 mmHg systolic BP ↑ 5–10 mmHg diastolic BP
Maternal gastrointestinal	↓ motility and absorption, aggravated by narcotics Nausea/vomiting – dehydration and ↓ plasma sodium and chloride levels
Foetal cardiovascular	Sometimes there is a slight fall in heart rate during contraction (type 1 dip) due to cord compression (see Ch. 20), cord stretch or foetal head pressure. Heart rate recovers at the end of the contraction

tions even though the cervix is not dilated to this level. Table 17.1 illustrates the physiological changes in the mother and foetus during labour.

What Causes the Spontaneous Onset of Labour?

The precise cause of the commencement of labour is still unknown. It is known that the uterus is capable of expelling its contents before term, as is demonstrated by miscarriage in early pregnancy, spontaneous premature labour or even by artificial induction of labour before term. The non-pregnant uterus is also capable of a strong contraction to expel a foreign body (e.g. an intrauterine contraceptive device) or a solid tumour such as a fibroid polyp.

The ultimate cause of labour is almost certainly a combination of factors and changes occurring throughout the pregnancy. These include:

- hypertrophy of myometrial cells;
- gradual formation of thick upper and thin lower uterine segments in the third trimester;
- rising oestrogen levels as the pregnancy progresses, stimulating myometrial sensitivity to oxytocin;
- release of prostaglandins from the myometrium, decidua and membranes, triggered by the rising oestrogen level.

The possible role of prostaglandins in the onset of labour has not been fully elucidated but it is proven that mechanical stimulation of the cervix (as in artificial rupture of the membranes) leads to local secretion of prostaglandins and that a prostaglandin pessary inserted at the vaginal vault at or near term can induce labour.

There is some evidence that the foetal adrenal gland may play a role in initiating labour. Animal studies by Liggins (1973) demonstrated a rapid increase in foetal cortisol production a few days before the onset of labour which suggests that a similar series of changes may enable the human foetus to initiate the onset of labour.

Two kinds of uterine contractions occur during pregnancy:

1. small contractions which remain localized to a small area of the uterus;
2. Braxton Hicks contractions which have a higher intensity and spread to a larger area of the organ but have a very low frequency.

With the onset of labour, strong, well-co-ordinated and rhythmical contractions are recorded.

Signs that Indicate that Labour is Imminent

Mucoid discharge and 'show'

With the movement of the lower segment of the uterus and cervix, the mucus plug which occludes the endocervical canal is released. The show of blood at this time is due to the detachment of membrane from the cervical wall.

Spontaneous rupture of membranes (SRM)

Rupture of the amniotic sac with loss of fluid usually occurs during or at the end of the first stage of labour. This can occur prior to the start of active labour. If there is a small loss of fluid some women may have difficulty in differentiating it from the loss of urine. The smell of liquor is sweet and quite unlike that of urine and this is a useful point to note. This loss should be reported even in the absence of contractions as there is a risk of ascending infection or the umbilical cord descending if the presenting part is not engaged. Wearing of a sanitary pad near term could avoid embarrassment if spontaneous loss occurred.

Rhythmic regular contractions

Rhythmic regular contractions progressing in amplitude, frequency and discomfort is the most significant sign, as it is noted that SRM often occurs after labour has begun and the mucoid plug can be released undetected.

Induction of Labour

Induction of labour is simply bringing about the onset of labour by artificial means. The decision as to when to carry out this procedure requires experience and judgement. Rates of induction quoted range from 5% to 25% (Beischer and Mackay, 1986) of deliveries in different centres. Considerations must include the risk of maternal and/or foetal complications if the pregnancy is allowed to continue compared with the risk of prematurity to the foetus and possible complications of the induction procedure itself. The question of induction gives rise to continual discussion and comment by some consumer groups who regard such procedures as too interventionist and too frequently performed for the convenience of the hospital or staff. It should be remembered, though, that requests from the mother to 'bring the baby on' (elective induction) are by no means rare or unknown.

Methods of induction

ARTIFICIAL RUPTURE OF THE MEMBRANES (ARM, KNOWN AS SURGICAL INDUCTION)

This involves stretching the cervix and stripping the membranes from the lower uterine segment and probably stimulates the release of the prostaglandins from the decidua which, together with rupture of the forewaters, increases the likelihood of success. It is important that the obstetrician checks after the procedure that cord prolapse has not occurred and that close observation is made of the foetal heart. This may be done via a foetal scalp electrode or by external monitoring (cardiotocograph).

OXYTOCIN

Oxytocin is now usually administered by intravenous infusion. This is much more effective if used in association with artificial rupture of the membranes, but an ARM is often successful without the addition of oxytocin, especially in multipara. Close monitoring of the foetal and uterine responses is required for an initial period and the procedure may have to be terminated because of foetal or maternal distress or unsatisfactory progress. Oxytocin infusion often produces severe pain associated with uterine contractions and adequate pain relief (e.g. epidural analgesia and support) is vital. Chapter 11 has explained that higher levels of oxytocin exist naturally at night and this raises the question of whether induction of labour should occur during the night.

PROSTAGLANDINS

Prostaglandins are divided into four basic-groups – A, B, E and F – each of which is then further subdivided into 1 or 2. The E1, E2 and F2 compounds have an intrinsic stimulating effect on the myometrium as well as causing oxytocin release from the posterior lobe of the pituitary gland. Prostaglandin is most commonly administered by high vaginal insertion, though it can be given orally or intravenously. It has certain advantages, in particular a specific ripening effect upon the cervix which makes it useful in those being induced at 36 weeks or less, and is not associated with water retention. Common side effects are nausea, vomiting, diarrhoea and hot flushes. Thus, in many cases a combination of methods of induction may be required to achieve the result, e.g. prostaglandins followed by artificial rupture of the membranes.

Indications for induction

Generally the conditions for elective induction should be favourable. These include:

- foetal head well applied to cervix;
- cervix effaced;
- certain gestation of 40–41 weeks.

Some 50% of inductions are done for one or more of the following reasons.

1. *Pre-eclampsia.* Moderate to severe degrees of this condition are uncommon in developed countries but induction is usually indicated when there is persistent proteinuria, persistent hypertension and indication of foetal growth retardation or placental insufficiency.
2. *Prolonged pregnancy.* There is a risk of placental insufficiency (reduced liquor, slower or fewer foetal movements) when gestation is 42 weeks or more. Observations which may assist in the decision to induce are cardiotocography and ultrasonography.
3. *Intrauterine growth retardation (IUGR).* This is usually accompanied by a failure of the normal maternal weight gain, fundal height significantly less than for dates and reduced liquor and foetal movement.
4. *Hypertension.* Most of these patients can be assisted with rest and antihypertensive medication and induction is usually performed only in those showing indications of placental insufficiency.
5. *Diabetes mellitus.* Induction is performed electively at 38 weeks gestation but delivery, usually by elective caesarean section, may be contemplated earlier if complications, particularly hypertension, present.
6. Other indications include rhesus immunization, foetal death in utero (IUFD), foetal malformations and acute polyhydramnios.

Contraindications to induction

- Cephalopelvic disproportion
- Abnormal presentation
- Unstable lie (because of the risk of prolapse of the umbilical cord)

Figure 17.1 The first stage of labour may be subdivided into a latent phase and an acceleration phase. The time of each phase varies from woman to woman.

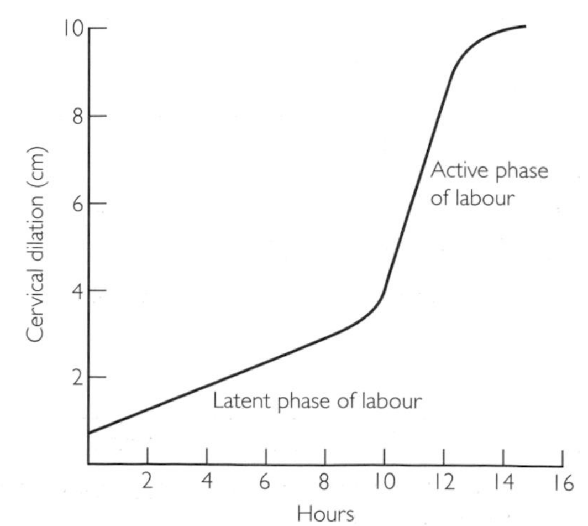

Figure 17.2 Effacement and dilation of the cervix – stage 1.

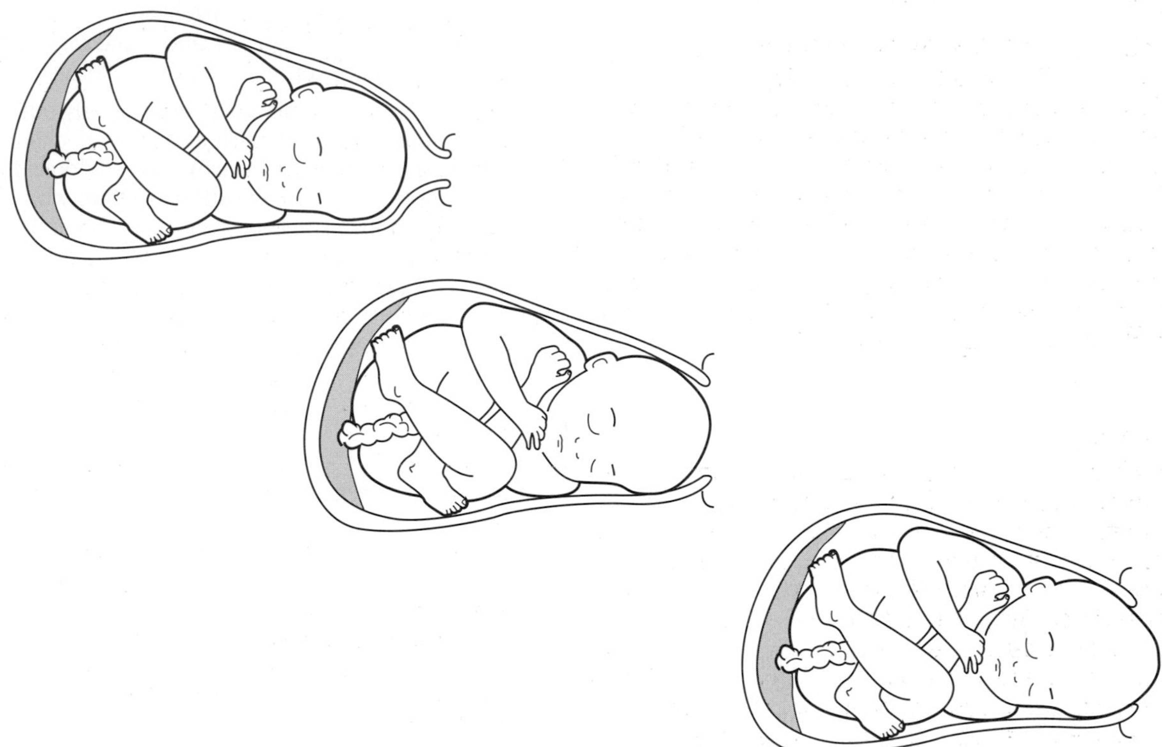

- Foetal distress, when urgent caesarean section is indicated
- Umbilical cord presentation

Complications of induction

Prolapse of the umbilical cord has been previously mentioned and other complications include foetal distress (requiring urgent caesarean section) precipitate delivery, ruptured uterus, amniotic fluid embolism (rare) and infection.

The Stages of Labour

Stage 1 is from the onset of labour until full dilation of the cervix.

Stage 2 is the stage from full cervical dilation to the expulsion of the foetus from the vagina.

Stage 3 is the expulsion of the placenta and membranes.

Stage 1

The uterus has certain important characteristics.

- It displays a resting tone between contractions which is referred to as basal activity.
- The ability to contract, usually in a co-ordinated and rhythmical manner, commencing in an area called the pacemaker in the region of the uterine horn and then spreading downwards to the lower segment.

If the fibres contract in concert the contraction is described as co-ordinate; if not, it is said to be inco-ordinate. The labour process is autonomous and depends on uterine contractibility versus cervical resistance.

During the latent phase (Fig. 17.1), the cervix becomes effaced (Fig. 17.2). Normally this phase accounts for about half the duration of labour, which in primigravidae averages 12–16 hours and in multigravidae 6–8 hours. However, there are infinite variations. When labour achieves a certain momentum, it is described as being in an acceleration phase with dilation of the cervix occurring at a rate of 1 cm $hour^{-1}$ or more. Spontaneous delivery is the outcome in over 95% of these labours (Beischer and Mackay, 1986).

Generally the cervix of a multipara begins to soften before the onset of labour and is less sensitive than that of a primipara. The intensity of uterine contractions in early labour tends to be higher in primiparae than in multiparae.

Intact membranes during labour act as a hydrostatic active wedge for early dilation, a protective cushion for the foetal head and a barrier to infection. During contractions the abdominal contour alters due to the rising forwards of the uterus so that the foetus approximates to the direction of the pelvic birth canal. This movement is easier if the woman is upright or in side lying. The progression of labour is mainly the result of the release of increasing quantities of

Figure 17.3 Characteristics of a uterine contraction: (1) early contraction, slow increment; (2) stronger contraction with short latent period, rapid increment, pain perceived earlier in contraction.

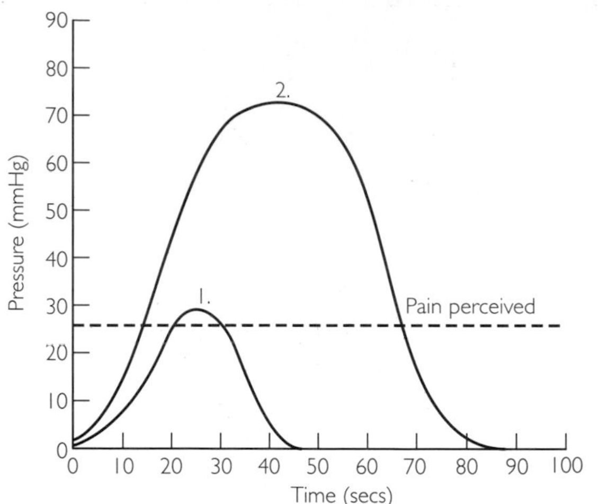

prostaglandin from the decidua and oxytocin from the posterior lobe of the pituitary gland.

The measure of the activity of the uterus is quoted in Montevideo units, which is the intensity of the contraction (measured in mmHg) multiplied by the number of contractions in a 10-minute period (e.g. if there are three contractions in a 10-minute period with an average intensity of 40 mmHg this equals 120 Montevideo units). In general the efficiency of the gravid uterus in labour depends upon:

- the strength of the contraction;
- the frequency of contraction (e.g. 2–3 every 10 minutes);
- the co-ordination or otherwise of contractions;
- the polarity of the contractions, i.e. fundal origin spreading downwards.

During each uterine contraction, normally, there are three phases (Fig. 17.3):

1. the *increment*, when pressure is rising within the uterus;
2. the *climax*, a comparatively short period of sustained maximum pressure;
3. the *decrement*, when the contraction is easing and the intrauterine pressure is falling.

PAIN IN LABOUR

Pain is a normal accompaniment of labour and delivery and is defined as 'the feeling which results from the noxious stimulation of special sensory receptors and nerves' (Beischer and Mackay, 1986, p. 350) but the exact neurophysiological and biochemical mechanism which produces pain during the various stages of labour and vaginal delivery has still not been conclusively determined (Bonica, 1980).

Individual tolerance to pain varies enormously but parturients often describe the severity of pain of childbirth as being like no other they have experienced. Individuals will find different ways of coping with pain either with or without the addition of modern pharmacological therapy. Analgesia for childbirth has certainly come a long way since Euphemia MacAlyane of Edinburgh was buried alive in 1591 on Castle Hill for seeking the assistance of Agnes Sampson for the relief of pain at the birth of her two sons.

Pain in stage 1

Most data suggest that the pain of the first stage of labour is primarily due to:

- the dilation of the cervix. Pain is influenced by the degree of dilation and the speed with which it is achieved;
- Contraction and distension of the uterine muscle itself. The specific stimulus has not yet been ascertained, but there is a correlation between the intensity and duration of the contraction and the intensity of the pain;
- pressure of the uterus on the surrounding sensitive structures (see Table 17.2 and Figs 17.4 and 17.5).

In early labour, if the intrauterine pressure during a contraction is less than 20–25 mmHg, no pain is felt. As the strength of the contractions increase, the build-up of pressure exceeds the pain threshold and pain is experienced (see Fig. 17.3).

With the early contractions this increment takes some time, but as the contractions become stronger the latent period decreases and pain is perceived earlier in the contraction. That is, contraction pain increases in intensity as the intrauterine pressure increases and the cervix dilates and stretches. Correlation between the onset of uterine contractions and the onset of pain, as noted by Caldeyro-Barcia and Poseiro (1960), has important implications when inhaled analgesia, such as nitrous oxide, is being used.

People vary enormously in their perception and response to pain during childbirth. Pain varies throughout the labour and from one labour to another in the same woman and can be influenced by many psychological as well as physical factors.

Table 17.2 Pain in labour during stage 1

Parturition pain pathway	Distribution of pain
Nerves from the uterus and cervix enter, primary to T11 and 12, secondary to T10 and L1. Important for placement of upper TENS electrodes	Diffused over a large area, lower abdomen and small of back. Later, more intense, including thigh and perineal area

Figure 17.4 Stage 1. Pain pathways from the uterus.

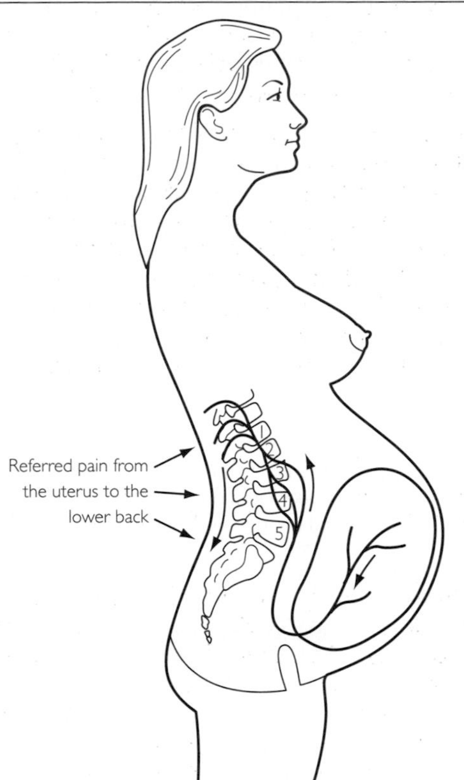

Anxiety and fear give rise to a higher perception of pain. These can be precipitated by:

- ignorance;
- previous adverse experience;
- cultural and social patterns and customs;
- psychological conditioning from childhood that parturition is very painful;
- negative approach to childbirth;
- hostility towards pregnancy and its outcome;
- hostile environment.

These attitudes can be significantly modified with effective ante-natal preparation which aims to make the experience of labour and delivery a positive and pleasurable one, in which pain relief is used if necessary. Response to pain, particularly of childbirth, can be modified by expectations. It has been said that one person's pain is another person's mild irritation (Norr et al, 1977).

Those observing the labouring woman cannot judge the severity of her pain. Only the woman herself knows the intensity she is experiencing. A pain gauge registering the intensity of what she is actually feeling would be very helpful to those in attendance, considering how differently they may view the situation.

Louise was experiencing very strong contractions of 50–60 seconds duration every three minutes.

Figure 17.5 Stage 1. Pain distribution. An increase in pain intensity over the lower abdomen, hips and lower back is common as labour progresses. Severe pain in the lower back is often experienced if an occipito-posterior position exists.

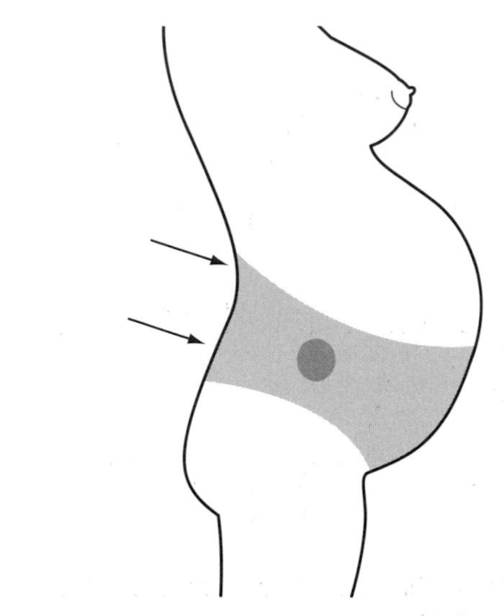

Figure 17.6 A pain gauge.

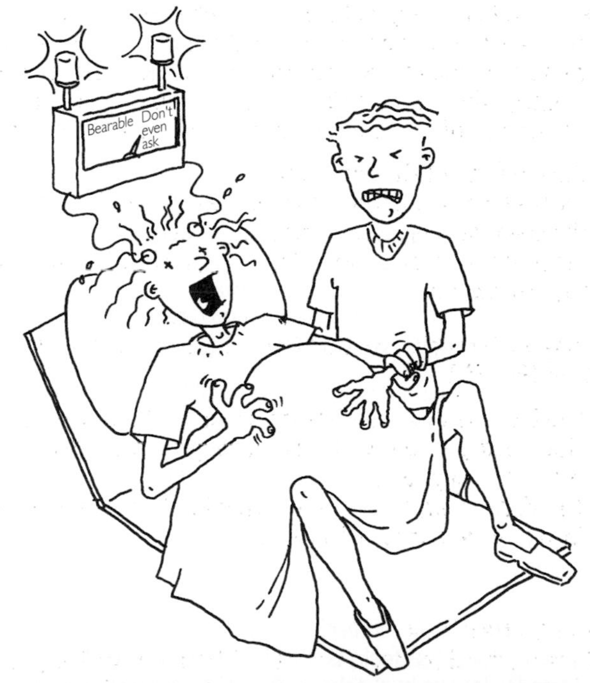

When last examined she was 8 cm dilated. She had attended ante-natal classes and was inhaling Entonox during each contraction; her appearance was calm and relaxed. John, her attentive partner, could smell the breakfast the staff had brought in for him and, on observing his wife in her relaxed state, said, 'I'll have my meal now so I'll be with her when things get tough!'

Women will rate pain of labour highest at the time of their labour, a little lower when it is over and lower still three months later. The perception of pain fades with time. In mothers who complained of severe pain, more than 90% viewed the experience with satisfaction in retrospect (Morgan et al, 1982).

Fiona's description of pain immediately after birth: 'At its worst, absolutely mind blowing' and at three months after birth: 'Not so bad for a first labour'.

The attitudes of ante-natal educators, attending staff, family and friends should not influence the woman's choice of pain relief. Ante-natally she needs to discuss the available options with her doctor (not all birth centres offer a full anaesthetic service). The ultimate decision about pain relief rests with the mother. Its use is not an indication of failure.

One study reported that women expecting their first babies were found not so much to underestimate the pain of labour as to overestimate their ability to cope with it. The number of mothers requesting epidurals during labour was four-times the number intending to do so and they were more likely to need epidural analgesia for the first, rather than subsequent labours (Rickford and Reynolds, 1987). However, fatigue, lack of sleep and concern for the foetus contribute to the mother's inability to cope with pain.

POSITIONS DURING FIRST STAGE OF LABOUR

In the early 19th century, Merriman (1816) stated that:

> . . . . the patient may be allowed to sit, stand, kneel or walk about as her inclination may prompt her; if fatigued, she should repose upon the bed or couch, but it is not expedient during (this) stage that she should remain very long at a time in a recumbent posture.

Women / couples arriving at ante-natal (AN) class are often surprised to learn that there are no formal positions for labour and delivery. Maternal comfort dictates choice but safety, progress of labour, state of the foetus and maternal well-being must be considered. If all is well ambulation is encouraged and at other times frequent changes of position are advocated.

What determines the mother's choice of position?

1. How does she feel? Is she fresh, is she restless, is she tired? Has she backache, indigestion, nausea or perhaps a heavy dragging sensation between her legs? In which position does she feel she can best cope with contractions?
2. What is the maternal and foetal status?
3. What resting supports are available? A bean bag, a stool, a birthing chair, a rocking chair or a bed?
4. Who is there to offer advice and assistance? Mothers often feel 'like a beached whale' and need assistance and encouragement to change from one position to another.
5. What pain relief is she using, if any? Nitrous oxide or low-dose epidurals may allow limited freedom of movement even though ambulation may be restricted in some incidences.
6. What is her cultural and social background?

All these aspects should be considered by the staff.

Physiological considerations affect the position adopted during labour (see Chapter 11). The supine position leads to the supine hypotension syndrome (SHS) which adversely affects mother and foetus and can delay labour (Caldeyro-Barcia, 1968, 1975). Maternal symptoms are alleviated by rolling onto the side. Some degree of compression of the vena cava still exists in the lateral position but is very much reduced (Kerr et al, 1964). Some women can compensate for

Figure 17.7 During contractions the abdominal contour alters due to the rising forwards of the uterus and it approximates to the direction of the pelvic birth canal. A woman may feel more comfortable upright and leaning forwards. Pelvic rocking and rotation movements are encouraged.

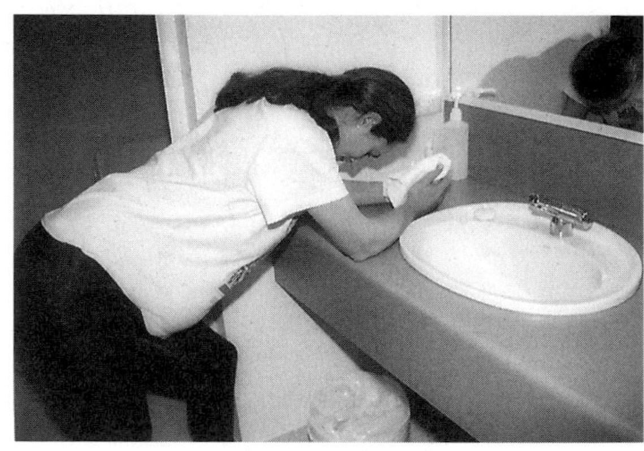

Figure 17.8 Comfortable position for women with back pain. A warm shower, hot packs, massage or counterpressure may be easily applied.

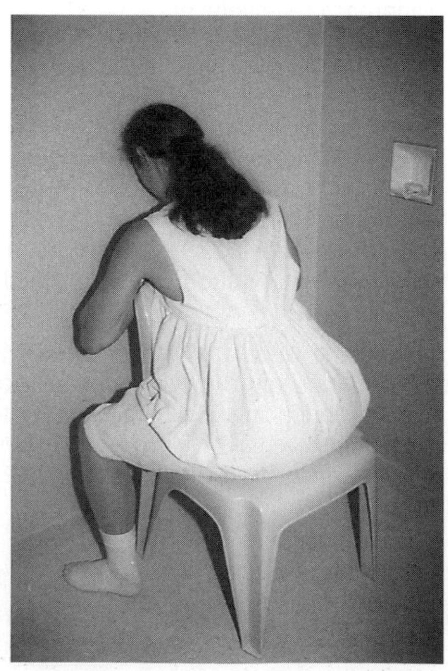

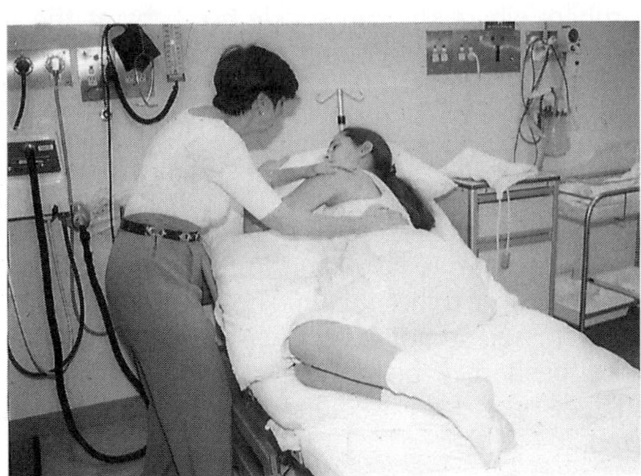

Figure 17.9 Women ofter prefer to be semirecumbent as labour progresses and resultant fatigue sets in. Liu (1974) indicated that women tolerated labour better in this position. Relaxation is reinforced by caress, touch and voice.

the reduction in venous return in the supine position by means of an increase in heart rate and development of a collateral circulation. This results in the 'concealed SHS', which in some ways is more hazardous to the foetus because of the absence of any warning maternal symptoms.

The supine position is 'the worst position during labour and delivery' (Caldeyro-Barcia, 1975). If the patient is examined in the supine position, a small pillow is placed under the right hip and she is encouraged to move into side lying immediately after the procedure. A lateral recumbent position is associated with uterine contractions which are of increased intensity and decreased frequency in comparison with supine, and potentially greater efficiency of labour (Caldeyro-Barcia et al, 1960; Hendricks, 1966).

PROGRESS AND SAFETY IN LABOUR

Various studies have looked at the benefits of the erect position in the first stage of labour (Chan, 1963; Flynn et al, 1978; Mendez-Bauer et al, 1975; Mitre, 1974).

Labour seemed to be shorter in the upright position, either sitting or ambulant. Standing was more efficient at dilating the cervix than sitting and this was more effective than supine (Mendez-Bauer et al, 1975). From clinical observation women appear to tolerate labour better if they are able to walk, stand or sit with the opportunity to lie down and rest when necessary. Recent work on maternal position during labour helps to substantiate these observations, showing that there was a significant difference in the duration of labour for primigravidae and women of mixed parity, with labour shorter in the upright position.

Other considerations will also influence maternal position. They are:

- premature or precipitate labour;
- effect of maternal medication;
- any vaginal bleeding;
- presentation of footling breech;
- a high presenting part with ruptured membranes.

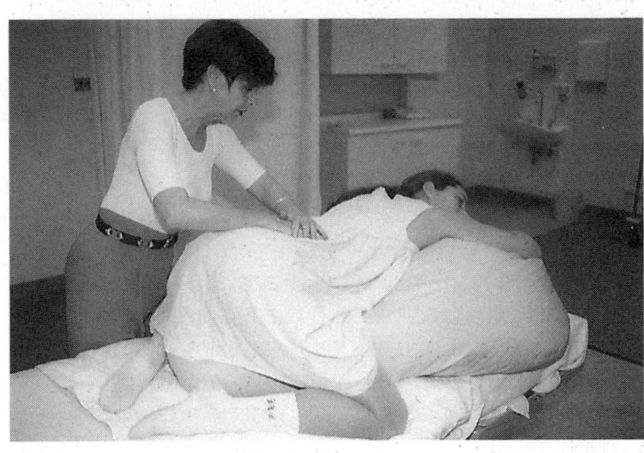

Figure 17.10 A tired mother fully supported over a bean bag alleviates the pressure on her back.

Stage 2

Once the cervix is fully dilated the labouring woman is said to have entered the second stage. The normal duration of this stage varies greatly, usually shorter in the multipara and up to two hours for primiparae. It is not uncommon at this time for the contractions, although intense, to become less frequent, causing alarm to the mother who may think she is 'going out of labour'. Parents must be reassured that this is a normal phenomenon of early stage 2, giving the body time to gather its resources for the intense work ahead.

The duration of the second stage is influenced by:

1. the size, presentation and position of the presenting part;
2. strength and co-ordination of uterine contractions;
3. the strength of the mother's voluntary bearing down efforts and the maternal pushing position;
4. the resistance of the birth canal, the resistance being lower in multiparae due to previous distension;
5. epidural anaesthesia effective in second stage.

Two phases of second stage are now recognized.

PHASE OF DESCENT

Phase of descent is described as an extension of the first stage where the head is high and there is no distension of the perineum. Pearson and Davies (1974) suggest that any active pushing at this time will introduce metabolic disturbances and mothers should not be encouraged to push vigorously until the baby is well placed for delivery. Bailey (1990), when discussing epidural analgesia and the management of second stage, states that it is acceptable to wait for perhaps an hour or two (if the mother has an epidural *in situ*) before instituting pushing, therefore extending stage 1, providing the foetus is continuously monitored and there are no signs of foetal distress. However, recent research shows that prolonged second stage with active epidural anaesthesia is a factor in the development of genuine stress incontinence (GSI) *de novo* in primiparae following delivery. Abolition of protective neuromuscular reflexes due to the epidural is a possible factor (Jackson et al, 1995; Viktrup and Lose, 1993).

As the foetus descends through the pelvis the head rotates and flexes so as to present in the optimal position for delivery (occipitoanterior (OA)). The suboccipital part of the foetal head pivots around the pubic arch and symphysis pubis and begins to extend upwards, following the curve of the pelvis (curve of Carus).

THE PERINEAL PHASE

A phase of stretching and bulging of the perineum occurs, forming an extended passage through which the head will pass. This passage bulges downwards and its initial antero-posterior length doubles, forming a gutter curved forward from the coccyx. The presenting part is now low in the birth canal and becomes visible at the vulva and expulsive efforts by the mother should now be encouraged. The head may still retreat a little between each contraction.

The possibility of an episiotomy is considered. This procedure has been described as the most common operative procedure during delivery. The incision in the perineum and vagina enlarges the introitus and lessens the curve of the birth canal. Exponents of this procedure believe it:

1. hastens the birth of the baby;
2. facilitates the delivery of premature, distressed and breech babies;
3. avoids excessive stretching or tearing of the surrounding tissues.

The head emerges, the perineum slips over the baby's face and the head extends. It is important that the accoucheur maintains some control over the emerging head to avoid sudden decompression and undue trauma to the maternal tissues. He/she may manually control the foetal head and the mother may be encouraged to cease her expulsive effort. Once the head has emerged and before the following contraction, the infant's neck is examined to determine whether the umbilical cord is wrapped around it. If so, a gentle attempt should be made to slip the umbilical cord over the head or the shoulder. Should this prove impossible the tight umbilical cord may be divided between two clamps.

The delivery of the baby's head is now greeted with jubilation, exhilaration or quiet relief; the hardest work is over and the pain has decreased. A slippery vernix-covered head may be felt by the mother. The eyes are swabbed and the nose cleared of mucus and suctioning may be initiated at this time.

The shoulders now begin to align with the AP axis of the pelvic outlet and the head rotates to realign with the shoulders; this is called restitution (see Chapter 11). The head flexes laterally towards the anus and the anterior shoulder releases from beneath the symphysis pubis. The posterior shoulder follows by lateral flexion in the opposite direction and the body usually emerges rapidly with the remaining amniotic fluid. The father may wish to cut the cord. (A description of this role should be included in an ante-natal class.) Depending on the warmth of the environment, the condition of baby and mother and the mother's preference, the baby may be assisted out by the mother and placed on her abdomen. Skin-to-skin contact with a warm blanket over mother and baby, especially in an air-conditioned labour ward, will maintain a warm and stable atmosphere where she can suckle her baby at the breast to serve the most immediate needs of both.

MATERNAL SENSATION AND PAIN

During the second stage of labour, a strong compelling urge to bear down is experienced by 85–90% of women. If the head is high there is no distension of the perineum and therefore no urge to bear down. Those with perineal analgesia (e.g. epidural) do not experience this urge. However, the urge to push may be present where selective epidural techniques have been used and perineal awareness is not affected.

The dilation, stretching and distension of the outlet and perineum cause the sharp pains described by parturients during second stage of labour. This pain increases in severity as second stage progresses, as the fascia, skin and subcutaneous tissue and other somatic structures which are pain-sensitive are stretched and torn. Pressure on and stretching of the bladder, urethra, rectum and other pain-sensitive structures in the pelvis, together with pressure on one or more roots of the lumbosacral plexus, must also contribute to the pain of childbirth (Figs 17.11, 17.12, 17.13). Stretching of tissue is likened to a burning sensation, 'a run of fire'.

EFFECTS ON MOTHER AND FOETUS

Throughout the second stage the foetal heart rate is monitored frequently, to assess any changes in placental function and consequential hypoxia. The mother must be observed closely for the effects of second stage exhaustion. These include:

- prolonged breath holding which causes a drop in oxygen levels;
- sustained blood pressure rise between contractions;
- a very obvious fall in blood pressure when the bearing down and exertion cease;
- maternal distress from fatigue and prolonged pain;
- dehydration.

The management of the second stage has changed little over the years and women are often encouraged to push hard; 'If you don't, you'll be here all day, dear!'. Beynon (1957) described three aspects of self-directed maternal effort in the second stage.

SECOND STAGE EFFORT

The amount of voluntary straining is slight until the head begins actively to distend the pelvic floor (second phase) but thereafter completely involuntary and irresistible straining efforts occur with a mechanism so similar to defaecation as to be almost indistinguishable from it. The straining mechanism does not come into play at the onset of each

Figure 17.11 Stage 2. Pain pathways. Nerves from the cervix and pelvic floor pass to sacral segments S2, S3 and S4.

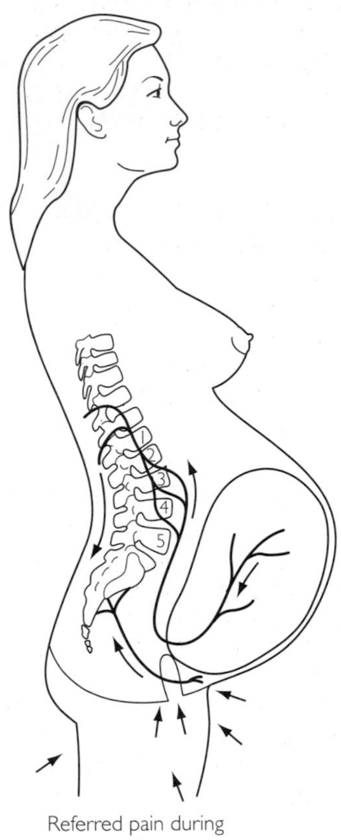

uterine contraction. There is a clear interval between the onset of the contraction and the patient's impulse to exert herself. There is often a considerable variation in the amount of push behind each pain, some being short and mild, while others are associated with a strong impulse and great progress.

Physiotherapists must be aware of the long-term effects of prolonged second stage on pelvic floor anatomy and innervation (see Chapter 23).

The AN instructions the physiotherapist can give on how to push, when to push and the appropriate positions for pushing are invaluable. Between contractions the mother is encouraged to rest and is kept cool by attending carers with a damp flannel, ice to suck and water to sip. If a mother's full bladder is obstructing progress an indwelling catheter may be inserted or an in/out catheter used. Rectal pressure and fear of faecal loss may inhibit maternal effort and the mother needs reassurance that this is normal. This is also a time of maternal exhaustion and confusion. A mother who is exhausted or confused may be assisted to direct her efforts with:

- a mirror, placed in position for her to see her baby's head and the progress achieved with each contraction. The sensation of pain may be replaced with a feeling of exhilaration and the release of the pelvic floor – 'opening the door for her baby and not fighting against the pain'.
- perineal pressure, which provides tactile feedback as to the direction of push – 'down and out'.

Figure 17.12 Early stage 2. Pain distribution. Intense pain in the lower abdomen.

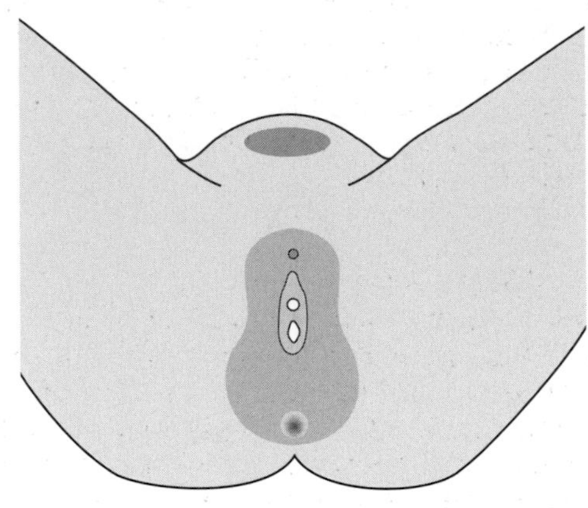

Figure 17.13 Late stage 2. Pain distribution. Intense localized perineal pain. Uterine pain decreasing.

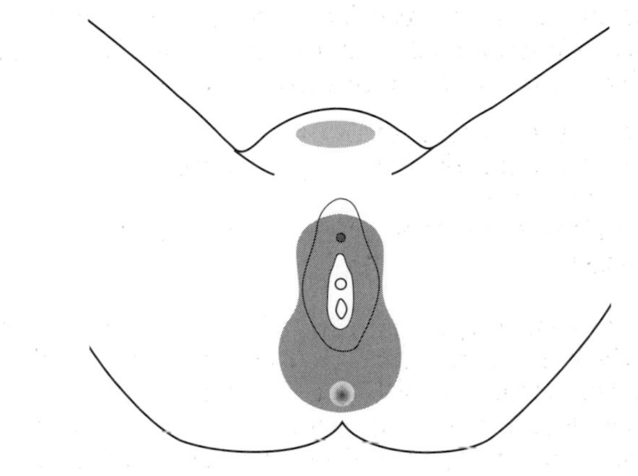

Figure 17.14 Direction of push.

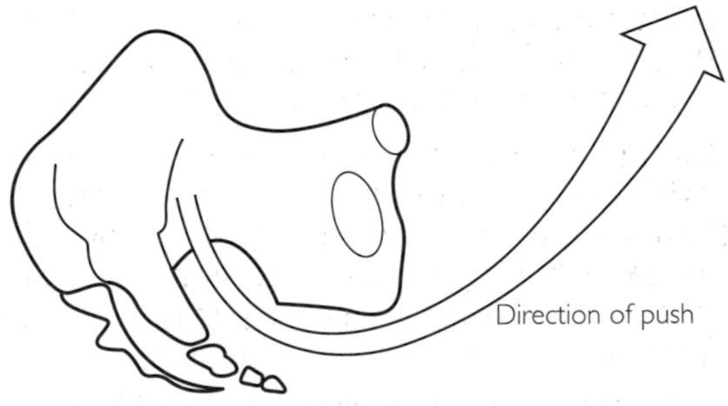

Abraham et al (1990), discussing recovery after childbirth, state that in many obstetrics units in Australia, Britain and the United States, between 60% and 90% of primigravida

Figure 17.15 Types of episiotomy incision. Mediolateral is recommended. J shaped avoids the anal sphincter.

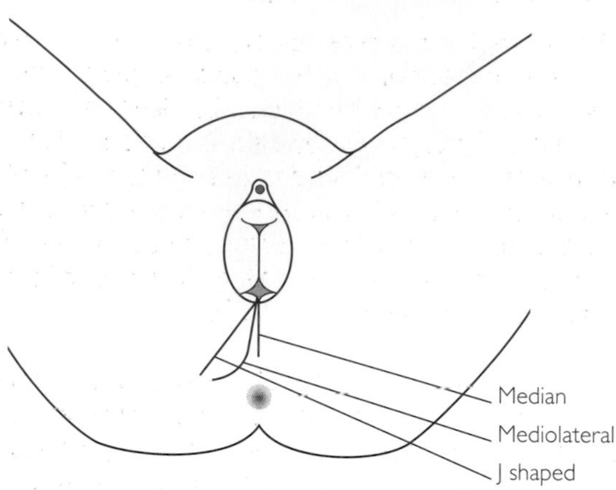

women who deliver vaginally will undergo an episiotomy. As the rate of episiotomies increased in modern obstetric care, so did the frequency of post-episiotomy discomfort and pain. Rochner et al (1989) concluded that there is little support for the claim that episiotomy prevents tears in normal deliveries and suggested the practice of episiotomy is in need of reappraisal. However, it has been suggested that there is reduced pelvic floor injury when an episiotomy is performed (Smith et al, 1989). Walker et al (1991) in fact demonstrated that the use of episiotomy increases the likelihood of major perineal trauma fourfold. Episiotomy is usually performed after infiltration with a local anaesthetic (Fig. 17.15). The tissues cut by episiotomy incision may be important in pelvic floor restoration and they are:

- vaginal epithelium and perineal skin;
- Colles fascia and bulbocavernosus muscle;
- superficial and deep transverse perineal muscles.

An extensive episiotomy may also include:

- external anal sphincter;
- levator ani muscle.

SECOND STAGE POSITIONS

History shows that virtually every 'conceivable' position has been used for labouring and delivery, including standing, squatting, semisitting and kneeling either with or without some sort of support. The final position for birthing is usually a compromise between the wishes and needs of the patient and those of the attendants. Today, the four most commonly used positions for delivery are lithotomy, dorsal (recumbent), lateral and semirecumbent (propped) – (Figs 17.16, 17.17). These positions allow easier access to the perineum and the abdomen for observation of the foetal heart rate and are generally more comfortable for the person who is carrying out the delivery. The supine positions may, however, produce adverse haemodynamic factors for the mother and the foetus.

Figure 17.16 A well-supported, semirecumbent, modified 'squat' position.

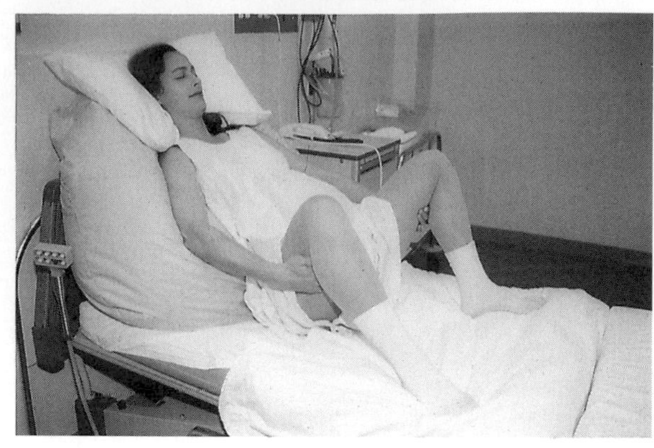

Figure 17.17 The lateral (SIMS) position avoids adverse haemodynamic factors and is comfortable for tired, nauseated women or those with back pain.

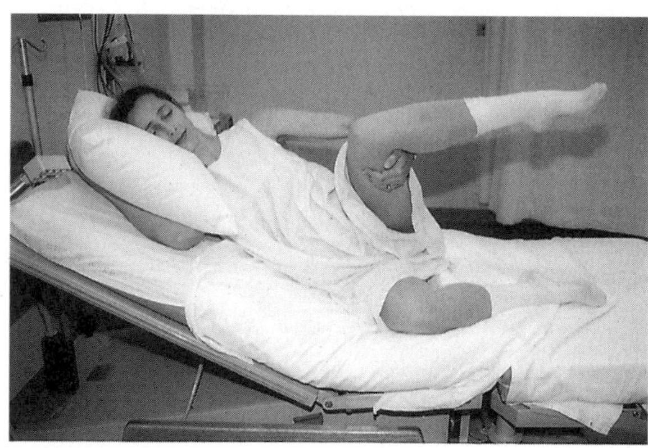

Figure 17.18 The upright position with abducted thighs increases both the transverse and the antero-posterior diameters of the pelvic outlet by up to 30% (Russell, 1982).

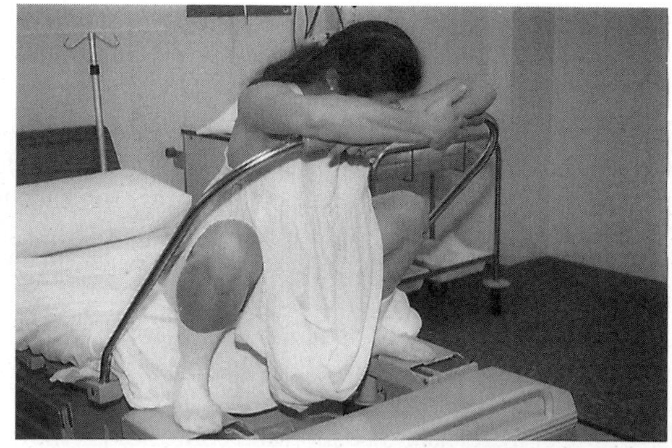

A controlled clinical trial encouraged women to adopt upright positions rather than be recumbent, e.g. squatting, kneeling, sitting or standing during second stage (Fig. 17.18) (Gardosi et al, 1989). These upright positions resulted in:

- a higher rate of intact perineums;
- apparent reduction of forceps deliveries;
- benefits if progress was slow.

Kneeling was the most favoured upright position. Squatting, although upright, is the least frequently used position. Its disadvantages include:

- increased vulval oedema;
- maternal fatigue;
- poor visibility and control of delivery;
- impossible if sedated.

Semisitting has been suggested as the optimum position for birthing, having the advantages of squatting but without the disadvantages (Roberts, 1989). A specially designed birth cushion (Gardosi, 1989) allows a modified squat position with most of the weight taken on the thighs. Trial results indicated:

- maternal comfort and ease of pushing;
- shorter stage;
- lower forceps rate;
- higher rate of intact perineum;
- higher rate of labial lacerations.

It would appear that women work more effectively in second stage if they are comfortable. Some women instinctively adopt the position that is right for them while others need to be encouraged and assisted to do so. Some women are too tired, too sedated or even too comfortable to move from a recumbent position.

INSTRUMENTAL DELIVERY

It may be necessary to assist the delivery of the baby in the second stage of labour. The two methods of intervention are forceps and vacuum extraction. Both instruments are widely used and are designed to expedite the safe delivery of the baby.

Common indications for instrumental intervention

1. Delay in stage 2 of labour; time limits of second stage depend on condition of the mother and foetus and the progress of labour.
2. Prevention of maternal stress and foetal distress.
3. Foetal distress.

Forceps Obstetric forceps consist of two metal pieces each with a handle and a blade which fit together. The blades are shaped to cradle the contour of the baby's head. Before application of the forceps, the mother is placed in the lithotomy position with adequate analgesia. The cervix must be fully dilated with the foetal head engaged or partially descended in the birth canal. Different types of forceps are used for different conditions, e.g. rotation or lift-out. Delivery is effected by steady traction with each uterine contraction.

Women having a forceps delivery usually require an episiotomy. Catheterization may be necessary. Epidural anaesthesia has been associated with a higher incidence of instrumental deliveries. The argument over the association of instrumental deliveries with epidural analgesia continues (see Chapter 10). Bruising of the bladder base and the presence of perineal trauma may cause urinary retention post-partum. Forceps deliveries are associated with a high incidence of occult anal sphincter tears (Sultan et al, 1993).

Vacuum extraction This is an alternative to forceps delivery. A metal or silicone rubber cap of the appropriate size is placed over or as near as possible to the posterior fontanelle, suction is applied and traction used with each uterine contraction. Once the head passes through the introitus the suction is released and the baby is delivered without any further suction assistance. As the foetal scalp has been sucked into the cup a red raised circular swelling will be evident after delivery. This abrasion (chignon) often takes several days to recede.

Stage 3

The third stage of labour is the time from the birth of the baby until delivery of the placenta. This stage usually takes place in the dorsal position. The contractions are often described by the mother as less painful and less frequent as the uterus expels the placenta from the uterine wall. As the uterus contracts at the end of the second stage, the great decrease in uterine wall size shears the placenta from its attachment and it is expelled into the lower uterine segment.

Expulsion of the placenta is often assisted by controlled traction on the remnant of the umbilical cord. Delivery of the placenta is followed by a rapid retraction of the uterus which becomes smaller and firmer. Placental separation exposes open blood vessels in the placental site, resulting in normal vaginal blood loss. Oxytocic drugs, e.g. syntocin, syntometrine or ergometrine, are usually administered to the mother during the third stage to stimulate uterine contraction and reduce the risk of post-partum haemorrhage. These drugs can be given intramuscularly or, for more rapid effect, intravenously.

Careful inspection of the placenta, membranes and cord ensures their completeness and checks for abnormalities. Blood loss is measured and episiotomy or tears are repaired. Third-degree tears (into the anal sphincter) may be repaired under anaesthesia in theatre. The mother is assessed for the following features before returning to the ward: blood pressure, pulse, ability to void, blood loss, uterine fundal position and state of contraction, perineum and general condition.

Disorders and Complications of Labour

Although modern obstetric practice continues to reduce the risks associated with childbirth, there are still many factors which can influence the conduct and outcome of labour. These include foetal distress, uterine dystocia, obstructed labour, prolonged labour, haemorrhage, manual removal of the placenta and maternal and foetal complications.

Foetal distress

Foetal distress is an acute, subacute or chronic impairment of oxygenation or nutrition to the foetus. It can occur in up to 30% of babies (Beischer and Mackay, 1986.). The causes can be considered as follows.

- Maternal – hypotension, cardiovascular disease, anaemia, respiratory depression, malnutrition, acidosis and dehydration, supine hypotension syndrome.
- Uterine – excessive or prolonged uterine activity.
- Placental – premature separation.
- Cord – compression (knot).
- Foetal – infection, haemorrhage.

DIAGNOSIS

- Intermittent or continuous monitoring of foetal heart rate. Electronic monitoring (cardiotocography) allows detailed observation of rate and rhythms.
- Presence of meconium staining (foetal gut contents) in the liquor. Asphyxia stimulates the gut.
- Increased foetal acidosis. Blood samples can be taken via the scalp electrode.

Uterine dystocia

Difficult or abnormal labour, which is usually prolonged, can be assessed by considering the strength of the uterine contractions, dilation of the cervix and descent of the presenting part.

UTERINE DYSFUNCTION

- Hypotonia – weak contractions, less than 30 mmHg, either throughout or later in labour.
- Hypertonia – strong co-ordinated (precipitate) or unco-ordinated contractions. 'Precipitate labour' can impede placental blood flow, exert high pressure on the foetal head and traumatize the birth canal.

DYSFUNCTIONAL VOLUNTARY MUSCLE

Weak abdominal and thin stabilizing muscles may affect the ability to expel the foetus. Strong and inflexible pelvic floor muscles may limit the relaxation and extensibility required to allow passage of the foetus. Patterns of pushing can also affect the ability of the pelvic floor to release (see Chapter 30).

CEPHALOPELVIC DISPROPORTION (CPD)

The bony pelvis may be narrow at the inlet, in mid-diameter or at the outlet (see Fig 10.6). A large foetus, due to genetic or medical factors (maternal pre-diabetic or diabetic conditions), or a less than optimal presenting part may not fit through the pelvis. Foetal presentation of face, brow, breech, transverse lie or persistent occipitoposterior (POP) may present too large a diameter at inlet or outlet.

Obstructed labour

Obstructed labour is usually diagnosed when two successive pelvic examinations, at least an hour apart, demonstrate that no progress in cervical dilation has occurred.

Prolonged labour

There now seems to be a general consensus of opinion that labour should not last longer than 24 hours. Diagnosis and proper management of prolonged labour is important because of the maternal and foetal risks.

Haemorrhage

Primary post-partum haemorrhage is usually due to:

1. uterine bleeding from the placental site, resulting from inadequate uterine contraction from hypotonia or retained placental tissue;
2. birth canal trauma including vaginal laceration and cervical tears.

Manual removal of the placenta

In up to 5% of cases (Beischer and Mackay, 1986) the placenta fails to separate from the uterine wall and manual removal of the placenta will be required under regional or general anaesthesia.

Maternal complications

These include metabolic disturbances such as oliguria, ketonuria and proteinuria, elevated pulse rate and temperature, possible uterine rupture, intrauterine infection and psychological effects due to anxiety, inadequate pain relief and exhaustion.

Foetal complications

Foetal complications are predominantly a result of the disturbance in the maternal physiology as well as mechanical effects resulting in hypoxia. The risk of intrauterine infection and its devastating effect on the foetus is also always present.

Although the physiological changes in the mother during normal labour have been described briefly, each change must be understood and considered if women are to be given safe advice on how best to cope during labour. The material presented at AN classes should be formulated in such a way as to be clearly relevant to these physiological changes and the techniques taught must have the potential to cope with these changes. These techniques are dealt with in the following chapter. While this chapter provides an overview of the physiology of labour, readers should refer to full obstetric texts for more detailed information.

References

Abraham S, Child A, Ferry J, Vizzard J and Mira M (1990) Recovery after child birth. *Medical Journal of Australia* **152**: 9–12.

Bailey P (1990) Epidural and spinal blockade. In: *Obstetrics* (F Reynold, ed.), pp. 59–71. London: Baillière Tindall.

Beischer N and Mackay E (1986) *Obstetrics and the Newborn*, 2nd edn. London: W.B. Saunders.

Beynon C (1957) The normal second stage of labour. *Obstetrics and Gynaecology of the British Empire* **64**: 815–820.

Bonica J (1980) *Obstetric Analgesia and Anaesthesia*, p. 174. New York: Elsevier.

Caldeyro-Barcia R (1975) Supine called worst position during labour and delivery. *Obstetric and Gynaecology News* **1**: 54.

Caldeyro-Barcia R and Poseiro J (1960) Physiology of the uterine contraction. *Clinical Obstetrics and Gynaecology* **3**: 386–408.

Caldeyro-Barcia R, Noriega-Guerra L, Cibils L et al (1960) Effect of position changes on the intensity and frequency of uterine contractions during labour. *American Journal of Obstetrics and Gynecology* **80**: 284–290.

Caldeyro-Barcia R, Bieniarz J, Crottogini J et al (1968) Aortocaval compression by the uterus in late human pregnancy. *American Journal of Obstetrics and Gynecology* **100**: 203–217.

Chan D (1963) Positions in labour. *British Medical Journal* **1**: 100–102

Flynn A, Kelly J, Hollins G and Lynch P (1978) Ambulation in labour. *British Medical Journal* **2**: 591–593.

Gardosi J (1989) Birth cushion trial. *Nursing Times* **85**: 58.

Gardosi J, Sylvester S and Lynch C (1989) Alternative positions in the second stage of labour: a randomised controlled trial. *British Journal of Obstetrics and Gynaecology* **96**: 1290–1296.

Hendricks C (1966) Amniotic fluid pressure recording. *Clinical Obstetrics and Gynaecology* **9**: 535–553.

Jackson S, Barry C, Davies G et al (1995) Duration of second stage labour and epidural anaesthesia: effect on subsequent urinary symptoms in primiparous women. *Neurourology and Urodynamics* **14**: 498–499.

Kerr M, Scott D and Samuel E (1964) Studies of the inferior vena cava in late pregnancy. *British Medical Journal* **1**: 532–533.

Liggins GC (1973) Foetal influence on myometrial contractility. *Clinical Obstetrics and Gynaecology* **16(3)**: 148–165.

Liu Y (1974) Effects of an upright position during labour. *American Journal of Nursing* **74**: 2202–2205.

Mendez-Bauer C, Arroyo J, Garcia-Ramos C et al (1975) Effects of standing position on spontaneous uterine contractility and other aspects of labour. *Journal of Perinatal Medicine* **3**: 89–100.

Merriman S (1816) Cited in Roberts J (1989) Alternative positions for childbirth. *Journal of Midwifery* **25**: 13–16.

Mitre N (1974) The influence of maternal position on duration of the active phase of labour. *International Journal of Gynaecology and Obstetrics* **12**: 181–183.

Morgan B, Bullpitt C, Clifton D and Lewis P (1982) Analgesia and satisfaction in childbirth. *Lancet* **i**: 808–810.

Norr K, Block C, Charles A, Meyering S and Myers E (1977) Explaining pain and enjoyment in childbirth. *Journal of Health and Social Behaviour* **18**: 260–275.

Pearson J and Davies P (1974) The effects of continuous lumbar epidural analgesia on foetal acid base status during second stage of labour. *Journal of Obstetrics and Gynaecology of British Commonwealth* **80**: 975–979.

Rickford W and Reynolds F (1987) *Expectations and Experiences of Pain Relief in Labour*, p. 163. Halifax, Nova Scotia: Society for Obstetric Anaesthesia and Perinatology (Abstracts).

Roberts J (1989) Alternative positions for childbirth. *Journal of Midwifery* **25**: 13–16.

Rochner G, Wahlberg V and Olund A (1989) Episiotomy and perineal trauma during childbirth. *Journal of Advanced Nursing* **14**: 264–268.

Russell J (1982) The rationale of primitive delivery positions. *British Journal of Obstetrics and Gynaecology* **89**: 712–715.

Smith ARB, Hosker GL and Warrell DW (1989) The role of partial denervation of the pelvic floor in the aetiology of genitourinary prolapse and stress incontinence of urine. A retrospective study. *British Journal of Obstetrics and Gynaecology* **96**: 24–28.

Sultan AH, Kamm MA, Hudson CN et al (1993) Anal-sphincter disruption during vaginal delivery. *New England Journal of Medicine* **329**: 1905–1911.

Viktrup L and Lose G (1993) Epidural anaesthesia during labour and stress incontinence after delivery. *Obstetrics and Gynecology* **82**: 984–986.

Walker MP, Farine D, Rolbin SH and Ritchie JW (1991) Epidural anaesthesia, episiotomy and obstetric laceration. *Obstetrics and Gynaecology* **77**: 668–671.

18

Coping with Labour: What are the options?

LURLENE LIVINGSTONE

Non-pharmacological Methods
•
Pharmacological Methods

Pharmacological and non-pharmacological methods of pain relief are complementary procedures which help a woman suffer less anxiety and pain during childbirth. Such approaches may enable the woman to state, 'I had a very dignified birth'.

Non-pharmacological Methods

Non-pharmacological methods may help to modify the woman's response to pain and enhance her coping mechanism, but studies show that the use of such pain control techniques in labour does not appear to reduce the intensity of labour pain (Copstick et al, 1986).

Non-pharmacological methods of pain management

- Antenatal preparation:
  - body awareness
  - relaxation
  - breathing awareness
  - positioning
- Partner support
- Congenial staff
- Music
- Warm baths
- Acupuncture
- Hypnosis
- TENS

Ante-natal preparation

RELAXATION AND BODY AWARENESS

Effective preparation for childbirth should give the mother accurate, honest information and teach her practical and positive management skills to use during labour. The poem by Kravette provides a reminder of the benefits of relaxation.

Relaxation

We learn how to be
By relaxing
a little bit at a time
By letting go of our tightness
and our tension
and our control
a little bit at a time
We learn how to be
By maintaining our awareness
and realizing:
That all of our actions are choices.

That all our choices are ours to make.
That given the choice
of being tense or of being relaxed,
the choice is obvious.
Steve Kravette (1979)

Relaxation may be defined as the 'diminution of tension; the restoration of equilibrium following disturbance' (*The Concise Oxford Dictionary*, 1982). This ability to diminish tension and restore equilibrium is the most important skill a woman can take with her into motherhood. The physical and emotional demands made on her during pregnancy, labour and in the post-partum period are more intense and complex than most have previously experienced and she requires help during ante-natal (AN) classes to understand these demands and assist her in coping with these stresses.

McKenna (1978) states:

> There have been many changes in AN preparation during the last 50 years – the programmes of exercises of the early days gave way to instructions for labour and concentration on emotional rather than physical aspects. The authoritarianism of psychoprophylaxis was rejected in favour of a more flexible type of teaching – the free discussion groups of today's psycho-physical preparation . . . Throughout all these changes and developments one factor has remained constant – the place of relaxation in the programmes of preparation. Indeed, many teachers consider it the most important component of their classes. (p. 234)

The statement is as relevant now as it was in 1978. The acquisition of this skill can give the woman the capability of her own self-management during the child-bearing year and beyond. It is a positive and essential approach to life.

Benefits for the mother

1. *During pregnancy.* Relaxation helps her to cope with the physical, psychological and emotional discomforts of pregnancy. It induces rest and reduces fatigue. As many of 'today's mothers' are continuing to work for most of their pregnancy, their use of relaxation will have an influence on their ability to deal with their busy lifestyle, thereby minimizing the effects of stress.
2. *During labour.* Relaxation is the single most important skill in the control and conduct of labour. It allows the body to function efficiently with the minimum of effort; energy is conserved and the pain threshold is said to increase. To impart this skill is to give the woman a sense of control over the pain. Between contractions, relaxation can give the woman the rest she deserves.
3. *During the puerperium and beyond.* After birth the new mother will continue to experience both physical and emotional stresses, e.g. putting the baby to the breast or trying to sit with a swollen perineum can evoke feelings of frustration, stress or in some cases pain. The benefits of her relaxation training can now be clearly seen and she can take responsibility for her own health and the well-being of her family. Vines (1978) refers to an old yet familiar quotation, 'The hand that rocks the cradle rules the world' (Wallace, 1865).

Clinical experience indicates that there is a drift away from AN classes which teach this self-management skill. Certain groups of pregnant women know that they will have instant access to regional pain relief and feel they have no need to learn and apply relaxation. It is important for physiotherapists to market and emphasize this concept of self-management, not only for use during labour but also because of its extraordinary potential for use during pregnancy, in the early discomfort phase of labour before the administration of pain relief, in the post-partum period and for life.

A woman preparing for an elective caesarean section may also not be aware of the benefits relaxation can offer her. She fails to attend AN classes as she is unaware of the benefits of relaxation during surgery and in the post-partum period when trying to mobilize with pain. It is difficult to remain calm in the operating theatre. Benson (1975) suggests that the relaxation response decreases blood pressure, respiration rate, muscle blood flow, metabolism and heart rate and counters the effects of stress.

> **Mary**: *As I lay on the operating table I could hear the beeps of the pulse oximeter decrease as I actively relaxed my body. I felt I was in control. I didn't think it possible.*

The early pioneer work by Dr Grantly Dick-Read in the 1930s introduced the concept of 'natural childbirth' and one's ability to interrupt the fear–tension–pain cycle. Jacobson (1938) developed the technique of progressive muscular relaxation, in which his subjects learnt to recognize a muscle contraction, usually initially with a resisted action, and then release it. His subjects were asked to practise for 1–2 hours per day and 50–200 sessions were required.

Over the years there have been many varied approaches to relaxation and many different techniques taught to elicit a relaxation response. They are well described by Polden and Mantle (1990a).

Childbirth educators have a captive audience in those attending AN classes, but unfortunately only have a very limited time to teach this most important skill. One full session in addition to short rehearsal periods throughout the course is usually all the time available.

Any new skill takes time to develop and become effective. The mother is not simply acquiring a new skill, but learning how to use this skill during times of stress and/or pain. Usually pain serves a useful function in warning her that something is wrong with her body and action must be taken. Not so in labour. The mother now has to change her normal and habitual response to pain by relaxing through the pain and not responding to it with repeated action which may lead to further stress. Some women find it easy to acquire this new skill, others find it very difficult to change their pattern of behaviour.

Therefore the role of the educator is not only to teach relaxation but to motivate the mother to practise regularly to perfect this self-help technique. The earlier the relaxation class is introduced in the pregnancy the more time the mother will have to perfect the technique and benefit from its use.

Mental relaxation techniques (e.g. use of imagery, calm music or thought blocking) are very useful for general relaxation to help reduce the level of alertness and promote sound sleeping habits. However, the labouring woman feels physically threatened and will therefore respond to this threat with an accumulation of physical tension, exhibiting all the bodily changes of the flight or fight response. It may therefore be appropriate to teach relaxation techniques which address this physical component, rather than the mental component of stress.

As Noble describes so well: 'Preparation for labour and delivery is assisted by the use of physical techniques to achieve relaxation, because this is a time of stress when the physical involuntary nature of the events is more significant' (1978, p. 124).

Teaching a new skill – recognizing tension The relaxation class may begin by asking the woman to explore and become aware of her behaviour when experiencing discomfort, pain or fear, sensations which accompany every birth.

Questions such as:

- How do you react when you are having a vaginal examination?
- What happens to your body when your baby kicks? Watch your hands, notice your breathing.
- How do you react when you have a cramp in your calf?

evoke discussion within the group and make each woman aware of the response. It is interesting to note that all will respond with similar observations, but will vary in the degree of response and where they perceived the cycle of tension to have commenced, i.e. their focal point of tension, the area where they react to stress first.

One mother may describe the way she clenches her hand and hugs her abdomen when her baby kicks and it becomes uncomfortable. Another will tighten her jaw and hold her breath. These are normal patterns of behaviour which she can be taught to modify if necessary. She may not be aware of her increased blood pressure and heart rate, increased blood flow to muscles or dilation of her pupils. However, she can be made aware of:

- changes in respiration: momentary breath holding or increased rate and irregularity of breathing;
- changes in body position, the 'flexor response': forehead frown, teeth clenched, shoulders elevated, arms adducted, elbows flexed, clenched fist, forward body lean, legs crossed or adducted and feet pulled up as when the body is drawn up into a position of defence;
- feeling hot and sweaty;
- increased heart rate;
- dryness of the mouth.

Discuss the fight or flight reactions and how important it is to evoke a relaxation response during pregnancy, labour and the post-partum period.

Releasing tension – the art of relaxation Mitchell's (1977) method of physiological relaxation is based on the principle of reciprocal relaxation. When a muscle contracts relaxation is always produced in the antagonist. By using this principle it is possible to release tension in the stressed muscle groups, generally those involved in the flexor response outlined above.

Instructions are precise and follow a set sequence. The sequence is: arms, legs, breathing, body, head and face. The orders to each joint are:

1. move and feel the result of the movement;
2. stop the movement;
3. feel the result of the 'letting go'. The feeling of ease (relaxation) is registered in the appropriate area of the joint and skin.

All movements are small and made by the tensor antagonist and once one body part has been released that part does not move again. Once the mother develops awareness of tension then she is able to mentally check through all the areas and release any perceived tension. Further details are contained in *Simple Relaxation* (Mitchell, 1977).

Before commencing a relaxation session consider the following

- Women need help to discover supportive comfortable positions of rest. Partners can assist. After they have mastered the relaxation technique they can vary their positions from time to time.
- *Avoid the supine position if pregnancy is advanced.*
- *A propped position may be more comfortable if women are experiencing bouts of indigestion.*
- *Room temperature should suit participants, not the instructor.*
- *Toilet facilities should be available.*

Simple relaxation has been used widely since its introduction and most physiotherapists find it enjoyable to use and very easy to implement. Whatever method of relaxation is taught, the mother must be aware of the way her body reacts to stress and the method must equip her with a technique to change tension to ease.

This total 'letting go' is a useful skill during pregnancy for maximizing rest periods. During labour it helps to conserve energy between contractions. Once the basic techniques for complete relaxation have been learnt and implemented the next step involves teaching selective relaxation.

Selective (differential) relaxation This is the method of implementing the new skill without disrupting activity. It is an active, everyday skill that can be used to cope with labour.

Mothers can now be introduced to the concept of 'active relaxation' in which they are able to function with calm efficiency, allowing only the muscles needed to perform the task to work while the others are placed at rest. Each woman is encouraged to watch the way she performs daily tasks and apply her skills of selective relaxation. Awareness of self-response and practice of selective relaxation during pregnancy are important and will better prepare the woman for her response to pain/discomfort during labour.

It is unfortunate that during pregnancy women are unable to practise relaxation while experiencing effective uterine pain. It is difficult to imagine how they will react under the circumstances as the sudden unexpected pain of childbirth cannot be related to any previous pain experienced. Meares (1968) introduced a method of self-management of pain which can be used in helping women condition themselves to be less disturbed by pain. By gradually exposing women to pain, they learn the need to relax more intensely to gain control over the pain. By increasing the intensity of the stimulus, women learn to increase relaxation and so increase the pain threshold. Gradual exposure to a painful stimulus, the step by step approach, is also beneficial in building up self-confidence.

As it is not possible to simulate a uterine contraction for 'rehearsal purposes', physical discomfort could be introduced in an area which is more sensitive to touch and which relates closely to the uterus. The medial surface of the the thigh is such an area. It often receives referred discomfort during contractions and will be exposed to touch from staff, who may be unknown to the woman, e.g. during perineal or vaginal examination. A normal response may be to tense this area and wait for the interference to 'go away', thereby feeling more discomfort.

To practise, the partner can apply pressure in the form of a pinch to this vulnerable area, gradually increasing its intensity over a 60–70-second period to simulate the pain of a contraction. The intensity of stimulus applied can be increased as the woman's ability to relax improves, thereby increasing the pain threshold and her self-management of that pain. During class sessions, ask the partner to commence the exercise gently. It is much better for the woman to ask for the pressure to be increased than for the whole class to be embarrassed by the weeping recipient of a strong first pinch.

Towards the end of the pregnancy, Braxton Hicks contractions or movements of the baby which cause discomfort will provide a perfect opportunity for practice.

Reinforcing relaxation During labour relaxation can be reinforced by some simple techniques taught to the partner and support persons.

Touch To touch the skin is to stimulate the largest and most sensitive organ of the body. Touch is a very powerful non-verbal form of communication between two people and can be used effectively in the labour ward to convey messages. It says:

- I am here.
- I understand.
- I can give you confidence and security.
- You can do it.
- Just release here!

Kitzinger (1977) describes touch relaxation as a mutual exercise in release between two people. When the loving relaxed hand of a partner rests upon his woman's contracted muscles, it gives her the ability to 'flow out' towards his touch and thus release her tension. She also teaches that the hand should move slowly, moulding well to the shape of the part. Partners may find this difficult to learn at first, but the image of 'stroking a cat or velvet fabric' often helps them to achieve the desired effect. The difference in skin pressure may make all the difference in the sensation experienced, giving either pain or pleasure. Beware of light quick movements that may lead to irritation. Firm consistent pressure over a painful site, as in back pain, can act as a counter-irritant and help reduce the intensity of the pain.

Couples in the labour ward often hold hands in readiness to share that special time together, but people show tension in their hands. They are often the first part to become tense when under stress. Hand holding can increase mother/partner tension levels very quickly (Fig. 18.1).

Figure 18.1 Tension cycle.

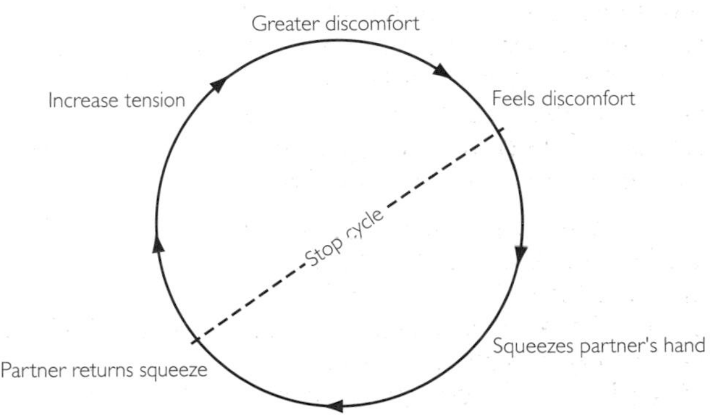

Suggest that the couple do not hold hands. A partner can place his hand gently and firmly over the top of her hand, conveying the non-verbal message 'I am here, I care, but I'm not encouraging you to tense up'. Occasionally, remind the women to shake hands loosely as if drying the finger tips.

Vicki was experiencing a long, strong labour and she found the touch of her loved ones a powerful reinforcing tool to help her cope. 'My mother and partner were both with me during labour, each playing a different role. Mother had a warm washer and she was stroking my face and playing with my hair. The comfort of her hands and the nurturing brought me back to my childhood. That was fantastic. Steve's hands were also wonderful, but firmer and different. What I got from both was different, but complementary.'

Verbal communication (often called verbal sedation): The voice, the choice of words and the tone used can be modified to instil in the woman a sense of confidence and reinforce the relaxation.

Choose words carefully. Simple descriptive instructions will be easier for the woman to follow. Keep instructions to a minimum with only one support person talking at a time. The words 'Flop' the part or 'Let go' of the part, when tension is obvious, will give her the positive cue to release that part. (The chosen word is the one used during pregnancy rehearsals.) Never ask her to 'relax'. Relaxation is what she is trying with great difficulty to achieve. She may respond to this command with irritation: 'That's what I'm trying to do, but the pains are very strong. *You* can have the next baby'.

Laura Mitchell tells us that 'Relaxation is the result of carefully selected orders, an end product. "Relax" can never itself be an order.' (Mitchell, 1977, p. 41).

The tone of voice must be calm and confident, never condemning and always encouraging and guiding.

BREATHING AWARENESS

Breathing

From the very first, there was breath.
You didn't have to think about it.
You just did it.
Life and breath came to you
at the same moment.
And that's all there was to it.
Steve Kravette (1979)

Why teach breathing for labour?

- To prevent the side effects of hyperventilation which are associated with pain/anxiety of labour.
- To reinforce relaxation.

During labour, when the woman is in a situation causing concern or is experiencing painful contractions, she instinctively reacts by unconsciously activating the 'fight or flight' response (Cannon, 1914). This is an emergency reaction which initiates a train of physiologic alterations in many organ systems – circulatory, respiratory, gastrointestinal, renal and endrocine – as well as changes in the musculoskeletal system. Excessive reactions can be potentially hazardous for both mother and foetus and should be carefully monitored. The mother does, however, have some voluntary control over the respiratory and musculoskeletal systems and behavioural adjustments are possible, to give her the ability to deal with the situation.

It should be noted that during labour the 'normal' hyperventilation of pregnancy is intensified, with an increase in oxygen consumption (this is more apparent in women who are very anxious or experiencing intense pain). The resultant hyperventilation decreases both maternal and foetal PO_2 and CO_2 and increases foetal acidosis. Hyperventilation can quickly lead to maternal CO_2 tensions as low as 10–15 mmHg (normal 40) (Wollman et al, 1964), which can cause maternal cerebral and probably placental vasoconstriction, reduced placental blood flow and thus reduced oxygen to the foetus, foetal hypoxia and acidosis. The apparent effects on the mother are likely to be increased apprehension, sweating, nausea, pallor of the skin and carpopedal spasm. Physiotherapists as teachers, therefore, have to be very aware of the problems associated with interfering with this finely tuned mechanism.

First stage of labour Over the years different methods of 'breathing' during labour have been taught in an attempt to cope with the contractions. Polden and Mantle (1990b) have set out a comprehensive table describing the different methods used by authors from 1942 to 1994. Many of these techniques have fallen into disrepute due to 'overbreathing' and resultant hyperventilation. They increased the mother's stress and left her with a sense of failure. Over the last few years there has been less emphasis on the AN teaching of any sort of control over breathing, with the assumption that women will instinctively do their own thing and give vent to their own emotions and feelings. Meares (1968), on the self-management of sudden unexpected pain, wrote:

> Be warned that there is a good deal of false teaching by psychiatrists and those who should know better that it is good to give vent to our emotions and feelings. If we give vent to our feelings of pain, we too easily become distressed, and the intensity of the pain is increased (p. 182).

Clinical experience confirms that the labouring woman equipped with tangible positive techniques is able to restore her composure more effectively and does not deplete her energy and tire as quickly. Tangible positive techniques give her quiet confidence in her *own ability* to cope. There is a close relationship between breathing and relaxation and this relationship should be explored if breathing techniques are to be used to reinforce the relaxation response. Introducing 'controlled breathing' without an understanding of physiological relaxation is a little like 'putting the cart before the horse'. Labouring women are frequently seen using strange and complicated breathing patterns but without the ability to relax, with shoulders raised, hands and jaw clenched.

The wonderful partnership of easy even breathing and the letting go of tension should not be underestimated or under-rehearsed. This harmony has helped many women keep in control of their labours and experience a happy, satisfying and dignified birth.

Becoming aware Each mother is asked to become aware of her normal breathing pattern and to note how it behaves during different activities or with different instructions.

- When she is at rest, is breathing easy and even?
- When she feels stress due to anger, fear or pain, is the breath held or quick and irregular?

- When asked to breathe deeply, is the breath forced with raised shoulders?
- When asked to breathe easy, is the rhythm comfortable?

Note the following.

- Rate of breathing (increase and decrease).
- Depth of breathing (Which part of the chest is working?).
- Rhythm (even, gasps, catches in breath, overbreathing).
- What are the positions of comfort for ease of breathing?

Discuss the woman's the ability to use the rhythm and the regularity of her breathing to reinforce relaxation. With each breath out the respiratory muscles relax and the body releases.

***Allison**: The first thing I do when I come home from work is to throw the car keys on the table and sigh out, saying to myself 'Thank goodness I'm home'. I feel an immediate sense of release.*

***Jill**: During the early part of my first labour I didn't think about my breathing as the discomfort was only slight. I was watching TV with Hue but as the pain became stronger I had to take control of my breathing – rather like a pilot taking control of a plane in rough weather – as it was no longer smoothly functioning on automatic and I didn't want to lose my way.*

Breath release The technique of breath release is taught to the mother as a cue to release tension from her body as soon as she feels her pain.

Her initial response to that pain is to take a spontaneous breath in as the body automatically adopts the position of stress. The instruction is 'Let that breath out slowly and easily and with it release the body'. With regular relaxation practice, the ability to 'let go' on one breath out can be perfected. Throughout the contraction she is taught to continue her easy, even breathing, continually scanning the body for tension spots, using each outward breath to reinforce the letting go of all the muscles.

The breathing rate often accelerates as contractions become stronger. This normal physiological response is discussed so that the woman does not try to resist this pattern but gently rides with her feelings, adapting the rhythm of her breathing to the strength of the contraction. Most people have watched a surf boat race and noticed the lifesavers paddle faster as they approach the top of a huge wave. They catch the wave and go over smoothly if they pull together evenly and easily even though the rate has accelerated. It is only when they lose their rhythm that they may founder. The use of such imagery can help women understand this physical experience and the work involved in coping with each contraction.

***Laurie**: I imagined a seagull hovering above the sea, as was suggested in the class. His wings rose and fell in a steady rhythm. I was breathing in time with the movements smoothly and evenly. As the contractions became stronger his wings moved faster and he soared to a greater height.*

***Annie**: During contractions I focused on my hands as they were my 'trigger spots' and when the contraction started I gave a deep sigh out and realeased my hands. The fingers flopped with each breath out and I imagined the pain dripping like rain out of my finger tips. I was able to combine my relaxation and breathing perfectly.*

Annie sat quietly with crossed legs, eyes closed, focusing within herself as she used 'breath release' to cope with her contractions. Other mothers feel the need to be more expressive: they sigh, moan and groan their breath out, keeping the rhythm of respiration flowing often in time with rhythmic body movements.

Working with a partner Effective breathing is an acquired skill and can improve with practice. Practice not only assists the mother to feel more confident but it also instils in the partner a feeling of competence in his ability to assist her if required. During AN classes the couple learn how to work together and co-operate as a team, finding what is acceptable and comfortable for them. For some women the confident touch of the hand on her ribs can reinforce her breathing rhythm, for others a confident soothing voice can be more effective.

Labour can be very stressful, particularly if prolonged and most definitely as it progresses. The end of the first stage is a most difficult time for the mother. She is tired, contractions are long, strong and painful. Most women 'lose their way' and need support.

Methods of reinforcing breathing rhythm and enhancing the relaxation response

1. Observe mother's respiration and body language.
2. A hand placed over the lower ribs encourages her 'to breathe into my hand' and discourages upper chest movement.
3. The hand mimics the rhythm of woman's breathing and is able to 'bring her back' to her rhythm if she loses her way – never dictating, only assisting. All women will find it very difficult to maintain control as the labour progresses.
4. Use the same verbal cues as practised antenatally, e.g. as contractions start, 'sigh out, let

go'. As contractions continue use easy even breathing. Remember the use of the word 'deep' may lead to forced breathing.

Second stage of labour Is instruction and guidance on breathing techniques appropriate for second stage or does the mother instinctively choose her own pushing/ breathing technique?

Clinical observation supports the theory that discussing, demonstrating and rehearsing techniques during AN classes helps the woman understand what is required of her and how she can effectively contribute to the birth at a time when she is very tired and finds it difficult to follow instructions. It is known that the maternal expulsive effort is supplementary to the expulsive effort of the uterus and unnecessary straining and exerting may not only exhaust the mother, but hinder this effort of the uterus. For a smooth descent, pressure must be exerted from above the fundus while the pelvic floor muscles relax completely. Co-ordination of her physical effort with the correct breathing pattern will result in the mother's available energy being used to its best effect.

Vocalization This is an important part of expressing feeling and can communicate this feeling to caregivers during labour and birth. Allowing the woman freedom of expression can give information about her needs and progress through labour. For example, expressive grunts may herald the second stage.

Breathing and pushing

- Ask the mother to place her index finger over her epigastrium, take a breath in and feel the expansion in this area.
- Fix the ribs and increase the intrathoracic pressure. With this inspiration, bear down and the diaphragm will then act as a piston directed downwards towards the fundus.
- Place the other hand on the waist, feel it expand sideways and become aware of the forward bulging (or releasing) of the lower abdominal muscles and the relaxation of the pelvic floor muscles. 'Open the door for the birth of the baby.'
- Note also the relaxation of the jaw. Lips are slightly parted and soft.
- Remind the woman of the direction of push. Downward, turn the corner (under the pubic bone) and out – the 'water slide' (see Fig. 10.12).
- Breath hold for only short periods (6–7 seconds has been suggested) to minimize any adverse effect on the foetus due to a prolonged pushing manoeuvre (Caldeyro-Barcia, 1979).
- Release breath and repeat pushing technique; several pushes may be necessary during a contraction.
- Between contractions sigh out, rest and relax.

As the baby's head crowns the mother is often asked to cease bearing down. This is a difficult instruction to follow as her whole body has now become involved in this expulsive effort. Her breath holding by now may be perfected and the urge to push is often uncontrollable. What can she do? If she replaces her breath holding with short, rapid, light breaths through her mouth (i.e. panting) she will release the downward pressure exerted by the diaphragm and allow more control over the baby's delivery. Panting is a very uncomfortable and unnatural breathing pattern and should only be utilized for a short period of time.

Partner support

***Louise**: Tim was helping me breathe through my contractions and assisting me with calm and confident words.*

In the Western world the father had been traditionally excluded from the labour and birth process and the importance of his participation during these events had received little or no attention. Women tended to support women in labour.

Recently, social attitudes have changed dramatically and fathers are now demanding to play a more positive role in supporting and encouraging their wives/partners during labour and sharing in the birthing experience. A father now needs to understand the process of management of labour and birth, what his partner may be feeling, how she may react to those feelings and what he can do to offer support.

In one study, women whose partners attended labour and birth reported less pain and had a significantly lower probability of receiving medication during labour and birth. These couples experienced more positive feelings about the total birthing experience (Henneborn and Cogan, 1975). Another study showed that support and encourage-

Figure 18.2 1950 – father waiting.

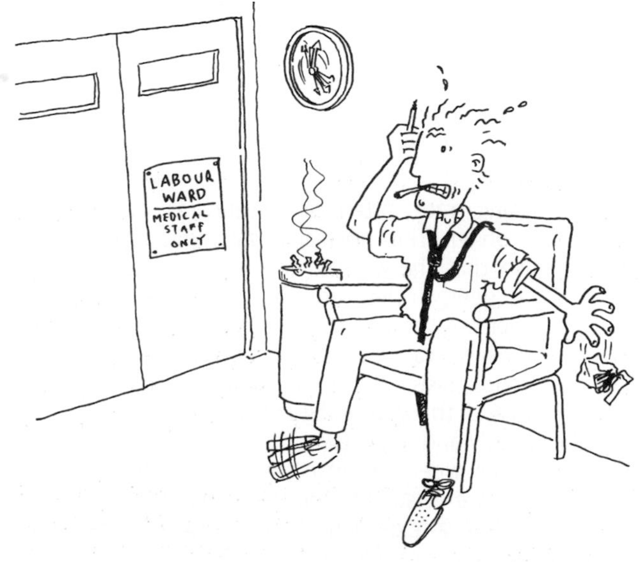

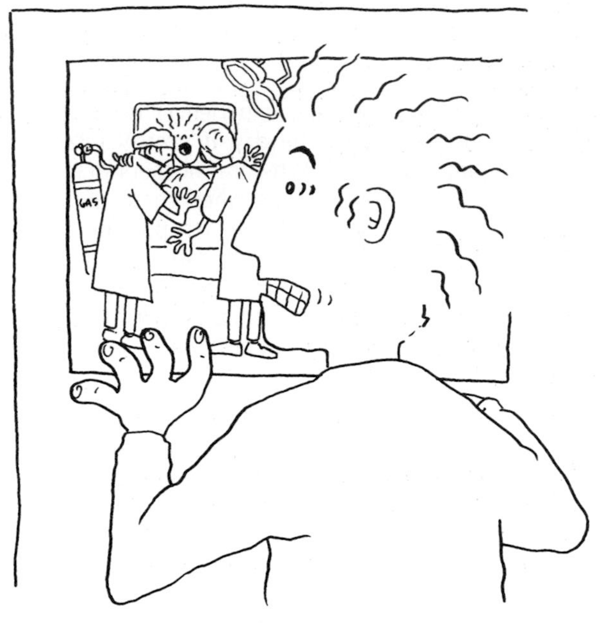

Figure 18.3 1970 – father as onlooker.

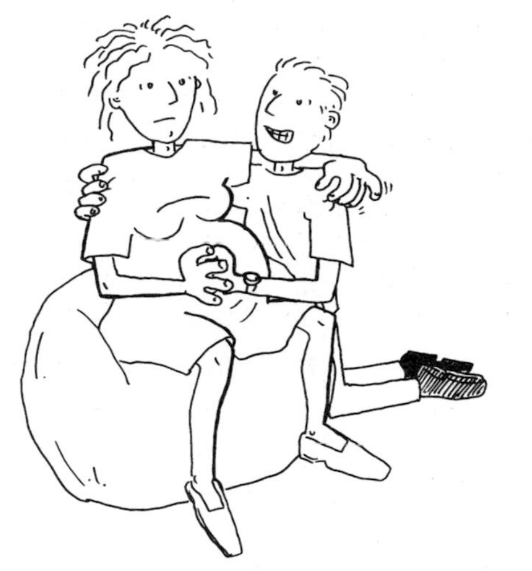

Figure 18.4 1990 – partner support.

ment in the use of pain control techniques was related to a significant reduction in frequency of epidurals, provided relatively good progress was made in labour (Copstick et al, 1985). These encouraging studies should make physiotherapists aware of how they structure AN classes. Is enough time devoted not only to educating partners, but also to teaching them practical skills with active participation, new skills which have to be reinforced time and time again, skills that they will need to use to help their women reinforce their learnt techniques?

However, Copstick et al (1985) said that women found it increasingly difficult to use their coping techniques as labour progressed. What a responsibility has now been placed on the new father's shoulders. Fathers also need support. The emotional factors he may experience include concern for his partner as labour progresses, perhaps doubts about his own ability to provide what is expected of him and a mounting concern about the outcome for the baby. These concerns, together with physical fatigue and hunger as a result of prolonged labour, must be considered by the attending staff. It must be remembered that not all fathers want to become involved during childbirth and not all mothers require their involvement. For example, different cultures vary in both the way they express their need for support and how they seek to satisfy it. Carers must be 'in tune' with each individual couple's needs and support their decision with due respect.

Congenial staff

If a mother is made comfortable, treated with respect and spoken to clearly with quiet confidence, she will respond better to directions given.

Kitzinger stresses the value of a supportive environment during the labour stages: 'The prospective parents, doctors, midwives and any other personnel in a maternity unit should be educated to be able to provide such an environment' (1978, p. 121). Relationships with the medical staff during this time have also been related to the degree of pain reported during labour and birth (Cherdok, 1969).

As mothers-to-be are usually admitted to the unit in an anxious state, the environment and the attending carers both play an important role in either contributing to or reducing her perception of pain. Factors which can influence a patient's sense of security include:

- *carer's behaviour.* Remember this is the couple's very special event, yet for the carer it is just another working day. Carers, leave your troubles at home;
- *continuity of care.* Continuity may be difficult in many maternity hospitals due to staff roster routines, but in some units a midwife may follow a woman throughout the course of her pregnancy, be present at delivery and care for her in the puerperium;
- *carer's own attitude to pain.* Any attempt to impose your own views onto the labouring woman should be guarded against;
- *carer's ability to offer support* to the woman who wishes to draw on her own resources. Is the carer familiar with techniques learnt ante-natally?
- *the experience and sensitivity of the carer.* With experience the valuable skills of touch and verbal communication act as efficient vehicles to convey security to the couple.

Music

Music is frequently used during ante-natal preparation to enhance relaxation as it both calms the mind and releases the body. Unfortunately, there is scant literature on the use of music for pain relief.

In one study, even though some women had rehearsed with music during their pregnancy and had intended to use it during labour, only half actually did so. Overall results demonstrated that music provided a positive adjunct to childbirth for some women, but was unappealing and inconvenient to others (Sammons, 1984). Music has the potential to:

- create a soothing atmosphere;
- assist relaxation of mind and body;
- reinforce breathing rhythms;
- act as an attention focus;
- be used as distraction.

Soothing music used in the operating room decreased minute oxygen consumption and basal metabolic rates, but high tempo music increased these (Metera, 1975). A conclusion was that soothing music would be helpful in clinical situations where reduction of the basal metabolic rate and relaxation was required, such as during labour.

Similarly, in a laboratory environment Melzack et al (1963) demonstrated that auditory stimulation provided an effective pain control strategy. They explained that auditory stimulation, in the form of stereophonic music and white noise, coupled with a strong suggestion that pain will be abolished is a contributing factor to an effective pain control strategy. However, to date, only a limited number of reports have attempted to relate Melzack's findings and recommendations to women in labour.

Pam*: I am a very fit girl, so I was completely devastated to be told my blood pressure was high and my labour was to be induced. I was to be confined to bed where the baby and I could be continually monitored. My physiotherapist suggested I take my music, a Walkman, into the labour ward with me and what a difference it made. Before the contractions became strong I was able to do a hundred exercises to music for my legs and my arms, the tempo was rhythmic and gentle, just perfect for my easy stretches and relaxes. Thank you Tom Jones. As the contractions became stronger the choice of music changed; with my favourite soft instrumental tape aboard, the rhythms helped me to relax. I was able to rock gently and breathe evenly in time with the music. I did move during my labour after all.*

Jenny*: I found music pleasant and relaxing when I was in early labour, but when things got tough the music irritated me, distracting me. I felt the need to focus totally on what I was doing with my hands and my jaw.*

Couples should choose their music thoughtfully, well before the birthing date. Coping techniques should be practised and the music should be used to enhance the skills in a happy atmosphere, making learning and moving more fun.

Warm baths

One of life's most pleasurable experiences is soaking in a warm bath at the end of the day. It greatly relaxes the body and calms the mind. Why are mothers denied this pleasurable experience at a time when these therapeutic effects would be most beneficial? At present there is scant research on bathing during labour, but clinical experience shows patient satisfaction when using this facility to help ease the pain associated with labour. The therapeutic effects of body immersion have long been known.

- The excellent distribution of heat promotes physical relaxation and reduces psychological tension.
- The immersed body is subject to the hydrokinetic effect and feels freer and buoyant.

Many birthing centres, unfortunately, do not have this facility available so mothers are encouraged to try this method of pain relief in early labour if they have a bath at home. Women are also encouraged to enjoy the warmth of a shower, under which they sit or stand, as they freely move their bodies.

Guidelines for body immersion

- Membranes intact.
- Water to be comfortably warm.
- Body fully immersed in a position of comfort. Four-point kneeling is the recommended position if back pain is severe.
- Stay in the bath for as long as comfortable, to help cope with labour pains.
- As labour progresses the patient needs to come out of the bath at regular intervals for monitoring.
- *Careful observations, noting signs of giddiness, faintness, nausea, pallor and changes in respiration, need to be made.*
- *Woman must never be left alone.*
- *Care should be taken to assist the woman in and out of the bath.*

Acupuncture

Acupuncture therapy has been used in traditional Chinese medicine for many centuries. It is now incorporated into Western physiotherapy and medical practice to provide analgesia. It must be provided only by those who have the appropriate training.

Acupuncture, like hypnosis, theoretically presents favourable advantages for use as an analgesic therapy during labour and childbirth since the technique is simple, inexpensive and there are no drugs to adversely affect the mother or the foetus. However, after a study, Abouleigh and Depp (1975) found the method had some disadvantages and its practicality was questionable for vaginal deliveries. Essentially, the study concluded:

1. acupuncture analgesia was incomplete, unpredictable and inconsistent;
2. it was time consuming;
3. needles were apt to become dislodged;
4. the woman's movements were restricted;
5. added wires and machinery were attached to the parturient;
6. there was interference with electronic monitoring of the mother and foetus.

Hypnosis

The main effect of hypnotherapy is to induce a high level of relaxation and consequently to eliminate or reduce the need for conventional analgesia. While some studies have found hypnotherapy to be of little benefit, one five-year study cited in Jenkins and Pritchard (1993) demonstrated the following practical benefits.

1. The use of analgesic agents was significantly reduced during labour.
2. Mean lengths of first stage of labour in primigravida women were less.

Hypnosis for obstetric anaesthesia has never been very widely applied. The woman must be suitable for hypnoanalgesia and well motivated. The conditioning sessions prior to labour are time and effort consuming, but once the patient has been trained for autohypnosis the instructor does not need to be present at the labour and delivery.

TENS

Transcutaneous electrical nerve stimulation (TENS) has been used for pain relief in labour since the 1970s. TENS is a non-invasive, self-controlled form of pain relief, free of any known side effects on mother or baby. See Chapter 24 for details relating to the use of TENS in labour.

Physiotherapist's role in the labour ward

The bells ring signalling the imminent birth of a baby and the scurry of feet can be heard in the maternity unit corridors as student midwives, doctors and physiotherapists all gather to witness the great experience of giving birth.

It is an exciting occasion and all the students walk away feeling their education is complete. But what of the preceding hours? What has led up to that climactic point? As educators, surely our interest should not only be in this terminal event but in the management of the total process of labouring.

It is only by being present during the entire experience that the physiotherapist can:

- assess the patient's needs;
- formulate an effective ante-natal programme;
- evaluate the effectiveness of the programmes.

Obstetric physiotherapists must be prepared to spend many hours in the labour ward to enhance their understanding of what real labour involves, to meet the staff and become familiar with their terminology and management of the labouring woman.

This acquired knowledge, coupled with the understanding of the physical and physiological changes of labour, enables the physiotherapist to become an accepted member of the obstetric team in the labour ward. Within this team the PT works with women who have attended ante-natal preparation classes and those who have not had the benefits of this preparation. Techniques used for pain control such as relaxation, breathing and massage can be reinforced. The physiotherapist's verbal and tactile communication skills are important. Positions of comfort can be encouraged and implemented.

> ***Louise**: We consider ourselves fortunate to have had our physiotherapist with us at Sarah's birth. Her hand resting on my stomach muscles helped concentration while her calm 'bear down' reminded me of what I had to do. With one leg pressed against her waist and the other against the midwife's, my hands held my inner thighs and I pushed my beautiful baby out into the world.*

Pharmacological Methods

Pharmacological methods of pain relief should be used to reinforce the acquired skills of relaxation and breathing. Therefore, the mother should not abandon her 'learnt' skills when other methods of pain relief are introduced, but use the pain relief to help her work with more comfort and efficiency and therefore maternal satisfaction.

Whatever method of pharmacological pain relief is employed, it must be remembered that virtually all drugs administered to the mother will gain access to the foetus. Some pass more readily and at a higher concentration than others and the traditional idea of the placenta acting as a 'barrier' is inaccurate.

The pharmacological methods of pain relief can be considered in four groups: oral, inhalational, parenteral and regional.

Oral

Oral medication is not commonly used by the labouring mother because of the unreliability of absorption from the gastrointestinal tract, often affected by nausea and/or vomiting. The usefulness of this route of administration is primarily for a mother in very early labour, who may already be tired from lack of sleep, when administration of a short-acting sedative or hypnotic drug may be useful.

Inhalational

The credit for the introduction of inhalational pain relief in labour is given to Sir James Young Simpson who first used ether in January 1847 and chloroform in November of the same year. It is interesting to reflect on the violent opposition and controversy this innovation generated amongst both physicians and the public, but particularly from members of the clergy.

This controversy continued unabated until 1853 when John Snow safely administered chloroform to Queen Victoria for the birth of her eighth child, Prince Leopold. Since then various inhalational anaesthetic agents have been tried in labour. Among them were trichlorethylene (Trilene) and methoxyflurane (Penthrane), usually administered in air. Both have now been discontinued. However, the agent which is still most commonly used is nitrous oxide (N_2O), first discovered by Priestley in 1775. It is administered in conjunction with oxygen as a 50/50 mixture known as Entonox. Some obstetric units have apparatus capable of delivering concentrations of nitrous oxide from 0% to 70% (i.e. from 100% oxygen to 30% oxygen).

The gases are absorbed from the lungs and reach the brain via the bloodstream.

ADVANTAGES OF NITROUS OXIDE

1. It is self-administered, intermittently, when pain relief is required.
2. It is readily available for the mother to use, attached to the wall in a delivery unit or from a portable cylinder.
3. The strength may be altered to suit individual needs, providing the apparatus is capable of this adjustment.
4. The onset is quick, with a latent period of 30–40 seconds before maximum effect (Fig. 18.5) and elimination via the lungs is rapid when administration is ceased.
5. It does not affect the progress of the labour.
6. It does not affect the foetal heart rate during labour.
7. It does not depress the baby's respiration at birth or the ability of the baby to suck.
8. It is also helpful as a supplementary method of pain relief combined with systemic opioids or low-dose epidurals.

DISADVANTAGES OF NITROUS OXIDE

1. Some women are averse to any form of inhalational therapy. They just don't like 'things over their face'. These women may feel more comfortable using a mouthpiece to administer the gas.
2. Some mothers experience nausea and/or vomiting. This is a common occurrence in labour as there is a delay in gastric emptying. Food remains undigested as a result of the effects of severe pain on the gastrointestinal tract and digestive processes.
3. The feeling of light-headedness, confusion and disorientation cannot be tolerated by some women, but these side effects are quickly reversed once the use of the gas is ceased.
4. Nitrous oxide/oxygen mixtures need to be used correctly and intelligently to be effective. Unfortunately, when a woman is in need of pain relief it is often too late to explain to her how to use it properly. It is therefore important that the woman has become familiar with its use before the onset of labour, preferably during antenatal classes. If possible, this teaching is reinforced before pain becomes uncomfortable. If it is used incorrectly, the woman may hyperventilate as she attempts to 'get the most out of' the gas with rapid gasping breaths.
5. It rarely relieves the pain of contractions completely. This can make a woman frustrated and further increase her tension, but it has the ability to change her perception of pain.

Figure 18.5 The effect of nitrous oxide on pain during uterine contraction.

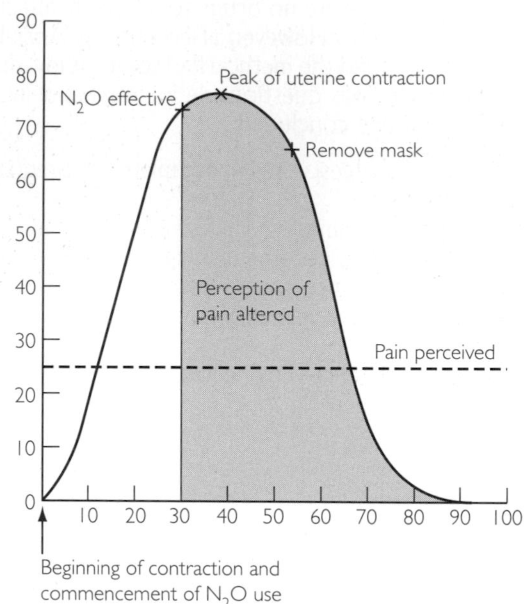

HOW TO USE NITROUS OXIDE

1. The woman must hold the mask firmly over her mouth and nose. Check that the mask fits well and forms an airtight seal (Fig. 18.6). The same principle applies to the mouthpiece.
2. As there is a latent period before the nitrous oxide reaches its maximum concentration, it is advisable to

Figure 18.6 Breathing nitrous oxide, releasing tension on each breath out. Note relaxation of the non-working hand.

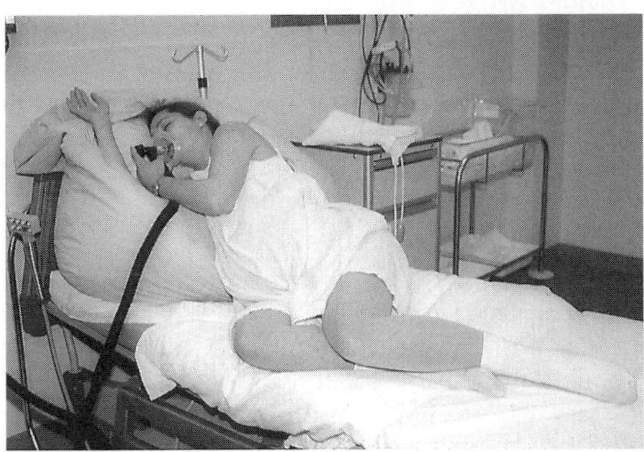

commence inhalation of the gas immediately the contraction begins or preferably before, not when the pain is intense. The mask should be removed after the contraction has reached its peak and the effects of the gas will help as the intensity of the contraction diminishes. Therefore, the N_2O is most effective when the woman is still able to anticipate her contractions and time the inhalation accordingly.

3. Inhale deeply, slowly and in a relaxed manner using each 'breath out' as a means of reinforcing relaxation.
4. Sips of water or ice between contractions may make the woman more comfortable, as there is often tingling and dryness around the mouth after inhalation.

Parenteral analgesics

For many years the opioid group of drugs, e.g. morphine and pethidine, has been the mainstay of analgesia for labour. These drugs, of which pethidine is the most popular, have the advantage that they are readily available and are simple to administer by intramuscular injection by nursing staff, without the need of medical staff. Both drugs are reasonably effective analgesics but care must be taken in administering a dose which takes into account the weight of the woman, severity of the pain, the stage of labour and any known allergies to drugs. The injections are of small volume (1–2 ml) and commonly given in the lateral compartment of the thigh. When given by this route the drugs take 15–30 minutes to reach a peak blood concentration where they become effective for up to two hours.

Morphine has a stronger analgesic effect than pethidine but because of its lower lipid solubility, it has a longer duration of onset of action. All narcotic drugs are associated with an incidence of nausea and vomiting and delay gastric emptying even further, increasing the hazards of administration of a general anaesthetic to the woman.

There is often a fear among mothers that opioid drugs will have an adverse effect on themselves and the foetus. For many years it was thought that administration of pethidine late in labour would be more likely to result in neonatal depression but Morrison et al (1973) showed that the depressant effects were greater when the maternal administration was several hours before delivery, because the drug itself and its active metabolites accumulate slowly in foetal tissues (Kuhnert et al, 1979).

Figure 18.7 The structure of the spinal cord and epidural space. (Reproduced from Brownridge (1994) with permission.)

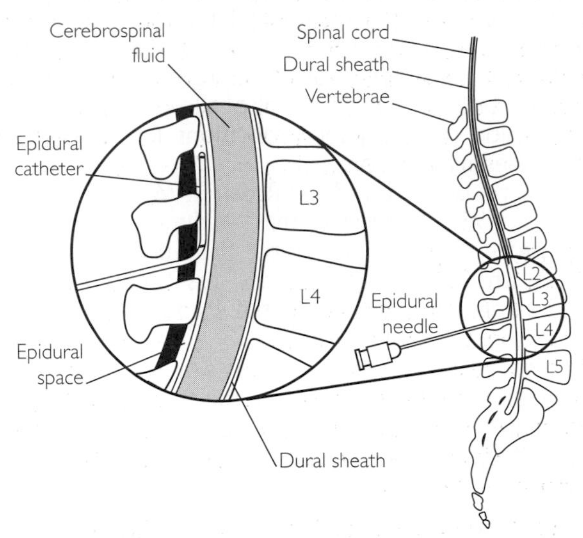

In recent years several investigators have looked at the possible effects of analgesics, including narcotics and local anaesthetic drugs, on the behaviour of the newborn and by performing certain neurological tests, have concluded that these drugs do have some effect on the newborn (Sopkoski et al, 1992; Wiener et al, 1977). The significance of these observations is not entirely clear, nor is their validity universally accepted.

Opioids have also been used via intravenous injection and Patient-controlled analgesia (PCA), but these are not in common use in obstetric pain relief.

Epidural analgesia

Epidural analgesia is the most effective form of pain relief for labour and over the last 20 years this technique has become more widely available.

Epidural analgesia is performed by a medical practitioner trained and skilled in the technique, which involves identification of the epidural space and injection of a local anaesthetic into it (Fig. 18.7). To enable the technique to be used continuously a very fine catheter is inserted into the space, through which intermittent injections of local anaesthetic may be given or, more commonly, it is attached to a syringe and an infusion pump for continuous administration.

INDICATIONS FOR EPIDURAL ANALGESIA

1. Pain.
2. Pregnancy-induced hypertension and toxaemia of

pregnancy. Epidural analgesia reduces the sympathetic/adrenal hyperactivity which is associated with pre-eclampsia and induces haemodynamic changes, giving an improvement in placental intervillous blood flow (Jouppila et al, 1982; Newsome et al, 1986). As well as allowing the progress of labour to be conducted in a more orderly fashion, it also allows for the rapid provision of satisfactory conditions for intervention, e.g. caesarean section.
3. Pre-term labour. David and Rosen (1976) and Osbourne et al (1989) suggested that epidural analgesia may improve the outcome for the baby because labour is less stressful and the delivery less traumatic. Similar advantages are claimed for the second twin in a twin pregnancy (Crawford, 1987).
4. There are many medical diseases where early use of an epidural is desirable to reduce the stress of labour and eliminate the risks associated with general anaesthesia should operative delivery be required.

CONTRAINDICATIONS TO EPIDURAL ANALGESIA

These are uncommon but must be carefully sought. The most important contraindication is an unexpected coagulopathy and sepsis which could result in epidural haematoma or abscess with consequential neurological effects.

LOCAL ANALGESIC DRUGS

The analgesic drug most commonly used for an epidural block is bupivacaine. When bupivacaine was first introduced it was commonly used in a concentration of 0.5%, but is now frequently used in a much weaker concentration, often in combination with a narcotic such as fentanyl (Chestnut et al, 1988; Justins et al, 1982).

However, nothing is perfect and epidurals, like all other modalities of therapy, have both advantages and disadvantages.

ADVANTAGES

1. A high degree of pain relief.
2. Prevents the adverse biochemical changes in the mother which may be associated with a painful and stressful labour.
3. Enables preparation for urgent intervention in a mother experiencing a complicated labour, e.g. forceps delivery, the following head of a breech delivery.
4. Benefits to the foetus by eliminating the adverse effects of maternal hyperventilation provoked by unrelieved pain resulting in reduction of placental oxygen exchange.

DISADVANTAGES

1. Compared with other methods of pain relief, epidural analgesia is an invasive technique and there are disadvantages associated with the procedure as well as risks, i.e. an intravenous infusion is a necessary part of the technique.
2. Postural hypotension may occur.
3. Weakness of the legs may make movement in bed difficult, let alone the prospect of walking.
4. Difficulty in passing urine.
5. Shivering, which can be extremely irritating and exhausting, though this may be reduced by using opioids in the epidural drugs.
6. Delay in the second stage and risk of forceps delivery. Controversy continues over this matter. In the last 10 years over 100 papers in the medical literature have considered this one aspect and, since this is responsible for a considerable proportion of consumer dissatisfaction, it is worth considering further.

Reynolds (1991) says that 'To minimize the possibility that epidural analgesia caused instrumental delivery, time and patience, possibly oxytocin and modest doses of local anaesthetic with early topping up and late pushing are necessary' (p. 144). She goes on to say: 'Because women at high risk of abnormal delivery tend to be over-represented in the epidural population, it is difficult to determine by comparison with a non-epidural group of mothers, if the forceps delivery rate is actually increased by epidural analgesia' (p. 144).

RISKS OF EPIDURAL ANALGESIA

1. *Infection.* As mentioned in the contraindications, infection remains a risk in any such medical procedure.
2. *Neural damage.* As can be appreciated, the insertion of a large needle in such close proximity to the central nervous system carries a risk of injury. Perusal of the medical literature suggests that the incidence of such damage is very low. Before attributing any symptoms or signs to the epidural procedure it is important also to consider a possible association with a number of other factors, including prolonged action of the local analgesic drug, possible injury during delivery, improper positioning of the mother during delivery and perhaps a coincidental prolapsed intervertebral disc. Macdonald (1994) claims that epidural analgesia is associated with less than one neurological complication per 11 000–20 000 blocks. Ong et al (1987) conducted a retrospective survey of the medical records of some 24 000 mothers at their hospital, delivered between 1975 and 1983, and found 45 cases of neurological defect, for an incidence of 19/10 000. They further noted that the incidence was significantly greater in primiparae, parturients who had assisted vaginal deliveries and those who received general or epidural anaesthetic, compared with those who had no assistance.
3. *Dural puncture.* Whenever epidural analgesia is administered there is a risk that the needle may be advanced too far and puncture the dura mater, resulting in a leak of cerebrospinal fluid. See Chapter 19 for further details on management of this risk factor.
4. Other *life-threatening complications* include: accidental subarachnoid (spinal injection) or intravenous injection of the local anaesthetic. Such complications are very uncommon and if properly managed, should not result in any long-term adverse effects.
5. *Backache.* Refer to Chapter 19.

Demonstration of the positions the women will be required to assume during this procedure (e.g. lying foetal-flexed position or sitting forward lean) should be included in ante-natal classes and the important role played by the support person in reinforcing relaxation should be emphasized and practised.

Clearly, pain is the most significant and often overwhelming accompaniment of labour. Various methods of pain control, from self-management to the more invasive forms of pharmacological pain relief, have been discussed. These methods can be complementary. The place of regional analgesia is clearly established but various aspects of this form of pain relief are still being refined. The effects of the method of pain relief on labour, mother and foetus will continue to be the subject for lively debate and ongoing research.

References

Abouleigh E and Depp R (1975) Acupuncture in obstetrics. *Anaesthesia and Analgesia* **54**(1): 83–85.

Benson H (1975) *The Relaxation Response*, pp. 16–19. New York: William Morrow.

Bortoluzzi G (1989) Transcutaneous electrical nerve stimulation in labour: practicability and effectiveness in a public hospital labour ward. *Australian Journal of Physiotherapy* **35**: 81–87.

Brownridge P (1994) *Pain Relief and Anaesthesia in Childbirth*. Victoria, Australia: Ashwood House Medical.

Caldeyro-Barcia R (1979) The influence of maternal bearing down efforts during second stage on foetal well-being. *Birth and Family Journal* **6**: 17–22.

Cannon W (1914) The emergency function of the adrenal medulla in pain and the major emotions. *American Journal of Physiology* **33**: 356–372.

Chestnut DH, Owen CL and Bates JN (1988) Continuous infusion epidural analgesia during labour: a randomised, double blind comparison. *Anesthesiology* **68**: 754–759.

Cherdok L (1969) *Motherhood and Personality: Psychosomatic Aspects of Childbirth*. Philadelphia: J. Lippincott.

Copstick S, Hayes R, Taylor K and Morris N (1985) A test of a common assumption regarding the use of antenatal training during labour. *Journal of Psychosomatic Research* **29**: 215–218.

Copstick S, Taylor K, Hayes R and Morris N (1986) Partner support and the use of coping techniques in labour. *Journal of Psychosomatic Research* **30**(4): 497–503.

Crawford JS (1987) A prospective study of 200 consecutive twin deliveries. *Anaesthesia* 42: 33–43.

David H and Rosen M (1976) Perinatal mortality after epidural analgesia. *Anaesthesia* **33**: 1054–1059.

Henneborn W and Cogan R (1975) The effect of husband participation on reported pain and probability of medication during labour and birth. *Journal of Psychosomatic Research* **19**: 215–216.

Jacobson E (1938) *Progressive Relaxation*. Chicago: University of Chicago Press.

Jenkins M and Pritchard M (1993) Hypnosis: practical applications and theoretical considerations in normal labour. *British Journal of Obstetrics and Gynaecology* **100**: 221–226.

Jouppila P, Jouppila R, Hollmen A and Koivula A (1982) Lumbar epidural analgesia to improve intervillous blood flow during labour in severe pre-eclampsia. *Obstetrics and Gynecology* **59**: 158–161.

Justins D, Francis DM, Houlton PG and Reynolds F (1982) A controlled trial of epidural fentanyl in labour, 1982. *British Journal of Anaesthesia* **54**: 409–414.

Kitzinger S (1977) *Education and Counselling for Childbirth*, p. 158–161. London: Baillière Tindall.

Kitzinger S (1978) Pain in childbirth. *Journal of Medical Ethics* **4**: 119–121.

Kravette S (1979) *Complete Relaxation*, p. 24. Rockport, Massachusetts: Para Research Inc.

Kuhnert BR, Kuhnert PM and Tu A-SL (1979) Meperidine and Normeperidine levels following Meperidine administration during labour. *American Journal of Obstetrics and Gynecology* **133**: 909–914.

Macdonald R (1994) Problems with regional anaesthesia: hazards or negligence? *British Journal of Anaesthesia* **73**: 64–68.

McKenna J (1978) The Mitchell method of physiological relaxation. *Physiotherapy* **64**: 234–235.

Meares A (1968) *Relief without Drugs*. Australia: Harper Collins.

Melzack R, Weisz A and Sprague L (1963) Strategems for controlling pain: contributions of auditory stimulation and suggestion. *Experimental Neurology* **8**: 239–247

Metera A (1975) Influence of music on the minute oxygen consumption and basal metabolic rate. *Anaesthesia, Resuscitation and Intensive Therapy* **3**: 259–264.

Mitchell L (1977) *Simple Relaxation*. London: John Murray.

Morrison JC, Wiser WL and Rosser SI (1973) Metabolites of Meperidine related to fetal depression. *American Journal of Obstetrics and Gynecology* **15**: 1132–1137.

Newsome LR, Bramwell RS and Curling PE (1986) Severe pre-eclampsia: haemodynamic effects of lumbar epidural anaesthesia. *Anesthesia and Analgesia* **65**: 31–36.

Noble E (1978) *Essential Exercises for the Child-Bearing Year*. London: John Murray.

Osbourne GK, Patel NB and Howat RCL (1989) A comparison of the outcome of low birth weight pregnancy in Glasgow and Dundee. *Health Bulletin (Edin)* **42**: 68–77.

Ong BY, Cohen MM, Esmail A et al (1987) Paraesthesia and motor dysfunction after labour and delivery. *Anesthesia and Analgesia* **66**(1): 18–22.

Polden M and Mantle J (1990a) *Physiotherapy in Obstetrics and Gynaecology*, pp. 165–168. London: Butterworth Heinemann Ltd.

Polden M and Mantle J (1990b) *Physiotherapy in Obstetrics and Gynaecology*, pp. 170–174. London: Butterworth Heinemann Ltd.

Reynolds F (1991) Pain relief in labour. *Progress in Obstetrics and Gynaecology* **9**: 144.

Sammons L (1984) The use of music by women during childbirth. *Journal of Nurse Midwifery* **29**: 266–269.

Sopkoski CM, Lester BM, Ostheimer GW and Brazelton TB (1992) The effects of maternal epidural anaesthesia on neonatal behaviour during the first month. *Developmental Medicine and Child Neurology* **34**(12): 1072–1080.

Vines L (1978) Stress management in early parenthood (audio cassette). Wollongong, Australia: Australian College of Recorded Education.

Wallace WR (1865) 'What rules the world' (poem).

Wiener PC, Hogg MJ and Rosen M (1977) Effects of naloxone on pethidine induced neonatal depression. *British Medical Journal* **2**: 228–231.

Wollman H, Alexander S, Cohen P et al (1964) Cerebral circulation of man during halothane anaesthesia: effect of hypocarbia. *Anesthesiology* **25**: 180–184.

19

Post-natal Management

LURLENE LIVINGSTONE

Immediately post-delivery, the woman is kept in the delivery ward until her vital signs are stable. The mother and baby will then be moved to the maternity unit where the changes of the early puerperium are noted and the role of mothering begins. The team of carers are there to help her to rest and recover her strength under their supervision.

The nursing team comprises an essential group of health professionals associated with the care of the woman. Their post-natal management includes such aspects as:

- regular monitoring of temperature, blood pressure, heart rate;
- assessment of position and consistency of the fundus of the uterus;
- assessment of the perineum (including episiotomy, grazes, etc.) and lochia;
- monitoring condition of the lower limbs, e.g. continuing oedema, redness, varicosities;
- monitoring of bowel function, especially in the presence of episiotomy or tear;
- inspection, care and advice on breast and nipple function. The stay in hospital can give the mother time to establish the baby's feeding routine, have early problems resolved and become aware of her baby's unique needs;
- education of mother in baby care, e.g. bathing, nursing, handling techniques. Group discussions and the viewing of videos help her to learn and gain experience in a relaxed unhurried manner.

The length of stay in hospital is variable. Some mothers who deliver in a hospital are discharged with their baby the same day if their vital signs are stable and baby is well. Others, though well, may stay until they feel competent in handling and caring for their baby, while others may need hospital care for some time.

There is a trend, however, towards early discharge, which appears to be growing rapidly and is principally related to economic factors for both public and private patients. In most units discharge takes place between the second and seventh day, depending on patient request and available follow-up home services.

Objectives of physiotherapy in the post-natal period include:

- assisting the new mother's physical recovery following pregnancy and the birth process, with a safe, effective and enjoyable exercise and relaxation programme;
- addressing any specific individual needs relating to the physical changes in the post-partum period.

The arrival of a new baby is a special event. During pregnancy the prevailing mood is usually one of euphoria associated with excitement and expectation of the coming event. After birth there are mixed emotions accompanied by mood swings – feelings of joy, apprehension, inadequacy and fatigue.

The physical and emotional stresses placed upon the body during pregnancy and labour have been so intense that expecting an immediate reversal to the pre-pregnancy state is unrealistic. In the third stage the placenta has been expelled, placental hormone production ceases and a decrease in the blood levels of oestrogen and progesterone is apparent. The withdrawal of these hormones allows for the phenomenon of involution, which occurs very dramatically now the baby is no longer dependent (see Chapter 10). The puerperium, the 6–8 weeks following delivery, is a very volatile and difficult time for the mother as she also is learning to care for her new infant.

She now has a different body – a new mother's body – and the woman will accept her new self more readily if these changes have been discussed during the ante-natal period. If the concept of a child-bearing year, nine months of pregnancy and at least three months of recovery, is introduced during classes both the woman and her partner will have a clearer picture of the length and intensity of the transition into parenthood, not expecting too much of themselves too soon.

> *When I visited Mary on day three post-natally she was very upset. She sobbed, 'I expected champagne, chocolates and flowers on my baby's arrival but all I have is a sore tail and sore breasts and I'm tired.'*

The immediate aim of the physiotherapist and the attending staff is to help this new mother adjust, both physically and emotionally, to her new role.

If she has a sore 'tail', begin there. Tl
and so help her over the first hurd
tact has been established with the
has been addressed and can now
effective programme to help hei
physical changes which are evolvin

Ideally, physiotherapy advice and assistance should be available as soon as possible following delivery. Unfortunately not all centres provide a physiotherapy service and the current trend of early discharge from hospital makes effective follow-up treatment difficult. Similarly, the practice of distributing exercise pamphlets without physiotherapy supervision does not address the physical and emotional needs of the post-natal woman, or her individual physical problems.

- Some women are not interested in body awareness and an appropriate exercise programme.
- Some women are interested but are overwhelmed with the amount of information they are receiving from carers, family and friends. As well as trying to absorb new information, they are trying to come to terms with caring for a new baby and the adjustment to their 'new self'.
- Some women are highly motivated but require direction on a safe and appropriate exercise programme to cater for the new demands on their body and to fit in with their new lifestyle.
- Some women are not aware of the availability, and benefits

Figure 19.1 Common post-natal 'at risk' areas.

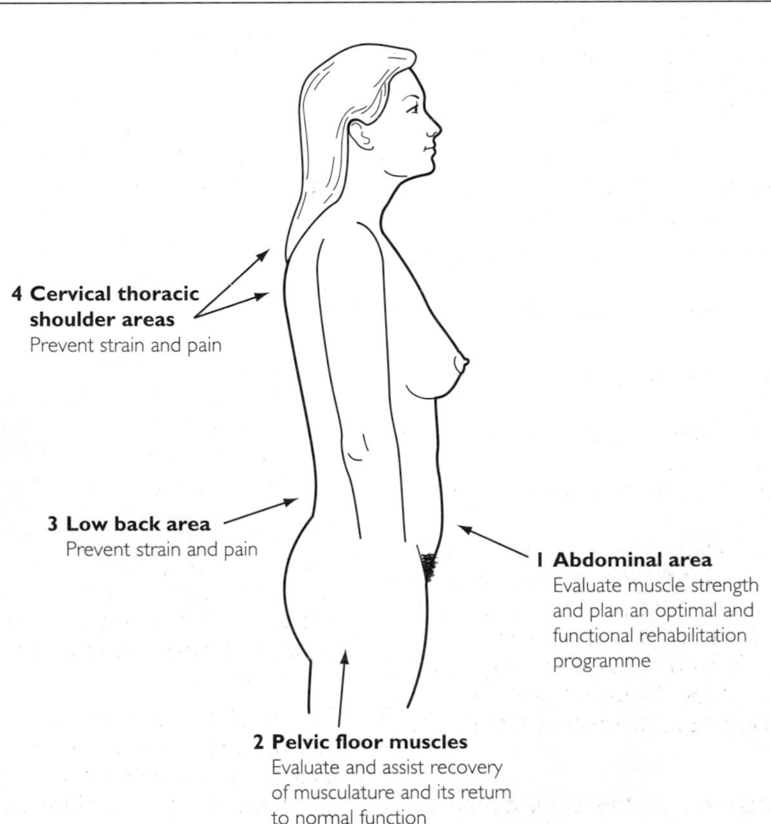

...a physiotherapy service. Information regarding the ...alue and type of post-partum treatments should be provided ante-natally through a variety of sources, e.g. the AN clinics, doctor's rooms, women's health services and AN classes. Physiotherapists must become more active in marketing their services.

- Some women have limited financial resources and are unable to afford the service offered.

It is important that the physiotherapist acts as an educator to increase the woman's body awareness and provide an appropriate exercise programme and as a motivator to explain the importance of this exercise regime to the new mother.

Development of Individual Physiotherapy Treatment Programmes

A treatment programme is formulated after assessing the common post-natal 'at risk' areas and specific post-natal problems.

The following illustrations demonstrate general exercises to include in a programme for the early post-natal woman. The exercises relate to the four 'at risk' areas and should be explained clearly and repeated slowly and frequently to facilitate an awareness of correct performance before progressing to a stronger exercise programme.

Area 1 Abdominals

Figure 19.2 Day 2 post-delivery. Standing, check posture and note weak abdominal muscles.

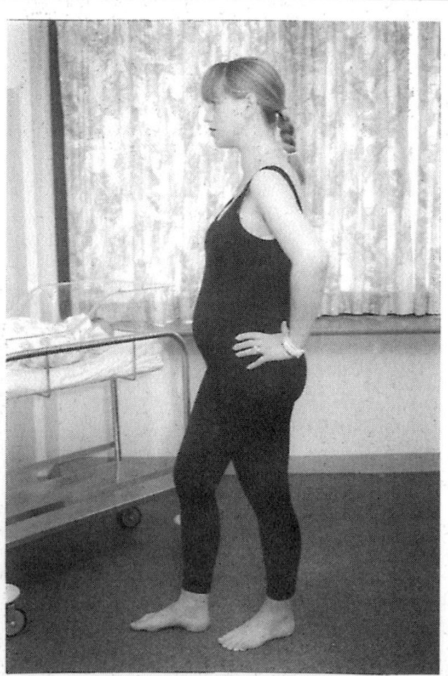

Figure 19.3 Standing. Becoming aware of the ability to contract (draw in) the abdominal muscles – transversus and internal oblique muscles (see Chapter 14 for specific details).

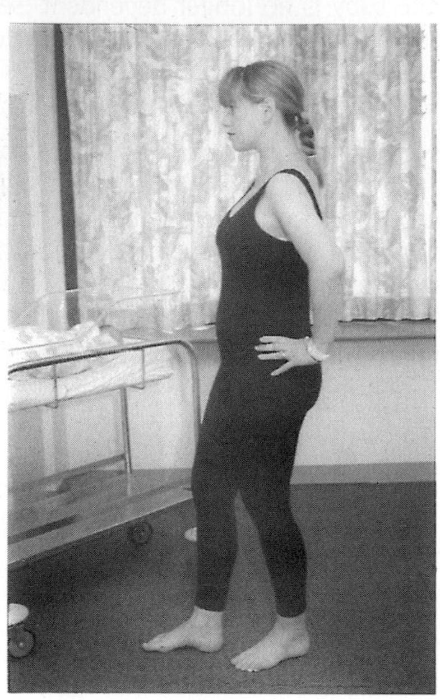

Figure 19.4 Standing. Maintain pelvic and spinal stability while adding movement of the lower limb. The woman must concentrate on performing the movement slowly and in a controlled manner.

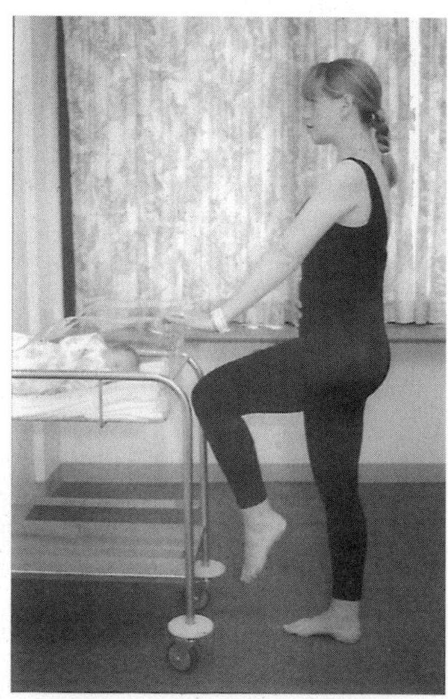

Area 2 Pelvic floor

Figure 19.5 Side lying with gravity eliminated is an effective position to re-establish a pubococcygeal lift. Hand pressure helps mother to localize area.

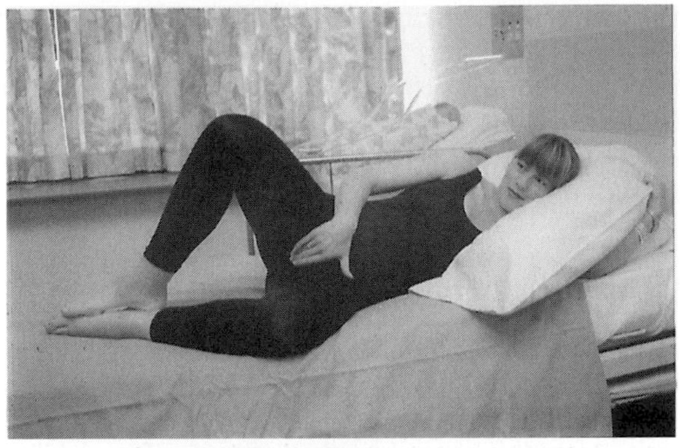

Area 3 Low back pain

Figure 19.6 Mother stands parallel to cot and leans forward with knees slightly bent. She may perform anterior and posterior pelvic rocks which will gently mobilize her lower back.

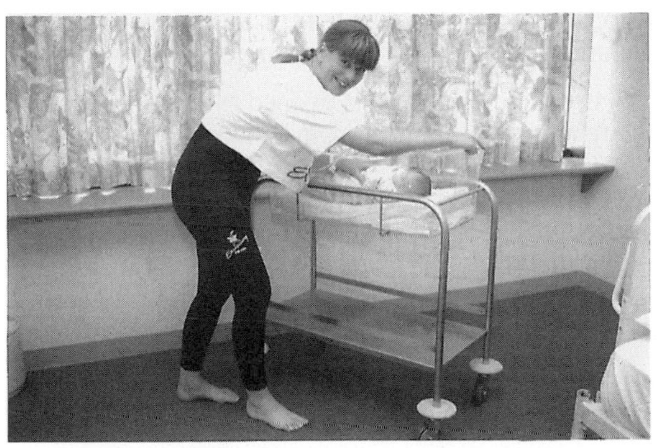

Figure 19.7 Before bending the mother stands close to and parallel to cot. She stabilizes her spine with abdominal control and lowers her body by hip and knee flexion (see Chapter 21 for further details).

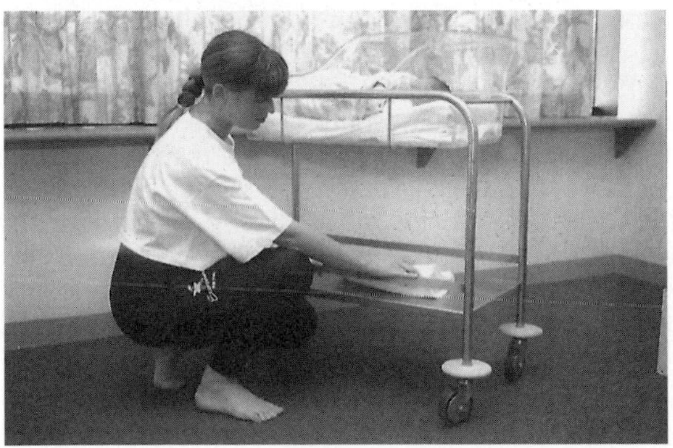

Figure 19.8 Strong quadriceps and good balance are essential for safe bending and lifting.

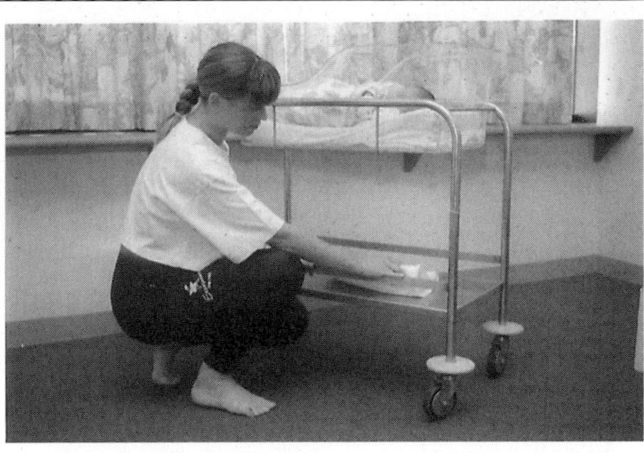

Area 4 Upper back

Figure 19.9 Sitting position with lumbar roll support. After nursing the baby, shoulder rolling and shoulder stretching followed by scapular retraction exercises are encouraged.

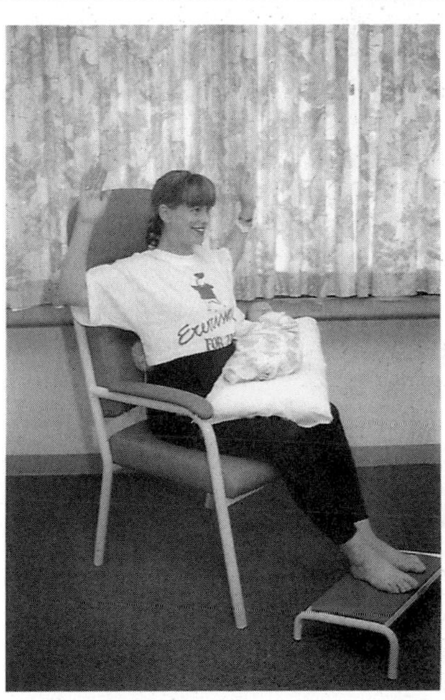

Figure 19.10 Resting in a well-supported position. An important pause in the day.

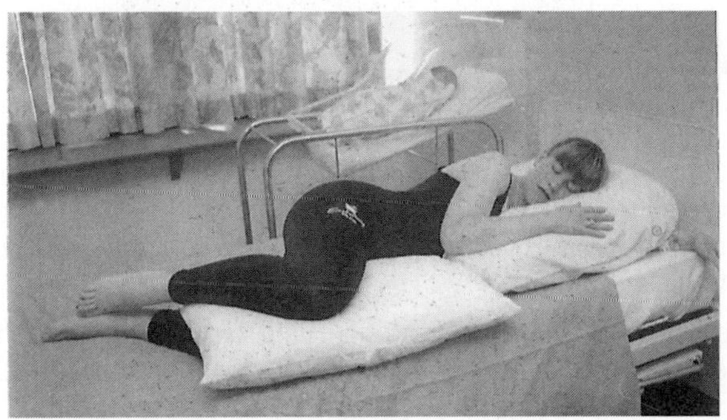

See the appendix on p. 244 for an example of an assessment form and a treatment outline.

Specific Post-natal Problems

Physiotherapy may be required post-natally for a wide range of problems that can present in this period. The following list comprises some of the more common problems for which physiotherapy attention may be beneficial.

1. Pre-existing conditions
2. Post-partum haemorrhage
3. Retained placenta
4. Painful perineum
5. Bladder control:
   urge incontinence
   stress incontinence
   retention of urine
6. Bowel control:
   incontinence
   constipation
7. Circulatory problems:
   varicose veins
   haemorrhoids
   oedema
   superficial vein thrombosis
   deep vein thrombosis
   pulmonary embolus
8. Afterpains
9. Breast engorgement, mastitis, tender and cracked nipples
10. Diastasis of recti abdomini muscles (DRAM)
11. Spinal pain:
    cervical
    thoracic
    low back
    Sacro-iliac joint (SIJ)
    coccyx
    epidural site
12. Pubic symphysis pain
13. Headaches
14. Fatigue
15. Concern for the baby
16. Carpal tunnel syndrome
17. De Quervain's tendonitis
18. Coccydynia

Post-partum haemorrhage (PPH)

Primary PPH is defined as bleeding from the genital tract of 600 ml or more in the first 24 hours following delivery and occurs in 3–5% of vaginal deliveries. Such bleeding usually occurs very unexpectedly due to retained placental tissue or birth canal trauma.

Secondary PPH, bleeding occurring from 24 hours after delivery until the end of the puerperium, occurs in 0.5–1.5% of vaginal deliveries (Beischer and Mackay, 1986).

The introduction of oxytocic drugs in the early 1950s dramatically improved the management of the third stage of labour and, in particular, has greatly diminished the incidence and severity of PPH. In the UK and Australia it has become standard teaching to advocate routine oxytocic drug (ergometrine and syntometrine) administration for managing the third stage of labour. This is usually administered by intramuscular injection (or intravenously (IV) if an infusion is *in situ*) during delivery of the anterior shoulder of the baby or, if it is a breech delivery, after the head has delivered. Following a PPH, the patient may be anaemic, may require a blood transfusion and is often very tired.

Retained placenta

This is described as a placenta still *in utero* one hour after birth of the baby and is a common cause of PPH. Manual removal of the placenta is usually carried out under anaesthesia. After this procedure the patient is often debilitated and, as with a PPH, physiotherapeutic progression of activity must be gradual and tailored to the individual's tolerance level.

Painful perineum

This is a result of trauma during childbirth, due to an episiotomy, a spontaneous tear or a combination of both. Lacerations may be classified in the following way.

1. First-degree laceration is defined as a perineal laceration extending through the vaginal mucosa and perineal skin only.
2. Second degree is one extending into the perineal muscles.
3. Third degree is one involving the external anal sphincter muscle.
4. Fourth degree is one involving the anal sphincter and anal mucosa.

The swelling and bruising which follow an episiotomy and repair or a tear produce a degree of pain. A haematoma may develop if the bleeding is into the tissues rather than externally. This causes very intense perineal pain and usually requires exploration and drainage under anaesthesia. Other causes of perineal pain may include wound breakdown, excessively tight sutures and infection (see Chapter 17). Various modalities have been used to relieve perineal pain post-delivery. They include ice, Epifoam (1% hydrocortisone and 1% local anaesthetic), cold baths, warm baths, saline baths, oral analgesia, ultrasound and pulsed electromagnetic energy. Cold baths are more effective than warm, but are generally unappealing. Warm baths, though initially helpful, tend to increase oedema and sensitivity to pain after treatment. Saline has little effect. Steroids are reported to impair wound healing, so their use appears to be inappropriate. Ice and local analgesics have been shown to be the most helpful (Hamis, 1992).

As with any traumatized tissue, oedema decreases with elevation and movement of the part. No wonder that most women who have experienced trauma to the perineum complain of increasing pain in the first few days after delivery. In most maternity units, if the new mother is medically well, she begins to care for her newborn very soon after delivery and is therefore on her feet for prolonged periods.

PHYSIOTHERAPY MANAGEMENT

1. Elevate the traumatized tissue, i.e. rest in bed frequently.
2. Apply ice to affected site immediately post-delivery for 10–15 minutes and repeat the application at regular intervals (every 2–4 hours for the first 24–36 hours). The most comfortable pack to apply to this difficult area is one which moulds to the part. Soft ice packs of cylindrical shape are ideal.
3. Commence pelvic floor exercises using a contract–relax technique as an efficient pump mechanism to increase circulation and decrease oedema. Exercise is the most efficient physiotherapeutic method of increasing blood flow (McMeeken, 1994). Many women find prone lying and side lying positions comfortable for both exercising and resting.
4. Firm-fitting underpants that hold the sanitary pad in place without movement will prevent 'rubbing' against the wound.
5. Electrotherapy (see Chapter 24).
6. Teach the correct defaecation technique and use of a pressure pad held against the wound during evacuation (see Chapter 30).
7. Use of an appropriate cushion when sitting.

Women often find it difficult to position themselves comfortably, requiring advice on getting into bed using one of these techniques:

- sitting on the side of the bed as if sitting 'side-saddle'; the weight is transmitted through the thigh and is followed by a roll onto the side in a lying position;
- crawling in and out of bed;
- sitting down slowly and carefully using hands to take weight.

Fortunately, there is a liberal blood supply to the area and episiotomy and laceration repairs have usually healed in 5–7 days. A preliminary prospective study (Abraham et al, 1990) looked at the recovery time after childbirth. Abraham found that even though the healing process is rapid, some women continue to experience perineal pain for several months following delivery and can take some months to experience comfort during sexual intercourse. Sleep and Grant (1987) found that perineal pain at three months post-partum was lessened in women who had performed more intensive pelvic floor exercises.

In Hay-Smith and Mantle's (1996) study, post-natal superficial dyspareunia was experienced by 60% of a sample of women following vaginal delivery. Many of them reported that pain had decreased sexual enjoyment, limited frequency of intercourse and prevented orgasm; 20% of the sufferers had not resumed intercourse within three months of delivery.

Bladder and bowel control

Functional problems related to bladder and bowel control are dealt with in Chapters 23, 28, 29 and 30.

Circulatory problems

The development of varicose veins during pregnancy appears to be related to the changes in the maternal blood circulation and the changes induced by the presence of progesterone on the smooth muscle of the venous walls, producing a degree of hypotonia, together with a raised intra-abdominal pressure. Usually these unsightly veins, which are often painful, fade post-delivery, although they may reappear and increase with subsequent pregnancies. If they are severe post-natally, compression stockings are applied before standing and worn during ambulation. Table 19.1 indicates some advice to be given with regard to stocking use.

During feeding the mother may spend long periods sitting so she is encouraged:

- not to sit with legs crossed or knees acutely flexed;
- to elevate legs when lying or sitting;
- to vigorously exercise her calf muscles during this time.

Haemorrhoids may have been present in the ante-natal period as a result of the vascular changes. During second stage the straining causes a ballooning and in some cases, a prolapse of these veins, resulting in excruciating pain in the perianal area. Surgical management may be necessary if the condition is severe. Steroid analgesic creams may ease the pain, as does the application of cold therapy. Unfortunately constipation is common in the early puerperium and straining to move the bowels can increase the risk of further ballooning. Oral analgesics containing codeine tend to increase constipation. Physiotherapy treatment similar to the care of the painful perineum and defaecation retraining should be implemented (see Chapter 30).

Venous thrombosis occurs most commonly in the superficial and deep veins of the lower extremities. Deep leg vein

Table 19.1 Frequent questions associated with compression stockings

Question	Answer
How can I most easily apply the thick compression stockings?	Apply with powdered rough rubber gloves
How frequently are they to be worn?	Before ambulation and throughout the day
Are compression stockings hot to wear?	As they assist the venous return and decrease the oedema, they make the legs feel cooler

thrombi are most likely to develop in the soleal arcade of the calf muscle. These conditions are discussed in the management of caesarean section. The one significant difference between the caesarean section and vaginal delivery patient is the earlier mobilization of the latter. Patient education on movement and positioning is important.

Afterpains

Oxytocin is released from the posterior lobe of the pituitary gland in response to the suckling of the baby. The role of oxytocin is to facilitate uterine contractions and assist with involution. If contractions are strong the patient will complain of abdominal 'cramp-like' pains and/or lower back pain. The pain is usually more intense in multiparae and may be relieved with analgesics, heat and movement.

Feeding difficulties

From clinical experience the most common problem experienced by mothers is the inability to breast feed with ease and comfort. The mother's anxiety can set in motion a circle which compounds the problem as she tries to establish lactation. In many cases mothers are overwhelmed with conflicting advice, not only from the ever-changing staff but also from relatives and friends, on how to position and attach their baby to the breast and even which breast to offer their baby. No wonder some women find those early breast-feeding days totally frustrating and confusing.

Physiotherapists should become more involved with lactation counselling. Their skills of palpation, positioning, relaxation and electrotherapy can all be used to assess and conservatively treat breast and breast-feeding problems. The physiotherapist is frequently asked to treat the conditions of breast engorgement and mastitis. Before treatment, *observe* the mother feeding the infant and this may give you an insight into the initial cause of the problem, why feeding is difficult, how the condition developed and where the solution may lie.

Observe baby

- Position – ventral surface of infant should be facing mother.
- Ability to attach to/suckle breast (Chapter 20).
- Whether wakeful/fussy.

Observe mother

- Position during feeding – note tension areas.
- Position of hand on breast – may be obstructing flow,
- Attitude to breast feeding.

Observe breast

- Size and shape.
- Nipple size and shape.
- Colour of breast.
- Texture of breast – hard/lumpy/soft.
- Over/low supply of milk.
- Milk flow.

You will need to interpret your findings and make a decision regarding the most appropriate treatment (see Chapters 10 and 24).

Diastasis of recti abdomini muscles (DRAM)

DRAM is a condition in which the rectus abdominis muscle separates in the mid-line at the linea alba. The diastasis is defined as a gap between the recti abdomini muscles of greater than 25 mm, palpated just superior to the umbilicus (Noble, 1995). The separation of the linea alba may occur during pregnancy or in the expulsive stage of labour.

Assessment of the DRAM can be performed by the physiotherapist or by a woman previously educated in the technique. The palpation should assess the following details:

1. width and length of any recti separation;
2. region of greatest diastasis;
3. bulge of the abdomen on recti contraction, when evident, and degree;
4. the woman's ability to activate abdominal musculature;
5. the endurance capacity of abdominal musculature.

Figure 19.11 Self-assessment of the extent of the DRAM width and length above and below the umbilicus.

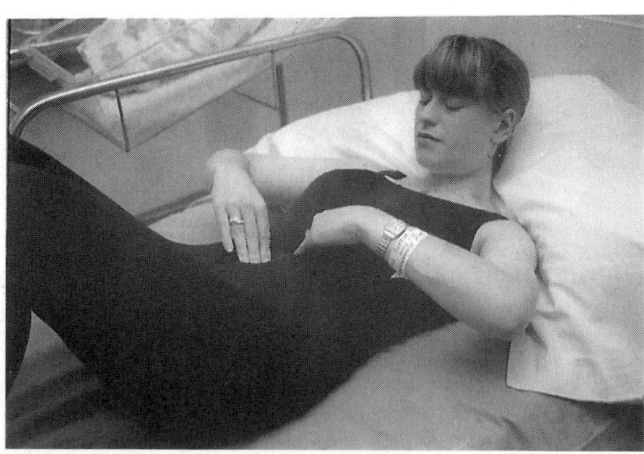

PHYSIOTHERAPY TREATMENT

This depends on the region and degree of the diastasis. The woman should start an exercise programme of hourly isometric abdominal exercises on expiration in all functional positions. Once movement is controlled and the pelvis stable, increase the level of difficulty by the following means:

1. repetition;
2. increase endurance;

3. add limb loading;
4. integrate these exercises into activities of daily living, e.g. sitting, lifting, loading the car.

If the diastasis is large the temporary use of an abdominal support is recommended. The binder is more effective if applied while the patient is supine. The woman is taught to continue to do her exercises within this support which helps to decrease the incidence of pain and discomfort while the recovery of abdominal control takes place. Some women have remarked on how effective the support is in providing them with a constant reminder to 'stand tall and draw the tummy in'.

After discharge the woman should return for a reassessment of the condition when the physiotherapist will monitor her progress, increase the intensity of her exercises and decrease the amount of external support required. For further details relating to abdominal muscle function, refer to Chapter 14.

Back pain

Hormones released in pregnancy lead to ligamentous laxity which affects the biomechanics of the pelvic girdle and the vertebral column. The laxity of these joints may remain for some time after delivery despite the decrease in hormonal levels at birth. It has been recorded that relaxin levels return to normal three days post-partum, but the effects of relaxin have been postulated to take up to three months to return to normal.

Back pain is a very common post-natal complaint. Östgaard and Andersson (1991) studied 817 women with post-partum back pain:

- 67% of the women experienced lower back pain at the time of delivery;
- 37% of the women were still experiencing some back pain 18 months post-delivery. Of these women, 26% were greatly improved, 4% somewhat improved and 7% were still experiencing serious back pain.

Although the pain was most frequently located in the posterior pelvic and lumbar areas, women also complain of both cervical and thoracic pain following delivery and in the immediate post-delivery period. Back pain is therefore a very significant condition and early treatment is recommended to avoid a chronic pain situation. See Chapter 14 for further information.

FREQUENT CAUSES OF POST-NATAL BACK PAIN

1. Altered physiological and biochemical state due to pregnancy. In the nine-month period, prevalence was 49% (Östgaard and Andersson 1990).
2. Trauma during labour and delivery.
3. Lack of postural control and stability during the early post-partum days.

Back pain can also be experienced due to post-delivery uterine contractions. These contractions, caused by the release of oxytocin, occur particularly during breast feeding. Urinary tract infection will also refer pain to this area. Explanation of the condition and the application of heat packs to the abdomen and the back can be of great comfort.

Every woman complaining of back pain should have a complete subjective and objective assessment to determine the exact cause of the pain and to ensure that the correct advice and treatment are dispensed. Using the body chart makes it easier to record your findings.

Subjective examination may include details on pain.

- Location of pain.
- Type of pain.
- Duration of pain.
- Onset of pain.
- What increases pain?
- What relieves pain?
- Which functional movements are resisted?
- Other associated symptoms.

Objective examination may include:

- observation of location of swelling, changes in skin colour, texture, muscle spasm;
- palpation, muscle spasm, wasting and tone, the reproduction of pain, bony abnormalities, skin temperature, joint mobility.

The present pain may be a continuation of back pain in the AN period, especially in sites such as the sacroiliac, lumbosacral and lumbar joints. Continuing treatment for any pre-existing conditions will be necessary (see Chapter 14) and in this period it is possible to expand the electrotherapy options to complement other modalities (see Chapter 24).

SIMPLE TREATMENT RATIONALE

If joint movement is restricted, gentle mobilization and movement is recommended. Weakness of muscles which would support the joint should be strengthened by low load, endurance exercises (minimal joint movement required). Hypermobility, causing discomfort, is best addressed by treatment measures to restrict excessive joint range.

Minimize the fatigue on the spine as much as possible, via advice on lifting and daily activities (see Chapter 21). During sitting, an inflatable cyclinder (Torso, Adelaide, Australia) is an effective back support which eases discomfort and enables active movement.

As with all home programmes in this population, exercise regimes are best related to activities of daily living. If the mother can incorporate activities with the infant then this is also useful (see Chapter 16).

Epidural site pain

Local pain can be present over epidural insertion sites. The mechanism of injury is probably due to the small amount of

Table 19.2 Post-natal spinal pain caused by joint, ligament and muscle strain

Probable cause and site of pain	Treatment of conditions: Posture correction	Suggested exercises	Other treatments/ modalities
Cervical joints 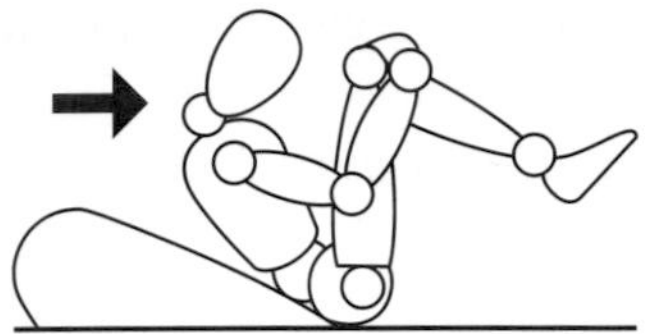 Unsupported stage 2 pushing position 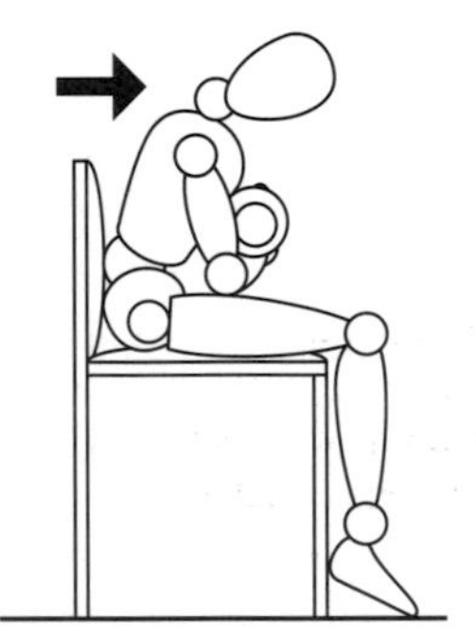 Poor feeding position	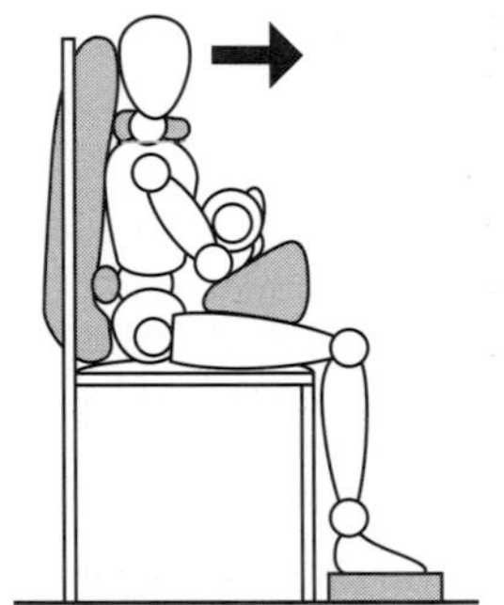	Gentle passive cervical traction. Gentle passive/active cervical movements. During feeding, frequent neck movements interrupt prolonged static holding in flexion rotation. Posture correction, chin retraction, cervical extension	Hot packs US therapy Soft collar during feeding When resting, check pillow and position Ergonomic advice
Thoracic joints 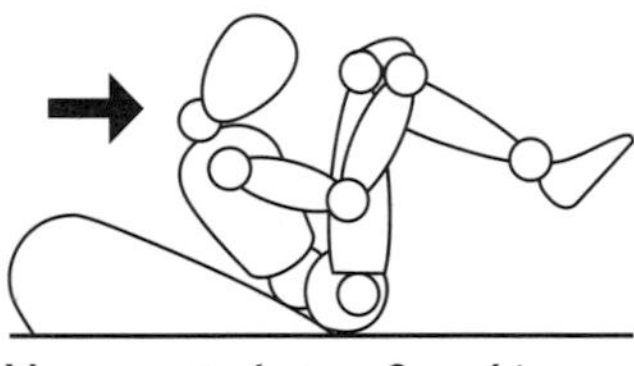 Unsupported stage 2 pushing position 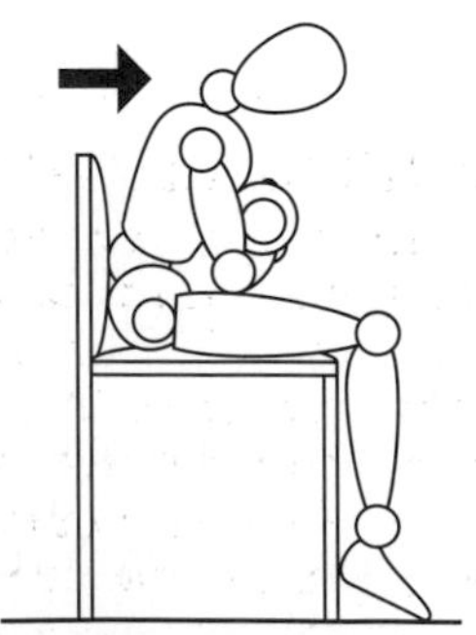 Poor feeding position	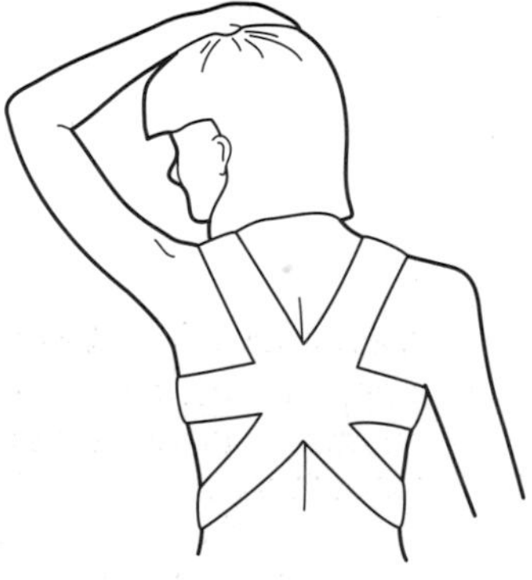	Shoulder and thoracic mobilizing exercises. Scapular retraction	Hot packs US, IF therapy Supportive bra Thoracic brace Ergonomic advice

Table 19.2 Continued

	Treatment of conditions		
Probable cause and site of pain	Posture correction	Suggested exercises	Other treatments/ modalities
Lumbar and lumbosacral joints			
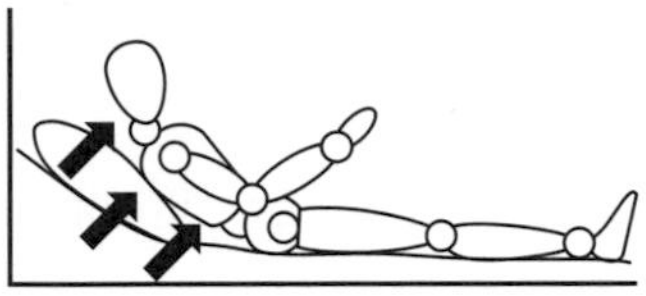 Poor bed position	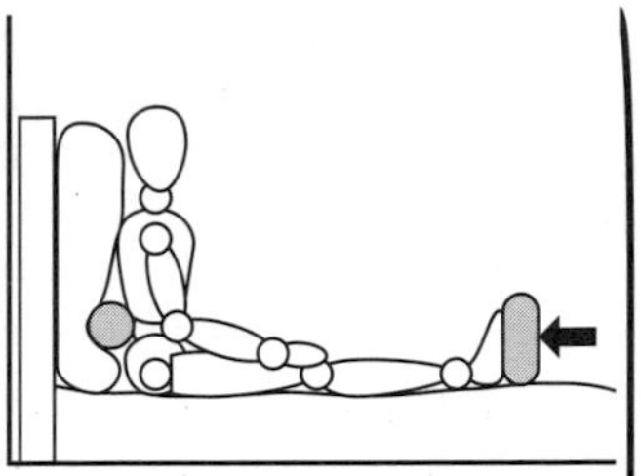		
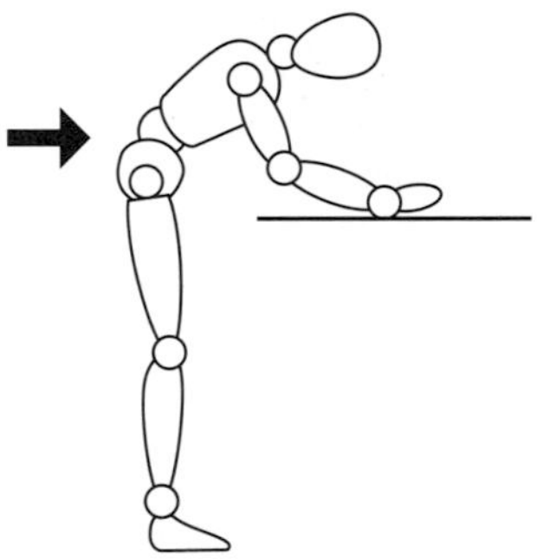 Incorrect working height	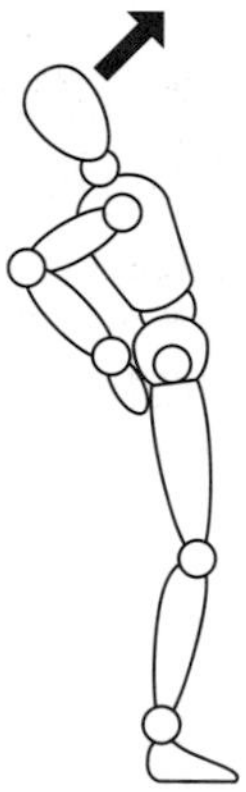	Back mobilizing exercises. Pelvic stability exercises. Corrective exercises after prolonged holding activities. Check posture, lifting during ADL	Hot packs US, IF therapy Lumbar support Ergonomic advice
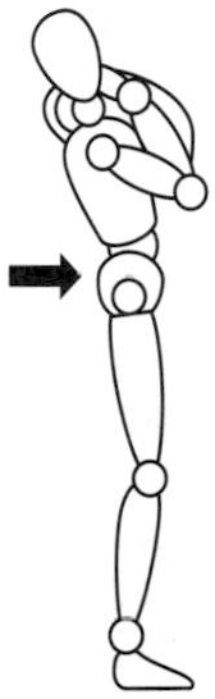 Lower back strain during nursing	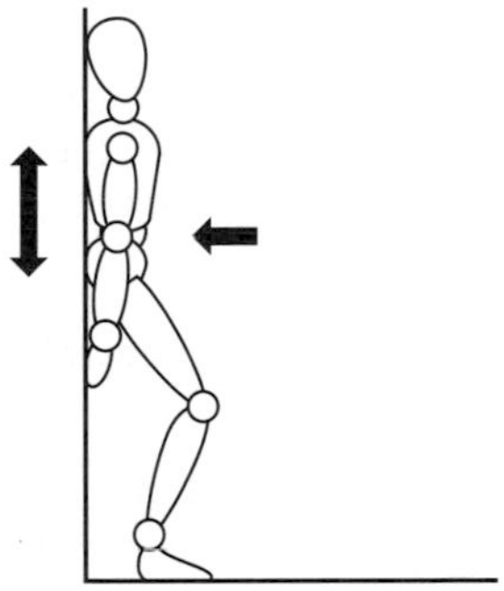		

haematoma present in the supraspinous ligament following the injection into body tissue (Crawford, 1985). The administration of an epidural injection is no different to any other injection into the tissues in this respect and usually settles after a few days.

PHYSIOTHERAPY MANAGEMENT

Aims of treatment are to decrease local swelling and to maintain mobility. This can be achieved by gentle controlled back-mobilizing exercises (e.g. pelvic rock, crook lying/hip rotation), heat/ice packs and electrotherapy including ultrasound and transcutaneous electrical nerve stimulation (TENS).

PERSISTENT BACK PAIN ATTRIBUTED TO EPIDURALS

At present there is no conclusive evidence to suggest that epidural analgesia is a significant cause of persistent back pain. MacArthur et al (1990), after a study of 11 701 women, concluded that the relation between backache and epidural anaesthesia is probably causal. It seems to result from a combination of effective analgesia and stressed posture during labour. They also state that further investigations on the mechanisms causing backache after epidural anaesthesia are required. Breen et al (1994) add to the debate by concluding that epidural anaesthesia for labour and delivery did not appear to be associated with back pain 1–2 months post-partum and suggest that the cause of post-natal back pain is musculoskeletal rather than iatrogenic.

The available data which implicate the administration of epidural as a cause of backache are yet to be substantiated. However, it is clear from the available data that physiotherapists ought to be investigating reasons other than administration of the epidural as a cause of major post-partum backache. It may be that loss of sensation as a result of the epidural curtails normal reactive responses to sustained or extreme musculoskeletal stress.

Physiotherapists may need to assume a more active role in ensuring that the positioning of the labouring woman affected by local anaesthestic is correct and that no strain is placed on her unstable musculoskeletal system. Attending staff should be made aware of this potential problem and, in turn, her partner should also be informed during ante-natal classes of correct handling and passive movement techniques so that he is able to help her into safe positions.

Symphysis pubis

The pubic symphysis (PS) is formed by the two pubic bones and held together by four ligaments: the anterior pubic (the strongest, its fibres forming an interlacing decussant structure), the posterior pubic (weakest), the superior arcuate and the inferior arcuate. The articular surfaces of the PS are covered by a thin layer of hyaline cartilage with an interspersed thick fibrocartilaginous interpubic disc.

The physiological widening associated with pregnancy is usually of small proportion and asymptomatic and it generally resolves within a few months after delivery. A separation of 4–9 mm has been recorded as normal (Abramson et al, 1934). Symptomatic pelvic girdle relaxation is defined as a condition in which pain develops at the sacroiliac joint (SIJ) and/or the pubic symphysis in connection with pregnancy or delivery (Ostergaard et al, 1992). See Chapter 14 for problems associated with the SIJ. Maclennan (1991) suggested that one of the roles of the hormone relaxin in pregnancy is to loosen connective tissue in the pelvic girdle. It is not yet possible to measure relaxin receptors in women exhibiting symptoms related to pelvic girdle relaxation, but high levels of relaxin or a susceptibility to relaxin may contribute to this problem. During pregnancy biomechanical factors may also contribute to the strain placed upon the pelvic joints (Kogstad and Biornstad, 1990).

The obstetrical literature pertaining to this syndrome is limited, merely recognizing its existence and rarity (Lindsey et al, 1988). However, physiotherapists working with pregnant women are aware of the frequency of the condition, usually beginning in the second trimester and becoming progressively more painful as the weight of the heavy gravid uterus is transmitted through the pubic rami. There has been a greater emphasis on these conditions in the 1990s.

SYMPTOMS

- Pain in the area of the symphysis pubis. It can be central, unilateral, radiating down medial thighs and accompanied by low back pain and SIJ pain
- Difficulty with walking or inability to walk.
- Difficulty with certain movements (e.g. rolling over in bed, low squatting movements, getting in/out of a car).

SIGNS

- Pain on palpation of the symphysis.
- Pain on unevenly applied pressure over both anterior superior iliac spines.
- Pain on unilateral weight bearing.
- Locomotion difficulty, waddling gait.
- Tight hip adductors (bi- or unilateral).
- Inability to freely flex hip.
- Pubic diastasis may be present but can be difficult to palpate if pain is severe.

TREATMENT IN THE ANTE-PARTUM PERIOD

Physiotherapy management is aimed at relieving symptoms and increasing patient comfort and, where possible, limitation of further widening.

Movement patterns which do not aggravate the condition include drawing in of the abdomen before movement and moving with thighs adducted if possible. A pillow placed between the thighs often makes rolling over more comfortable. Treatment options for this condition can incorporate:

1. stabilization of the joint or limitation of joint translation:
    - via a trochanter support (it may be difficult to find a comfortable support if the woman is large, as a belt must be firm to stabilize the symphysis) (Fig. 19.12);
    - via an auxiliary support for SIJ stability and abdominal support control if necessary;
    - decreasing the distractive forces associated with muscle shortness by lengthening of tight hip

Figure 19.12 Trochanter belt fitted to stabilize the symphysis pubis.

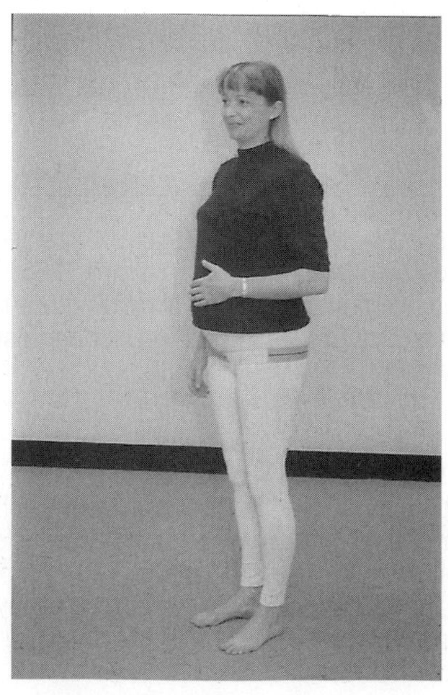

adductors which originate from the pubic rami (a gentle contract–relax technique may be used);

2. pain management:
   - ice therapy: if pain is severe and accompanied by swelling, suggest crook lying with thighs well supported in abduction and apply a soft ice pack for 10–20 minutes;
   - a walking stick or orthopaedic frame for ambulation, if waddling gait and/or pain persists;
   - rest;
3. activities to be avoided include:
   - asymmetrical weight bearing: this should be minimized where possible so modify or cease existing exercise programme if it encourages asymmetrical weight bearing;
   - long strides when walking, walking on uneven surfaces and excessive use of steps.

Consider the following case history of Marian who suffered an injury to the symphysis pubis at 31 weeks gestation.

The injury I sustained to my symphysis pubis joint occurred spontaneously as I twisted and ran from a stationary standing position. The pain and discomfort was immediate and acute. The pain to the area seemed to be exacerbated when getting into and out of a car, wheeling a not very co-operative shopping trolley, walking long distances or activities which required uneven weight distribution, i.e. trying to put on pants, trousers, shoes, etc. while standing up.

Caution

Careful positioning of the woman during labour and delivery is essential if she is unable to monitor her position and movement due to use of regional analgesia for pain relief.

Elective caesarean section may be the delivery of choice if the condition is severe. Symptoms may cease after delivery but in some cases it takes several months for the pain to subside.

Taylor and Sonson (1986), in their retrospective review of symphysial separations during pregnancy, report that the condition is an under-recognized peripartum complication revealing an incidence more frequent than the current literature suggests. Any physiotherapist working with pregnant women would agree. All of their cases (11) occurred following spontaneous non-operative vaginal deliveries and the rapid descent of the presenting part in the second stage was a common feature.

The rupture of the joint during delivery may result in a widening of the gap by more than 1 cm and be associated with considerable complications. The width of the separation does not correlate with the severity of the symptoms. This condition and the diagnosis, confirmed by diagnostic radiology, requires prompt treatment (Fig. 19.13).

Anna delivered a healthy, 8 lb 8 oz boy vaginally and felt a snap during second stage. After delivery, any movement caused excruciating pain and brought tears to her eyes. An X-ray two days post-delivery revealed a disruption of the PS. The physiotherapist had been called in by staff to get this lady moving as she was reluctant to do so – no wonder! Rest and support were required, not ambulation.

Dhar and Anderton (1992) reported two cases of spontaneous rupture of the PS. Both patients were treated conservatively with bed rest, mostly in the lateral decubitus position, within pelvic binders and were asymptomatic after several months. In the author's experience women with severe PS pain find side lying a difficult and painful position and have to be nursed supine. Patients with less pain may find comfort in side lying on the unaffected side, if pain is unilateral.

It is interesting to note that Driessen (1987) described 11 patients with a syndrome of post-partum pelvic arthropathy. All complained of pain located in the PS and were unable to walk and all were symptom free for an interval of 1–2 days after delivery. It is speculated that the symptoms described in these cases were not caused by rupture of the symphysis or softening under the influence of hormones, but by swelling inside the intact fibrous confines of the joint. In view of these findings it appears that not all patients who complain of these symptoms may have either a partial or complete rupture.

TREATMENT IN THE POST-PARTUM PERIOD

Post-partum management must be initiated early to bring about the closure of the symphysis and prevent the

Figure 19.13 Anteroposterior radiography of the pelvis demonstrates gross disruption of the symphysis pubis.

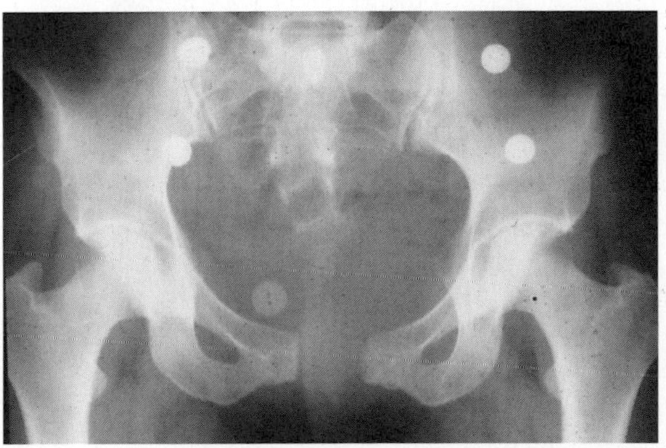

development of a condition of chronic pelvic girdle relaxation and, subsequently, chronic back pain. Early post-partum immobilization is important. The woman has a newborn infant to look after and she is usually very concerned about how she will attend to its needs now and in the immediate future. She is usually very frustrated and distressed and requires the help of supportive staff to care for the baby and help her into a comfortable position for such activities as feeding. As the pain decreases the patient will be able to sit for short periods with the application of the 'Back-Up' support (Fig. 19.14).

Treatments used ante-natally can now be supplemented by other measures.

1. Stabilization of the joint to limit joint translation:
   - trochanter belts or a full pelvic binder are easier to apply;
   - abdominal drawing in is encouraged before movement around the bed. A pillow may be placed between knees to make rolling over more comfortable.
2. Reduction of pain:
   - electrotherapy agents can be used (TENS, low-dosage US or laser) followed by a rest period;
   - orthopaedic aids may be necessary;
   - a re-education board to assist with gravity-eliminated hip movement may be helpful in the early stages of mobilization for the patient who is confined to bed.

Using an alternative form of management, Schwartz et al (1985) treated 13 post-partum women by intrasymphysial injection of a combination of hydrocortisone, chymotrypsin and lignocaine. Immediate relief was obtained in all cases after the first injection and all symptoms disappeared after treatment was completed. Is it the effect of decrease of inflammation by electrotherapy which makes that an effective treatment modality?

Figure 19.14 'Back-Up' support (Nada-Chair, USA) used to maintain the correct sitting posture.

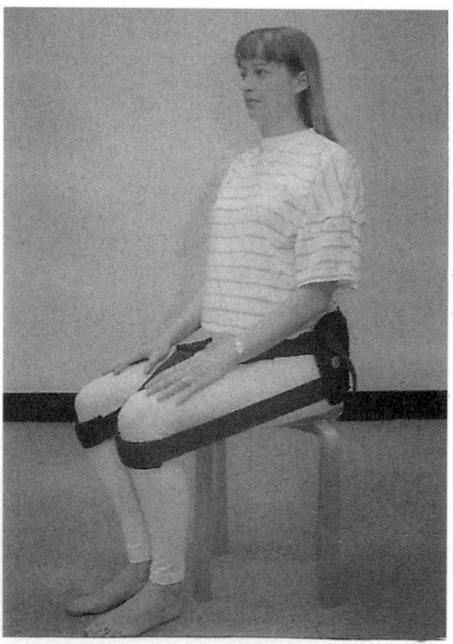

Surgical intervention (i.e. fusing and plating of the PS joint) is a very rare procedure.

There is no indication that the condition progresses with successive pregnancies.

Headaches

SPINAL HEADACHES

The accidental puncture of the dura and the resultant leaking of the cerebrospinal fluid (CSF) into the epidural space can give rise to a severe headache. Symptoms are aggravated by the upright position and relieved when the patient lies down. A mother who experiences a spinal headache is very distressed by this condition, as it has a spontaneous onset and she is unable to respond immediately to her baby's needs. She has to rely on the attending staff for all her baby's and her own personal care. When treating this condition, the physiotherapist must be aware of the patient's despondency and feelings of inadequacy. Assure her the condition is temporary and plan an exercise programme that she can commence in the supine phase. Emphasize just how much she can do in this position, not how little. She may have to remain flat for 48–72 hours.

Physiotherapy treatment goals include:

- decrease the risk of deep venous thrombosis (DVT) and pulmonary complications (PE) due to enforced bed rest;
- show the patient how to facilitate movement around the bed without head raising and position herself and the baby for the feeding;
- keep her physically comfortable;
- commence a muscle-strengthening programme in supine.

The suggested treatment programme includes:

- lower limb movements hourly;
- deep-breathing exercises;
- back-mobilization exercises;
- abdominal drawing-in exercises;
- pelvic floor exercises;
- crook lying, buttock lifts to facilitate movement around the bed.

If the condition is severe or does not resolve spontaneously by 48 hours post-partum, the anaesthetist may inject 10–20 ml of venous blood into the epidural space at the site of the puncture (blood patch). This is the most effective form of treatment (Figure 19.15).

NON-SPECIFIC HEADACHES

These may be described loosely as tension headaches. It is not uncomon for post-partum women to complain of headaches in the first few days. Many new demands, both physical and emotional and within a strange environment, have been placed upon them. Medical investigation may be required if the attacks are frequent, severe and persistent. A neurological consultation may be necessary. If asked to manage this condition, a physiotherapist must be aware of

Figure 19.15 The mechanism of a spinal headache. (Reproduced by permission of P. Brownridge).

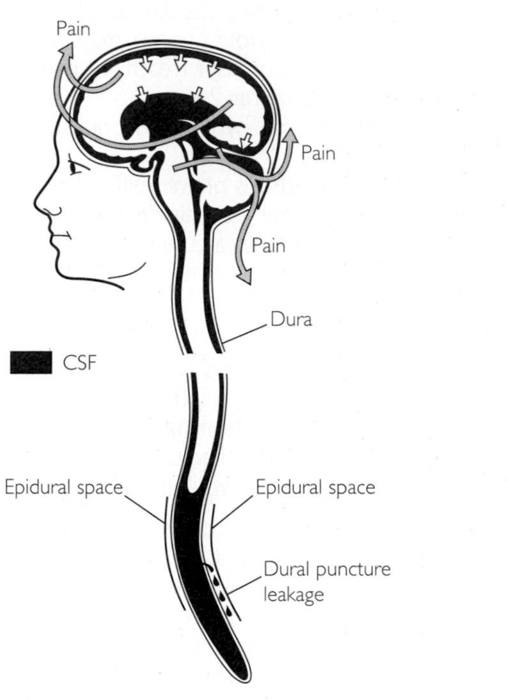

the factors that could be contributing to the condition and not only manage the symptoms as they present. Figure 19.16 indicates some of the more common causes of headache to be considered in the assessment.

Treatment should include management of these basic causes. If the patient has spent the past three days in a small, isolated air-conditioned room, she could be encouraged to take a walk in the garden, have morning tea with another mother or gather with other mothers to discuss the joy and anxiety of parenting.

Specific treatment for the headache could include:

- application of hot or cold packs;
- gentle cervical mobilizing exercises may be combined with gentle, passive, manual cervical traction;
- upper trapezius and cervical massage;
- relaxation instructions.

Maternal fatigue

The demands on an inexperienced mother are many and give rise to nervous tension and fatigue. Labour and delivery can also be an exhausting experience, draining the patient of all her strength, both physically and emotionally, and leaving her with little reserve to respond to her baby. Alternatively, some mothers are overzealous in their concern for the baby's well-being, leaving little time to think of or care for

Figure 19.16 Factors contributing to tension headaches.

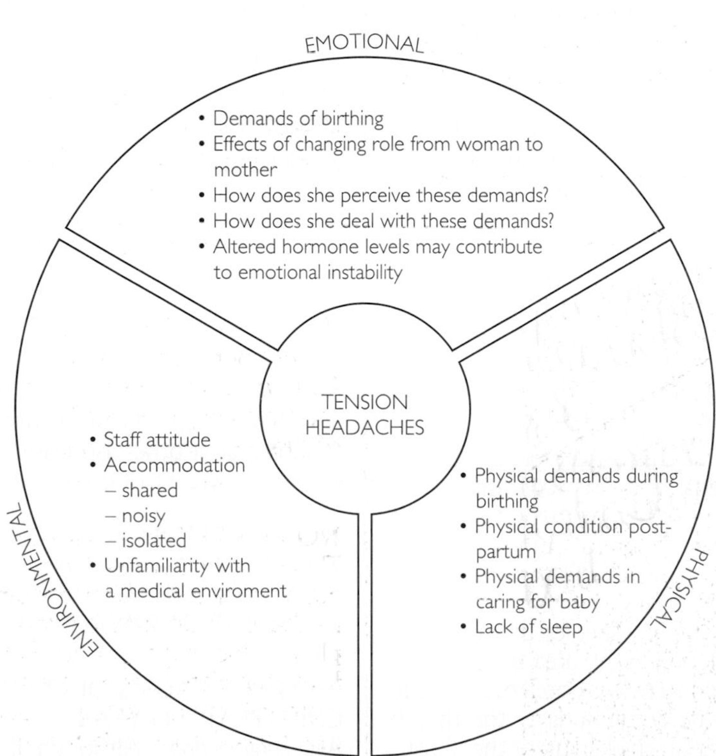

themselves. Relaxation and mother massage sessions may help to alleviate the tension, resulting in a refreshed patient.

Concern for the Baby

The health needs of the newborn baby must be taken into consideration when treating the mother. The mother may be preoccupied and unable to absorb direction if the baby is upset. Her attention span and concentration could be diminished if her baby is unwell. Ensure you are aware of the baby's condition before treating the mother. For example, taking a woman who has had a caesarean section for a walk to the special care nursery to visit her baby may be the appropriate treatment. During the walk, advice and practice related to posture, gait and abdominal support are relevant.

Carpal tunnel syndrome

Rarely do post-partum women develop carpal tunnel syndrome (CTS). Those complaining of the condition in the early days post-delivery have usually been troubled by it during pregnancy as a result of fluid retention and oedema.

The woman should continue her previous management, i.e.:

1. refrain from sleeping on the affected side if the condition is unilateral and elevate the part if possible;
2. wear a night splint to maintain a neutral position of the wrist;
3. exercise the wrist and hand after a period of rest to increase the circulation and reduce oedema;
4. use ice therapy to decrease the oedema;
5. massage;
6. electrotherapy.

If symptoms of tingling, numbness and pain persist, they can make it very difficult for the mother to perform even simple tasks such as fastening a nappy for her newborn. Performing any fine movement becomes difficult. Hydrocortisone injected into the retinaculum is often effective in relieving these frustrating symptoms. Surgical intervention to relieve the pressure on the median nerve is the treatment of choice if the condition persists.

De Quervain's tendonitis

In the author's opinion, the painful wrist condition most frequently seen in the late post-partum period after the mother has been caring for her baby for some time is De Quervain's tendonitis. This is characterized by pain over the styloid process of the radius. Certain recurrent movements of the wrist, for example wringing nappies or carrying a baby, may cause excessive friction in this area and resultant pain. On examination, local tenderness is noted over the site where the extensor and abductor tendons of the thumb cross the radial styloid process. If thickening of the fibrous sheaths has occurred, a nodule may be palpated.

TREATMENT

- Resting of the wrist is advised, but when caring for a baby this is difficult and impractical.
- The use of a splint during the day to minimize movement and friction at the styloid process may be effective.
- Electrotherapy and/or laser treatment may give symptomatic relief (see Chapter 24)
- A local injection of hydrocortisone sometimes gives relief.
- If conservative methods prove ineffective and the condition is severe, surgery to divide the offending tendon sheaths usually provides a cure.

Coccydynia

Coccydynia is the term used to describe a painful coccyx and neighbouring sacral area. Little has been written about it in association with child bearing but physiotherapists are often aware of it, and are called upon to treat it in the post-partum period and even several months later.

The coccyx is loosely articulated with the lower border of the sacrum via a fibrocartilaginous disc supported by the lateral, ventral and the dorsal sacrococcygeal ligaments. This laxity allows the coccyx to move backwards as parturition takes place. The mobility is said to increase during pregnancy, unless the joint is ankylosed due to a previous condition. The coccyx is described as having four segments and the fourth segment is called the 'tip' or the 'apex'. Similarly, these coccygeal joints show variation and ossify with advancing years. Four types of configuration of the coccyx were identified by Postacchini and Massobrio (1983). They found that most of their subjects (68%) had a type 1 configuration. Key (1937) reported that he found no two coccyges were alike in position or form and the gross form or position of the coccyx had nothing to do with the syndrome of coccydynia.

As clinicians, physiotherapists must therefore be careful not to attribute current symptoms and signs to any seemingly unusual configuration of the coccyx in the absence of any prior radiographic comparison. Figure 19.17 illustrates a range of normal presentations of the coccyx.

Thiele (1963) made some interesting observations after studying the case records of 324 patients complaining of coccydynia, 275 women and 49 men.

- Eighty percent of cases were caused by poor sitting or by anorectal or other associated infection.
- Twenty percent of cases were caused by direct trauma.

He also found that coccydynia was more frequent in women than in men (5 : 1) and commented that, '. . . except in patients with coccydynia of acute traumatic origin, pressure on the tip of the coccyx is not painful'.

PROBABLE CAUSES OF COCCYDYNIA DURING THE CHILD-BEARING YEAR

Ante-natal period Although it is often stated that the condition is rare during this period, clinical experience

Figure 19.17 Four types of coccyx structure.

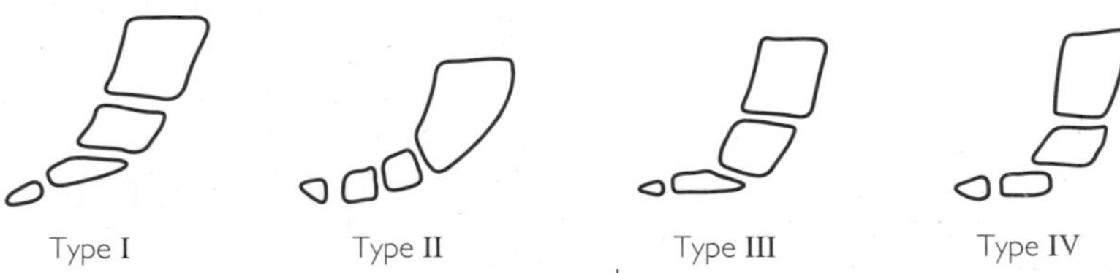

contradicts this. In fact, many pregnant women complain of discomfort as early as the first trimester. It has been suggested that the hormonal changes of pregnancy, together with the ligamentous traction on the coccyx, cause strain and resultant pain. As early as the mid 1800s it was recorded that when the coccyx or coccygeal joints have been injured or when the surrounding structures are the site of inflammation, any contraction of the muscles connected with the coccyx would excite the characteristic pain of coccydynia.

Nowadays many women have jobs which require prolonged sitting, e.g.: computer operators, and many stay at work during most of their pregnancy. These women will benefit from treatment, which can include:

- lower back examination and assessment. Coccygeal pain may be referred from the lumbar region;
- advice on sitting positions – see post-natal advice;
- cessation of heavy lifting;
- frequent pause activities in standing;
- ice/heat packs;
- TENS.

Pain can often be related to a previous injury or an acute injury during the pregnancy.

The post-natal period The passage of the foetus through the birth canal can cause acute trauma to the region. This can be further aggravated by forceps delivery. Types of problems include:

- stretching and/or rupture of the supporting ligaments, with or without posterior displacement of the coccyx;
- fracture of the ankylosed sacrococcygeal joint, with or without displacement of the coccyx;
- exacerbation of a previous coccygeal injury;
- soft tissue damage, including neuritis of the coccygeal plexus.

It is not unusual for a mother who has had a caesarean section to complain post-natally of pain, as her coccyx has also been subjected to the physiological reaction to pregnancy and her resting posture is often less than perfect.

CLINICAL FINDINGS

Subjectively, the patient complains of tailbone pain on:

- sitting;
- arising from chair after prolonged sitting;
- changing position, particularly getting in and out of bed;
- standing, walking and forward flexion movements;
- defaecation and coughing;
- feeding both herself and her baby.

Objectively, the patient sits down slowly and carefully, often shifting her weight from one buttock to the other. Usually the sitting posture is poor, with a slumped position, and the mother may just stand, being too frightened to try and sit down. Pain is increased on palpation over the sacrococcygeal or coccygeal joint sites.

Figure 19.18 Coccyx wedge pillow allows weight transmission through thighs with no direct pressure on coccyx.

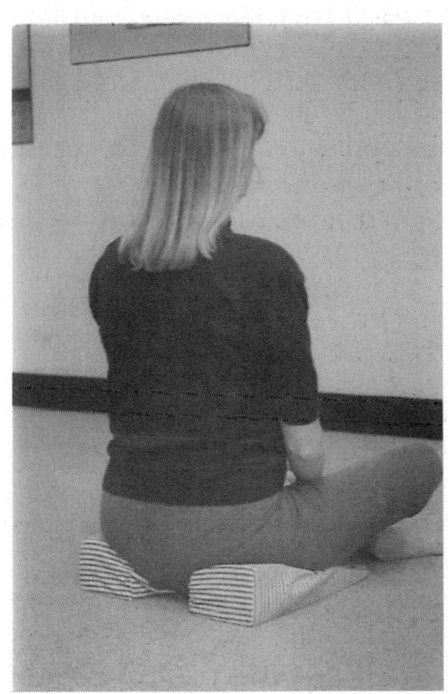

TREATMENT

Differential diagnosis is important before treatment commences. Women are frequently nursed in a 'propped' hospital bed position. Review this situation immediately and place the bed flat. The patient should sit erect, maintaining the normal concavity of the lumbosacral spine with the body weight being transmitted through the ischial tuberosities. The use of a coccygeal cushion (a ring cushion does not relieve coccygeal pressure) (Fig. 19.18) and a lumbar roll helps the woman maintain this position for prolonged periods, for example when feeding baby or entertaining visitors in hospital. Sitting in the acute phase may need to be discouraged. Caldwell (1951) states, '. . . that the severity of pain is in direct proportion to the amount of time spent sitting'.

Management includes the following modalities

1. Demonstrate techniques for getting in and out of bed:
   - side sitting with weight transferred through thighs to side lying;
   - crawling in and out of bed.
2. Demonstrate comfortable positions for resting:
   - side lying (this is also a good position for feeding);
   - prone lying is also a good position to perform gluteal and pelvic floor exercises and for the application of ice and electrotherapy treatments.
3. Ice or hot packs. Ice is usually more appropriate, as this condition is usually associated with pain and trauma of the perineum.
4. Laser, US and TENS applications are all useful.
5. Pelvic floor exercises may decrease symptoms. Discontinue if symptoms increase.
6. Advice on bowel habits, particularly prevention of constipation.
7. Avoid forward flexion movements and lifting.

However, this condition is difficult to treat and often takes a long time to resolve. It is not uncommon for women to return some months after delivery, complaining of a painful tailbone.

Questions such as the following may indicate the direction of management.

1. Are you feeding the child in a different chair now? Maybe her confidence as a nursing mother has taken her from the nursing chair to the TV lounge.
2. Have you returned to a sedentary work situation where the coccyx is continually abused?
3. Have you finished breast feeding and has your period recommenced?

Thiele (1963) suggests that, almost without exception, women complain that all coccydynia symptoms are greatly increased just before and during the menstrual period.

Always be aware that there may be some other non-pregnancy-related cause for this condition which will require further medical investigation.

Follow-up Care, Physiotherapy Plus

In the first few weeks after discharge from hospital, the new family can feel most vulnerable. The physical and emotional demands placed upon the parents at this time are enormous. The mother, the primary health carer in the family, is often experiencing overwhelming tiredness. Her partner may be at work and she may feel isolated and unhappy. It is little wonder that a new mother learning to care for her unpredictable and demanding infant has little time to care for herself, that is, to gain rest and restoration.

There is no doubt that the combination of fatigue and poor physical strength can give rise to her lack of feeling of control, a sense of failure and low self-worth. She certainly needs support and stamina during this busy time.

Where is her support to come from?

Physiotherapists have the ideal opportunity to provide an environment to encourage both rest and restoration through contact with the new mother after birth. She needs support, she needs to communicate, and she needs to have realistic expectations of her new role. She also needs physical activities to increase strength, decrease fatigue, increase emotional well-being and decrease aches and pains. These can help her adjust most positively to this new role.

Physiotherapists can provide information about activities the mother can access after discharge, motivate her and discuss with her and the family the value of joining in activities and have the ability to assess, plan and implement a safe and effective exercise programme. This leads to a physical awareness which recognizes the value of exercise and could lead to a lifetime commitment to physical care.

Group activities help the new mother keep 'in contact', increasing her physical and emotional well-being. Mothers can be introduced to the group circle via different activities and encouraged to move around the circle sharing their experiences. For example, a mother who feels uncomfortable about exercise may enter the circle via the baby massage class, start to feel more comfortable, then move to the mother / baby exercise class, PN exercise class or Exercises for Life. A pattern has been established to promote a healthy lifestyle.

Heather and her baby, Mack, attended the baby massage class. Throughout the session Mack cried constantly. Heather looked worn out. She was upset and embarrassed. She said Mack had been crying continually, refusing the breast and did not appear to be putting on weight. She did not want to trouble her paediatrician, as her next appointment with him was two weeks away. The physiotherapist suggested she see her paediatrician immediately. An appointment was made, the paediatrician was visited and a diagnosis made: Mack had oral thrush. Appropriate medication was given and the problem solved.

Group classes give mothers the opportunity to share their experiences with other women. They may need to talk of:

- their birthing experience;
- their coping ability or inability;
- their feelings of fatigue, joy and frustration;
- their concern about their body shape;
- how they are establishing their new lifestyle.

Figure 19.19 The contact circle.

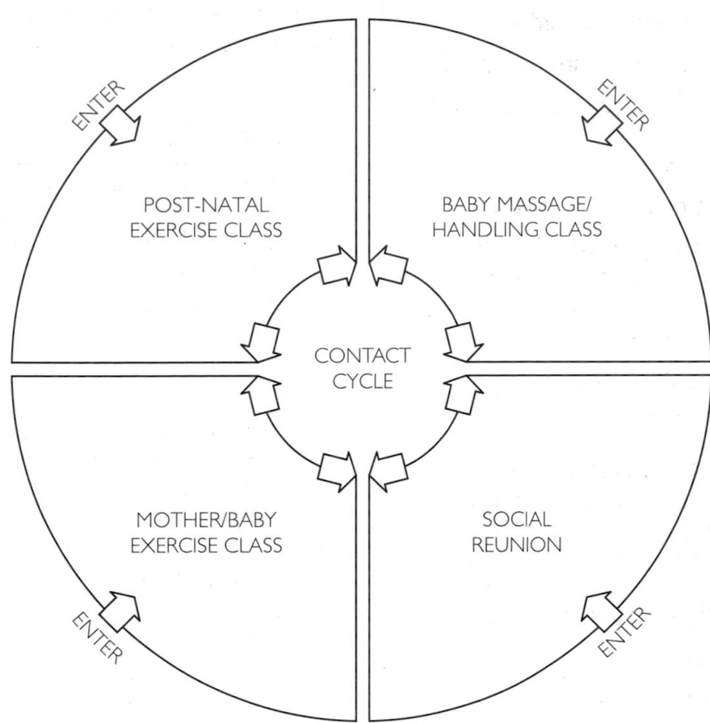

These classes provide an opportunity for the physiotherapist to discuss specific problems, reinforce correct posture/lifting techniques during activities of daily living, identify associated problems of mother and baby and refer mothers to the appropriate help organizations.

Caesarean Section

It has been said that a woman does not become pregnant in order to have a vaginal delivery but to bear a healthy child.

Caesarean section (CS) is the surgical technique whereby the foetus is delivered through incisions in the uterus and the abdomen. The surgical approach is usually made transversely through the lower uterine segment (lower segment caesarean section – LSCS). Rarely, a vertical incision is made in the upper body of the uterus (classic caesarean section). For further reading see Beischer and Mackay (1986).

The CS rate varies between countries, cities and hospitals. The increase in CS rate which has occurred in most centres over the last three decades is a result of the increasing safety of the operation and a desire for optimum outcome for mother and baby, although the maternal mortality rate is increased with CS. These deaths generally result from surgery-related complications. Improved quality of infant survival is difficult to document. Infant perinatal mortality figures (24 in 1000) do not truly reflect CS outcome, as more at-risk foetuses (from prematurity, APH, severe pre-eclampsia, etc.) are contributing to the increased CS rate (Beischer and Mackay, 1986).

Much concern has been expressed about the rising CS rate. In 1989, the CS rate in the USA had reached nearly one in five deliveries (Taffel et al, 1991). This figure was not significantly different from those for the years of 1986–1988, which seems to suggest that the rate may have peaked. In fact, Taffel et al offer some evidence that the rate may have begun to fall by showing a significant increase in the percentage of vaginal births after a previous CS for a non-recurrent condition. However, there is some evidence from other sources that in some specific groups of patients, for example those who have experienced a prolonged period of infertility and those who are on IVF or GIFT programmes, the rate is increasing. Venn and Lumley (1993) quote a CS rate of 41% for such patients, more than double the rate of 16% in the rest of the studied population.

CS may be performed as a planned procedure (elective) or an emergency procedure prior to or during labour. If it is an elective procedure the patient may be admitted to hospital the day or a few hours before the scheduled time for her pre-operative preparation.

An anaesthetist examines the patient and discusses the types of anaesthesia available and appropriate for her. The patient is then able to make an informed decision on the preferred method of anaesthesia.

The nursing staff offer patient preparation in the following way.

1. Familiarization with ward layout and the various facilities available.
2. Recording of a concise obstetric and relevant medical history and baseline observations on the mother and foetus, e.g. temperature, blood pressure, foetal heart rate, position of foetus, etc.
3. Explanation of the pre-operative preparation, including antisepsis of the operation site, shave (if any), insertion of IDC if indicated, period of starvation and administration of the anaesthetic medication, e.g. antacids.

CS are performed using general anaesthesia or regional anaesthesia, i.e. spinal or epidural. Regional anaesthesia is increasingly used for CS as it allows the mother to be aware of the birth of her infant. In some centres the partner is encouraged to be present during such a procedure, providing psychological support and helping to decrease the feelings of anxiety which may be present in the strange environment of the operating theatre. He shares with her the first precious moments of the baby's birth and is there to offer support should the outcome be less than perfect.

Immediately post-operatively the patient remains in a recovery area. Observations are made of her level of consciousness, blood pressure, heart rate, respiration and vaginal loss. Once these are stable and satisfactory pain relief has been established, the patient is returned to the ward, where ward nursing care will include regular assessment of:

- temperature;
- blood pressure, heart rate and colour;
- uterine position and consistency (i.e. firm or soft);
- lochia;
- wound appearance, bleeding, ooze, function of drains;
- bladder function and urine output;
- oral fluid intake;
- effectiveness of analgesia, the need for antiemetics and the maintenance of IV therapy and administration of medications.

Physiotherapy management

PRE-OPERATIVE MANAGEMENT

Pre-operative physiotherapy for all elective CS should be the physiotherapist's goal.

Prior to surgery the mother is pain free and alert and therefore has time to prepare emotionally and physically for her delivery and the post-operative period. Involving her partner at this time may help him overcome any fear of the surgical delivery of their baby and give him the confidence to assist his partner with her early mobilization.

Therefore the following aspects should be covered.

- Discussions to minimize or eliminate negative feelings about this method of delivery and fears about the surgical procedure and the post-operative period. A positive approach is necessary. Videos and/or pictures of a CS may be helpful in this process to illustrate to the patient the unfamiliar surroundings of an operating theatre, how she will be positioned (e.g. in a lateral tilt position on the operating table to avoid supine hypotensive effects) and the position of the screen to obstruct her view of the operation site. Videos and pictures should be used with discretion as some patients are fearful of seeing an operation and would prefer only to view the procedure from their perspective and not that of the surgeon.
- Medical conditions such as respiratory problems may require attention by the physiotherapist prior to surgery. Patients with a history of previous or current circulatory problems should be advised on the post-operative use of antithromboembolic stockings by the obstetrician or physiotherapist.
- Mobilization techniques. At this time the physiotherapist should also demonstrate to the patient how she can mobilize early with the minimum amount of strain and pain. Early mobilization may help to prevent post-operative complications (e.g. deep venous thrombosis and pulmonary complications). In the early post-operative period, almost any movement will increase the pain from the wound, but certain movements reduce strain on the wound and allow more comfortable mobility. (see Fig. 19.22).

Abdominal supports are useful to control a floppy abdomen when moving. Discuss the types and benefits of their early post-surgical use.

- Tubigrip – width and size.
- Firm pants.
- Abdominal binders.
- Cycling shorts may also be useful in decreasing

Table 19.3 Main obstetrical indications for caesarean section

Elective caesarean section	Emergency caesarean section
Cephalopelvic disproportion (CPD)	Obstructed labour
Placenta praevia	Foetal and maternal distress
Malpresentation (e.g. unstable lie, breech)	Ante-partum haemorrhage
Previous CS – depending on its indication	Placental abruption
Previous classic incision	Prolapsed cord
Active genital herpes	Failed trial of forceps
Pre-eclampsia and eclampsia	Failed trial of previous CS scar
Multiple births	
Low birth weight	

excessive abdominal movement, resulting in increased patient comfort.

A handout listing useful items to assist the comfort of the woman who has had a CS whilst in the hospital should include:

- short night attire – to allow more freedom of movement;
- safe slip-on footwear – to prevent the unnecessary struggle to fasten footwear and provide security during ambulation;
- small soft pillow to support abdomen when side lying, to prevent the dragging sensation of a swollen abdomen;
- feeding pillow to support baby (e.g. A-frame to prevent pressure of baby on wound site);
- supports for abdomen as previously described above.

POST-OPERATIVE MANAGEMENT

> Precautions, such as the wearing of gloves, should be taken by the physiotherapist for her own protection when handling surgical patients where there is the possibility of contact with body fluids.

Prior to treating the patient a review of her medical history is essential. The following details from the medical chart are relevant.

- The indications for a CS.
- Any relevant previous and current treatments.
- Condition of the baby and mother.

When meeting the patient it is important to observe:

- level of alertness;
- resting posture.

Physiotherapy assessment of the following is essential.

- Degree and sites of pain.
- Patient's mobility.

Only then can an effective treatment plan be formulated.

PHYSIOTHERAPY TREATMENT

A supervised programme within the first 24 hours is advisable and this should be reinforced every two hours by the attending staff.

- Assisted active and active movement of the limbs to help prevent venous stasis, joint stiffness and peripheral oedema.
- Encourage movement around the bed, using crook lying, feet placement, bottom lift techniques (see Fig. 19.21).
- Encourage deep-breathing exercises. Aim to keep the lungs well ventilated to decrease the risk of mucus accumulation and increase the venous return.
- Encourage gentle exercises, such as crook lying/pelvic rock, crook lying/knee rolls from side to side, abdominal contraction on expiration, gluteal contractions and pelvic floor exercises.

Ambulation is the next step in the process of recovery, which often occurs after the removal of the IDC and IVT. The appropriate abdominal support may now be fitted to enhance patient comfort during movement. Demonstrate in and out of bed techniques and in and out of a chair (Figs 19.22–24).

In many hospitals, rooming in of the baby begins very soon after delivery. Mothers have to attend to the needs of their baby and therefore movement techniques must also relate to the functional activities associated with these. It is a difficult procedure to get in and out of a feeding chair whilst nursing a baby. As some mothers have found themselves marooned and unable to move after feeding, always position the feeding chair close to the buzzer so that the patient is able to call for assistance if necessary.

Figure 19.20 Marooned!

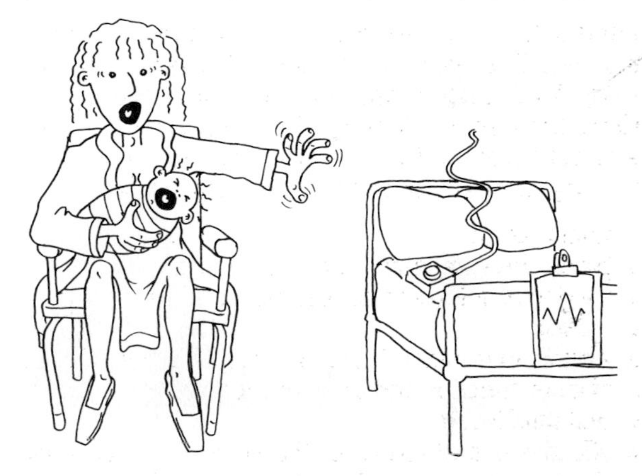

Effective post-operative pain relief which allows the patient to mobilize early can also be responsible for the woman overestimating her capabilities. Once pain relief is decreased or withdrawn, it is not uncommon for the woman to feel she has gone backwards, experiencing fatigue and despondency. She must be reassured that these feelings are normal and aim to progress slowly. Carers must be sensitive to these feelings.

An active exercise programme to strengthen the abdominal muscles is cautiously introduced (refer to the section on abdominal exercises in Chapter 14). The intensity of this programme will depend on the recovery rate of the patient.

Be prepared to answer questions such as:

1. How soon can I drive a car?
2. Can I hang the washing out?
3. When can I return to the gym?

The physiotherapist must be familiar with all the situations encountered in these activities. Involvement in a motor vehicle accident, if driving early post-operation, may compromise insurance, as the subject may be deemed not to have the strength and flexibility for optimum control. Guidelines for return to driving should be defined by the medical adviser.

Ideally, on discharge, a follow-up physiotherapy appointment should be made to monitor the patient's progress and increase the intensity of the original programme. Some centres have established post-natal exercise classes conducted by a physiotherapist to guide the woman through these early weeks and back to her former level of activity. These classes are also useful in providing a forum for the new mothers to gather and share their experience of mothering.

***Julie**: After my first caesarean section I stayed on my feet all day, frightened to get in and out of bed due to the pain. I was exhausted. This method of crawling into bed was so comfortable that I was able to get into bed and rest more frequently (see Fig. 19.23).*

Figure 19.21 Moving around the bed while concentrating on control of the spine and pelvis using 'abdominal drawing in' and 'lift bottom' techniques.

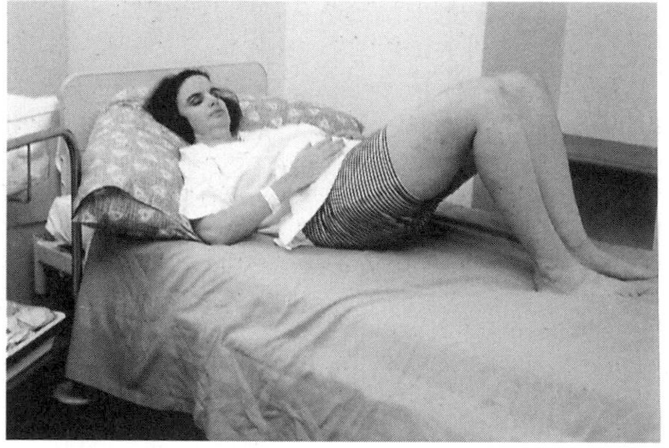

POST-OPERATIVE PROBLEMS

In many ways the post-operative complications are similar to those associated with any other lower abdominal surgery in the female. These include respiratory problems, excessive abdominal pain, wind pain, DVT, PE, back pain and dependent oedema. In addition, the CS patient may experience other problems related specifically to her pregnancy, such as afterpains, problems associated with caring for a new baby, breast problems, fatigue (particularly if CS followed long labour), medical problems associated with indication for CS such as congenital or acquired cardiac disease/asthma/diabetes mellitus, obstetric problems associated with indication for CS (pre-eclampsia) and musculoskeletal problems experienced during pregnancy (e.g. carpal tunnel, sacroiliac joint and pubic symphysis pain).

Respiratory problems The physiological changes in the respiratory system in pregnancy (see Chapter 11) are further affected by the inhibitory effects of pain and immobilization post-caesarean section. These may render the woman more susceptible to respiratory problems.

She may even present for her CS with a pre-existing chest condition. Deep breathing, huffing and effective coughing are encouraged. Deep breathing and coughing are very painful activities after surgery and the weakened abdominal muscles can make the cough ineffective. Help the patient into an upright position with legs over the side of the bed or into a chair with feet firmly supported. Support the abdomen with a towel 'binder' placed over the lower abdomen – the physiotherapist applies traction to the binder during the expulsive effort (Fig. 19.25). A pillow held firmly over the CS site may be used but it is a less effective support. Abdominal and pelvic floor sustained contractions are encouraged during the expulsive effort.

Figure 19.22 (a,b) To stand from supine lying position, bend knees, roll onto side with lower arm well tucked under body. While dropping lower legs over side of bed, push up using arms. Reverse technique to get into bed. To assist patient to stand upright, exercises to relax the body are introduced, e.g. in standing, loosen up with gentle knee bends, shoulder rolls and relaxed breathing.

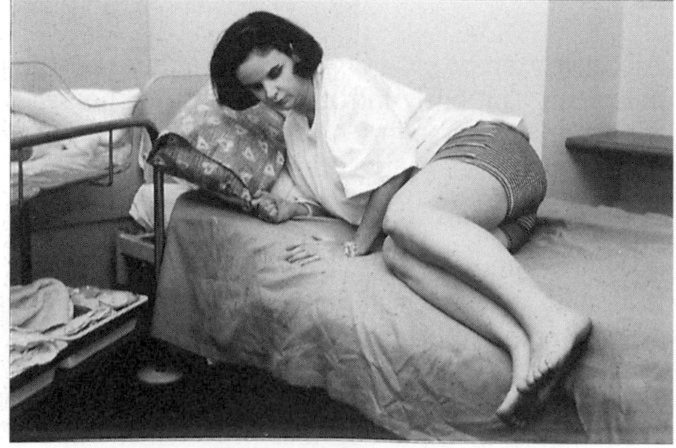

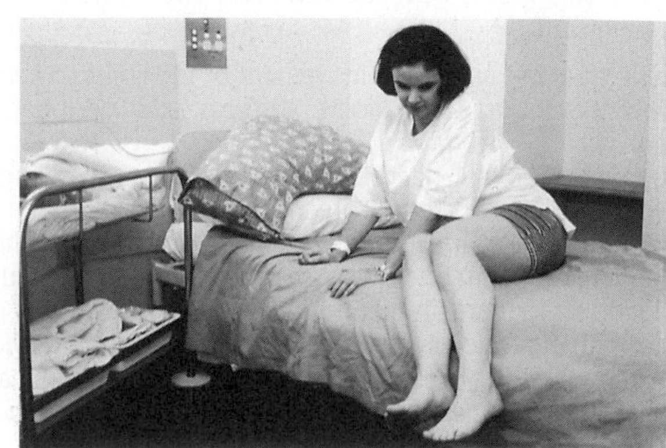

Excessive abdominal pain Most women complain of abdominal wall pain following a CS. Usually the pain resolves spontaneously over a couple of days provided that due care is taken with movements. The following conditions will increase pain at or around the CS site and require special attention.

- *Wound infection.* If the wound becomes infected antibiotics are prescribed. The patient may be febrile, listless and tired. A prophylactic programme to minimize the development of other complications such as stiffness, DVT and pulmonary complications is instigated. The wound must be kept dry and airy and it may be necessary to support a pendulous abdomen with Tubigrip or binder to lift it off the wound.
- *Haematoma* – a bleed into the tissues post-surgically. The degree of discomfort to the patient is proportional to the size of the haematoma. In some circumstances surgical drainage is required. Therapeutic ultrasound may accelerate resolution and increase the patient's comfort.
- *Excessive localized oedema.*
- *Nerve entrapment syndrome.* Occasionally a patient will complain of atypical lower abdominal pain following surgery. The syndrome of ilioinguinal or iliohypogastric nerve entrapment was described as early as 1942 and has been described as a complication of a Pfannenstiel incision (as used in LSCS).

Figure 19.23 Crawling into bed to sit upright.

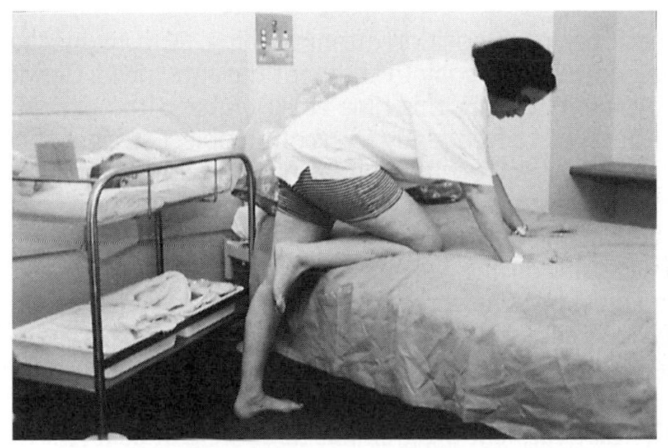

Symptoms include pain in the anatomical distribution of the ilioinguinal nerve (Fig. 19.26), a combination of pain and hyperaesthesia and pain increased with movement. Challis and Bennett (1994) set out the diagnostic criteria for the condition and the surgical management. They reported complete resolution of symptoms in all patients operated on.

The pain may only be due to swelling in the region of the nerve and subsequently resolve with conservative management.

Wind pain Wind pain is experienced by some mothers and described as a severe intermittent colic type pain. The abdomen is usually very distended, painful to touch and may be accompanied by referred shoulder tip pain.

- Deep breathing is often restricted as pain increases with diaphragmatic descent. This activity may need to be encouraged.
- The patient is also encouraged to draw in her abdominal muscles so as to increase intra-abdominal pressure.
- Early ambulation is also helpful.
- Massage in a clockwise direction along the line of the colon appears to help movement of the gas.
- Many patients find the use of heating pads very soothing.

Deep venous thrombosis (DVT) and pulmonary embolism (PE) Venous thrombosis and pulmonary thromboembolism are potentially lethal conditions in pregnancy and the puerperium. Several changes occur during pregnancy which may also expose the patient to this condition in the early post-delivery period. These changes cause hypercoagulability. They are venous stasis, increased levels of clotting factors and decreased fibrinolytic activity. Decreased venous tone and venous flow in the extremities occur during pregnancy, both of which can contribute to venous stasis and increase the

Figure 19.24 **(a)** Getting in and out of a chair. Space feet asymmetrically apart. Contract abdominal and back muscles, lean body forwards, place one hand on support and one on thigh. Press through back foot and both hands and slowly rise. Gradually stand tall after several knee bends. Reverse this technique when lowering to sit. (b) Getting in and out of a chair with the newborn.

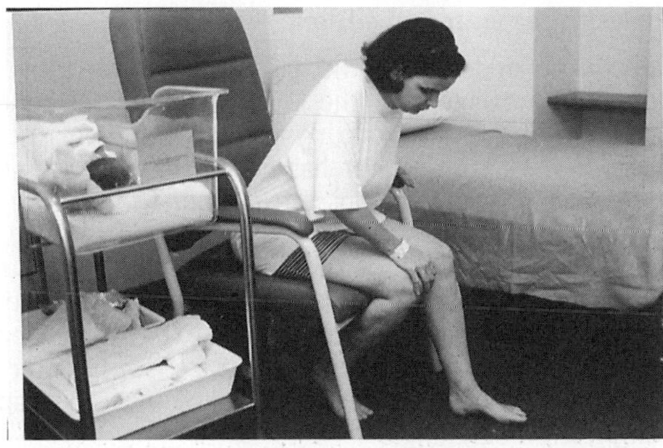

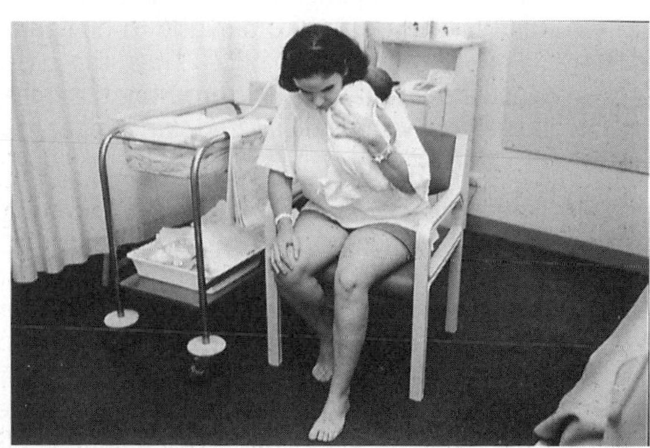

Figure 19.25 Effective supportive coughing position using a towel as a binder. Treatment sessions should be short, handled with sensitivity and only after pain relief has been administered and seen to be effective.

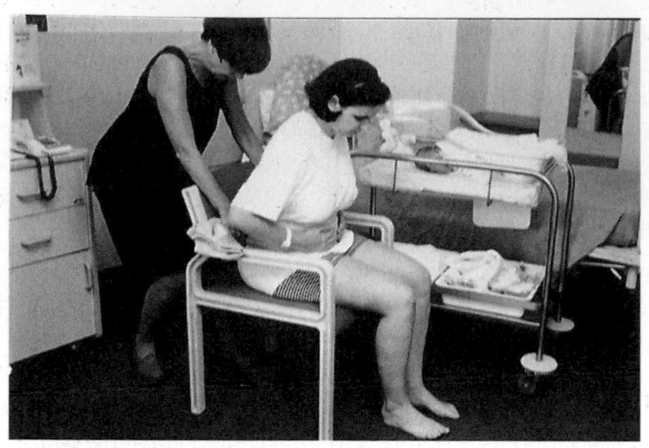

Figure 19.26 Pain in the anatomical distribution of the ilioinguinal nerve.

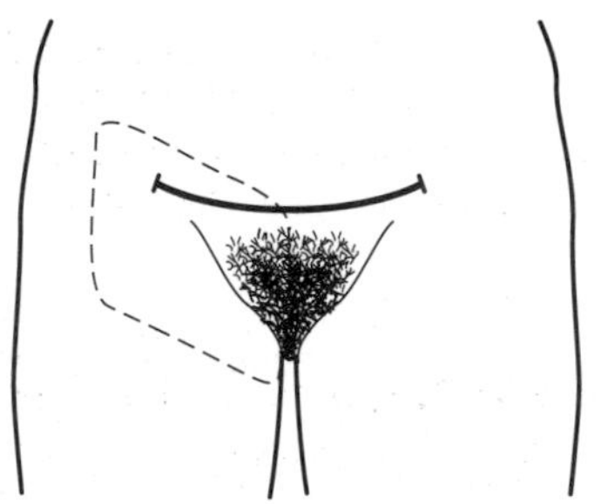

likelihood of venous thrombosis. In addition, venous outflow obstruction may occur during pregnancy as a consequence of obstruction of the inferior vena cava and left iliac vein by the gravid uterus.

Pelvic surgical procedures are among the group of procedures that are associated with the highest incidence of DVT (Gray and Graor, 1992). Symptoms, when they occur, often do not manifest until 4–5 days after surgical treatment. The peak incidence of *symptomatic* pulmonary embolism occurs 7–10 days post-operatively. The practice of early discharge of CS patients now presents a problem with detection of these conditions.

It must also be noted that the signs and symptoms of DVT are absent in about 50% of patients who are later shown to have the condition. They range from subtle to obvious in the other 50% (Gray and Graor, 1992). Thus, the classic signs of an oedematous limb with erythrocyanotic appearance, dilated superficial veins and elevated skin temperature may be absent.

The physiotherapist must be aware of these elusive clinical signs and the difficulty in diagnosing thromboembolic disease after surgery. Become suspicious if the patient complains of pain in the calf of the leg when the foot is dorsiflexed (Homan's sign) or of shortness of breath. The medical staff should be notified. Venography is the most accurate confirmation test. Once diagnosed, anticoagulant therapy is usually commenced, antiembolic stockings fitted and the foot of the bed elevated. Ambulation of the patient depends on the medical management and the physiotherapy aim is to encourage venous blood return with:

- deep breathing exercises;
- all lower limb movement especially dorsi- and plantarflexion and gluteal contractions.

For pregnant women with high-risk profiles, the likelihood of developing DVT post-surgically is significantly reduced by prophylactic anticoagulant therapy prior to delivery.

For all surgical patients prophylaxis of DVT should begin at the time of hospital admission, continuing until the patient is ambulatory. Prevention includes:

- application of compression stockings;
- early mobilization;
- avoidance of pressure under thighs and calves;
- avoidance of sitting with knees acutely flexed;
- encouragement of deep breathing and movement.

Back pain It is not uncommon for the CS patient to complain of back pain in the early post-operative period. Since the surgery, she may have been placed in the half lying or semirecumbent position (Fig. 19.27), moving as little as possible while learning to feed her new baby.

Check her neck position during feeding, as many mothers look down at the baby throughout the entire feed. Cervical movements during this time are useful and the patient is encouraged to frequently focus on an object straight ahead of her. Correct positioning combined with general back mobility exercises and the application of heat is often efficacious. If a patient has a history of back pain, including pelvic pain, during her pregnancy this pre-existing condition must be considered and treated. Pain referred from the pelvic viscera can also present as lower back pain and will subside gradually. Adequate medication for this pain relief is important as this will facilitate the implementation of the physical treatment programme. Be aware that pain-relieving medication which contains codeine will slow gastrointestinal motility and cause constipation.

Dependent oedema Generalized retention of fluid during pregnancy takes some time to resolve following delivery. This is often a surprise for new mothers who expect thin ankles to reappear immediately.

Dependent oedema of the legs is aggravated by the decreased movement of the lower limb muscles and the condition of the veins, occurring often in the presence of varicose veins. The author has noted that the degree of swelling can be unequal in distribution. The swelling will take longer to resolve if the patient has had toxaemia of pregnancy. Vigorous foot and ankle exercises plus gluteal contractions should be carried out every half hour. Lower limbs should be elevated while resting and a partner shown the technique of lymphoedema massage (see Chapter 35) to decrease the discomfort of swelling. If severe, apply compression stockings.

Figure 19.27 Poor resting position – note strain on cervical, thoracic and lumbar area. As soon as practical, encourage patient to sit upright against top end of the bed with a lumbar support.

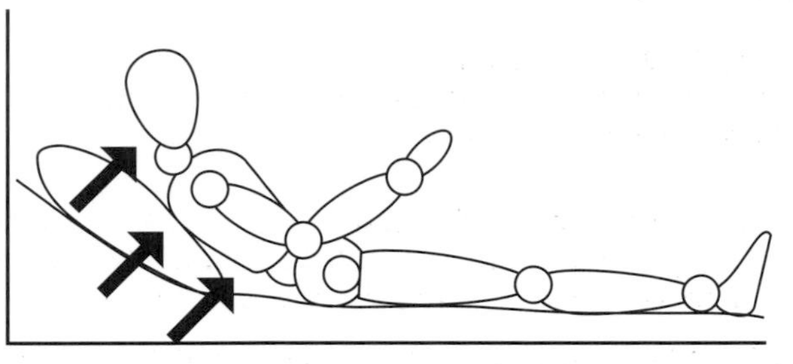

Figure 19.28 Well-supported sitting posture.

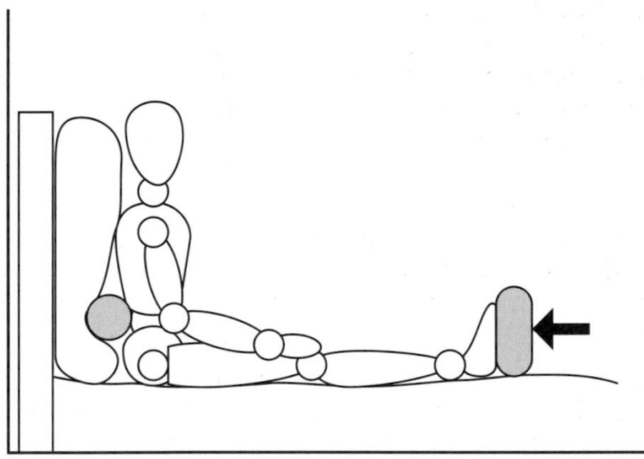

After pains Oxytocic drugs are commonly added to the intravenous infusion to maintain haemostasis for up to 24 hours after surgery and may result in afterpains (i.e. the pain resulting from uterine contractions which are more intense than those after vaginal deliveries).

Gentle physiotherapy exercises, oral analgesics and heat are useful in reducing pain. In severe cases TENS applied over the nerve roots innervating the uterus (T10–L1) may help to reduce the painful cramp-like sensations.

Tiredness Many women experience an overwhelming feeling of tiredness after their surgery. No doubt this is a result of a long and stressful labour before an emergency CS or a high level of anxiety accompanying a pre-existing medical condition (e.g. pre-eclampsia) before an elective CS. A low haemoglobin following excessive blood loss results in a feeling of profound listlessness. Sleep may be difficult due to the strange environment, regular interruptions for feeding and nursing observations, as well as the day-time demands placed upon the mother. One mother counted 20 intrusions during her day, from the early morning tea lady to the cleaners, the paper boy, the photographer, the visitors, the doctors and even the physiotherapist. No wonder she was exhausted by these while learning to care for her new baby with the inconvenience of drips and drains still in place.

The experience of a CS is not only physically but also emotionally draining for most women. The surgery is often unanticipated and though discussion about the likelihood of a CS takes place during the AN preparation classes, couples never think it will happen to them. A woman who has experienced a trouble-free pregnancy and is fit and active often finds it difficult to accept the fact that she has not delivered 'naturally' and is often the most disappointed. She will need time to work through her experience before she can come to terms with this unexpected method of birthing.

Margaret *(mother of James, 4010 g): I felt robbed of my birth experience and very angry with my husband who kept smiling and showing off our baby to the adoring visitors while I was feeling uncomfortable and detached.*

Not all women have a negative reaction to this method of delivery. Those with a positive attitude are often easier to motivate, usually finding it easier to make the transition to motherhood and caring for their dependent baby.

Before treatment, do you know:

1. the patient's attitude to CS?
2. whether it was elective or emergency, if it was preceded by a long labour and if there are any medical problems?
3. if the baby is well or in SCN/ICN?
4. if there is easy access for the mother to those units?
5. what nursing support she has?
6. what family support she has?

A better understanding of the circumstances surrounding her delivery will give a holistic approach to your treatment of this patient.

On discharge, community services are available to all women entering motherhood. Specialized support groups are established in the USA and UK but in some countries the development of these groups is limited. In Australia, the Childbirth Education Association (CEA) distributes pamphlets on request and has a telephone counselling service.

Physiotherapists have an ideal opportunity to contribute to optimum post-natal recovery, with the provision of an appropriate exercise regimen, treatment of specific problems and education for a healthy lifestyle.

Appendix – Example of a Post-natal Assessment and Outline of Treatment

OBSTETRIC RECORD

SURNAME: M.

GIVEN NAMES: L. H. DOB: 13.3.59

DOCTOR: P.D.L.

OBSTETRICAL HISTORY				COMPLICATIONS			GRIVIDA		PARA:
No.	Date	Type of Delivery	Gest'n	Pregnancy	Labour	Puerperium	Sex	Birth Weight	Foetal Outcome Method of Feeding
1.									
2.									
3.									

RELEVANT MEDICAL HISTORY: (Illnesses, Operations) NIL

ANTENATAL COMPLICATIONS THIS PREGNANCY: NIL

DELIVERY SUMMARY

Date of Delivery: 21.8.95

Stages of labour
- 1st: 3 hours
- 2nd: 1.5 hours
- 3rd: 10 mins

DESCRIPTION OF DELIVERY:

Labour: Spontaneous (Induced:) Type Prostin

Type of delivery: S.V.D.

Reasons: (If other than spont) K-42

Complications:

Perineum: (Epis) (Laceration:) Degree 1°

Pain Relief: Pethedine

NEONATAL DETAILS

Name: H.	(Male:)	Female:	Gest'n Age: 42.	Wt: 3740	Medical Status: good condition

PREVIOUS LEVEL OF ACTIVITY: Very fit lady. Marathon runner
No physical ass. during A N period

AREAS TO ASSESS
- Abdomen — see notes
- Pelvic Floor ✓
- Lower Back ✓
- Upper Back ✓
- Neck/Shoulders ✓
- Others
- Breasts

lumpy sites + total breast engorgement

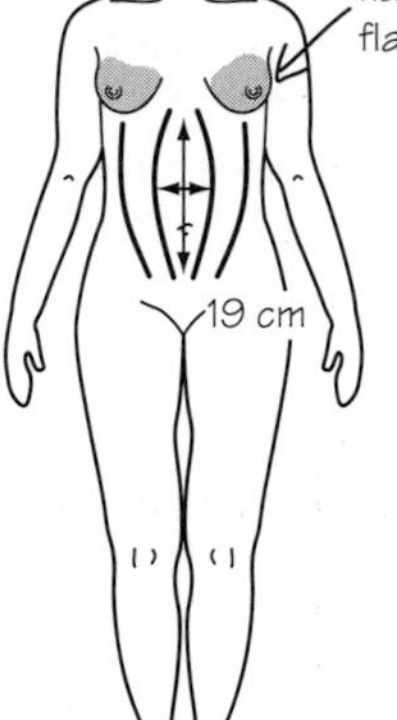

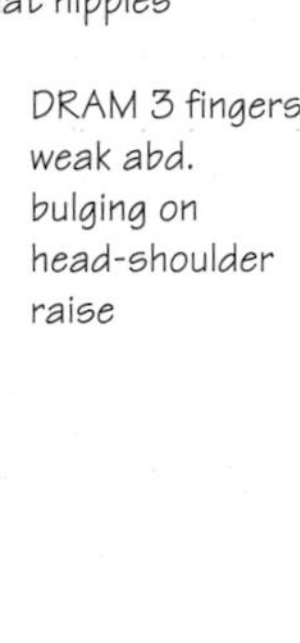

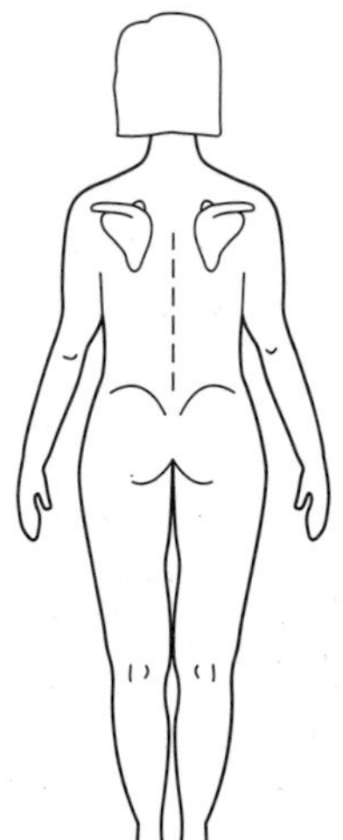

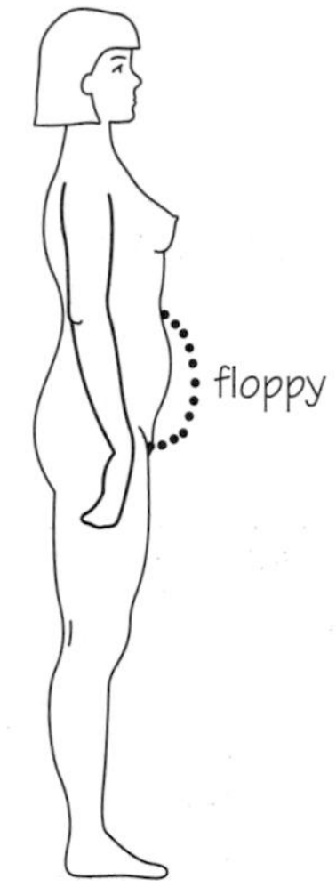

DATE	PATIENT'S CONCERN	CLINICAL ASS.	TREATMENT
24.8.95	floppy abdomen	as above	• Abdominal cont. isometrically obliques + transversus x 5 times. Hourly in all positions • Back mobilizing exs • P.F. exs • Posture correction
25.8.95	painful breasts	as above	• Check abdominal exs + add 'lower limb loading' in sitting. DRAM – now 2 fingers' • Bending v lifting techniques • U.S. to lumpy breast sites • Massage to breast → baby feeding Check. sucking technique → after feed check breast
26.8.95	tiredness	breasts settled	• Shoulder mobilization + scapular retract • Relaxation back massage in prone ly • DRAM now 1.5 fingers
27.8.95	nil	–	• Check all previous programs + inc. intensity + frequency of exs relating them to A.D.L.

FOLLOW UP ADVICE:
1. 2 week follow up prog. necc. to check extent of DRAM + reass ex programme
2. 6 week VAG. ASS. of P F muscles
3. On going group activities – baby massage class
   – P.N ex class
4. To ring for app + if any problem arises before this time

References

Abraham S, Child A, Ferry J et al (1990) Recovery after childbirth: a preliminary prospective study. *Medical Journal of Australia* **152**: 9–12.

Abramson D, Roberts S and Wilson P (1934) Relaxation of pelvic joints in pregnancy. *Journal of Surgery, Gynecology and Obstetrics* **58**: 595–613.

Beischer N and Mackay E (1986) *Obstetrics and the Newborn*, 2nd edn. Sydney: W.B. Saunders.

Breen T, Ransil B, Groves P and Oriol N (1994) Factors associated with back pain after childbirth. *Anesthesiology* 81: 29–34.

Caldwell G (1951) Minor injuries of the lumbar spine and coccyx. *Surgical Clinics of North America* **31**: 1345.

Challis D and Bennett M (1994) Nerve entrapment – an important complication of transverse lower abdominal incisions. *Australian and New Zealand Journal of Obstetrics and Gynaecology* **34**: 594–595.

Crawford JS (1985) Some maternal complications of epidural analgesia for labour. *Analgesia* **40**: 1219–1225.

Dhar S and Anderton J (1992) Rupture of the symphysis pubis during labour. *Clinical Orthopaedics and Related Research* **283**: 252–257.

Driessen F (1987) Postpartum pelvic arthropathy with unusual features. *British Journal of Obstetrics and Gynaecology* **94**: 870–872.

Gray B and Graor R (1992) Deep venous thrombosis and pulmonary embolism. *Postgraduate Medicine* **91**: 207–218.

Hamis M (1992) The impact of research findings on current practice in relieving post-partum perineal pain in a large district general hospital. *Midwifery* **8**: 125–131.

Hay-Smith J and Mantle J (1996) Surveys of the experience and perceptions of post-natal superficial dyspareunia of post-natal women, general practitioners and physiotherapists. *Physiotherapy* **82**: 91–97.

Key J (1937) Operative treatment of coccygodynia. *Journal of Bone and Joint Surgery* **19**: 759.

Kogstad O and Biornstad N (1990) Pelvic girdle relaxation. *TidssKr-Nor-Laegeforen* **110**: 2209–2211.

Lindsey R, Leggon R, Wright D and Nolasco D (1988) Separation of the symphysis pubis in association with childbearing. *Journal of Bone and Joint Surgery* **70**: 289–292.

MacArthur C, Lewis M, Knox E and Crawford J (1990) Epidural anaesthesia and long term backache after childbirth. *British Medical Journal* **301**: 9–12.

Maclennan A (1991) Role of the hormone relaxin in human reproduction and pelvic girdle relaxation. *Scandinavian Journal of Rheumatology* **88**: 7–15.

McMeeken J (1994) Tissue temperature and blood flow: a research based overview of electrophysical modalities. *Australian Journal of Physiotherapy* 40th Jubilee Issue: 49–57.

Noble E (1995) *Essential Exercises for the Childbearing Year*, 4th edn. Harwich, MA: New Life Images.

Ostergaard M, Bonde B and Thomsen B (1992) Pelvic insufficiency during pregnancy. *Ugeskr-Laeger* **154**: 3568–3572.

Östgaard H and Andersson G (1990) Prevalence of back pain in pregnancy. *Spine* **16**: 549–552.

Östgaard H and Andersson G (1991) Postpartum low-back pain. *Spine* **17**: 53–55.

Postacchini F and Massobrio M (1983) Idiopathic coccygodynia. *Journal of Bone and Joint Surgery* **65**: 1116–1124.

Schwartz L, Katz Z and Lancet M (1985) Management of puerperal separation of the symphysis pubis. *International Journal of Gynaecology and Obstetrics* **23**: 125–128.

Sleep J and Grant A (1987) Pelvic floor exercises in post-natal care. *Midwifery* **3**: 158–164.

Taffel SM, Placek P, Moien M and Kosary C (1991) 1989 US cesarean section rate studies – Vx BAC rate raised to nearly one in five. *Birth* **18**: 73–77.

Taylor R and Sonson R (1986) Separation of the pubic symphysis. *Journal of Reproductive Medicine* **31**: 203–206.

Thiele G (1963) Coccygodynia: cause and treatment. *Diseases of the Colon and Rectum* **6**: 422–435.

Venn A and Lumley J (1993) Births after a period of infertility in Victorian women 1982–1990. *Australian and New Zealand Journal of Obstetrics and Gynaecology* **33(4)**: 379–384.

20

Assessment and Handling of the Newborn

CATHERINE BAGLEY

Assessment of the Newborn
•
Baby Handling and Parent Education
•
Other Problems
•
Grief

Some mention of the baby and common problems and management strategies relevant to physiotherapists is warranted in a text such as this. The following chapter will briefly outline assessment of the newborn, including general physical assessment, musculoskeletal, respiratory and neurological assessments. Advice to parents regarding developmental handling, baby massage and positions for feeding and comfort are included as well as some discussion on SIDS, bonding and grief.

The physiotherapist working with new parents should have a basic knowledge of these topics, as the well-being of the baby has a significant impact on the recovery and well-being of the mother. For more details regarding management of specific disabilities, a general paediatric text is recommended, e.g. Burns and MacDonald (1996).

Assessment of the Newborn

The medical examination of a newborn baby consists of four stages associated with the progression of the child's development.

1. The ante-natal assessment.
2. Intrapartum monitoring of the baby during labour.
3. The examination at delivery (the transitional period).
4. The clinical assessment, usually performed within hours of delivery. This includes:
   - the general physical examination;
   - the respiratory assessment;
   - the musculoskeletal assessment;
   - the neurodevelopmental appraisal.

The ante-natal assessment

The normal uninterrupted growth and development of the foetus is dependent on many factors. The mother's health and well-being have a significant effect on the foetus and its development. A mother with diabetes, renal disease, respiratory problems or cardiovascular disease may have complications with pregnancy and the risks of negative health effects on the foetus are increased in these cases. Smoking and consumption of large amounts of alcohol or other drugs during pregnancy affect the foetus who is 'at risk for a plethora of structural, functional and development problems' (Merenstein and Gardner, 1993). Infections such as rubella, cytomegalovirus and toxoplasmosis and toxins such as lead or mercury are also known to have adverse effects on foetal development.

During pregnancy, progressive assessment of foetal development and monitoring of foetal well-being is usually standard practice. Investigations such as ultrasonography, amniocentesis, chorion villus sampling, foetal blood sampling, Doppler flow velocity analysis and foetal radiography can be helpful in identifying foetal abnormalities.

Accurate, comprehensive documentation of maternal history is an important prerequisite to the assessment of the newborn.

Intrapartum monitoring of the baby during labour

The foetus is monitored during labour to ascertain its state of well-being. Signs of foetal distress include:

- abnormal heart rate;
- passage of meconium;
- decreasing foetal movement;
- scalp electrode registering a pH of less than 7.20.

Foetal heart rate during labour is monitored either externally, using a cardiotocograph, or by attaching a foetal scalp electrode. The behaviour of the heart rate is related to the degree of stress of the foetus and will affect the delivery outcome.

A slowing of the heart rate with uterine contractions can occur normally and is usually due to compression of the foetal head. Generally this does not indicate hypoxia and is classified as *early deceleration* (type I). If the heart rate drops after the contraction peak and continues to fall after the contraction subsides, it is an indication of foetal hypoxia. Such a situation is classified as *late deceleration* (type II). The term *variable deceleration* refers to the situation where the heart rate drops, usually with compression of the cord during a contraction. If the occlusion is severe, recovery may be slow and the baby may become distressed.

The passage of meconium before delivery, and hence meconium-stained liquor, not only signifies foetal distress but also increases the risk of meconium aspiration as the baby gasps.

These signs alert the attending staff to the possibility of a baby requiring resuscitation, so enabling the appropriate preparation to take place.

Examination of the baby at the time of delivery

The successful transition between intrauterine and extrauterine life relies on the immediate onset of independent respiration and newborn circulation (rather than foetal circulation). Other adaptations are those of independent thermoregulation and oral feeding.

The assessment of the infant's condition at birth is commenced almost immediately. An apparently well infant will usually have gentle pharyngeal suctioning in order to clear the airway of blood, mucus, vernix or meconium and is kept warm while the heart is auscultated. Oxygen may be administered via a face mask if the baby is slow to 'pink up'; vitamin K is administered and cord blood is sampled in case further investigations become necessary. Immediately post-partum, any gross abnormalities will be identified and appropriate treatment and parent counselling commenced.

The quantitative assessment described by Apgar in 1953 is still in use and grades essential functions of the infant from 0 to 10 (Table 20.1). Assessments are performed at one, five and 10 minutes post-partum and a score out of 10 allocated for each time frame. Table 20.2 indicates the relevant medical management of the infant in this early period, dependent on the Apgar score.

Table 20.1 The Apgar score

Sign	0 points	1 point	2 points
Heart rate	Absent	$< 100\ \text{min}^{-1}$	$> 100\ \text{min}^{-1}$
Respiratory effort	Absent	Weak cry	Strong cry
Muscle tone	Limp	Some flexion	Good flexion
Reflex irritability (suctioning)	No response	Some motion	Cry
Colour	Pale, generalized cyanosis	Centrally pink, peripherally blue	Pink

Table 20.2 Relevant medical management associated with Apgar score

Apgar score	Baby's status description	Medical management
7–10 points	Normal	Routine care
4–6 points	Moderately depressed	Oxygen via bag and mask
0–3 points	Severely depressed ('flat') baby	Active resuscitation, intubation, assisted ventilation, external cardiac massage, sodium bicarbonate, adrenaline

'Vigorous resuscitation is attempted on all babies who are believed to have been alive immediately prior to birth' (Levene and Tudehope, 1993). Yeo and Tudehope (1994) stated that 'One-third of successfully resuscitated, apparently stillborn infants were normal at follow-up assessment'.

In circumstances such as those listed in the box, the baby is transferred into the intensive care nursery (ICN) or the special care nursery (SCN). Treatment may include assisted ventilation, intravenous therapy, nursing in an isolette (to maintain a neutral thermal environment and to reduce heat and fluid loss) or merely close observation for a few hours by specialized staff.

Possible reasons for admission to ICN or SCN

- Pre-term birth (<35 weeks)
- Poor thermoregulation
- Respiratory distress
- Serious birth defect
- Diabetic mother
- Caesarean section
- Assisted delivery (forceps, vacuum extraction, etc.)
- Major feed intolerance
- Low blood glucose estimations

Physiotherapists are active in the intensive care and special care nurseries as they have a role to play in respiratory, developmental and musculoskeletal care. For babies with retained secretions or who, on X-ray, demonstrate evidence of collapse and/or infiltrate (meconium aspiration, pneumonia, respiratory distress syndrome), physiotherapists are involved in the respiratory care. The role may range from overseeing positioning and suctioning techniques to the active treatment of respiratory disorders.

In addition, many babies requiring intensive or special care are at risk of developmental disabilities (e.g. pre-term babies, babies with cerebral pathology or babies who have undergone surgery necessitating prolonged stay in hospital). It is the role of the physiotherapist to initiate and oversee neurodevelopmental programmes, which may consist of:

- positioning to promote comfort, containment (as *in utero*) and to enhance quiet sleep;
- filtering noxious stimuli (light, sound);
- appropriate stimulation (tactile, vestibular, visual, auditory and oral);
- education of parents and staff in handling techniques to encourage appropriate development and behaviours.

The physiotherapist routinely performs neurodevelopmental assessments (including feeding assessments) in order to plan programmes and assist with diagnosis and outcome. Should the baby be hospitalized for musculoskeletal conditions, the physiotherapist has an important role as part of the orthopaedic team.

Clinical assessment of the new-born

A general paediatric physical examination usually occurs within 24 hours of delivery or sooner if warranted, in order to assess the baby's general health and identify any defects.

Careful, clinical examination carried out by an experienced practitioner will reveal most defects. However, early symptoms such as cyanosis, jaundice, vomiting, failure to pass meconium or urine or unusual behaviours may alert the practitioner to other problems.

During examination, observation of the baby's behavioural state is essential. Prechtl (1968) and Brazelton (1973) have both highlighted the relationship between the level of alertness and agitation of the baby and the neurological assessment. Ideally, during the examination, the baby should be in a quiet alert state and fully undressed in a warm, well-lit room. Most clinicians reserve the assessments which may cause discomfort (such as of the hip) to the last moment.

A general observation of the baby's appearance, size (recording length and weight), colour, posture, nutritional status, spontaneous movement and level of alertness is usually done first. A thorough examination follows in a cephalocaudal direction, examining the head (circumference, anterior and posterior fontanelles, suture lines and moulding or elongation due to pressure during birth), eyes, ears, mouth, nose, abdomen, spine and cry (which should be vigorous) (Fig. 20.1). Within 24 hours the baby will pass meconium and urine.

ASSESSMENT OF THE RESPIRATORY SYSTEM

Of particular relevance to physiotherapists is the assessment of the chest and the respiratory status of the newborn. For an adequate assessment to be carried out, knowledge of the four stages of foetal lung development is essential.

Foetal lung development This includes the *embryonic stage* (up to five weeks post-ovulation), where the lung develops as an outpouching of the primitive foregut, and the *pseudoglandular stage* (5–16 weeks gestation) where budding and branching of the lung bud occurs, so that by 16 weeks a primitive tracheobronchial tree has been formed. The *canalicular stage* (16–24 weeks gestation) occurs with the development of a network of capillaries which at times interact with the epithelium. By 24 weeks, respiration is possible. It is not realistically possible for a baby born at less than 24 weeks to survive and active resuscitation is rarely attempted on a baby so young.

The fourth respiratory development stage is the *terminal sac stage* (24–40 weeks gestation). When differentiation of the lung continues, terminal airways (called saccules) develop and it is from these saccules that alveoli are formed. Gas exchange is possible across respiratory bronchioles, saccules and the few alveoli present by 40 weeks.

At about 30 weeks, the consistent production of surfactant (produced by alveolar type II cells) occurs and enables the distal airways to retain air, thus maintaining the functional residual capacity.

Characteristics of newborn respiration

- The baby has horizontal ribs and the diaphragm is the principal muscle of respiration.
- The airways are narrow, so that small quantities of secretions may cause occlusion and atelectasis.

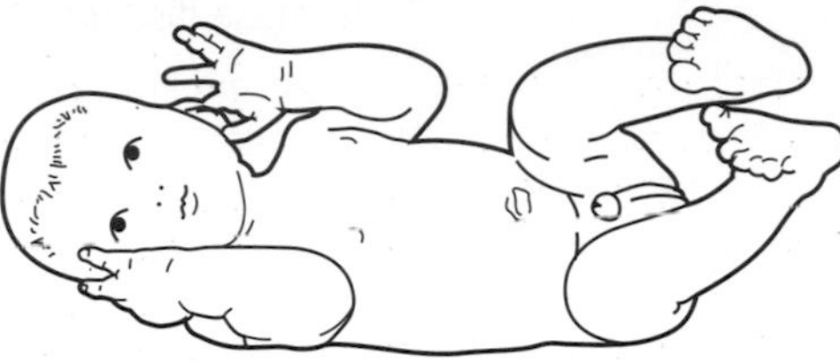
General appearance: size (length and weight); colour; posture; nutritional status (well hydrated and sufficient subcutaneous fat); spontaneous movement (for all four limbs); level of alertness
Eyes: checked for movement, colour and reaction to light
Ears: size, shape and position
Mouth: oral reflexes checked, presence of cleft palate or neonatal teeth
Cry: should be loud and vigorous
Nose: patency assessed
Occipitofrontal circumference measured
Anterior/posterior fontanelles and suture lines palpated
Moulding of the head: elongation (due to normal birth process); flattening at brow (due to breech position); asymmetry (plagiocephaly – usually due to positioning in utero); caput succadaneum (oedema due to birth process, subsides in 48 hrs); cephalohaematoma (bleeding under the periosteum)
Spine: in prone lying, evidence of scoliosis or a cleft or sinus in the low back is determined
Abdomen: contour, colour observed. Number of umbilical vessels counted (usually 2 venous and 1 arterial)

Figure 20.1 General assessment of the neonate.

- The baby has a soft compliant rib cage and respiratory distress will often cause marked recession.
- The baby is a preferable nasal breather.
- When distressed, the neonate breathes more rapidly, not more deeply, thus increasing the work of respiration.
- The percentage of fatigue-resistant fibres in the newborn is much lower than in an older baby (10% at 24 weeks, 50% at eight months). Newborns are susceptible to fatigue from the increased work of breathing and respond by becoming apnoeic.
- The normal respiratory rate of a newborn is 30–40 breaths per minute.
- Normal arterial oxygen level is 9.5 kPa (71 mmHg)

Causes of respiratory distress The most common causes of respiratory distress in the newborn are retained foetal lung fluid, meconium aspiration and hyaline membrane disease. There are many other causes of respiratory distress and the reader should refer to texts in the reference list for more information.

Signs of respiratory distress

- Increased respiratory rate
- Grunting on expiration
- Cyanosis
- Nasal flaring (dilator nares is an accessory muscle of respiration)
- Head bobbing (due to the use of accessory muscles)
- Apnoea

Retained foetal lung fluid (transient tachypnoea of the newborn) The lungs of the foetus are fluid filled. During the descent through the birth canal, most of the fluid is squeezed out or absorbed by pulmonary lymphatics or capillaries. In the event of this clearing process not being completed, the baby presents with tachypnoea and an increased oxygen requirement.

As the condition is usually self-limiting, management consists of nursing the baby in an isolette, in a prone position with the head elevated. Oxygen is administered either into the cot or via a headbox. Intravenous fluids and careful monitoring are usually necessary for several days.

Meconium aspiration The passage of meconium *in utero* or at birth is associated with foetal distress. Aspiration of meconium can readily occur when the baby attempts to gasp. The baby is usually term or post-term.

Treatment at delivery consists of direct suction of any meconium from the mouth, nasopharynx and trachea. If the baby then appears well, close observation alone is required for a few hours. However, if the baby has respiratory distress, humidification of inspired oxygen-enriched air (via headbox or endotracheal tube), active physiotherapy with suction and treatment with antibiotics are indicated.

Hyaline membrane disease (respiratory distress syndrome) Hyaline membrane disease is the most common cause of respiratory distress in the newborn infant (more commonly the pre-term infant). It is caused by inadequate synthesis of surfactant and results in progressive atelectasis. Treatment may consist of the administration of mechanical ventilation, surfactant and oxygen. Physiotherapy is often indicated as the resolution stage involves the production of excess secretions.

Chest physiotherapy is indicated in most conditions where there are excessive secretions and/or evidence of atelectasis or infiltrate on X-ray. See Burns and MacDonald (1996) for more details of specific physiotherapy management techniques.

MUSCULOSKELETAL ASSESSMENT

Generally, term babies demonstrate a flexed posture, with a kyphotic spine easily able to actively extend with stimulation. The hips and knees are also slightly flexed, lacking full extension. When the infant is relaxed, the hips will fully abduct from a flexed position. Range of motion of the ankle is large with full dorsiflexion (little toe touches the lateral border of the fibula) and 15–30° of plantarflexion. An infant will have flexed and adducted arms with loosely fisted hands which relax periodically.

There are a number of common orthopaedic conditions (e.g. congenital dislocation of the hip, congenital talipes equinovarus, metatarsus adductus, talipes calcaneovalgus, brachial plexus injuries and sternocleidomastoid tumour) for which physiotherapy plays an active role. See MacDonald (1996) for further reading on the management of the orthopaedic problems that are included in this chapter.

Common musculoskeletal disorders

Congenital dislocation of the hip (CDH). CDH describes the abnormal relationship between the femoral head and the acetabulum. The direction of dislocation is posterior, with some hips sitting in a dislocated position and others which can be fairly easily dislocated during examination manoeuvres. The incidence is approximately four in 1000 and is more frequently seen in full-term babies and those babies born by breech presentation. It is commonly the left hip in baby girls.

Identification is usually made by physical examination. The importance of gentle examination in a relaxed infant is stressed by many authors, including Beverly and Nathan (1995). X-ray is not appropriate until 3–4 months as the femoral epiphyses do not begin to ossify until that time. Real-time diagnostic ultrasound may be used to confirm clinical findings or to help in the diagnosis if the clinical examination has been inconclusive (Holen et al, 1994).

The hip may be subluxed, dislocated, dislocatable or teratologically dislocated.

1. The subluxed hip occurs when the femoral head can be partially displaced on testing, but there is no dislocation.
2. The dislocated hip (commonly posterolaterally) is diagnosed using Ortolani's manoeuvre. With the hip and knees flexed to 90°, thigh abduction and traction along the length of the femur are applied to the tested hip, while an anteromedially directed pressure is applied over the greater trochanter using the index or middle finger. A reducible dislocation will result in a 'clunk' that is felt by the tester, but not necessarily heard or seen (Fig. 20.2a). Signs of dislocation may include apparent leg shortening and/or asymmetrical thigh creases.
3. The dislocatable hip is detected with the hip in flexion by adding gentle adduction and downward and outward pressure (posterolaterally directed) along the length of the femur. The hip is felt to dislocate posteriorly over the edge of the acetabulum. This test is termed Barlow's test (Barlow, 1962) (Fig. 20.2b).
4. The teratological hip is fixed in dislocation. The leg appears shorter and cannot be abducted. The Ortolani manoeuvre fails to relocate the hip.

The management of the unstable or dislocated hip is supervised by the orthopaedic surgeon and consists of immobilizing the reduced hip in a position of flexion and abduction for 6–12 weeks. The splints most commonly used are the von Rosen splint, the Pavlic harness or the Denis Brown harness.

There is a place for physiotherapy involvement in the management of neonatal CDH. While the baby is splinted the parents may benefit from advice regarding handling and positioning for comfort and general stimulation, such as the following.

- The use of a pillow for changing and sleeping.
- The encouragement of prone lying during waking hours (over a pillow).
- The use of massage to enhance tactile responses.
- Techniques for carrying and lifting the baby (a possum pouch can be helpful).

Figure 20.2 (a) Ortolani test. This figure illustrates therapist performing test on the baby's right hip. Therapist's left thenar surface directs a gentle longitudinal traction while slowly abducting the hip. The therapist's index finger palpates the greater trochanter for signs of reduction of dislocation. (b) Barlow test. The therapist's right hand is assessing the baby's left hip, a gentle longitudinal compression posterolaterally directed is applied to the hip during slow adduction.

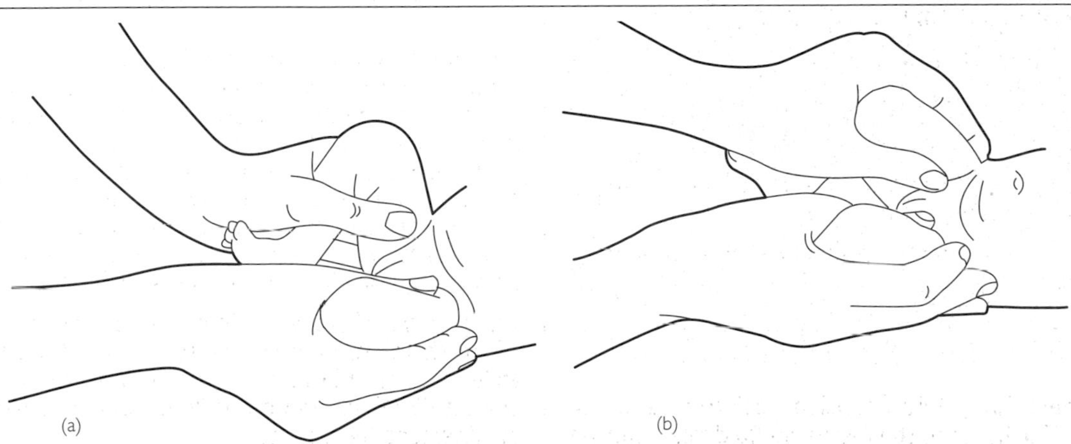

- Use of a carrycot rather than a capsule for travelling in the car.
- Care of the splint to protect the baby's skin and maintain a good position, i.e. maintaining a clean dry splint and overseeing the correct fitting, between visits to the orthopaedic surgeon.

After the splint is removed, the baby may require encouragement to move and begin exploring the environment. The physiotherapist gradually introduces positions such as side-lying and sitting, while continuing to reinforce prone as a necessary position.

Massage is often beneficial and the baby should begin to enjoy deep baths which encourage movement and relaxation. The baby can often be reluctant to commence rolling and by five months, if this is so, some facilitated rolling might be of benefit. Babies who have been immobilized in splints or plaster are more at risk of motor delays and the physiotherapist should be available for advice.

Talipes equinovarus There are four types of talipes equinovarus (TEV).

1. Rigid/structural congenital TEV (club foot).
2. Postural TEV.
3. TEV associated with muscle imbalance secondary to an upper motor neurone disorder (e.g. spina bifida, cerebral palsy) and muscular disease (e.g. muscular dystrophy).
4. Congenital TEV in association with other significant teratological malformation.

Both congenital and postural TEV will be briefly discussed.

Congenital TEV (club foot) occurs in 1–2 per 1000 births and is more common in boys (Hesinger and Jones, 1986). It may affect one or both feet with varying degrees of severity. The primary deformity is one of plantarflexion at the ankle joint and inversion at the subtalar, talocalcaneal, talonavicular and calcaneocuboid joints. Varus displacement (adduction) occurs at the mid-tarsal joints (Fig. 20.3).

While postural TEV presents with no other complicating factors, in the structural varieties, bony and soft tissue changes are evident. The calcaneum is tilted into equinus and may be felt as a small bony prominence under a soft tissue heel area. The medial deviation of the neck of the talus is 45–65° compared to 25–30° in the normal foot (Irani and Sherman, 1963). The navicular is displaced medially on the head of the talus and indeed, Williams and Cole (1991) believe that the 'primary deformity is a dislocation of the talonavicular joint so that the forefoot is mounted on the hindfoot at almost a right angle'. The other bones follow the pattern of medial deviation. The muscles of the calf are wasted and the foot tends to be shorter.

In all but the mild postural varieties, management is overseen by an orthopaedic surgeon and varies considerably, according to local preferences. In many cases the physiotherapist carries out the treatment and educates the parents. Table 20.3 presents some guidelines on the management of TEV.

Caution

Before undertaking treatment of club foot, the physiotherapist should ensure that he or she has a sound working knowledge of the condition and has received specific training by a physiotherapist experienced in the management of club foot. Passive movements of the infant's foot should be done with great care.

Serious damage to small joints (in particular to tibial and fibular epiphysial growth plates) may occur if the treatment force is poorly applied and inappropriately directed. Overstretching of the

Figure 20.3 Talipes equinovarus deformity.

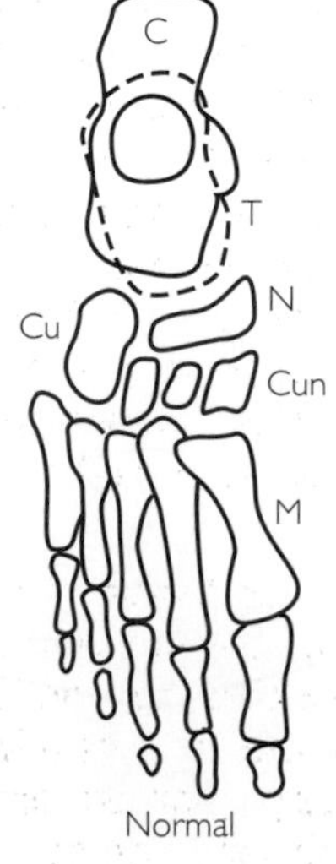

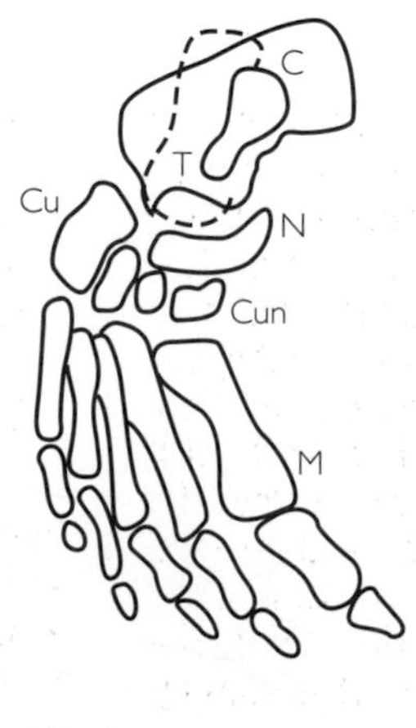

C = calcaneum
T = talus
N = navicular
Cu = cuboid
Cun = cuniform
M = metatarsal

Table 20.3 Guidlines for the management of congenital talipes equinovarus

Type	Early treatment (0–4 weeks)	Further treatment (4 weeks–4 months)	Possible sequelae
Mild postural deformity Foot rests in a position of plantarflexion, inversion and adduction Easily overcorrected with active and passive movement	'Unpack' the baby to allow normal movement Educate the parents in tactile stimulation of eversion and dorsiflexion	No further treatment	No sequelae Normal foot
Significant postural deformity Foot rests in the abnormal position May correct to neutral or slightly more with passive movement. Poor active correction. No bony changes evident	Strapping Passive movements Parent education Stimulation Stretches Care of strapping	Passive movements Exercises	No sequelae Normal foot
Structural deformity Foot fixed in the abnormal position Little correction possible Evidence of bony and soft tissue changes.	Serial plasters until foot corrected to neutral	Strapping Passive movements Exercises	Night splints (Denis Brown) Stretching Exercises (throughout growth) Surgery The foot often looks good but can remain 'stiff'

mid-foot on the hindfoot causes soft tissue damage, often referred to as a 'broken foot'.

The aim of conservative treatment is to gently encourage the foot into a position of 'over correction' (i.e. full dorsiflexion and eversion), while maintaining the integrity of the structures in the foot. Correction is achieved by the use of serial plasters, strapping or splinting and passive movements and exercise. Surgery is required if conservative management fails to correct the foot.

- *'Unpack' the baby.* This occurs naturally as the baby moves in the more spacious extrauterine environment. Although swaddling of newborns is encouraged, it is best to leave the baby with foot deformities some freedom to kick the legs and move the feet.
- *Exercises and stimulation.* The muscle groups that require exercising and stimulating are the dorsiflexors and evertors. Muscles can be stimulated by pressure and movement on specific parts of the skin, facilitating appropriate muscle activity via reflex responses. Dorsiflexion can be stimulated by eliciting a placing reaction. By stroking the dorsum of the foot, it will move actively into dorsiflexion. It is important to stimulate eversion simultaneously with dorsiflexion. Eversion can be facilitated by tickling the lateral border of the foot or stroking the anterolateral surface of the lower leg to encourage contraction of the evertors. The therapist moves from the dorsum of the foot quickly to the lateral border of the foot then runs up the anterolateral surface of the leg.
- *Passive mobilization/lengthening of short soft tissues.* Passive mobilization is directed at movement into abduction, eversion and dorsiflexion at the mid-tarsal, subtalar and talocrural joints, respectively. With one hand (the therapist's right hand on the baby's left leg), the knee is flexed and the lower leg stabilized while the calcaneus is held at neutral. With the other hand, the forefoot is first abducted to neutral and the inversion corrected as far as comfortable. Provided the mid-foot and forefoot are corrected at least to neutral and held firm, an attempt may be made to gently take the foot towards dorsiflexion. The corrected position should be maintained for 20 seconds (Fig. 20.4). These movements can be performed during day-time nappy changes when the baby is calm. Such a routine should ensure that passive movements occur at least five times daily. It is important to review the parents'/caregivers' passive movement skills on each attendance at the clinic.
- *Strapping.* Rigid strapping tape provides a means of maintaining the foot in a corrected position. Strapping methods for TEV vary between centres. Commonly used approaches are the Robert Jones strapping for club feet, the Denis Brown splints and strapping and the buckle and strap method (Fig. 20.5).

Metatarsus adductus This deformity consists of adduction of the forefoot and slight varus of the mid-foot. Medial tibial torsion is often present. Mild deformities that can be passively corrected tend to resolve spontaneously (Ponseti and Becker, 1966). However, if the deformity cannot to be corrected fully, a

Figure 20.4 Stretch for talipes equinovarus deformity.

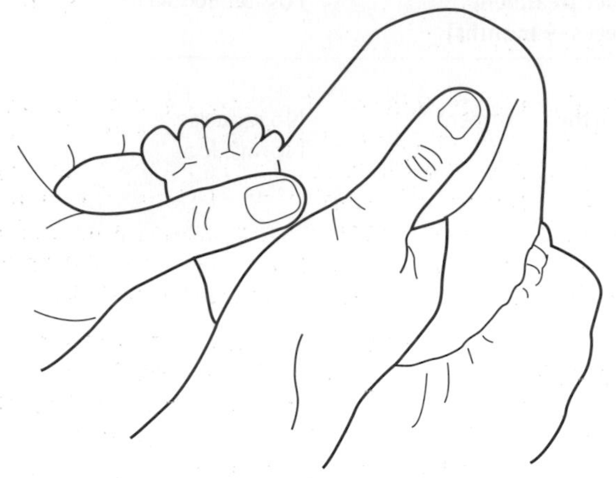

Figure 20.5 Strapping in place for talipes equinovarus deformity.

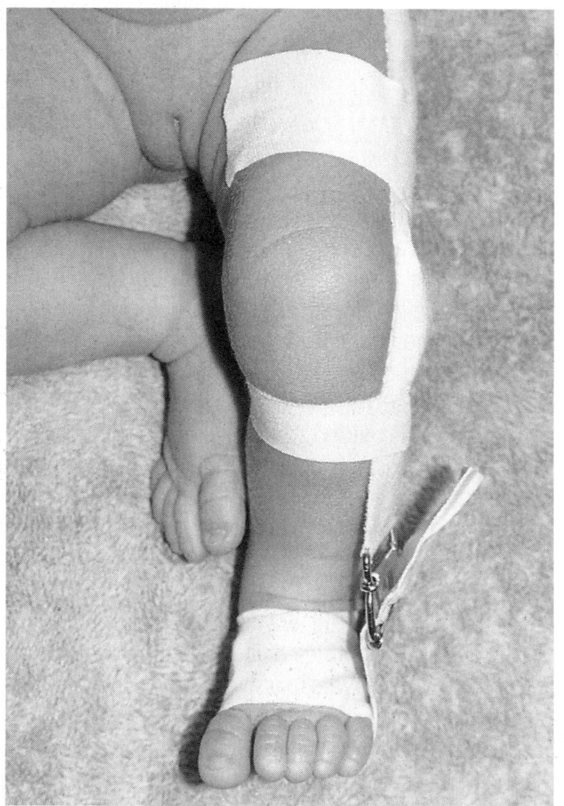

programme of passive movements and exercising is initiated by the physiotherapist.

Passive movements (at day-time nappy change) for a foot with metatarsus adductus can be performed as follows. One hand is placed on the calcaneus and cuboid to stabilize these bones and the baby's hip and knee are flexed. With the other hand, the thumb is moved along the medial border of the forefoot (or over the medial aspect of the first metatarsal head) and a lateral pressure applied slowly and gradually. The therapist should aim to increase the distance between the stabilized hindfoot and the forefoot (Fig. 20.6).

Figure 20.6 Stretch for metatarsus adductus.

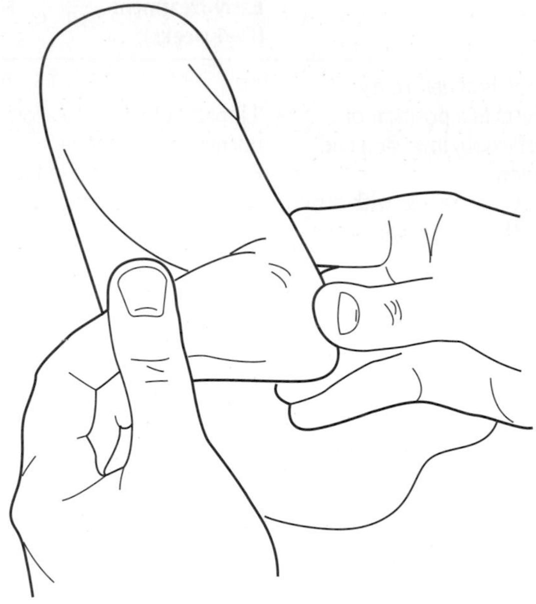

The corrected position is held for 20 seconds and repeated 2–3 times. All lengthening techniques need to be followed by active contraction of the muscles through the new range. The therapist should concentrate on facilitating action of the everters through stroking or other tactile facilitatory techniques.

Babies whose feet do not respond to passive movement or to the passage of time may require plasters or surgery (Lloyd-Roberts and Fixsen, 1990; Williams and Cole, 1991).

Talipes calcaneovalgus Talipes calcaneovalgus (TCV) is a postural deformity in which the foot is held in dorsiflexion and the heel in a valgus position (Hesinger and Jones, 1986) (Fig. 20.7). The range of plantarflexion is usually no greater than to neutral. There is an increased incidence of hip instability in babies with TCV and hips should always be examined. This may be due to the forces *in utero* that combine to generate this deformity, where the foot presses on the uterine wall (Bernhardt, 1988).

Although this condition will resolve in time as the baby kicks in a less restricted environment, gentle passive movements can be shown to the mother.

The baby's heel is held at neutral with one hand and with the other a gentle downward massage stroke is applied to the lateral aspect of the lower leg and foot, aimed towards moving the foot into plantarflexion and inversion (Fig. 20.8). The action is performed for 20 seconds. A massage oil suitable for babies can be used (peanut oil, almond oil, etc.) as the skin is often dry and cracked on the dorsum. Once again, the passive movements should be firm but gentle and the baby should not cry.

The regime of passive movements and exercising postural foot deformities in neonates is continued until the foot rests in a neutral position and can actively and passively overcorrect. While many of the postural deformities may correct spontaneously, some do not. These resistant deformities require invasive intervention at a later stage. The feet may become difficult to fit into shoes or cause the toddler to trip and fall.

Figure 20.7 Talipes calcaneovalgus.

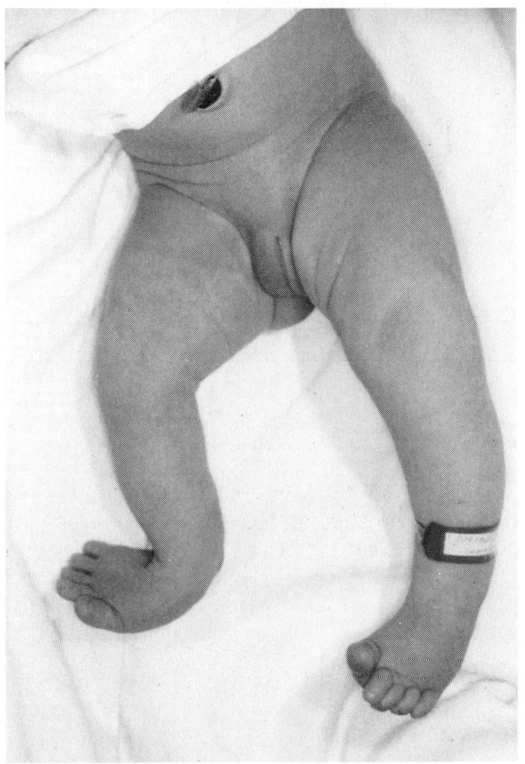

Parental instruction in giving gentle exercise and passive movements in the neonatal period is considered to be of benefit (Levene and Tudehope, 1993; Lloyd Roberts and Fixsen, 1990; Tecklin, 1992).

Brachial plexus injuries Birth-related brachial plexus lesions occur in approximately one per 1000 births. They include conditions such as Erb's palsy, Klumkpe's paralysis and total brachial plexus lesions. The injury is caused by traction on the brachial plexus during delivery. A common history is that of a vertex presentation with shoulder dystocia in a large infant (often >4000 g).

A baby with Erb's palsy (C5, C6) is reluctant to move the arm at birth and holds it in a position of shoulder adduction, elbow extension and wrist pronation and flexion (Fig. 20.9). A lesion of C7, C8 and T1 nerves is called Klumkpe's paralysis and is less common. It involves wrist drop and hand paralysis. Total brachial plexus lesions involve paralysis of the whole arm.

With respect to Erb's palsy, the most prevalent brachial plexus condition, an initial brief, gentle assessment should be made as the baby is often experiencing pain. An X-ray is taken to exclude any fractures (especially a fractured clavicle) and to detect the presence of diaphragmatic paralysis. Muscle groups commonly affected in Erb's palsy are:

- shoulder elevators, external rotators and abductors;
- elbow flexors;
- wrist extensors and supinators.

Initially, the baby is left to rest and given pain relief as necessary. The baby should be swaddled to keep the arm comfortable and nursed either supine or on the unaffected side. As the baby will often prefer to turn away from the affected side, the use of a peanut pillow during nappy change, to prevent soft tissue contracture, may be helpful

Figure 20.8 Stretch for talipes calcaneovalgus.

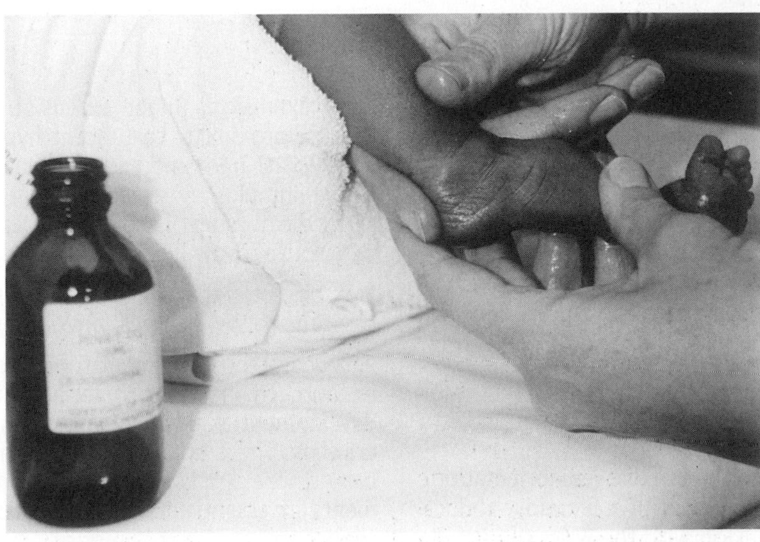

Figure 20.9 Typical posture of Erb's palsy.

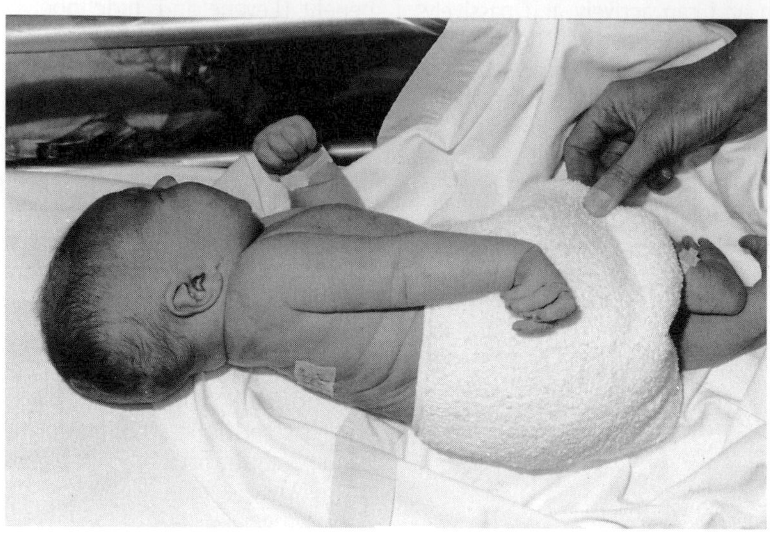

Figure 20.10 Use of a peanut pillow.

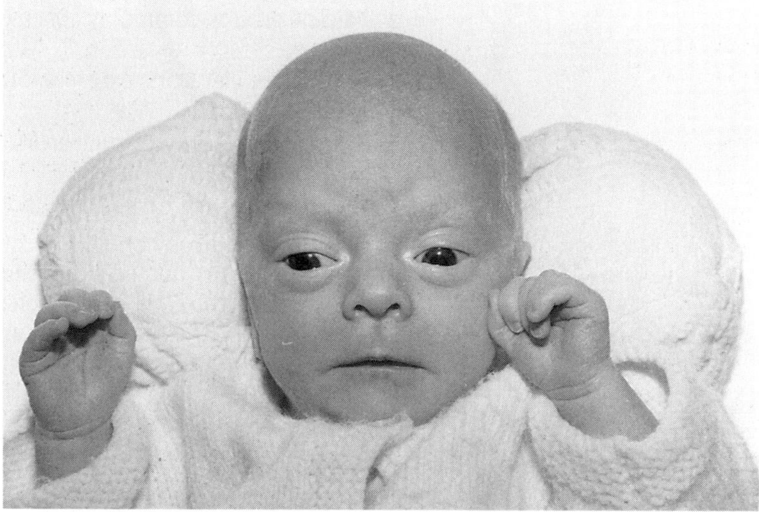

(Fig. 20.10). Dressing should be a gentle affair, slipping the affected arm into a shirt or dress first.

Passive movements *should not be attempted* in the first few days. They cause unnecessary discomfort and are not useful in affecting the outcome.

Mild injuries will recover in a few days and most brachial plexus injuries (92%) have fully recovered by 12 months (Gordon et al, 1973). However, for those babies who show few signs of recovery by discharge (five days), parents should receive a positioning, passive movement and stimulation programme to carry out at home.

Using a peanut pillow to maintain mid-line orientation, gentle passive movements are performed. Shoulder abduction and elevation, elbow flexion with the wrist supinated, wrist extension, finger extension and thumb abduction (abduct proximally to prevent hyperextension at the first MCP joint) are combined and repeated slowly. In addition, tactile stimulus by stroking along the belly of biceps and along the dorsum of the hand (placing reaction) may encourage active elbow flexion and wrist and finger extension.

It is suggested that these movements be carried out during day-time nappy changes, provided the baby is relaxed.

A general programme of positioning and handling is encouraged in order to facilitate age-appropriate motor development, e.g. hands to mouth, prone play, rolling and crawling. These tasks in particular may not be achieved in a baby whose arm is not moving normally. Follow-up assessments are essential for progression and to provide parental support.

In severe cases, surgical exploration and repair is attempted in some centres and results to date have been promising (Mutimer, 1994).

Sternocleidomastoid tumour A sternocleidomastoid (SCM) tumour is a hard lump occurring in the SCM muscle at about the level of the angle of the jaw. It is usually felt when the baby is about two weeks old. Two main theories are suggested as to the cause. Firstly, malpositioning *in utero* may lead to local ischaemic changes. Secondly, direct trauma during a difficult delivery may cause local damage. In both situations, the tumour usually shortens the sternomastoid muscle, causing the baby to tilt its head towards the affected side and to rotate it to the opposite side. Plagiocephaly, i.e. flattening of the occipital region on one side (called a parallelogram head), if not present at birth, will often be acquired as the baby persistently lies on one side of the head.

The management of sternomastoid tumour consists of instructing the parents in a stimulation, positioning and handling programme. The aim of the programme is to encourage active, full range movement of the head to maintain good length of the sternomastoid muscle while the lump resolves and to prevent further soft tissue contractures.

Should the neck remain tight, passive lengthening techniques are necessary and, at 12 months, surgery may be performed.

Encouragement of head movements is helped by:

- prone lying encouraging a head-up position and head turning towards the affected side;
- visual stimulation to encourage head turn;
- the use of a peanut pillow for changing and for travel in the baby capsule and stroller (often the baby has difficulty maintaining mid-line orientation);
- sleeping the baby on the less preferred side to encourage symmetry;
- carrying the baby prone over the arm (Fig. 20.11);
- picking the baby up from side lying on the affected side, to encourage lateral head righting to the opposite side.

If the neck is still tight after two weeks, the following lengthening programme could be performed at the daytime nappy change. Lengthening requires a combination of movements, directed at increasing the distance between the origin and insertion of the affected muscle. This is achieved when the baby is supine by:

- stabilizing the shoulders with one hand across the shoulder girdle (i.e. stabilizing the insertion of the muscle);
- laterally tilting the baby's head away from the affected side (ear to shoulder);
- then maintaining the lateral tilt, rotating the head towards the affected side (chin to same shoulder);
- hold for five seconds.

Muscle stretches should not be performed if the baby is crying as unnecessary force may be required to achieve the range of movement and soft tissue damage may result. The baby will usually tolerate one or two repetitions before showing signs of discomfort. Lateral tilt can be achieved by carrying the baby in side lying with the head held in a position of stretch. Rotation can be achieved by carrying the baby in the prone position, resting on the operator's forearm (see Fig. 20.11). These carrying stretches can often be maintained for longer than formal stretches, i.e. 30 seconds to a few minutes, depending on the baby's tolerance.

Figure 20.11 Carrying infant in prone position.

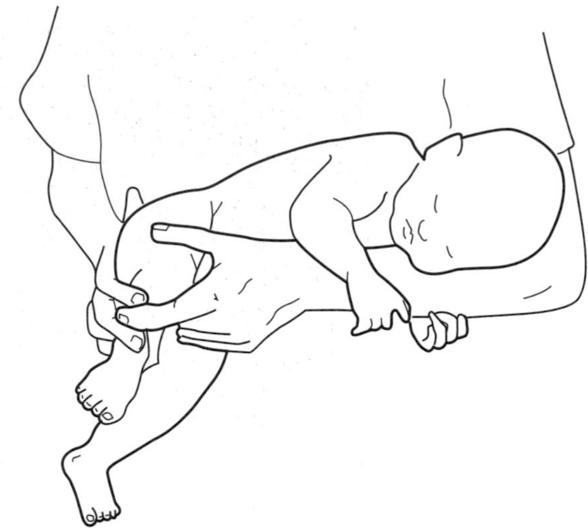

Treatment continues until the baby has good active rotation, is able to hold the head up in the mid-line and head-righting reactions are symmetrical. This may take several months.

The neurodevelopmental appraisal

Careful assessment of neurodevelopmental status is necessary in the examination of the newborn. The results of the assessment provide a reliable indicator of the integrity and maturity of the baby's nervous system and are useful in the prediction of developmental outcomes.

Dubowitz and Dubowitz (1981) have described a comprehensive method of assessing neurodevelopmental status in the pre-term and full-term infant. This assessment is now widely used. The test items, which are clearly described and therefore relatively easy to administer, consist of habituation, movement and tone, reflexes and neurobehavioural items. The test is administered between feeds so that the baby is comfortably alert. A healthy full-term baby will score most items towards the middle of the chart. Poorly responsive or pre-term infants will score to the left while hyper-responsive, irritable babies will tend to score further to the right of the chart.

The infant's state of alertness is documented, as is the time after a feed and the presence of any medical condition or musculoskeletal abnormality which may affect the outcome.

For a clear explanation of how to elicit reflexes and reactions in the newborn, the work of Prechtl (1968) is recommended.

Early identification of neurological dysfunction assists in the implementation of appropriate management programmes, as well as guiding parent counselling and education. The importance of follow-up assessment and review cannot be overemphasized. A 'one-off' assessment should never be used as a predictor of disability. Some babies who score poorly in the original assessment may proceed to developmental normality at a later stage.

A useful format for assessment during follow-up is the Neurosensory Motor Developmental Assessment (NSMDA) (Burns, 1992).

Baby Handling and Parent Education

A prerequisite for successful, confident handling of the newborn by both parents is the initiation and continuation of the bonding process.

Bonding

Klaus and Kennell (1982) describe nine steps in the process of forming a maternal-infant attachment. These steps start prior to pregnancy and are complete with the role of care taking.

1. Planning the pregnancy
2. Confirming the pregnancy
3. Accepting the pregnancy
4. Foetal movements
5. Accepting the baby / foetus as an individual
6. The birth process
7. Seeing the baby
8. Touching the baby
9. Care taking

In the event of a planned, uneventful pregnancy, the steps of attachment usually occur spontaneously. If the pregnancy was unplanned or unwanted or if the baby or mother becomes ill and they are separated at birth, the attachment process can become interrupted and at times irretrievably lost.

Members of the medical team who are in contact with the mother ante-natally and post-natally need to be aware of the situations where extra support may need to be offered. These include:

- very young parents;
- a single mother;
- a mother who has been abused during childhood;
- battered mother;
- ill mother, separated from the baby;
- premature, ill, congenital malformations in the baby;
- a mother involved with alcohol or substance abuse;
- a mother who has had no ante-natal care;
- marital conflict;
- a difficult labour;
- post-natal depression;
- some cultural differences (see Chapter 22).

Some signs of failure to bond

- Reluctant or rough handling
- Refusal to care for baby
- Poor interation between mother and baby – no eye contact or verbalizing
- Ignoring the baby's cries
- Mother's preoccupation with her own health or discomfort

It is clear that the outcome of poor mother–infant bonding may lead to developmental difficulties for the infant. Both the physiotherapist and the nursing staff are involved with parent education in baby handling and are often able to identify problems early. Prompt intervention and support may well improve the outcome and possibly prevent some instances of child abuse and neglect.

Handling the newborn

VISION AND HEARING

The 'born at term' baby responds to eye contact at a distance of 15–25 cm (Sheridan, 1982), soft singing, light music and occasionally to a mobile (black and white) fluttering in the breeze.

When quietly alert, the baby responds to soft sounds and diffuse light by 'freezing' to the sound (light bell or murmuring voice) and quietly regarding the light, often drifting the eyes towards a window or dim lamp. He or she will also enjoy close eye contact.

Bright lights and sudden loud noises stimulate varying degrees of distress, ranging from a startle reaction to crying.

Parents are encouraged to speak softly to their newborn and, as much as is practical, avoid bright lights and loud noises. This is especially relevant for babies in special care nurseries, where excessive environmental noise and light has been shown to distress babies and delay recovery.

POSTURE AND MOVEMENT

The posture of the newborn is predominantly one of flexion. The newborn displays a repertoire of reflexes which demonstrate the integrity of the nervous system and careful assessment of these reflexes and other postural reactions is carried out soon after birth. For a more detailed explanation of reflexes and testing procedures, the work of Prechtl (1968) and the Dubowitz and Dubowitz (1981) neurodevelopmental scheme are recommended for reading. Once the baby reaches one month of age, ongoing assessment as necessary is recommended, using the NSMDA (Burns, 1992).

Spontaneous movements are usually gross and purposeless, being more common in the supine position, where the newborn is less 'contained'. These large movements can at times distress the baby and cause a startle reaction.

When advising parents on handling and settling techniques, the aim is to encourage postures which will assist motor development as well as those which might provide comfort. The use of prone for play and dressing (not for sleeping) and side lying encourage motor development. Swaddling and firm cuddling is considered useful for settling newborns, not used to an unconfined environment. Prone bathing has been advocated to provide gentle movement through the water, thus enhancing relaxation.

When it is necessary to lie the baby supine (as for nappy change), the use of a large pillow to promote some flexion and mid-line orientation will facilitate eye contact, which calms and focuses the baby, and will inhibit uncontrolled head and trunk rotation, which may be unsettling. As much socializing between parent and infant occurs at change time, it is more comfortable for the parent to be looking at the baby who is elevated, rather than having to lean further forward into flexion, thus compromising the neck and back.

Picking the baby up from prone or side lying (Fig. 20.12) avoids supine, facilitates righting reactions, as minimal head support is required, requires less effort on the part of the parent, as the arms are closer to the body, and sets the pattern for the development of rotation responses in the baby in preparation for later development.

The physiotherapist has a role in teaching parents the benefits of using a variety of carrying and nursing positions. The use of different positions for carrying is recommended as it gives the baby the opportunity to respond to gravity in different ways, using a variety of postural reactions and muscle groups.

Figure 20.12 Picking up an infant from side lying.

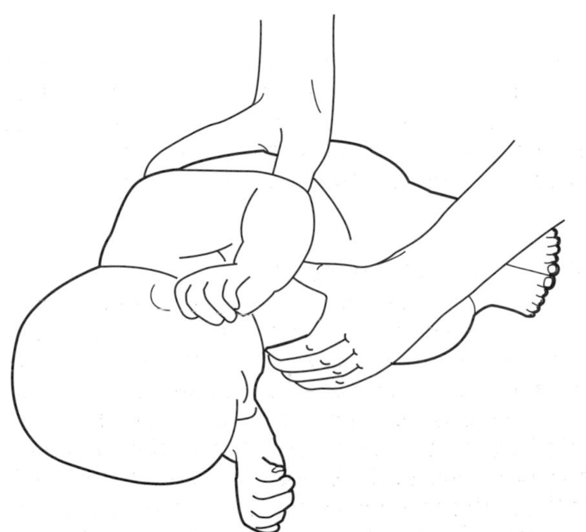

Some recommended positions are

- over the arm (prone) (see Fig. 20.11);
- high up over the shoulder;
- upright over the arm, facing outwards;
- prone over the knees, with the parent in sitting;
- possum pouch or sling (the unsettled baby will especially enjoy spending time in a pouch).

A variety of carrying positions will also be beneficial for the parent, as the load is spread over several joints and muscles, minimizing the development of fatigue.

The newborn usually spends most of the time feeding and sleeping. However, behavioural and personality differences may often be reported at this stage (Sheridan, 1982). When hungry or uncomfortable, the baby will cry in protest. Most will settle temporarily with attention, but the hungry baby will continue to cry. A high-pitched cry or a continuous whimper which does not respond to attention or feeding should be investigated by a doctor. In such a case, it is more than likely that the baby is unwell.

FEEDING

Provided that the baby's oral responses and anatomy are normal, feeding should be a fairly straightforward process in the normal healthy neonate. Although breast feeding is to be encouraged, the choice is entirely up to the mother and she should be fully supported in whatever choice she makes.

At the initial physical examination, the anatomy of the baby's mouth, tongue and palate is checked and the reflexes associated with feeding are assessed.

Stimulating the cheek with the nipple, teat or finger will elicit the rooting reflex. The baby will turn towards the stimulus and open the mouth and lower the lip on that side in preparation for attachment.

Circling the baby's lips may elicit the mouthing response, where the baby 'smacks' the lips in anticipation. Stimulation of the palate will result in a strong sucking motion. The tongue remains down and forward over the lower gum line and curves around the teat. Suction is maintained while the baby compresses the nipple with the tongue from front to back in a wave like pattern (Marmet and Shell, 1984). The jaw moves rhythmically up and down and it is said that the jaw movement actually milks the breast (Ardran et al, 1958). The lips are rotated up and out and a suck / swallow action, with occasional pauses to breathe, is the common mechanism involved in neonatal sucking. As the baby matures, a suck, suck, suck, swallow pattern emerges.

The gag reflex is stimulated by passing a catheter into the posterior oropharynx. This reflex should be assessed before commencement of breast or bottle feeding, particularly in the case of a baby who has been ill or is showing signs of neurological impairment.

Positions for feeding The mother should be comfortably supported and the baby held close, establishing eye contact if possible. 'The mother holds her infant at approximately a 45° angle with the baby's face and body turned towards the mother (cradle position), (Marmet and Shell, 1984). The head is supported in neutral flexion and in the mid-line (Fig. 20.13).

The baby may feed better if firmly swaddled. This helps to focus the baby on the task at hand and prevents interference from wayward hands.

Some babies feed better if gently rocked in a rocking chair.

The upright position is considered preferable for several reasons:

- sucking and swallowing are more efficient (Ingle, personal communication);
- gravity assists the settling of the milk in the stomach and air is more easily expelled upwards (burping);
- the principal muscle for respiration in the neonate is the diaphragm, so feeding upright ensures less work of breathing, which in turn improves the energy reserves remaining for feeding. This is especially relevant for babies who have lung pathology or who are frail because of illness;
- the upright position reduces the risk of gastro-oesophageal reflux.

Gastro-oesophageal reflux (GOR) is described by Shepherd (1991) as the retrograde movement of gastric contents into the oesophagus due to dysfunction of the distal oesophagus and is a common event which can occur repeatedly throughout life without disability but which can result in serious morbidity and even mortality. It is particularly common in infants, where repeated regurgitation of milk is said to occur in up to 40% of infants less than three months of age. Symptoms range from the occasional posset in a happy baby to excessive irritability in a baby with feeding problems, extensor posturing with reluctance to being placed horizontal and failure to thrive. A careful medical assessment is required and often a trial of medication is recommended. Parents should seek help when the baby is behaving in this manner. A persistently unhappy baby causes a great deal of stress both to the baby and the family and instances of child abuse associated with the problem have been reported (Shepherd, 1991). GOR not only causes distress but may cause respiratory symptoms resulting from milk aspiration.

In the event of a baby experiencing feeding difficulties, some basic guidelines are provided. However, further expert advice may be obtained from a speech pathologist and/or a lactation consultant.

As with any problem encountered with the baby, a thorough physical examination should be performed by the doctor in order to rule out the possibility of an underlying medical condition causing the poor feeding (e.g. septicaemia, jaundice).

Some of the following suggestions can assist the development of feeding in neonates.

- Apply pre-feeding exercises involving one minute of stimulation of the oral reflexes of rooting, mouthing and sucking, as well as rubbing the gums.
- Express or drop some milk onto the finger and the lips of the baby before performing the pre-feeding exercises.
- Swaddle the baby, maintaining neutral head flexion and midline orientation.
- Hold the baby upright.
- Support the jaw once the nipple or bottle is in place.
- Make gentle circles under the chin as this will often stimulate a suck if the baby is reluctant to do so.

Figure 20.13 (a) Mother breast feeding. (b) Mother bottle feeding.

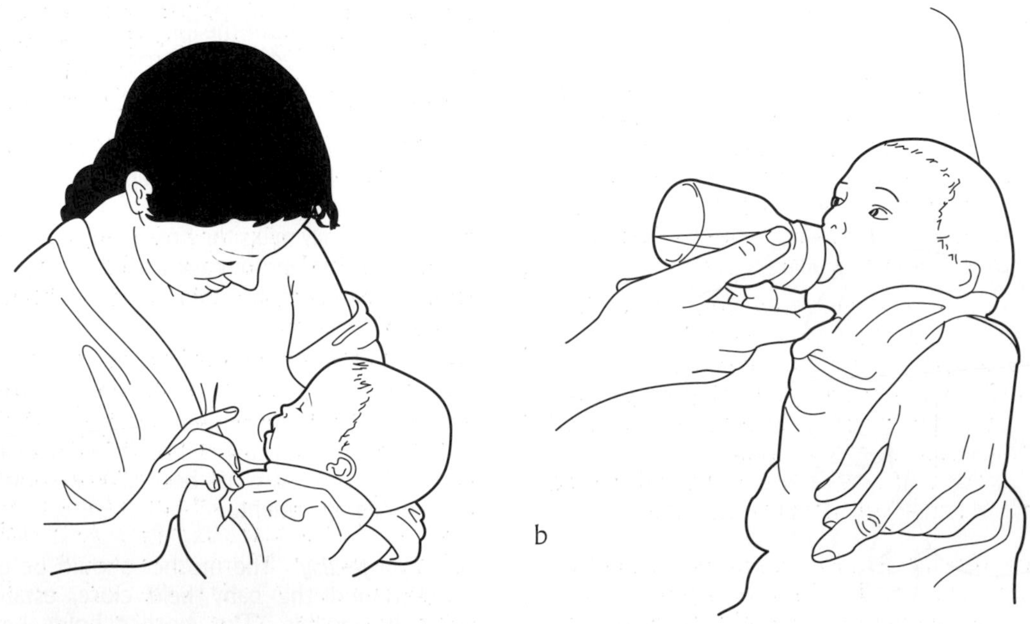

- Apply gentle traction, as this will often stimulate the baby to hold on to the nipple or teat and recommence sucking.
- Vocalize or sing, as this will sometimes help to maintain an alert state in the baby, as will a gentle tickle of the foot.
- Try using a 'NUK' teat or a nipple shield for the baby with a high palate as this reaches up to the palate to stimulate a suck.
- Experiment with a variety of teats.

Bringing up wind (some ideas) With the baby sitting upright, extend the spine with the heel of the hand while supporting under the arms with the other hand. Take care not to flex the hips too much, as pressure on the abdomen might cause vomiting.

SLEEPING

There is widespread awareness and concern in the community about sudden infant death syndrome (SIDS). Education of parents regarding sleeping positions cannot exclude discussion on the subject of SIDS. As a result of research presented by the SIDS Foundation, recommended positions for sleeping now include side lying or supine on a firm mattress, with no pillow and a minimum of extra bedding, duvets, bumpers or soft toys. A separate section has been allocated to SIDS later in this chapter.

If the baby is slept on the side, care must be taken to position the dependent arm well forward to prevent the baby rolling into prone. Alternating the sides will prevent asymmetrical head moulding and soft tissue tightening which occurs if the baby sleeps exclusively on one side. If the baby is slept supine, care must be taken to ensure that the head rotates both ways. This avoids head moulding and asymmetries. Should asymmetries be present, attending to the sleep position will often assist the problem.

Handling the older baby

SIX WEEKS AND ONWARDS

By six weeks, there is a weakening of the flexed postures and extensor responses become evident. Prone lying has an essential role in the development of the infant. Parents are encouraged to place their baby in prone several times a day. If they have not been doing so since birth, the six-week-old baby will not enjoy the position and may need to be coaxed. Some suggestions to encourage prone include:

- lie the baby over the forearm in prone (see Fig. 20.11);
- lie the baby on the parent's chest while reclining;
- place the baby across the knees, with head up to facilitate head control (Fig. 20.14). The baby will enjoy this position especially if given a rocking movement and if provided with entertainment by an older sibling;
- lie the baby prone over a large pillow. This assists head control and provides a more comfortable surface.

From prone, the baby has a varied view of the world and is given the opportunity to lift the head against gravity, straighten the legs and, by three months, to prop onto the forearms. From this position, the baby learns to roll (at about five months) and to creep and crawl (at 7–10 months). As most parents are advised not to sleep their babies in prone, many are reluctant to place them prone at any time. It is not uncommon for developmental delays to occur as a result of this lack of stimulus and this would require intervention by a physiotherapist.

Figure 20.14 Prone lying over lap.

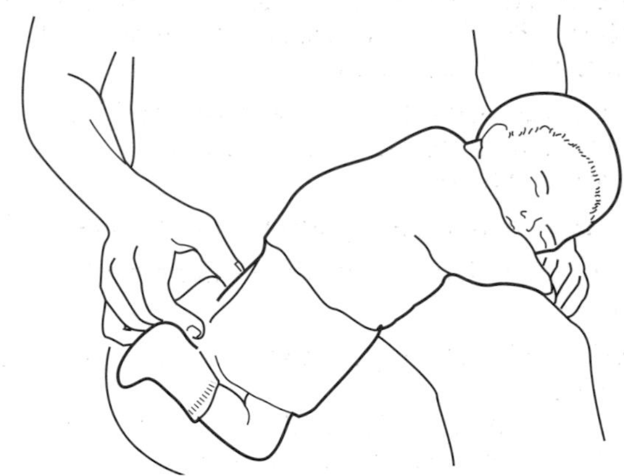

Advice to parents regarding the need for frequent use of prone positions should be given early, even ante-natally if possible.

By three months, the smiling, sociable baby watches the movements of his or her own hands (Illingworth, 1975) and parents report seeing the baby gazing fixedly at them. In prone, the baby extends the whole body easily and props on the forearms. He or she can be held in sitting by supporting the trunk, leaving the head to turn freely. The hands are held open and the baby spends time clutching at clothing, bringing the hands together, regarding the hands and sucking the hands and fingers. The baby will hold an object if placed in the hand, but rarely maintains the grasp and the object will fall away or onto the face. In supine, the baby is able to maintain mid-line orientation, kick freely and with more purpose and will show little head lag when pulled to sitting.

The three-month-old baby can be placed in the following situations during wakeful hours.

- Prone play – the baby should be happy to spend time on the floor or in the cot while on the tummy.
- Sitting in the stroller (semireclined) or sitting supported on the parent's lap.
- Swing. The three-month-old baby is almost ready to sit in a bucket swing (supported with cushions) gently swinging. Allowing the swing to move as the baby moves will provide some vestibular input and if the swing can be moved, the baby can accompany the parent to the washing line, the verandah or into the kitchen where the swing can be hooked up to the door jamb. As the baby becomes older, the swing will become an enjoyable location while the parents are busy with other activities. The use of a swing is preferable to a baby walker or jolly jumper.

Baby walkers are *not* recommended for babies of any age, under any circumstances. The growing injury statistics and concerns regarding the effects on early locomotor development (Banco and Powers, 1991; Canadian Medical Association, 1987; Fazen and Fielizerto, 1982; Simpkiss and Raikes, 1972) have resulted in calls to ban the sale of baby walkers. Education for parents against their use is a necessary inclusion in any programme.

In addition, when carrying and lifting, it is no longer necessary to support the head, unless the baby is asleep or unwell. At three months, the baby will enjoy a massage, responding happily to the interaction. Bath time is an enjoyable experience, with a great deal of happy interaction between baby and parent.

Physiotherapists can provide parents with guidelines for stimulating the baby's development. Their knowledge of the neurodevelopmental stages and relevant milestones can help to guide parents to appropriate play. General advice to parents should suggest that baby development proceeds according to a loose plan. Various stages are achieved as the baby's nervous system reaches sufficient maturity to cope with that stage and as the muscles and joints strengthen to support the new independence. However, before a new stage occurs, a great deal of training is necessary. Most of this training is performed by the baby him/herself, but it will not proceed smoothly if the baby is not given opportunities to develop.

The baby who is overprotected by oversupporting or restricted in pieces of equipment (e.g. chairs, bouncers or baby walkers) will find it difficult to progress developmentally, as will the baby whose parents fully support the head and trunk for many months as they handle it. The baby who is not placed in prone will be fearful and poorly equipped to roll, creep and crawl.

Advice to parents should consist of encouragement to:

- provide the baby with opportunities for learning and training, whether on the floor, out and about in the stroller or in the cot on the tummy with lots of toys to handle;
- support only if the baby cannot maintain a position independently;
- withdraw head support as the baby takes over;
- provide semisupported sitting as soon as the baby enjoys that position;
- remove hands if the baby holds him/herself up;
- replace hands if needed.

A high chair and car seat should be used as soon as the baby is able to sit with support (usually 4–6 months). Make the home environment as safe as possible and give the mobile baby freedom to run. General safety precautions for infants are listed in Table 20.4.

Table 20.4 General safety precautions for infants

Bassinette and cot	No pillow for child ≤12 months (SIDS Foundation) Non-rocking cradles Firm mattress with minimum of extra bedding Cot sides 500 mm high, 50 mm bars, spaced 85 mm.
Stroller	Firm harness Difficult to tip Free-running wheels
High chair	Wide, stable base Full harness
Car restraint	Approved brand If second hand, ensure restraint has not been in a previous accident Never leave child alone in the car
Clothes	Close fit with no ribbons
Water	Hot water system no hotter than 50°C Cold tap on first, off last Never leave baby alone in the bath Remove wading pools, nappy buckets, fish ponds to avoid drowning
Stairs	Barricade stairs
Baby walkers	Do not use
Sun exposure	Hat and full sun screen when outside
Food temperature	Always pre-test food temperatures
First aid	Have a recent first aid certificate.

Baby massage

For centuries, parents, grandparents, aunts and other carers have been massaging babies. The therapeutic application has been used especially by the Chinese and they claim success in treating a range of illnesses in infants from colic to colds by this method. Indeed, they offer it as a drug-free alternative in the treatment of infant illnesses (Tiguia, 1986). Although many Western cultures are embracing more natural therapies, the use of massage in infants remains largely a means of creating a loving touch and is a bonding, calming exercise for both parent and baby.

Massage opens doors to communication and can lead to the development of a special relationship between parents and babies. Parents are encouraged to touch and stroke their baby from the moment of birth. In fact, most parents need no encouragement to do this. It seems instinctive to commence stroking the newborn's head and to fondle little hands and feet. Fingertip circles around the head, gentle strokes behind the ears and the use of thumbs to work across the forehead, easing away little frowns, can be used, as may a cupped hand, commencing at the eye brows and stroking up and over the head.

With the baby in supine, propped up on a pillow or on the parent's lap and using a little natural oil (such as almond oil), the baby may be stroked diagonally across the chest, alternating right to left, left to right. The stroke can be extended across the shoulder and down the arms, later moving across the abdomen and along the legs, using a hand-over-hand motion.

With the baby prone across the knee or on a comfortable surface, the hand can commence the massage stroke at the forehead and then can sweep up across the head and down the back, gradually moving down each leg.

Auckett (1982) recommends an abdominal massage to assist in relieving the pain of colic. Using flat fingertips, circle the umbilicus in ever-widening circles, in a clockwise direction.

Massage can be used at any time. However, it is wise if the first few sessions are tried when the baby is calm and relaxed. The baby then associates touch with pleasant feelings. As the parents and baby become familiar with massage, it can be used to calm and settle at stressful times. Older babies and children enjoy massage and, if encouraged, children will enjoy massaging each other and their parents.

Other Problems

Sudden infant death syndrome

Sudden infant death syndrome (SIDS), commonly known as 'cot death', is the term used to describe 'the sudden, unexpected death of an infant who has seemed well or almost well and whose death remains unexplained after the performance of an adequate post-mortem investigation including an autopsy' (National SIDS Council of Australia, n.d.). The diagnosis is therefore one of exclusion. No sufficient explanation of death can be given after other causes have been ruled out such as accidental asphyxia, homicide, metabolic disorders, infection or other lethal disorders. The incidence of SIDS is approximately 1 : 1000. The incidence has dropped significantly since the 1980s and this could be attributed to the 'Help Reduce the Risk of SIDS' campaign. In particular, avoidance of the prone sleeping position seems to have been a significant factor in reducing the incidence of the syndrome.

Involvement of the police and the coroner and the need for probing questions, as well as a thorough investigation of the death scene, causes significant distress for the family. Once the findings of 'cot death' have been officially presented, the family is left with intense grief reactions, in particular, anxiety, questioning and guilt.

Epidemiological studies have identified some possible risk factors.

- Co-sleeping (Byard, 1994; Scragg et al, 1993).
- Non-attendance at a baby clinic.
- Babies who have had a febrile illness (Byard, 1991).
- Lower socioeconomic status.
- Babies exposed to maternal smoking, both *in utero* and in the home environment (Scragg et al, 1993).
- Indigenous families (Alessandri et al, 1994).
- Cooler climates (National SIDS Council, n.d.).
- Babies who are slept in the prone position (Beal and Finch, 1991; Ponsonby et al, 1993; Ramanthan et al, 1993) and especially babies who are slept prone on soft bedding, such as fibre or Teatree mattresses, quilts or duvets or on free-flowing water beds (Ponsonby et al, 1993; Ramanthan et al, 1993).

Compelling evidence is now available to recommend against sleeping babies prone. Prone positioning for sleep is postulated to lead to hyperthermia, rebreathing of CO_2 or obstructive apnoea due to pressure of bedding on immature airways. It is also said that babies sleeping prone spend more time in deep sleep than in rapid eye movement (REM) sleep, so that arousal states could be affected.

In The Netherlands, the SIDS rate fell by 40% in 1987–1988 when parents were advised against prone lying for sleep. In Tasmania, Australia, the SIDS rate fell from 3.8/1000 in 1975–1990 to 1.6/1000 in 1995 after the same advice was given to parents. Similarly in New Zealand, the incidence dropped from 6–8/1000 to 0.8/1000 after parents were cautioned against sleeping their babies in prone.

In spite of prone not being particularly associated with an increased incidence of SIDS in the USA, both the American and Canadian Pediatric Associations have now advocated abandoning the prone sleeping position for infants, as have health authorities in Australia, France, The Netherlands, United Kingdom, Northern Ireland, Belgium, Hong Kong, New Zealand and Germany.

The cause of SIDS is by definition unknown. However, Ponsonby et al (1993) suggest that SIDS appears to be a biphasic event, with a possible combination of ante-natal factors making an infant vulnerable and with environmental loading factors being required to trigger the death.

The significant environmental factors seem to be the prone position for sleeping, hyperthermia caused by either a febrile illness or environmental conditions such as overwrapping, soft bedding or co-sleeping and parental smoking. The factors which identify a baby as vulnerable in the first instance are the subject of much debate. The possibilities include:

- surfactant deficiency resulting in a prolonged expiratory apnoea, which does not reverse. This may be a result of high temperatures;
- obstructive apnoea due to soft upper airways collapsing when asleep, especially in prone;
- brainstem dysfunction occurring during sleep, which leads to cardiorespiratory instability. This in turn leads to a failure to arouse under stress;
- the dive reflex. Lobban (1991) hypothesized that the human dive reflex may be responsible for SIDS.

Recommendations for parents and caregivers

- Sleep the baby on the back, on a firm mattress, with a minimum of extra soft bedding, toys or bumpers
- Avoid overwrapping the baby, especially if unwell. Leave the head uncovered. The head is an efficient thermoregulatory area.
- Avoid smoking during pregnancy and in the home.
- Avoid co-sleeping.
- Breast feed if possible, as some studies have suggested the possibility of a protective effect from breast feeding.

PHYSIOTHERAPY

It is the role of the physiotherapist to support the education of parents in the risk factors associated with cot death or SIDS. However, parents should be encouraged to ensure that the baby spends some time each day in the prone position when awake.

Physiotherapists working with babies and young children are noticing an increase in referrals for developmental dysfunction related to the avoidance of the prone position at any time (awake or asleep). In the more recent publications by the SIDS Council, special mention has been made of the importance of the experience of prone in the development of young babies.

Other factors worth considering are the importance of alternating the sides when side sleeping. Physiotherapists are also well qualified to educate parents on the risks associated with smoking, not only in regard to SIDS but also in regard to childhood respiratory infections.

The physiotherapist working with women in the child-bearing years is in an ideal position to include education on baby handling and development and it should be obligatory for the education of parents and health professionals to include instruction on how to minimize the risks of SIDS when caring for babies.

Neurological disorders

A useful way of classifying neurological disorders is that used by Levene and Tudehope (1993) outlined in Table 20.5.

A baby significantly affected by any of the neurological conditions listed will show disorders of posture, movement, behaviour and autonomic homoeostasis. The assessment and management of these conditions is discussed in depth in the text *Physiotherapy and The Growing Child* (Burns and MacDonald, 1996) and this should be referred to for further information.

Table 20.5 Origin of neurological disorders of the neonate

Pre-natal – 70–75%	Down syndrome and other chromosomal disorders Neural tube defects, e.g. spina bifida Viral infections, e.g. cytomegalovirus Toxins and drugs
Perinatal – 20% 10% pre-term babies 10% full-term babies	Perinatal asphyxia Intracranial haemorrhage Periventricular leukomalacia Ototoxic drugs Kernicterus Hypoglycaemia
Postnatal – 5–10%	Hypothyroidism Meningitis Trauma Metabolic disorders

Table 20.6 Causes of pre-term labour and delivery

The mother	Diabetes Renal disease Cardiorespiratory disease Reproductive tract abnormalities Smoking Age (very young or ageing) Urinary tract infection Premature rupture of membranes Polyhydramnios
The baby	Multiple pregnancy Anomalies Intrauterine foetal death Infection

The pre-term baby

If a baby is born before 37 weeks of gestation it is considered to be pre-term. Possible causes of pre-term labour and delivery are included in Table 20.6.

Because many organ systems are still developing, the baby born pre-term may have some trouble adapting to extra-uterine life. The baby can present with heart and lung problems, food intolerance, poor immunity, poor thermoregulation, CNS insults, kidney immaturity and metabolic disturbances. It may show developmental and behavioural dysfunction at a later stage.

Physiotherapists are not only involved in the critical care of the pre-term baby, especially respiratory care, but also in the developmental and musculoskeletal care. Graduates from intensive care/special care nurseries have been shown to exhibit musculoskeletal and developmental differences compared with their term counterparts (see Table 20.7). Some babies go on to develop chronic neonatal lung disease (if they are still receiving supplemental oxygen after 28

Table 20.7 Developmental differences of pre-term neonates

Musculoskeletal differences	Increased extension – especially hips Increased occipitofrontal head moulding Increased external rotation of the hips Less ankle dorsiflexion Higher arched palates
Behavioural differences	Less time in quiet sleep Attentional disorders Increased activity levels
Intellectual differences	Learning difficulties
Motor disorders	Fine motor delays Gross motor delays Poorer postural responses
General health	More frequent ill health

days). These babies are at risk of long-term respiratory and developmental problems.

Physiotherapists implement and oversee programmes aimed at optimizing development by positioning and handling and provide appropriate stimulation programmes.

Grief

Many families experience grief over the loss of a baby. The process of grieving was described by Freud in 1917 as necessary in order to return to a normal life. This grief process and the importance of working through the stages has also been supported by Kübler-Ross (1969), Culberg (1972) and Kennell et al (1970). The grieving process usually proceeds as follows.

1. Shock and disbelief.
2. Anger.
3. Disorganization.
4. Resolution.

The time span is very variable and some people dwell on one stage for a lengthy period. There may be times when all seems to be proceeding well and then the person returns unexpectedly to an earlier stage, perhaps when faced with a birthday or a reminder of the dead baby.

A pathological reaction to grief (i.e. when the mother's health and well-being are seriously affected) has been reported in up to 30% of mothers (Tudehope et al, 1986). Factors adversely affecting the resolution of the grief process have been found to be:

- a crisis during the pregnancy (e.g. the death of a loved one);
- seeing the dead baby, but not touching it;
- an unsupportive partner or family.

The grief reaction is seen not only in the event of neonatal death but also if the baby is born pre-term or malformed or after a miscarriage or a failure to conceive. The parents grieve for the imagined perfect baby and a sensitive and caring attitude is important in any staff member in attendance. Some parents may grieve when the baby is not of the preferred gender.

For staff, the overanxious angry parent is often difficult to relate to. However, it is helpful to realize that anger and anxiety are part of the normal grief process. Inexperienced staff may require some support from colleagues at this stage.

Khong et al (1993) showed that presenting the mother with a package of mementos (photo, hair, hand or foot prints) helped with the grieving process. Giving the parents time alone with the dead baby or foetus and encouraging them and other family members to hold and touch the baby (Rafael, 1986) or even to take it home for a while has been shown to help.

Allowing the mother every opportunity to talk about the death is important. In the event of an intrauterine foetal death, miscarriage or stillbirth, well-meaning people will often prefer not to mention it and encourage her to forget about it, to get on with her life and perhaps to 'try for another one'. Some women have been known to welcome the opportunity to grieve over the loss of a baby perhaps 30–40 years earlier.

Children express their grief in different ways including withdrawal, disruption, nightmares, reverting to younger stages such as bed wetting, using baby talk or demanding the long forgotten dummy or bottle. Children need special understanding and reassurance that they will be cared for in a secure environment by both parents if possible. They need to be permitted to grieve along with the family and should not be excluded in any way. Attendance at funerals and opportunities to express their feelings should be encouraged. This is often difficult for parents experiencing their own grief, so help from others in the extended family or community is particularly useful here.

Physiotherapists working in the area of women's health may find that they can provide the opportunity for grief communication. Details of early pregnancies and losses required for the assessment of the woman who has come for assistance for physical problems may provide a trigger for grief expression.

Warning signs

A parent experiencing a prolonged grief process showing no signs of resolution and exhibiting depression, anxiety, continuing ill health or anger directed obsessively at one person or a group of people requires referral to a qualified, experienced psychiatrist, psychologist or doctor.

The physiotherapist caring for the mother at a later stage will often have the opportunity to detect the warning signs. The paediatric physiotherapist caring for the baby who is malformed or ill will have the same opportunity, as it must be remembered that parents and families of babies with disabilities or illnesses all go through a grieving process.

This chapter has provided an overview of management of the neonate that enhances the understanding of physiotherapists working in women's health. Physiotherapists working in obstetric hospitals, who are rostered to all areas, will need to study this topic in greater detail to provide effective treatments in special care and intensive care nurseries.

References

Alessandri LM, Read AW, Stanley FJ et al (1994) Sudden infant death syndrome in Aboriginal and non-Aboriginal infants. *Journal of Paediatrics and Child Health* **30**: 234–241.

Apgar V (1953) A proposal for a new method of evaluation of the newborn infant. *Current Research in Anesthetics and Analgesia* **32**: 260.

Ardran GM, Kemp FH and Lind J (1958) A radiographic study of breast feeding. *British Journal of Radiology* **31**: 156.

Auckett AD (1982) *Baby Massage.* Melbourne: Hill of Content.

Banco L and Powers A (1991) Hospitals: unsafe environments for children. *Paediatrics* **82**: 794–797.

Barlow TG (1962) Early diagnosis and treatment of congenital dislocation of the hip. *Journal of Bone and Joint Surgery* [Br] **44**: 292–301.

Beal SM and Finch CF (1991) An overview of retrospective case-control studies investigating the relationship between prone sleeping position and SIDS. *Journal of Paediatric Child Health* **27**: 334–339.

Bernhardt DB (1988) Prenatal and post-natal growth and development of the foot and ankle. *Physical Therapy* **68**: 1831–1839.

Beverly M and Nathan S (1995) Diagnosing developmental dysplasia of the hip (DDH). *Maternal and Child Health* **20**: 122–124.

Brazelton TB (1973) *Neonatal Behavioural Assessment Scale.* Clinics in Developmental Medicine No. 50. London: Heinemann.

Burns Y (1992) *N.S.M.D.A. Physiotherapy Assessment for Infants and Young Children.* Brisbane, Copyright Publishing.

Burns Y and MacDonald J (eds) (1996) *Physiotherapy and the Growing Child.* London: W.B. Saunders.

Byard RW (1991) Possible mechanisms responsible for the sudden infant death syndrome. *Journal of Paediatric Child Health* **27**: 147–157.

Byard RW (1994) Annotation: 'Is co-sleeping in infancy a desirable or dangerous practice?' *Journal of Paediatric Child Health* **30**: 198–199.

Canadian Medical Association (1987) Ban sale of baby walkers CMA urges (Newsbriefs). *Canadian Medical Association Journal* **136**: 57.

Culberg J (1972) Mental reactions of women to perinatal death. In: Morris D (ed) *Psychosomatic Medicine in Obstetrics and Gynaecology,* pp. 326–329. New York: Karger.

Dubowitz L and Dubowitz V (1981) *The Neurological Assessment of the Pre-term and Full-Term Newborn Infant.* Spastics International Medical Publications, 5a Netherhall Gardens, London NW3 5RN.

Fazen LE, and Fielizerto PI (1982) Baby walker injuries. *Paediatrics* **70**: 106–109.

Gordon M, Rich M, Deutschberger J and Even M (1973) The immediate and long term outcome of obstetric birth trauma, brachial plexus paralysis. *American Journal of Obstetrics and Gynecology* **117**: 51.

Hesinger RN and Jones ET (1986) Developmental orthopaedics. 1 The lower limb. *Developmental Medicine and Child Neurology* **24**: 95–116.

Holen KJ, Terjesen T, Tegnander A et al (1994) Ultrasound screening for hip dysplasia in newborns. *Journal of Paediatric Orthopaedics* **14**: 667–673.

Illingworth RS (1975) *The Normal Child: Some Problems of the Early Years and Their Treatment,* 6th edn, London: Churchill Livingstone.

Irani RN and Sherman MS (1963) Pathological anatomy of club foot. *Journal of Bone and Joint Surgery* 45A: 45.

Kennell JH, Slyte H and Klaus MH (1970) The mourning response of parents to the death of a newborn infant. *New England Journal of Medicine* **283**: 344–349.

Khong TY, Hill F, Chambers HM et al (1993) Acceptance of mementos of foetal and perinatal loss in a South Australian population. *Australian and New Zealand Journal of Obstetrics and Gynaecology* **33**: 392–394.

Klaus MH and Kennell JH (1982) *Parent–Infant Bonding,* 2nd edn. St Louis: C.V. Mosby.

Kübler-Ross E (1969) *On Death and Dying.* New York: Macmillan.

Levene MI and Tudehope D (1993) *Essentials of Neonatal Medicine.* Oxford: Blackwell Scientific Publications.

Lloyd-Roberts GC and Fixsen J (1990) *Orthopaedics in Infancy and Childhood,* 2nd edn. London: Butterworth Heinemann.

Lobban CDR (1991) The human dive reflex as a primary cause of SIDS. A review of the literature. *Medical Journal of Australia* **155**: 561–563.

MacDonald J (1996) Physiotherapy management of musculo-skeletal anomalies – neonates and infants. In: Burns Y and MacDonald J (eds) *Physiotherapy and the Growing Child,* pp. 267–290. London, W.B. Saunders.

Marmet C and Shell E (1984) Training neonates to suck correctly. *American Journal of Maternal and Child Nursing* **9**: 401–410.

Merenstein GB and Gardner SL (eds) (1993) *Handbook of Neonatal Intensive Care,* 3rd edn. St Louis: Mosby Year Book.

Mutimer K (1994) *Birth-related brachial plexus injuries in infants: modern management.* Royal Children's Hospital report, Brisbane, Australia.

National SIDS Council of Australia (n.d.). Information Kit for Health Professionals. Brisbane.

Ponseti IV and Becker JR (1966) Congenital metatarsus adductus: the results of treatment. *Journal of Bone and Joint Surgery* **48A**: 702–711.

Ponsonby AL, Dwyer T, Cribbons LE et al (1993) Factors potentiating the risk of sudden infant death syndrome associated with the prone position. *New England Journal of Medicine* **329**: 377–382.

Prechtl H (1968) The neurological examination of the full-term newborn infant. *Clinics in Developmental Medicine* 63: 1–57.

Rafael B (1986) Grieving over the loss of a baby. *Medical Journal of Australia* **144**: 281–282.

Ramanthan R, Chandra S and Barnesse G (1993) *Report of the Chief Medical Officers*

Expert Group on the Sleeping Position of Infants and Cot Death. London: Department of Health.

Scragg R, Mitchell EA, Taylor BJ et al (1993) Bed sharing, smoking and alcohol in the sudden infant death syndrome. *British Medical Journal* **307**: 1312–1318.

Shepherd R (1991) The diagnosis and managment of oesophageal reflux in infancy. *Modern Medicine Reprint* **34**: 80–86.

Sheridan M (1982) *From Birth to Five Years.* Windsor: NFER Publishing.

Simpkiss MJ and Raikes AS (1972) Problems resulting from the excessive use of baby walkers and baby bouncers. *Lancet* **1**: 747.

Tecklin JS (1992) *Paediatric Physical Therapy.* Philadelphia: J. Lippincott.

Tiguia R (1986) *Chinese Infant Massage.* Richmond: Greenshouse.

Tudehope DI, Iredell J, Rogers D et al (1986) Neonatal death: grieving families. *Medical Journal of Australia* **144**: 290–292.

Williams PF and Cole WG (1991) *Orthopaedic Management in Childhood,* 2nd edn. London: Chapman and Hall Medical.

Yeo C and Tudehope D (1994) Outcome of resuscitated apparently stillborn infants: a ten year review. *Journal of Paediatric Child Health* **30**: 129–133.

21

Women in the Workplace: Ergonomic Control of Musculoskeletal Injuries

JOANNE BULLOCK-SAXTON

A woman's work is never done! So goes the age-old saying. Although in today's world there are many labour-saving devices, the modern woman often carries responsibilities involving long hours of duty. Women employed in industry or with major home-care responsibilities can be involved in a variety of tasks requiring strong mental, physical, emotional and social abilities. For many, additional burdens exist. The career woman with a family, the pregnant woman with several children, the woman caring for a disabled child or an ageing parent and the wife and mother confined to a wheelchair are all faced with the challenges of coping with prolonged demands on both their energy and time. Some traditionally female jobs in the workforce are also susceptible to special stresses. These include nursing, computer operation or repetitive work on an assembly line.

There are many tasks performed by women in which the sitting or standing position is maintained for long periods and where, if correct height relationships have not been observed, the posture assumed is inadequate and static work by specific muscle groups must be sustained for prolonged periods. Where household or industrial tasks require that the head, trunk or arms be held in antigravity positions, strain and aching of the muscles of the shoulder girdle, neck and upper back may soon result.

The frequency of task repetition in industry varies according to job requirements. In many instances, a frequency of thousands of times a day has been reported and it is not unusual to find that the task is 'paced' by the speed of the machine, so adding to the strain imposed on the woman. Many industrial tasks require repetitive small movements involving the elbow, forearm, wrist and fingers. Where there is insufficient time for relaxation, muscles are liable to fatigue and other soft tissues to injury. Surveys have shown that the shoulder is particularly susceptible to such conditions as subdeltoid bursitis following the use of machines involving repetitive shoulder motion, the elbow to contusions and bursitis due to rapid, repetitive forearm rotation and the wrist to tendonitis from repetitive movements of the hand. Prolonged standing with poor posture can also lead to the development or aggravation of leg pain, foot pain, arthritis and varicose veins.

Low back pain in women is also common. Epidemiological studies show that lifetime prevalence of low back pain can be as high as 60–80% (Biering-Sorensen, 1984; Svensson and Andersson, 1982). However, Biering-Sorensen (1984) has shown that while the prevalence rate for men decreases after 50 years, it increases for women in this age group. Chaffin (1987) refers to a National Institute of Occupational Safety and Health (NIOSH) study in which it was shown that overexertion was claimed as the cause of lower back pain by over 60% of people suffering from it and that approximately two-thirds of overexertion injury claims involved lifting loads. While such studies have focused on surveys of industry, Grandjean (1973) has suggested that considering the unnatural attitudes of the spine often required for household activities, it is reasonable to believe that home makers are likely to suffer in this way as often as do other people.

As Egan (1975) pointed out, women are not as strong physically as men, they cannot lift the same weights, stretch or reach as far, nor can they stand as straight. Yet they often work under the same conditions and use exactly the same equipment as men. It is not surprising that Egan's analysis of injuries at work showed that in the area of manual handling, women incurred more work injuries (e.g. sprains and strains) than men. Further, far more women than men appear to be involved in repetitive tasks and they are thus at greater risk for some forms of musculoskeletal injury than men because of the overuse of muscles involved and the muscle strains associated with the sustained posture.

As the well-being of the home maker indirectly affects her entire family, the consequences of poor working conditions are considerable.

To a large extent, the reasons for the occurrence of injuries or the development of specific symptoms such as fatigue or pain can be found in the neglect of personal requirements in design of the machine, workplace or task. It is therefore important to examine the risks to which women are exposed, to consider the areas presenting those risks and to apply principles which would ensure resolution of potential problems to health and welfare. Such an approach is embodied in the practice of ergonomics.

Ergonomic Analysis for Risk Assessment

Ergonomics is concerned with ensuring that the workplace is so designed that work-induced injuries, disease or discomfort are prevented and safety is ensured and that efficiency and productivity are maintained or increased.

Through ergonomic analysis, those aspects of the work situation which represent a risk to the worker can be identified and assessed, so that areas of risk can be placed according to priority and control can be implemented effectively. Discussion with the personnel involved often helps to reveal problem areas. Ergonomic analysis includes, on the one hand, an assessment of the workplace and the work environment in terms of the risks they present and on the other, a survey of the load imposed on the worker, a comprehensive evaluation of the worker's method of performing the task and their capacity to cope with the particular demands of the task. These categories of 'work' and 'effect of work' often overlap and analysis of one may confirm findings relating to the other. The most common and difficult form of harmful workload is continuous, slightly overloading work. The short-term effects of this are usually temporary fatigue experienced as unpleasant feelings or discomfort. It is important to recognize the factors causing fatigue, as their control could prevent the possible production of pain which often follows fatigue.

Risk factors

To introduce some form of risk control and protection of the woman against musculoskeletal and postural load, it is important to evaluate the risk in the workplace. Analysis of workplace characteristics and identification of risk factors involve consideration of the many factors which could influence workload. These could include:

- the general layout;
- the design of implements;
- the task itself;
- the person's working technique;
- the general organization.

It is important to note that evaluations must be comprehensive and multifaceted because factors influencing workload are often inter-related.

Minimizing the risks for low back pain

As one of the major effects of poor work methods in women is low back pain, likely causes need to be appreciated. Although low back pain is undoubtedly multifactorial, some of the workplace factors which have been found to be associated with it and which frequently exist in home-related tasks include:

- jobs with high physical demand, including frequent heavy lifting in combination with stooped postures (in flexion and rotation) or in a cramped space;
- occasional heavy lifting;
- sudden unexpected movements;
- sustained postures, including bent-over working positions, prolonged sitting and prolonged standing.

In addition to the more obvious physical risks for injury, organizational factors can also play a part in creating stress for women and must be considered in a comprehensive review of potential risk factors. In particular, peaks of activity need to be identified, and the time allowed for certain tasks determined, so that undue pressures can be avoided.

In seeking to identify risk factors associated with a woman's work in the home or in industry, particular attention should be paid to the following.

- Space and access.
- Static work postures (which involve consideration of height relationships).
- Dynamic work postures (which include movements restricted by clothing or some other factor).
- Stooped positions.
- General physical demands (which includes consideration of factors associated with lifting).
- Overall organization and control of demands.

HIGH-RISK AREAS AND HIGH-RISK TASKS

It is important to identify **high-risk areas.** Depending on the woman's circumstances in the home, these could be the kitchen, the bathroom, the laundry and the bedroom.

High-risk tasks involve lifting (for example, a heavy household implement, loads of washing or a small child), reaching

Figure 21.1 (a–e) Frequent demands of daily work combined with poor motor patterns for bending and lifting increase the risk of injury. Solutions to minimize risk need to be found for the woman (c, d and e) and correct movement patterns practised, to establish improved habits to decrease risk.

a

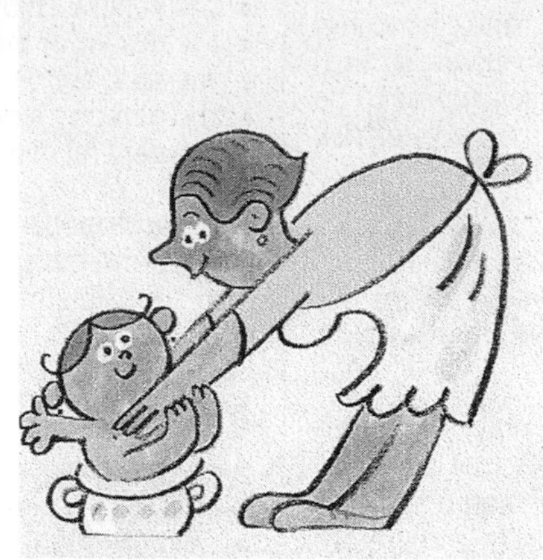

b

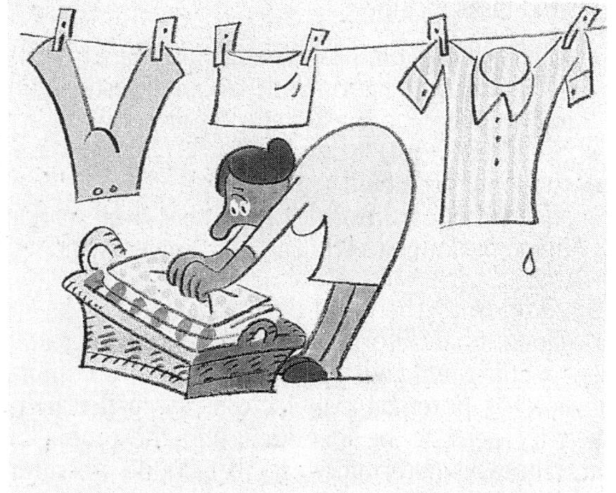

c

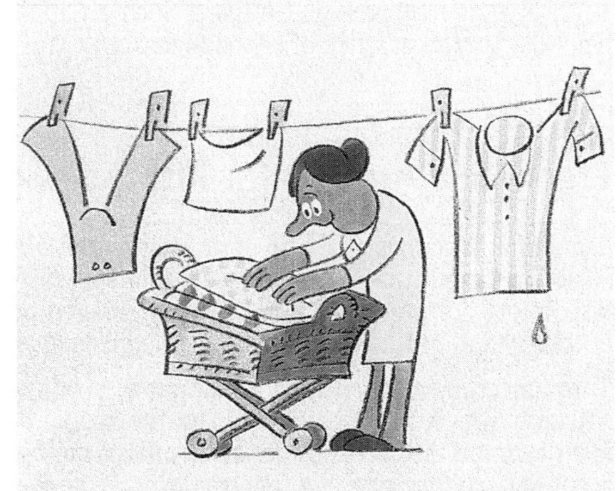

d

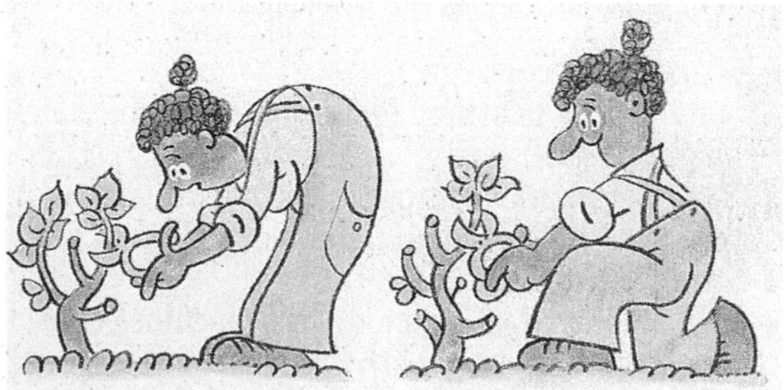

e

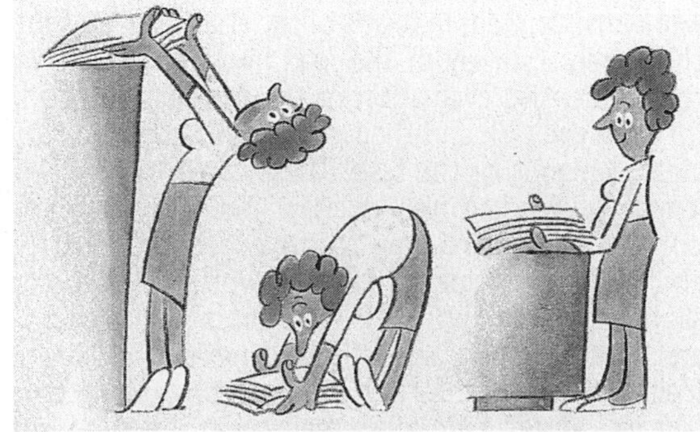

to high storage levels, stooping to do the gardening, to reach low storage or low electrical outlets or to manipulate household objects, placing an infant into a car seat, bending over a bath or cot, standing at the kitchen sink or at the ironing board.

Justification for considering these factors, areas and tasks as sources of risk is found in the fact that common precipitating events of female back injury include working in confined spaces (such as toilet or bathroom), moving heavy objects with insufficient assistance, carrying out tasks which are beyond the woman's capacity, acting hastily without consideration of safety measures and transferring young or disabled children or elderly parents from one position or level to another.

Risks associated with lifting

The high incidence of low back pain in women emphasizes the need to consider closely the particular risks associated with lifting.

As the spine or the muscles supporting it are most commonly affected in lifting tasks, it is important to understand the external factors which influence the load on the spine. These include:

- the weight of the object to be lifted;
- the horizontal distance from the body from which or to which it is lifted;
- the body posture of the worker;
- the duration or period of lifting;
- the frequency of lifting;
- the size and bulk of the object lifted;
- the height or vertical distance of the lift;
- the speed of the lift;
- the stability and steadiness of the load.

There are also internal factors associated with spinal stability and these are discussed in Chapter 14.

Vulnerability to risk for injury

While it is not uncommon for the able-bodied woman to develop fatigue when doing housework, problems exist to a greater degree for women during pregnancy, women caring for small infants, those with a disability or using a wheelchair, women caring for disabled children and also for the frail elderly. In each case, risks for injury and design to control such risks need to be considered.

THE PREGNANT WOMAN

Fatigue is commonly associated with pregnancy, especially in the first trimester and at term. Nicholls and Grieve (1992) suggest that carrying loads and walking up slopes are examples of activities which cause the fatigue. Fatigue can also affect posture (Oliver, 1994) and quite possibly influence the stability of the spine (Richardson et al, 1992). In turn, poor postural control may influence protection of the spine (Hodges and Richardson, 1995). A variety of approaches, such as relaxation programmes which include breathing exercises and awareness of specific muscle activation for the maintenance of stability (Gleeson and Paul, 1988), may help the woman to cope with demands more effectively.

Nicholls and Grieve (1992) suggest that together with many other physiological changes, a pregnant woman's weight gain and increase in abdominal depth can impose increased demands for postural alignment and can limit performance and endurance of everyday activities and tasks. A greater degree of difficulty is experienced in carrying out tasks and a greater risk for musculoskeletal injury exists.

THE ELDERLY

Fatigue can also increase the risk of accidents and injury in the elderly. Ageing is often associated with a decline in health, physical ability and sensory capacities, all of which can affect the elderly person's ability to function effectively and safely within the home environment.

For the elderly, natural degenerative changes such as muscle weakening, joint instability, decreased functional reach, increased postural sway and decreased visual ability can influence equilibrium when standing (Kelly and Kroemer, 1990). This possible instability affects safety in reaching to high shelves, removing food from the oven or items from a low cupboard. Any tasks which demand twisted or awkward postures could affect stability and increase risk for injury. In addition, forces required for such tasks as tap turning or jar opening may be beyond the capacity of the elderly woman and aids should be provided.

WOMEN WITH DISABILITIES

Women are subject to the whole range of disabilities existing in the adult population. A proportion of women handle their home tasks from a wheelchair, in some cases because of a stroke resulting in hemiplegia, through traumatic accident and a resulting paraplegia or from development of a disabling neurological disorder. It is essential that risks for fatigue and injury be identified for disabled women, so that appropriate modification to the home can be made. For the paraplegic population, upper extremity pain is a realistic concern (Sie et al, 1992). Gellman et al (1988) reported that 67.8% of their subjects experienced pain in one or more areas of the upper limb which, for 30% of the subjects, limited function or caused pain during two or more activities of daily living.

To the physically handicapped woman who may have successfully coped with a career before marriage, the additional role of housewife and mother may prove a traumatic experience. Whereas her work skills may have allowed her to be an equal partner with her fellow workers, she may now feel it necessary to perform certain physical feats in order to maintain her self-respect at home. The longer the history of her disability, the more likely is she to try and prove her physical prowess as a housewife. Weeks or years later, the accumulated fatigue may overtake her. Fatigue-producing stresses can often lead to erratic choices of expending energy. The needs of her husband and children often weigh heavily upon the physically handicapped woman's shoulders and, seeing no resolution, depression often becomes a natural state of being.

The individual nature of each woman's circumstances and relevant risks for injury need to be considered to ensure her long-term safety and well-being in the home.

NURSING

While risks associated with stooping and lifting exist for most women, those caring for the disabled, the elderly in the home or nurses involved in patient care within hospitals or institutions are particularly vulnerable. The majority of tasks causing injury in nursing homes are concerned with the handling of people rather than of inanimate objects. Elderly patients can exhibit unpredictable behaviour and combativeness, which increases the risk to the nurse. A decrease in the patient's balance and co-ordination, as well as a generally lowered level of ability to help themselves, are other risk factors.

A study by Stobbe et al (1988) revealed that the frequency of lifting patients is a significant causative factor in producing low back injuries. In addition, Baty and Stubbs (1987) suggest that for nurses, the postural stress of standing and stooping may be associated with a higher risk of back pain than dynamic activities. The high-risk areas for back pain problems in nursing have been identified by various investigators as being associated with patient transfers involving the bed, toilet, weight scale chair and bathing, or in repositioning patients in the bed or wheelchair, stooping to tend patients, adjusting the bed or picking up objects from the floor.

Application of ergonomics for risk control

Once a risk has been identified, it is important to decide whether it can be eliminated or minimized. The preference is to eliminate the risk and this could be achieved by changing the work process to remove the need for the activity creating the hazard. This often requires considerable adaptation, since most people develop patterns of behaviour and work which can be difficult to change.

In her comprehensive text, Bullock (1990) has outlined the many-faceted role of the physiotherapist in controlling risks. To be effective, prevention strategies should initially focus upon some organizational change whereby the woman herself will learn to identify and control risk factors in her own work situation. Without this participation, it is unlikely that preventive processes will be successful. Where stress is high, improved organization through long-term planning can often minimize the problem. Usually, peak demands are well known. In an office, stress could be alleviated during periods of peak demand by diverting telephone calls to an answering service at those times. This may also be appropriate within the home where severe stresses from many quarters are often placed on the woman. Her careful planning of priority tasks for these periods could help to alleviate difficulties. This is particularly important for the woman with a new baby or several school-aged children or the woman with a disability where more time needs to be allocated for completion of tasks.

DESIGN APPROACHES TO RISK CONTROL

Ergonomic solutions to control the risk for injury in women in the home or in industry may be developed according to relevant design principles, as suggested by Bullock and Bullock-Saxton (1994). Those applicable to the risks enumerated above consider space requirements, dynamic and static posture, the physical workload, the work environment and organizational factors pertaining to efficiency and stress reduction. One of the most important aspects of the ergonomic approach is the concern for careful specification of the worker–task relationship within the design process, so that the load on the locomotor system is reduced. In particular, it is important to design the process to avoid peak strains and static loads.

TASK RATIONALIZATION AND IMPLEMENTATION

A question normally asked by an ergonomist after reviewing components of a work process is 'Is the task necessary?'. Not infrequently, modification to a process or a change of attitude towards priorities may lead to elimination of a stressful or hazardous task.

Task simplification and improvement of efficiency are important goals in the control of risks associated with fatigue. Task simplification is a useful approach for all women and is particularly essential advice for the disabled housewife. It involves:

- separation of a task into its basic components;
- using both hands;
- positioning equipment effectively for transferring between surfaces;
- designing more efficient and effective storage spaces.

The principle of using a 'working triangle' formed by the stove, sink and refrigerator (as advocated by Kantowitz and Sorkin, 1983) is important for the efficiency of all women in the kitchen, but more so for the disabled or elderly woman (Fig. 21.2).

CONSIDERATION OF MOVEMENTS

Because repetition of certain movements can lead to fatigue, strain or specific injury, the design of workplaces should be guided by principles advocating avoidance of any undesirable features of movements. For example:

- the components of the task should be arranged to permit a natural rhythm of motion, since flowing dynamic movements are less fatiguing than rigid stilted movements;
- where tasks involve a transfer of material, movements

Figure 21.2 An example of the work triangle for the kitchen environment. Such design considerations may be applied to a wide variety of workplaces.

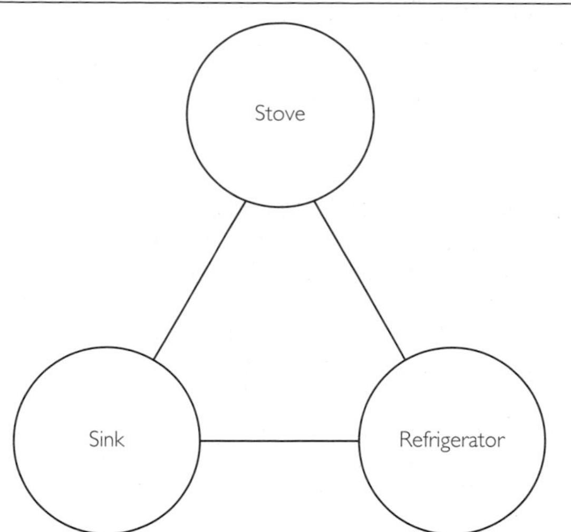

should be towards rather than away from gravity, so that weights are not lifted unnecessarily;

- materials, tools and equipment should be arranged efficiently and located close to the site of use and at comfortable heights in order to eradicate unnecessary movements, to permit the most appropriate sequence of movements and to avoid repeated asymmetrical reaching;
- consider the floor surface – hard floors have large reactive forces transmitted back to the body. Fatigue is often associated with prolonged standing on hard surfaces. Anti-fatigue mats, often used in factories, are available in domestic sizes and can be placed in areas of more prolonged sustained activity.

WORK LEVEL

Many household activities, constrained by current designs and by traditions of practice, involve repetitive or a prolonged stooping posture which, owing to the weight of the trunk, causes considerable strain on the musculature.

The suitability of work level in relation to the woman's body dimensions is important where sustained postures or lifting activities are unavoidable. The workplace and the equipment within it need to be at an appropriate height relative to the woman so that her posture can remain upright and so that excessive static muscle work of the head, trunk or shoulder girdle can be avoided. The woman caring for an infant or small child must be aware of the need to adjust work surfaces to suit her own dimensions or to modify the way a task is carried out to avoid excessive stooping when attending to the child. The infant's cot should not be too low and the mother should remember to drop the cot side when reaching to lift or lower her infant. Tables and benches positioned a little below the level of the elbow are desirable for general activities. Figure 21.3 illustrates a changing table designed to provide suitable support and storage for safe and efficient dressing of an infant.

Although the equipment, storage and work surface requirements for a workplace must be determined primarily by the nature of the activity, they must be tempered by the work requirements if the design is to be truly functional. If the work calls for the application of considerable force, then the bench top must be considerably lower than the level of the elbows so that the force may be directed downwards through the elbow joint. For manual operations which do not require much strength, the bench top should generally be no more than 10–15 cm below elbow height while, to relieve the muscles of the back during work requiring precision handling, a bench top above elbow level, to allow the elbows to be rested during the activity, is more suitable. Where possible, it is wise to have home facilities designed to match the particular requirements, demands and dimensions of the woman using them. Where the facilities are to be shared by others, some form of height adjustment should be provided to ensure that no individual person is disadvantaged.

Elizabeth and James had decided to remodel their kitchen and as Elizabeth had recently been attending her physiotherapist for low back pain she was aware of the importance of considering design to minimize stress. Elizabeth was a tall woman of 1780 mm and James was 1850 mm. They both enjoyed working in the kitchen and agreed to design the work benches to suit various functions.

Standard kitchen benches were 800 mm high which was 350 mm and 440 mm below Elizabeth's and James' elbow height respectively (1150 mm and 1240 mm). They decided on a general bench height of 960 mm and in addition, they had a mobile bench at 850 mm, with a board on top for cutting which required greater force to be directed downwards. There was no extra cost for the higher benches, as the kitchen makers were able to make the cabinets the standard dimensions. The compensation for the height was in the level of the kickboard.

They chose a cork surface for the floor which was less hard than their previous ceramic tiles. In addition, James purchased an anti-fatigue mat to place in front of the sink and adjacent bench as this was where they estimated the majority of their static standing postures would be maintained.

Bending to pick up a low placed object or reach a low control switch also occurs frequently in household activities. Storage sites need to be considered with care, while electrical outlets should be positioned at a level for easy access and reach without undue bending.

MAINTENANCE OF STABILITY

The design of tasks to ensure maintenance of stability is particularly important for the pregnant woman whose

Figure 21.3 A design for a baby change table considering safety and the anthropometric dimensions of the worker and child. Designed by Scott Bullock, Brisbane, Australia.

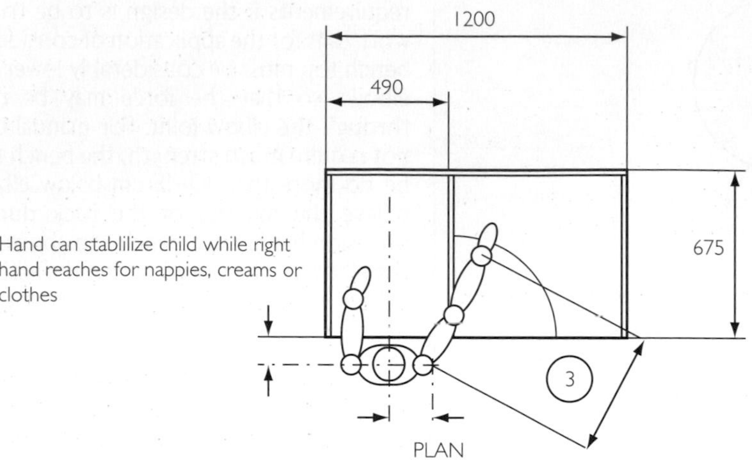

1. Height from floor to wrist
2. Height from floor to elbow in flexed to 90° position – 100mm
3. Length from shoulders to wrist with arm extended

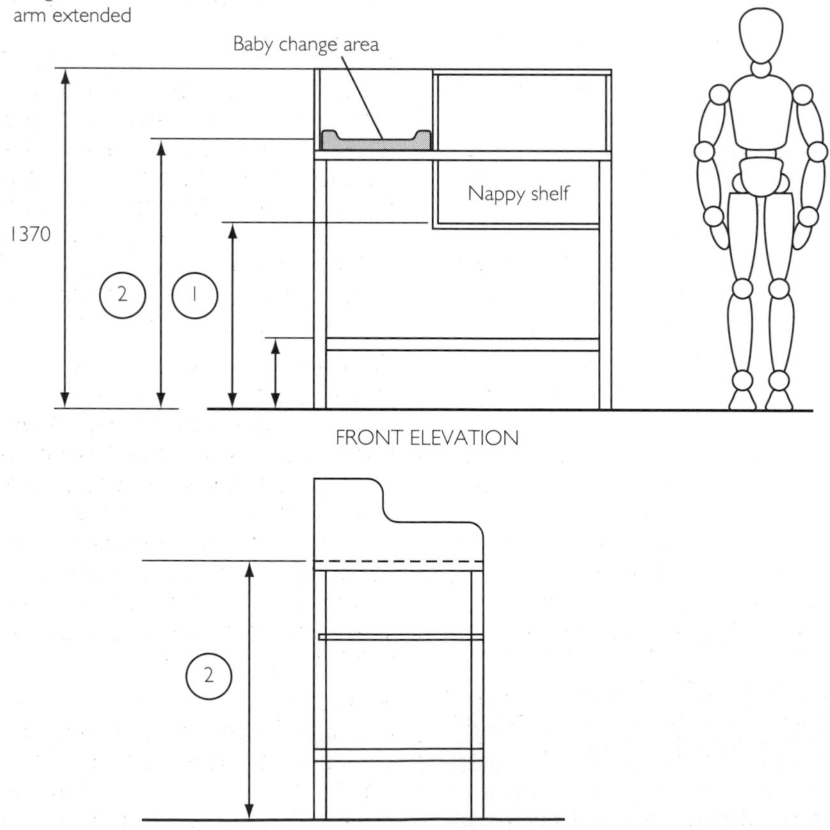

equilibrium may be influenced by altered mass distribution (Paul et al, 1995).

Where reduced stability or decreased muscle strength exist as risk factors (as for a pregnant woman, the elderly or disabled), it is important to avoid storage on high or low shelves. For safety reasons, the stove hotplates should also be regarded as a work surface and should be at the same height recommended for other benches, with a free bench area next to the hotplate so that food may be slid off directly onto a heat-resistant bench.

The elderly, whose stability is often impaired, tend to have accidents because of slower reactions and poor eyesight and hearing. Bright lighting, grab-rails in the bathroom and toilet and non-slip floor surfaces can help to reduce this problem.

Planning lifting activities

The woman involved in lifting children, frail elderly or patients who are disabled has persistent demands placed on her spine and needs to be shown an appropriate and safe method of handling, which will ensure maintenance of balance, postural control and avoidance of stress on the spine.

The physiotherapist advising on correct lifting procedures should recommend the following practice.

- Plan ahead.
- Avoid lifting heavy objects alone; seek assistance.
- Ensure adequate space is available.
- Use a wide base of support.
- Keep the weight close to the body.
- Bend the knees and hips comfortably and maintain normal spinal curvatures where possible.
- Avoid lifting combined with rotation.
- Minimize the distance over which the load is carried.

While everyone agrees that these recommendations are useful, there is often great difficulty in putting theory into practice. The physiotherapist needs to assess the factors that prevent the woman developing a new pattern of behaviour. One of these may be a poor motor plan for bending, which involves trunk and hip flexion with little knee flexion. Adequate muscle strength and flexibility of the knees need to be developed and the woman needs to repeat the movement of hip and knee flexion while maintaining trunk alignment. Only after the poor motor programme has been interrupted can any long-term change in behaviour be successful.

In relation to women involved in patient care, Garg and Owen (1992) have observed that some patient-handling tasks are so stressful that back injuries result even when staff have been educated in proper handling techniques. This highlights the view that control of risks for injury must be comprehensive, covering a range of preventive measures, including re-design. Several studies (for example, those by Dehlin et al, 1976; Garg and Owen, 1992; Greenwood, 1986; Owen and Garg, 1993; Wood, 1987) have reported on the inadequacy of education alone as a mechanism to diminish risk of musculoskeletal injury in nursing staff.

It should also be remembered that alternative equipment and procedures are available to substitute for manual lifting. These include walking belts, gait belts, the use of slings for hand gripping, mechanical hoists (for example the Hoyer, Trans-aid, Ambulift) and power-driven overhead lift systems. These have been described by Bell (1984), Garg et al (1991a, b), Holiday et al (1994) and Owen and Garg (1993). Other simple equipment which could provide assistance to the nurse in the nursing home or hospital situation includes bath and shower grab-rails, sliding boards, overhead trapezes, hand blocks and drag sheets, as described by Bell (1984, 1987) and Takala and Kukkonen (1987). Of the hoists available, studies undertaken to evaluate patient comfort and ease of use of the various hoists have revealed that the Ambulift is the most effective (Garg et al, 1991a, b; Garg and Owen, 1992; Owen and Garg, 1993). While principally developed for patient care in hospitals and institutions, many of these items may be used to provide lifting assistance for special circumstances in the home.

As an alternative to lifting, pulling methods have been recommended by Garg et al (1991a), following a biomechanical evaluation. These authors suggest that both one- and two-person pulling methods of transferring patients are significantly less stressful than the two-person manual lifting method.

Women need to receive advice and education on ergonomic principles which they can apply to their own work situation, using appropriate self-assessment guides.

Design for Special Populations

Redesign of the task and the workplace can have a lasting effect on the control of risks and, depending on the particular circumstances, structural redesign of a task or of a workplace should be considered. For example, redesign is essential where a woman acquires a disability and wishes to be independent within the home or the workplace. It is also necessary for the ageing person where capacities are diminishing but an independent spirit remains. Without redesign, frustration and stress could lead to an exacerbation of risks and almost inevitably to injury.

Generally, the design of houses and equipment should enable a person handicapped by age, injury, illness or pregnancy to move about freely. However, the redesign of a home or a work situation to cater for the special needs of a physically handicapped woman is essential for her safety and well-being. If the woman is in a wheelchair, architectural barriers must be removed. Remodelling and building alterations may be costly and often the family decides to make only minimal changes. Such decisions should be taken only after careful consideration of the long-term effects on the well-being of the woman.

A number of recommendations exist for developing an optimum design for those who use a wheelchair. For example, sufficient room must be available for manoeuvring the wheelchair in the kitchen, as the person must be able to move freely from one position to another. Goldsmith (1976) recommended an 'L' or 'U'-shaped layout in the kitchen with an unobstructed space of 1.4 m × 1.4 m when toe recesses were present and 1.5 m × 1.5 m when they were not. While the height of the work surface is important for all women, it is particularly important for the woman in the wheelchair. The bench height needs to be at an appropriate level for the wheelchair user, so that the arm rests may fit easily under it. O'Sullivan and Schmitz (1988) have recommended a bench height of 800 mm with a knee clearance of approximately

700 mm. Higher levels could place additional stress on the shoulder joints. Pull-out boards are also useful for wheelchair users. An adjusting device could ensure that the board could be fixed at heights lower than bench height for tasks requiring application of greater force (for example, when cutting objects).

Ease of reach is an important consideration. Goldsmith (1976) considers that the maximum reaching height of a person in a wheelchair is approximately 1.3 m and this should be the upper limit for any storage unit, so as to minimize the need to reach over the head, a movement which could irritate the shoulder complex. As for the able-bodied housewife and worker, heavy objects should be stored at approximately waist height. O'Sullivan and Schmitz (1988) recommend that for a woman in a wheelchair, if shelving is placed above the counter top, it should be no higher than 400 mm. The depth of a bench is also important, as the ability to reach forward from a wheelchair is curtailed. Goldsmith (1976) recommends that benches be no deeper than 0.6 m to ensure adequate and safe reaching from the wheelchair.

The placement of a bench alongside special storage units (e.g. ovens, refrigerators and cupboards) needs careful thought. This bench should have unrestricted knee access below the work surface, so that the woman may reach into the unit with safety. It is also desirable to have lateral access to these particular units.

Similarly, a bench placed next to a wall oven is essential for safety. A bench-height sink with shallow depth (e.g. 120–150 mm) is optimal to ensure knee clearance below the sink (O'Sullivan and Schmitz, 1988). For the wheelchair user, a narrow sink (e.g. not greater than 0.7 m) would allow the person to reach to either side of it without undue stress being placed on the back or shoulder.

An essential item for any housewife with strength or stability limitations is a trolley on wheels, which may be used to transport household articles from one place to another, so improving safety, reducing energy demands and increasing efficiency.

The psychological effects of disability must be remembered when considering the control of risks in the home. The physically handicapped woman under stress may adapt to fit her environment by developing negative attitudes, goals and behaviour. It is particularly important in these circumstances to change the environment to suit her physical capacities. By adopting more positive attitudes and rearranging priorities, some of the problems may be resolved. She must be assisted to understand that changing attitudes to housework can be of benefit and she should be educated to conserve energy, pace her activities and develop alternative ways of performing functional tasks, as recommended by Sie et al (1992). Certain household tasks could be eliminated and some of her physical energies could be applied to more fulfilling and relaxing leisure activities.

The current availability of telecommuting, whereby clerical work can be undertaken in the home, or of participating in modern education through various forms of media could provide important stimuli for women confined to the home for a large part of the day.

Summary

In considering the range of demands on a woman in the home or at work, it is essential that risks for injury be identified and appropriate steps be taken to control them. It is of the utmost importance that the relationship of the woman to all aspects of her task be considered, so that she may carry out her work more effectively, with less fatigue and less strain. In the long run, any action taken to ensure her physical safety and well-being must also lead to more effective use of her time and to a more contented home maker.

References

Baty D and Stubbs DA (1987) Postural stress in geriatric nursing. *International Journal of Nursing Studies* **24**: 339–344.

Bell F (1984) *Patient Lifting Devices in Hospitals.* Beckenham: Croom Helm.

Bell F (1987) Ergonomic aspects of equipment. *International Journal of Nursing Studies* **24**: 331–337.

Biering-Sorensen F (1984) A one year prospect of study of low back trouble in a general population. *Danish Medical Bulletin* **31**: 362–374.

Bullock MI (1990) Ergonomics – a broad challenge for the physiotherapist. In: Bullock MI (ed) *Ergonomics: The Physiotherapist in the Workplace*, pp. 3–12. Edinburgh: Churchill Livingstone.

Bullock MI and Bullock-Saxton JE (1994) Low back pain in the workplace: an ergonomic approach to control. In: Twomey LT and Taylor JR (eds) *Physical Therapy of the Low Back*, 2nd edn, pp. 305–328. Edinburgh: Churchill Livingstone.

Chaffin DB (1987) Occupational biomechanics – a basis for workplace design to prevent musculoskeletal injuries. *Ergonomics* **30** (2): 321–329.

Dehlin O, Hedenrun B and Horal J (1976) Back symptoms in nursing aides in a geriatric hospital. *Scandinavian Journal of Rehabilitation Medicine* **8**: 47–53.

Egan DP (1975) Health promotion in industry and occupational hazards. In: *Women's Health in a Changing Society*, Proceedings of a Conference on Women's Health. Commonwealth Department of Health, August, Brisbane.

Garg A and Owen B (1992) Reducing back stress to nursing personnel: an ergonomic intervention in a nursing home. *Ergonomics* **35**: 1353–1375.

Garg A, Owen B, Beller D and Banaag J (1991a) A biomechanical and ergonomic evaluation of patient transferring tasks: bed to wheelchair and wheelchair to bed. *Ergonomics* **34**: 289–312.

Garg A, Owen B, Beller D and Banaag J (1991b) A biomechanical and ergonomic evaluation of patient transferring tasks: wheelchair to shower chair and shower chair to wheelchair. *Ergonomics* **34**: 407–419.

Gellman H, Sie I and Waters R L (1988) Late complications of weight bearing upper extremity in the paraplegic patient. *Clinical Orthopaedic Related Research* **233** (8): 132–135.

Gleeson PB and Paul JA (1988) Obstetrical physical therapy. *Physical therapy* **68** (11): 1699–1702.

Goldsmith S (1976) *Designing for the Disabled.* London: RIBA Publications.

Grandjean E (1973) *Ergonomics of the Home.* London: Taylor and Francis.

Greenwood JG (1986) Back injuries can be reduced with worker training, reinforcement. *Occupational Health and Safety* **55**: 26–29.

Hodges PW and Richardson CA (1995) Neuromotor dysfunction of the trunk musculature in low back pain patients. Proceedings of the World Confederation of Physical Therapists Conference, Washington.

Holiday PJ, Ferniew GR and Plowman S (1994) The impact of new lifting technology in long term care, a pilot study. *AAOHN Journal* **24**: 582–589.

Kantowitz BH and Sorkin RD (1938) *Human Factors – Understanding People–System Relationships.* New York: John Wiley and Sons.

Kelly P and Kroemer H (1990) Anthropometry of the elderly: status and recommendations. *Human Factors* **32** (5): 571–595.

Nicholls JA and Grieve DW (1992) Performance of physical tasks in pregnancy. *Ergonomics* **30** (3): 301–311.

Oliver J (1994) *Back Care: An Illustrated Guide.* Oxford: Butterworth Heinemann.

O'Sullivan J and Schmitz TJ (1988) *Physical Rehabilitation: Assessment and Treatment.* Philadelphia: F.A. Davis.

Owen B and Garg A (1993) Back stress isn't part of the job. *American Journal of Nursing* **93**: 48–51.

Paul JA, Frings-Drsen MHW, Salle HJA et al (1995) Pregnant women and working surface height and working surface areas for standing manual work. *Applied Ergonomics* **26** (2): 129–133.

Richardson CA, Jull GA, Toppenberg R et al (1992) Techniques for active lumbar stabilisation for spinal protection: a pilot study. *Australian Journal of Physiotherapy* **38**(2), 105–112.

Sie H, Waters RL, Adkins RH et al (1992) Upper extremity pain in the post rehabilitation spinal-cord injured patient. *Archives of Physical Medicine and Rehabilitation* **73** (1): 44–48.

Stobbe TJ, Plummer RW, Jensen RC et al (1988) Incidence of low back injuries among nursing personnel as a function of patient lifting frequency. *Journal of Safety Research* **19**: 21–28.

Svensson HO and Andersson GBJ (1982) Low back pain in 40–47 year old men. Frequency of occurrence and impact on medical services. *Scandinavian Journal of Rehabilitation Medicine* **14**: 47–53.

Takala EP and Kukkonen R (1987) The handling of patients on geriatric wards: a challenge for on-the-job training. *Applied Ergonomics* **18**: 17–22.

Wood DJ (1987) Design and evaluation of a back injury prevention program within a geriatric hospital. *Spine* **12**: 77–82.

22

Women with Special Needs

ZOE McLACHLAN

There are a number of groups within the community who need particular care during the child-bearing year. Identification of these women and attention to their needs will help them cope more effectively with pregnancy and motherhood.

Adolescent Mothers

Pregnancy often comes as a shock both to teenage girls and to their families. There will be many issues to be explored by the girl, her partner, if he is involved, and by their families. Most of these issues will not involve the physiotherapist specifically, unless there are separate physical problems. These girls usually need early contact with hospital or community social workers to help them work through their issues. The types of issues to be confronted include deciding whether or not to keep the baby, options if they do not, continuing education, financial support and relationship issues. It is a time of great change and stress for all concerned with huge implications for the rest of their lives.

Many young girls/couples may not fit into routine ante-natal education classes. They may feel very different to other class members and, indeed, their needs and experiences will be quite different. These girls may need individual education or, if appropriate, education in groups together. Some hospitals run groups for 'Young Mums', which may include slightly older girls, if their circumstances and needs are similar. This is probably the ideal as it fosters group support, learning and sharing. These girls are likely to need more educational input on baby needs, e.g. awareness of babies' abilities, limitations and dependence. They will appreciate the opportunity to observe other young mothers handling their babies. In these classes, the physiotherapist will become an important member of the team which will usually consist of a parent education midwife, a social worker and a physiotherapist but may include input from other professionals.

The role of the physiotherapist will be as for other ante-natal education, but with particular emphasis on parenting and baby handling skills. These young girls should be given more explanation and suggestions of how to cope physically and emotionally with the demands that a baby places upon them. They also need information on baby handling, developmental stages and ways to play with a baby to enhance its development.

In some places programmable doll babies (Baby Think It Over) are used to help adolescents learn mothering skills. The 'baby' is programmed to cry at intervals and its crying is only settled when it receives the appropriate handling and care. Microprocessors record what type and how much handling is given. This introduction to the challenge of caring for a baby was piloted at one Brisbane high school in 1997, in the hope that the reality of parenting, rather than a glamourous view, is brought home to adolescents (Koch, 1997).

Written and verbal information will need to be in language understood by the young girls, possibly using colloquial terms. To aid this communication some hospital groups may encourage the new mums to return to the group after the baby's birth so that the peer support can continue and ideas and practicalities can be shared.

Apart from the emotional factors, pregnancy and labour during adolescence present no more problems than in a normal group in the community (Bradford and Giles, 1989). The tendency to low birth weight in some studies probably reflects poor sociodemographic and ante-natal care status in this group.

The Older Primipara

Women at the other end of the child-bearing age range may also present with special needs. These days, as many women delay their child-bearing, the older mother does not usually present as a 'special need'. However, some women in their 40s may feel they are different and conspicuous in clinics and ante-natal classes. Medically, they are usually managed most carefully as statistics show they have an increased risk of complications and interventions. There is often the 'precious baby' phenomenon in the older woman, i.e. the woman with infertility problems who finally conceives, often with the help of modern technology – IVF (*in vitro* fertilization), GIFT (gonad interfallopian transfer – placing semen and/or ovum into the fallopian tube and letting fertilization happen naturally) and ovulation stimulation. These pregnancies are more carefully nurtured and monitored and the woman may be advised against much physical activity although this is not as common now as it was in the earlier stages of such technology. Now, once the pregnancy has been firmly established at 15 weeks, women are usually advised to act 'normally'.

Some of these women are intelligent, motivated career women who are used to having a very organized life. They may appreciate discussion during pregnancy to help prepare them for the disorganization a baby is likely to bring into their lives. They often have unrealistic expectations regarding the demands a baby will make and their ability to return to their careers as planned. They may need to be encouraged to plan more flexible programmes.

Pregnancy and Already Existing Medical Conditions

Consideration of the effects of pregnancy on already existing diseases and conditions is paramount for those women involved. Many are worried about the effect of the disease on their pregnancy and child and the effects of the pregnancy on their condition. Some of these effects, in conditions relevant to physiotherapy, are detailed here but more comprehensive material is to be found in obstetric reference texts.

Autoimmune disease

Women who have *rheumatoid arthritis* experience moderation of their disease during pregnancy; 75% will improve during the first and second trimester, with maximum improvement in the third trimester. However, 90% of these patients will have a flare-up in the puerperium. It is thought that hormones are responsible for the ameliorating effects of pregnancy, as the contraceptive pill also seems to have that effect (Hutchinson, 1993).

However, women with *systemic lupus erythematosus* (SLE) have less likelihood of improvement during pregnancy and a higher probability of a flare-up in the puerperium.

Neurological disease

Many studies have retrospectively looked at *multiple sclerosis* and pregnancy and it appears that pregnancy does not alter the risks of long-term disability (Hutchinson, 1993). There seems to be evidence that the disease stabilizes during pregnancy but there is an increased risk of relapse in the three months of the puerperium (Albert and Morrison, 1992; Roullet et al, 1993).

Respiratory disease

With better treatment for cystic fibrosis (CF), many patients are surviving into their 30s and 40s and some will become pregnant. They have a 20–25% increased risk of a pre-term delivery (Kent and Farquaharson, 1993). One of the possible causes is thought to be the potential effect of chronic hypoxia on the foetus. A predictor of a successful outcome to the pregnancy in a CF woman is a 50% or greater functional vital capacity (FVC) in comparison with predicted levels or a reasonable time of stable pulmonary condition preceding the pregnancy. During pregnancy intensive surveillance of mother and foetus is necessary. Breast feeding is not contraindicated in these conditions.

Women with chronic respiratory conditions apart from CF, such as *severe asthma* and *bronchiectasis*, may need more help during pregnancy. Some may find their asthma less stable during pregnancy and also that they are prone to acute exacerbations needing hospitalization. Hypoxia for any length of time needs to be avoided because of the effects on the foetus. All respiratory patients find diaphragmatic excursion curtailed late in pregnancy by the gravid uterus. Positioning for removal of secretions will need to be limited to the horizontal as tipping will be impossible from about 6–7 months gestation. Many women find it harder to recover from respiratory infections later in pregnancy and may need to be hospitalized for rest, medical management and physiotherapy.

Women with Physical Disabilities

Many women with physical disabilities have babies and physiotherapy may be an important element in their care. The physical disabilities may range from relatively minor (e.g. scoliosis) to severe (e.g. paraplegia or multiple sclerosis). For all these women the physical changes of pregnancy can have a major impact on them physically and their ability to cope independently.

Women with the milder problems like *scoliosis* or other *pre-existing spinal problems* may need advice and monitoring from the physiotherapist. They need to be made aware of the body changes to expect, education concerning safe exercise, treatment for any symptoms arising from the pregnancy and adaptation or prescription of braces or corsets, etc. to help support their backs during the pregnancy. They should be encouraged to change their lifestyle to include more rest. Emphasis should be on prevention of problems from early in the pregnancy. Abdominal exercise, good lifting techniques, pelvic floor exercise and posture correction will be very important components of their care. Encouragement of regular exercise, preferably swimming, will be beneficial. Swimming will exercise back and abdominal muscles and provide safe aerobic exercise. Walking may exacerbate spinal problems during pregnancy.

Women with *spinal injuries* have increased risks of anaemia, decubitus ulcers, urinary tract infections, deep vein thrombosis (DVT) and pulmonary complications. Any respiratory problems will need earlier and more aggressive treatment as the woman may have increased difficulty removing secretions because of the pregnancy, especially in the third trimester. These spinal patients have the added complications of being unable to feel uterine contractions so they may not realize when labour has started.

Women with a greater level of physical disability should be monitored throughout pregnancy by the physiotherapist.

Conditions like multiple sclerosis, neurological disorders and paraplegia are difficult enough at any time, but pregnancy and birth are times of special concern for women sufferers. Weight gain and ligamentous laxity may cause problems with walking or transferring independently. The physiotherapist may need to help them adapt. They require education on the possible effects of the pregnancy on their bodies, encouragement to exercise to maintain muscle strength within their capacity and possibly more help with walking aids. Many of these women have concerns about the labour and may appreciate help in preparing for this. They may have fears about being stranded and helpless and unable to move during labour. Reassurance and suggestions for positioning for labour and delivery and education of support people will be beneficial. They should be aware that there will be an increased likelihood of a forceps-assisted delivery. If abdominal muscles are weakened, the woman is limited in her ability to push effectively and she may have difficulty in achieving a gravity-assisted position. The need for extra rest will also have to be emphasized as pregnancy and birth are likely to take a greater toll on their limited physical resources.

These women may need a longer hospital stay to recover or some form of mother and baby centre to enable them to recuperate gradually, before resuming independent living, if that is possible. Physiotherapy can assist with the normal post-natal problems of weakened abdominal and pelvic floor muscles and lax ligaments. Breast feeding may prove a challenge and the physiotherapist can help the woman to solve problems of positioning and safety.

Women using walking aids such as crutches or walking frames and those using wheelchairs face problems of transporting their babies safely. They can use a sling or use the baby's bassinette or pram as a support for themselves for short distances if it is stable. They may need encouragement to get extra help and social workers and occupational therapists may become involved.

Women who are *visually or hearing impaired* may need special help during pregnancy, delivery and the post-natal period. It is usually more satisfactory to provide individual sessions for education and preparation. With visually impaired women, the professional should put more emphasis on verbal communication and use of three-dimensional models. Hospitals may have to allow access to guide dogs, even for inpatients. It is important that the visually impaired person is not left without their support and it allows the guide dog to be familiar with the baby from the beginning. For the hearing-impaired woman, a sign language interpreter may be necessary and she should be encouraged to read as much information as possible.

Certain conditions requiring physiotherapeutic rehabilitation can result from an event during pregnancy. *Bell's palsy* has a sevenfold increase in pregnancy and presents more commonly in the third trimester (Albert and Morrison, 1992). Peripheral palsies include carpal tunnel-induced median nerve palsy and brachial nerve palsy.

According to Albert and Morrison (1992) *cerebrovascular accidents* occurred in a small percentage of pregnant women (less than 0.1%) but accounted for 8% of maternal deaths in the US in 1980–1985.The chance of ischaemic stroke is increased in pregnancy. Risk factors include hypertension, diabetes mellitus or hyperlipidaemia. Haemorrhagic strokes are likely to result from aneurysms, arteriovenous malformations or chronic hypertension. Surgery may be necessary to repair the defect.

Bed Rest during Pregnancy

There are a variety of problems associated with pregnancy that may mean a woman is confined to bed or hospital for long periods. The types of problems that may necessitate this are:

- threatened premature labour;
- hypertension/pre-eclampsia;
- premature rupture of membranes;
- ante-partum haemorrhage (APH);
- placenta praevia;
- intrauterine growth retardation (IUGR);
- diabetes mellitus.

These are the most common but there are many others, e.g. coincidental heart and lung problems and DVT. The prolonged bed rest brings with it many emotional and physical problems. Women are naturally anxious about the pregnancy and its outcome and if hospitalized, they are separated from their families and main means of support. While in hospital the women can become bored and may need some activities to keep them occupied. Being in a ward or sharing a room can be both helpful and stressful: stressful because they see other women coming and going and they wonder about their outcomes; helpful because they have company and can talk to other mothers who are experiencing similar problems.

The physiotherapist is often asked to help these women. This has to be done within the confines of her condition and there should be full consultation with medical staff, as there is some difference of opinion about the safety of abdominal and pelvic floor exercises for these women. According to Mayberry et al (1992), exercising in side lying during bed rest (e.g. breathing and isotonic/isometric exercise for neck, shoulders, upper and lower limbs) did not increase maternal heart rate above 104 beats a minute or increase uterine activity. Advice on suitable sitting positions when watching TV or doing handicrafts may be needed and also for suitable sleeping positions. Hot packs can be of great comfort, relaxation is beneficial and can be encouraged in many situations. Childbirth preparation can be done individually or in a group on the ward.

After delivery these women often feel very weak and unfit and need advice about a gradual return to fitness. A graduated walking programme will help. As abdominal exercises are often prohibited ante-natally if the pregnancy is at risk (e.g. placenta praevia, threatened premature labour, hypertension, APH), most will have less than normal abdominal tone. The women must be encouraged to do their exercises and take extra care with their backs in the initial post-partum period.

If a woman delivers her baby prematurely, she is usually discharged long before her baby. This brings advantages and disadvantages. She is still very busy expressing breast milk regularly, looking after other members of the family and coming in to visit her baby. This leaves little time for her to exercise and rest. It may be a worrying time, as most premature babies experience fluctuations in well-being. Bonding with such a baby may not be as easy. It may also be a time of coming to terms with the fact that the baby may not be perfect (see Chapter 20 for more details).

Women of Non-English-Speaking Backgrounds (NESB)

This category of women now form probably the most statistically significant group of women with special needs in many countries. In 1991, in the state of Victoria, Australia, 4.7% of the female population was of Asian origin and 6.9% of births were to Asian women (Rice, 1994).

There are women from many different cultures giving birth in Westernized countries. Those of European extraction may experience some difficulties with language but culturally are less likely to have problems. The groups likely to have cultural as well as language problems are the Asians and women of Muslim backgrounds, predominantly from the Middle East, North and Central Africa.

Professionals dealing with NESB women will find it invaluable to have some ideas of their cultural beliefs about birth and confinement. This can avoid misunderstanding and upset to the women and their families. Social workers usually have access to relevant literature. To scientifically trained professionals, many of these beliefs and practices seem to have little basis in anatomical or physiological fact. Some may seem amusing, some fanciful and some dangerous. The challenge for the professional is to understand and be tolerant of these cultural attitudes but to encourage practices which are beneficial.

Based on clinical experience over many years, the author has developed an awareness of some of the different attitudes of NESB women to pregnancy and parturition. Many Asian beliefs revolve around food. For example, Cambodian women eat different foods for the three trimesters of pregnancy and they believe that drinking beer makes the body beautiful. All Asian cultures try to avoid a big baby, no doubt for the good reason that big babies traditionally meant difficult labours. Cambodian women avoid showers and baths at night to keep the baby small and Vietnamese women keep active all through pregnancy, as they believe that an afternoon rest will lead to a big baby. Of interest to the physiotherapist is that Cambodian women think exercises during pregnancy are unnecessary and harmful to the pregnancy and 'look silly'. It is stated in the book *Asian Mothers and Australian Births* (Rice, 1994) that Cambodian women 'do not see the value of physiotherapy but would attend if referred by the doctor. However, they tend to abandon it if their condition does not show improvement' (p. 43). Asian women in general appear to have different concepts of body awareness to other cultures and tend to see the body more as a whole, influenced by food, temperature and spirits. Careful explanations are needed if physiotherapists are to be effective in educating and managing the treatment of individuals with such attitudes.

The birth process is considered best if it is as short as possible, but many Asian women believe they should be quiet and not complain about labour pain. Staff need to be careful not to underestimate pain in these women. It is often considered preferable that men are not present, but most want the support of their mother or other female relative or friend. However, during hospitalization in Westernized countries, many women prefer to have their husbands present as well and he may be a valuable interpreter.

The cultural practice of Asian and Muslim women has been to have a confinement period after delivery, that is, a period of 30–40 days when the mother rests, is looked after, eats the 'right' foods, keeps warm and does not bath or shower for several days (Rice, 1993). This is considered necessary to avoid problems later in life. These problems include bloated and wrinkled skin, prolapse and incontinence. The rest period is valuable for pelvic floor healing. However, it is difficult for Westernized health professionals to comprehend their belief that eating sour food causes incontinence. Chinese women believe they must lie flat in bed during this period to allow the back to straighten after pregnancy and prevent the stomach from sagging.

The establishment of breast feeding can cause many problems in the hospital situation. Many Asian women believe colostrum is 'bad milk' and should be discarded, so will tell staff they do not wish to breast feed initially. Then, after three days, when the milk comes in, they want to begin breast feeding.

One of the big issues with NESB women is the sex and age of their carer. Muslim women will often refuse to be examined by a male. Asian women prefer a female doctor, but may not insist and may subsequently feel humiliated after examination by a male doctor. They may also feel they should only be examined internally 'if something is wrong' and not routinely.

Indigenous aboriginal women

Aboriginal women in Australia have problems with some modern birth practices. Urban Kooris/Murris expect to deliver their babies in a hospital but generally dislike hospitals and miss their families. They dislike filling in forms and answering questions and feel they are being judged by appearances rather than as individuals. They feel uncomfortable having many people looking after them but are receptive to any procedure or examination if given a good explanation. Tribal aboriginal women may have to stay in a hostel in town prior to the delivery of their babies and they pine for their families.

The Koori (aboriginal) community is generally supportive of women during their pregnancy and post-natal period. The pregnant women expect to gain most of their education from other women in the community. From the physical aspect, women are unlikely to do specific exercises during pregnancy or to do general exercise such as walking or swimming. Sport is popular but is usually ceased later in pregnancy. It is unlikely that they would seek help for back pain or other musculoskeletal problems but would rather endure it. There is a higher incidence of gestational diabetes amongst aboriginal women than in the general population and so they may need education about diet (Cutter, 1989).

Indigenous women of other countries, such as Maoris or North American Indians, will have attitudes to health and childbirth that vary from the white populations. Every effort should be made to understand their needs whilst encouraging good health practices.

This is a brief background of cultural differences and the listed references will provide a more detailed picture.

Language can be a major problem. Hospitals need to provide interpreters as much as possible and telephone interpreters can be accessed out of hours. Families can be used, but only if necessary, as they will often answer for the patient and not interpret literally.

One answer to some of these issues is the training of professionals from the various ethnic backgrounds and having them available to work with their own people. At one Melbourne hospital, childbirth education for Vietnamese women is conducted by a Vietnamese midwife and Vietnamese physiotherapist. These professionals are uniquely placed to bridge the gap between cultures and promote a two-way flow of information.

References

Albert JR and Morrison JC (1992). Neurological diseases in pregnancy. *Obstetrics and Gynecology Clinics of North America* **19**: 765–781.

Bradford JA and Giles WB (1989) Teenage pregnancy in western Sydney. *Australian and New Zealand Journal of Obstetrics and Gynaecology* **29**: 1–4.

Cutter T (1989) *A Clinician's Diabetic Manual.* Victorian Aboriginal Health Service, Melbourne.

Hutchinson M (1993) Pregnancy in multiple sclerosis. *Journal of Neurology, Neurosurgery and Psychiatry* **56**: 1043–1045.

Kent NE and Farquaharson DF (1993) Cystic fibrosis in pregnancy. *Canadian Medical Association Journal* **149** (809): 228–229.

Koch J (1997) New 'mum' trial no child's play. *Sunday Mail*, Brisbane, 23rd February.

Mayberry LJ, Smith M and Gill P (1992) Effect of exercise on uterine activity in the patient in preterm labour. *Journal of Perinatology* **12**: 354–358.

Roullet E, Verdier-Taillefer M-H, Amarenco P et al (1993) Pregnancy and multiple sclerosis; a longitudinal study of 125 remittent patients. *Journal of Neurology, Neurosurgery and Psychiatry* **56**: 1062–1065.

Rice PL (1993) *My Forty Days.* Melbourne: The Vietnamese Antenatal/Postnatal Support Project.

Rice PL (Ed) (1994) *Asian Mothers and Australian Births.* Melbourne: Ausmed Publications.

23

Pelvic Floor Dysfunction in the Perinatal Period

RUTH SAPSFORD AND SUE MARKWELL

Pregnancy
•
Parturition
•
Puerperium
•
Summary

The perinatal period is a time of extreme change for the pelvic floor as well as other parts of the female body. Pregnant women have always been encouraged to maintain PFM strength and PF exercises are considered by some as the most important aspect of rehabilitation post-partum. While abdominopelvic floor coactivation occurs in normal women, how well this continues in pregnancy, particularly later pregnancy, and early post-partum is not known.

Trauma to the pelvic floor occurs during the birth process and whether this can be reduced by different positions for pushing, better pushing techniques and earlier intervention for prolonged second stage is still unclear. Also, whether more intensive and early muscle rehabilitation can make a difference to long-term outcomes has yet to be discovered.

However, for those women without obvious trauma following vaginal delivery it seems that focusing on gaining and maintaining lumbopelvic stability by using transversus abdominis (initially for endurance and later for strength – see Chapter 14) plays a major part in restoration of post-partum PFM strength. Isometric abdominal exercises, using transversus abdominis and the obliques, have been shown to activate pubococcygeus, the principal muscle of the pelvic floor (Sapsford et al, 1997). For others, vaginal delivery can be the catalyst for lifelong change in bladder and bowel function. This chapter outlines the processes of functional change specific to the perinatal period.

Pregnancy

Increased blood flow to the kidneys during pregnancy results in increased filtration and greater urine volumes. Hormonal influences – progesterone and relaxin – decrease ureteric tone and this relaxed state, combined with elongation and distortion around the enlarging uterus, provides greater opportunities for infection to ascend to the kidney. Urinary tract infections during pregnancy require early intervention and follow-up testing to prevent upper urinary tract involvement.

Changes to the bladder and urethra in normal pregnancy include

- an increase in total bladder and maximal urethral pressures (probably due to direct uterine pressure);
- a small increase in urethral closing pressure;
- a small increase in anatomical and functional urethral length;
- a marked increase in collagenous fibres;
- an increase in blood flow to the urethra, which tapers off in the last trimester of pregnancy.

However, no hormonal effect on the anal sphincters has been demonstrated during pregnancy (Sultan et al, 1993a).

The types of urinary dysfunction related to child bearing and their causes are listed in Table 23.1, but a full description

Table 23.1 Prevalence of urinary dysfunction during first trimester and at term in nulliparae and multiparae

	Frequency		Nocturia		Stress incont.		Urge incont.	
	Nulli.	Multi.	Nulli.	Multi.	Nulli.	Multi.	Nulli.	Multi.
Ist trimester	49.3%	41.3%	19.2%	23.9%	6.1%	26.5%	2.4%	5.1%
Term	95%	76.1%	72.5%	55.7%	34.1%	38.1%	5%	18.6%

Figures from Stanton et al (1980). Overall, women in their first pregnancy had greater day frequency and nocturia, but less stress and urge incontinence than those in second or subsequent pregnancies.

of the conditions and management is contained in Chapters 28 and 30.

Day frequency of more than seven voids a day occurs in almost 50% of women during the first trimester of pregnancy and increases in the last trimester to be almost universal, especially in nulliparae (Stanton et al, 1980). Early in pregnancy increased frequency is probably due to increased urine production and later it may be related to increased uterine size and restriction of bladder expansion. Being woken from sleep to void two or more times a night is generally regarded as frequent night voiding – nocturia. Symptoms of stress incontinence, urgency and urge incontinence (see Chapter 28) begin early in pregnancy and persist and increase throughout. Table 23.1 details the incidence of these conditions. The onset of stress incontinence in pregnancy, unless pre-existing, is hormone related. Decreased smooth muscle tone in the urethra and the supporting fascia and increased ligamentous laxity contribute to this.

Urinary urgency, independent of urge incontinence, is very common in the first trimester of pregnancy, with a prevalence of 57% at 11 weeks gestation (Cutner et al, 1990). Urodynamic studies (see Chapter 28) confirmed detrusor instability in 28% of those tested, but symptoms of urgency and urge incontinence occurred independent of proven instability. Women who had hesitancy in initiating voiding prior to pregnancy continued to have problems during pregnancy, but post-partum there was a definite improvement.

Women with uterovaginal prolapse prior to pregnancy experience some improvement in symptoms once the uterus enlarges and becomes an abdominal organ and the low-lying cervix and upper vagina are elevated. Cystocoeles also improve.

Gastrointestinal motility

Gastrointestinal (GI) tract disorders are common in normal pregnancies. Changes in circulating sex hormones are considered causal. Secretion and absorption are not affected, but motility may be slowed considerably (Baron et al, 1993). Oestrogen and progesterone receptors have been demonstrated in intestinal smooth muscle (Kamm, 1994) but their functional relevance is not yet fully understood.

Increased levels of circulating progesterone and oestradiol affect the upper GI tract, causing uncomplicated gastro-oesophageal reflux in pregnancy. Avoidance of substances thought to have a lowering effect on cardiac sphincter tone may be useful. These include chocolate, coffee, fried and fatty foods, alcohol and cigarettes. Simple pillow support to elevate the head and thorax during rest is helpful rather than using supine or side lying.

Nausea is a normal variant and occurs in 50–90% of all pregnancies. Vomiting is present in 25–55% (Baron et al, 1993). Symptoms will be more severe and prolonged in those women who have existing dysmotility (see Chapter 29). Delayed gastric emptying with early 'fullness' may occur in nauseated pregnant women (Koch and Stern, 1993). Dietary manipulation, with small frequent meals high in carbohydrates and low in fats, is helpful. Vitamin B6 and medication may be necessary (Baron et al, 1993).

In hyperemesis gravidarum, abnormal levels of progesterone, oestradiol, HCG and the thyroid hormones are implicated (Baron et al, 1993). Of particular interest to physiotherapists is the slowing effect on small bowel and colon transit. Bloating and constipation are frequently reported in the first and third trimesters. This is probably due to a combination of dysmotile and mechanical factors associated with the gravid uterus. Long-term hingdgut (left colon) dysmotility has been shown to occur after parturition (MacDonald et al, 1993).

Of clinical interest, rectal outlet disorders involving incoordination (see Chapter 29) often improve during pregnancy. Women who suffer from obstructed defaecation prior to pregnancy may find it easier to evacuate later in pregnancy when the enlarging abdomen alters abdominal muscle patterns during defaecation. This may be a transient state only and patients may have to be retrained during the puerperium. In addition to dietary advice, attention must be given to ante-natal evacuation techniques and positioning, to avoid straining at stool. During pregnancy, iron supplements, antacids containing aluminium and medications containing codeine may affect motility. Bulking agents may be used safely in pregnancy and the puerperium. In conjunction, safe use of osmotic or stimulant agents may be necessary (see Chapter 29).

How can rectal outlet disorders, uterine dystocia and optimum muscle co-ordination be linked?

A recent report described a 17-year-old primigravida who chose to defaecate at monthly intervals and who underwent a caesarean section because of persistent faecal impaction (Joels and Manyonda, 1994). Many factors lead to severe constipation and faecal impaction, but a psychiatric history is often associated with gross faecal impaction causing uterine dystocia, i.e. disordered uterine action (Joels and Manyonda, 1994). Devroede (1996) has noted forms of uterine dystocia relating to the pelvic floor. Anecdotal evidence suggests women may unconsciously retain the baby as a result of uteropelvic dyssynergia (muscle inco-ordination). The delay of the presenting part may be due to unconscious inco-ordination of the pelvic floor. Other examples of pelvic organ and pelvic floor dyssynergia include difficulty in voiding and 'anismus' (inability to release the anus) (see Chapters 28 and 29). Many workers have noted the prevalence of past sexual abuse with pelvic outlet disorders. Kumar et al (1989) showed that psychological stress and physical pain increased both the resting pressure of the internal anal sphincter and external anal sphincter activity. This factor may not be recognized in labouring women.

What is the common link? How should physiotherapists be involved?

Expulsion of both foetus and faeces requires the same co-ordinated activity. Physiotherapists are the ideal obstetric team members to assess dysfunction. They help patients recruit specific abdominopelvic floor muscles required for pelvic organ function, before labour begins. Sitting or squatting with a normal lumbar curve and fully flexed hips and knees promotes more efficient rectal emptying. However, squatting in this way may not be easy for Westernized women. Scott (1995) noticed that by encouraging a similar position in pregnancy and labour an occipito-anterior presentation was more common. Clinical observation in midwifery (Scott, 1995) and in defaecation disorders (Markwell and Sapsford, 1995) has led to identification of 'at-risk' groups in both categories. Persistent posterior pelvic tilting as a postural habit in standing and sitting is considered a significant factor. Elite athletes and those who over-develop their abdominal muscles, particularly the rectus abdominis, have difficulty in co-ordinating levator support with sphincter release (Sapsford et al, 1996).

Parturition

The most obvious and immediate effect of vaginal delivery and its management on the pelvic floor is the presence of an episiotomy or perineal tear. Depending on its extent, an episiotomy cuts through vaginal epithelium and perineal skin, fascia and bulbospongiosus muscle, superficial and deep perineal muscles, external anal sphincter (sometimes) and the levator ani (if the incision is extensive). However, the levator ani muscle is usually displaced upwards away from the scissors as the head stretches the perineum. The ischiorectal fossa fat may be cut in deep incisions (Beischer and Mackay, 1986). A tear can extend towards the urethra or, more commonly, posteriorly and if extensive, into the anal muscle and mucosa.

These lesions are usually sutured in the labour ward under top-up epidural or local analgesia. The type of suture material, the method of suturing used and the skill of the clinician can all play a part in minimizing postpartum perineal pain (Harris, 1992). In some centres tears into the anal sphincter are repaired under anaesthesia by an experienced surgeon. See Chapter 19 for immediate post-partum management of perineal trauma and pain.

The effects of vaginal delivery on PFM function have been the focus of recent investigations in an attempt to establish the causes of prolapse and functional bladder and bowel disorders. Up to 80% of women sustain PFM damage during their first vaginal delivery (Allen et al, 1990). Though many conditions present clinically later in life, the basis can often be traced back to an obstetric event, whose effect has been compounded by further parity and age. Studies show that those women who have elective ceasarean sections are spared this damage (Allen et al, 1990; Sultan et al, 1993b; Wynne et al, 1996).

Modern investigative techniques enable precise definitions of defects, but most conditions arise from a combination of factors. Anal endosonography, EMG, nerve conduction and muscle fibre density studies have all provided enlightening information. However, prevention and remediation still present great challenges.

Anal sphincter tears

The anal sphincter is the most accessible part of the striated pelvic floor and often presents the most obvious defect at the time of delivery. Open (overt) sphincter tears (third degree external sphincter, fourth degree external sphincter and mucosa) occur in 0.7% of women who have posterolateral episiotomies (Sultan et al, 1993b). Women who have had a complete anal tear and repair are generally allowed to have a vaginal delivery in a subsequent pregnancy. However, those who have experienced transient anal incontinence after the tear are at risk of permanent anal incontinence after a subsequent vaginal delivery (Bek and Laurberg, 1992). The sphincter can also suffer hidden (occult) disruption. Anal ultrasound has been used to discover partial or complete tears in the internal or external sphincter or both, as a result of a

Table 23.2 Prevalence of anal sphincter defects, detected by anal endosonography, at 34 weeks of pregnancy and six weeks after delivery (Sultan et al, 1993b)

	Ante-natal	Six weeks post-natal
Primigravidae	0%	35%
Multigravidae	40%	44%

vaginal delivery. Shearing forces created by the descent of the foetal head are considered responsible. Figures indicate a high incidence of sphincter disruption without recovery six months post-partum.

Denervation of external anal sphincter and the pelvic floor

Increased nerve conduction times are indicative of denervation. Pudendal nerve terminal motor latency (PNTML) measures conduction time in the inferior haemorrhoidal branch of the pudendal nerve supplying the external anal sphincter. This time was lengthened at 48–72 hours following vaginal delivery in comparison with controls, being longer in multipara and those who had forceps deliveries. By two months post-partum there had been significant recovery, indicating that much of the damage was reversible (Snooks et al, 1984).

PNTML compared ante-natally and 6–8 weeks post-partum in the same subjects showed a significant increase in conduction time with greater damage on the left side. When retested at six months post-partum, two-thirds had recovered. Birth weight of >4000 g and an active second stage of >30 minutes in primiparae were significant factors in this damage (Sultan et al, 1994).

Measurement of motor unit potentials of the pubococcygeus indicated partial denervation of the pelvic floor in 80% of primiparae delivering vaginally. The length of the second stage and weight of the baby were significant factors (Allen et al, 1990).

Perineal descent

The position of the perineum (anal verge) in relation to the ischial tuberosities at rest and on straining indicates the extent of soft tissue laxity. Descent on straining below the level of the ischial tuberosity is considered abnormal (Fig. 23.1). Both planes (rest and straining) were lower and the extent of the descent greater after the first vaginal delivery. Abnormal perineal descent on straining was frequently accompanied by increased nerve conduction times. Three-quarters of the multiparae tested had abnormal descent on straining (Sultan et al, 1994).

Figure 23.1 Weakness of the muscles of the pelvic floor and fascial stretching is disclosed by a 'descending perineum'. (Reproduced from Kiff (1993) with permission.)

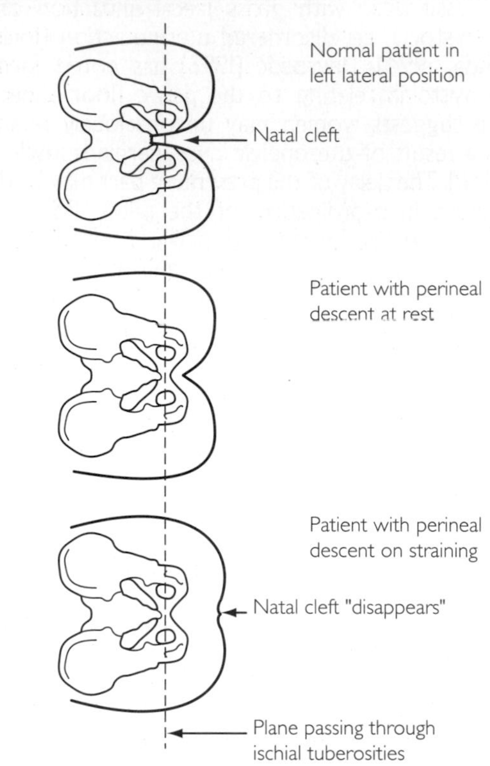

Local anorectal pathology

HAEMORRHOIDS

Haemorrhoids may cause symptoms for the first time during pregnancy. They have a familial incidence and may be graded by severity of symptoms. In the pregnant or parturient female the interaction of follicle-stimulating hormone, prolactin and glucocorticoids may play a causative role (Thompson et al, 1992). They may result from or be aggravated by maternal expulsive effort during the second stage of labour. In one series they occurred in 35% of women early post-partum (Thomas et al, 1993). They usually cause pain, itching and bleeding. Advice regarding soluble dietary fibre intake, perianal support during defaecation and the use of optimum defaecation dynamics can be helpful. Use of a special cooling device had little effect in reducing pain (Thomas et al, 1993). Ice provides temporary relief and rectal ointments may be helpful. Referral to a surgeon may be necessary.

FISTULAE

Obstetric rectovaginal fistulae are uncommon. They may arise from incomplete healing of a perineal body laceration. Fistulae may occur above the puborectalis and the anal sphincters, with discharge being able to seep through the opening in the posterior vaginal wall (Hudson, 1992). Trauma due to poorly managed labour has significant morbidity and mortality and is common in developing countries. In any obstetric setting gross tissue destruction, extensive haematomata and adherent scar tissue may necessitate a temporary colostomy while rectovaginal and vesicovaginal fistulae are repaired.

Prolapse

Second- and third-degree post-partum prolapse, as a result of a difficult or precipitate second stage of labour, is unusual. The fascial supporting tissues are stretched and torn and it has been suggested that there can be some recovery from the immediate post-partum condition, once healing occurs and connective tissue and hormones have had time to return to their pre-pregnancy status. Sometimes a pessary has been used post-partum to retain the cervix above the pelvic floor muscles until recovery is maximized. It is not considered helpful before six weeks. In severe cases surgery may be required within a few months of parturition. Rest in supine and pelvic floor muscle strengthening are very important aspects of early rehabilitation.

Effect of epidural anaesthesia

Prolonged epidural anaesthesia during the second stage of labour, allowing the foetal head to descend by uterine contraction alone without active maternal effort, has been advocated as a possible method to avoid pelvic floor damage. Two recent studies have shown that stress incontinence has occurred *de novo* post-partum in women who had an epidural-induced prolonged second stage. A possible explanation is that the epidural abolishes the protective neuromuscular reflexes (Jackson et al, 1995; Viktrup and Lose, 1993).

Pubococcygeal muscle strength

A comparison of digitally tested PF strength, perineometer pressure and the extent of PF lift was carried out ante-natally, 3–7 days post-delivery and six weeks post-partum. There was a drop in all three early post-partum, but by six weeks digitally assessed strength and PF lift had recovered to ante-natal levels. Passive mobility of the bladder neck and relaxation of the bladder base increased early post-partum and even further at six weeks (Peschers et al, 1994). Allen et al (1990) measured pubococcygeal strength in primiparae, using vaginal squeeze pressures. The low levels at 2–5 days post-partum had improved at two months but were still approximately two-thirds of ante-natal pressures.

Marie, a 27-year-old primipara, was referred to physiotherapy by her obstetrician six weeks post-partum with some bladder prolapse but no urinary or faecal symptoms. On vaginal digital examination no muscle contraction in either the puborectalis or pubococcygeus was detected on voluntary contraction. However, there was some contraction of the pubococcygeus detected vaginally during a transversus abdominis contraction. Marie was given a vaginal weight to use initially in supine (see Chapter 30) and an exercise programme for the transversus abdominis (Richardson and Jull, 1995) as well as pelvic floor muscles. When she returned for follow up after two weeks, the pubococcygeus was able to lift weakly and hold for five seconds and the transversus abdominis was improving. Her rehabilitation programme continued, eventually achieving a strong pubococcygeal co-contraction with active transversus abdominis work.

Puerperium

Many women complain of urinary symptoms immediately post-partum (up to 48–72 hours post-delivery) but they are frequently short-lived.

Women can report:

- inability to initiate micturition;
- total lack of awareness of the bladder and desire to void;
- loss or dribbling on walking to the toilet;
- full bladder loss without warning, on standing;
- full bladder loss in the shower;
- lack of sensation of urine flow and completion of voiding.

The pressure of the foetus on the bladder and urethra, the stretch on fascia, muscle and nerve in both spontaneous and forceps deliveries, pain of a tear or episiotomy and swelling around suture lines can all contribute to the above conditions. Urinary dysfunction can create anxiety and apprehension, especially in primipara and even in multipara if their first confinement was problem free. There is often a perception that once labour is over problems should resolve. In all of these cases the physiotherapist working with these women should be aware of the problem, provide reassurance and support, institute appropriate treatment and make sure that follow-up is provided. If dysfunction has not resolved by the day of discharge, continued exercising should be encouraged and an appointment made with the pelvic floor physiotherapist for follow-up at six weeks. By that time much of the neuropraxia will have reversed, lochia ceased, episiotomy soreness lessened and the mother will have had time to adapt to the demands of her newborn. An earlier appointment may be necessary. With ever-shortening post-partum hospital stays, it may be difficult to decide who needs further help so follow-up by phone may be useful.

Symptoms of genuine stress incontinence existing after childbirth can be a continuation of those during pregnancy or can occur *de novo* after the event. Obstetric factors such as length of second stage of labour, head circumference, birth weight and episiotomy seemed to be associated with the development of stress incontinence after the delivery. However, episiotomy was performed more frequently with a longer second stage of labour (Viktrup et al, 1992). Viktrup et al (1992) noted that by 12 months after the delivery much of the intrapartum and post-partum stress incontinence had disappeared.

There is a lower incidence of anorectal disturbances but faecal urgency (unable to hold on for five minutes) and incontinence of wind (flatus) are not uncommon. Like urinary problems, functional anorectal upsets are frequently transient, but weakness remains. This is particularly so in vaginal deliveries following a previous third-degree tear.

Studies vary in measurements made and timing and definition of problems, hence comparisons between them can be difficult. Some figures on the incidence of problems are shown in Table 23.3.

Table 23.3 Prevalence of urinary and faecal incontinence following vaginal deliveries

Author	Post-partum	Numbers	Urinary incontinence	Faecal incontinence / urge	Details
Allen et al, 1990	8 weeks	75 primiparae	26 (35%)		With baby >3.4 kg and active 2nd stage >83 minutes, UI in 55%.
Sleep and Grant, 1987	12 weeks	1609 mixed	355 (22%)	43 (2.7%)	13.3% urine loss <1/week FI occasional loss
Sultan et al, 1993b	7 weeks	79 primiparae	2 (3%)	10 (13%)	F urgency 10%, FI 5%
		48 multiparae	10 (21%)	11 (23%)	19% F symptoms AN 6% new symptoms
Viktrup et al, 1992	5 days	305 primiparae	19% GSI		Daily loss figures much lower
	3 months	293 primiparae	6% GSI		
	1 year	292 primiparae	3% GSI		

UI = urinary incontinence, F = faecal, FI = faecal incontinence, AN = ante-natal, GSI = genuine stress incontinence.

None of the studies documenting urinary incontinence 2–3 months post-partum commented on whether subjects were breast feeding. The hormonal variations may affect continence. Genuine stress incontinence is considered to be the most common urinary problem affecting women post-partum, but in one study at 3–4 months post-delivery more women complained of symptomatic urgency and urge incontinence than of stress incontinence (Sapsford, 1989). Management of different types of dysfunction is covered in Chapter 30.

Sharon, a 29-year-old primipara, was referred to physiotherapy by her obstetrician with poor PF muscle tone and a lax vagina seven weeks after a forceps delivery of a 3680 g baby. She had occasional urge incontinence. She commented that she had always had urinary urgency. On examination, the introitus and vagina were wide open with no detectable superficial perineal muscle activity and the pubococcygeus (R>L) was weak (grade 2) with a seven-second hold. Bladder volumes during the day were mostly in the region of 100–150 ml. She was anxious to return to aerobics. She was given a PF exercise programme and urge control techniques, encouraged to use her PF during effort activities and to defer aerobics.

At follow-up there was a marked improvement in her pubococcygeal strength and endurance (25-second hold) but no change in the introitus. She was given a vaginal weight (30 g) to use in standing. She was able to retain this for two minutes initially and three weeks later could retain it for almost an hour. At this visit the introitus was well closed. She still experienced occasional urinary urgency with the sound of running water, but no loss. She was encouraged to increase her level of activity around the house while using the weight for the next month, to add strong five-second PF holds to her programme, continue with urge control, defer voiding to improve bladder capacity and then grade through low-impact exercising into fitness activities.

Sexual dysfunction

Many factors contribute to interrupted or prolonged avoidance of coitus post-partum. Local factors may be obvious, e.g. traumatized perineum, poorly healing stitches. Exhaustion, preoccupation with the baby, post-natal depression and poor body image, especially if this combined with urinary or faecal loss, are global factors. Pelvic floor dyssynergia in the form of vaginismus (Devroede, 1996), vestibulitis or decreased vaginal sensation may follow delivery. These are discussed in Chapters 9, 13 and 29.

Anal fissures

Anal fissures commonly occur in women. They are associated with compromised blood supply allowing anterior or posterior splitting of the anal canal from the anal verge to the dentate line (Hancock, 1993). Anal fissures may occur after prolonged straining at stool early in the puerperium and may become chronic (Fig. 23.2). High resting pressures of the internal anal sphincter with an associated protective reflex spasm of the external anal sphincter are implicated.

Pruritis ani (itchy anus)

Simple pruritis ani may be associated with mechanical disturbances of the anorectal mechanism, e.g. fissures, fistulae, skin tags, haemorrhoids and rectal mucosal prolapse. The inability to fully evacuate soft pasty faeces causing external seepage or even the residue of small particles remaining after attempts at cleaning, along with the highly irritating mucosal leak accompanying prolapsed tissue, can cause considerable distress. Simple management techniques are shown in the box.

Figure 23.2 Anal fissure – a vertical split in the squamous-lined lower half of the anal canal. (Reproduced from Hancock (1993) with permission.)

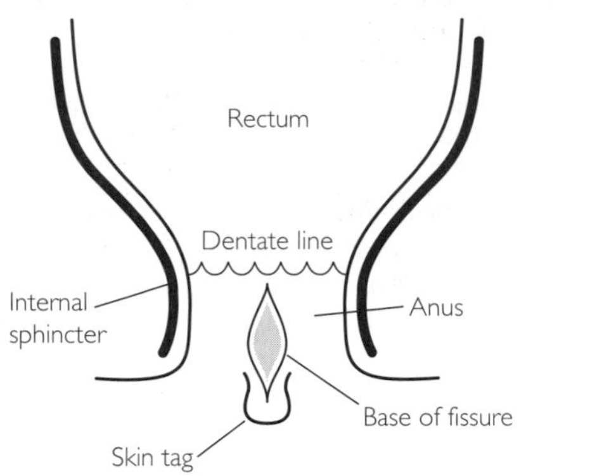

Simple measures for pruritis ani

- Replace toilet paper with non-alcohol baby wipes.
- Wash perineum after defaecation (use a non-soap substitute).
- Apply a barrier cream, e.g. zinc and caster oil, several times a day after defaecation.
- Attend to diet – avoid known irritants.
- Optimize defaecatory effort.

Faecal incontinence

PRESENTING SYMPTOMS

In the general population incontinence of flatus and faeces affects up to 11% of adults (Kamm, 1994). Faecal loss has been classified into two categories (Engel et al, 1995).

1. Rectal urgency or urge incontinence indicates fatigue or poor EAS recruitment. This may be due to denervation or sphincter disruption or both.
2. Passive or insensitive loss of contents is associated with poor internal anal sphincter function. This indicates denervation of smooth muscle. Both categories may present after parturition. Voluntary contraction of the external anal sphincter (EAS) is required to generate enough pressure in order to defer defaecation.

Squeeze pressures decreased significantly following vaginal delivery in primiparae and multiparae and remained lower than ante-natal levels at two months post-partum (Sultan et al, 1993b). A fall in resting pressures (internal anal sphincter) has also been recorded early and at two months post-partum (Wynne et al, 1996). In a similar study Sultan et al (1993b) noted no improvement at six months.

Much research has been directed to the aetiology of faecal incontinence related to childbirth.

PREVALENCE

Thirteen percent of women having their first vaginal delivery develop urgency or incontinence (Kamm, 1994). Sultan et al (1993b) found that there was a high incidence of anal sphincter defects after delivery (see Table 23.2). Permanent flatus incontinence has been shown to be more common following the third vaginal delivery in young premenopausal women (Ryhammer et al, 1995).

Prevalence of third-degree tears:

- 0.5–2% of vaginal deliveries result in overt tears in one or both sphincters;
- 85% of these tears show persistent defects following repair;
- 50% of sufferers continue to have symptoms despite repair.

Risk factors include:

- primiparae;
- occipitoposterior position (Kamm, 1994).

Predictors of faecal incontinence include:

- forceps delivery;
- large baby;
- long second stage;
- precipitate delivery (Allen et al, 1990; Kamm, 1994; Snooks et al, 1990).

Hidden anal sphincter defects occurred in primiparae in:

- 81% of forceps deliveries;
- 24% of vacuum extractions;
- 36% of unassisted deliveries (Sultan et al, 1993c).

In primiparae who had a forceps delivery, 38% developed faecal urgency or incontinence to flatus or liquid (Sultan et al, 1993c).

PROGNOSIS

Sangwan et al (1996) found that both pudendal nerves must be intact to achieve normal continence after sphincter repair. This may explain why 50% of women continue to have symptoms after their sphincter repair. Future implications must include improved methods of rehabilitation.

During the middle years progression of nerve damage partly due to the normal ageing process may occur. This may lead to decreased IAS pressure, increase in rectal and anal sensory thresholds and increasing pudendal nerve terminal motor latencies. Hormonal changes may make previously symptom-free women conscious of dysfunction for the first time (see Chapter 29 for further details).

The descending perineum syndrome

This broad term encompasses disruption to the integrity of support and its effect on function of the anorectum. It implies denervation and reinnervation of levator and sphincter muscles, fascial stretching and tearing and rectal wall mucosal prolapse and rectocoele, with or without faecal incontinence. Ineffective and incomplete rectal emptying and associated bladder dysfunction may be accompanied by pelvic, perineal and perianal pain. Associated uterovaginal prolapse is made worse by straining at the toilet (Spence-Jones et al, 1994). This syndrome can be the aftermath of difficult vaginal deliveries.

Summary

Identification and management of urinary and sexual dysfunction related to the perinatal period continues to expand. For many women this period marks the turning point in their ordered pattern of bowel function.

Decreased gastrointestinal motility during pregnancy, combined with local trauma during delivery and events postpartum are all significant. Pelvic organ dysfunction may result from acquired pathology or may exacerbate existing problems. Sensory, motor and proprioceptive changes associated with denervation occur, but are often unrecognized. Insidious change over time leads to functional bladder and bowel disorders presenting later in life.

Pelvic floor dysfunction seems to be an occupational hazard of motherhood (at least of vaginal deliveries). Education combined with exercise and functional use of the pelvic floor can help prevent later problems. Women are generally anxious to regain a svelte figure. It is now realized that pelvic floor and the deep abdominal muscles can be strengthened and maintained with functional exercise which combines both muscle groups.

References

Allen RE, Hosker GL, Smith ARB et al (1990) Pelvic floor damage and childbirth: a neurophysiological study. *British Journal of Obstetrics and Gynaecology* **97**: 770–779.

Baron TH, Ramirez B and Richter JE (1993) Gastrointestinal motility disorders during pregnancy. *Annals of Internal Medicine* **188**: 366–375.

Beischer NA and Mackay EV (1986) *Obstetrics and the Newborn*, 2nd edn. Sydney: W.B. Saunders.

Bek KM and Laurberg S (1992) Risks of anal incontinence from subsequent vaginal delivery after a complete obstetric anal sphincter tear. *British Journal of Obstetrics and Gynaecology* **99**: 724–726.

Cutner A, Cardozo LD, Benness CJ et al (1990) Detrusor instability in early pregnancy. *Neurourology and Urodynamics* **9**: 328–329.

Devroede G (1996) Front and rear. *Proceedings Controversies in Colon and Rectal Surgery*, Nijmegen.

Engel AF, Kamm MA, Bartram CI et al (1995) Relationship of symptoms in faecal incontinence to specific sphincter abnormalities. *International Journal of Colorectal Disease* **10**: 152–155.

Hancock BD (1993) Anal fissures and fistulae. In: Jones DJ and Irving MH (eds) *ABC of Colorectal Diseases*, p. 26. London: BMJ Publishing.

Harris M (1992) The impact of research findings on current practice in relieving post-partum perineal pain in a large district general hospital. *Midwifery* **8**: 125–131.

Hudson CN (1992) Gynaecological conditions and coloproctology. In: Henry MM and Swash M (eds) *Coloproctology and the Pelvic Floor*, 2nd edn, pp. 459–469. Oxford: Butterworth Heinemann.

Jackson S, Barry C, Davies G et al (1995) Duration of second stage of labour and epidural anaesthesia: effect on subsequent urinary symptoms in primiparous women. *Neurourology and Urodynamics* **14**: 498–499.

Joels LA and Manyonda IT (1994) Chronic faecal impaction impairing vaginal delivery at term, and first trimester termination of pregnancy. *British Journal of Obstetrics and Gynaecology* **101**: 168–169.

Kamm MA (1994) Obstetric damage and faecal incontinence. *Lancet* **344**: 730–733.

Kiff ES (1993) Faecal incontinence. In: Jones DJ and Irving MH (eds) *ABC of Colorectal Diseases*. London: BMJ Publishing.

Koch KL and Stern RM (1993) Electrogastrography. In: Kumar D and Wingate DL (eds) *An Illustrated Guide to Gastrointestinal Motility*, 2nd edn, p. 303. Edinburgh: Churchill Livingstone.

Kumar D, Waldron D, Wingate DL and Williams NL (1989) Does psychological pain and stress affect anorectal motility and external sphincter activity in humans? *British Journal of Surgery SRS Abstract* **76**: 636.

MacDonald A, Baxter JN and Findlay IG (1993) Anorectal manometry in patients with postchildbirth / hysterectomy constipation. *Gut* 34 (Suppl. 4): F190.

Markwell SJ and Sapsford RR (1995) Physiotherapy management of obstructed defaecation. *Australian Journal of Physiotherapy* **41**: 279–283.

Peschers U, Schar G, Anthuber C et al (1994) Post partal pelvic floor damage: is connective tissue impairment more important than neuromuscular changes? *Neurourology and Urodynamics* **13**: 376–377.

Richardson CA and Jull GA (1995) Muscle control – pain control. What exercises would you prescribe? *Manual Therapy* **1**: 2–10.

Ryhammer AM, Bek KM and Laurberg S (1995) Multiple vaginal deliveries increase the risk of permanent incontinence of flatus and urine in normal premenopausal women. *Diseases of Colon and Rectum* **38**: 1206–1209.

Sangwan YP, Coller JA, Barrett RC et al (1996) Unilateral pudendal neuropathy. Impact on outcome of anal sphincter repair. *Diseases of Colon and Rectum* **39**: 686–689.

Sapsford RR (1989) Post partum urinary problems. *Australian Physiotherapy Association National Women's Health Journal* **8**: 4–7.

Sapsford RR, Markwell SJ and Richardson CA (1996) Abdominal muscles and the anal sphincter: their interaction during defaecation. Proceedings of the Australian Physiotherapy Association National Congress, Brisbane, pp. 103–104.

Sapsford R, Hodges PW, Richardson CA et al (1997) Activation of pubococcygeus during a variety of isometric abdominal exercises. Conference Abstract, *International Continence Society*, Yokohama, p. 115.

Scott P (1995) Optimal foetal positioning. Making childbirth easier. *Birth Issues* **4**: 5–10.

Sleep J and Grant A (1987) Pelvic floor exercises in post natal care. *Midwifery* **3**: 158–164.

Snooks SJ, Setchell M, Swash M et al (1984) Injury to innervation of pelvic floor sphincter musculature in childbirth. *Lancet* **2**: 546–550.

Snooks SJ, Swash M, Mathers SE et al (1990) Effect of vaginal delivery on the pelvic floor: a 5-year follow-up. *British Journal of Surgery* **77**: 1358–1360.

Spence-Jones C, Kamm MA, Henry MM et al (1994) Bowel dysfunction: a pathogenic factor in uterovaginal prolapse and urinary stress incontinence. *British Journal of Obstetrics and Gynaecology* **101**: 147–152.

Stanton SL, Kerr-Wilson R and Harris VG (1980) The incidence of urological symptoms in normal pregnancy. *British Journal of Obstetrics and Gynaecology* **87**: 897–900.

Sultan AH, Kamm MA, Hudson CN et al (1993a) Effect of pregnancy on anal sphincter morphology and function. *International Journal of Colorectal Disease* **8**: 206–209.

Sultan AH, Kamm MA, Hudson CN et al (1993b) Anal sphincter disruption during vaginal delivery. *New England Journal of Medicine* **329**: 1905–1911.

Sultan AH, Kamm MA, Bartram CI et al (1993c) Anal sphincter trauma during instrumental delivery. *International Journal of Gynecology and Obstetrics* **43**: 263–270.

Sultan AH, Kamm MA and Hudson CN (1994) Pudendal nerve damage during labour: a prospective study before and after childbirth. *British Journal of Obstetrics and Gynaecology* **101**: 22–28.

Thomas IL, Erian M, Sarson D et al (1993) Postpartum haemorrhoids – evaluation of a cooling device (Anurex) for relief of symptoms. *Medical Journal of Australia* **159**: 459–460.

Thompson JPS, Leicester RJ and Smith LE (1992) Haemorrhoids. In: Henry MM and Swash M (eds) *Coloproctology and the Pelvic Floor*, 2nd edn, p. 376. Oxford: Butterworth Heinemann.

Viktrup L and Lose G (1993) Epidural anesthesia during labour and stress incontinence after delivery. *Obstetrics and Gynecology* **82**: 984–986.

Viktrup L, Lose G, Rolff M et al (1992) The symptom of stress incontinence caused by pregnancy or delivery in primiparas. *Obstetrics and Gynecology* **79**: 945–949.

Wynne JM, Myles J, Jones I et al (1996) Disturbed anal sphincter function following vaginal delivery. *Gut* **39**: 120–124.

24

Electrotherapy Options for the Perinatal Period and Beyond

ZOE McLACHLAN

Treatment in the Ante-natal Period Using Therapeutic Agents

The principal reasons for using therapeutic agents are for pain relief, muscle stimulation / strengthening or promotion of healing of either acute or chronic soft tissue problems. Patients presenting for treatment in the ante-natal period have a variety of complaints which could include spinal pain, pelvic pain, oedema and fluid retention and any pre-existing musculoskeletal conditions aggravated by the pregnancy. The physiotherapist treating any of these problems may wish to use therapeutic agents as an adjunct to manual therapy, exercise and support devices. When the patient is a pregnant woman (or potentially pregnant woman), the therapist should carefully consider the following factors before using any treatment.

1. What is the desired effect of the proposed treatment?
2. What are the known physiological effects of that treatment, i.e. what will be achieved?
3. Will there be any detrimental effects on the developing foetus?

Questions 1 and 2 are essential for consideration for all patients and all treatments. They form the basic underlying rationale for treatment. However, it is vital to consider question 3 when treating any potentially pregnant female. Detrimental effects on the foetus could fall into the following categories:

1. increase of maternal core temperature (see Chapter 16);
2. increased uterine muscular activity;
3. decreased placental blood flow.

> The student is reminded that a thorough understanding of the effects that any therapeutic agent may have on the physiological functions is essential before considering any application. In addition, appropriate skin testing and safety precautions should always be applied. For knowledge of electrotherapy agents refer to Lehmann and de Lateur (1982) and Low and Reed (1994).

If there is a clear answer to questions 1 and 2 and a clear no to question 3, the therapist should feel free to use a therapeutic agent. If there are any slight doubts about the effect on the foetus, or if the effects are not known, the therapist should err on the side of caution and not use the therapeutic agent.

Electrotherapy treatment has been used by physiotherapists for many years. Much of this has been theoretically based and some of it has been confirmed or disproved more recently. Much more needs to be known. Muscle, nerve and cardiac function are all controlled by intrinsic electrical activity and the introduction of an electrical current from outside must affect intrinsic functioning. The contraindication to use of any stimulating treatment for people with pacemakers is well known. But if untoward effects, either short or long term, result from other situations, they are unknown.

Modalities which should not be used in the pregnant or potentially pregnant female include short-wave diathermy, pulsed short-wave diathermy and microwave therapy. This is due to the presumed deep-heating effect of these modalities and in the case of pregnancy, such modalities could adversely affect the foetus. Recommendations that these modalities should not come within 30 cm of the pregnant uterus are commonly given (Lehmann and de Lateur, 1982).

Modalities that have been claimed to be useful in ante-natal management include:

- moist heat;
- ice;
- transcutaneous electrical nerve stimulation (TENS);
- co-planar interferential;
- ultrasound (US) – continuous (thermal) and pulsed (non-thermal);
- laser.

As a general rule, no electrotherapy should be used over or be able to pass through the pregnant abdomen. All treatments, including the physiological effects, should be explained carefully to the patient. Pregnant women are often very concerned that any treatment should have no deleterious effects on the foetus and may prefer to use an alternative to electrotherapy. Remain with the patient or within call during the treatment.

Pain relief

In management of pain relief in spinal, pelvic or pre-existing musculoskeletal disorders applications of the modalities are primarily influenced by the positioning adaptations which will be required as the pregnancy develops, as well as the precautions of various modalities. The benefits and precautions for these various applications will be outlined.

MOIST HEAT

Moist heat in the form of hot packs is safe, effective, readily accessible and appropriate for home use. Hot packs can be applied prior to manual therapy or exercise to encourage muscle relaxation and reduction of spasm.

The physiological effects of superficial heat on tissues are:

- an increase in skin temperature which decreases in inverse proportion to the depth;
- local skin vasodilation occurs which dissipates the heat. There is some temperature increase in deeper levels.

The physiological processes associated with pain relief from superficial heating are explained as follows.

There is stimulation of sensory afferent receptors, which activates the pain gate mechanism. There is usually relaxation of muscle spasm. It is thought that increased circulation may contribute to movement of pain-producing metabolites. There is also an unspecified 'sedative' effect noted from the use of superficial heat both during and after treatment. Patients report being able to sleep more easily. It could be just pain relief, but it has been noted that there is naturally an increase in skin temperature prior to sleep. Therefore the increased skin temperature provided by a hot pack could trigger a reflex phenomenon (Lehmann and de Lateur, 1982). In addition, due to a reflex phenomenon there is usually a cutaneous vasoconstriction followed by vasodilation which occurs as a result of local heating in other parts of a limb.

Healing is also thought to be encouraged as a result of superficial heating. It is suggested that mild inflammation will benefit from rises in temperature of between 2° and 5°C, as this will increase phagocytosis and improve absorption of exudate.

Increases in joint mobility are possible following heating due to the analgesic effects of the application, so women should rest for 20 minutes following a heat application before leaving. Some care must be taken in post-application mobilization for the pregnant woman who will have increased joint mobility from the effects of relaxin.

ICE

Ice can be used safely during the pregnancy for pain relief on a local lesion. Cooling of skin stimulates temperature receptors and decreases conduction rates of nerve fibres. Enough cooling will cause numbness. Ice applications have also been used to decrease muscle spasm.

It is essential that ice be applied only after appropriate skin testing and explanation to the patient. Care should be taken to ensure that any ice packs left in contact with the skin have a moist layer between the ice and skin to avoid ice burns.

CO-PLANAR INTERFERENTIAL AND TENS

These two modalities are both considered useful in the treatment of pain. Both applications generate an electrical current at specific frequencies which is considered to provide an analgesic effect to the area of application. The physiology of the pain relief is explained as follows.

- Activation of pain gate mechanism due to stimulation of large-diameter, low-threshold nerve fibres with high frequencies (100–200 Hz).
- Activation of A delta fibres and C fibres enhances release of the body's natural pain inhibitors, endorphin and encephalin, at low frequencies (10–25 Hz).
- Temporary block of finely myelinated and non-

myelinated nocioceptive fibres at frequencies above 50 Hz (Low and Reed, 1994).

In addition to these physiological responses, it is considered that the placebo effect may be significant. Interferential/ TENS machines look and feel impressive and many patients feel they have had a more thorough treatment if they have been applied. It is the role of the physiotherapist to ensure that appropriate education on the nature of these applications is provided.

Interferential machines function by the interference of two medium-frequency currents placed around the area to be treated. A carrier wave of 4000 Hz is preferable for pain relief. The therapist then selects the desired treatment frequency for pain relief. The advantage of this method is the minimal skin resistance offered at the medium-frequency range. TENS, on the other hand, uses direct application of the current at the chosen frequency. The name TENS is commonly used for small battery-powered machines which patients can use for extended periods, often at home, for chronic conditions.

Co-planar interferential may be used with two or four electrodes on either side or on all sides of the painful area. As the current takes the shortest, well-conducting pathway between two electrodes it has a shallow depth of spread over muscular areas. A co-planar interferential application is one option in the treatment of lumbosacral pain during pregnancy.

Physiotherapists should place electrodes for co-planar applications for lumbosacral pain close to the vertebral column, so that there is no risk of current spread to the abdomen.

Larger electrodes ensure greater comfort at higher intensity and may be beneficial. If side lying is used for comfort, electrodes may need to be secured with Velcro straps. Alternatively, a vacuum suction system can be used if available. This has a massaging effect that may add to the effectiveness of the treatment by aiding muscle relaxation.

Frequency for pain relief should be between 80 and 150 Hz. If available, a sweep mode is best. This prevents nerve habituation and increases the range of nerve types that can be stimulated, thus maximizing effectiveness.

Intensity is increased slowly to allow for accommodation and set at a comfortably low level of perception.

Precaution

Do not use interferential on the thoracic area with an intensity above 50 mA. This has been shown to cause ventricular fibrillation in some instances.

Practical application of TENS for pain relief is by the use of rubber electrodes which may be attached to the skin with micropore tape. Electroconducting gel is placed on the electrode surface against the skin and the skin checked regularly in the first 4–6 hours for any signs of aggravation. After use, the electrodes must be washed well and more gel is applied before each application. The skin should be washed with warm soapy water before and after each application. Alternatively, disposable adhesive electrodes may be used. These will have a definite 'life' and will need to be replaced when they no longer adhere properly. It often helps to moisten the skin slightly before application.

Reduction of oedema

Some therapeutic agents may be useful adjuncts to treatment by elevation, firm continuous pressure (distal to proximal) and massage. These include ice and ultrasound (Fig. 24.1). A common condition associated with oedema and often occurring in pregnancy is carpal tunnel syndrome. Apart from splinting which limits wrist flexion, and elevation during rest, ultrasound or contrast bathing are therapeutic interventions that have been considered useful.

ULTRASOUND

When ultrasound waves are absorbed in the tissues immense mechanical forces are working. Alternation of positive and negative pressures at the frequency of the machine cause the micromassage effect of ultrasound. One of the effects of ultrasound is heating. Any medium exposed to ultrasound will undergo heating proportional to the energy absorbed, the time isonated and the specific frequency of the machine (Wadsworth and Chanmungam, 1980).

Figure 24.1 Ultrasound to the cervical area in sitting.

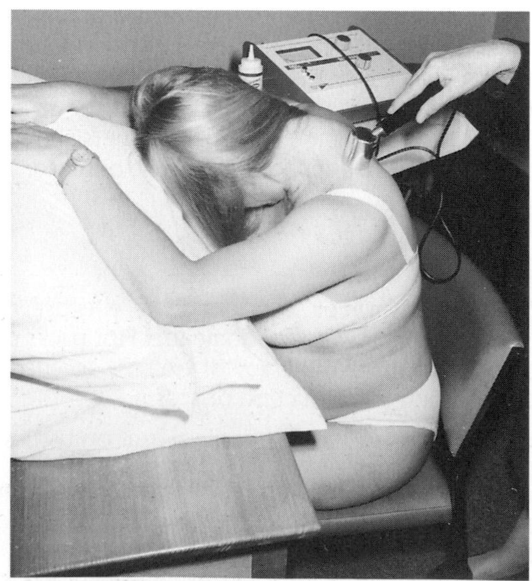

Precaution

The use of ultrasound therapy (US) is contraindicated in any area in the proximity of the pregnant uterus. Continuous or thermal US may produce heating that could have a teratogenic effect on the foetus. It is known that an increase in the core temperature of 1 °C can affect the foetus, especially in the first 12 weeks. Artal and Buckenmeyer (1995) have stated that a possible maternal threshold for teratogenesis is 39.2°C. Even though US does not penetrate through bone, there is a scatter effect and some could pass around to the pelvic/abdominal cavity. It would be hard to prove beyond doubt that no waves passed the pelvis.

Pulsed US causes acoustic streaming and cavitation. There would be a small risk (in theory) that incorrect application of US, by minimal movement of the sound head, could set up collapse cavitation in tissue, which is very damaging. The fundal height at 24 weeks corresponds with T12–L1 and at 36 weeks with T10.

CO-PLANAR INTERFERENTIAL

The effect of interferential on oedema is considered to be related to an increased circulation and fluid exchange because of vasodilation which occurs especially close to the electrodes (Currier et al, 1986). Savage (1984) states that frequencies of 10–150 Hz stimulate parasympathetic nerves leading to increased blood flow. There is possible stimulation of autonomic nerves which will help remove chemical irritants from nerve endings. This effect of increased circulation is challenged by Nussbaum et al (1990) who found no supporting evidence using thermography.

ICE

Ice has been considered to cause vasoconstriction of the area being iced, which will decrease the rate of swelling and production of irritants and so alleviate pain.

The Use of TENS in Labour

Transcutaneous electrical nerve stimulation (TENS) has been used for pain relief in labour since the 1970s. TENS is a non-invasive, self-controlled form of pain relief, free of any known side effects on mother or baby. It is not suitable for all women. The theory of pain relief by TENS is as outlined briefly below.

1. Activation of pain gate mechanism due to stimulation of low-threshold nerve fibres, mechanoreceptors and A beta fibres which reduces the excitability of A delta and C pain fibres. This stimulation 'takes up space' and reduces the amount of pain messages passing up the spinal cord (Melzack and Wall, 1982). This stimulation is provided by low-intensity, high-frequency stimulation at 100–200 Hz.
2. Activation of A delta and C fibres enhances release of the body's natural pain inhibitors, endorphin and encephalin. This occurs best with low-frequency high-intensity stimulation at 2–10 Hz.

Application

Placement of electrodes for TENS is usually over the site of pain or paravertebrally over the corresponding nerve roots. The preferred site for pain relief in labour is paravertebrally. Usually two sets of electrodes are used as obstetric machines have dual channels (Fig. 24.2). The top set is attached either side of the vertebral column from the level of T10–L1. This corresponds to the area that provides the uterine nerve supply, so is effective in reducing pain in the first stage of labour. During the first stage, women may also experience severe back pain centred over the sacral area, so the lower set of electrodes placed over S2–S4 can be helpful in first and second stage labour. It has been reported by women as being effective in relieving back pain and the pain of stretch to the pelvic floor and perineum in the second stage. Most women find TENS more helpful when started early in labour.

Figure 24.2 Placement of electrodes for TENS in labour.

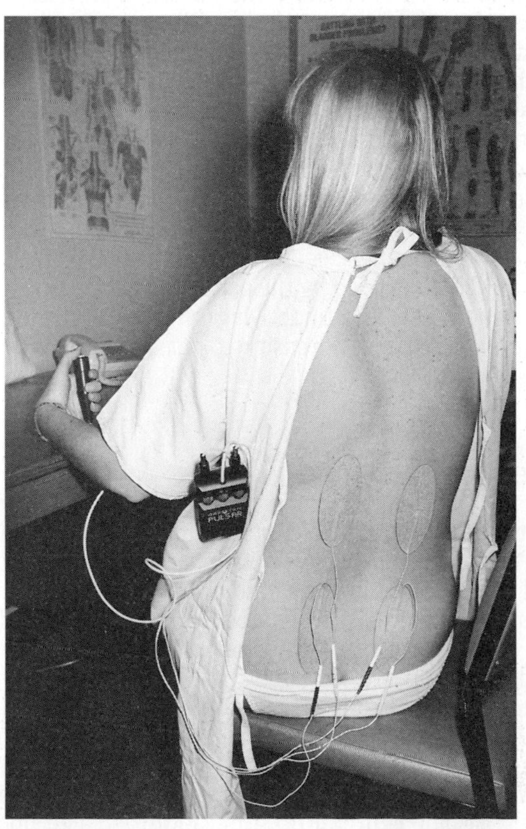

Technique

The most effective technique developed for labour has been use of constant low-intensity stimulation from reasonably early in the first stage of labour with the addition of boosted, higher intensity stimulation during contractions. This boost is usually provided by pressing a 'boost' button to turn the higher intensity on and off. This means that the patient has control of the machine and administration of stimulation herself. This has proved to be a very positive aspect of the system. As any underlying discomfort increases, the patient can increase the lower level of intensity to provide more relief. The dual channel system enables her to have different levels of underlying stimulation from the two sets of electrodes.

The electrodes are easy to apply. Usually adhesive disposable electrodes are used on washed skin. Normal, large rubber electrodes may be used, approximately 8 × 3 cm. Conducting gel should be put under the electrodes and renewed after 4–6 hours. The electrodes are firmly attached to the skin by adhesive tape and removed for showering. The partner, support person or midwife can help apply the electrodes after being taught the correct positions. The stimulation may affect foetal monitoring equipment and may need to be removed if that happens.

Guidelines for application

Obstetric TENS machines are conveniently small machines powered by a 9 V battery. They usually have a clip to be attached to the patient's clothes. The pulse width may be fixed or variable and is usually in the range 0.1–0.2 ms. The machine should provide a biphasic pulse. The frequency is usually presented as 'RATE' on obstetric machines and is controlled by the patient via a dial marked 1–10. The range of frequency is usually 1–100 Hz, but is non-linear. It is suggested to the patient that she choose a comfortable sensation usually at the upper end of scale, around 6–8 on the dial, as lower frequencies are less comfortable. Intensity (0–100 mA) is controlled by the patient via a dial marked 1–10. The patient sets the underlying intensity and the boost button will increase intensity to maximum if pushed all the way.

Effectiveness

Many studies have looked at the effectiveness of TENS as pain relief in labour, with very varying results. Augustinsson et al (1977) found in their study of 147 women that 44% considered pain relief to be good and 44% had moderate pain relief. Bortoluzzi (1989) found in her study that the group of 'prepared' or educated TENS users reported a higher degree of satisfaction with TENS and used significantly less narcotics than a matched comparison group. Crothers (1994) conducted a trial comparing three groups of women: a group using TENS, a group using placebo TENS (flashing light but no stimulation) and a group using drugs. There was no prior knowledge of TENS in the women taking part. The results showed no differences in perceived levels of pain experienced by the women as labour progressed, but 50% of all groups felt they had received some benefit from their 'intervention'. Crothers went on to investigate the relationship between endorphin levels and 'ability to cope' during labour and found a correlation.

In many of the studies TENS was introduced to women who were already in labour. Physiotherapists advocating TENS for pain relief have always found it was more successful when the patient was well educated in its use. Post-operative pain relief is clinically more successful when the patient is introduced to the concept pre-operatively and familiarized with the machine and its sensation. It has never seemed logical to introduce a device requiring compliance and understanding when the patient is already in a stressful situation.

Many hospitals that offer TENS as pain relief in labour run special TENS classes, which enable the physiotherapist to explain the theory and allow the woman to become familiar with the sensation and the machine. Women and partners need to know that TENS can be used in conjunction with gas and pethidine, but is redundant if an epidural is needed. Some patients choose to hire their own TENS machine. This ensures availability and also allows them to start using TENS reasonably early in labour without having to come to hospital at this stage. There is generally good acceptance from midwives who find that educated patients can look after their own unit.

Women must have realistic expectations of TENS and a clear understanding that it will not eliminate pain. They need to know that labour pain is likely to be stronger than any previous experience of pain. However, for the motivated woman educated in its use, it would seem a valuable addition to the range of pain relief media for labour.

TENS has been used in some instances for management of after-birth pain, especially for multiparae. The obstetric TENS is ideal to use.

Placement of electrodes is suprapubically adjacent to the uterus, frequency 80–120 Hz, intensity to comfort. Use would be either just during feeding or on low intensity constantly and boosted as needed.

There is no research on its efficacy.

Use of Electrotherapy for Post-natal Conditions

Acute perineal trauma

Electrotherapy is an option the physiotherapist may consider in the post-natal period for perineal pain. Women who deliver vaginally may have an episiotomy or tear involving stitches. The rate varies from about 50% upwards. Many will also have swelling and bruising as a result of trauma, not to mention overstretching and possible neurological damage to the pelvic floor muscles. All of this results in much pain for some women, interfering with their ability to move easily and sit comfortably during breast feeding.

ICE

Ice should be the first and most easily applied form of treatment (see Chapter 19).

ULTRASOUND (US)

If the perineum remains very bruised and painful, the physiotherapist may wish to provide further pain relief with ultrasound.

Position the patient in side lying with lower leg straight and upper limb bent up. The patient can hold up her top buttock. Strict hygiene and sterilization procedures need to be followed in relation to infection. The head of the US should be washed in soap and water prior to treatment. There are two methods of administering treatment.

1. A condom filled with water so that when ultrasound is applied, the depth is about 10 mm. Gel is applied to upper and lower surfaces and held in place by an assistant, is usually a more comfortable way, especially over sutures (Fig. 24.3).
2. The head of the US is covered with a condom, gel is applied to the inside and outside of the condom and treatment given directly over the bruised area.

Following treatment, the condom is disposed of and the treatment head washed in soap and water. If any contact is made with the body surface, the treatment head should be soaked in 1% glutaraldehyde for 10 minutes.

Ultrasound parameters Using a pulsed mode with ratios of 1:3 or 1:4, Table 24.1 illustrates the suggested dosages which can be applied for an acute injury.

Despite the use of ultrasound treatment, there are few studies looking at the effects of US on the perineum after childbirth. Creates (1987) showed a significant positive effect with regards to pain. This was a randomized double blind trial using pulsed US versus a placebo involving 76 patients. However, the significant effect as measured by visual analogue scale was not reflected in analgesic use. Most patients only had one treatment and so longer term effects were not expected or evaluated. Grant et al (1989) did a

Table 24.1 Suggested ultrasound parameters for treatment of acute perineal trauma

Frequency	1 or 3 MHz	3 MHz half value depth – 25 mm 1 MHz half value depth – 40 mm
Intensity	0.75–1 W cm^2	3 MHz intensity needs to be increased by 30% through 10 mm water
	0.5–0.75 W cm^2	1 MHz
Time	1–2 minutes/10 cm^2	Total of 4–5 minutes should be sufficient
No. of treatments	2–3	Should benefit initial healing

Ward and Robertson (1996); Robertson, VJ (personal communication)

Figure 24.3 Ultrasound for acute perineal trauma. A water-filled condom, gelled on both surfaces, is used for comfort. This also avoids sound head contamination.

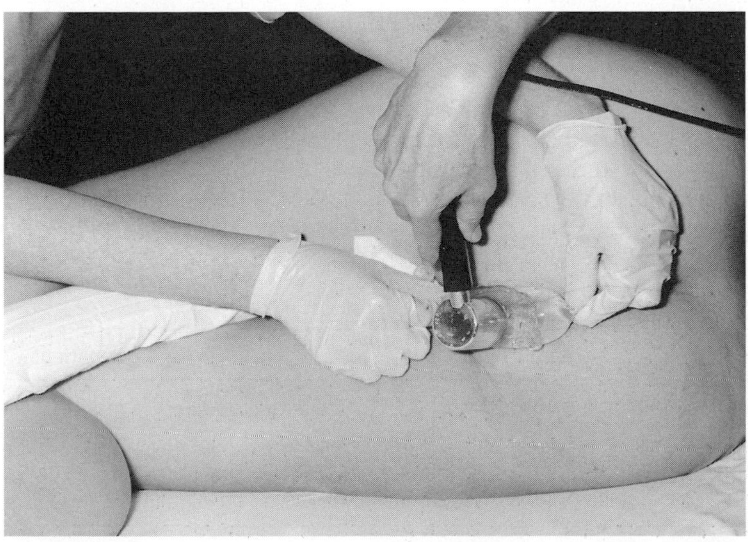

much larger study comparing pulsed electromagnetic energy (pulsed SWD), US and placebo of both, involving 414 women. In this study, neither treatment had a statistically significant effect compared with placebo treatment. Patients in each group had three treatments within a 36-hour period. The US was pulsed, frequency 3 MHz, intensity 0.5 W cm^2, for three minutes for each area of treatment equal to the size of the transmitting head (average eight minutes) and assessment made at two hours post-treatment, 10 days and three months. US appeared to spread bruising immediately after treatment, but it was better dispersed after 10 days. However, these effects were not statistically significant.

The research to date therefore would not indicate wholesale use of US and more positive effects would be needed to justify the time involved.

PULSED ELECTROMAGNETIC ENERGY (PEME)

This is often known as pulsed short-wave and is another modality that can be used to promote healing of the perineum. This has been more widely used in hospitals in the UK, where the equipment is more readily available. The physiological effects of PEME are basically:

- decrease in swelling and inflammation;
- reabsorption of haematoma;
- increase in rate of fibrin and collagen deposition and organization.

As there are no heating effects, it would seem to be ideal for promoting wound healing and this has been shown in studies. It has also been shown to increase nerve growth and repair (Raji, 1984; Wilson and Jagadeesh, 1976) – perhaps food for thought regarding damaged PF muscles.

Position the patient in side lying as for US. The single head monoplode is used and positioned very close to the perineum. However, there should be no skin contact.

- Frequency – 27 MHz
- Pulse rate – 100 pulses / second
- Pulse width – 65 μs
- Time – 10 minutes

This regime is the same as that used by Grant et al (1989) and is similar to that used widely in the UK. It should be remembered, however, that the study by Grant et al (1989) failed to demonstrate any objective benefit as far as pain and healing were concerned. No studies have considered any possible effect on a neurologically impaired pelvic floor.

LOW-LEVEL LASER THERAPY (LLLT)

Laser has been used in some centres to promote perineal healing. LLLT is used therapeutically for tissue healing and pain relief. Laser radiation is principally absorbed in the dermal layer (80–99%), so a very small amount penetrates to subcutaneous tissue. Young et al (1989) demonstrated that using wavelengths of 660, 820 and 870 nm encouraged macrophage activity, but that the wavelength of 880 nm was inhibitory to this activity. The claims made about the pain-relieving characteristics of LLLT are predominantly anecdotal and no clear physiological explanation has been given.

A small hand-held continuous-wave laser, usually either helium–neon (632.8 nm) or gallium–aluminium–arsenide (fixed wavelengths in the range 630–904 nm) and an output of up to 50 mW, could be used. Many of the current laser models use a pulsed wave. The patient should be positioned in side lying with the perineum exposed. If a large area is being treated, it should be divided into sections and each treated separately.

Technique The probe should be held as close as possible to the target tissue without making contact. Irradiation should occur at 1 cm intervals along the episiotomy wound. The laser probe tip should be cleaned with alcohol wipes before and after treatment. Skin testing is not necessary prior to treatment.

Dosage The dosage depends on the aim of the treatment. In those women predisposed to keloid scarring or in those with keloid scars, laser treatment can be beneficial (Table 24.2).

Caution

Both the patient and therapist should wear goggles to protect their eyes from accidental exposure to the laser beam.

To date, no research trials of LLLT for episiotomy healing have been cited in the literature. Beckerman et al (1992) undertook a meta-analysis of randomized clinical trials and found very mixed results. Their reviews showed that many of the trials were poorly designed, but found some evidence of therapeutic value for post-traumatic joint disorders, myofascial pain and rheumatoid arthritis. More recently levels of beta-endorphins and adrenocorticotrophic

Table 24.2 Dosage for laser treatment of the perineum

Purpose	Wavelength	Dosage per patient	Pulse frequency
Wound healing	600–750 nm	0.5–4 J cm^2	< 1000 Hz
Inhibition / treatment of scar tissue	750–905 nm	4–6 J cm^2	>1000 Hz
Pain relief	Short or long wavelength	0.5–4 J cm^2	Maximal

hormone (ACTH) have been shown to be increased following laser treatment in patients with chronic pain (Laakso et al, 1994).

INFRARED/SURFACE HEAT

Infrared lamps were commonly used for episiotomy healing years ago but are used far less frequently today. However, they are used for promotion of healing of cracked nipples. The therapeutic effects are surface vasodilation and pain relief. An argument could be made that vasodilation and the subsequent increased circulation leads to improved healing to surface wounds. With episiotomies, it may help surface healing and dry the wound for a short period but is unlikely to effect healing of deeper levels. Infrared is contraindicated if haemorrhoids are present.

Hairdryers have previously been suggested by some paramedical staff for drying episiotomy sites after showering or bathing. However, it is recommended by physiotherapists that they should not be used because of the danger of air entering the body via the lax vagina and creating an air embolus through an open placental site.

Chronic perineal pain

Perineal pain persisting over weeks or months has been treated by physiotherapists with ultrasound, particularly over the scar area. US has been shown to increase the extensibility of collagen tissue bands on the surface of a scar (Bierman, 1954). Stretch should be applied during treatment to help break up the scar. In a small trial by Everett et al (1992), ultrasound was found to have no real benefit over a placebo in reducing perineal pain. The results showed some trend towards better outcomes amongst the trial group, but the numbers were too small to demonstrate significance. The application regime used in this trial was a frequency of 3 MHz pulsed (1:1), with an intensity of 0.5 W cm^{2}', applied for five minutes over eight treatment sessions.

Both US and PEME have seemed clinically effective and hence are used by physiotherapists. However, the research to date does not appear to substantiate this clinical success rate. More research is needed to test other regimes and dosages. If only some temporary relief is afforded to women, it may make treatment worthwhile in some cases.

Pubic symphysis diastasis

Some women experience severe pain in the pubic symphysis post-natally. This may occur because of softening of ligaments and separation of the joint during pregnancy plus joint oedema and the impact of delivery, particularly with a large baby or shoulder dystocia. Ice provides pain relief and assists in reduction of oedema. An ice pack (readily available in post-natal wards) wrapped in damp gauze or a flannel can be placed over the symphysis pubis for 10–15 minutes every 1–2 hours in the first 24 hours (see Chapter 19 for more information).

Ultrasound is another option, especially if an acute injury is obvious (Fig. 24.4). Suggestions for a therapeutic application are found in Table 24.3.

Figure 24.4 Ultrasound treatment to the pubic symphysis for acute post-natal pain.

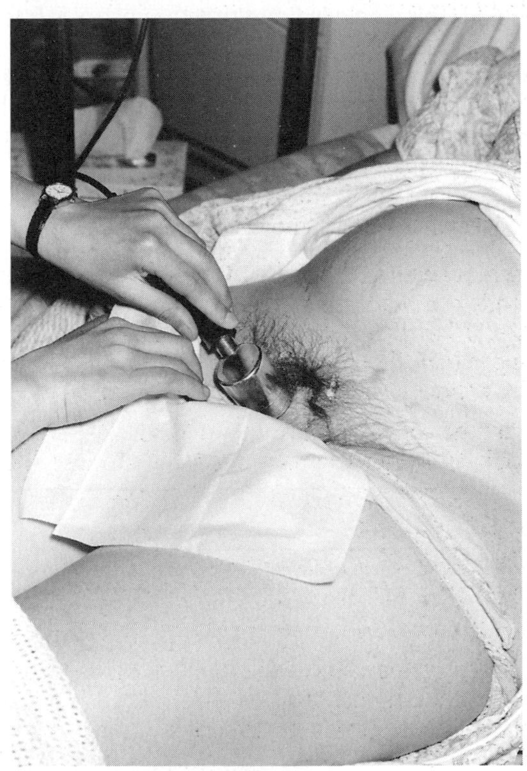

Table 24.3 Suggested ultrasound parameters for pubic symphysis diastasis

Mode	Pulsed 1:1
Frequency	3 MHz if available (half value depth is 25 mm) or 1 MHz (half value depth is 40 mm)
Intensity	3 MHz, 0.5 W cm^2 or 1 MHz, 0.5 W cm^2
Time	3–4 minutes (1 minute for every 10 cm^2 of surface covered)
No. of treatments	2–3
Position	Woman in supine position. US head can be used directly over symphysis coated with gel. If this is too painful, a water-filled condom or other water-filled plastic bag could be used with gel on both upper and lower surfaces of bag.

Following treatment by ultrasound, the patient should be advised to rest for at least 20 minutes. The US effects may include increased elasticity of collagenous tissue which is already softened from the effects of relaxin. The sound head of the US needs to be cleaned after this application.

Sacroiliac joint pain / coccydynia

The physiotherapist may encounter a woman with either acute SIJ pain or coccydynia. The damaged ligaments will often respond to treatment with electrotherapy. In the first 24 hours, ice can help by reducing swelling and providing pain relief, particularly for coccydynia. An ice pack can be applied over the coccyx for 10–15 minutes every 2–3 hours as needed. Ultrasound can also be helpful. Table 24.4 sets out the various parameters for treatment.

For coccydynia, increase the ultrasound intensity slowly and cease treatment immediately if acute pain is produced (Fig. 24.5). This would indicate that the coccyx is fractured and in this case ultrasound will be too painful in the acute period. If a fracture has occurred there is usually a loud crack at delivery, heard by all present. The patient should also be advised to rest for 20 minutes following treatment for reasons explained previously.

Electrotherapy for Post-partum Breast Problems

Breast problems occur at any stage of lactation. Engorgement generally occurs in the first few days post-partum, while blocked ducts or mastitis present later. The physiology of the breast and normal lactation are covered in Chapter 10.

Engorgement

Engorgement is defined as an uncomfortable swelling of the breasts associated with increased milk secretion and usually occurs from the second to fourth day post-natally. There may be lymphatic and vascular congestion and possible interstitial oedema, causing swelling and tenderness. This exacerbates the tension of milk in the ducts and may cause stasis of the milk, resulting in inability of the milk to flow. This swelling and hardness may make it difficult for the baby to attach to the nipple and problems can be further aggravated by nipple soreness. The resultant inhibition of the let-down reflex can lead to incomplete emptying and decreased milk supply.

Table 24.4 Ultrasound parameters for treatment of sacroiliac joint pain or coccydynia

Mode	Pulsed 1:1 or less	Acute injury
Frequency	1 or 3 MHz	Close to surface so small penetration is needed
Intensity	0.5–1 W cm^2	Greater after first treatment if little effect is noted
Time	5 minutes approximately	Dependent on the area to be treated
No. of treatments	3–4	

Figure 24.5 Ultrasound treatment for coccydynia. The patient lies prone over pillows.

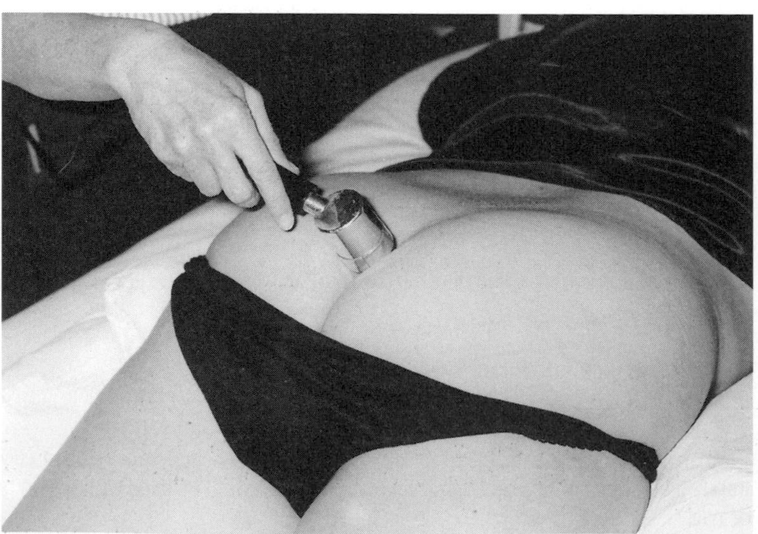

Unrelieved pressure on alveoli can ultimately cause atrophy of alveoli and basket cells, leading to failure of lactation. Engorgement is usually relieved by demand feeding. Heat and cold can be used to relieve symptoms – heat to increase blood flow to help movement of fluids prior to a feed and cold between feeds to reduce congestion.

The application of cold cabbage leaves to the breast was a popular treatment for breast engorgement and is still used in some hospitals. The theory is that the leaves produce an enzyme that passes through the skin and is effective in reducing swelling. However, clinical trials have failed to provide a basis for their use and this treatment has largely passed out of favour. It is thought that the cold was the most effective agent in the treatment.

PHYSIOTHERAPY TREATMENT

Ultrasound has been used as a treatment for severe post-partum engorgement. Both continuous (thermal) and pulsed (non-thermal) parameters have been used. The effects of continuous US are heating and acoustic streaming. The heating occurs quite deeply within the tissues of the breast. As attenuation (scatter) is increased with the amount of structural protein in the tissue and decreased with water content in the breast, there is good penetration and very little scatter. Half value depth of penetration for skin and fat is 40 mm for 1 MHz and 16.5 mm for 3 MHz. Therefore, for breast treatment 1 MHz frequency will provide the best penetration.

The effects of heating will be increased circulation of venous and lymphatic fluids and this leads to decreased pressure on milk ducts and improved flow. The pain relief will enhance the let-down reflex. The non-thermal effects of acoustic streaming increase the permeability of the cell membrane and promote movement of fluid at the molecular level. The treatment also provides a pleasant massage effect. There are psychological benefits in receiving pleasant treatment in a comfortable position. It often gives the mother much needed rest and relaxation. Table 24.5 details parameters for the US treatment of breast engorgement.

APPLICATION

The patient should be made comfortable in supine, with the arm of the treated side placed behind the head. A pillow under the knees may be helpful to relieve any tension on sutures. The physiotherapist passes the head of the ultrasound firmly over the breast from the periphery towards the areola, lightly back to the chest and firmly down again to the areola, gradually working around the breast. This action gives a good massage effect and is very soothing. Ideally, the baby should breast feed soon after treatment (within 20 minutes) to gain maximum benefit. The improved circulation and relief of pressure on ducts will allow good milk flow during this feed. Two to three treatments should be enough to break the cycle. In the McLachlan et al (1991) trial, the average number of treatments was 2.8.

STERILIZATION

Milk will often flow during treatment and will mix with the gel, so the US head must be carefully sterilized following treatment. It is known that some viruses and bacteria exist in and can be transmitted via breast milk. These include cytomegalovirus (CMV), HIV, herpes and staphylococci (Lawrence, 1989, p. 142). The US head should be washed in soap and water, dried well and soaked in glutaraldehyde for 10 minutes following treatment. Another method is to place a condom over the sound head during treatment. Adequate coupling medium needs to be placed on both surfaces of the condom, i.e. internal and external. After treatment and disposal of the condom, the US head is washed in soap and water.

RESEARCH

US treatment for breast engorgement was started in the 1980s and was perceived to be clinically successful. However, the only known trial conducted to date showed that while the treatment was indeed successful, it was not the US component that was significant. The trial (McLachlan et al, 1991) was a randomized double blind clinical trial comparing continuous US with a placebo machine adapted to provide warmth but with the crystal removed. This trial did not look at pulsed US and was limited to early post-partum problems of engorgement. As a result of this trial, US is not widely used by physiotherapists for treatment of engorgement. It is felt that the warmth and massage effects can be provided by other means. A single case experimental study demonstrated the effects of therapeutic ultrasound on the composition of breast milk (Luscombe et al, 1995).

Mastitis

Mastitis, another breast-feeding problem, generally occurs after the first week post-partum. Mastitis is a clinical term which describes a range of inflammatory disorders of the

Table 24.5 Parameters for US treatment of breast engorgement

Mode	Continuous or pulsed
Frequency	1 MHz
Intensity	1 W cm^2 – this would produce 0.5 W cm^2 40 mm within the breast
Time	This is difficult to estimate if treating the whole breast, as estimating the surface area of the breast is awkward. Bra cup size was used in one study (McLachlan et al, 1991): A cup – 10 minutes; B cup – 12 minutes; C cup – 14 minutes; D cup – 15 minutes

breast. Infective mastitis is most commonly caused by the bacteria *Staphylococcus aureus*. It causes cellulitis of interlobular connective tissue resulting in pain, swelling, redness and fever (Beischer and Mackay, 1986; Lawrence, 1989, in the further reading list). It is often associated with cracked and fissured nipples, allowing bacteria to enter the breast from the nipple. There is a peak of occurrence before the end of the second week post-partum and another peak at 5–6 weeks. Pathophysiological mechanisms of mastitis are ill understood. Apparently, extraductal breast tissue is colonized from the nipple by bacteria shared with the baby's oropharynx and bacteria have been shown to be present in milk from both breasts. Because the site of the infection is extraductal, continued breast feeding is recommended as any bacteria is common with the baby. The best and most common treatments include antibiotics, continued breast feeding and pain relief to improve let-down. There is no record of a baby becoming sick as a result of the mother having mastitis. Ultrasound could have a role in pain relief.

Blocked ducts

Obstruction of ducts can occur at any time in the breast-feeding period. Anything that disrupts normal breast drainage can be a risk factor, e.g. bruising, finger compression and hurried or infrequent feeds. It usually occurs as a tender lump and erythema and may be called non-infective mastitis. Some women seem prone to developing the problem in the same area of the breast. Treatment includes feeding from the affected breast first, massaging the area during the feed, nursing frequently and positioning the mother during the feed to encourage drainage from the affected area.

Ultrasound has also been used as a treatment for blocked ducts. It is theorized that continuous US would help by the effects of heat and micromassage to open the ducts and increase circulation, thereby assisting in movement of milk through the area. There are no studies to date proving the efficacy of US for treatment of mastitis or blocked ducts, but clinically both have appeared successful (Riddoch and Grimmer, 1993). The positive effects would enhance healing properties. Table 24.6 gives US treatment parameters for mastitis.

Precaution

Care should be taken by the physiotherapist using US in the case of active infective mastitis. Theoretically, increased circulation could lead to increased spread of organisms through the breast, but this is unlikely not to have occurred already.

APPLICATION

If a smaller area is being treated on the superior, lateral or medial surface, the patient may be made comfortable in sitting. However, it may be better to give treatment with the patient in a position that will encourage drainage of the breast from the affected area. The patient should also be encouraged to feed her baby in that position after treatment. Discussion with a lactation consultant is recommended for breast-feeding problems. She would be able to advise the physiotherapist about positioning.

Contraindications

Patients who have had silicone breast implants should not be treated with ultrasound. The effects of US on silicone are not known and could be potentially harmful. Patients who have had breast cancer should not be treated with US without consultation with their physician.

Electrotherapy for the Pelvic Floor

The main indications for use of electrotherapy for problems of pelvic floor dysfunction are to stimulate weak muscles, to inhibit detrusor instability and to aid cortical awareness of an isolated pelvic floor muscle (PFM) contraction.

Muscle strengthening

Before using electrotherapy to stimulate PFM, thought must be given to the cause of muscle weakness, the degree of weakness and what will be achieved by stimulation. Weak-

Table 24.6 US parameters for the treatment of mastitis

Mode	Mastitis – pulsed Blocked ducts – continuous Breast abscess	Acute problem – non-thermal best Chronic problem – thermal best US treatment not appropriate
Frequency	1 MHz	Half value depth 40 mm – good penetration
Intensity	Mastitis – 1 W cm^2 Blocked duct – 1.5–2 W cm^2	Acute condition Chronic condition
Time	1–2 minutes per 10 cm^2	

ness results from lack of use or nerve or muscle damage. Weakness from lack of use of PFM occurs frequently, but is unlikely to result in muscles weak enough to need stimulation. These muscles will benefit most from re-education and an exercise regime. The muscles may not have been used voluntarily, but will generally achieve a reflex response. Gains made by electrostimulation would be equalled or exceeded by voluntary exercise. Lack of the ability to voluntarily contract PFM will be discussed later under biofeedback (BFB).

Weakness from nerve or muscle damage can be the result of birth trauma, chronic constipation and constant straining at stool and extensive surgical damage, though this is rare.

Types of nerve damage include:

- neuropraxia of pudendal or pelvic nerves or some of their branches by pressure of the foetal head as it passes through the pelvis;
- disruption to the neuromuscular junction leading to partial denervation of PFM caused by overstretching of muscles as the baby's head passes through them.

This damage has been correlated with a long second stage of labour (over two hours), a big baby and use of forceps, but similar damage can occur with any birth (Smith et al, 1989b; Snooks et al, 1984). Constant straining at stool with perineal descent damages the pudendal and perineal nerves and causes similar problems (Kiff and Swash, 1984). The resultant denervation and reinnervation changes can be demonstrated by single-fibre EMG (Fig. 24.6) and nerve conduction studies. The following changes have been demonstrated.

- Increased perineal and pudendal nerve latencies (Smith et al, 1989b). This shows an increased time between nerve stimulation and muscle response.
- Increased fibre density of the pubococcygeus (Smith et al, 1989a).
- Increased polyphasia in the pubococcygeus (Allen et al, 1990).
- Clumping of fibre types in the pubococcygeus (Dubowitz, 1970). This showed a decreased proportion of fast-twitch fibres in the posterior pubococcygeus.
- Increase in percentage of slow-twitch fibres in the pubococcygeus (Gilpin et al, 1989).

These changes are highly correlated with the incidence of genuine stress incontinence (Gilpin et al, 1989). Damage can also occur within the muscle fibres and this can result in smaller fibres with central nuclei and/or muscle tissue being replaced by scar tissue.

Stimulation

What effect will electrostimulation have on these changes? It will have no effect on the reinnervation changes of increased nerve latency, fibre density and polyphasia. However, stimulation can have an effect on muscle fibre type, depending on the frequency used. This will be discussed in the section on current frequency. Therefore, stimulation will be used to maximize the 'normal' muscle component of PFM. It is thought that electrical stimulation is not an alternative for voluntary exercise (Lloyd, 1986). However, some studies have shown that stimulation combined with exercise leads to greater strength gains (Hon Sun Lai et al, 1988).

PFM strength gain has always been considered important in the treatment of genuine stress incontinence, but Laycock et al (1995) showed similar improvement in function in three groups: PF exercise and BFB; PF exercise, BFB and chronic stimulation; PF exercise, BFB and acute maximal stimulation.

Figure 24.6 (*left*) Normal muscle innervation; (*right*), axon sprouting that occurs in reinnervation after nerve damage to striated muscle. Some muscle fibres die.

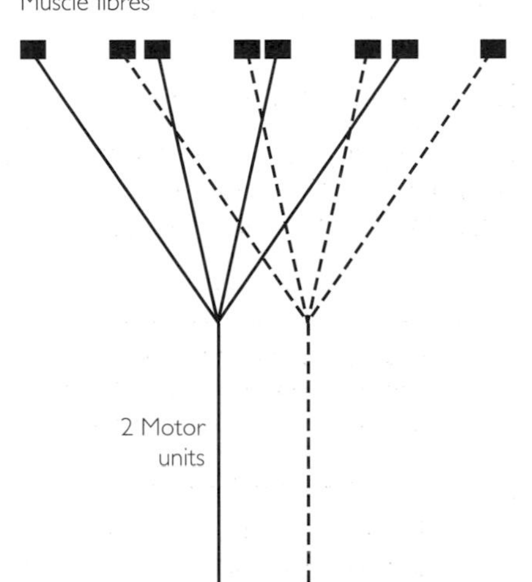

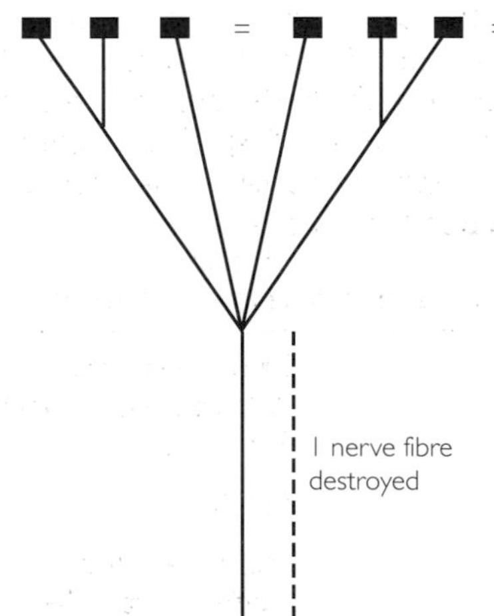

Those who received acute maximal stimulation to the PFM had a significantly greater increase in strength over the other two groups, but no real advantage in function.

A patient with very weak PFM should be offered electrical stimulation together with an exercise programme to optimize her recovery.

The physiotherapist must always be aware that the physiological effects of any neuromuscular electrical stimulation (NMES) are as yet only partially understood. Every effort must be made to keep abreast of the research literature. Unless the therapist is involved in a verified research study, the clinical parameters used should be those from published studies that have proved to be effective. Stimulation of the PFM during treatment of incontinence has been used for many years utilizing many different parameters (Tables 24.7, 24.8) and no deleterious effects have been reported so far. Some studies had a follow-up of six or more years.

When the decision to use stimulation has been made, factors to consider are:

- the type of machine;
- frequency;
- pulse width and shape;
- intensity;
- electrodes;
- duty cycle.

TYPE OF MACHINE

Any muscle stimulation machine that provides low- or medium-frequency currents can be used. Machines with alternating or biphasic current will provide comfortable treatment and eliminate any possibility of burns from chemical build-up over a sensitive part of the body. Many companies have small take-home machines available for PFM stimulation. The physiotherapist needs to check the parameters set by the machine and devise a programme that will benefit each patient individually.

FREQUENCY

This needs to be chosen to stimulate both fast- and slow-twitch fibres. PFM have a predominance of slow-twitch fibres. In women with symptomatic genuine stress incontinence, the posterior pubococcygeus has 90% slow-twitch fibres and the anterior pubococcygeus has 61% (Gilpin et al, 1989) (see Chapter 7 for normal fibre distribution). The distribution is probably dependent on lifestyle but PFM are predominantly postural muscles with the added ability to contract quickly to counteract sudden increases of intra-abdominal pressure. Slow-twitch fibres are stimulated at 8–20 Hz and 10 Hz is usually used. Fast-twitch fibres are stimulated at 20–60 Hz and for PFM 35–40 Hz is commonly used. Both frequencies should be used to prevent fibre type conversion if using chronic stimulation (see below).

Table 24.7 Chronic stimulation for stress incontinence

Author	Freqnency	Duration	Results
Farragher (1990)	5–10 Hz 35–40 Hz	1 hr/day for 28 days, then add 15 minutes/day for 14–28 days	Not available
Fall (1984)	20–50 Hz	10–12 hr/day for 2–14 months	80% cure or improvement
Blowman et al (1991)	10 Hz 35 Hz	1 hr/day for 28 days then add 15 minutes/day for 14 days	100% cure or improvement (small numbers)
Laycock et al (1995)	10 Hz	3+ hours a day for 6 months	83% greatly improved or cured
Erikson and Eik-Nes (1989)	25 Hz	'As much as possible' every day, 3–6 months	66% cure or improvement

Table 24.8 Acute stimulation for stress incontinence

Author	Frequency	Duration	Results
Laycock and Jerwood (1993) Trial 1 Trial 2	1 Hz 10–40 Hz 40 Hz	30 minutes × 2–3/week × 10 sessions	Trial 1 43% cured or improved Trial 2 73% cured or improved
Laycock et al (1995)	35 Hz	30 minutes – 16 treatments in 6 months	85% greatly improved or cured
Haig et al (1995)	10–40 Hz	20 minutes × 3 times/week for 4 weeks	Small numbers. Significant improvement in treated and placebo groups
Plevnik et al (1986)	20 Hz	20 minutes/day for 30 days	56% cure or improvement

PULSE WIDTH AND SHAPE

If the machine used provides the ability to choose pulse width and shape, thought should be given to the most effective parameters. Factors to consider are the following.

1. The cutaneous sensory nerves will be affected first and higher intensities will affect motor nerves supplying PFM. To avoid pain, a smaller pulse width should be used – 0.05–0.4 ms. The current needs to be increased rapidly to prevent accommodation, so a square waveform is best to stimulate nerves. Many muscle stimulators use either 0.25 or 0.3 ms.
2. Skin impedance is decreased with a shorter pulse duration of 0.1 ms or less, so the current penetrates deeper and spreads more evenly.

INTENSITY

Once a nerve has been stimulated, a higher intensity will not make the muscle fibres work harder. However, it will spread the current and stimulate more nerves, therefore causing more muscle fibres to contract. There are two ways to stimulate PFM:

1. chronic stimulation or long-term, low intensity (sometimes called trophic stimulation);
2. acute stimulation or short term, maximal intensity.

Both types of stimulation have been used effectively for PFM. Chronic or so-called eutrophic stimulation was begun in the 1980s for treatment of people with Bell's palsy and hand problems from arthritis (Farragher et al, 1987). The effects are to maintain or build up bulk in muscle that has been weakened by denervation or lack of use. There is an increase in capillary bed density and levels of oxidative enzymes after 10–28 days of stimulation. As a muscle takes its properties from the nerve supplying it, i.e. the electrical messages received, care must be taken with chronic stimulation. Stimulation at one frequency (e.g. 10 Hz) has been shown in the laboratory to convert fast-twitch fibres to slow. However, if stimulation at 35 Hz is added for just a short time, fast-twitch fibres will retain their properties (Salmons and Vrbova, 1969).

Chronic stimulation can be used over 1–6 months for daily treatments of one hour or longer. Acute stimulation can be used in the clinical situation if take-home machines are unavailable or too expensive for patients to hire.This uses higher intensities of 60 mA or greater for 20–30 minutes, 2–3 times per week for 5–6 weeks. At home, use of acute stimulation can be carried out daily. Careful attention must be given to the stimulation programme. Both types of stimulation have been successful in studies (see Tables 24.7, 24.8).

DUTY CYCLE

The duty cycle or on:off ratio allows the therapist to ensure the muscle is not stimulated to the point of fatigue. To achieve maximum contraction rest is needed to allow the muscle time to recover. For a weak muscle a longer duty cycle of 1:4 or 1:3 is preferable and this can be reduced gradually as the muscle improves.

ELECTRODES

Both internal and external electrodes can be used. It is generally accepted that internal electrodes are more successful, if tolerated, as the current is delivered in close proximity to the pubococcygeus muscle. These electrodes need to be single patient vaginal or anal electrodes which have both positive and negative nodes incorporated. Most women find these electrodes acceptable and comfortable. Consideration needs to be given to the following points.

1. The older and sexually inactive woman may have an atrophic or sensitive vagina and find that anything internal is uncomfortable. This can sometimes be overcome by the use of topical oestrogen creams to rejuvenate vaginal mucosa. The presence of an intact hymen would be an obvious contraindication to use of an internal electrode.
2. The size of the vagina and the size of the electrode need to match. Smaller electrodes will not provide good contact in a woman with a large vagina and in the opposite situation, discomfort will be caused. Sometimes use of an anal electrode will overcome these problems. Anal electrodes can be successfully used for stimulation of the male pelvic floor.
3. Lifestyle needs to be considered. Use of an internal electrode requires the patient to be supine for the duration of the treatment, so privacy and time must be available (see Chapter 30).

External electrodes are an alternative and can be used on small home machines, as well as extending the possibilities in the clinic. Higher intensities will need to be used to ensure spread of current from the more superficial perineal muscles to the deeper pubococcygeus. The electrodes will either have to be multiuse single patient electrodes or covered by individual or disposable covers. Wet 'Chix' nappy liners can be used to cover rubber electrodes. After use, the Chix covers should be discarded and the rubber electrodes washed in soap and water.

Electrode placement varies. With the Laycock 2 position (Laycock and Green, 1988) the patient sits with a larger electrode placed horizontally across the anus/perineal body and a smaller electrode placed vertically just below the pubic bone. There is a concentration of current towards the smaller electrode and this follows the line of the pubococcygeus and offers lower impedance. An alternative application is to use two small electrodes paravaginally or anterior and posterior to the anus. Adhesive gel pads over small rubber electrodes are suitable for these latter placements and can be used repeatedly by patients. Some patients will need to remove perineal hair in the area of the electrode site.

REGIMES AND RESULTS

Some routines for chronic and acute stimulation that have been used successfully and are published in the literature are given in Tables 24.7 and 24.8. Some therapists would argue that the benefits can be attributed to increased sensory awareness rather than an increase in muscular strength. It is difficult to separate out the effects of electrotherapy and exercise but some studies have tried to do this (Laycock and Jerwood, 1993). Many patients have reported significant improvement in function that is not matched by an increase in muscle strength. In the clinical situation the aim is to optimize treatment for each patient so the therapist may opt for the added benefits of electrotherapy.

STIMULATION OF DAMAGED MUSCLE

Care must be taken if a physiotherapist is treating post-natal weakness of PFM. It is possible that the muscle fibre itself may be damaged as well as being temporarily denervated. Stimulation can have negative and positive effects on this healing muscle. It can encourage axon sprouting.

Precaution

Stimulation at >60 Hz and intensities of >80 mA will kill denervated muscle fibre. Stimulation at lower intensities can damage the recovering muscle fibres which results in maintenance of an immature muscle cell with a central nuclei (Jones, personal communication). Physiotherapists working with post-natal women usually take the conservative approach and do not use electrotherapy until damage is healed and mature muscle cells formed, i.e. at least eight weeks post-partum.

STIMULATION OF DENERVATED MUSCLE

It is unlikely that a physiotherapist would wish to stimulate a totally denervated PFM. No benefit is apparent as any effect of building up or maintaining muscle bulk would disappear soon after ceasing stimulation. One exception would be stimulating in the presence of a severe pudendal nerve neuropraxia whilst awaiting full recovery after allowing at least eight weeks for muscle healing. For stimulation of denervated muscle, different pulse widths and shapes are needed. Muscle is less accommodating than nerve, so slow rising triangular pulses or low-intensity wide pulses are preferred.

STIMULATION TO INHIBIT THE DETRUSOR

Electrotherapy has provided an alternative way to help people with incontinence caused by an unstable detrusor (motor urgency). Other forms of treatment are bladder training and drug therapy (see Chapter 30).

How does electrotherapy work? Bladder control is a complex mixture of inhibitory and facilitatory reflexes (see Chapter 7). Urge incontinence results from a breakdown in this reflex control. This occurs either in the bladder itself, the spinal centres (sacral and hypogastric) or in the brain (pontine and cerebral centres). It is hypothesized that the bladder overexcitability needs to be balanced by increased inhibition from another source.

Effects of sensory stimulation to achieve detrusor inhibition Inhibition of detrusor muscle instability is achieved by stimulation of sensory afferent fibres of the pudendal and other nerves. The effect is achieved via stimulation of sensory fibres of the bladder or S3 dermatome to modify the output from the sacral micturition reflex centre (S2,3,4) to the detrusor (bladder). The rationale for this approach is an attempt to facilitate more appropriate detrusor activity (Fall and Lindstrom, 1991; Janez et al, 1981).

Method Stimulation is produced by a similar method to that used for muscle strengthening. Frequency used is 5–10 Hz. However, the physiotherapist must be aware that the PFM will be stimulated too, so consideration will need to be given to looking after the fast-twitch fibres. A short time for stimulation of fast-twitch fibres, i.e. 35–40 Hz for 10–15 minutes, should always be included.

Some therapists have used stimulation over the S3 dermatomes to achieve inhibition via the sacral micturition reflex centre S2,3,4 (Webb and Powell, 1992). Table 24.9 details applications and results.

Cortical awareness

The principal form of electrotherapy used to teach PFM contraction is electromyography (EMG), commonly referred to as biofeedback (BFB). This can be used in the absence of a voluntary conscious contraction or to assist in learning to isolate a contraction to reduce use of accessory muscles. EMG can be used with internal or external electrodes though each has disadvantages. Internal electrodes are superior for isolating the pubococcygeus muscle but are not so extensively available, are fairly expensive and of course must be single patient use or sterilized according to accepted standards. External electrodes, whilst cheaper and more readily available, are not as selective in isolating the pubococcygeus. Placement can be either over the perineal body (probably most successful), laterally over

Table 24.9 Stimulation for detrusor instability

Author	Frequency	Duration	Results
Erikson et al (1989)	5–10 Hz	20 minutes 1–2/week × 7 sessions	50% cure and 33% improvement
Fall (1984)	8–10 Hz	All day 1–6 months	56% cure or improvement
Plevnik et al (1986)	20 Hz	20 minutes/day for 30 days	56% cure or improvement

the pubococcygeus, where stimulation will occur first in the superficial perineal muscles, or either side of the anus.

Simpler forms of biofeedback include pressure biofeedback machines (perineometers such as the Peritron) which are readily available, inexpensive, simple to use and can be used with a condom (see Chapter 30). Any muscle-stimulating machine that can produce a palpable contraction can also be used as a teaching device. The patient can be asked to try to work with the machine as it produces the contraction and then try to reproduce it herself. Expensive equipment is not generally needed to achieve effective results.

Contraindications to electrotherapy for PFM

Accepted contraindications for use of electrotherapy on the pelvic floor are the following.

- Acute inflammation of the perineum or vagina.
- Pacemaker.
- Pregnancy.
- Excessive bleeding and danger of haemorrhage. (Normal menstruation is not a contraindication for use of external stimulation if the patient is using a tampon.)
- Poor skin condition
- Lack of internal or external sensation.
- Pelvic malignancy. The effect of stimulation on malignant cells is not known. Some doctors and physiotherapists have used it following radical surgery. Extreme caution is recommended and consultation with doctor and patient prior to use in these circumstances would be mandatory.
- Immediately post-natal (see above).
- Inability to understand or tolerate treatment

Gynaecological Conditions

In past years, pelvic inflammatory disease has been treated in the chronic phase with short-wave diathermy (SWD). It was thought to reduce inflammation and hence pain. It is rarely used now, but some women find it beneficial. Continuous or pulsed SWD can be used.

TENS has also been used for treatment of menstrual cramps with postioning and parameters used as for after-birth pain.

Electrotherapy modalities can be helpful in the overall physiotherapy management of women's health problems. It is sometimes difficult, however, to convince patients that exercise is generally the best way to improve circulation and muscle strength. Everyone likes to believe in that magic machine. It is the responsibility of all physiotherapists to provide accurate information, optimum treatment and motivate the patient to contribute to her own recovery and well-being.

References

Allen RE, Hosker GL, Smith ARB et al (1990) Pelvic floor damage and childbirth: a neurophysiological study. *British Journal of Obstetrics and Gynaecology* **97**: 770–779.

Artal R and Buckenmeyer PJ (1995) Exercise during pregnancy and postpartum. *Contemporary Obstetrics/Gynecology* **40**(5): 62–90.

Augustinsson LE, Bohlin P, Bundsen P et al (1977) Pain relief during delivery by transcutaneous electrical nerve stimulation. *Pain* **4**: 59–65.

Beckerman H, de Bie RA, Bouter LM et al (1992) The efficacy of laser therapy for musculoskeletal and skin disorders: a criteria based meta-analysis of randomised clinical trials. *Physical Therapy* **72**: 483–491.

Beischer NA and Mackay EV (1986) *Obstetrics and the Newborn*, 2nd edn. Sydney: WB Saunders.

Bierman W (1954) Ultrasound in the treatment of scars. *Archives of Physical Medicine* **35**: 209–213.

Blowman C, Pickles C, Emery S et al. (1991) Prospective double blind controlled trial of intensive physiotherapy with and without stimulation of the pelvic floor in treatment of GSI. *Physiotherapy* **77**: 661–664.

Bortoluzzi G (1989) Transcutaneous electrical nerve stimulation in labour: practicability and effectiveness in a public hospital labour ward. *Australian Journal of Physiotherapy* **35**: 81–87.

Creates V (1987) *A study of ultrasound treatment to the painful perineum after childbirth. Physiotherapy* **73**: 162–165.

Crothers E (1994) Labour pains: a study of pain control mechanisms during labour. *Journal of Association of Chartered Physiotherapists in Obstetrics and Gynaecology* **74**: 4–9.

Currier DP, Petrilli CR and Threlkeld AJ (1986) Effects of medium frequency electrical stimulation on local blood circulation to healthy muscles. *Physical Therapy* **66**: 937–943.

Dubowitz V (1970) Cited in Gilpin et al (1989) The pathogenesis of genitourinary prolapse and stress incontinence of urine – a histological and histochemical study. *British Journal of Obstetrics and Gynaecology* **96**: 15–23.

Erikson BC and Eik-Nes SH (1989) Long term electrostimulation of the pelvic floor: primary therapy in female stress incontinence? *Urology International* **44**: 90–95.

Erikson BC, Bergmann S and Eik-Nes SH (1989) Maximal electrostimulation of the pelvic floor in female idiopathic detrusor instability and urge incontinence. *Neurourology and Urodynamics* **8**: 219–230.

Everett T, Macintosh J and Grant A (1992) *Ultrasound therapy for persistent post-natal perineal pain and dyspareunia. Physiotherapy* **78**: 263–267.

Fall M (1984) Does electrostimulation cure urinary incontinence? *Journal of Urology* **131**: 664–667.

Fall M and Lindstrom S (1991) Electrical stimulation: a physiologic approach to the treatment of urinary incontinence. *Urologic Clinics of North America* **18**: 393–406.

Farragher DJ (1990) Trophic stimulation. *Nursing Standard* **5**(8): 10–11.

Farragher DJ, Kidd GL and Tallis RC (1987) Eurotrophic electrical stimulation for Bell's palsy. *Clinical Rehabilitation* **21**: 256–271.

Gilpin SA, Gosling JA, Smith ARB et al (1989) The pathogenesis of genitourinary prolapse and stress incontinence of urine – a histological and histochemical study. *British Journal of Obstetrics and Gynaecology* **96**: 15–23.

Grant A, Sleep J, McIntosh J et al (1989) Ultrasound and pulsed electromagnetic energy treatment for perineal trauma – a randomised placebo-controlled trial. *British Journal of Obstetrics and Gynaecology* **96**: 434–439.

Haig L, Mantle J and Versi E (1995) Does interferential therapy (IFT) confer added benefit over a pelvic floor muscle exercise program (PFMEP) for genuine stress incontinence (GSI)? Proceedings of the Conference of the International Continence Society, pp. 36–7.

Hon Sun Lai, de Domenica G and Strauss GR (1988) The effect of different electromotor stimulation training intensities on strength improvement. *Australian Journal of Physiotherapy* **34**: 151–164.

Janez J, Plevnik S, Korosec L et al (1981) Changes in detrusor receptor activity after electric pelvic floor stimulation. *Proceedings of the Conference of the International Continence Society*, pp. 22–23.

Kiff ES and Swash M (1984) Slowed conduction in the pudendal nerves in idiopathic (neurogenic) faecal incontinence. *British Journal of Surgery* **71**: 614–616.

Laakso EL, Crammond T, Richardson C et al (1994) Plasma ACTH and beta endorphin levels in response to low level laser therapy for myofascial trigger points. *Laser Therapy* **6**: 133–142.

Lawrence RA (1989) *Breast Feeding – A Guide for the Medical Profession*, 3rd edn. St Louis: C.V. Mosby.

Laycock F and Jerwood D (1993) Does pre-modulated interferential therapy cure genuine stress incontinence? *Physiotherapy* **79**: 553–560.

Laycock J and Green RJ (1988) Interferential therapy in the treatment of incontinence. *Physiotherapy* **74**: 161–168.

Laycock J, Knight S and Naylor D (1995) Prospective, randomised, controlled clinical trial to compare acute and chronic electrical stimulation in combination therapy for GSI. *Neurourology and Urodynamics* **14**: 425–426.

Lehmann JF and de Lateur BJ (1982) Therapeutic heat. In: Lehmann JF (ed) *Therapeutic Heat and Cold*, pp. 404–562. Baltimore: Williams and Wilkins.

Lloyd T, de Domenica G and Strauss GR et al (1986) A review of the use of electromotor stimulation in human muscles. *Australian Journal of Physiotherapy* **32**: 18–30.

Low J and Reed A (1994) *Electrotherapy Explained – Principles and Practice*, 3rd edn. London: Butterworth Heinemann.

Luscombe D, Jones S, Cox D et al (1995) The effects of therapeutic ultrasound on breast milk composition: a single case experimental study. *Australian Physiotherapy Association, National Women's Health Journal* **14**: 48.

McLachlan Z, Milne J, Lumley J and Walker B (1991) Ultrasound treatment for breast engorgement: a randomised double blind trial. *Australian Journal of Physiotherapy* **37**: 23–28.

Melzack R and Wall P (1982) *The Challenge of Pain*. Harmondsworth: Penguin Books.

Nussbaum E, Rush P and Disenhaus L (1990) The effects of interferential therapy on peripheral blood flow. *Physiotherapy* **76**: 803–807.

Plevnik S, Janez J, Vrtacnik P et al (1986) Short term electrical stimulation: home treatment for urinary incontinence. *World Journal of Urology* **4**: 24–26.

Raji AM (1984) An experimental study of the effects of pulsed electromagnetic field (diapulse) on nerve repair. *Journal of Hand Surgery* **9B**: 105–111.

Riddoch S and Grimmer K (1993) Developing a clinical indicator for obstructive mastitis. *Australian Journal of Physiotherapy* **39**: 321–322.

Salmons S and Vrbova G (1969) The influence of activity on some contractile characteristics of mammalian fast and slow muscles. *Journal of Physiology* **210**: 535–549.

Savage B (1984) *Interferential Therapy*. London: Faber and Faber.

Smith ARB, Hosker GL and Warrell DW (1989a) The role of partial denervation of the pelvic floor in the aetiology of genitourinary prolapse and stress incontinence of urine: a neurophysiological study. *British Journal of Obstetrics and Gynaecology* **96**: 24–28.

Smith ARB, Hosker GL and Warrell DW (1989b) The role of pudendal nerve damage in the aetiology of genuine stress incontinence in women. *British Journal of Obstetrics and Gynaecology* **96**: 29–32.

Snooks SJ, Swash M, Setchell M and Henry M (1984) Injury to innervation of pelvic floor sphincter musculature in childbirth. *Lancet* **8**: 546–550.

Wadsworth H and Chanmungam APP (1980) *Electrophysical Agents in Physiotherapy*. Sydney: Science Press.

Ward AR and Robertson VJ (1996) Dosage factors for subaqueous application of 1 MHz ultrasound. *Archives of Physical Medicine and Rehabilitation* **77**: 1167–1172.

Webb RJ and Powell PH (1992) Transcutaneous electrical nerve stimulation in patients with idiopathic detrusor instability. *Neurourology and Urodynamics* **11**: 40.

Wilson DH and Jagadeesh P (1976) Experimental regeneration in peripheral nerves and the spinal cord in laboratory animals exposed to a pulsed electromagnetic field. *Journal of the International Medical Society of Paraplegia* **14**: 12–20.

Young SR, Bolton P, Dyson M et al. (1989) Macrophage responsiveness to light therapy. *Lasers in Surgery and Medicine* **9**: 497–505.

Further reading

Beischer NA and Mackay EV (1986) *Obstetrics and the Newborn*, 2nd edn. Sydney: W.B. Saunders.

Beischer NA, Mackay EV and Purcal NK (1989) *Care of The Pregnant Woman and Her Baby*, 2nd edn. Sydney: W.B. Saunders / Baillière Tindall.

Health and Community Services, Victoria (1994) *Promoting Breast Feeding – Victorian Breast Feeding Guidelines*. Melbourne: Victorian Government Publications.

Hecox B, Mehreteas TA and Weisberg J (1994) *Physical Agents – A Comprehensive Text for Physiotherapists*. Norwalk: Appleton and Lange.

Jones DA and Round JM (1992) *Skeletal Muscle in Health and Disease*. Manchester: Manchester University Press, 221p.

Neville MC and Neifert MR (1983) *Lactation – Physiology, Nutrition and Breast Feeding*. New York: Plenum Press.

Schussler B, Laycock J, Norton P and Stanton S (1994) *Pelvic Floor Re-education*. New York: Springer Verlag.

Part Three

The Mature Woman

25

Physiological and Endocrine Changes of the Menopause

YVONNE KIRKEGARD

The menopause is a physiological event that occurs in all women living beyond the age of 60 years (Whitehead and Godfree, 1992a). Menopause, the very last menstruation, denotes the end of the reproductive period of life and the beginning of a new era.

The perimenopause or climacteric is the transition time leading up to the menopause, when endocrinological, biological and clinical features of the menopause first become manifest. For most women the perimenopausal transition lasts four years (McKinlay et al, 1992). During this period the menstrual cycle may increase to any duration (28 days to many months), anovulation cycles occur and menstrual loss varies (Whitehead and Godfree, 1992b). Post-menopause is usually determined by 12 months of amenorrhoea or complete lack of monthly menstruation (Khaw, 1992).

The average age of menopause (median age of last menstrual period) is 51 years, occurring typically between the ages of 49 and 55 (Wren and Eden, 1994). An earlier menopause is associated with living at high altitudes, with undernourished and thinner women and with cigarette smoking (Midgette and Baron, 1990). About 1% of women will experience menopause before the age of 40 (Speroff et al, 1994b).

Peri- and post-menopausal women are a rapidly growing proportion of the population and in several countries already constitute 15–20% of the population as a whole (Berg and Hammar, 1994).

Women can expect to spend over one-third of their lives after the menopause. At present the average female life expectancy is approximately 80 years (Fig. 25.1). Because of the growing number of older women in the community, a greater number of diseases such as osteoporosis and cardiovascular disease are occurring which are directly related to the post-menopausal loss of sex hormone activity (Diczfalusy, 1986; Wren and Eden, 1994).

When the ovary no longer produces adequate amounts of oestrogen, a complex series of vasovagal, physical, psychological and biochemical symptoms occur (Wren and Eden, 1994). Three out of every four women experience climacteric symptoms to a varying degree (Whitehead and Godfree, 1992b).

Sex Steroid Hormones

Oestrogens

The main source of oestrogen for reproductive females is the ovary. The normal human ovary produces all three classes of sex steroids: oestrogens, progestins, androgens and inhibin (Burger, 1994).

Oestradiol is the major oestrogen secreted by the human ovary. In the normal pre-menopausal non-pregnant female, oestradiol production varies throughout the menstrual cycle. The range varies from 90 to 1390 pmol/l per day (Whitehead and Godfree, 1992b).

Figure 25.1 Increase in female life expectancy from the years 1900 to 2000. (Reproduced from Speroff et al (1994b) with permission of L Speroff and the publishers.)

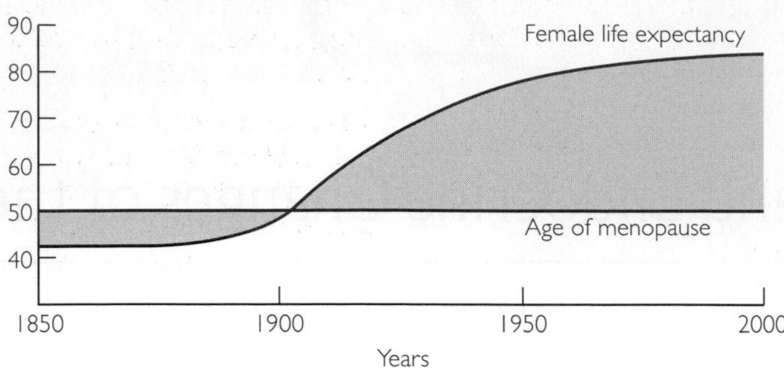

Figure 25.2 Scheme of the hormone production of the ovary and adrenal glands before and after menopause. (Reproduced with permission of JLH Evers and MJ Heineman (1990) and Wetenschappelijke Uitgeverij Bunge, Utrecht, Netherlands.)

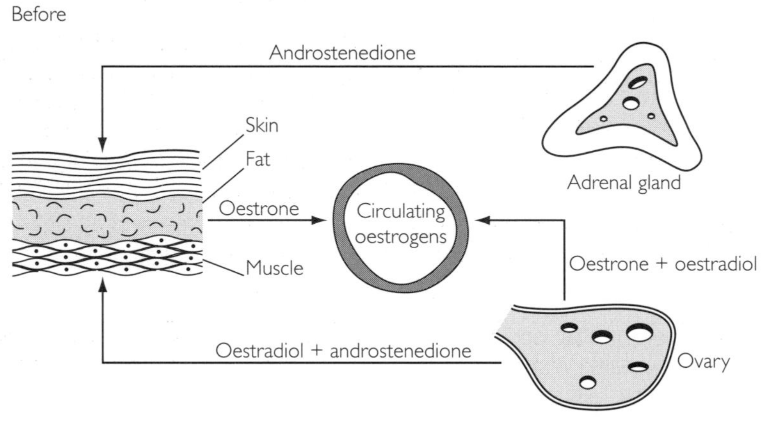

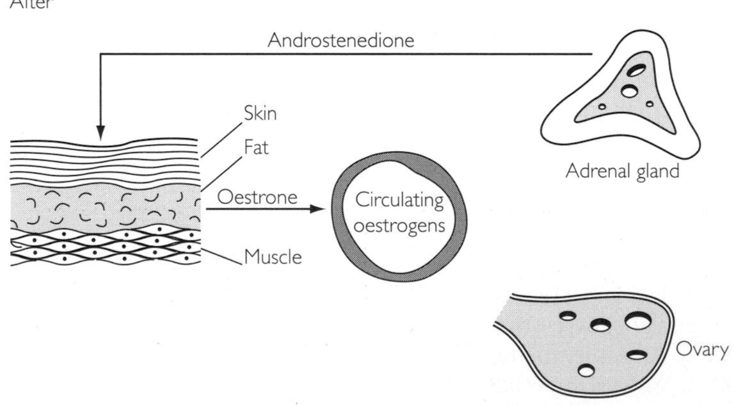

Androgens are the common precursors of oestrogens. Free androgens are peripherally converted to free oestrogens in skin and adipose tissue. In women, the adrenal gland is the major source of circulating androgens, particularly androstenedione (Siiteri and McDonald, 1973). Androstenedione is converted to oestrone and accounts for 20–30% of the oestrone produced per day. Circulating oestrogens in the female are predominantly the sum of direct ovarian secretion of oestradiol and oestrone (Siiteri and McDonald, 1973).

In the post-menopausal ovary oestrogen production ceases (Fig. 25.2). Oestrogen is derived post-menopausally from the peripheral conversion of androstenedione and testosterone to oestrogen via oestrone and this is less biologically active than oestradiol. Increased production of oestrogen from androstenedione with increasing body weight is probably due to the ability of fat to aromatize androgens. Body weight therefore has a positive correlation with circulating levels of oestrone and oestradiol (Speroff et al, 1994b). The oestradiol to oestrone ratio is reversed after the menopause. The decline in oestrogen production leads to a relative excess of androgens in the post-menopause, giving rise to androgenic features such as greasy skin, acne and facial hair as well as adverse changes in lipid profiles, which may influence the long-term risk of cardiovascular disease (Whitehead and Godfree, 1992b).

Androgens

Androgens in the female are produced by both the ovaries and by the adrenal cortex. The adrenal gland produces testosterone, androstenedione, dehydroepiandrosterone sulphate (DHEAS) and dehydroepiandrosterone (DHEA) (Fig. 25.3). The ovary produces testosterone, androstenedione and DHEA (Speroff et al, 1994a).

Fifty percent of testosterone in women is derived from peripheral conversion of these compounds (androstenedione, DHEA and DHEAS), and the ovaries and adrenals each contribute 25% (Sherwin, 1994).

At the menopause, there is a subtle change in testosterone (Roger et al, 1980). Over the years preceding the menopause there is a gradual decline of testosterone levels. Some authors suggest that this reflects waning ovarian function. The plasma testosterone levels are lower in menstruating women over 40 than in younger menstruating women (Roger et al, 1980). Testosterone decreases about 20% and androstenedione decreases about 50% after the menopause (Davis, 1995).

The post-menopausal ovary continues to secrete testosterone in about 50% of women but at lower concentrations (Longcope, 1992). The other 50% have no significant ovarian testosterone production and on examination, many have quite fibrotic ovaries (Sherwin, 1994).

Progesterone

Progesterone is produced by the ovaries after ovulation. The blood production rate of progesterone in the preovulatory phase is less than 1 mg per day, rising to 20–30 mg per day in the luteal phase (Carr, 1992).

The function of the ovaries changes more quickly after the age of 35 (Evers and Heineman, 1990). At the menopause there are about 2000 follicles and these continue to develop in more or less monthly waves for another year or two, occasionally leading to an ovulatory cycle and, rarely, a pregnancy (Jansen, 1995) (Fig. 25.4). Contraception for women in this age group should therefore be continued for a year after the last menstrual period.

Figure 25.3 Source of testosterone. (Reproduced from Speroff L et al (1994a) with permission of L Speroff and the publishers.)

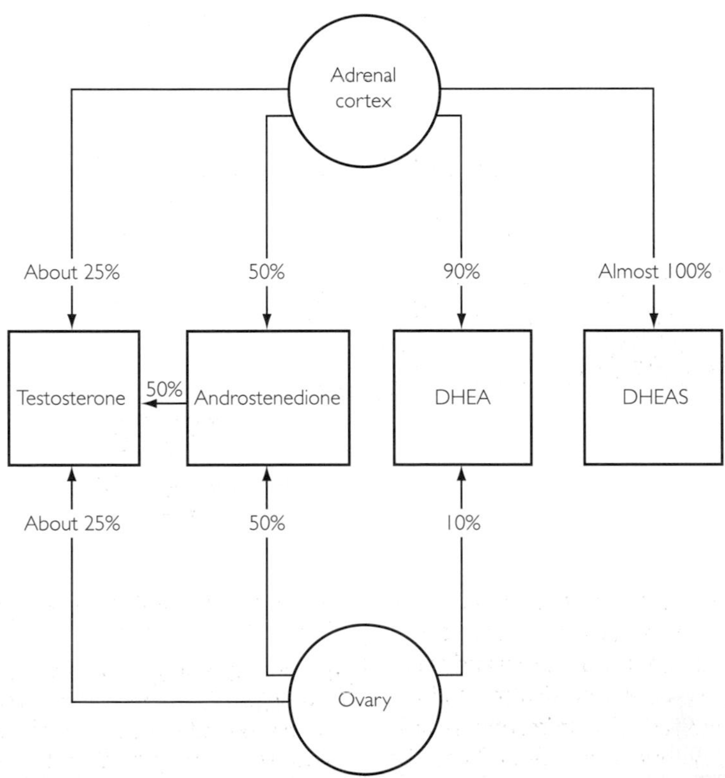

Figure 25.4 Scheme of the number of oogonia (follicles) in the ovaries and the gradual decrease in these numbers between birth and menopause. (Reproduced with permission of JLH Evers and MJ Heineman (1990) and Wetenschappelijke Uitgeverij Bunge, Utrecht, Netherlands.)

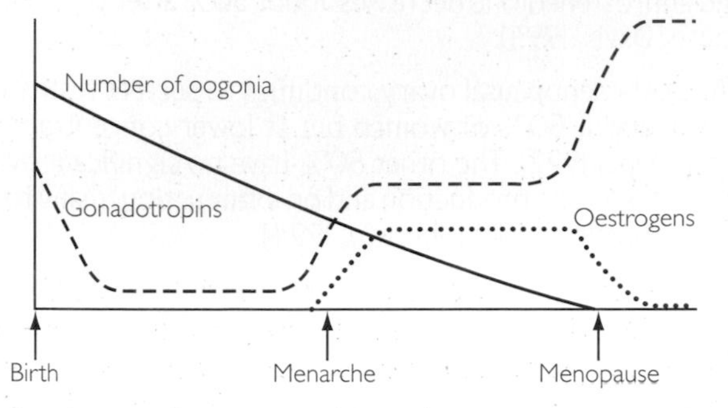

Symptoms Associated with Oestrogen Deficiency

Vasomotor symptoms

The flush is the most common symptom that women complain about during the menopause (Speroff et al, 1994b). The onset of flushing may be pre- or post-menopausal and the duration can be months to years. Some women never experience a flush whereas others have frequent flushes during the day and night.

The exact mechanism of the flush is still unknown. The disturbance responsible for flushing and sweating episodes apparently originates in the hypothalamus (Speroff et al, 1994b). The flush is described as an unpleasant sensation of heat beginning in the face, head or chest and spreading in any direction, sometimes over the whole body. It may be accompanied by palpitations, dizziness, nausea, headaches or fainting. Flushes are aggravated by hot weather, hot drinks, alcohol, stressful situations and by environmental temperature changes. For most flushes, however, the trigger is not known (Whitehead and Godfree, 1992c). Frequent night sweats may lead to chronic sleep deprivation and fatigue which may result in irritability, mood swings, indecisiveness and difficulties in concentration (Whitehead and Godfree, 1992c).

Urogenital tissue

The urogenital tract includes the vagina, urethra and bladder. Oestrogen receptors have been identified in these tissues (Iosif et al, 1981) and oestrogen deficiency will result in their atrophy.

Atrophic vaginitis is characterized by vaginal dryness and soreness, vaginal infections and dyspareunia (Speroff et al, 1994b; Whitehead and Godfree, 1992c). Atrophy of the bladder and urethra lead to symptoms of urinary frequency, dysuria, urgency, incontinence and recurrent urinary tract infections. A more detailed discussion of urogenital atrophy appears in the section on the aged (Chapter 36).

Loss of libido and sexual changes commonly occur at this time. The most prevalent sexual problem is dyspareunia. The majority of women going through the menopause report adverse changes in sexual function that affect sexual interest, sexual activity and the sexual response cycle. Oestrogen deprivation at menopause has been shown to adversely affect a number of physiological functions including lubrication, clitoral sensitivity, expansion of the vaginal barrel, labial colour changes and length of orgasm (McCoy, 1992).

Connective tissue

Consequences of ageing and oestrogen deficiency include musculoskeletal aches and pains, skin thinning, uterovaginal and bladder prolapse. Collagen changes may be implicated in some of these.

Skin changes associated with the menopause include thinning and dryness of the skin, increased skin fragility and decreased sensory perception. Some women complain of a sensation of ants crawling over them (formication) and this is possibly a consequence of peripheral neuropathy (Gilchrest, 1987).

Atrophic changes occur in other oestrogen target organs such as the breasts, uterus, ovaries and vulva (Whitehead and Godfree, 1992c).

Other Changes Associated with the Post-menopause

The buccal mucosa is affected by post-menopausal changes and reported symptoms include a dry mouth, difficulty with eating and speech and an increase in oral infections (Wren and Eden, 1994). There is some evidence that the occurrence of dry mouth progressively increases with age (Screebny, 1993).

Post-menopausal thinning of hair is common and is caused by changes in the synchronization of hair loss, due to oestrogen deficiency and a relative excess of androgens. Apart from a generalized thinning of hair, some elderly females also have areas of baldness (Rietschel, 1990). Axillary and pubic hair may also be lost.

Other changes that occur include muscle slackening as a result of loss of myocytes and decrease in type II fibres. The subcutaneous fat also disappears (Evers and Heineman, 1990).

Dryness of the eyes is considered to be another menopausal disorder (Whitehead and Godfree, 1992c).

Psychological symptoms

These reach a peak prevalence immediately prior to the menopause, occurring in 25–50% of women. Women often have a depressed mood accompanied by feelings of worthlessness, anxiety, crying, fatigue, loss of drive, aches and pains and headaches (Whitehead and Godfree, 1992c). Long-term consequences of oestrogen deficiency are discussed in subsequent sections.

Clinical Assessment for Menopause

The menstrual cycle changes prior to menopause are shown by elevated follicle-stimulating hormone (FSH) levels and decreased levels of inhibin, but with normal levels of oestradiol and luteinizing hormone (LH). Inhibin has an inverse relationship to FSH. The decrease in inhibin secretion by the ovarian follicles begins early (around age 35) but accelerates after 40 years of age. This is reflected in the decrease in fecundity that occurs with ageing (Speroff et al, 1994b).

If a woman presents with menopausal type symptoms and is still menstruating and it is suspected that she is perimenopausal, there are two approaches that may be taken (Eden, 1995). The first includes hormone assays.

Serum FSH values

- Best time is between days 1 and 7 of cycle.
- FSH should be measured more than once.
- Normally FSH <10 U/l, never >20 U/l.
- Perimenopausal FSH may be normal at times, but is typically 20–60 U/l.
- There is a 10–20-fold increase in FSH and a three-fold increase in LH, over time.
- A maximal level is reached 1–3 years after menopause.
- Long after menopause there is a gradual, but slight decline in both gonadotropins.

In the middle years, elevated levels of both FSH and LH are conclusive evidence of ovarian failure (Speroff et al, 1994b). The post-menopausal period is characterized by amenorrhoea, with low oestradiol and elevated FSH and LH levels.

In the second approach, it is often simpler for the woman over 40 years to be given a trial of HRT and see if symptoms improve. If there are no contraindications, 1–2 months of an oral contraceptive pill (OCP) is considered as it is simple, easy and convenient. Symptoms should be relieved within a month. Apart from relief from menopausal symptoms, the assessment of efficacy of hormone replacement includes assessment of vaginal acid–base balance. The oestrogenized vagina is acid (pH 3.8–4.5) and this can be assessed easily with simple pH test strips. This may be a reliable guide to adequacy of oestrogen dose.

Symptoms associated with oestrogen deficiency and their occurrence during menopause are outlined in Figures 25.5 and 25.6.

Figure 25.5 Relationship between hormone changes and symptoms during the menopause. Reproduced from WHO (1981) with permission.

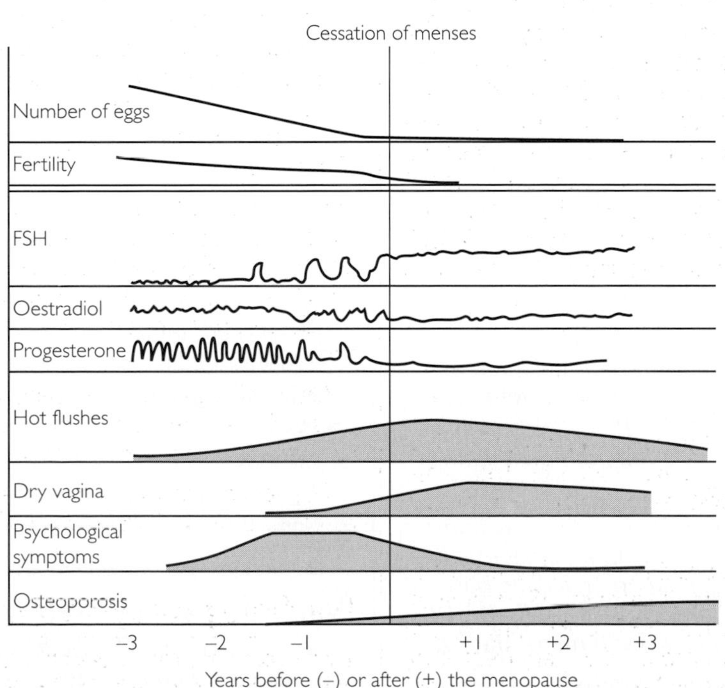

Figure 25.6 Acute, intermediate and long-term symptoms associated with oestrogen deficiency. (With permission: Whitehead M, Godfree V (1922c)

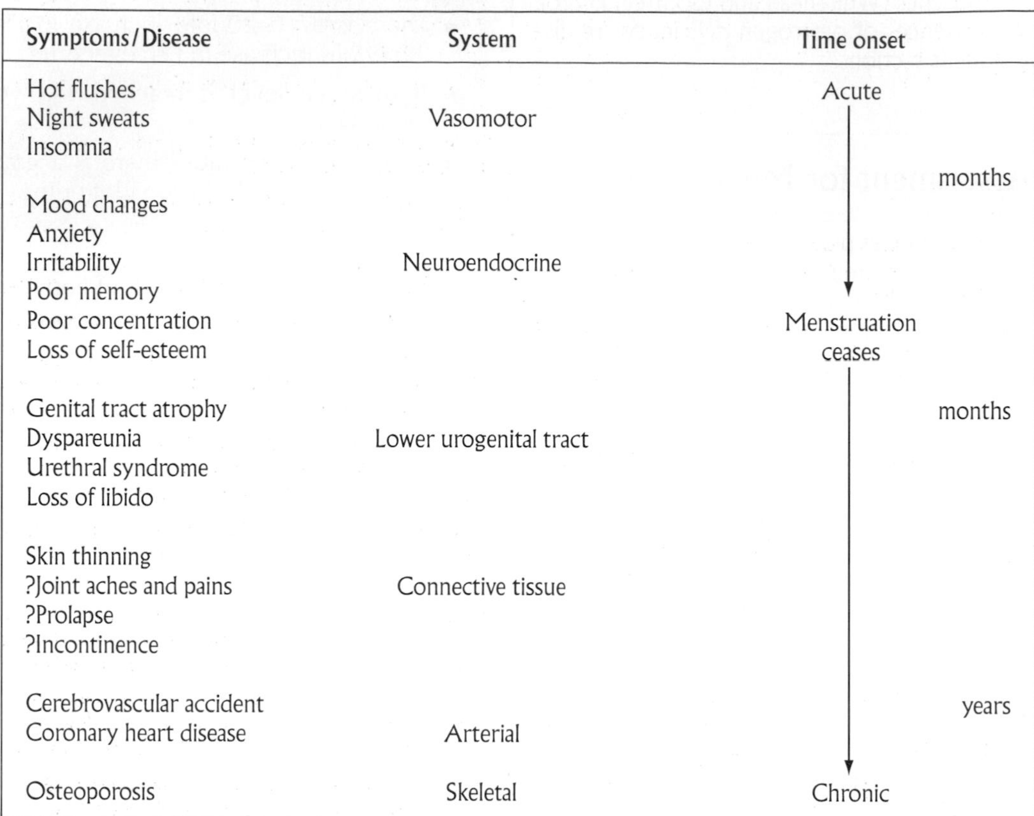

Symptoms/Disease	System	Time onset	
Hot flushes Night sweats Insomnia	Vasomotor	Acute	months
Mood changes Anxiety Irritability Poor memory Poor concentration Loss of self-esteem	Neuroendocrine	Menstruation ceases	
Genital tract atrophy Dyspareunia Urethral syndrome Loss of libido	Lower urogenital tract		months
Skin thinning ?Joint aches and pains ?Prolapse ?Incontinence	Connective tissue		
Cerebrovascular accident Coronary heart disease	Arterial		years
Osteoporosis	Skeletal	Chronic	

Physiotherapists have contact with many women in their menopausal years and beyond. An understanding of menopausal symptoms, sequelae and their possible hormonal management is essential if the physiotherapist is to provide optimum care and advice for her patients. The case histories which follow illustrate the medical management of some perimenopausal problems.

Mary, a 49-year-old housewife, presented to the doctor with the following complaints: night sweats, muscle aches, vaginal dryness and stress incontinence. Her periods were regular. A FSH taken on the fifth day of her menstrual cycle was 42 U/l (menopausal range 20–140). Her past health was good, but there was a significant family history of heart disease on her paternal side and her mother had osteoporosis. Her weight was 66 kg, height 162 cm and BP 130/90. Pelvic examination revealed cystocoele, rectocoele and first-degree uterine prolapse.

Contraception was not required so she was commenced on an oral cyclical hormone replacement therapy regimen (oestrogen taken on a daily basis, progestogen taken for a number of days, e.g. 10–12 days every 28 days) as she was still menstruating.

After six months therapy she reported:

- *that she had a sense of well-being;*
- *the condition of her skin had improved;*
- *there were no night sweats or hot flushes;*
- *no muscle aches,*
- *her memory had improved,*
- *she had lost 10 kg in weight.*

Gay, aged 44, was troubled by shortening of her menstrual cycle from every 28 days to 25 days, recent onset of heavy menstrual blood loss sufficient to induce iron deficiency and worsening of premenstrual symptoms (PMT), e.g. irritability, emotional lability, tiredness, tearfulness and a sense of heat.

Her management involved treating her iron deficiency and she was commenced on an oral contraceptive pill (OCP). There were no contraindications to the use of the OCP.

After three months she reported that:

- *her periods were now every 28 days;*
- *her menstrual blood loss was lighter;*
- *the duration of blood loss was less (originally six days, now three days);*

- *PMT symptoms were less;*
- *there was no sense of heat;*
- *she felt emotionally better;*
- *she was less tired.*

References

Berg G and Hammar M (1994) Preface. In: Berg G and Hammar M (eds) *The Modern Management of the Menopause: A Perspective for the 21st Century*, pp. xiii–xiv. London: Parthenon Publishing Group.

Burger HG (1994) Reproductive hormone measurements during the menopause transition. In: Berg G and Hammar M (eds) *The Modern Management of the Menopause: A Perspective for the 21st Century*, pp. 103–107. London: Parthenon Publishing Group.

Carr BR (1992) Disorders of the ovary and female tract. In: Wilson JD and Foster DW (eds) *Williams Textbook of Endocrinology*, 8th edn, pp. 733–798. Philadelphia: W.B. Saunders.

Davis S (1995) Androgens in the post-menopausal woman. Proceedings of the 5th Congress of the Australian Menopause Society, Hobart, Australia.

Diczfalusy E (1986) Menopause, developing countries and the 21st century. *Acta Obstetrica et Gynecologica Scandinavica* **134**(Suppl): 45–57.

Eden JA (1995) The menopause. In: Eden JA (ed) *Women's Hormone Problems*, 3rd edn, pp. 45–58. Sydney: Dezini.

Evers JLH and Heineman MJ (1990) Gynaecology of the climacteric and the menopause. In: Evers JLH and Heineman MJ (eds) *Gynaecology – A Clinical Atlas*, pp. 130–141. Antwerp: Koninklijke Smeets Offset, Organon.

Gilchrest BA (1987) Aging of skin. In: Fitzpatrick TB, Eisen AZ, Wolf K (eds) *Dermatology in General Medicine*, 3rd edn, pp. 146–153. New York: McGraw-Hill.

Iosif CS, Batra SC, Ek A and Astedt B (1981) Estrogen receptors in the human female lower urinary tract. *American Journal of Obstetrics and Gynecology* **14**: 817–820.

Jansen RPS (1995) Older ovaries: ageing and reproduction. *Medical Journal of Australia* **162**: 623–624.

Khaw KT (1992) The menopause and hormone replacement therapy. *Postgraduate Medical Journal* **68**: 615–623.

Longcope C (1992) Metabolic clearance and blood production rates of estrogen in post-menopausal women. *American Journal of Obstetrics and Gynecology* **111**: 779–785.

McCoy NL (1992) Menopause and sexuality. In: Sitruk-Ware R and Utian W (eds) *The Menopause and Hormonal Replacement Therapy: Facts and Controversies*, pp. 73–100. New York: Marcel Dekker.

McKinlay SM, Brambilla DJ and Posner JG (1992) The normal menopause transition. *Maturitas* **14**: 103–115.

Midgette AS and Baron JA (1990) Cigarette smoking and the risk of natural menopause. *Epidemiology* **1**: 474.

Rietschel RL (1990) Hair loss in woman. Proceedings of the 9th Regional Conference of Dermatology, Kuala Lumpur, Malaysia. Hong Kong: Excerpta Medica.

Roger M, Nahoul K, Scholler R and Bagrel D (1980) Evolution with aging of four plasma androgens in post-menopausal women. *Maturitas* **2**: 171–177.

Screebny LM (1993) Xerostomia, xerosis and systemic disease. *Female Patient* **3**: 9–21.

Sherwin BB (1994) Hormonal influences on sexuality in the post-menopause. In: Berg G and Hammar M (eds) *The Modern Management of the Menopause: A Perspective for the 21st Century*, pp. 589–598. London: Parthenon Publishing Group.

Siiteri PK and McDonald PC (1973) Role of extraglandular estrogen in human endocrinology. In: Astwood EB and Greep RO (eds) *Handbook of Physiology*, pp. 615–629. Washington DC: American Physiological Society.

Speroff L, Glass RH and Kase NG (1994a) Hirsutism. In: Speroff L, Glass RH and Kase NG (eds) *Clinical Gynecologic Endocrinology and Infertility*, pp. 483–513. Baltimore: Williams and Wilkins.

Speroff L, Glass RH and Kase NG (1994b) Menopause and postmenopausal hormone therapy. In: Speroff L, Glass RH and Kase NG (eds) *Clinical Gynecologic Endocrinology and Infertility*, pp. 583–649. Baltimore: Williams and Wilkins.

Whitehead M and Godfree V (1992a) The menopause – a growing problem. In: Whitehead M and Godfree V (eds) *Hormone Replacement Therapy – Your Questions Answered*, pp. 1–6. Edinburgh: Churchill Livingstone.

Whitehead M and Godfree V (1992b) The climacteric: definitions and endocrinology. In: Whitehead M and Godfree V (eds) *Hormone Replacement Therapy – Your Questions Answered* pp. 7–11. Edinburgh: Churchill Livingstone.

Whitehead M and Godfree V (1992c) Consequences of oestrogen deficiency. In: Whitehead M and Godfree V (eds) *Hormone Replacement Therapy – Your Questions Answered*, pp. 13–36. Edinburgh: Churchill Livingstone.

WHO (1981) Research on the menopause. Technical Report Series, No. 670. Geneva: World Health Organization.

Wren BG and Eden JA (1994) Hormone replacement therapy: a review. Part 1. *Female Patient* **4**: 5–16.

26

Menopausal Systemic Changes and Their Management

YVONNE KIRKEGARD

The perimenopausal and menopausal years may be unsettling to a vast majority of women. Women may feel this is a time to redirect their lifestyles and careers and yet they are often confused and 'let down' by changes in bodily appearance and function. Extra weight gain alone may prompt medical consultation at this time. This universal desire to improve appearance may lead to the identification of factors causing an increased risk of cardiovascular disease.

Cardiovascular and coronary heart disease are now considered to be major causes of female mortality. Early identification of those at risk and early intervention may do much to reduce morbidity.

This chapter will cover cardiovascular disease, weight, skin and musculoskeletal responses to ageing. Psychological symptoms and depression are expanded. A consideration of standard hormone replacement therapy and its role in ameliorating the disease and dysfunctional states induced by the menopause is included.

Weight Problems

Most women are concerned about their weight and this is especially important for the woman entering the middle years. There is a natural tendency for weight to increase and shape to change as a woman becomes older, irrespective of changes in hormone levels and medical treatments.

Before the implications of excess weight are discussed there needs to be some consideration of basal metabolic rate (BMR), body mass index (BMI) and waist to hip ratio (WHR).

> BMR – when a subject is at complete rest and no physical work is being carried out, energy is required for the activity of the internal organs and to maintain the body temperature (Passmore and Eastwood, 1986).

The BMR is best correlated with lean (or fat-free) body mass, so a reduction in muscle mass will result in a slower metabolism. Women have a higher ratio of fat tissue to lean muscle tissue than do males and usually have a lower BMR than males. The BMR decreases with age; the lower the BMR, the greater the problem there is with weight control. Exercise increases the BMR (Passmore and Eastwood, 1986).

> BMI is the ratio of weight divided by height squared and is expressed as kg m^2 (see Chapter 5). The average adult has a BMI of 25. A body mass of about 30 is roughly equivalent to 30% excess body weight usually stored as fat.

WHR is the waist to hip ratio and is a good indicator of central obesity, i.e. android distribution of fat. A high WHR predisposes one to a number of diseases. A high WHR in males is >0.90 and in females >0.80

To assess the WHR, measure the waist circumference by taking the narrowest diameter between the 12th rib and the superior border of the iliac crest. Then measure the hip circumference at the broadest circumference around the buttocks posteriorly and the symphysis pubis anteriorly (ASSO, 1995a).

- Obesity (BMI greater than 30 kg m^2) is an excess of body fat.
- Overweight (BMI greater than 25 kg m^2 but less than 30 kg m^2) is a body weight in excess of a standard or ideal weight.
- Obesity and overweight have serious medical implications.

The prevalence of overweight and obesity

The prevalence of overweight or obesity in Australia appears to be similar to the USA and Western Europe. In urban Australia, 40% of adults are overweight or obese. At all ages the prevalence of overweight and obesity combined is greater among men than women. However, obesity alone is more prevalent among women (11%) than males (9%), particularly in older groups. In women, the proportion who are overweight or obese rises steadily from just under 20% in those aged 20–24 years to slightly less than 60% among women aged 65–69 years (ASSO, 1995b; *Heart Facts*, 1992) (Fig. 26.1).

Women tend to gain weight several years before they reach menopause and weight begins its steepest rise after 40 (*Heart Facts*, 1992).

Diseases associated with overweight and obesity

Overweight and obesity are recognized by health professionals as predisposing factors for cardiovascular disease (CVD), hyperlipidaemia, non-insulin-dependent diabetes mellitus (NIDDM), osteoarthritis, gall bladder disease and some sex hormone-sensitive cancers such as breast and endometrial cancer, and sleep apnoea (ASSO, 1995a).

There is convincing evidence for the association between high WHR (android or central obesity) and NIDDM, hypertension, hypertriglyceridaemia and incidence of myocardial infarction and stroke in both sexes (ASSO, 1995a). Upper body fat localization in women is also associated with an increased prevalence of gall bladder disease (Schapira et al, 1991).

Figure 26.1 Proportions of overweight or obese women in the 20–69-year age groups. (Reproduced from *Heart Facts* (1992) with permission of the National Heart Foundation of Australia.)

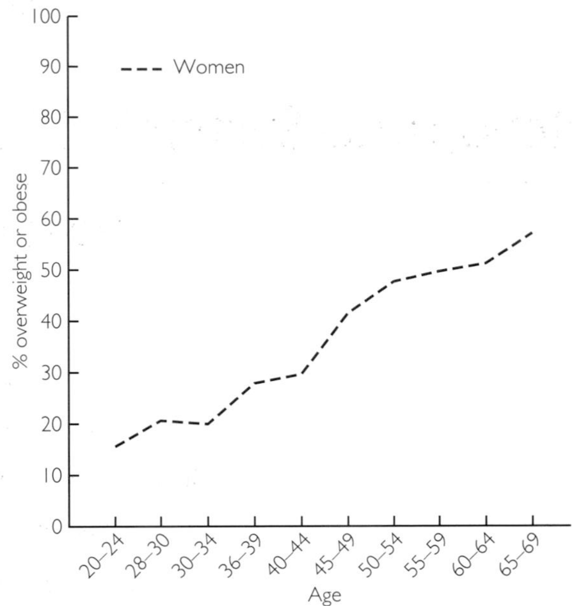

Breast cancer is higher in post-menopausal women who gain weight, especially of the male distribution type (central obesity). Endometrial cancer is linked to the amount of fat gained rather than to distribution of fat (Brzezinski and Wurtman, 1993).

Even mild to moderate overweight increases the risk of coronary disease in middle-aged women (Manson et al, 1990).

Menopausal weight problems

The so-called 'apple' or abdominal adipose deposition is characteristic of male obesity; pre-menopausal (reproductive) women tend to have a 'pear' or gluteofemoral pattern of fat deposition (Brzezinski and Wurtman, 1993) (Fig. 26.2).

Menopause is now thought to be associated with a shift to an android or male-pattern adiposity (Brzezinski and Wurtman, 1993). There is a redistribution of body fat from thighs and buttocks to the anterior abdominal wall to give the middle-aged spread.

Some studies show that administration of oestrogen post-menopausally reverses this type of distribution of fat from the anterior abdominal wall to buttocks and thighs (Haarbo et al, 1991; Jensen et al, 1986). During post-menopause, lean body mass (muscle) decreases and fat mass increases (Svendsen et al, 1995). Consequently the BMR decreases which adds to the problem of weight control.

Figure 26.2 The so-called 'apple' or abdominal adipose deposition of male and post-menopausal female obesity. Pre-menopausal women tend to have a 'pear'-shaped distribution. (Reproduced from Brzezinski and Wurtman (1993) with permission.)

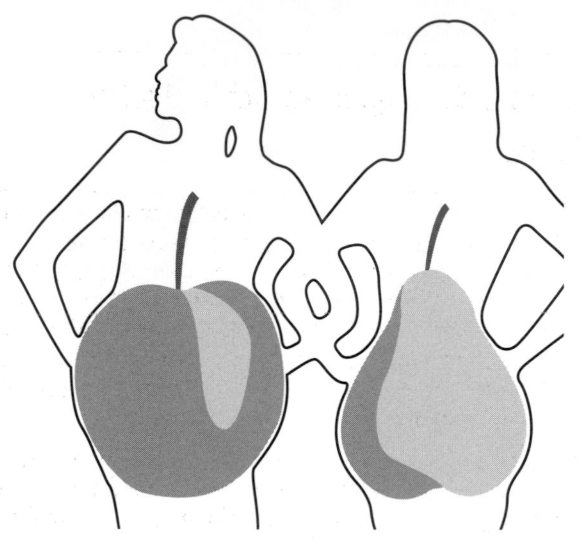

A common perception among women at menopause is that hormone replacement therapy (HRT) causes weight gain. There is little evidence to support this belief. In a large controlled trial, the placebo group gained more weight than those receiving HRT, although all gained weight over three years (PEPI Trial, 1995).

Summary

Approaching mid-life, women experience:

- a falling BMR;
- an increase in body fat;
- a decrease in lean body mass (muscle);
- a redistribution of body fat which in turn leads to the middle-aged spread.

If a woman wishes to minimize the impact of these bodily changes she may:

- exercise regularly;
- reduce her fat intake;
- increase her complex carbohydrate and fibre intake;
- have at least three meals per day;
- balance calcium intake/loss.

Exercise is the only course of therapy that can preserve and increase muscle mass and minimize the muscle loss which occurs with ageing (Shangold, 1990).

Musculoskeletal Changes

Musculoskeletal changes in the menopausal years have been described in detail in Chapter 32, which highlights the muscular deficits and skeletal changes associated with ageing. However, there are some features of the musculoskeletal system which are apparently related to a decrease in the oestrogen levels and which are worthy of mention.

Articular and muscular changes

Common presenting complaints around the transition to menopause are muscle aches and joint pains. Joint pains may occur due to a decrease in the collagen of ligaments and articular soft tissues (Whitehead and Godfree, 1992a). In addition, rheumatoid arthritis is more prevalent in women of this age group and Hall and Spector (1994) have commented on the usefulness of HRT as a therapeutic adjunct in the treatment of rheumatoid arthritis. This point is somewhat controversial, as van den Brink et al (1993) were unable to demonstrate any beneficial effects.

Muscular changes relate to an overall decrease in muscle mass. This decline can be attributed to a decrease in both strength and endurance of the muscle. Factors associated with these declines are height changes, weight increases and a decreased level of activity (Speroff et al, 1994a). The result of these changes is inevitably a higher risk of falls and subsequently of fractures (see Chapter 32) as well as a decrease in fitness levels.

Fitness changes

Lack of physical activity is linked to clinical problems associated with ageing, including decreased cardiovascular fitness, elevated blood pressure, bone loss, movement impairments, sleep disorders, depression and diabetes (Lampman and Savage, 1988).

Numerous studies have confirmed a progressive decline in women's physical fitness with time, a factor that has been attributed both to the natural process of age-related deterioration and a decrease in activity (Notelovitz, 1994).

With inactivity there is loss of muscle tissue and loss of muscle strength which is responsible for the weakness women develop with ageing. Inactivity also slows the metabolism. Regular physical training retards and reduces these changes (Fiatarone et al, 1994; Shangold 1990).

TYPES OF EXERCISE

Exercise involves both aerobic and muscle-strengthening activity. Aerobic exercise can be practised five days per week and muscle-strengthening exercises 2–3 times a week (Notelovitz, 1994).

Exercise accelerates the metabolic rate in several ways and different types of exercise accomplish this by various mechanisms. Strength training adds muscle tissue while increasing the resting metabolic rate. Aerobic exercises such as jogging, brisk walking, dancing, bicycling and swimming induce increased metabolic rate even after the exercise has ended (Shangold, 1990).

BENEFITS OF EXERCISE

Increased exercise has been found to be directly related to symptom reduction for a variety of disorders including obesity (Rauramaa, 1984), coronary artery disease (Rigotti et al, 1983) and depression (Klein et al, 1984).

Recent studies have confirmed that as physical fitness of women improves, so the risk for all causes of mortality, especially from cardiovascular disease and cancer, decreases (Notelovitz, 1994).

Lord and Castell (1994) showed that a progressive exercise programme among older women (mean age 62.5 years) resulted in improvements in reaction time, neuromuscular control, body sway and muscle strength. Strength training in post-menopausal and elderly, frail women was effective in increasing muscle strength (Fiatarone et al, 1994; Heislein et al, 1994).

A regular pattern of physical exercise reduces the risk of myocardial infarction in all people (Paffenberger et al, 1978). Both weight loss and increased physical activity, through an unknown mechanism, lower the level of low density lipoprotein cholesterol (LDL-C) and increase the level of high density lipoprotein cholesterol (HDL-C) (Weisweiler, 1987). Appropriate exercise is associated with an increase in the resting metabolic rate for 2–48 hours (Speroff et al, 1994b).

Physical activity (weight bearing) for as little as 30 minutes a day for three days a week will increase the mineral content of bone in older women (Chow et al, 1986; Smith et al, 1991).

There is little doubt that the incidence of osteoporotic bone fractures in elderly persons could be reduced substantially if exercise levels were generally maintained into retirement. This reduced risk of fracture may relate as much to the maintenance of muscle strength and neuromuscular co-ordination as to the associated maintenance of bone mass (Twomey and Taylor, 1984).

Exercise helps with:

- weight control and hence the diseases associated with obesity;
- preservation of muscle mass;
- stabilization of bone mass;
- reduction of mortality from cardiovascular disease;
- the reduction of adverse psychological symptoms.

Exercise also reduces serum lipid levels and the insulin resistance associated with obesity. There is an improvement in reaction time and neuromuscular control with exercise, especially in elderly women.

Vascular Changes Associated with Menopause

Cardiovascular disease (CVD) is the most common cause of death in the Western world and is responsible for 46% of all female deaths. Of these, 50% are due to coronary heart disease (CHD), a condition which presents differently in women and men (Collins, 1994). In the US 500 000 women die each year of cardiovascular disease (Wenger et al, 1993), with 36% of women presenting with sudden cardiac death or fatal myocardial infarction.

Most cardiovascular disease results from atherosclerosis in major vessels. The risk factors are the same for men and women: high blood pressure, smoking, diabetes mellitus and obesity (Speroff et al, 1994b).

Atherosclerosis

Atherosclerosis eventually causes narrowing of the arteries. The resultant effect is an inadequate blood supply to the target organs, e.g. narrowing of coronary arteries causes damage to the cardiac muscle, which results in angina or myocardial infarction.

Associated conditions are listed below.

HYPERTENSION

Hypertension accelerates atherosclerosis by increasing infiltration of lipids through the arterial wall. It also thickens the arterial walls and eventually progressive narrowing of the lumen occurs.

The hallmark of the atherosclerotic plaque is lipid accumulation and lipid usually constitutes a large volume of the lesion. Gradual plaque enlargement producing lumen narrowing (greater than 80%) may give rise to symptoms such as angina. Acute myocardial infarction has a different pathogenesis. It relates to thrombus formation at a site of plaque rupture, which occurs in lipid-rich plaques associated with a thinned fibrous cap. The degree of lumen narrowing is typically only 30–40% (Simons, 1994).

BLOOD LIPIDS AND OTHER PHYSIOLOGICAL CHANGES

The blood lipids are triglycerides (TG) and total cholesterol (TC), which includes LDL-C and HDL-C.

HDL-C is antiatherogenic whereas LDL-C is atherogenic, as are the triglycerides. Lowering LDL-C reduces the risk of future coronary heart disease. Between the ages of 48 and

56 the average cholesterol level rises more in women than in men as the HDL-C declines and LDL-C increases (Mathews et al, 1989). Lipoprotein (a) [LP(a)] is an independent risk factor for human atherosclerosis. Its concentration increases after the menopause.

HYPERTRIGLYCERIDAEMIC STATES

Hypertriglyceridaemic states are often associated with abnormal glucose intolerance, ranging from chemical glucose intolerance to frank diabetes mellitus. Atherosclerosis risk increases with moderate hypertriglyceridaemia, especially when other risk factors are present such as associated elevated LDL-C and low HDL-C.

UPPER ABDOMINAL OBESITY

Android distribution of weight leads to hyperinsulinaemia, hypertension, hypertriglyceridaemia and a low HDL-C level. Frequently these conditions are complicated by diabetes (Piziak, 1993).

INSULIN RESISTANCE

Insulin resistance describes the phenomenon of a minimal fall in blood glucose with the administration of insulin. It is seen in non-insulin-dependent diabetics (NIDDM), close relatives of diabetic subjects and in the obese person (Campbell, 1992). It is considered widely to be a predisposition to vascular disease. This is probably as a result of the growth-promoting effects of the associated high concentrations of insulin on smooth muscle and other cells in the arterial wall (Newnham and Burger, 1992). As a result the cells accumulate lipid due to increased lipogenesis.

Coronary heart disease (CHD) in females

CHD in pre-menopausal women is uncommon, the mortality rate being about 1.5 per 100 000 at the age of 30 years. Risk factors include hypercholesterolaemia, cigarette smoking and the addition of the oral contraceptive pill. Bilateral oophorectomy at a young age results in the premature development of atherosclerosis and its clinical outcomes (Ross, 1994). At any given age, post-menopausal women have a higher risk of cardiovascular disease than pre-menopausal women, with 10 per 100 000 dying of CHD at the age of 55. Eventually the rates for women and men become almost equal (*Heart Facts*, 1992; Kalin and Zumoff, 1990) (Figs 26.3, 26.4).

Figure 26.3 Coronary heart disease death rates according to age and gender in Australia (1988–1992). (Reproduced from *Heart Facts* (1992) with permission of the National Heart Foundation of Australia.)

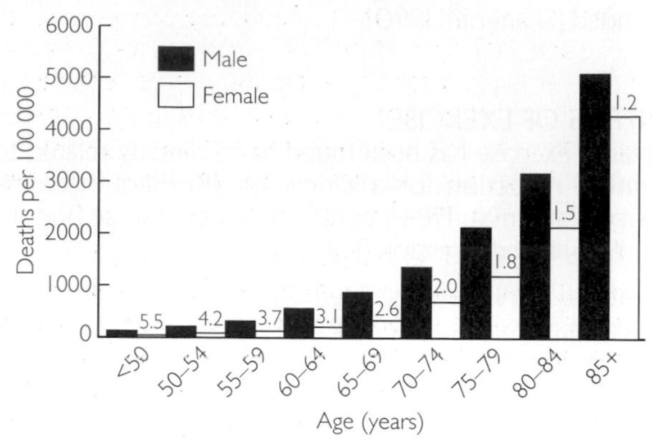

Figure 26.4 Age-specific mortality for coronary heart disease according to age and gender. (Reproduced from *Heart Facts* (1992) with permission of the National Heart Foundation of Australia.)

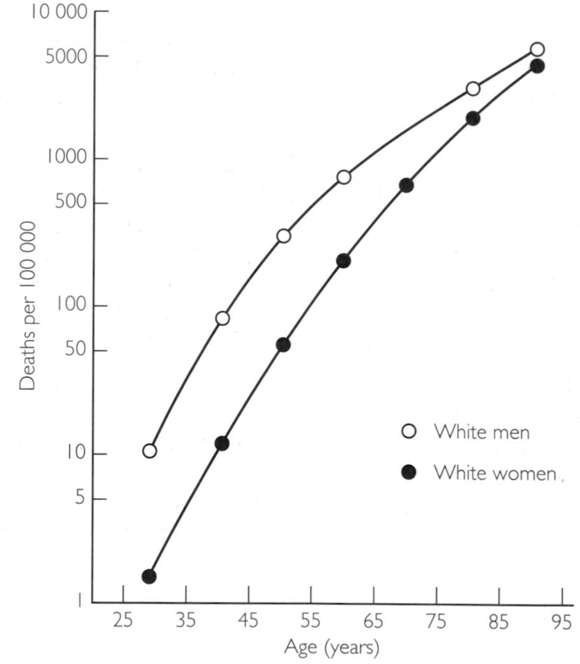

Risk factors for coronary heart disease in women

1. Family history of CHD
2. Smoking
3. Hypertension; ↑ systolic BP
4. Elevated total cholesterol and LDL-C; reduced HDL-C.
5. Hypertriglyceridaemia
6. Hyperinsulinaemia
7. Diabetes
8. Overweight/obesity – BMI above 27
9. Waist to hip ratio (WHR) >0.8 (central or abdominal obesity)
10. Increasing age up to 75 years
11. Other medical conditions such as abnormal immune and coagulation factors

Risk factors for CHD are qualitatively similar for women and men, although diabetes mellitus and elevated triglyceride

(TG) levels may be more atherogenic in women than men (Kalin and Zumoff, 1990). However, women have more severe disease despite milder symptoms and are less likely to be referred for investigation than men. Women have a worse prognosis for both medical and surgical therapies for heart disease (Wenger et al, 1993). They have increased mortality after myocardial infarction, more congestive heart failure and more strokes. They have a higher incidence of reinfarction and are less likely to return to the workforce than men. It has been suggested that the disease process may be different in females (Collins, 1994).

On the other hand, chest pain in women is often non-cardiac in origin and angiography more often reveals normal anatomy than in men. Cardiac flow disturbances, including coronary artery spasm (part of a little understood symptom cluster known as syndrome X), are often the causes of chest pain (Craig, 1995). Hormonal status is implicated in these cardiac conditions.

HORMONE REPLACEMENT THERAPY AND CORONARY HEART DISEASE IN POST-MENOPAUSAL WOMEN

Considerable evidence indicates that the increased post-menopausal risk from coronary artery disease is related to oestrogen deficiency and can be ameliorated by HRT (Burger, 1992).

Studies have shown that CHD events, stroke and mortality rates may be reduced by up to 50% in HRT users compared to non-users (Kalin and Zumoff, 1990; Paganini-Hill et al, 1988). Oestrogen replacement appears to be particularly effective in preventing CVD in post-menopausal women who are at high risk because of hyperlipidaemia, hypertension and smoking (Newnham and Burger, 1992) (Table 26.1).

The addition of progestogens to oestrogen therapy apparently attenuates the favourable increase in HDL-C but, at this stage, is thought to have little impact on the other beneficial cardiovascular effects. An epidemiological study from Uppsala (Falkeborn et al, 1992) and a randomized hormonal intervention trial (PEPI Trial, 1995) did not show any adverse effect from the addition of progestogens.

SUMMARY

Coronary heart disease is still the major cause of mortality and morbidity in Western communities. There is good evidence that control of risk factors and oestrogen replacement therapy can reduce CHD risk in women (Craig, 1995).

Skin, Menopause and Ageing

The female skin experiences both chronological (natural) ageing and accelerated ageing (associated with menopause and sun exposure). Women are disadvantaged as their skin is thinner (Shuster et al, 1975) and provides less protection from the sun, with fair skin more easily damaged by exposure to sunlight than dark skin. The earliest natural ageing events not caused by sunlight are loss of skin elasticity, loss of subcutaneous fat and thinning of the skin (Okun et al, 1988b). There is no doubt that sun exposure is the single most important environmental factor responsible for accelerating ageing of skin (Kuhl, 1994; Okun et al, 1988b).

Skin histology

The skin is composed of three layers. The two outer layers, the epidermis and the dermis, are firmly attached to one another. Beneath these two layers is the fatty layer called the subcutaneous tissue.

The dermis is composed of a dense network of collagen and elastin fibres. The other major constituent of the dermis is water. The collagen and elastin fibres are set into a jelly-like

Table 26.1 Beneficial effects of oestrogen replacement therapy on heart disease

Process	Effect
1. Lipid profile	• ↑ HDL, ↓ LDL, ↓ TC • Direct antiatherosclerotic effect in arteries
2. Carbohydrate metabolism	• ↓ Insulin resistance • ↓ Incidence of non-insulin-dependent diabetes mellitus
3. Cardiac output	• Direct inotropic action on cardiac muscle ↑ output • ↓ Blood pressure (selected forms of ORT)
4. Blood flow	• Vasodilation in atherosclerotic and non-atherosclerotic arteries • Reduction in peripheral vascular resistance • ↑ Exercise tolerance in post-menopausal women • Has a beneficial effect on vasoactive substances
5. Coagulation (vascular and non-vascular tissue)	• Platelet adhesion (protective anticoagulatory and fibrinolytic effects)
6. Obesity	• Redistributes central or android fat

HDL = high density lipoprotein cholesterol; LDL = low density lipoprotein cholesterol; TC = total cholesterol; ORT = oestrogen replacement therapy.

tissue called ground substance (Okun et al, 1988a). Collagen comprises 50–75% of the total protein in skin and oestrogen receptors are present in both the epidermis and dermis (Kuhl, 1994).

Changes in the epidermis with ageing

Gradual atrophy of the epidermis begins after the age of 30 and is intensified between 40 and 50 years (Kuhl, 1994; Gilchrest, 1987). There is an overall thinning of the epidermis to give the thin, shiny appearance of aged skin. Roughness and dryness of the skin surface occur due to a reduction in the moisture and oil content of the skin and the irregular, mottled pigmentation is due to a decline in the number of melanocytes (pigment cells) (Gilchrest, 1987).

Epidermis

- Thinning – shiny appearance.
- Roughness and dryness.
- Mottled appearance.

Dermis

- Loss of subcutaneous fat.
- Decline in the number of sweat glands and a decrease in sebum production.
- Nerve endings responsible for touch and pressure perception also decline in number to give decreased sensory perception.
- There are also fewer blood vessels and hair follicles.

Changes in the dermis with ageing

The dermis decreases in thickness and density after the age of 20. This is more evident in the thinner dermis of the female. The total amount of collagen in the dermis decreases steadily throughout adult life and elastin fibres thicken and degenerate. The skin loses its elasticity and a decrease in dermal ground substance may adversely affect skin turgor, tension and resilience (Gilchrest, 1987).

Changes in the skin with sun exposure

In addition to causing skin cancers, ultraviolet light has a similar effect to age on all skin layers. Thus in sun-damaged skin, wrinkles will appear earlier and be deeper than would be expected just with time. The skin thus becomes prematurely aged, wrinkled, wizened and leathery and may have a yellowish colour (Okun et al, 1988b).

Changes in the skin at menopause

In post-menopausal women there is a continuous decline of skin collagen during the first 15 years after the menopause, after which time it stabilizes. The average loss of dermal collagen is 2.1% per post-menopausal year and there is also a linear decline in skin thickness (Brincat et al, 1983, 1987; Castelo-Branco et al, 1992). This decline can be ameliorated by post-menopausal oestrogen to reverse the changes of oestrogen deficiency, i.e. decreased water, collagen and elastin. Due to loss of water storage there is subsequent dehydration of tissue. Thus oestrogen deficiency enhances the age-dependent degenerative changes in the skin and the skin becomes thin, dry and flaky and easily bruised (Kuhl, 1994). Concomitant thinning of hair and nails may also occur (Gilchrest, 1987). There is also a general thinning of other collagen-containing connective tissues throughout the body. It is lost from between the organs and from bone (Castelo-Branco et al, 1992). Peripheral neuropathy is believed to be the cause of the altered skin sensations experienced by many perimenopausal women (Gilchrest, 1987). Some describe it as 'ants crawling on the skin' (formication) or 'worms under the skin' or 'intense itchiness'.

Psychological Aspects of Menopause

It has been well established that specific receptors for oestrogen, progesterone and testosterone are found in areas of the brain that subserve emotion, memory and sexuality (McEwen et al, 1979). Sex hormones may also have an indirect effect on central nervous system morphology and physiology (Sherwin, 1994b). It has been shown in well-controlled studies that hormone replacement therapy (HRT) effectively reverses minor psychological symptoms such as dysphoria, irritability and mood swings but does not by itself alleviate depression (Sherwin, 1994a).

Psychological symptoms

Clearly a number of women find mid-life a difficult time. Psychological symptoms reported by perimenopausal and menopausal women include moodiness, anxiety, irritability, tiredness, headache, difficulty in sleeping, depression, memory and sexual problems.

Studies of menopausal women who seek help at special clinics have shown similar symptom profiles. Three large-scale studies indicated an increase in psychological symptoms just before menopause, when women were still menstruating. These symptoms were shown to decrease in the post-menopausal period (Ballinger, 1985; Bungay et al, 1980; Jaszmann et al, 1969). Similar results were found in studies based on symptom-related attendance at gynaecology clinics (Greene, 1976; Hunter et al, 1986).

However, large-scale random surveys of the general population of mid-life women in Sweden, England, the

USA and Canada all suggested that there was no increase in psychological symptoms at menopause (Garth et al, 1987; Hallstrom and Samuelsson, 1985; Kaufert et al, 1988; McKinlay et al, 1987). Dennerstein et al (1994), in their study on Australian women, confirmed these findings.

The problems that appear to be most directly related to the decreased levels of oestrogen accompanying the peri-menopausal and post-menopausal period are vasomotor symptoms (night sweats and hot flushes) and vaginal symptoms (Kaufert, 1984; McKinlay and Jefferys, 1974). Vaginal symptoms are identified as vaginal dryness, dyspareunia, dissatisfaction with sexual relationships and loss of sexual interest (Hunter et al, 1986).

A population-based study of urban Australian-born women found that current health status, psychosocial and lifestyle variables were significantly related to mood swings and overall well-being. Menopausal status was not related to mood measures or overall well-being (Dennerstein et al, 1994). Avis and McKinlay (1991) found that psychological and physical symptom reporting was highly related to attitudes towards menopause.

Depression

Both somatization disorder and depression are diagnosed more commonly in women (Raphael and Martinek, 1994).

Somatization has been defined as 'the tendency to experience and communicate psychological distress in the form of physical symptoms and to seek medical help for them' (Samuels, 1995).

Some of the symptoms of depression include: loss of interest in activities once enjoyed; sleep problems; loss of appetite; irritability; feeling low, sad or tearful; loss of sexual drive; tiredness; impaired concentration and inability to make decisions; feelings of worthlessness, helplessness and hopelessness; thoughts of suicide; withdrawal from social events.

Most depression in middle-aged women is associated with prior depression, personal health problems and stresses such as death and illness of family members, rather than the menopause itself (Avis et al, 1994; Kaufert et al, 1992).

Avis et al (1994) found that women who experience a long perimenopausal period (at least 27 months) have an increased risk of depression. The observed increase in depression during a lengthy perimenopause appears to be transitory.

Hormone replacement therapy does not by itself alleviate clinical depression (Sherwin, 1994a). Severe depression may be a very disabling condition and its management requires appropriate medical attention. This may include the use of antidepressant therapy and adequate support from trained therapists and family members.

Hormone Replacement Therapy

Hormone replacement therapy (HRT) refers to the prescribing of replacement doses of any one of the three steroid hormones produced by the ovary prior to the menopause: oestrogen, progesterone and testosterone (Darling and Davis, 1994). The benefits of HRT have been well established since the 1950s when oestrogen supplementation was first used to treat the symptoms associated with the menopause (Wren and Eden, 1994b).

Orally active oestrogens include both natural and synthetic preparations. Synthetic oestrogens are potent compounds and are not appropriate in routine hormone replacement therapy. Progestogens are added to oestrogens to protect against endometrial stimulation by oestrogen. It is not required for those women who have had a hysterectomy. Testosterone is given in selected cases of diminished libido.

Hormone replacement therapy (HRT) is not a contraceptive and there are no absolute contraindications to HRT (MacLennan, 1993).

Parenteral oestrogens bypass the gastrointestinal tract and avoid the first-pass effect through the liver. They provide more constant serum levels of oestrogen and are useful for women with liver disease, with a past history of thromboembolism, with inflammatory bowel disease, malabsorption or nausea associated with oral oestrogens (MacLennan, 1993).

Regimens of HRT

CYCLICAL REGIMENS

In all HRT regimens oestrogens are used in a continuous fashion without breaks. The continuous or cyclic regimens refer to the length of the progestogen therapy and are for non-hysterectomized women only.

As a general rule combined cyclic therapy is suitable for the perimenopausal woman and the progestogen is given for 12–14 days duration. Toward the end of the course of progestogen the woman has a predictable withdrawal bleed. The low-dose oral contraceptive pill is very useful for perimenopausal women, providing symptom relief

Table 26.2 Routes of oestrogen administration currently used (Whitehead and Godfree, 1992b)

Route	Preparation
Oral	Tablets
Parenteral	Percutaneous cream Subcutaneous implant Transdermal patches
Local	Vaginal creams Pessaries or vaginal tablets Flexible vaginal rings

Table 26.3 Objectives of HRT (Mahmoud, 1995)

Short term
Immediate relief from:
- vasomotor symptoms
- psychological symptoms
- genitourinary symptoms
- symptoms associated with premature, surgical or natural menopause

Long term
Protection from:
- cardiovascular disease
- osteoporosis
- possibly Alzheimer's disease
- selected cancers

and contraception if needed (Whitehead and Godfree, 1992b; Wren and Eden, 1994a, b).

CONTINUOUS COMBINED

In the continuous combined therapy both oestrogen and progestogen are given continuously. Eventually, within a year no withdrawal bleeds occur.

If a woman commencing HRT is 10–15 years post-menopausal it is preferable for her to be given a low dose of oestrogen at first to avoid side effects such as breast tenderness, irregular bleeding and bloating.

Women who suffer from urogenital symptoms and who prefer not to take systemic oestrogens can benefit from the use of local vaginal creams and pessaries or an oestrogen-releasing vaginal ring (Whitehead and Godfree, 1992b; Wren and Eden, 1994b).

Benefits of HRT

OSTEOPOROSIS PREVENTION

In the long term HRT is used to prevent osteoporosis (Barzel, 1988). The most common cause of osteoporosis is oestrogen deficiency associated with the post-menopausal state.

PREVENTION OF CARDIOVASCULAR DISEASE

Oral, unopposed oestrogen replacement therapy has a role in primary prevention of cardiovascular disease in selected women and there is consistent evidence to support the protective effect of oestrogen in women with established coronary heart disease (Lobo and Speroff, 1994).

Common problems associated with HRT

Initially some women may experience breast tenderness, nausea, fluid retention and bloating and skin irritation (Whitehead and Godfree, 1992c).

Table 26.4 Recommended duration of HRT (Darling and Davis, 1994; MacLennan, 1993)

Purpose of therapy	Duration
Relief of systemic symptoms	Up to five years
Relief of vaginal or urinary symptoms	Lifelong
Prevention of osteoporosis	10–15 years
Prevention of coronary heart disease	10–15 years or lifelong

Risks / benefits ratio

Different studies on HRT have shown an increased risk, a decreased risk or no effect on breast cancer (Petitti, 1995). Many of these studies have statistical flaws, making cause and effect relationship difficult to establish.

There is now evidence that women taking HRT have a lower incidence of Alzheimer's disease than those not taking any HRT (Paganini-Hill and Henderson, 1994).

It is predicted that ischaemic heart disease will kill 20%, stroke 13% and breast cancer 3.4% of women over 55 years of age. HRT reduces the risk of heart disease (Stampfer and Colditz, 1991; Stampfer et al, 1991) and stroke by 50% (Paganini-Hill et al, 1988). By the age of 85 years nearly 50% of women will have experienced an osteoporotic fracture (MacLennan, 1992). Long-term hormone therapy also significantly reduces the risk of fractures of the hip, spine and wrist by 50–70% (Consensus Development Conference, 1991).

Lower bowel and rectal cancers appear to be reduced by approximately 50% in oestrogen users (Chute et al, 1991) and where progestogen is appropriately prescribed, the spontaneous incidence of endometrial cancer is also reduced significantly (MacLennan, 1992).

Mortality and morbidity from oestrogen deficiency diseases such as osteoporosis, cardiovascular diseases, urogenital atrophy and possibly dementia make the risk / benefit ratio strongly in favour of HRT use. The final decision to commence (or cease) HRT rests with the woman concerned.

Hormone replacement therapy represents the greatest breakthrough in the health care of women during and after the menopause. When this treatment is combined with positive changes in lifestyle, a healthy diet, adequate and appropriate exercise and good medical advice, women can look forward to many fulfilling and happy years in the post-menopause.

References

Australasian Society for the Study of Obesity (ASSO) (1995a) Part One: Understanding the problem: defining and classifying overweight and obesity. In: *Healthy Weight, Australia*, pp. 7–11. Sydney: Department of Public Health.

Australasian Society for the Study of Obesity (ASSO) (1995b) Part Two: Understanding the problem: the costs and prevalence of overweight and obesity in Australia. In: *Healthy Weight, Australia*, pp. 13–16. Sydney: Department of Public Health.

Avis NE and McKinlay SM (1991) A longitudinal analysis of women's attitudes toward the menopause: results from the Massachusetts Women's Study. *Maturitas* **13**: 65–75.

Avis NE, Brambilla D, McKinlay SM and Vass K (1994) A longitudinal analysis of the association between menopause and depression. Results from the Massachusetts Women's Health Study. *Annals of Epidemiology* **4**(3): 214–220.

Ballinger S (1985) Psychosocial stress and symptoms of menopause: a comparative study of menopause clinic patients and non-patients. *Maturitas* **7**: 315–327.

Barzel VS (1988) Estrogens in the prevention and treatment of post-menopausal osteoporosis – a review. *American Journal of Medicine* **85**: 847–850.

Brincat M, Moniz CF, Studd JWW et al (1983) Sex hormones and skin collagen content in postmenopausal women. *British Medical Journal* **287**: 1337–1338.

Brincat M, Kabalan S, Studd JWW et al (1987) A study of the decrease of skin collagen content, skin thickness and bone mass in the postmenopausal woman. *Obstetrics and Gynecology* **70**: 840–845.

Brzezinski A and Wurtman JJ (1993) Managing weight through the transition years. *Menopause Management* **11**(10): 18–23.

Bungay GT, Vessey MP and McPherson CK (1980) Study of symptoms in middle life with special reference to the menopause. *British Medical Journal* **2**: 181–183.

Burger HG (1992) The menopause: implications for coronary disease. In: Kelly DT (ed) *Women and Coronary Disease*, pp. 15–21. Sydney: Excerpta Medica.

Campbell V (1992) Syndrome X and coronary disease. In: Kelly DT (ed) *Women and Coronary Disease*, pp. 47–50. Sydney: Excerpta Medica.

Castelo-Branco C, Duran M and Gonzalez-Merlo J (1992) Skin collagen changes related to age and hormone replacement therapy. *Maturitas* **15**: 113–110.

Chow RK, Harrison JE, Brown et al (1986) Physical fitness effect on bone mass in postmenopausal women. *Archives of Physical Medicine and Rehabilitation* **67**: 231.

Chute CG, Willett WC, Colditz GA et al (1991) A prospective study of reproductive history and exogenous oestrogens on the risk of colorectal cancer in women. *Epidemiology* **2**: 201–207.

Collins P (1994) Clinical problems of coronary heart disease in post menopausal women. In: Stevenson J (ed) *Hormone Replacement Therapy and the Cardiovascular System*, pp. 30–32. Abingdon, Oxon: The Medicine Group.

Consensus Development Conference (1991) Prophylaxis and treatment of osteoporosis. *American Journal of Medicine* **90**: 107–110.

Craig IH (1995) Women and coronary heart disease. *Current Therapeutics* **3**: 69–72.

Darling G and Davis S (1994) Hormone replacement therapy: logical prescribing. *Modern Medicine Australia* **37**: 57–66.

Dennerstein L, Smith MA and Morse C (1994) Psychological well-being, mid-life and the menopause. *Maturitas* **20**: 1–11.

Falkeborn M, Persson I, Adami HO et al (1992) The risk of acute myocardial infarction after oestrogen and oestrogen–progestogen replacement. *British Journal of Obstetrics and Gynaecology* **99**: 821–828.

Fiatarone MA, O'Neill EF, Ryan ND et al (1994) Exercise training and nutritional supplementation for physical frailty in very elderly people. *New England Journal of Medicine* **330**: 1669–1675.

Garth D, Osborn M, Bungay G et al (1987) Psychiatric disorder and gynecological symptoms in middle aged women: a community survey. *British Medical Journal* **294**: 213–218.

Gilchrest BA (1987) Aging of skin. In: Fitzpatrick TB, Eisen AX, Wolf K et al (eds) Dermatology in General Medicine, 3rd edn, pp. 146–153. New York: McGraw-Hill.

Greene JG (1976) A factor analytic study of climacteric symptoms. *Journal of Psychosomatic Research* **20**: 425–430.

Haarbo J, Marslew U, Gotfredsen A et al (1991) Postmenopausal hormone replacement therapy prevents central distribution of body fat after menopause. *Metabolism* **40**: 1323–1326.

Hall G and Spector T (1994) The use of estrogen replacement as an adjunct therapy in rheumatoid arthritis. In: Berg G and Hammar M (eds) *The Modern Management of the Menopause: A Perspective for the 21st Century*, pp. 369–375. London: Parthenon Publishing Group.

Hallstrom T and Samuelsson S (1985) Mental health in the climacteric: the longitudinal study of women in Gothenburg. *Acta Obstetrica et Gynecologica Scandinavica* **130**(Suppl): 13–18.

Heart Facts (1992) Canberra: National Heart Foundation of Australia.

Heislein DM, Harris BA and Jette AM (1994) A strength training program for postmenopausal women: a pilot study. *Archives of Physical Medicine and Rehabilitation* **75**(2): 198–204.

Hunter M, Batterby R and Whitehead M (1986) Relationships between psychological symptoms, somatic complaints and menopausal status. *Maturitas* **13**: 217–228.

Jaszmann I, van Lith N and Zaat J (1969) The perimenopausal symptoms: the statistical analysis of a survey (Part A & B). *Medical Gynaecology and Sociology* **4**: 268–277.

Jensen J, Christiansen C and Rodbro P (1986) Estrogen-progestogen replacement therapy changes body composition in early postmenopausal women. *Maturitas* **8**: 209–216.

Kalin M and Zumoff B (1990) Sex hormones and coronary disease: a review of the clinical studies. *Steroids* **55**: 330–352

Kaufert P (1984) Women and their health in the middle years: a Manitoba project. *Social Science and Medicine* **18**: 279–281.

Kaufert P, Gilbert P and Hassard T (1988) Researching the symptoms of menopause: an exercise in methodology. *Maturitas* **10**: 117–131.

Kaufert PA, Gilbert P and Tate R (1992) The Manitoba Project: a re-examination of the link between menopause and depression. *Maturitas* **14**(2): 145–155.

Klein M, Greist J, Gurman A et al (1984) A comparative outcome study of group psychotherapy versus exercise treatments for depression. *International Journal of Mental Health* **5**: 148–176.

Kuhl H (1994) Ovarian failure and the skin. In: Berg G and Hammar M (eds) *The Modern Management of the Menopause: a Perspective for the 21st Century*, pp. 381–391. London: Parthenon Publishing.

Lampman RM and Savage PJ (1988) Exercise and aging: a review of benefits and a plan for action. In: Sowers JR and Felicetta JV (eds) *The Endocrinology of Aging*, pp. 307–335. New York: Raven Press.

Lobo RA and Speroff L (1994) International consensus conference on postmenopausal hormone therapy and the cardiovascular system. *Fertility and Sterility* **51**: 502–505.

Lord S and Castell S (1994) Effect of exercise on balance, strength and reaction time in older people. *Australian Journal of Physiotherapy* **40**: 83–88.

MacLennan A (1992) Hormone replacement therapy: the evidence on primary and secondary prevention of coronary disease: a gynaecologist's viewpoint. In: Kelly DT (ed) *Women and Coronary Disease*. Sydney: Excerpta Medica.

MacLennan A (1993) HRT regimens for the menopausal woman. *Current Therapeutics* **34**: 43–48.

Mahmoud F (1995) Problems in the management of hormone replacement therapy. *Current Therapeutics* **36**: 37–43.

Manson JE, Colditz GA, Stampfer MJ et al (1990) A prospective study of obesity and risk of coronary heart disease in women. *New England Journal of Medicine* **322**: 882–889.

Matthews KA, Meilahn E, Kuller LH et al (1989) Menopause and risk factors for coronary heart disease. *New England Journal of Medicine* **321**: 641.

McEwen BS, Davis P, Parsons B and Pfaff D (1979) The brain as target for steroid hormone action. *Annual Review of Neuroscience* **2**: 65–74.

McKinlay JB, McKinlay SM and Brambilla D (1987) The relative contributions of endocrine changes and social circumstances to depression in mid-aged women. *Journal of Health and Social Behaviour* **28**: 345–363.

McKinlay S and Jefferys M (1974) The menopausal syndrome. *British Journal of Preventive Medicine* **28**: 108–115.

Newnham HH and Burger HG (1992) Cardiovascular issues in the menopause. *Australian Prescriber* **15**(3): 60–62.

Notelovitz M (1994) Non-hormonal management of the menopause. In: Berg G and Hammar M (eds) *The Modern Management of the Menopause: A Perspective for the 21st Century*, pp. 513–523. London: Parthenon Publishing Group.

Okun MR, Edelstein LM and Fisher BK (1988a) Normal histology of the skin. In: Okun MR, Edelstein LM and Fisher BK (eds) *Gross and Microscopic Pathology of the Skin*, 2nd edn, pp. 13–82. Canton, MA, USA: Dermatopathology Foundation Press.

Okun MR, Edelstein LM and Fisher BK (1988b) Degenerative dermatoses. In: Okun MR, Edelstein LM and Fisher BK (eds) *Gross and Microscopic Pathology and the Skin*, 2nd edn, pp. 608–609. Canton, MA, USA: Dermatopathology Foundation Press.

Paffenberger RS Jr, Wing AL and Hyde RT (1978) Physical activity as an index of heart attack risk in college alumni. *American Journal of Epidemiology* **108**: 161.

Paganini-Hill A and Henderson VW (1994) Estrogen deficiency and risk of Alzheimer's disease in women. *American Journal of Epidemiology* **140**(3): 256–261.

Paganini-Hill A, Ross RK and Henderson BE (1988) Postmenopausal oestrogen treatment and stroke: a prospective study. *British Medical Journal* **297**: 519–522.

Passmore R and Eastwood MA (1986) Energy. In: Passmore R and Eastwood MA (eds) *Davidson and Passmore Human Nutrition and Dietetics*, 8th edn, pp. 14–28. Edinburgh: Churchill Livingstone.

PEPI Trial Writing Group (1995) Effects of estrogen or estrogen/progestin regimens on heart disease risk factors in post menopausal women: the Postmenopausal Estrogen/Progestin Intervention (PEPI) Trial. *Journal of the American Medical Association* **273**(3): 199–208.

Petitti DB (1995) Hormone replacement therapy: risks and benefits. *Female Patient* **1**: 23–27.

Piziak V (1993) Lipid disorders in women. *Female Patient* **3**: 17–23.

Raphael B and Martinek N (1994) Social contexts affecting women's well-being in pregnancy and post-partum. *Medical Journal of Australia* **161**: 463–470.

Rauramaa R (1984) Relationship of physical activity, glucose tolerance and weight management. *Preventive Medicine* **13**: 37–46.

Rigotti NA, Thomas GS and Leaf A (1983) Exercise and coronary heart disease. *Annual Review of Medicine* **34**: 391–412.

Ross RK (1994) Impact of hormone replacement therapy on coronary heart disease. In: Stevenson J (ed) *Hormone Replacement Therapy and the Cardiovascular System: Recent Advances.* Abingdon: The Medicine Group (Journals) Ltd.

Samuels AH (1995) Somatisation disorder: a major public health issue. *Medical Journal of Australia* **163**: 147–149.

Schapira DV, Nagi B, Kumar RD et al (1991) Upper-body fat distribution and endometrial risk. *Journal of the American Medical Association* **266**: 1003–1011.

Shangold MM (1990) Exercise in the menopausal woman. *Obstetrics and Gynecology* **75**: 538.

Sherwin BB (1994a) Sex hormones and psychological functioning in postmenopausal women. *Experimental Gerontology* **29**(3–4): 423–430.

Sherwin BB (1994b) Hormonal influences on sexuality in the post-menopause. In: Berg G and Hammar M (eds) *The Modern Management of the Menopause: A Perspective for the 21st Century*, pp. 589–598. London: Parthenon Publishing Group.

Shuster S, Black MM and McVitie E (1975) The influence of age and sex on skin thickness, skin collagen and density. *British Journal of Dermatology* **93**: 639–643.

Simons LA (1994) *The Clinicians Handbook on Lipids.* Sydney: Aids International Pty.

Smith EL, Reddan W and Smith PE (1991) Physical activity and calcium modalities for bone mineral increase in aged women. *Medicine and Science in Sports and Exercise* **13**: 60–64.

Speroff L, Glass RH and Kase NG (1994a) Menopause and postmenopausal hormone therapy. In: Speroff L, Glass RH and Kase NG (eds) *Clinical Gynecologic Endocrinology and Infertility*, pp. 583–649. Baltimore: Williams and Wilkins.

Speroff L , Glass RH and Kase NG (1994b) Obesity. In: Speroff L, Glass RH and Kase NG (eds) *Clinical Gynecologic Endocrinology and Infertility*, pp. 651–666. Baltimore: Williams and Wilkins.

Stampfer MJ and Colditz GA (1991) Estrogen replacement therapy and coronary heart disease: a quantitative assessment of the epidemiological evidence. *Preventive Medicine* **20**: 46–63.

Stampfer MJ, Colditz GA, Willet WC et al (1991) Postmenopausal estrogen therapy and cardiovascular disease. *New England Journal of Medicine* **325**: 756–762.

Svendsen OL, Hassager C and Christiansen C (1995) Age- and menopause-associated variations in body composition and fat distribution in healthy women as measured by dual-energy X-ray absorptiometry. *Metabolism: Clinical and Experimental* **44**(3): 369–373.

Twomey LT and Taylor JR (1984) Old age and physical capacity. *Australian Journal of Physiotherapy* **30**: 115.

Van den Brink HR, van Everdingen AA, van Wijk MJ et al (1993) Adjuvant oestrogen therapy does not improve disease activity in postmenopausal patients with rheumatoid arthritis. *Annals of Rheumatic Disease* **52**(12): 862–865.

Weisweiler P (1987) Plasma lipoproteins and lipase and lecithin: cholesterol acyltransferase activities in obese subjects before and after weight reduction. *Journal of Clinical Endocrinology and Metabolism* **65**: 969.

Wenger NK, Speroff L and Packard B (1993) Cardiovascular health and disease in women. *New England Journal of Medicine.* **329**: 247–255.

Whitehead M and Godfree V (1992a) Consequences of oestrogen deficiency. In: Whitehead M and Godfree V (eds) *Hormone Replacement Therapy: Your Questions Answered*, pp. 13–36. Edinburgh: Churchill Livingstone.

Whitehead M and Godfree V (1992b) Types of HRT available. In: Whitehead M and Godfree V (eds) *Hormone Replacement Therapy: Your Questions Answered*, pp. 93–122. Edinburgh: Churchill Livingstone.

Whitehead M and Godfree V (1992c) Side effects of HRT. In: Whitehead M and Godfree V (eds) *Hormone Replacement Therapy: Your Questions Answered*, pp. 123–134. Edinburgh: Churchill Livingstone.

Wren BG and Eden JA (1994a) Hormone replacement therapy: a review. Part I. *Female Patient* **1**: 5–16.

Wren BG and Eden JA (1994b) Hormone replacement therapy: a review. Part II. *Female Patient* **4**: 5–14.

27

Health Promotion and Gynaecological Problems in the Middle Years

VIVIENNE O'CONNOR

Women's health encompasses the full range of health issues which affect women; they experience particular health problems and health service needs arising from their roles, responsibilities and position in society and from specific biological differences. Women's health differs in other respects. Women experience problems which may present and respond to treatment differently (e.g. coronary artery disease and alcohol abuse); some medical problems are more common in women (e.g. gall stones and osteoporosis), and some problems occur exclusively to women (e.g. obstetric and gynaecologic problems).

A number of other factors make the health and health care needs of women different from those of men. Some of these factors (such as poverty, poor housing, caring responsibilities, family violence, hormonal changes associated with the menstrual cycle, pregnancy and menopause) exert a combined effect on the emotional well-being of women and a disproportionate number of women are affected by depression, anxiety and eating disorders. Although all women are affected by these issues, those in the lower socioeconomic groups and minority groups, such as the disabled and women from non-English-speaking backgrounds, require special consideration and have specific needs. The meaning of health, well-being and quality of life will vary with the individual and her cultural background; it will also alter throughout a person's life and with her changing health status.

The development of medicine should be viewed in the context of the history of social attitudes. It is now apparent that with the changing role of women in society, there should to be parallel changes in teaching. Medical and allied health professions should now encourage their students to take a broader view of women's health and take into account the complexities of a woman's biologic, emotional and social functioning rather than the organ system approach of traditional care.

Mortality

The average life expectancy for white women in developed countries in 1900 was about 50 years; today these women can expect to live into their 80s. The leading cause of death for women in Australia, the USA and UK is heart disease, followed by cancer. Combined with cerebrovascular disease, these disorders account for 70% of all female deaths. In the 15–34-year age group accidents, homicide and suicide account for over half of all deaths. Cancer is the leading cause of death in the 35–74 year age group, after which death from heart disease predominates. Women are protected from heart disease by natural oestrogens during child-bearing years when the ratio of male to female deaths from coronary heart disease is 4.4:1; by 69 years this ratio is 2.5:1. At any age men have the same coronary death rate as women 10 years older.

Morbidity

The main cause of death in the 1800s and even the early part of the 20th century was infectious disease. Many factors have played a part in the eradication of these causes of death, including better nutrition and housing, public health measures, contraception and the development of antibiotics. Only a few women survived long enough to experience the effects of the menopause and diseases of older age. Since 1900 not only have the causes of death changed, but there are now more chronic illnesses causing debilitation. With longevity increasing, the accompanying debility can affect quality of life. This is of particular concern to women as they live longer than men; the predominance of women in the over-75s is just over 2:1. Older women have to deal with health issues of arthritis, osteoporosis, incontinence and dementia and related issues of isolation and lack of social support.

Cancer

Since the 1940s there have been reductions in the deaths attributable to cancer of the uterus, stomach and liver and, to a lesser extent, colorectal cancer. The deaths from breast and ovarian cancer have remained fairly stable. In contrast is the increase in mortality from lung cancer in women.

Smoking

The prevalence of cigarette smoking among men has decreased since the 1960s. In women the level has decreased little and recent studies suggest an increase in teenage and young women. Smoking has a profound impact on women's health. It affects reproduction, increasing the chance of infertility, spontaneous abortion, bleeding in pregnancy and low birth-weight babies. Young women using the oral contraceptive pill (OCP) increase their chance of developing a thromboembolic complication if they also smoke. Smoking is a risk factor for cardiovascular disease, osteoporosis and a number of cancers and affects a woman's skin, leading to discoloration, wrinkling and early ageing.

Depression

Female gender is one of the primary risk factors for depression. The current prevalence is between 5% and 10%, compared with a male prevalence of 2–3%. Depressive disorders are the most prevalent psychiatric diagnoses in women. Less than half of depressed patients are properly diagnosed. A number of medical conditions may include depression as a symptom, including alcohol and substance abuse, cancer, chronic fatigue, diabetes and dementia; it is important to exclude these. The family and relationship issues throughout a woman's life cycle are intricately involved in a woman's development. These and issues of work must be placed at the centre of any management programme.

Domestic Violence

Domestic violence is a leading cause of morbidity and mortality in women. Domestic violence has been defined as an ongoing debilitating experience of physical, psychological and/or sexual abuse in the home. This is associated with increasing isolation from the outside world and limited personal freedom and accessibility to resources. Although domestic violence can occur across all social and cultural groups, some women may be more at risk than others. Barriers to identification of domestic violence include a woman's feelings of shame, guilt, embarrassment or that her doctor has no interest in this area. A woman may fear the partner's reprisals, threats to the children and her own safety. The doctor or health worker may feel inadequately educated to identify and deal with the issues. Once identification can take place, the woman needs to be referred to an appropriate network for help.

Women at risk of domestic violence

- Single women
- Recently separated or divorced women
- Ages 17–28 years
- Partner with alcohol, substance abuse

- Pregnancy
- A history of childhood abuse

National Women's Health Policy

This was proposed in Australia in 1989 to advance women's health. It continues to be developed by the commonwealth, state and territorial governments (Commonwealth Department of Community Services and Health, 1989). The policy recognized priority health issues for women: reproductive health and sexuality, health of ageing women, women's emotional and mental health, violence against women, occupational health and safety, the health needs of women as carers and the health effects of sex role stereotyping on women. Key areas for action were identified. However, policy development and research are only of value to women if implemented and this involves improving the education of health professionals from the undergraduate level and thereafter.

Key action areas in the health-care system to improve women's health

- Improvements in health services
- Affordable, acceptable, accessible and appropriate services
- Provision of health information for women
- Research and data collection on women's health
- Women's participation in decision making on health
- Training of health-care providers

Health Promotion, Disease Prevention and Education for the Asymptomatic Woman

Health is not just the absence of disease but prevention of illness and the promotion of activities to achieve good health and well-being. The middle years are an ideal time for a review of health. The multiple roles that women play tend to give low priority to personal time. Exercise, relaxation and health care are likely to be at the bottom of the priority list as women place the needs of others before themselves. A medical consultation at this time of life allows a woman to reflect on her health status; it is never too late to modify health risks by changes in lifestyle. Women need to be provided with information to empower decision making about their own health. A review of past and current health events in the life of the woman and her family provides a background on which advice and information can be based (Fig. 27.1). It is useful

Symptoms suggestive of gynaecological disease

- *Bleeding*: too much; too little; intermenstrual; post-coital; post-menopausal
- *Pain*: Chronic pelvic pain; dyspareunia; dysmenorrhoea
- *Abdominal swelling*
- *Urinary symptoms*: dysuria; haematuria; incontinence
- *Vulval irritation and discomfort*
- *Vaginal discharge*
- *Breast symptoms*: tenderness; irritation; 'lump'

Figure 27.1 Changes for the woman in her middle years.

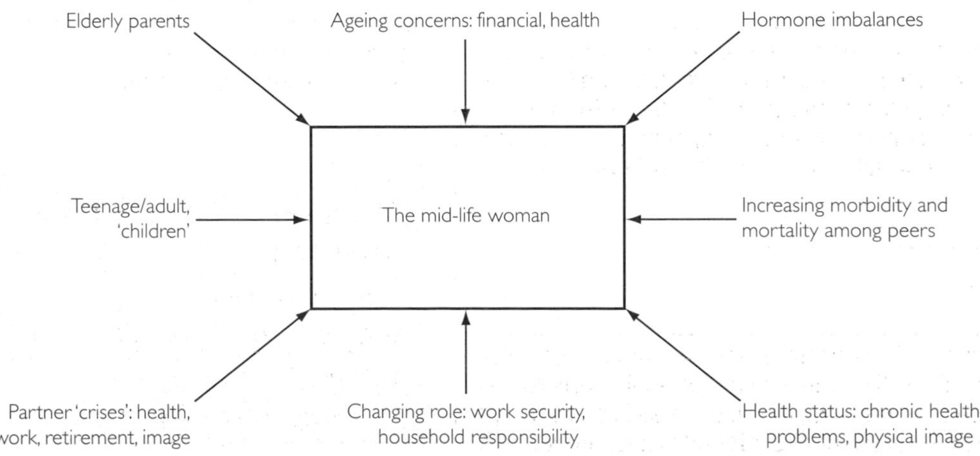

to reflect on lifestyle factors which affect health both positively and negatively. Symptoms may indicate gynaecological disease and the need for investigation.

Stress affects all ages and everyone suffers from short-term stress, such as taking exams. Chronic stress is different and can look very much like depression. This occurs when there is 'overload', extra demands and expectations which take extra energy and the body switches to 'emergency supply'. This is usually held in reserve for 'fight or flight' situations and is not designed for continued use. Eventually messages are sent from the body in the form of psychological or physical symptoms (e.g. pelvic pain). The psychological symptoms – a sense of anxiety and, finally, mental exhaustion – become stronger as the problem continues. Counselling, rest, relaxation and support of family and friends are required initially; it is then important to address the stressors which initiated the process. The importance of stress on health cannot be overemphasized and needs to be considered in all health consultations.

A 'social drug' is an unfortunate label as it implies harmless pleasure and relaxation, which is now known to be far from the truth. The role played by *smoking* in the development of heart disease, lung, mouth and throat cancers is beyond dispute. Similarly, smoking *marijuana* is also associated with oral cancers and is implicated in other disorders. Other aspects about smoking important to women are its role as a risk factor for cervical cancer and the long-term effects on the skin, leading to an early ageing appearance with lining and discoloration of the skin. Interestingly, *alcohol* gives a mixed picture with one to two drinks a day having long term benefits on the cardiovascular system but with an increasing number of drinks, these benefits are outweighed by possible harmful effects elsewhere in the body, such as the liver.

Women are fortunate in having a number of conditions that can be identified by a *screening test* early in their course and which are amenable to treatment. A test would ideally be able to detect two distinct populations – the healthy and the diseased. An arbitrary figure has to be set – the cut-off point – to divide the test results into two. In practice, the tests are not perfect and the two groups overlap. This means that some healthy people will be screened as having the disease – false positive – and some people with the disease are screened as healthy – false negative. A variety of screening tests are recommended at different ages (Hart and Burke, 1992). These screening tests include the cervical or Papanicolaou (Pap) smear test, mammography, skin examination and blood pressure testing. Other tests may be indicated for an individual woman from the history obtained (e.g. a woman with a family history of bowel cancer would be advised to have a colonoscopy). However, the cost effectiveness and psychological sequelae need to be factored into any screening programme before it is instigated.

Prophylactic treatments available against the development of future disease should also be discussed with each woman; for example, this may, involve the use of hormone replacement therapy to prevent osteoporosis or low-dose aspirin to decrease the risk of cardiovascular disease. A complete social history is essential to provide the context in which a woman is offered advice. Whether working outside and/or inside the home, women psychologically organize their lives around family and relationship issues.

Any pregnancy after the age of 40 years has risks in addition to those found in all age groups. The most important is an increased incidence of a chromosomal abnormality (Table 27.1). Where this is severe enough to cause death of the embryo, a miscarriage (abortion) occurs within the first 12 weeks of pregnancy. Other embryonic abnormalities which are not incompatible with life also increase with maternal age. Chromosomal and some of the other abnormalities can be diagnosed early in the pregnancy and termination of pregnancy offered to the couple.

Gynaecological Conditions and Treatment

Changing menstrual patterns

The normal menstrual cycle for the individual woman is assessed on the cycle frequency and the quantity or amount of bleeding.

FREQUENCY

During the menopause the normal menstrual cycle (range 21–35 days, average 28 days) may follow the woman's usual pattern and stop abruptly at menopause, become longer with less frequent periods or become shorter with more frequent periods.

Based on these patterns, a woman's menopausal status is described as pre-menopausal while the periods continue the same pattern; perimenopausal once a new irregular pattern develops or post-menopausal once she has not experienced any vaginal bleeding for 12 months or more.

QUANTITY

At the same time the amount of bleeding with each period may stay the same, increase or decrease. The period is said to be heavy if 80 ml or more of blood is lost (menorrhagia). In practice, this amount is assessed from the history by the number of pads or tampons used over a 24-hour span; passage of clots, their size and frequency; occurrence of

Table 27.1 Risk of chromosomal abnormality at mid-trimester amniocentesis

Maternal age (yrs)	Trisomy 21 (Down syndrome)	All abnormalities
35	1 : 263	1 : 110
40	1 : 75	1 : 43
45	1 : 22	1 : 15

'flooding' – sudden loss of a large amount of fresh blood; presence of pain or effect on lifestyle, e.g. prevents her leaving the house.

MENOPAUSE

The average age for a woman to pass through the menopause is 50 with a wide range between 40 and 60 years. Before 40 the menopause is said to be premature and should be investigated for other pathological conditions and hormone replacement therapy recommended. Today women can expect to spend one-third or more of their lives in the post-menopausal years (see Chapters 25 and 26 for further information). Bleeding occurring after a gap of a year is termed post-menopausal bleeding. The causes of post-menopausal bleeding are numerous (see box), but 10–20% of patients with this complaint have a gynaecologic malignancy, usually endometrial carcinoma. Some conditions which are related to oestrogen or the menstrual cycle may improve after menopause. These conditions include both endometriosis and fibroids (both of which may grow under the influence of oestrogen), menstrual migraine and pre-menstrual syndrome.

Aetiology of post-menopausal bleeding

Oestrogen therapy

Cancer: endometrium, cervix

Atrophic vaginitis

Endometrial polyps

Cervical polyps/cervicitis

No pathology

Heavy, prolonged or post-menopausal bleeding in all women in the middle years should be investigated

Menorrhagia

This term describes heavy or prolonged bleeding different from the woman's usual cycle. Objectively it is defined as a loss of 80 ml or more. In this age group there may be a variety of possible underlying pathological causes (see box) but cancer (either pre-malignant or invasive) is more likely than in younger age groups.

Causes of menorrhagia

Uterine pathology:
- Endometrial polyps
- Adenomyosis
- Fibroids
- Sarcoma

General medical:
- Thyroid disease
- Systemic lupus erythematosus

Dysfunctional uterine bleeding

Investigation includes a full blood count, thyroid function tests (abnormal thyroid function can cause bleeding problems in this age group), a luteal phase progesterone (to check whether or not the woman is ovulating), pelvic ultrasound, endometrial biopsy and hysteroscopy. If the investigation has excluded any specific underlying pathology the bleeding is termed dysfunctional uterine bleeding. This designates it as unusual but caused by no pathological process currently recognized and this probably accounts for more than half of the women with menorrhagia. The treatment offered will depend on the underlying cause and may be medical, with hormone management, or surgical (e.g. endometrial ablation or hysterectomy). In all treatment options it is important that the choice takes into account both immediate side effects and possible long-term risks and benefits.

MEDICAL OPTIONS

1. The non-steroidal anti-inflammatory drugs (NSAIDs) may reduce bleeding in up to 50% of women with menorrhagia and are only taken at period times. They also reduce dysmenorrhoea, headaches and diarrhoea associated with menstruation.
2. The low-dose OCP will induce regular shedding of a thin endometrium and inhibit ovulation. It therefore produces a light, regular period with contraceptive cover.
3. The progestogens can be useful in the ovulatory woman and increase the predictability of bleeding. Medicated intrauterine devices which release progesterone locally are the most recent development which may prove to be the ideal long-term medical solution for menorrhagia. They provide local treatment without systemic side effects.
4. The antifibrinolytics can reduce the loss by up to 50%.

SURGICAL OPTIONS

Endometrial ablation provides an alternative surgical management to hysterectomy in carefully selected women with menorrhagia, who have completed child bearing and are resistant to medical treatment. This method also provides a surgical option for women who may be medically unfit for abdominal surgery or general anaesthesia. The techniques used involve a method of destroying (ablating) the endometrium. The technique requires heat in the form of laser or cautery or the lining is removed with a resectoscope. Complications include haemorrhage and infection, as in other surgical procedures;

also uterine perforation and fluid overload (used to distend the uterine cavity during the procedure) can be potential problems. The long-term morbidity is as yet unknown, particularly with respect to the chance of unwanted pregnancy and potential malignant change within the uterine cavity.

Abdominal hysterectomy A total hysterectomy is the removal of the uterus, body and cervix, either through an incision in the abdominal wall or through the vagina. If the cervix is not removed (unusual) the procedure is termed a subtotal hysterectomy (Figs 27.2, 27.3). The ovaries will continue to produce hormones if the woman is pre-menopausal and she may still experience cyclical hormone changes even though there is no period.

Vaginal hysterectomy This procedure involves removal of the uterus, with or without the ovaries, using the vaginal route and not involving any abdominal incisions. The main contraindications to this route include a uterus equivalent to more than a 12-week pregnancy size, restricted uterine mobility and adnexal pathology. The mortality of vaginal hysterectomy is less than 0.1%.

Laparoscopic-assisted vaginal hysterectomy A combination of the two methods above (the abdominal part, employing only the small incisions required for the laparoscopy, forms the basis of this procedure). This method can be undertaken as day or short-stay surgery.

Wertheim hysterectomy Employed for surgical treatment of cervical cancer, this procedure involves removal of the uterus, tubes, ovaries, parametrium and upper one-third of the vagina. It is usually performed with a pelvic lymph node dissection via an abdominal incision. The major disadvantages are bladder and bowel problems due to partial denervation. Other complications can include fistula formation and other general post-operative surgical problems.

Caesarean hysterectomy There is sometimes, albeit rarely, an occasion when hysterectomy is undertaken at the time of a caesarean section. This is most likely to occur in a situation where life-threatening bleeding cannot be

Figure 27.2 Uterus and upper vagina: coronal section.

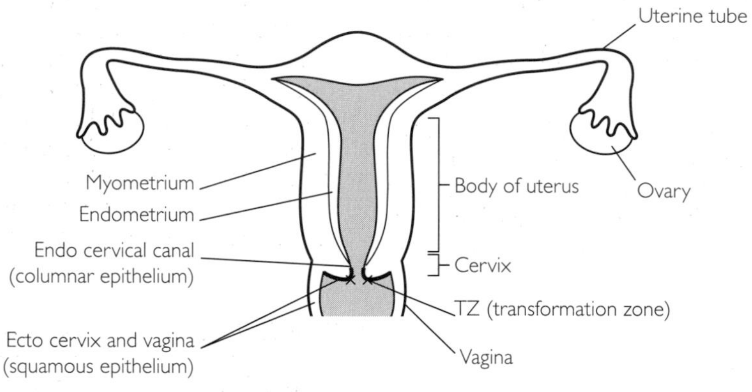

Figure 27.3 Anatomy after total hysterectomy with conservation of the ovaries.

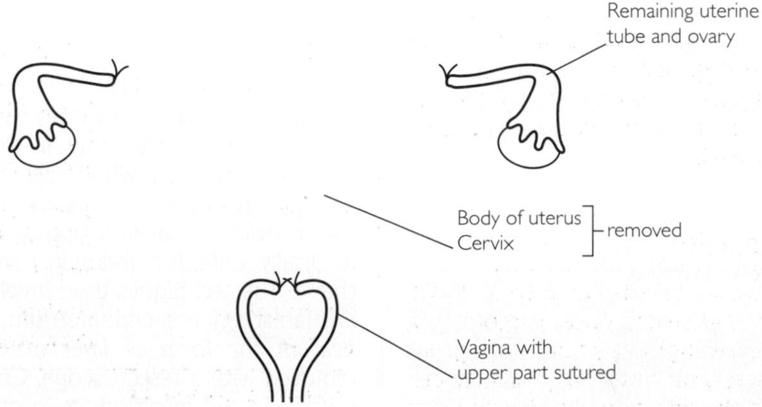

controlled by any other means, including tying the internal iliac vessels. The tissues have been stretched during the pregnancy and care must be taken that the vagina is not left too short.

COMPLICATIONS OF HYSTERECTOMY

No surgery or anaesthetic is without risks. These may be greater for women who smoke, are overweight or have other medical problems, such as diabetes or hypertension. Myths abound about the consequences of hysterectomy and the procedure will not cause a woman to put on weight, become hairier or develop a psychological impairment. As some women get older some of these changes may occur, with or without a hysterectomy.

Immediate damage Bowel and bladder damage can occur at hysterectomy. Ureteral injuries may occur, two-thirds at abdominal and one-third at vaginal hysterectomy. Any surgical procedure may be complicated by bleeding, infection, deep venous thrombosis (DVT) or pulmonary embolism.

Long-term effects These effects of hysterectomy are not well understood but appear to be limited to psychological, sexual and cardiovascular sequelae. Epidemiological studies have suggested that the relative risk for cardiovascular outcomes, including coronary artery disease and hypertension, is increased in women undergoing pre-menopausal hysterectomy with or without removal of the ovaries.

Careful preparation, counselling and identification of problems before embarking on surgery are essential to minimize later complications. Women choosing hysterectomy for a problem that has interfered with their lifestyle who receive thorough explanation and preparation achieve excellent and satisfying results.

Post-coital bleeding

Bleeding after coitus (sexual intercourse) is abnormal. Possible underlying causes may include a friable area on the cervix or vagina resulting from inflammation, a polyp (outgrowth of normal mucosal tissue), pre-cancer or cancer. An initial examination, taking a cervical swab to exclude infection and cervical smear test for dysplasia are indicated. Other causes in the upper genital tract, such as pelvic inflammatory disease, should be considered. Subsequent referral to a specialist for further tests, such as colposcopy and hysteroscopy, may be advised.

Intermenstrual bleeding

Bleeding between periods may be attributed to a physiological cause (hormone imbalance) once pathology is excluded (see post-coital bleeding). In a younger age group a sexually transmitted disease, such as chlamydia, may present with this symptom; it should also be considered in the older woman, particularly if a new relationship has recently occurred for either partner.

Pain

DYSMENORRHOEA (PERIOD PAIN)

This is a common complaint in young women in the early years following the menarche and results from events intrinsic to normal ovulation. It is termed primary dysmenorrhoea. Pickles et al (1965) first suspected that the pain of dysmenorrhoea was related to the release of prostaglandins F2a and E2. This occurs as a result of the fall in progesterone towards the end of the menstrual cycle and is accelerated by the tissue trauma and necrosis associated with endometrial shedding. Prostaglandin release leads to myometrial (uterine muscle) contraction and vasoconstriction (narrowing of the blood vessels) which causes ischaemia. Both the contractions and ischaemia result in pain. Dysmenorrhoea may also occur in an older woman and may suggest an underlying pathological condition. It is then termed secondary dysmenorrhoea.

CHRONIC PELVIC PAIN

This is an enormous and important problem. It is more common in women in the child-bearing years but may present or continue into the middle years. It has been cited as a major symptom among one-third of women attending gynaecology outpatients. A small number of women may have a gynaecological disease, a medical disorder or a surgical problem (see Table 27.2). Investigation includes diagnostic laparoscopy and pelvic ultrasound. However, treatment for the majority of women is unsatisfactory. Psychotherapy, medical suppression of ovarian activity, pain management

Table 27.2 Causes of chronic pelvic pain

Gynaecological	Pelvic venous congestion Inflammation: pelvic inflammatory disease (PID), endometriosis Hormonal: mittelschmerz Neoplasia: benign – fibroids malignant – ovarian cysts
Medical	Irritable bowel syndrome Diverticulitis Urinary tract infection Lumbosacral osteoarthritis Spondylolithiasis
Surgical	Bowel malignancy Subacute intestinal obstruction Renal calculus
Psychological/ psychiatric	Anxiety Depression

This is not a complete list

and surgical management (hysterectomy, oophorectomy and ligation of pelvic veins) may be options for discussion. This complicated area is in great need of more research into both causes and management.

DYSPAREUNIA

Pain during sexual intercourse (dyspareunia) is termed deep, related to pelvic organ disease such as PID, or superficial, signifying pain at the vaginal entrance with local causes such as inflammation. Vestibulitis is characterized by burning and severe entry dyspareunia at the introitus (vaginal opening). Aetiology is uncertain.

Pelvic floor dysfunction

This term describes conditions which adversely affect urinary and faecal voiding and continence mechanisms and may be associated with pelvic organ prolapse. These conditions are inter-related and may require a multidisciplinary approach to management. Combined urinary and faecal incontinence is five times more common than faecal incontinence alone. Of women with faecal incontinence, over 50% have been noted to have pudendal neuropathy (Vernava et al, 1993). See Chapters 28, 29 and 30 for further reading on conditions and conservative management.

URINARY INCONTINENCE

Defined by the International Continence Society, urinary incontinence is a condition in which involuntary loss of urine is a social or hygienic problem and is objectively demonstrated. Genuine stress incontinence (GSI), the mechanical stress-induced involuntary loss of urine occurring in the absence of detrusor contraction, accounts for about 50% of cases of incontinence. There are many different operations for genuine stress incontinence (Bergman et al, 1989). The three most commonly performed are the anterior colporrhaphy (Beck and McCormick, 1982), the vaginal retropubic procedures (Pereyra et al, 1982; Stamey, 1980) and the abdominal retropubic operations (Burch, 1968; Parnell et al, 1982) (Fig. 27.4). An adverse surgical outcome is more likely with increasing age, previous incontinence surgery, the presence of detrusor instability and a low maximum urethral closing pressure. The role of oestrogen to improve local tissues in GSI is probably one of supplementation to surgery or physiotherapy.

UTEROVAGINAL PROLAPSE

The majority of women with this problem complain of 'something coming down'. Uterovaginal prolapse is a common problem of middle and older age. The damage originates at the time of childbirth and is further compromised at the menopause with the deprivation of oestrogen. It is exacerbated in situations where the intra-abdominal pressure is raised, such as coughing and obesity. A number of obstetric factors, such as prolonged second stage labour and forceps delivery, have been identified in the aetiology of uterovaginal prolapse. It remains to be seen whether active management of labour (fewer women with long labours and more undergoing caesarean section) will eventually result in fewer women with prolapse problems.

The pelvic organs are suspended by the pelvic ligaments and supported by the levator ani muscles. Neuromuscular damage and breaks in the connective tissue affect the pelvic floor and lead to prolapse of the pelvic organs (Benson, 1994; DeLancey, 1994). The number and site of abnormalities is diverse and may cause specific defects in pelvic organ supports, cystocoele (bladder prolapse), rectocoele or uterine descent (Fig. 27.5).

This diversity has necessitated the development of a number of operative procedures to correct specific problems.

Figure 27.4 Surgical correction of urethrovesical angle. (a) Loss of the urethrovesical angle; increases of intra-abdominal pressure are applied to the bladder and not to the urethra. (b)The effect of a sling procedure is to elevate the urethrovesical junction within the body cavity. (Reproduced from Nichols DH and Randall CL (1989), *Vaginal Surgery*, 3rd edn. Baltimore: Williams and Wilkins, with permission of Professor DH Nichols and the publisher.)

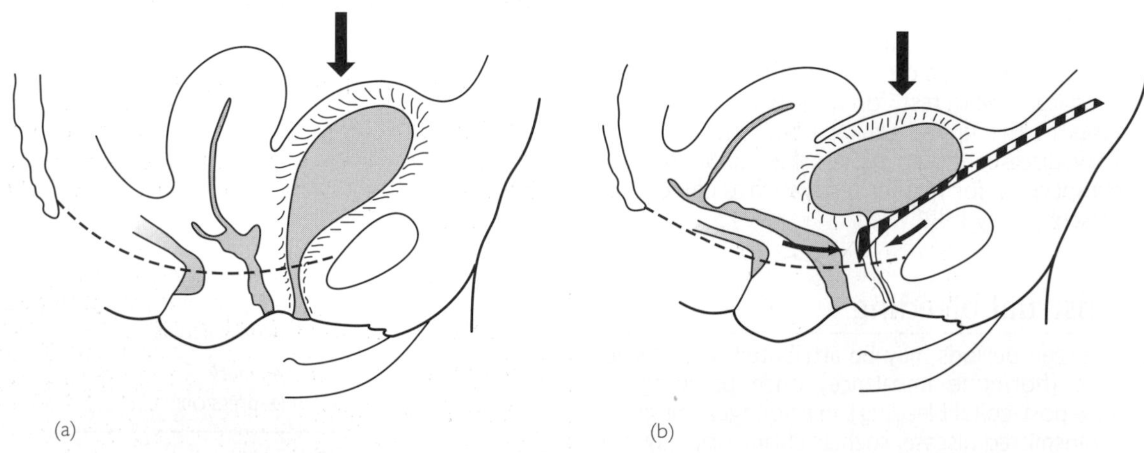

Figures 27.5 (a) Diagram showing prolapse of upper anterior and posterior vaginal walls. (b) Degrees of uterine prolapse. 1. First degree: descent within the vagina. 2. Second degree: the cervix protrudes through the introitus. 3. Third degree: the vagina is completely everted; there is a cystocoele, rectocoele and entercocoele. (Reproduced from Mackay EV, Beischer NA, Pepperell RJ and Wood C (1992) *Illustrated Textbook of Gynaecology*, 2nd edn. Philadelphia: W.B. Saunders, with permission of Professor EV Mackay and the publisher.)

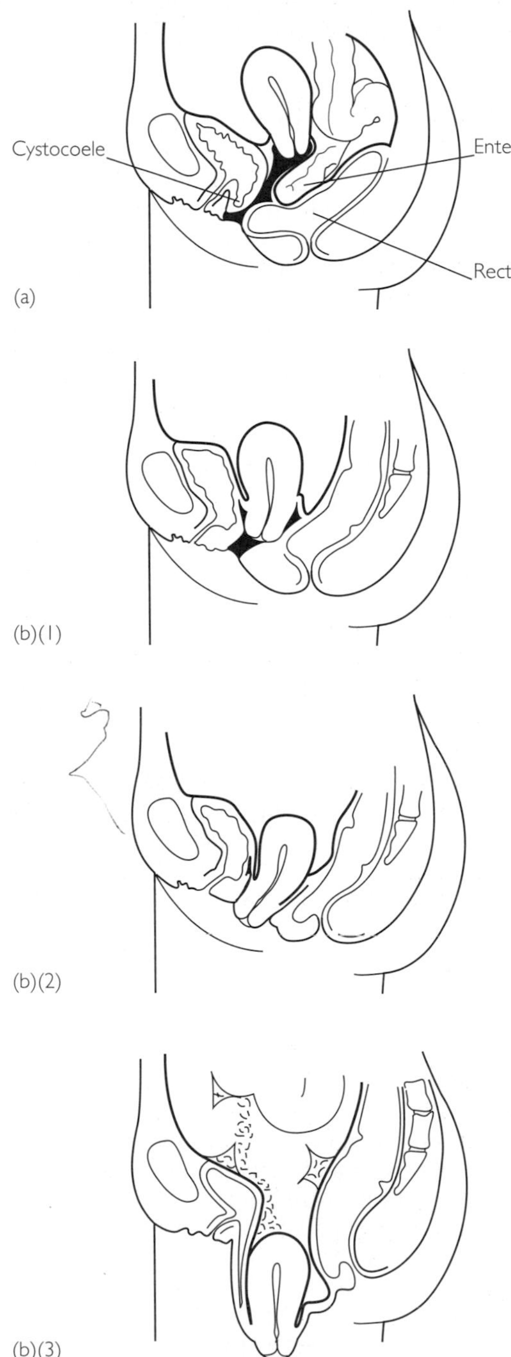

The most common operation is that of vaginal hysterectomy, combined with vaginal vault support using the transverse cervical or uterosacral ligaments, anterior colporrhaphy and approximation of the uterosacral ligaments to reduce the chance of post-operative enterocoele formation. Treatment with ring pessaries or other supporting devices have a limited place but may be useful in the elderly woman who declines or is unfit for surgery. The pessaries require changing a few times a year and vaginal ulceration can be minimized if a vaginal oestrogen cream is also used.

COMPLICATIONS OF REPAIR OPERATIONS

Initial assessment, investigation and performance of the most appropriate operation is essential if the woman is to be relieved of her symptoms and not have a worse post-operative urinary problem than her initial complaint. Dyspareunia may result if the vagina is either too tight or too short. Vaginal prolapse after hysterectomy is a distressing problem and correction involves an abdominal procedure which anchors the vaginal vault to the sacral promontory using an artificial mesh.

Vaginal discharge

This is the second most common gynaecological problem after menstrual disorders. The discharge may be normal or it may be pathological. It may arise from the vagina itself or be a symptom of a disorder of the cervix or body of the uterus. The commonest vaginal infection is *Candida albicans* (thrush); other agents are *Trichomonas vaginalis*, *Gardnerella vaginalis*, *Chlamydia trachomatis* and *Neisseria gonorrhoeae* (see Chapter 9). Although more common in younger women, sexually transmitted diseases should be considered in any sexually active woman.

In the post-menopausal woman the vaginal mucosa becomes thin and atrophic from the lack of oestrogen. Less mucus is produced and the vagina becomes more susceptible to infection. Local non-specific vaginitis can be treated with oestrogen cream. Post-menopausal purulent, blood-tinged discharge may indicate an endometrial carcinoma or pyometra (pus inside the uterine cavity).

Vulval irritation (pruritus)

Vulval irritation is a common complaint but underlying pathology should always be sought (see box). The presentation may be acute or the woman may have a chronically symptomatic vulva.

Causes of pruritus

Vaginal discharge/yeast infection
Vulval dystrophy

Pre-cancerous changes – vulvar intraepithelial neoplasia (VIN)
Skin conditions – dermatitis, allergic reaction
Cancer
Condylomata (warts)
Human papilloma virus infection (HPV)
Hypo-oestrogenic tissue

Pathological Gynaecological Conditions

Inflammatory disease

ENDOMETRIOSIS AND ADENOMYOSIS

Islands of endometrial tissue can occur between the muscle fibres of the myometrium. This condition is termed *adenomyosis*. It can cause dysmenorrhoea, pelvic pain and bleeding problems. Hysterectomy is often required for the symptoms produced and often the diagnosis may not be made until the histology is reported.

Endometriosis denotes the presence of endometrial glands and stoma outside the endometrium. Sampson's theory suggests that retrograde menstruation and implantation of viable endometrial tissue may be a likely cause.

Signs and symptoms The spectrum of disease ranges from asymptomatic haemosiderin pigmentation of the peritoneum to severe disease associated with dense adhesions and fibrosis, endometriomas and invasion of bowel and bladder. The woman may present with infertility or the pelvic pain syndromes (dysmenorrhoea, chronic pelvic pain or dyspareunia). The incidence in the general population is not known.

Treatment goals include management of pelvic pain, prevention of progression or recurrence of lesions and restoration or preservation of fertility. Expectant management (i.e. no therapy) is certainly an option, particularly for infertile patients with minimal endometriosis, and may offer similar results to treatment. Evidence is accumulating that endometriosis may be a self-limiting disease in many women.

Medical therapy has been shown to be effective for many women. The NSAIDs are effective for dysmenorrhoea; significant relief may be obtained for pelvic pain using a variety of treatments which suppress ovulation, e.g. oral contraceptive pill, progestogens, danazol and gonadotropin-releasing hormone analogues.

Surgical treatment involves ablation of lesions and division of adhesions through the laparoscope. Women who have completed their child bearing may be offered the option of hysterectomy, with or without removal of the ovaries, and hormone replacement therapy.

Future research and current debate includes the following areas.

- Is the presence of some viable endometrial tissue in the pelvis a 'normal' physiological variant?
- When does 'normal' become pathological?

PELVIC INFLAMMATORY DISEASE (PID)

Pelvic inflammatory disease describes infection involving one or more of the upper genital tract organs – uterus, tubes and ovaries. Once the area involved has been identified by diagnostic laparoscopy, a more specific term can be used (e.g. salpingitis to indicate only uterine tube infection).

Pathogenesis PID can be caused by a variety of organisms and different combinations of organisms can be present at different times during the course of the disease (e.g. *Chlamydia trachomatis* and *Neisseria gonorrhoeae*). These are thought to ascend from the vagina, possibly with spermatozoa as carriers. The time of menstruation is often associated with the development of PID.

An initial infection of the endometrial lining of the uterus occurs which passes to the tubes. An inflammatory exudate is produced which leaks from the ends of the tubes and leads to inflammation of other pelvic structures, with the tissues sticking together. This can result in the tubes becoming sealed, with permanent damage and resultant infertility. With a single episode of pelvic infection, about 10–15% of women are subsequently infertile; after three episodes nearly 75% may be infertile.

Diagnosis The clinical features may range from no symptoms to a severely ill woman. The fact that probably up to one-third of acute infections are undiagnosed means that preventing the sequelae, particularly ectopic pregnancy, chronic pelvic disease and infertility, is a difficult problem. Treatment is by antibiotics. Prevention of this disease, by screening sexually active young women under 25 years for *Chlamydia trachomatis*, should be considered. The use of barrier contraception is advised, particularly with new or casual partners (see Chapter 9).

Benign disease

FIBROMYOMAS (FIBROIDS, MYOMAS, LEIOMYOMAS)

Fibromyomas are tumours of smooth muscle, which contain some fibrous tissue and occur in the muscle wall of the uterus. The tumours are usually multiple and develop within the muscle wall (intramural) or can extend into the endometrial cavity (submucous) or peritoneal cavity (subserosal) (Fig. 27.6). Their size can vary from a few millimetres to 15 cm or more in diameter. One in five women can expect to develop fibroids and malignant (sarcomatous) change can occur, although this is rare. Clinical features depend on the size, number and position of the fibroids. Symptoms include menorrhagia, dysmenorrhoea, vaginal discharge, pelvic pain and abdominal swelling. Treatment may be conservative, if

Figure 27.6 Leiomyomata (fibroids) of the uterus.

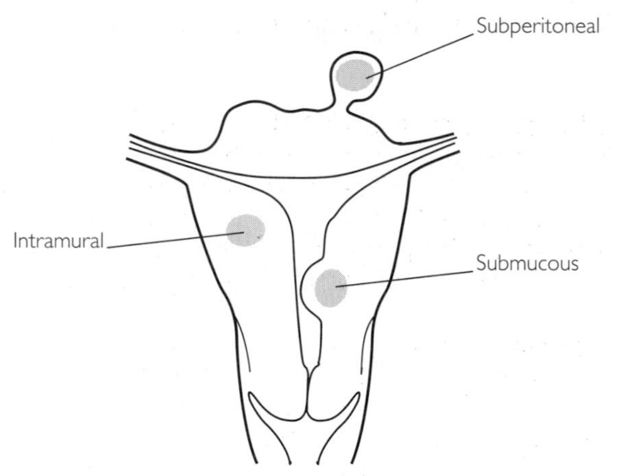

there are no symptoms or infertility, or surgical. Surgical options include a myomectomy (removal of the fibroids with conservation of the uterus) or hysterectomy. The choice depends on the woman's age and desire to maintain her uterus.

OVARIAN CYSTS

While the woman is still having a menstrual cycle, ovarian cysts can occur and are related to hormonal fluctuations. Follicular cysts occur in the first part of the cycle, may often be multiple and do not require any treatment. The woman's age provides a clue to the nature of an enlargement of the ovary. During child-bearing years the ratio of benign to malignant tumours is about 20 : 1. Symptoms are usually related to the pressure effects of the enlarging ovary or to rupture, torsion or haemorrhage into the cyst, all of which cause abdominal pain. In the older woman the major problem is recognition of malignancy at an early stage. Surgical removal is indicated for all solid tumours and cystic tumours >5 cm. Persisting or enlarging cysts are usually removed.

VULVAL DYSTROPHY

Vulval dystrophy mainly affects post-menopausal women but can occur in the young pre-menopausal woman. The skin may show thinning and loss of structure (lichen sclerosis) or thickening (hyperplasia) or may be mixed. The skin may appear red or white and the woman complains of pruritus. Treatment is with steroid cream. Careful follow-up is essential as some of these conditions may develop cancerous changes.

VULVODYNIA

This refers to symptoms of vulvar burning or raw sensations. Aetiologic or exacerbating factors include the dermatoses (such as contact dermatitis), yeast or HPV infections, oestrogen deficiency or pudendal neuralgia. Treatment may include local steroid ointment, oral anticandidal agents or amitriptyline, an antidepressant useful for some neuralgias.

Figure 27.7 Cervical smear changes.

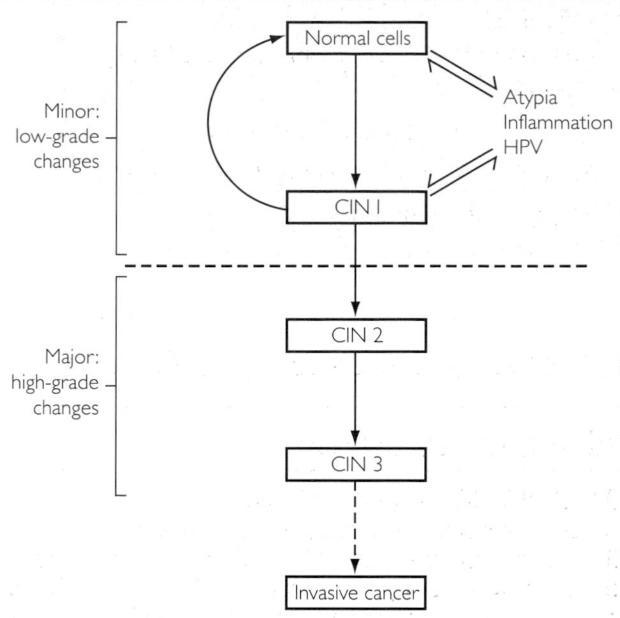

CIN = cervical intraepithelial neoplasia
HPV = human papilloma virus

Pre-malignant disease

Pre-malignant disease refers to tissue changes preceding the development of a 'true' invasive cancer. Disease detected at this stage is amenable to treatment and this may therefore prevent an invasive cancer developing in the future.

THE CERVIX: CERVICAL INTRAEPITHELIAL NEOPLASIA (CIN)

The incidence of these pre-malignant changes has more than doubled in the past decade and is becoming more common in younger women (Draper and Cook, 1983; Wolfendale et al, 1983). It is believed that if CIN is detected and treated, the number of deaths from cervical cancer can be reduced. A significant number of women will ultimately progress to invasive cancer if CIN is untreated (Fig. 27.7). All CIN II and III (termed high-grade lesions) should be treated by some form of local destructive treatment or local excision. If a high-grade cervical smear abnormality cannot be confirmed on colposcopy or the lesion extends into the cervical canal, a cone biopsy may be recommended. This procedure removes the lining of the endocervical canal and may be all the treatment that is required. All women require follow-up after treatment with Pap smears and possibly colposcopy. Treatment of CIN I and other minor abnormalities, with or without associated HPV infection, is more controversial. All women with any cervical smear abnormality must receive

Figure 27.8 The changing cervical cell puzzle: risk factors

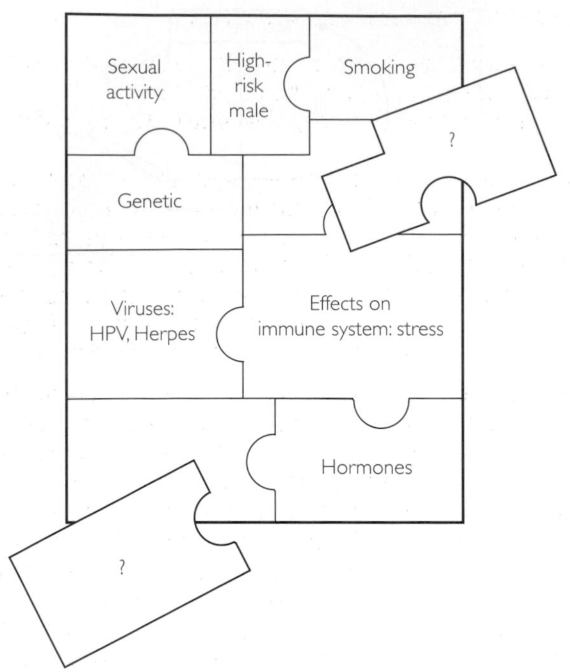

explanation and counselling about contributing factors (Fig. 27.8) and follow-up required.

THE UTERUS: ENDOMETRIAL HYPERPLASIA

The effect of oestrogen on the uterus is increased growth of the endometrial lining if there is either prolonged or unopposed use (without progestogen). This occurs largely at the extremes of life (the adolescent or menopausal woman) when anovulation is common. It can also occur from the use of unopposed exogenous oestrogens. As in the breast, the hyperplasia often results in cystic enlargement of the glands. There can be progression from glandular hyperplasia to atypical hyperplasia and to frank adenocarcinoma of the endometrium for some women. Progestogen can be used to treat hyperplasia but follow-up is essential and hysterectomy may be advised or preferred by some women.

THE VAGINA AND VULVA

The conditions of vaginal intraepithelial neoplasia (VAIN) and vulval intraepithelial neoplasia (VIN) usually occur at a younger age compared with invasive malignant lesions. The principal symptom is pruritus (itching). Women who have a squamous cell abnormality at one site are more likely to develop one at another site; for instance, women with CIN III (cervix) are at increased risk of a vulval lesion. These lesions appear to be increasing in frequency and this may reflect the increased incidence of papillomavirus infections, which many of these lesions contain. Treatment is conservative with local excision or laser therapy. Women with VAIN or VIN are at risk of developing a recurrence of *in situ* disease or invasive disease and require careful follow-up.

Cancer

The behaviour of cancer cells distinguishes it from normal cells.

1. *Aberrant growth* – normal cells come under the control of a number of checks and balances to control growth, while the cancer cell does not respond to these control signals.
2. *Invasion* – the cancer induces the development of new blood vessels and then invades them.
3. *Metastasis* – this is the ability for cells to break away from the parent growth, spread to other parts of the body by the blood or lymphatic systems and establish a new growth.

In most cancers several errors in the genetic machinery are necessary for malignant transformation. Two classes of genes are associated with development of neoplastic tumours. The first are oncogenes which are derived from activated normal cellular genes; the presence of two or more may lead to malignant transformation. The second are the tumour suppressors, present in normal cells, whose inactivation may also lead to malignant transformation. This transformation is facilitated under conditions that depress immune function, such as viral infections, drugs or stress.

Clinical diagnosis of cancer occurs when the cell population is between 10^{10} and 10^{12} cells, towards the end of the tumour life cycle. Research is focusing on ways to detect cancers before this time. The prevalence of cancers of the cervix, body of the uterus and ovary is about 10–30 per 100 000 women per year. Vulval and vaginal cancers are uncommon and uterine tube cancer rare. Cancers of the body of the uterus, vulva and vagina occur mainly after the menopause; cervical cancer occurs from 25 years onwards and the ovary is unique as cancers occur throughout life.

MANAGEMENT

It is essential that women with cancer are assessed and treated by a multidisciplinary team including a gynae-oncological surgeon, chemotherapist, radiotherapist and support staff of psychologist, psychiatrist, physiotherapist and social worker. The team approach will ensure that all aspects of the woman's treatment, health and well-being are taken into consideration and that the family also receive adequate counselling.

Staging of gynaecological cancers facilitates planning of treatment, assists in predicting the likely result of treatment and permits exchange of information between individuals and centres to compare the results of different managements. The classification is based on the examination of the woman under anaesthetic by an experienced examiner.

Radiotherapy Radiotherapy is used in the treatment of gynaecological cancers, often complementary to surgery. It also has a useful role in palliation with the relief of distressing symptoms such as pain, bleeding and urinary obstruction. Cancer cells are more sensitive to the radiation than is surrounding normal tissue, termed a favourable therapeutic ratio. The higher the dose tolerated by the normal tissue, the more lethal the effect on the cancer cells and the more radiocurable the tumour. Counselling of women before treatment is essential as there may be initial side effects and later problems. Early reactions of malaise, nausea, anorexia and diarrhoea usually subside after treatment is completed. The major complications are due to post-treatment ischaemia (lack of blood supply) of the pelvis involving the vagina (leading to sexual problems), the rectum (proctitis producing diarrhoea sometimes with blood loss) and the small bowel (leading to necrosis (tissue death) months or years later with bowel perforation). Scar formation (fibrosis) and atrophy of connective tissue and its supportive elements (blood vessels and nerves) can lead to serious sequelae to the organ involved, months or years later.

Chemotherapy Chemotherapy involves the use of drugs which aim to kill the rapidly dividing cancer cells. Many factors affect the sensitivity of the neoplastic cells to these drugs, including the proportion of tumour cells in a resting phase, the concentration and adequate exposure time of the drug. The use of these drugs will be limited by adverse effects such as depletion of white blood cells and platelets (affecting resistance to infection and haemorrhage) and systemic effects such as nausea, vomiting and diarrhoea.

BREAST CANCER

In Australia breast cancer is the most common cancer for women, accounting for more than a quarter of all malignancies in females. The incidence rate (number of new cases per year) is 21 per 100 000 women, and one in 13 women will develop breast cancer by the age of 75 years.

Women are advised to perform breast self-examination (BSE) monthly (after a period, if still menstruating) and consult their general practitioner for an annual examination. Whether the detection of a breast lump by BSE ultimately affects the outcome has still to be determined. Screening for breast cancer is recommended for women from 50 years of age or for those with a family history from 40 years. Screening will diagnose eight out of 10 breast cancers and is more effective in the older woman in whom the breasts are less dense.

> The greatest risk factor for breast cancer is getting older – 92% cancers occur over 40 years of age.

Most breast cancers occur without any family history. There are some which have a genetic component and a family history does give an increase in risk, according to the relationship.

Treatment

Surgery The method of surgery advised depends on the size of the breast and of the tumour.

1. Conservation of the breast with lumpectomy, axillary clearance of lymph nodes and radiotherapy.
2. Mastectomy with axillary clearance of lymph nodes.

The tissue is evaluated for the oestrogen receptor status which provides additional information to advise on subsequent treatment. Life expectancy is the same for both methods and follow-up is essential for all women; 1% of women per year with conservative treatment will develop a new cancer in that breast requiring treatment. Early treatment of this cancer gives the same long-term outcome.

Either surgical procedure can be followed by tamoxifen or chemotherapy. Tamoxifen is an adjuvant systemic therapy which reduces growth rate of any micrometastases present. Benefits include antioestrogenic effects, binding to the oestrogen receptor site and oestrogenic effects. In post-menopausal women with breast cancer, it reduces the incidence of future problems by 20%.The oestrogen effect may cause growth of the endometrial lining, in some women producing hyperplasia or cancer. Any woman on tamoxifen who experiences vaginal bleeding requires investigation.

Chemotherapy Chemotherapy is used for treating metastatic disease and for women who may have micrometastases. It will reduce the relative risk of death by about 20%.

Breast reconstruction This can be done for women after mastectomy and may be important for some women to improve their self-esteem. It does not increase the risk for recurrence of breast cancer.

Physiotherapy management Physiotherapy can play an active role in the post-surgical management of breast cancer. Chapter 33 covers this area in detail.

Hormones and breast cancer The main regulators of growth and differentiation of normal breast tissue are the endogenous oestrogens. Many of the established risk factors are related to an increased length and intensity of exposure to natural oestrogens – early menarche, late menopause. The role of exogenous oestrogens is more complex. The OCP taken for many years before a first pregnancy may slightly increase the risk of developing breast cancer under 40 years. However, the OCP will offer protection against ovarian and endometrial cancers. In the case of hormone replacement therapy (HRT) used in the post-menopausal period, it is possible that with prolonged use of more than 10 years there may be a slight increase in the risk of developing breast cancer. It is essential that risks are weighed against the benefits, the prevention of osteoporosis and cardiovascular disease and quality of life for the individual woman. Different oestrogen types, doses, regimens and methods of administration and the use of progestogens may produce different effects. The final conclusions have not yet been reached.

CERVICAL CANCER

The peak age for occurrence of cervical cancer is 45–55 years. When the diagnosis of cervical cancer is established 20% of women are asymptomatic. Those with symptoms experience abnormal bleeding (80–90% of women) or abnormal discharge. The bleeding problems are often related to periods which may be too long, too heavy or too frequent. The cervix may look normal (if the cancer is small or in the endocervical canal) and the cervical smear test may also be normal or the cervix may show an obvious growth. Diagnosis is made using cervical cytology, colposcopy, biopsy and endocervical curettage. Direct spread of the cancer cells occurs mostly along the lymphatic/vascular channels that run in the uterosacral and cardinal ligaments. Spread to the body of the uterus and lymph nodes occurs progressively with increasing stages of the disease. Management of women with this disorder, like that of all other cancers, should involve an experienced team consisting of gynaecologist, oncologist, radiotherapist and pathologist. Treatment is usually by radical radiotherapy and/or radical surgery – a Wertheim hysterectomy. The overall survival for all stages is 60–65%.

OVARIAN CANCER

The ovary gives rise to more varieties of neoplasm with a greater diversity of histologic appearance and biologic behaviour than any other organ. The ovary is also often the target for metastases from malignant tumours in other organs, especially the gastrointestinal tract, the genital tract and the breast. The tumours of epithelial origin are the largest group, with some risk factors identified in Table 27.3. The two characteristics of primary ovarian cancer which paint a particularly bleak picture are, firstly, that it is a disease which presents late, with approximately 75% of cases having advanced disease at initial laparotomy. Secondly, the success of treatment of disseminated disease is extremely poor, with a five-year survival of about 10% among women presenting with disease outside the pelvis. Abdominal pain or swelling is a sign of late disease. Early non-gynaecological complaints account for the fact that 50% of women with ovarian cancer present to a non-gynaecological specialist in the first instance.

Table 27.3 Risk factors for epithelial ovarian cancer

Age	>45 years (median age 6th decade)
Race	Caucasian, Jewish
Distribution	Northern European, industrialized nations
Reproductive history	Late age 1st pregnancy, low parity
Past medical history	Primary of breast, endometrial, colon cancer = 2–4-fold risk
Family history	Ovarian: mother or sister = 18-fold risk Endometrial cancer
Cosmetic talc	Regular use on vulva, perineum, sanitary pads

Screening The use of clinical examination, tumour markers or ultrasound has not as yet been shown to fulfil the requirements of a good screening test.

Treatment Treatment is primarily surgical with removal of as much cancer tissue as possible (debulking), including the uterus, tubes, ovaries and omentum. Surgery is usually followed by chemotherapy which may be oral and/or intravenous.

Prophylactic oophorectomy Hysterectomy is performed for 20–30% of women between 45 and 55 years, mostly for bleeding problems. If the ovaries are not diseased, the woman has the choice of whether to keep or lose the ovaries. If not removed, there is a small chance that further surgery will be required, for benign disease, pain or suspected malignancy. There may also be morbidity from abnormal ovarian function (attributed to compromised blood flow after hysterectomy) which may result in an earlier menopause than expected. These facts must be balanced against the efficacy of hormone replacement therapy and psychological sequelae for the individual woman should prophylactic oophorectomy be performed.

ENDOMETRIAL CARCINOMA

Approximately 75% of endometrial cancers occur in the post-menopausal age group and in more than 90%, the initial complaint is vaginal bleeding. A smaller proportion of women present with a purulent discharge and pain, the latter generally associated with metastatic disease. There is a propensity for even early endometrial cancer to invade the lymphatic system. Eighty percent of primary endometrial cancers are either pure or mixed adenocarcinomas and have a relatively good prognosis; the five-year survival rate for all stages of the disease is 70%.

Treatment Treatment is primarily surgical. Traditionally a total abdominal hysterectomy, a bilateral salpingo-oophorectomy (BSO) with a cuff of vagina (taken to prevent early recurrence in the vaginal vault) has been performed. However, approximately 15% of patients with clinical stage I disease have lymph vascular invasion. Wertheim's hysterectomy, which includes the removal of the uterus, BSO, vaginal cuff and lymph nodes, is indicated for the more advanced stages of endometrial cancer. Radiotherapy may be employed post-operatively to the vaginal vault and the pelvic or para-aortic lymph nodes. Surgery and radiotherapy together may increase the risk of complications.

CANCER OF THE VULVAL AND VAGINAL AREAS

Vaginal malignancy is often asymptomatic in the early stages; eventually vaginal discharge or post-coital bleeding may develop. The most common invasive malignancy in this area is squamous cell carcinoma. The most important predictor of survival is the stage of the disease (Table 27.4) and treatment includes radical surgery and radiotherapy.

Table 27.4 Clinical staging for vaginal cancer

Stage	Description
1	Limited to the vaginal wall
2	Paravaginal extension but not to the side wall
3	Extension to the pelvic side wall
4	Distant metastasis: (a) adjacent organs (b) distant organs

Squamous cell carcinoma is found in 85% of cases of vulval malignancy. The usual symptom is that of persistent irritation. The spread of disease is first to the superficial inguinal lymph nodes and then the pelvic lymph nodes. Haematogenous spread occurs late in the course of this disease and standard treatment is surgical with vulvectomy and lymph node dissection. Earlier diagnosis has led to less radical surgery in recent years. A combination of radiation and extensive surgery may be required for more advanced disease.

Vulvectomy Treatment of vulval cancer is planned according to the size of the lesion, whether there is lymph node or metastatic involvement, the woman's age, general health and her views on treatment options. As the primary lesion becomes larger, the surgery by necessity needs to be more extensive. Extension of the lesion to the urethra, anal sphincter, rectal wall and vagina can be treated with a combination of surgery and radiotherapy. In this situation the treatment is mutilating to the woman. Approximately half the women undergoing radical surgery will have one or more major complication (the majority not life threatening). The most difficult problems include wound infection and breakdown, lymphoedema, urinary incontinence, sexual dysfunction and numbness of the anterior thighs. Deaths may occur from pulmonary embolus, myocardial infarction and stroke.

A 60-year-old woman, Mrs AG, presents to her GP for a cervical smear test. On checking his records the GP notices that her last cervical smear was four years ago. The GP tells Mrs AG that he is delighted that she has come for a check and wonders what has prompted her action. She states that the previous week she had one day of vaginal spotting, sufficient to wear one panti-liner. She was in excellent health with no pain or any other symptoms. However, she mentioned the bleeding to her daughter who reminded her about the cervical smear test. Her menopause had been at 54 years of age.

On examination, Mrs AG was overweight at 95 kg, breast and abdominal examination revealed no abnormality. A vaginal speculum examination showed atrophic changes in the vagina and a cervix which looked normal with a closed cervical os. The GP took a routine smear test. The pelvic examination revealed a small uterus with no abnormal masses in the pelvis. The GP explained to Mrs AG that, although there was no abnormality on his examination, he was unable to exclude a problem within the uterus and advised referral to a gynaecologist for investigation. The gynaecologist performed a D&C and hysteroscopy. The histology of the endometrial curettings showed a well-differentiated endometrial carcinoma. Mrs AG underwent a total abdominal hysterectomy. There was no involvement of the pelvic or aortic nodes and the tumour invaded less than half of the myometrium. Early, prompt detection and treatment of the tumour produced a favourable prognosis – the tumour was graded as 1b, which gave Mrs AG a nearly 80% five-year survival rate.

Gynaecological Surgery – Avoiding Pre- and Perioperative Problems

The abdominal incision used may vary according to the procedure being undertaken and the woman's preference (Fig. 27.9). Vaginal oestrogen cream can be used for 2–3 weeks before vaginal surgery to improve the tissues.

Chest infection

Pre- and post-operative physiotherapy including early mobilization is invaluable in the prevention of chest infection, the minimization of 'wind' pain and the prevention of DVT. Further details about specific treatment goals can be found in Chapter 34.

Figure 27.9 Incisions for abdominal surgery.

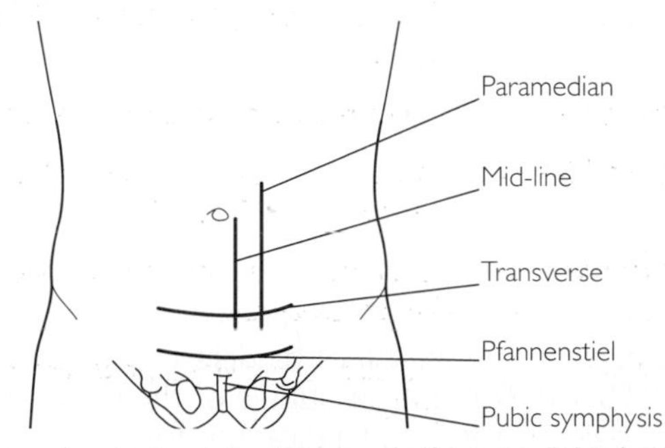

Infection and bleeding

The common complications of any surgical procedure are bleeding and infection. Careful attention to haemostasis during surgery is essential although some post-operative bleeding may be secondary to infection. A closed suction drain may be placed in the pelvic cavity and/or the wound. These are left *in situ* for 24 hours or until blood stops draining. Wound infection may occur early, from bacterial contamination, or some days later, sometimes secondary to a wound haematoma. A vaginal pack (a long gauze roll soaked in an antiseptic solution or cream) may be inserted into the upper vagina after some procedures (e.g. cone biopsy, vaginal repair, vaginal hysterectomy) to assist post-operative haemostasis. The pack is usually removed after 24 hours. Antibiotics, started at the time of pre-medication and continuing for a further 48 hours or until a urinary catheter is removed, will reduce the incidence of post-operative infections. The use of a suprapubic catheter adds to the patient's comfort and avoids repeated urethral catheterization and possible infections. Continuous catheterization may be used for the first 24 hours post-operatively or for several days if a repair procedure is undertaken.

Deep venous thrombosis and pulmonary embolism

Deep venous thrombosis and pulmonary embolism are serious complications. Preventive activities include avoiding excessive pressure on the woman's legs during surgery, the use of graduated supportive stockings, intermittent compression to calf muscles during surgery, early mobilization and physiotherapy. Prophylactic subcutaneous heparin can be used for all women, although some surgeons consider that this will increase pre- and peri-operative bleeding and post-operative haematoma formation. It may be preferred to keep this option for women at increased risk of thrombosis, such as the obese or those with a past history of thromboembolic disease.

Ileus of the bowel

Ileus of the bowel may occasionally occur when the bowel is slow to resume function after surgery. The woman may require continuation of intravenous fluids and nasogastric suction until the bowel starts to work again. This may be associated with 'wind pain' requiring analgesia.

Fertility

Any operative procedure which removes the uterus or both ovaries or both uterine tubes renders the woman sterile. Tables 27.5 and 27.6 give an outline of the most common gynaecological surgery and indications for it.

Conclusion

A careful assessment of a woman before operation can avoid many post-operative problems. The assessment should be based on the woman's current medical state, past history and family history. Specific problems may require an opinion, advice or investigation by a consultant anaesthetist or physician.

Glossary of Terms, Procedures and Investigations

Ablation

Destruction of cervical lesions may be used to treat pre-cancer and inflammation. The methods of tissue destruction used involve heat (cautery, laser), cold (cryosurgery), excision (cone biopsy) or a combination of heat and excision.

Biopsy

A biopsy is the removal of a tiny piece of tissue for histology to define the cytologic abnormality precisely.

Colposcopy

This is a means of inspecting the cervix under magnification with a strong light source. It identifies the location and extent of a cytological abnormality detected on a cervical smear. It is also used for investigating symptoms such as abnormal bleeding.

Hysteroscopy

Hysteroscopy is the visualization of the uterine cavity with a 4 mm diameter telescope within a sheath. The telescope can be further enclosed in an operating sheath through which a variety of surgical instruments can be used. The gas used for uterine distension is carbon dioxide, which is easily absorbed and inert. Fluid distension is achieved with high molecular weight dextran, dextrose saline or saline. The light source is provided by a fibreoptic cable or xenon and the procedure is monitored on closed circuit television. The procedure can be carried out under a local or general anaesthetic. Hysteroscopy is indicated to investigate menstrual irregularities due to post-coital, intermenstrual, post-menopausal and dysfunctional uterine bleeding.

Laparoscopy

Laparoscopy is an exploratory surgical procedure which allows the gynaecologist to see the organs inside the pelvis

Table 27.5 Common gynaecological operations

Name of operation	Procedure	Useful notes
D & C (dilation and curettage)	Cervix gradually dilated and uterine lining (endometrium) removed	Uterine perforation (more likely if uterine wall is soft – pregnancy or malignancy) is a complication
Bartholin's marsupialization	The dilated duct from Bartholin's gland is opened and the edges stitched to surrounding tissue	If infected, a small ribbon gauze pack is left *in situ* for 24 hours. Defect heals over several days
Laparoscopy	To investigate abdominal symptoms or masses or for sterilization (dividing or sealing the uterine tubes)	Discomfort under ribs, shoulders and neck for 24 hours (from CO_2 gas in abdominal cavity). 2–3 $\times$ 1 cm abdominal scars
Myomectomy	Fibroids shelled out of uterine muscle wall and defects repaired	
Ovarian cystectomy	Cyst shelled out of ovary and remaining ovarian tissue repaired and conserved	Ovary retains normal function
Ventrosuspension	Round ligaments between upper uterine angles and pelvic side walls are shortened.This lifts the uterus out of the pouch of Douglas	Useful if pathology (endometriosis or PID) in pouch of Douglas. Prevents dyspareunia by lifting ovaries away from pouch of Douglas
Abdominal hysterectomy + bilateral salpingo-oophorectomy (BSO)	• Removal of uterus and cervix • Removal of both tubes and ovaries as well	Removal of both ovaries in the pre-menopausal woman requires discussion on HRT
Vaginal hysterectomy (+/– BSO)	Uterus and cervix removed via vagina. No abdominal scar	May be combined with bladder or posterior vaginal wall repair
Laparosopically assisted vaginal hysterectomy	Upper pedicles divided via laparoscope. Uterus removed via vagina	Combination of laparoscopy and vaginal hysterectomy
Marshall Marchetti, sling operation, Burch colposuspension	Elevating and fixing bladder neck to pubic symphysis or nearby tissue	Bladder catheterization for 3–7 days post-operation
Manchester repair	Cervix amputated and lateral uterine ligaments shortened. Used for uterovaginal prolapse preserving the uterus	Often performed with anterior and posterior vaginal repair

and abdomen. It is usually performed under general anaesthesia for a variety of indications. Diagnostic indications include:

- to investigate abdominal pain;
- to determine causes of infertility;
- to examine cysts and tumours;
- to obtain biopsies;
- to detect an ectopic pregnancy.

Indications for treatment include:

- sterilization;
- ectopic pregnancy;
- adhesions/endometriosis.

Carbon dioxide gas is introduced through a needle into the abdominal cavity to provide a space to view and carry out procedures. The laparoscope is a narrow telescope and is inserted just below the umbilicus. Other instruments may be introduced through small incisions near the pubic hair line. Complications are rare but may include bleeding within the abdomen or damage to bowel or adjacent organs and this may require further surgery.

Recovery is usually rapid but there may be some initial symptoms:

1. pain at the incision site and aches in the shoulder, neck and under the rib cage due to gas under the diaphragm. This usually settles within 24 hours as the gas is absorbed;
2. abdominal cramps similar to period pain;
3. a sensation of swelling in the abdomen;
4. light bleeding/vaginal discharge for a few days.

Laser

Laser is an acronym for light amplification by stimulated emission of radiation. The carbon dioxide laser produces electromagnetic irradiation of high intensity by controlled discharge of a mixture of carbon dioxide, nitrogen and helium. This energy, in the form of an infrared light,

Table 27.6 Indications for gynaecological operations

Operation	Indications
Abdominal hysterectomy	Bleeding problems; pelvic pain; cancer of endometrium, cervix, ovary
Cone biopsy	Diagnostic – adenocarcinoma cervix, microinvasive or invasive squamous carcinoma cervix Therapeutic – CIN in endocervical canal
Dilation and curettage (D & C)	Diagnostic – abnormal bleeding Pregnancy complications – abortion, hydatidiform mole
Examination under anaesthesia	Forms part of assessment for staging gynaecological cancer and exploring uterine cavity after a post-partum haemorrhage
Laparoscopy	Diagnostic – acute and chronic abdominal pain, infertility Procedural – sterilization; ovarian cysts; ectopic pregnancy; endometriosis – staging and ablative treatment
Manchester repair	Prolapse, retaining the uterus
Marshall Marchetti Burch colposuspension	Stress incontinence
Myomectomy	Fibroids, conserving the uterus
Oophorectomy	Endometriosis; PID; ovarian cysts (after accident, torsion, rupture); cancer
Ovarian cystectomy	Benign ovarian cysts, conserving the ovary
Salpingectomy	Ectopic pregnancy; PID; cancer
Salpingostomy	Ectopic pregnancy, PID, conserving uterine tube
Vaginal hysterectomy	Bleeding problems
Vaginal repair: anterior posterior perineal	Cystocoele; cystourethrocoele Rectocoele; enterocoele Perineal body laxity
Ventrosuspension	Retroverted uterus; endometriosis and PID (to prevent the uterus adhering to pouch of Douglas)
Vulvectomy – simple/radical	Cancer; pre-cancer
Radical hysterectomy, e.g. Wertheim's	Cancer of cervix

vaporizes tissue by raising the temperature of the cell until the intracellular water turns into steam.

Prevalence

This is the probability of having a condition. It is calculated as:

$$\frac{\text{The number of persons with the condition}}{\text{The number of those examined}}$$

Screening test

This is a test performed in a well person to detect a disease at a stage before symptoms develop and when treatment will prevent future problems. The test must be comfortable, convenient, easy to perform, be cost effective and have a low incidence of side effects. It must combine a high specificity (to avoid further investigation of a large number of individuals without disease) and high sensitivity (to prevent failure of detection of pre-clinical disease).

Sensitivity

Sensitivity is defined as the proportion of people *with* the condition who are correctly identified on being screened, i.e. the probability that a test result will be positive when the condition is present.

Specificity

Specificity may be defined as the proportion of people *without* the condition who are correctly identified on being screened, i.e. the probability that a test result will be negative when the condition is absent.

Tumour markers

A blood test detecting a substance biochemically, such as a protein, hormone or enzyme, or immunologically, such as an antigen. The test should have sufficient sensitivity and specificity to detect a particular disease.

Ultrasound

A short pulse of ultrasound is transmitted into the body via a small probe. In gynaecology it may be used to check the pelvic contents and provide information about the nature and size of an abdominal mass. The examination may be performed transabdominally or transvaginally.

References

Beck RP and McCormick S (1982) Treatment of urinary stress incontinence with anterior colporrhaphy. *Obstetrics and Gynecology* **59**: 269–270.

Benson JT (1994) Neurophysiology of the female pelvic floor. *Current Opinion in Obstetrics and Gynecology* **6**: 320–323.

Bergman A, Ballard CA and Koonings PP (1989) Comparison of three different surgical procedures for genuine stress incontinence: prospective randomised study. *American Journal of Obstetrics and Gynecology* **160**: 1102–1106.

Burch JC (1968) Cooper's ligament urethrovesical suspension for stress incontinence. *American Journal of Obstetrics and Gynecology* **100**: 764–766.

Commonwealth Department of Community Services and Health (1989) *National Women's Health Policy.* Canberra: Australian Government Publications.

DeLancey JOL (1994) The anatomy of the pelvic floor. *Current Opinion in Obstetrics and Gynecology* **6**: 313–316.

Draper GJ and Cook GA (1983) Changing patterns of cervical cancer. *British Medical Journal* **287**: 510–512.

Hart CR and Burke P (eds) (1992) *Screening and Surveillance in General Practice.* Edinburgh: Churchill Livingstone.

Parnell JP, Marshall VF and Vaughan ED (1982) Primary management of urinary stress incontinence by the Marshall-Marchetti-Krantz vesicourethropexy. *Journal of Urology* **127**: 697–700.

Pereyra AJ, Lebberz TB, Growden WA et al (1982) Pubourethral support in perspective: modified Pereyra procedure for urinary incontinence. *Obstetrics and Gynecology* **59**: 643–648.

Pickles VR, Hall WJ, Best FA et al (1965) Prostaglandins in endometrium and menstrual fluid from normal and dysmenorrhoeic subjects. *British Journal of Obstetrics and Gynaecology* **72**: 185.

Stamey TA (1980) Endoscopic suspension of the vesical neck. In: Stanton SL and Tanagho EA (eds) *Surgery of Female Incontinence*, pp. 77–91. Berlin: Springer-Verlag.

Vernava AM, Longo WE and Daniel GL (1993) Pudendal neuropathy and the importance of EMG evaluation of fecal incontinence. *Diseases of Colon and Rectum* **36**: 23–27.

Wolfendale MR, King S and Usherwood MM (1983) Abnormal cervical smears: are we in for an epidemic? *British Medical Journal* **87**: 526–528.

Further reading

DiMona L and Herndon C (1994) *Women's Sourcebook*. Boston: Houghton Mifflin.

National Health and Research Council (1995) *Guidelines for the Management of Women with Screen Detected Abnormalities*, pp. 1–36. Canberra: Australian Government Publishing Service.

Smith ARB (1995) *The Investigation and Management of Urinary Incontinence in Women.* London: RCOG Press.

Spector RE (1991) *Cultural Diversity in Health and Illness*, 3rd edn. Norwalk, Conn: Appleton and Lange.

28

Urogenital Dysfunction

RUTH SAPSFORD

A woman may present at any stage of her adult life complaining of a problem associated with bladder, bowel or genital function. Problems are frequently multifactorial, involving one or more of the following components – bladder, urethral and anal smooth muscle, urethral, anal and PF striated muscle and endopelvic fascia.

Causes of pelvic floor dysfunction

- Genetic factors
- Connective tissue quality
- Parturition
- Perimenopausal changes
- Prolonged heavy lifting
- Defaecation straining
- Surgery
- Ageing

Connective Tissue Changes

Endopelvic fascia and fascia over the pelvic floor muscles differ in their structural components and biomechanical properties. In both, collagen is a major structural protein. PFM fascia is similar in composition to rectus sheath fascia. During pregnancy, rectus fascia becomes weaker and more elastic and is more easily damaged or ruptured. Components in fascia may change in type and proportion in response to injury. Stronger type 1 collagen may be replaced by weaker type 3 collagen during recovery post-partum. Smith (1994) questioned whether pelvic floor fascia would rehabilitate more effectively post-partum if PFM rehabilitation was more effective.

In women with stress incontinence the skin has less collagen and the rectus sheath is stiffer and more brittle than in normals. When stress incontinence is combined with bladder neck prolapse, the pubocervical fascia has been found to be weaker and abdominal striae are significantly greater than in those without prolapse (Sayer et al, 1990).

Other fascial variations occur in women with genitourinary prolapse. They have a significantly greater prevalence of joint hypermobility than those without prolapse (Norton et al, 1995) and a significant reduction in total collagen in vaginal tissues (Jackson et al, 1995).

Connective tissue quality is probably an inherited characteristic and these women are likely to be at greater risk of pelvic floor dysfunction. Education and prevention should be approached more vigorously in this group.

Bladder Dysfunction

Normal bladder and urethral function are discussed in Chapter 7. An understanding of all aspects of dysfunction is essential if patients are to be treated satisfactorily. Definitions relating to urethrovesical dysfunction are contained in the International Continence Society's publication Standardization of terminology of lower urinary tract function (Abrams et al, 1988). These are the accepted definitions used throughout the medical literature and are usually followed by the acknowledgment 'ICS definition'.

In normal bladder filling, there should be little or no increase in intravesical pressure with increasing volumes of urine, even when there are changes in intra-abdominal pressure (IAP). The bladder is said to be stable and compliant. With an *overactive bladder* there are involuntary detrusor contractions during filling, occurring spontaneously or provoked by increases in IAP or movement. This is said to be an *unstable detrusor* and may be termed *detrusor instability*, as involuntary contractions occur when the subject is trying to inhibit voiding. Overactivity occurring in neurological disorders is termed *detrusor hyper-reflexia*. During voiding the detrusor should contract on command and continue until empty or until voiding is interrupted. When the contraction is not strong enough, nor sustained for long enough to empty the bladder in a reasonable time, this is called *detrusor underactivity*. When no contraction is observed during urodynamic assessment of voiding (see p. 354) the patient is said to have an *acontractile detrusor*. In neurological disorders this may be called *detrusor areflexia*.

Urethral Dysfunction

The normal bladder neck and urethra remain closed during bladder filling, even when the IAP is raised. With an *incompetent urethra* urine often enters the proximal section when the bladder is not contracting. Thus urethral closing pressure may not be great enough to prevent loss of urine when the IAP is raised. There may also be a transient involuntary fall in urethral pressure which allows urine to escape. This is called *urethral instability*.

Urethral instability has been defined as a spontaneous fall in maximal urethral pressure of one-third or more (Wise et al, 1993) or of >15 cmH_2O pressure (Vereecken et al, 1985). This drop in pressure is accompanied by a decrease in EMG activity in the external anal sphincter and the periurethral sphincter musculature (Vereecken et al 1985). The sound of running water induced a 30% or greater drop in urethral closing pressure in 25% of patients having bladder cystometry as part of the investigation for incontinence (Skehan et al, 1990).

During voiding the urethra opens and allows complete bladder emptying. If relaxation does not occur with attempted voiding, there is said to be *urethral overactivity*. Synchronous bladder and striated urethral sphincter contraction is termed *detrusor–sphincter dyssynergia* and is generally associated with neurological conditions. *Voiding dysfunction* can occur when the striated sphincter mechanism or the pubococcygei are overactive during attempted voiding in the absence of neurological disease. Mechanical factors, such as scarring and strictures, are uncommon in women but can interfere with urine flow.

Urinary Incontinence

Accidental loss of urine is termed *incontinence*. Incontinence is a condition in which an involuntary loss of urine is a social or hygienic problem and is objectively demonstrable (ICS definition). Many studies and surveys define incontinence as any urine loss or loss two or more times a month. A small, occasional loss may not be a social or hygienic problem. When pad tests are used to quantify urine loss only loss greater than 2 g is classified as incontinence.

Conditions Associated with Urethrovesical Dysfunction

- *Day frequency* – voiding more than 7–8 times a day.
- *Nocturia* – waking from sleep to void two or more times at night in women less than 70 years.
- *Urgency* – a very strong urge to void. This is often perceived as a perineal sensation, not a suprapubic bladder fullness sensation. Sensory urgency relates to bladder mucosal hypersensitivity as it occurs with inflammation. Motor urgency is related to detrusor overactivity. Recently, more sensitive monitoring in sensory urgency has detected frequent unstable detrusor contractions (Kolton et al, 1995).
- *Hesitancy* – slow start to voiding.
- *Straining* – use of raised IAP to expel urine. This may produce an intermittent flow and incomplete emptying.
- *Poor stream* – continuous but very slow flow.
- *Intermittent flow* – when flow starts and stops several times during voiding.
- *Urethral syndrome* – frequency, urgency, dysuria and sometimes suprapubic and back pain.

- *Urinary retention* – when urine remains in the bladder at the end of micturition. Retained volumes increase in the aged. Volumes of <100 ml are generally considered acceptable for daily function. See Table 28.1 for causes of urinary dysfunction.
- *Urge incontinence* is an involuntary loss of urine associated with a strong desire to void (ICS definition). It can result in the loss of a large volume of urine, when a detrusor contraction follows urethral relaxation.
- *Genuine stress incontinence* is an involuntary loss of urine, occurring in the absence of a detrusor contraction, when the intravesical pressure exceeds the maximal urethral pressure (ICS definition). This results in a small volume loss, frequently a spot, and occurs at the same time as the increase in IAP.
- *Nocturnal enuresis* is an involuntary loss of urine during sleep (ICS definition). It can be primary or secondary (see Chapter 8).
- *Overflow incontinence* is an involuntary loss of urine associated with overdistension of the bladder (ICS definition). It may or may not be associated with a detrusor contraction. There tends to be a continuous leakage both day and night.
- *Reflex incontinence* is a loss of urine due to detrusor hyper-reflexia and/or involuntary urethral relaxation in the absence of the sensation usually associated with the desire to micturate (ICS definition). A sudden loss of a large volume of urine occurs.
- *Giggle incontinence* is said to occur when urine loss is preceded by prolonged and often hysterical laughter. It may be a small leakage or a full loss (see Chapter 8).
- *Post-micturition loss* or dribble is the loss of a small volume of urine after voiding appears to be complete. Causes of urinary incontinence are outlined in Table 28.2.

Causes of urinary incontinence can be grouped into urological, obstetric, gynaecological, medical, pharmacological, neurological, psychological and environmental. Urine can be lost other than through the urethra due to structural defects or damage, as in fistulae and ectopic ureters. This is termed *extraurethral incontinence.* A fistula between the bladder and vagina can develop after severe childbirth trauma. It is uncommon in Western societies, but occurs quite frequently in third World areas. The Fistula Hospital in Addis Ababa repairs hundreds of fistulae a year. Ectopic ureters, which connect to the vagina, are usually detected in childhood.

Other Factors Affecting Urinary Control

Hormonal status

- Sufferers often complain that genuine stress incontinence is worse a few days before a period, in the luteal phase of the menstrual cycle.
- Low oestrogen levels post-menopausally result in mucosal thinning and decreased vascularity in the submucosal urethral tissues, thus reducing urethral closure.
- Genuine stress incontinence can worsen during the cyclical progesterone phase of hormone replacement therapy.
- Prolonged breast feeding has been mentioned as a factor in genuine stress incontinence.

Prolapse

Stretching of the vagina and endopelvic fascia allows sagging of the vaginal walls and organs prolapse into the vagina. This usually follows vaginal delivery, especially of a large baby and forceps delivery, and can be aggravated by heavy lifting or straining at defaecation. Prolapse of the bladder into the vagina is called a *cystocoele* (see Chapter 27) and the degree to which this occurs, first, second or third, can affect the ability to empty the bladder. If the posterior bladder sags below the urethral opening, complete emptying may only be achieved if the bladder is pushed back into place.

Table 28.1 Causes of urinary dysfunction

Problem	Causes
Frequency	UTI, small bladder, large fluid intake, anxiety, habit, drugs, alcohol
Nocturia	Small capacity, late intake, ↑ diuresis due to ↑ venous return in supine or inadequate antidiuretic hormone = nocturnal polyuria, bladder overactivity
Urgency	UTI, bladder stones, tumours. See urge incontinence
Hesitancy	Detrusor underactivity, slow sphincter relaxation
Straining	Outlet obstruction, acontractile detrusor
Intermittent flow	Voiding dysfunction, voiding by ↑ IAP
Poor stream	Detrusor underactivity, outlet obstruction, incomplete sphincter relaxation
Urethral syndrome	Recurrent infection, inflammation, low-level bacterial pathogens, fastidious organisms, poor bladder neck suppor
Urinary retention	Detrusor underactivity, urethral obstruction, large cystocoele

Table 28.2 Causes of urinary incontinence

Problem	Causes
Urge incontinence	• ↓ neurological control – cortical, pathways • ↑afferent input – epithelium: infection, inflammation – detrusor: tumour, prolapse, constipation, surgery, caffeine, increases in IAP • Deconditioned voiding reflex – anxiety, frequency, ↓ capacity, ↑ bladder wall thickness, urgency • Urethral instability – spontaneous, running water. May trigger bladder instability
Genuine stress incontinence	• Hypermobile urethra – vaginal delivery (large baby, forceps delivery, long active 2nd stage); long-term straining at defaecation; prolonged heavy lifting • Poor urethral pressure – pregnancy (hormonal); striated muscle weakness – parturition, atrophy; low oestrogenization – post-menopause; scarring – post-surgery, 'lead pipe urethra'; ageing
Nocturnal enuresis	• Small functional bladder capacity, low levels of antidiuretic hormone, detrusor overactivity, abnormal sleep patterns (see Chapter 8)
Overflow incontinence	• Bladder outlet/urethral obstruction – stricture • Acontractile detrusor – overstretch, neuropathy
Reflex incontinence	• Neurological conditions – multiple sclerosis, spinal injuries, etc.
Giggle incontinence	• Detrusor instability, genetic factors (see Chapter 8)
Post-micturition loss	• Possible cause – lax bladder base which allows urine to remain below the outlet level

Surgery to correct a cystocoele has been known to be followed by urinary incontinence. The surgery changes the position of the bladder and the posterior urethrovesical angle. Perhaps the urethral kink caused by the cystocoele was enough to reinforce weak urethral closing pressure. With the bladder restored to a normal position, the pressure may be inadequate for continence.

Medical and neurological conditions

Acute-stay hospital patients, medical and surgical, have a high incidence of urinary incontinence, often associated with their current morbidity. Much of this is transitory. However, reliance on others for toileting needs can mean a long wait and accidents do occur, especially in those where rapid toilet access is a prerequisite for continence. Neurological diseases, conditions and neuropathies are the principal causes of problems – CVA, MS, parkinsonism, etc. – and these tend to be compounded by age.

Ageing

Ageing affects all body systems. Changes occurring in the urogenital system are outlined in Chapter 36.

Drugs

Many medications prescribed for unrelated conditions can compromise continence and these tend to have more influence as the woman ages. The box contains functional aspects to consider in relation to drug ingestion. A detailed knowledge of these drugs is not the province of physiotherapists, but it is important to be able to ascertain the effect of specific drugs, prescribed for unrelated conditions, on urinary function. Referral of the woman back to her medical adviser for further management may be appropriate. Access to a drug reference text is invaluable. Some of the drugs which affect urinary function are listed in Table 28.3.

Functions to be considered in relation to drug ingestion

Urine volumes

Urethral closure

Detrusor contractility

Awareness

Gastrointestinal function

Lifestyle Factors which Compromise Continence

Smoking is implicated as a cause of genuine stress incontinence, as chronic coughing strains pelvic supporting tissues. The prevalence of smokers and reformed smokers

Table 28.3 Some drugs that affect urinary function

Drug group	Indication	Example	Effect
Diuretics	Cardiac-related oedema	Frusemide	Frequency, urgency, especially fast-acting loop diuretics
alpha blockers	Hypertension	Prazosin	alpha adrenergic antagonist – decreases UCP, leads to GSI (Mathew et al, 1988)
NSAIDs	Arthritis, inflammatory conditions	Tiaprofenic acid	Frequency, nocturia, urgency, dysuria, suprapubic pain – severe cystitis (O'Neill, 1994)
Antidepressants	Depression	Imipramine	Anticholinergic effect, decreased bladder contractility – retention, overflow. Decreased GI motility – constipation
Opioid analgesics	Pain	Codeine	Decreased GI motility – constipation
Prokinetic	GI dysmotility	Cisapride	Bladder overactivity – frequency, incontinence (Boyd and Rohan, 1994)
Alcohol	Social		Diuresis
Caffeine	Social	Coffee, tea, cola	Detrusor overactivity

GSI = genuine stress incontinence; UCP = urethral closing pressure; NSAID = non-steroidal anti-inflammatory drugs; GI = gastrointestinal. Drugs have been listed using generic terms as many drugs have different proprietary names in different countries. Drugs which have an adverse effect can also have positive effects in women who suffer from the opposite conditions, e.g. imipramine is frequently used in the treatment of detrusor overactivity.

amongst an incontinent group was significantly greater than in a continent group (Bump and McClish, 1991).

Obesity leads to a decrease in fascial strength and an increase in tissue stiffness. Tissue failure occurs more easily (Sayer and Smith, 1994).

Diets low in fibre can lead to slow gastrointestinal motility, constipation and 'straining at stool', which have adverse effects on pelvic supporting tissues and continence (Spence-Jones et al, 1994).

Anxiety can lead to frequency, urgency and small bladder capacity and a vicious circle evolves.

Injury and Disuse in Striated Muscle

Disuse, injury, disease and age can impair striated muscle function and this is very obvious in the pelvic floor, which is predominantly a slow-twitch tonic muscle.

After injury, slow-twitch fibres tend to lose their tonic ability and act more phasically, rather than provide ongoing support (Richardson, 1987). Weakness and disuse lead to diminished levels of afferent impulses which are necessary for tonic muscle activity. If afferent impulses are blocked muscle motor unit recruitment order is disturbed and the pattern of activity resembles that of fast-twitch phasic muscles rather than tonic muscle activity (Grimby and Hannerz, 1976). Jager et al (1996) found that the number of slow-twitch fibres, taken from three sections of the levator ani, decreased after vaginal delivery and with ageing.

Sexual Activity and Urinary Incontinence

Loss of urine during sexual activity is information not often volunteered by women seeking treatment for urinary incontinence. Though causing distress to women, many partners are not perturbed by the loss. Of sexually active women seeking treatment for incontinence, 34% reported symptoms during sexual activity (Vierhout and Gianotten, 1993). Provocation has been divided into mechanical factors – abdominal pressure, penile entry and deep penetration – and non-mechanical factors – arousal, orgasm and clitoral stimulation.

In those women who suffered loss with penetration, there was a high incidence of stress incontinence, whereas loss associated with orgasm occurred with both stress incontinence and detrusor instability (Hilton, 1988). It has been noted that urine loss does affect sexual function. Detrusor instability and sensory urgency had a particular impact, leading to loss of sexual interest, decreased activity and subsequent interpersonal problems (Kelleher et al, 1992). Urinary incontinence can also be used as an excuse to avoid intercourse in those with pre-existing relationship problems (Hilton, 1988).

Research Findings

Research into urinary incontinence is extensive. Histology, pharmacology, neurophysiology, kinesiology and many other aspects have been investigated. While it would be impossible to review all the literature and undesirable to include much here, some studies provide facts which are of interest to physiotherapists and will influence treatment decisions and outcome expectations.

The short-term effect of vaginal delivery on PFM has been reviewed in Chapter 23. Other studies have looked at pathology in specific conditions, particularly genuine stress incontinence and detrusor instability. A summary of some of the findings appears below.

- *PFM damage.* Pathological changes have been demonstrated in muscle fibres of posterior pubococcygeus in women with genuine stress incontinence and genitourinary prolapse. There was evidence of denervation and reinnervation and in some patients only slow-twitch fibres were present (Gilpin et al, 1989). Fibres of anterior pubococcygeus did not demonstrate such differences between subjects and controls. Heit et al (1996) demonstrated similar findings in anterior pubococcygeus.
- *Delayed nerve conduction.* Prolonged pudendal and perineal nerve conduction times to the external anal sphincter and the urethral sphincter have been demonstrated in women with genuine stress incontinence (Mallet et al, 1994).
- *Denervation.* Single-fibre EMG studies show that one nerve axon has 'sprouted' to supply more than one muscle fibre (Chapter 24). Living nerves reinnervate muscle fibres whose nerve supply has died. One nerve can supply up to eight fibres. Averaging over 20 samples provides more accurate single-fibre EMG figures. Increased fibre density has been shown in women with genuine stress incontinence (Smith et al, 1989).
- *PFM weakness.* This has been detected on vaginal pressure measurements in subjects with genuine stress incontinence and/or urge incontinence (Deindl et al, 1994; Gunnarson and Mattiason, 1992).
- *Urinary incontinence.* Five-year follow-up studies after early post-partum investigation demonstrated the development of urinary incontinence in multiparous women who had experienced unassisted vaginal deliveries. Five out of 14 had developed clinical symptoms of stress incontinence (Snooks et al, 1990).
- *Detrusor instability.* When this is present prior to surgery for genuine stress incontinence, it persists afterwards. There also appears to be a *de novo* increase in detrusor instability post-operatively which may be directly related to the type of surgery undertaken (Heslington and Hilton, 1995).
- Operative results were especially good in patients who had PFM training prior to surgery for genuine stress incontinence (Klarskov et al, 1986).

Urinary incontinence is very prevalent amongst the female population, with varying prevalence in different studies. The figures stated may also reflect different definitions of urinary incontinence as applied by different researchers. Some figures are included in Table 28.4.

Uterovaginal Dysfunction

Over-stretching of the vaginal tissues and the endopelvic fascia that supports the female pelvic organs leads to problems associated with the genital tract. These structural changes are termed *prolapses.* Obstetric trauma has long been thought to be the most important causative factor. More recently, a history of straining at defaecation prior to the development of the prolapse has been shown to be common. In a group of women with uterovaginal prolapse, 61% had a history of defaecation straining compared with 4% of controls and 95% were constipated at the time of consultation (Spence-Jones et al, 1994).

The site of the prolapse, whether bladder (*cystocoele*), cervix and uterus (*uterovaginal prolapse*), small intestine (*enterocoele*) or rectum (*rectocoele*), depends on the section of the endopelvic fascia that is stretched and torn. Prolapses are generally classified according to severity from first to third degrees (see Chapter 27). A new method of prolapse evaluation has recently been proposed by an International Continence Society committee dealing with pelvic organ prolapse and pelvic floor dysfunction. This involves objective measurement of a range of variables,

Table 28.4 Prevalence of urinary incontinence in females

Author	Number	Type	%	Comments
Thomas et al, 1980	6205 1562	Unspecified	8.5% 11.4%	15–64-year-olds – regular incontinence 65 and over – regular incontinence Moderate to severe in 1/5 Occasional loss (<2 × month) in twice as many
Millard, 1983	651	Unspecified	33%	Much of it minor – GSI in younger, urge incontinence in older women
Kondo et al, 1990	181 122	GSI Handwash	43% 16%	50–59-year-olds 60–69-year-olds
Kok et al, 1991	719	Unspecified	23.5%	60 years and over

GSI = genuine stress incontinence

thus providing accurate detail on site-specific PF relaxation (Athanasiou et al, 1995).

A degree of rectocoele (prolapse of the posterior vaginal wall) is very common in multiparae and minor rectocoeles have even been shown in 81% of nulliparae (Shorvon et al, 1989). Symptoms of obstructed defaecation only occur in a minority of these subjects (Lubowski and King, 1995).

Women with prolapse may complain of a heavy dragging feeling, which worsens as the day progresses. At a later stage, the dragging discomfort eases and the patient can be left with a sensation of bulging in the vagina, made worse with squatting. If the prolapse protrudes from the vagina it tends to rub on underwear. Many women are unaware that they have minor prolapses.

Another problem which affects some women is that of *vaginal flatus.* Air is drawn into a dilated upper vagina, above the pelvic floor, and often escapes noisily, causing great embarrassment. The vagina is dilated during the delivery of a large baby and the stretched smooth muscle vaginal walls do not recover their previous dimensions. The problem worsens as the day progresses and more air is drawn in as the subject moves.

It is important for physiotherapists dealing with PF dysfunction to realize that structural changes attributed to smooth muscle and fascial defects are not likely to change greatly with rehabilitation of striated muscles. Improving weak muscles can provide a certain amount of support but structural damage which affects function needs surgical repair. However, the role of physiotherapists in these cases is important. They should teach muscle rehabilitation, defaecation retraining to limit PF and organ descent while evacuating and reinforcement of the PF during functional activities. These measures maintain the status quo and can prevent the condition worsening. When muscles are rehabilitated prior to surgical repair, good support for the repositioned organs is available immediately post-operatively.

Investigation of Urethrovesical Dysfunction

Urinary incontinence is a symptom. It has an underlying cause and the physiotherapist has to decide on the best management for each case.

There are a number of investigations which can be carried out by medical personnel. A general practitioner will test a mid-stream urine specimen for infection, check on general health, drugs and perhaps do a vaginal examination. Further investigations such as a micro-urine or a urine culture may be necessary. Other investigations of function are carried out by specialists. The most valuable, to assess lower urinary tract function, is *urodynamic evaluation.* If damage to the kidneys is suspected an *intravenous pyelogram (IVP)* may be done. Contrast medium, injected intravenously, outlines the renal pelves and ureters and fills the bladder. A *cystoscopy* to examine the bladder and urethra may be necessary to eliminate local pathology. *Ultrasound* scanning is used to detect residual urine, which can also be checked clinically by catheterizing after voiding.

Urodynamics

Urine flow rate involves emptying a full bladder, in private, into a flow meter. In normals the flow should be continuous. The rate varies with urine volume, but it is usually at a maximum of 25–30 ml per second. Graphically the flow rate presents as a bell-shaped curve.

Cystometry is an invasive test measuring bladder behaviour and pressures on filling, voiding and during provocative actions, such as coughing. Pressures are recorded graphically and video display units can be used to visualize changes in bladder shape and incontinence. Testing is carried out in supine and later in standing.

Measurement of the *urethral pressure profile* is made at rest along the length of the urethra, by withdrawing a transducer from the bladder and recording pressures at intervals. Pressure can also be measured, in the region of greatest pressure, during voiding, coughing and a PF contraction and a profile of pressures can be mapped.

Urethral sphincter EMG may be measured. However, evidence of denervation has been found in both normals and those with stress incontinence, so its diagnostic value has been questioned (Barnick and Cardozol, 1989).

Stress tests measure the transmission of abdominal pressure to the proximal urethra during effort, e.g. cough. A positive stress test indicates that transmitted abdominal pressure to the urethra plus the urethral closing pressure is greater than the combined bladder and abdominal pressure during the stress.

Other tests

Other tests for nerve conduction (perineal nerve terminal motor latency) and muscle denervation (single-fibre EMG) are not used in clinical evaluation. The introduction of ambulatory bladder monitoring in the last decade, made possible by modern electronics, allows natural bladder filling and a record of bladder activity during everyday living. Generally detrusor instability occurs more often, voiding pressures are higher and voided volumes less in comparison with conventional cystometry (Robertson et al, 1994). This occurs even in asymptomatic volunteers (Heslington and Hilton, 1996). However, the irritant effect of the monitoring catheter must be taken into account.

PAD TEST

This is a valuable way to quantify urine loss and to assess improvement at the end of treatment. Tests can be for one, two, 24 or 48 hours. Obviously longer tests are more

Table 28.5 Example of a urinary frequency/volume chart with fluid intake.

Urine output				Fluid intake		
Time	Volume	Wet/dry?	Comments	Time	Amount	Type
8.30am	710 ml*	D	On waking	10.25	250 ml	Juice
9.50	100 ml	D	With defaecation	10.50	150 ml	Milk
11.30	280 ml	D	Need – moving around	12.00	260 ml	Tea
12.55	200 ml	D	Going out	4.30pm	280 ml	Cordial
4.25pm	450 ml	Spot loss	Urge – home coming	5.05	260 ml	Tea
9.30	320 ml	D	Need	8.00	250 ml	Water
11.30	390 ml	D	Before shower/bed	9.00	250 ml	Tea
				10.00	250 ml	Tea
8.00am	750 ml*	D	On waking	8.30am	260 ml	Juice
10.15	250 ml	D	With defaecation	9.50	150 ml	Milk
1.50pm	410 ml	D	Need	10.15	280 ml	Tea
3.10	200 ml	D	Going out	1.15pm	250 ml	Tea
9.20	320 ml	D	Need	3.10	200 ml	Tea
12.00	200 ml	D	Before bed	7.50	250 ml	Soup
				9.00	250 ml	Tea
				10.30	260 ml	Tea
7.15am	660 ml*	D	On waking	12.00	70 ml	Milk

* Note large bladder volumes.

accurate, but they are difficult for the patient. In some cases tests are carried out with the bladder filled by catheter to two-thirds capacity.

In a one-hour test (ICS recommended) pads are weighed before and after testing. The test begins without voiding, with drinking 500 ml, waiting 1/2 hour, being active for 1/2 hour including walking up stairs, handwashing, bending, coughing, running on the spot. Loss of <2 g of urine is considered dry. These tests are not regularly used in clinical practice, only in studies, but some investigators consider such short tests unreliable.

FREQUENCY/VOLUME CHART

This test is non-invasive, can be carried out at home and does not require any special equipment. It is the most useful test that the clinician can do. It is a record of how often and how much is voided. Simultaneous recording of fluid intake may be done. A container is placed in the toilet, the patient sits to void (sitting allows more complete bladder emptying in women), volume is measured and the patient records the data. Comments include triggers for loss and the reason for voiding. Voiding can be initiated at will and there are many occasions when women void without the stimulus of a full bladder. Table 28.5 gives an example of a frequency/volume chart.

Measuring is continued for every void day and night for at least 24 hours and preferably for longer. Not everyone is able to manage this, particularly the elderly. For them, counting the day and night voids may be all that they can manage. Information gained from the chart includes the number of day and night voids, functional bladder capacity, triggers for voiding and episodes of loss. These all provide a useful base for a management programme. A repeat chart after a period of treatment can be used to assess progress. A frequency/volume chart should be completed when bladder instability and overactivity are suspected, but not generally for stress incontinence.

Problems of urinary dysfunction may not occur in isolation. They are frequently accompanied by some disruption of anorectal function, sometimes difficult evacuation or, less frequently, faecal incontinence. The patient may present with poor urinary control, but be unaware that her difficulty in defaecation is the major causative factor of her urinary problem. The physiotherapist working with pelvic floor dysfunction needs a good understanding of anorectal dysfunction as well as of urogenital dysfunction. Anorectal dysfunction may be a new topic for many physiotherapists and it is outlined in Chapter 29. Physiotherapy management of the problems outlined in this chapter is contained in Chapter 30.

References

Abrams P, Blaivas JG, Stanton SL et al (1988) The standardisation of terminology of lower urinary tract function. *Scandanavian Journal of Urology and Nephrology* **114**: 5–19.

Athanasiou S, Hill S, Gleeson C et al (1995) Validation of the ICS proposed pelvic organ prolapse descriptive system. *Neurourology and Urodynamics* **14**: 414–415.

Barnick CG and Cardozol L (1989) Electromyography of the urethral sphincter in genuine stress incontinence: a useless test. *Neurourology and Urodynamics* **8**: 318–319.

Boyd IW and Rohan AP (1994) Urinary disorders associated with cisapride. *Medical Journal of Australia* **160**: 579–580.

Bump RC and McClish DK (1991) Cigarette smoking and urinary incontinence in women. *Neurourology and Urodynamics* **10**: 333–334.

Deindl FM, Vodusek DB, Hesse U et al (1994) Pelvic floor activity patterns: comparison of nulliparous continent and parous urinary stress incontinent women. A kinesiological EMG study. *British Journal of Urology* **73**: 413–417.

Gilpin SA, Gosling JA, Smith ARB et al (1989) The pathogenesis of genitourinary prolapse and stress incontinence of urine. A histological and histochemical study. *British Journal of Obstetrics and Gynaecology* **96**: 15–23.

Grimby L and Hannerz J (1976) Disturbances in voluntary recruitment order of low and high frequency motor units on blockades of proprioceptive afferent activity. *Acta Physiologica Scandanavica* **96**: 207–216.

Gunnarson M and Mattiasson A (1992) Defective function of the circumvaginal musculature not only in stress but also in urge incontinence. *Neurourology and Urodynamics* **11**: 436–437.

Heit M, Benson JT, Russell B et al (1996) Levator ani muscle in women with genitourinary prolapse: indirect assessment by muscle histopathology. *Neurourology and Urodynamics* **15**: 17–29.

Heslington K and Hilton P (1995) The incidence of detrusor instability by ambulatory monitoring and conventional cystometry pre and post colposuspension. *Neurourology and Urodynamics* **14**: 416–417.

Heslington K and Hilton P (1996) Ambulatory monitoring and conventional cystometry in asymptomatic female volunteers. *British Journal of Obstetrics and Gynaecology* **103**: 434–441.

Hilton P (1988) Urinary incontinence during sexual intercourse: a common, but rarely volunteered, symptom. *British Journal of Obstetrics and Gynaecology* **95**: 377–381.

Jackson S, Avery N, Eckford S et al (1995) Connective tissue analysis in genitourinary prolapse. *Neurourology and Urodynamics* **14**: 412–414.

Jager C, Schmidt M, Muller-Felber W et al (1996) Histomorphology of the pelvic floor muscles under specific consideration of age and parity. *Neurourology and Urodynamics* **15**: 333–334.

Kelleher CJ, Cardozo LD, Wise BG et al (1992) The impact of urinary incontinence on sexual function. *Neurourology and Urodynamics* **11**: 359–360.

Klarskov P, Belving D, Bischoff N et al (1986) Pelvic floor exercise versus surgery for female urinary stress incontinence. *Urology International* **41**: 129–132.

Kok ALM, Burger CW, Voorhorst FJ et al (1991) Prevalence of urinary and faecal incontinence and independent risk factors for incontinence in community-residing elderly women. *Neurourology and Urodynamics* **10**: 416–417.

Kolton D, Monga A and Stanton SL (1995) Does sensory urgency exist? *Neurourology and Urodynamics* **14**: 576–577

Kondo A, Kato K, Saito M et al (1990) Prevalence of handwashing urinary incontinence in females in comparison with stress and urge incontinence. *Neurourology and Urodynamics* **9**: 330–331.

Lubowski DZ and King DW (1995) Obstructed defaecation: current status of pathophysiology and management. *Australian and New Zealand Journal of Surgery* **65**: 87–92.

Mallet V, Hosker G, Smith ARB et al (1994) Pelvic floor damage and childbirth: a neurophysiological follow up study. *Neurourology and Urodynamics* **13**: 357–358.

Mathew TH, McEwan J and Rohan A (1988) Urinary incontinence secondary to prazosin. *Medical Journal of Australia* **148**: 305.

Millard RJ (1983) *Incidence of Urinary Incontinence in Australia.* Sydney: Department of Urology, Prince Henry Hospital.

Norton PA, Baker JE, Sharp HC et al (1995) Genitourinary prolapse and joint hypermobility in women. *Obstetrics and Gynecology* **85**: 225–228.

O'Neill GFA (1994) Tiaprofenic acid as a cause of non-bacterial cystitis. *Medical Journal of Australia* **160**: 123–125.

Richardson C (1987) Atrophy of vastus medialis in patello-femoral pain syndrome. *Proceedings of the International Congress of World Confederation of Physical Therapists*, Sydney, pp. 400–403.

Robertson AS, Griffiths CJ, Ramsden PD et al (1994) Bladder function in healthy volunteers: ambulatory monitoring and conventional cystometry. *British Journal of Urology* **73**: 242–249.

Sayer T and Smith T (1994) Pelvic floor biopsy. In: Schussler B, Laycock J, Norton P and Stanton S (eds) *Pelvic Floor Re-education*, pp. 98–101. London: Springer-Verlag.

Sayer TR, Dixon JS, Hosker GL et al (1990) A study of paraurethral connective tissue in women with stress incontinence of urine. *Neurourology and Urodynamics* **9**: 319–320.

Shorvon PJ, McHugh S, Diamant NE et al (1989) Defecography in normal volunteers: results and implications. *Gut* **30**: 1737–1749.

Skehan M, Moore KH and Richmond DH (1990) The auditory stimulus of running water: its effect on urethral pressure. *Neurourology and Urodynamics* **9**: 351–353.

Smith ARB (1994) Role of connective tissue and muscle in pelvic floor dysfunction. *Current Opinion in Obstetrics and Gynecology* **6**: 317–319.

Smith ARB, Hosker G and Warrell D (1989) The role of partial denervation of the pelvic floor in the aetiology of genitourinary prolapse and stress incontinence of urine. A neurophysiological study. *British Journal of Obstetrics and Gynaecology* **96**: 24–28.

Snooks SJ, Swash M, Mathers SE et al (1990) Effect of vaginal delivery on the pelvic floor: a 5 year follow up. *British Journal of Surgery* **77**: 1358–1360.

Spence-Jones C, Kamm MA, Henry MM et al (1994) Bowel dysfunction: a pathogenic factor in uterovaginal prolapse and urinary stress incontinence. *British Journal of Obstetrics and Gynaecology* **101**: 147–152.

Thomas TM, Plymat KR, Blannin J et al (1980) Prevalence of urinary incontinence. *British Medical Journal* **281**: 1243–1245.

Vereecken RL, Cornelissen M, Das J et al (1985) Urethral and perineal instability. *Urology International* **40**: 325–330.

Vierhout ME and Gianotten WL (1993) Mechanisms of urine loss during sexual activity. *European Journal of Obstetrics and Gynecology and Reproductive Biology* **52**: 45–47.

Wise BG, Cardozo LA, Cutner A et al (1993) Prevalence and significance of urethral instability in women with detrusor instability. *British Journal of Urology* **72**: 26–29.

29

Functional Disorders of the Anorectum and Pain Syndromes

SUE MARKWELL

Colon Motility
•
Constipation in Females
•
Gastrointestinal Dysfunction in Young Women
•
Obstructed Defaecation
•
Bowel Dysfunction in the Mature Woman
•
Clinical Investigation
•
Faecal Incontinence
•
Biofeedback in Defaecation Disorders
•
The Role of Physiotherapy
•
Pain Syndromes

This chapter introduces a new concept, disordered bowel function. It briefly considers recent advances in the aetiology and management of rectal outlet disorders, faecal incontinence and non-organic pain syndromes involving pelvic floor dysfunction. Books on the suggested reading list are recommended for further understanding beyond the scope of this chapter.

Constipation, obstructed defaecation and faecal incontinence cause much morbidity in the community and physiotherapists are not exempt. In constipation there is abnormal colonic transport. Obstructed defaecation refers to the inability to fully empty the rectum with or without straining. Faecal incontinence is the accidental loss of contents per anum (flatus, liquid or solid).

Physiotherapy has a role in the rehabilitation of those who suffer from anorectal dysfunction. This focuses on striated muscle activity. Straining at stool is one sign of anorectal dysfunction and Markwell and Sapsford (1995a) have noted that in a physiotherapy population this dysfunction conforms to the community norm.

Recent definition of a pattern of straining and the widespread application of specific retraining without biofeedback have ensured a role for physiotherapists as part of a multidisciplinary team. While physiotherapists do not specifically treat smooth muscle dysfunction, it is important to have a basic understanding of this, and how it impacts on anorectal function.

Colon Motility

This refers to the movement of contents from caecum to rectum.

The average length of the human colon is 1.5 metres. Colon length increases progressively with age and its function has evolved as an adaptation to terrestrial life (Christensen, 1994).

There are two important aspects of colorectal motility: motor activity (co-ordinated muscle contraction); and transit (movement of contents through the colon) (Kellow, 1990). Normal motor function depends on the combined interaction of myogenic and neurogenic factors and chemical/hormonal gut substances. This relies on intact

Table 29.1 Causes of constipation in females

Category	Precipitating factors
Behavioural	Faulty diet, dehydration, rushed lifestyle, travel, institutional living, immobility
Psychological	Altered motility due to neurotransmitter response to stress; cerebral inhibition of motility; somatization (depression, trauma, past history of sexual violation or abuse) (Devroede, 1996b) Impaired intellect, cognition
Hormonal	Pregnancy; symptomatic bowel dysfunction during luteal phase; oral contraceptives and progesterone used in HRT
Medication	Iron, opioids, antacids, anticholinergics, antidepressants, other
Endocrine	Hypothyroidism, ovarian disorders, other
Metabolic	Diabetes, chronic renal failure
Other	Scleroderma
Neurological	Parkinson's disease, multiple sclerosis *Colonic factors*: • neuronal dysfunction of neurotransmitter substances; decreased response to stimulant laxatives • smooth muscle dysfunction • visceral myopathy – multivisceral – panenteric • pseudo-obstruction *Extracolonic factors*: • spinal, cauda equina trauma, degeneration, inflammation or congenital malformation • pelvic surgery (e.g. hysterectomy) • disruption to parasympathetic nerve supply • effect of haematoma or disruption to surgical tissue planes • local neuropathy associated with childbirth
Obstruction	*Mechanical*: • adhesions, tumours, strictures, diverticulitis *Functional*: • ileus (metabolic, post-surgery, etc.)
Dysmotility	Irritable bowel syndrome (IBS) Diverticulosis Associated gall bladder dysfunction Normal diameter colon and rectum Acquired megacolon, megarectum (male and female prevalence equal) Idiopathic slow-transit constipation, colon inertia, hindgut inertia
Anorectal outlet disorders	Local anal conditions, trauma, e.g. fissure, haemorrhoids

Anorectal outlet dysfunction	Hirschsprung's disease (more common in males) Disruption to integrated smooth and striated muscle activity* Pelvic floor inco-ordination* • never learnt • acquired (e.g. specific abdominal muscle overdevelopment) • pelvic floor/organ dyssynergia • 'anismus' (abuse?) Pelvic floor neuropathy/fascial disruption – descending perineum syndrome (DPS)*: • childbirth • straining at stool • lifestyle, e.g. prolonged heavy lifting WITH • blunted rectal sensation • rectal inertia • associated structural defects, rectocoele, rectal lining/rectal wall prolapse • mechano/inflammatory conditions – solitary rectal ulcer, proctitis cystica profunda • terminal reservoir syndrome • any combination of the above (the elderly) This is not a complete list.

* indicates the most important causes.

central, autonomic and enteric nervous systems and the ordered interaction between them. Motility is affected by the physical and chemical make-up of the contents. The incompletely understood complex chemical and hormonal neurotransmitter substances and enzymes affecting gut function, e.g. amines, peptides, prostaglandins and sex hormones, all play a part. Many of these chemical and hormonal substances are active as a response to eating. Emotional disturbances and stress may profoundly affect transit.

Colonic muscle has both cholinergic and non-cholinergic excitatory nerve receptors but the principal one is cholinergic (Christensen, 1994). Noradrenaline, rather than adrenaline, has the major inhibitory effect. Mass movements of the colon represent disinhibition. Thus electrical slow waves exert a pacing ('stop/go') action within the smooth muscle and complex mass movements occur briefly, with long rest periods in between.

Constipation is the main symptom of disordered colon function and is the term given to delayed or abnormal transport of colon contents (see Table 29.1 for the causes of constipation). Human motility displays a wide fluctuation during a 24-hour period (Bassotti et al, 1995). Profound inactivity leads to constipation, while marathon runners frequently complain of diarrhoea. The role of exercise on colon transit is not clear, but intense activity is more likely to accelerate transit (Bassotti et al, 1995).

Normal transit time, as measured by the orderly ingestion of radio-opaque markers, is 33 hours at the upper limit in men and 47 hours in women (Fig. 29.1). When isotope scanning is used, 70% of the tracer should be defaecated in 48 hours (Bassotti et al, 1995).

Figure 29.1 Well-distributed colon transit markers still obvious after 96 hours, indicating colon inertia.

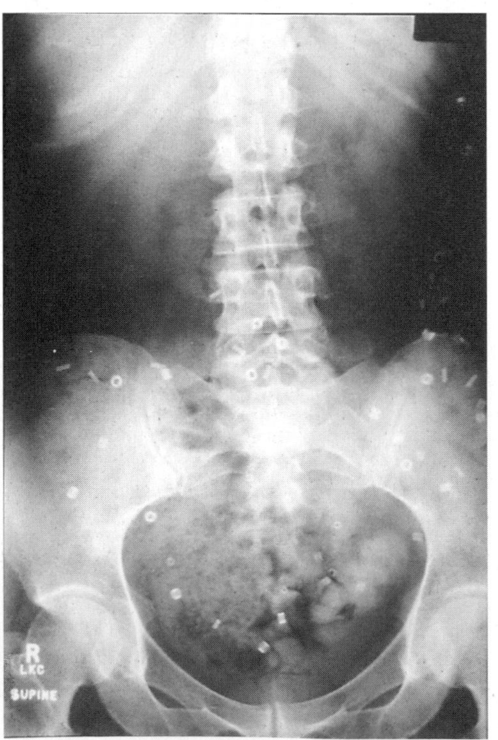

Table 29.2 Drugs and their effects on colonic motility

Enhance	Inhibit
Bulking agents	Antihypertensives
Softening agents	beta blockers
Stimulants	Ca channel blockers
Osmotic agents	Antiarrhythmics
Prokinetics:	Hypolipidaemics
cholinergic agonists	Diuretics – non-K-sparing
opiate antagonists	Iron
dopamine antagonists	Antineoplastics
motilin agonists	Opioid analgesics
indirect cholinergic stimulants	Antihistamines
acting through release of ACH	Antidepressants (tricyclic)
in intramural plexus – cisapride	Tranquillizers
	Anticholinergics
	Antiparkinsonians
	Antacids

Probert et al (1993), in a community-based study looking at reasons why females have longer transit times than males, concluded the following. Alcohol hastened transit in both sexes and women using the oral contraceptive had significantly longer colon transit. They concluded that these two factors had a greater effect than dietary fibre and helped to explain the sex differences. Various drugs have an effect on colonic motility and may be used to enhance it (Table 29.2). The side effects of prescribed drugs on motility must be considered when treating patients with constipation.

Constipation in Females

Constipation, the symptom or sign of delayed colonic motility, is approximately three times more prevalent in females. It is usually considered to occur when stool frequency is less than three times a week or straining to evacuate occurs more than 25% of the time (Drossman et al, 1982). In the United States constipation accounts for 2.5 million physician visits each year and more than $400 million is spent annually on over-the-counter laxatives (Harris, 1994). The prevalence in both men and women increases with advancing age. It may be mild, moderately severe or intractable. Many aetiological factors must be considered. There are distinct age- and lifestyle-related aetiological factors in female constipation.

Recent understanding has led to a broad division of functional constipation into psychophysiological and psychoneuroimmunological categories (Devroede, 1996a). Trauma, adverse life events and grief have often been implicated in slowing of colon transit. In the light of present knowledge, constipation is considered a symptom or a sign, not a disease (Devroede, 1996a). Common symptoms of constipation are listed in the box.

Figure 29.2 Megacolon and megarectum. Symptoms include marked discomfort with bloating.

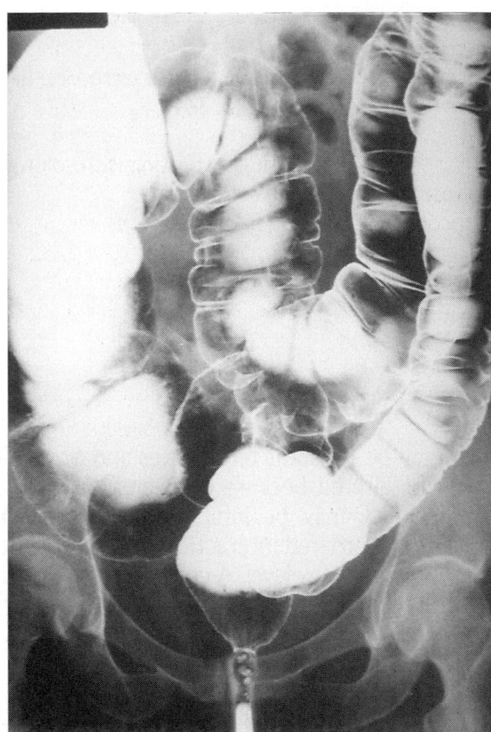

Symptoms of constipation

Abdominal distension/bloating (see Fig. 29.2)

Abdominal pain

Backache

Nausea

Headache

Difficult defaecation

Although aetiology may be confusing there are certain symptom clusters that must be understood by the physiotherapist. The onset of functional constipation, symptoms and the severity of the problem and past management must indicate to the physiotherapist the level of multidisciplinary intervention to be undertaken. It may be considered that there are distinct age- and lifestyle-related aetiological divisions of constipation.

1. Idiopathic constipation of childhood:
   - onset before age 10;
   - more boys affected than girls;
   - characterized by faecal impaction and overflow soiling.
2. Idiopathic slow-transit constipation in young women:
   - onset between 10 and 20 years;
   - characterized by bloating and diminished rectal urge;
   - may be complicated by anismus.
3. Irritable bowel syndrome:
   - all ages; predominantly females.
4. Mature age onset:
   - descending perineum syndrome (DPS);
   - as a result of hysterectomy or pelvic surgery;
   - may be combined with 1, 2 or 3.
5. Elderly:
   - slowing of colon transit;
   - global features more important, e.g. immobility;
   - terminal reservoir syndrome with faecal impaction;
   - overflow incontinence (Bartolo et al, 1992).

The irritable bowel syndrome (IBS) may be a common cause of constipation in females. Characteristics of IBS are included in the box.

Irritable bowel syndrome (IBS)

Irritable bowel syndrome is a collection of symptoms, common in the 15–40-year age group and more common in females

Aetiology

- Disturbance in visceral pain perception associated with impaired motility.
- Associated psychosocial and gender features occur with impaired gut transit in IBS (Bennett et al, 1996).

Altered anorectal physiology in IBS

- Rectal contractions are induced at abnormally low rectal distension.
- ↑ rectal contractions and external anal sphincter relaxation occur in response to diarrhoea.
- Rectal compliance is reduced.
- Pain at lower volumes of rectal distension.

The international definition is abdominal pain relieved by defaecation or associated with changes of frequency or consistency of stool and/or disturbed defaecation (two or more of):

- altered stool frequency;
- altered stool form (hard or loose/watery);
- altered stool passage (straining, urgency, feeling of incomplete evacuation);
- passage of mucus

usually with:

- bloating or feeling of abdominal distension (Wingate, 1993).

Diverticulosis is considered to be caused by changes in motility, in which the colonic muscle layers are functionally shortened. Inflammation of the diverticulum is termed

Table 29.3 Management of constipation

Surgery		No surgery
Slow-transit constipation	**Obstructed defaecation**	
Megacolon subtotal colectomy: iliorectal anastomosis total colectomy: ileal pouch (neorectum) ileostomy continent colonic conduit (Williams et al, 1994)	Surgical procedure for Hirschsprung's disease (p. 364) Proctectomy with coloanal anastomosis for isolated acquired megarectum Surgery for anatomical anorectal abnormalities associated with obstructed defaecation: • mucosal banding for anterior rectal wall prolapse • peranal modified Delorme procedure for rectocoele, intussusception (p. 368) • rectopexy (abdominal repair, p. 367) for moderate to severe rectal prolapse • anterior resection for entrapped / redundant sigmoid colons, sigmoidocoeles	Anismus (p. 364) DPS without functional rectocoele or rectal wall prolapse (p. 364) IBS Slow-transit constipation with colon of normal diameter Combination of the above

Figure 29.3 Megarectum following colectomy with ileorectal anastomosis.

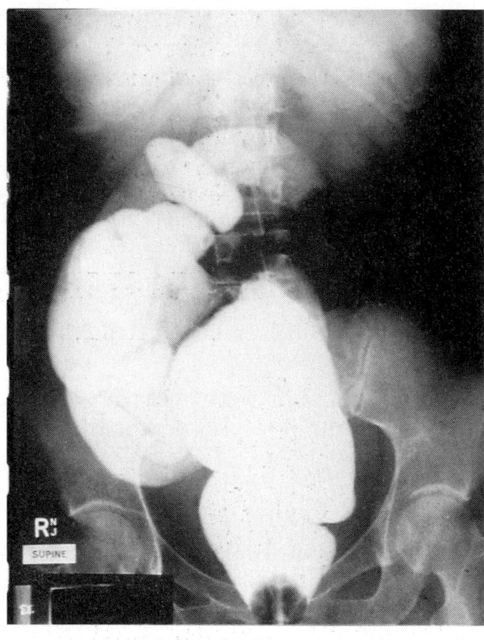

diverticulitis. Many patients will have this process of diverticular inflammation associated with anorectal dysfunction.

Management

Constipation is managed by dietary modification, a regimen of medication, defaecation retraining and surgery. This is outlined in Table 29.3.

Platell et al (1996), in a recent study, noted that the majority of patients who underwent resectional colonic surgery for chronic idiopathic constipation were improved, but surgery was associated with considerable morbidity (see Fig. 29.3).

Constipation implies a decreased frequency of bowel emptying which may be associated with considerable bloating and which may be resistant to laxatives and fibre. Colonic transit may be altered because of decreased mass movements or motility may be inhibited at a cerebral level. Disruption of the ordered interaction of the three nervous systems may occur at any level. A common cause of hindgut delay in young women is pelvic floor inco-ordination.

Gastrointestinal Dysfunction in Young Women

Gastrointestinal dysfunction may be characterized by abnormally slow transit. From puberty onwards (10–20 years), colon transit in many young women may slow profoundly. Idiopathic slow-transit constipation commonly starts at this time and may dramatically worsen when a woman reaches her 30s and 40s. In 1909 Arbuthnot Lane noted that a syndrome of 'chronic intestinal stasis' was found in women under the age of 35. It was associated with sex hormone-related dysfunction and included a high incidence of ovarian cysts. Colectomy (surgical removal of the colon) was the treatment of choice. This was never fully accepted by the medical profession and it soon fell out of favour (Preston and Lennard-Jones, 1986).

During the 1980s there was renewed interest in the cause of disabling intractable constipation in young women with a stool frequency approximating one a week. Preston and Lennard-Jones (1986) noted a combination of slow total gut transit with a colon of normal diameter and this was associated with abdominal, anorectal, gynaecological and somatic symptoms. Hesitancy in voiding was also noted.

Other aetiological factors in intractable slow-transit constipation include:

- multisystem visceral myopathy (Watier et al, 1983);
- axonal and neuronal abnormality of the myenteric plexus (Krishnamurthy et al, 1984);
- alteration of neurotransmitter substances (decreased vasoactive intestinal polypeptide) (Milner et al, 1990);

- reduced substance P (Hutson et al, 1996);
- associated visceral neuropathy in most patients (Schouten et al, 1993).

Extra factors commonly found in female adolescents include the effect of dietary fads and eating disorders which, if continued, delay colon transit. It has been shown in recent studies (Leroi et al, 1995) that past sexual abuse is causative in functional bowel disorders. Increased stress and other psychological manifestations have a positive correlation with constipated patients who have normal transit. Those with slow-transit constipation were shown to have low levels of stress (Agachan et al, 1996; Heyman, 1996; Wald et al, 1989).

Associated bladder dysfunction

Bannister et al (1988) described analogous abnormalities of bladder and rectal function in constipated patients. Voiding volumes and maximum tolerable capacities were increased in both organs, suggesting sensory blunting, but compliance was considered to be normal. Rectal sensory blunting may occur as an adaptation to rectal distension caused by outlet obstruction.

Women with urinary retention commonly have bowel symptoms. Abnormal EMG activity of the urethral sphincter was shown by Lemieux et al (1993). This may help to explain the observed urinary hesitancy noted by Preston and Lennard-Jones (1985) and shown by Fowler et al (1988) in women with polycystic ovaries and voiding dysfunction. Refer to Chapter 7 for normal bladder function.

How are dysfunctional patterns acquired?

During adolescence integrated function of the abdominal and pelvic floor muscles develops. The lumbar curve becomes concave and puborectalis (PR) separates from pubococcygeus (PC) to develop posteriorly in a plane inferior to PC and iliococcygeus (Lansman and Robertson, 1992). At this time PR adapts to its function of maintaining the anorectal angle, one of the factors in maintaining faecal continence. Lansman and Robertson (1992) noted that in amphibians the primitive recti and puborectalis were in alignment, separated only by os pubis. Social and cultural determinants are instrumental in shaping anorectal function at the time of adolescence. A naturally assumed neutral or anterior pelvic tilt in sitting indicates that the person is probably able to achieve lumbar stability and effective bladder and bowel emptying.

- The male evacuation position of forward lean with legs abducted is not favoured socially by females, so a lifelong ineffective position on the toilet may unconsciously develop. 'Kangarooing' (crouching over) on public toilets is equally ineffective. Rectal emptying may be inhibited on a toilet other than at home.
- During a simulated defaecation pattern, bulging of the abdomen, in addition to abdominal bracing, decreases the activity of the external anal sphincter (Sapsford et al, 1996) Fig. 29.4a).

Figure 29.4 (a) Correct defaecation pattern – spine straight and rectus abdominis held at its greatest length. (b) Incorrect pattern of defaecation, showing a slumped spine with concentric rectus abdominis activity. Forward pelvic tilting enhances the defaecation process.

a

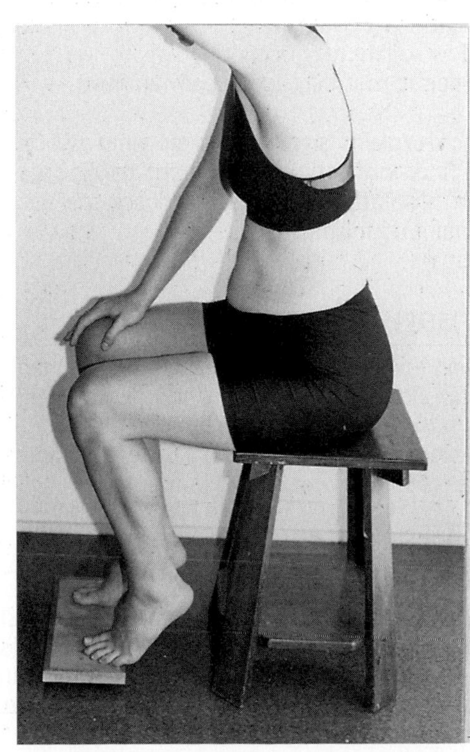

b

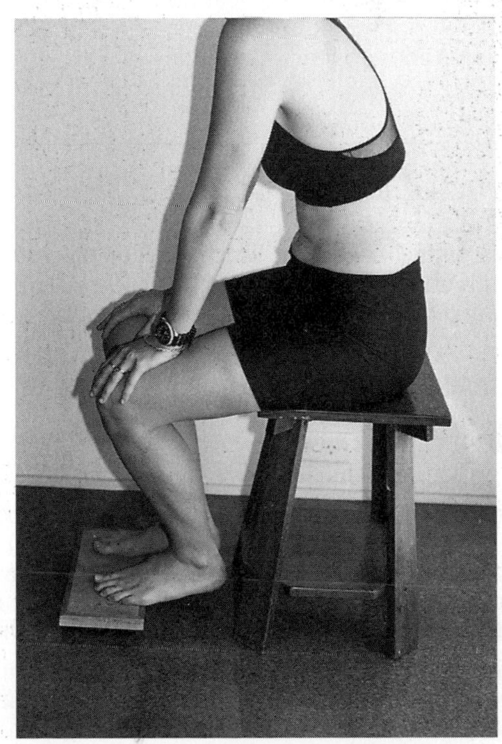

- Conversely, clinical experience has shown that repeated contractions of rectus abdominis with posterior pelvic tilting, or by selective overdevelopment during abdominal 'crunches', appear to increase PR and EAS tone. These crunches are still a measure of fitness in the defence forces and have questionable functional sequelae.
- Inco-ordination may be encouraged by sporting and artistic activities that increase development of the pelvic floor. Ballet, swimming and wind instrument playing enhance levator support and sphincter closure.
- However, raised intra-abdominal pressure *without* lateral levator development may lead, over time, to dysfunctional pelvic floor patterns involving lack of muscle and fascial support. Martial arts devotees and inexperienced weightlifters or those in occupations where heavy lifting is expected are commonly affected, e.g. nurses or defence forces personnel.

Adolescents with 'anismus' may have never learnt to co-ordinate their abdominopelvic floor muscles to release contents (Fig 29.4b). Should a dyssynergic pattern of function occur as a result of adverse life events, functional retraining often facilitates the way to future counselling, leading to ultimate recovery.

Early childhood and puberty are crucial stages of development in mastering co-ordinated defaecation and enhancing the defaecation reflex. Foot support when on the toilet, to provide trunk stability, will facilitate the pattern. Hormonal changes at puberty or the use of the oral contraceptive pill at this time may affect colon motility. This, combined with rectal outlet obstruction as a result of muscle dissociation, may lead to hindgut inertia. Education during these stages may prevent future anorectal and urogenital morbidity.

Obstructed Defaecation

There are several conditions which fall into this category. Simply, this may be considered as having the urge to empty, but having difficulty in getting the contents out.

The descending perineum syndrome (DPS)

In this syndrome, usually confined to mature women, the perineum descends below the plane of the ischial tuberosities at rest or during straining (Parks et al, 1966). On examination, the perineum 'balloons' below the bony outlet of the pelvis during a straining effort (see Fig. 23.2). Table 29.4 outlines the pathogenesis and management of DPS.

As DPS is a very common condition, further reading is strongly recommended (Allen-Mersch et al, 1987; Bartolo et al, 1983; Henry et al, 1982; Pemberton, 1990).

Table 29.5 explains the signs and symptoms of DPS in the different pelvic organs.

Prevalence of DPS

In a major study to assess bowel dysfunction in healthy women, 387 women admitted to symptoms of constipation, bloating, obstructed defaecation, pelvi/perineal pain and associated urinary symptoms. 267 (67%) were aged between 40 and 60 years. Of the 387 women, 342 (88.4%) were parous. The descending perineum syndrome (93.3%) was the most significant finding. Most patients (77.5%) responded to education, muscle rehabilitation and defaecation retraining. 89 (22.5%) were referred to a colorectal unit. Of these, only 31 patients (8%) needed surgical intervention; the remainder returned for conservative care (O'Neill et al, 1993).

Figure 29.5 illustrates the pelvic floor extensibility seen in DPS.

Anismus

This is the failure of co-ordinated release of the levator and sphincter muscles. Rectal emptying does not occur normally. It is a form of pelvic floor / pelvic organ dyssynergia. Puborectalis fails to relax or may actually contract during the defaecation attempt. Other factors include:

- inability to initiate defaecation;
- evacuation is incomplete;
- overflow soiling may occur;
- dyssynergic pain may accompany anismus.

Table 29.6 explains signs and symptoms associated with anismus (inco-ordination) in different pelvic organs. Conventional physiotherapy or biofeedback are used in the management of anismus.

Hirschsprung's Disease

This refers to an ultrashort aganglionic segment of the myenteric plexus at the anorectal junction (see Chapter 7). It is not commonly seen in females. It may cause considerable morbidity, hindgut inertia, megarectum or megacolon. Surgery is almost always indicated.

Surgery in obstructed defaecation – DPS

Surgery is part of colorectal management for obstructed defaecation and includes the Delorme procedure (see box and Fig. 29.6). Rectal intussusception is a common finding in obstructed defaecation and the modified Delorme procedure is often indicated (Berman et al, 1990).

Table 29.4 Pathogenesis and management of descending perineum syndrome

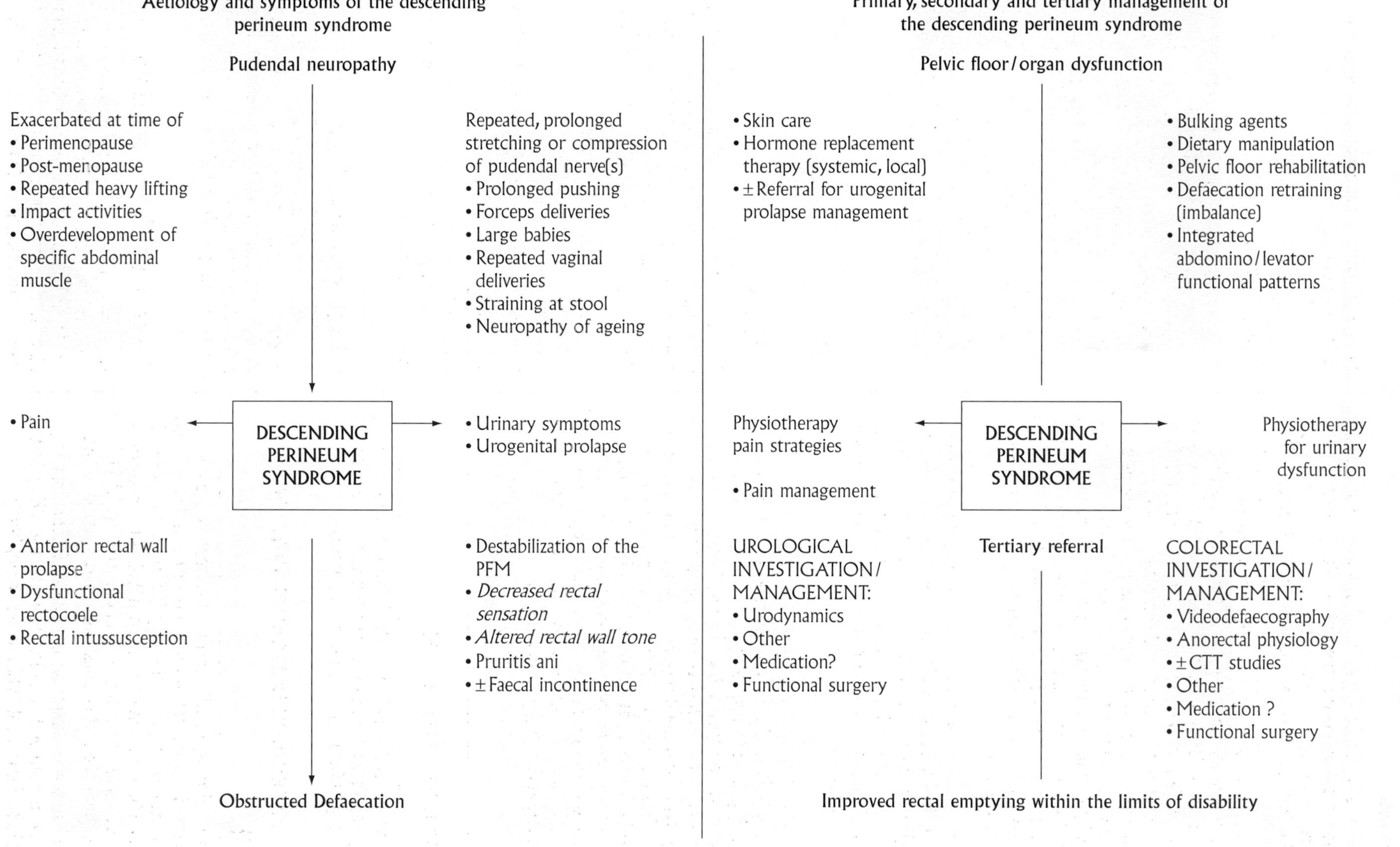
Aetiology and symptoms of the descending perineum syndrome
Pudendal neuropathy
Exacerbated at time of
• Perimenopause
• Post-menopause
• Repeated heavy lifting
• Impact activities
• Overdevelopment of specific abdominal muscle
Repeated, prolonged stretching or compression of pudendal nerve(s)
• Prolonged pushing
• Forceps deliveries
• Large babies
• Repeated vaginal deliveries
• Straining at stool
• Neuropathy of ageing
• Pain
DESCENDING PERINEUM SYNDROME
• Urinary symptoms
• Urogenital prolapse
• Anterior rectal wall prolapse
• Dysfunctional rectocoele
• Rectal intussusception
• Destabilization of the PFM
• *Decreased rectal sensation*
• *Altered rectal wall tone*
• Pruritis ani
• ± Faecal incontinence
Obstructed Defaecation
Primary, secondary and tertiary management of the descending perineum syndrome
Pelvic floor / organ dysfunction
• Skin care
• Hormone replacement therapy (systemic, local)
• ± Referral for urogenital prolapse management
• Bulking agents
• Dietary manipulation
• Pelvic floor rehabilitation
• Defaecation retraining (imbalance)
• Integrated abdomino / levator functional patterns
Physiotherapy pain strategies
• Pain management
DESCENDING PERINEUM SYNDROME
Physiotherapy for urinary dysfunction
UROLOGICAL INVESTIGATION / MANAGEMENT:
• Urodynamics
• Other
• Medication?
• Functional surgery
Tertiary referral
COLORECTAL INVESTIGATION / MANAGEMENT:
• Videodefaecography
• Anorectal physiology
• ± CTT studies
• Other
• Medication ?
• Functional surgery
Improved rectal emptying within the limits of disability

Figure 29.5 Videodefaecograms of a subject with DPS and nerve entrapment pain. Extensibility can be assessed against the scale. The position of the anorectum is shown (a) at rest; (b) with a contracted pelvic floor; (c) on straining (minimal anal opening) ; (d) on straining harder; (e) with patient relaxed; (f) on straining again; (g) at rest after emptying.

a

b

c

d

e

f

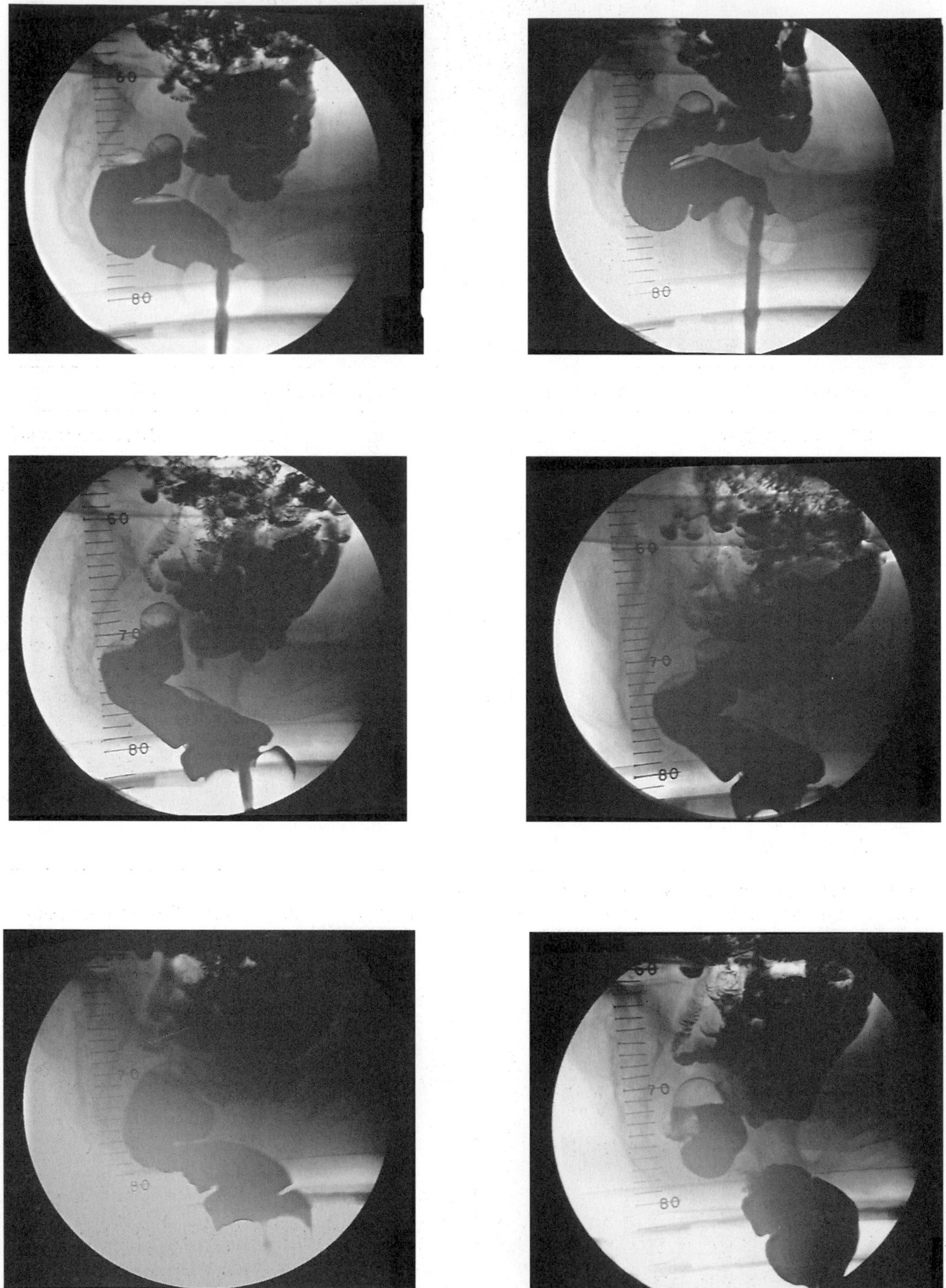

Figure 29.5 Continued

g

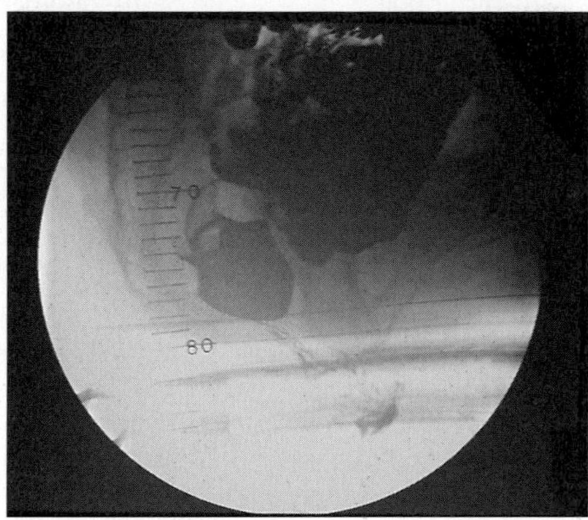

Table 29.5 Obstructed defaecation – 'imbalance' – combined pelvic organ dysfunction

	Defaecation	Micturition	Sexual disorders	Pain
Symptoms	DPS – poor support Outlet obstruction ↓ colon motility Neuropathic FI Anal pruritis Bloating Hindgut pain	Stress incontinence Bladder instability Mixed incontinence Overflow incontinence Incomplete bladder emptying	Lack of sensation Deep discomfort on penetration Exquisite pain superficially on entry No penetration	Nerve trunk pain (toothache quality) Worsened by gravity and defaecation Relieved in lying Burning pain Proctalgia fugax
Signs	DPS Megacolon / rectum Mucosal prolapse Rectal prolapse Solitary rectal ulcer Inflammatory rectal conditions (PCP) Enterocoele Anal fissures, IAS / EAS tears	Lax anterior vaginal wall Cystourethrocoele Hypermobility of urethra Poor urethral closing pressure	Lack of PC bulk Organ prolapse Pressure over pudendal nerve Vestibulitis Combination	Stretching / compression of pelvic / pudendal / perineal / perianal nerves Destabilization of PFM Unilateral nerve trauma Trauma to coccyx Result of surgery Sacral nerve pathology

Imbalance-type obstructed defaecation is usually associated with neuropathy.
DPS = descending perineum syndrome; FI = faecal incontinence; I = incontinence; PFM = pelvic floor muscles; PC = pubococcygeus; PCP = Proctitis cystica profunda.

Intussusception of the rectum

- Internal intussusception of the rectum may be defined as the funnel-shaped infolding of the rectum during straining to defaecate.
- Rectum descends from the sacrum (stretched mesentery).
- There is no overt prolapse.
- Results from impaired pelvic floor function.
- Faecal incontinence may occur after prolonged straining if the sphincter is compromised.
- Multiple symptoms include rectal pressure, pain in association with obstructed defaecation and straining.
- Treatment: medical; pelvic floor physiotherapy; surgery.

The modified Delorme procedure

- Per anal approach to reduce rectocoele and rectal capacity.

Table 29.6 Obstructed defaecation – 'inco-ordination' – combined pelvic organ dysfunction

	Defaecation	Micturition	Sexual disorders	Pain
Symptoms	Bloating/pain Hindgut and colonic inertia	Voiding dyssynergia Overflow incontinence ↑ UTIs	Vaginismus No penetration	Pain during defaecation Pain on sitting (sits on one cheek) Pain unrelieved on lying Burning pain (perianal, perineal) Proctalgia fugax Hindgut pain
Signs	Normal diameter colon Megacolon and/or megarectum over time May lead to DPS over time and mucosal and structural prolapse Fissures	Lax anterior vaginal wall Can cause urethral hypermobility	Destabilization of PFM ↓ PC bulk Hyperaemia – with vestibulitis, vaginismus Overactive urethral, anal, and PR muscles	Overactive PR, ilio/ischiococcygeus – may be unilateral Anal spasm, spasm of lateral levators Result of rectal or coccygeal surgery Local anal trauma (List not exhaustive)

In inco-ordination-type obstructed defaecation ('anismus') neuropathy is not usually a feature. There is little perineal descent and no sphincter release. I = incontinence; UTI = urinary tract infection; DPS = descending perineum syndrome; PFM = pelvic floor muscles; PC = pubococcygeus; PR = puborectalis.

Figure 29.6 Delorme procedure. Rectal muscle is vertically 'ruched', partially or completely around the lower rectum, to improve the function of the anorectal funnel.

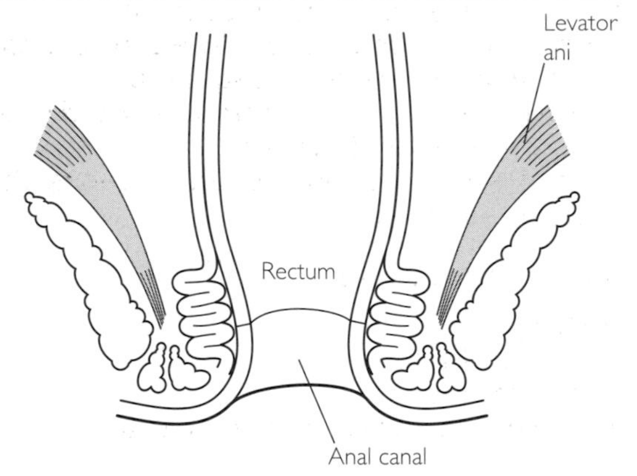

- Affords direct access above the sphincter.
- Anterior or circumferential repair of prolapsed mucosa.
- Allows good support using rectal wall folds as 'doughnut ring pessary'.

Both the distressing symptoms of obstructed defaecation and faecal incontinence and pruritis ani caused by IAS relaxation due to mucosal prolapse are helped by the modified Delorme procedure. However, ring banding may be a simple solution for mild symptoms. Abdominal rectopexy is used for more severe cases when the rectum has pulled away from the sacral mesentery. However, it must be considered with care, as severe constipation may be an unwanted side effect (Janssen and vanDijke, 1994; Kuijpers, 1992; Mumme and Markwell, 1994; vanTets and Kuijpers, 1995).

Pelvic floor rehabilitation and defaecation retraining have been shown clinically to enhance the role of surgery and improve function.

Local anorectal pathology

Local anorectal pathology coexisting with obstructed defaecation includes the solitary rectal ulcer syndrome (SRUS) and proctitis cystica profunda (PCP). These reflect ischaemic and/or inflammatory changes that may result from repeated mechanical trauma to the mucosal wall of the rectum during defaecation. They are mechano-inflammatory rectal conditions.

SOLITARY RECTAL ULCER SYNDROME (SRUS)

Aetiology Most common in the third and fourth decades, SRUS occurs as a result of frequent prolonged straining due to pelvic floor inco-ordination (Snooks et al, 1985c; Van Laarhoven, 1996) or secondary to prolapse or intussusception of the rectal mucosa (Rutter and Riddell, 1975). It predominantly occurs on the anterior rectal wall, but posterior SRUS may occur; rectal valve ulceration and ischaemia are common.

SRUS may present with pain, bleeding and discharge with/without difficult defaecation. Histological changes are identified at biopsy.

Treatment Dietary modification and physiotherapy defaecation retraining is usually successful (Stitz, personal communication). Surgery may be required, e.g. abdominal rectopexy.

PROCTITIS CYSTICA PROFUNDA (PCP)

Aetiology PCP has a similar aetiology to solitary rectal ulcer syndrome (SRUS). Mucosal oedema and erythema of the anterior rectal wall include cysts, polyps, mucosal friability, ulcers and masses.

Treatment Dietary modification, stool bulking agents and defaecation retraining are useful. Surgery may be required for haemorrhage, pain and stenosis (Bentley et al, 1985; Binnie et al, 1992; Kuijpers et al, 1986; Rutter and Riddell, 1975; Snooks et al, 1985c; Womack et al, 1987).

RADIATION PROCTITIS

A distressing complaint associated with both obstructed defaecation and faecal incontinence is radiation proctitis.

- A common primary cause is treatment for cervical, uterine and vaginal cancers in women.
- Relationship of low splanchnic blood flow and radiation injury to lower GIT. Blood flow may be compromised by hypertension, diabetes, hysterectomy.
- Radiation injury to the rectum is reasonably common.
- Damage is usually an ulcer or stricture occurring within five years of therapy.
- There may be decreased rectal compliance altering rectal sensory volumes. If the sphincter is compromised both pathologies may occur.

Anorectal conditions associated with high resting pressures of the IAS often coexist with poor defaecation dynamics. These include anal fissures and haemorrhoids. Both conditions are very common in the community. Table 29.7 gives details of anal fissures.

Table 29.7 Anal fissures

Definition	Split in the anoderm extending externally from the dentate line Usually occurs in the mid-line posteriorly Heals poorly
Symptoms	Acutely painful during defaecation and up to two hours post-defaecation Pain may only *follow* defaecation
Pathogenesis	Stress contributes to hypertonia of the IAS. Increased IAS pressure reduces blood supply to the anoderm and any minor lacerations present heal poorly (Schouten, 1996)
Treatment	Local application of nitroglycerine Lateral internal sphincterotomy Defaecation retraining is complementary

HAEMORRHOIDS

Haemorrhoids cause much misery and symptoms may vary in severity. In women, they often present for the first time during pregnancy or following labour.

Haemorrhoids are displaced anal cushions. Anal cushions help seal the upper anal canal and contribute to continence. During straining or prolonged bearing down the cushions become displaced. As part of this process venous spaces in the cushions distend and congest, as the area is well supplied by arterial blood flow. High pressures of the internal anal sphincter may aggravate this mechanism during repeated straining at stool and prolapse of the cushions may occur outside the anal canal (Hancock, 1993).

Contributing factors include:

- ageing;
- pregnancy;
- chronic diarrhoea;
- obstructed defaecation – imbalance and inco-ordination.

External haemorrhoids may arise from the inferior haemorrhoidal plexus distal to the dentate line. They may swell, thrombose, ulcerate and bleed. Moderate discomfort is common and severe pain indicates thrombosis, prolapse or fissure. Skin tags may follow thrombosis. Itching, burning and soiling are due to mucus discharge.

Internal haemorrhoids are divided into:

- first degree – submucosal vascular tissue above the dentate line; they bleed with defaecation;
- second degree – protrude on defaecation but spontaneously return on cessation of straining;
- third degree – protrude with straining outside the anal verge, may be reduced manually;
- fourth degree – haemorrhoids are irreducibly thrombosed and prolapsed.

Treatment options include:

- injection;
- rubber band ligation;
- haemorrhoidectomy;
- defaecation retraining complements surgery.

Obstructed defaecation requires a multidisciplinary approach to management.

Bowel Dysfunction in the Mature Woman

The changes in bowel function experienced by the older woman are a reflection of life events, particularly past obstetric and surgical history, straining at stool and inappropriate heavy physical activity (O'Neill et al, 1993). These factors will affect the ability of the striated PFM to function adequately.

A common precipitant of altered bowel function is hysterectomy, following which, women reported difficulty with bowel function when compared with controls (Taylor et al, 1990). Smith et al (1990) concluded that disruption of the autonomic innervation of the hindgut resulted in severe constipation in some patients following surgery.

Urinary symptoms were similarly noted. While Smith et al (1990) found their subjects had increased rectal compliance and decreased rectal sensory function, these anorectal changes were not found by MacDonald et al (1993a). Christensen and Schulze-Delrieu (1985) have suggested the autonomic supply may be compromised by mechanical trauma. This may be due to the surgical procedure in radical cases or as a result of haematoma between the tissue planes during healing. MacDonald et al (1993b) proposed that some women post-hysterectomy develop distinct hindgut delay. Prior et al (1992) also reported alterations in bladder and bowel sensitivity. To avoid such complications, subtotal hysterectomy is now regaining favour in some centres (Wood et al, 1992).

Structural abnormalities, commonly presenting as a result of childbirth or previous gynaecological history, ± pelvic floor dysfunction that affects bowel function include rectocoele, enterocoele and sigmoidocoele. Smith (1994) stresses that muscle and fascia are interdependent for pelvic floor integrity. Spence-Jones et al (1994) suggested that uterovaginal prolapse was more common in women who had a prolonged history of straining at stool. They considered this factor to be highly significant in the development of symptoms and urogenital dysfunction.

Rectocoele denotes a herniation of the anterior rectal wall which pushes through the posterior vaginal wall into the vagina. It may provide a sizable and significant barrier to the normal passage of faeces. Yoshioka et al (1991) found that increased pelvic floor descent was the only significant physiological change associated with rectocoele. However, there may be many symptoms, e.g. difficult defaecation, pain, proctitis, faecal soiling and associated urogenital prolapse in the presence of a rectocoele.

Janssen and vanDijke (1994) found that anterior rectal wall repair improved rectal sensation in patients with obstructed defaecation, affected by rectocoele or anterior rectal wall prolapse. Endoanal repair is an alternative to posterior vaginal repair. Where anorectal function is compromised modified 'prolapse' operations, e.g. Delorme can be very helpful. Results have shown that rectal stabilization may also affect bladder function when the pelvic floor and pelvic organs are destabilized in DPS (Mumme and Markwell, 1994). Pruritis ani may also be helped, as the production of mucus perianally is eliminated following repair of the anterior rectal wall.

A sigmoidocoele is an enlarged or redundant segment of colon displaced in the pelvis, affecting the clear passage of contents from the descending colon to rectum (Jorge et al, 1994). This is usually managed surgically, with complementary physiotherapy. However, an enterocoele is a hernia of the small intestine into the pouch of Douglas. Many follow vaginal or abdominal hysterectomy (Holley, 1994; Mellgren et al, 1994). They frequently occur with prolapse of the vaginal vault and general destabilization of the pelvic floor.

Common symptoms are difficult defaecation and low back pain. Rectocoeles may occur due to a weakness in the rectovaginal septum as well as with pelvic floor and fascial weakness. Rectal intussusception (that is, telescoping of the rectal wall) can be associated with rectocoele. Complex pelvic and vaginal surgery is often required.

Thorpe et al (1993) stressed that pelvic floor dysfunction may be the causal factor of both urinary and defaecatory symptoms. In a group of constipated subjects, inappropriate muscle function, e.g. non-relaxing puborectalis during micturition, was associated with rectocoele, obstructed micturition and straining at stool. Some patients had a previous history of failed repair for stress urinary incontinence. These combined symptoms may be seen in milder forms in a number of women.

By far the most common cause of obstructed defaecation in the mature to older woman is the descending perineum syndrome. Other factors are covered in the box.

Summary of bowel dysfunction in the mature woman

- IBS with or without rectal outlet disorder.
- IBS with rectal urgency and faecal soiling (Houghton et al,1995).
- Slow-transit constipation with rectal outlet disorder.
- Gall stones associated with slow-transit constipation (Heaton et al, 1993).
- Obstructed defaecation:
  - (a) DPS with or without prolapse
    anterior rectal wall prolapse
    rectocoele
    intussusception
    enterocoele with associated urogenital prolapse
    sigmoidocoele;
  - (b) dyssynergia 'anismus' often with failed bladder repair;
  - (c) post-surgery, e.g. hysterectomy.
- Faecal incontinence.
- Pain syndromes.
- Combinations of all the above.

Clinical Investigation

When continence and defaecation, the complementary functions of the anorectum, are compromised, integrated medical assessment may be required. Functional evaluation frequently involves specific investigations.

Investigation may include assessment of intestinal motility and function, after eliminating the possibility of structural abnormalities. Tests commonly used are listed below.

Investigation of colorectal dysfunction

Panenteric dysmotility:

- gastric emptying scan;
- small bowel transit:

Colon transit studies:

- radiotracer study
- radio-opaque markers

} These studies can differentiate between colon, hindgut and outlet disorders

Colorectal investigations:

- proctoscopy;
- rigid sigmoidoscopy.

Colon imaging:

- flexible sigmoidoscopy;
- colonoscopy;
- plain X-ray of the abdomen;
- barium enema – megacolon/rectum is determined if the width of the bowel is >6.5 cm at the pelvic brim (Preston et al, 1985).

When bowel dysfunction involves the outlet mechanism, that is, the anus and rectum, anorectal physiology studies are required. These are the most useful tests for clinical management and are outlined in the box. Normal rectal sensation is the most important indicator of present, and predictor of future, function.

Anorectal physiology tests

Sphincter manometry

Anal manometry provides useful information about the sphincters in constipation and incontinence and is useful prior to colorectal and sphincter surgery. Pressure measurements within the anal canal quantify the function of the internal and external anal sphincters.

- IAS is responsible for 85% of the resting pressure and is under autonomic control; it is measured 1–2 cm from the anal verge.
- EAS tone is maintained during the day and is present during sleep. It is responsible for voluntary or squeeze pressure and 15% of resting pressure.

Anal manometry

Resting pressure – lowest limit for continence – is approximately 35 mmHg. Squeeze pressure is usually double the resting pressure. The *transducer system* can provide a continuous pull-through pressure profile of the anal sphincters. These measurements are reproducible and accurate. The length of the sphincters and rectal pressure can also be measured.

Rectoanal inhibitory reflex (RAIR)

This reflex is the relaxation response of the IAS to rectal distension. It is absent in Hirschsprung's disease (paediatric and adult short segment – aganglionosis).

- Distension is produced by inflating a balloon in the rectal ampulla.
- The presence of the RAIR is quantified by the transducer system.

Rectal sensation and compliance

The first awareness of rectal filling occurs at the same distending pressure as that which first elicits the rectoanal inhibitory response.

- This is called the sensory threshold and the norm is 30 ml or less.
- The defaecation threshold is 80–120 ml.
- The maximum tolerable volume is 180–240 ml. Upper limit is 320 ml in women.

Blunted rectal sensation may accompany pelvi/perineal neuropathy.

While anorectal physiology studies provide quantified parameters, videodefaecography gives an accurate picture of the evacuation process and its deficiencies (Fig. 29.5).

It is useful in determining anorectal outlet obstruction and may show the following.

- Perineal descent, which is defined as a greater than 2 cm drop in the anorectal junction below the pubococcygeal line, during attempted defaecation.
- Rectal intussusception / instability.
- Dysfunctional rectocoele.
- Megarectum.
- Rectal motility.
- Pelvic floor inco-ordination or imbalance.

When the specific action of striated muscle needs to be determined, a form of electromyography (EMG) is the appropriate modality.

Percutaneous insertion of a concentric needle EMG electrode into the external anal sphincter or puborectalis enables the electrical activity of these muscles to be monitored at rest, on contraction, during coughing and straining. It is useful in determining:

- neuropathic faecal incontinence;
- external anal sphincter defects;
- 'mapping' prior to sphincter surgery, e.g. external anal sphincter repair;
- non-relaxing puborectalis on attempted defaecation. This is also referred to as 'anismus' or dyssynergia.

Much of the research literature involves other investigation procedures. These are not generally used in clinical practice and are outlined in the box. However, many consider pudendal nerve terminal motor latency (PNTML) an important test in determining neuropathy following childbirth.

Investigations with limited clinical use

Nerve conduction studies

Pudendal nerve terminal motor latency (PNTML)

Strength – duration test of EAS

Transcutaneous spinal stimulation

Sacral evoked response

Mucosal sensitivity

Manometry

Balloon expulsion

Saline continence

Ambulatory monitoring

Faecoflowmetry

Imaging

Multiple monitoring:

- colpocystodefaecography (Hock et al, 1993)
- cinedefaecography and electromyography (Jorge et al, 1992)
- defaecography and peritoneography (Bremmer et al, 1995)

Magnetic resonance imaging

Electromyography

Concentric needle

Single fibre

While the physiotherapist will see a number of patients with mild problems, those with ongoing and more complex pathology will often require some of the investigations described above. It is suggested that the reader refer to the following references for a fuller understanding: Bartolo et al (1985); Bartram et al (1988); Farouk and Bartolo (1993); Papachrysostomou et al (1992, 1993); Preston et al (1985).

Faecal Incontinence

The prevalence of faecal incontinence (FI) is difficult to assess accurately. In the past patients disclosed the information to medical personnel with great reluctance. Kamm (1994) considers that loss of gas or faeces can affect up to 11% of adults, with 2% frequently troubled. However, a recent survey of 1000 men and women showed that 20% of Australian males complained of faecal incontinence. Lubowski, as quoted in Margo (1996), suggested that blunted rectal sensation in association with raised intra-abdominal pressure (IAP) caused anal seepage.

Common causes of faecal incontinence are listed in Table 29.8. Pudendal neuropathy is one of the most common aetiological factors in female faecal incontinence (Roig et al, 1995; Snooks et al, 1985b, 1990; Womack et al, 1986). Haphazard denervation and reinnervation of the levator ani and sphincter muscles may also result from frequent or prolonged straining at stool (Snooks et al, 1985a).

Obstetric trauma is a gender-selective causative factor of faecal incontinence. Forceps delivery is associated with a high incidence of incomplete sphincter tears (Sultan et al, 1993). Wynne et al (1996) found that the first vaginal delivery causes a permanent lowering of anal resting pressures. In the middle years in females, faecal incontinence may occur for the first time. This is caused by the cumulative effects of the climacteric, neuropathy and muscle loss when the damaged sphincters can no longer compensate (Bartram and Sultan, 1995).

The physiology, pathogenesis and symptomatology of the common aetiological factors of faecal incontinence are included in Table 29.9. A basic understanding of the mechanisms of faecal incontinence must include the following topics.

- Rectal pressure must *exceed* anal pressure for faecal incontinence to occur. This is common with brisk rises in intra-abdominal pressure with compromised EAS activity or a prolonged reflex response to coughing (Duthie et al, 1993; Margo, 1996; Meagher et al, 1993).
- *Passive faecal incontinence* (anal loss without knowledge) is related to IAS dysfunction.
- *Urge faecal incontinence* (anal loss with awareness) is related to EAS dysfunction (Engel et al, 1995)

For clinical diagnosis, investigation is **mandatory**. This may include the following **integrated investigations**:

- Anorectal physiology
- Endoanal ultrasound
- EMG sphincter mapping
- Video defaecography
- ± Colon transit studies
- PNTML

Mucosal sensitivity tests are not used routinely.

ANAL SONOGRAPHY

This recent test uses high-frequency transducers to provide an image of the sphincter layers. This is based on the acoustic reflections from the tissue interfaces which have different impedance (Bartram and Sultan, 1995). Much has been said about the relative thickness of the IAS and EAS (Gantke et al, 1993; Papachrysostomou and Smith, 1994). Bartram and Sultan (1995) consider the IAS to be a hypoechoic ring 1–3 mm in thickness. Connective tissue replaces smooth muscle with increasing age. Anatomical gender differences in the EAS makes imaging more difficult in females. The results of surgical and obstetric trauma can be demonstrated with anal ultrasound.

Management

Faecal incontinence predominantly due to IAS dysfunction is managed by dietary modification, bulking agents, defaecation retraining and levator muscle rehabilitation. The use of antidiarrhoeal medication may be most helpful, with its effect on IAS resting pressure. With poor EAS recruitment and levator ani destabilization due to neuropathy, intensive physiotherapy, again directed to the supporting muscles, is indicated (Bannister et al, 1989). Hormone replacement has a complementary therapeutic role.

Surgery may be indicated. The overflow incontinence of the aged is best treated by agents to keep the rectum empty, defaecation retraining, behaviour modification and mobility aids. Biofeedback may be used alone, with conservative medical management, after surgery or to complement combined management. Physiotherapy and biofeedback have a complementary role in both increasing levator support and modifying sphincter function.

SURGICAL MANAGEMENT OF FAECAL INCONTINENCE

Surgery may be required to correct an underlying anal defect. Trauma to the anal canal without neuropathy is most effectively managed. Sangwan et al (1996) showed that even unilateral pudendal neuropathy compromised the results of sphincter repair. When faecal incontinence is associated with destabilization of the pelvic floor and descent of the perineum, it is often connected with anterior rectal wall prolapse. This may effectively keep the anus partially relaxed, with resultant mucus seepage. Surgical management of the prolapse is useful. This may also be undertaken with sphincter surgery, the two having a combined effect of increasing the functional sphincter length (Mumme, personal communication).

Procedures *Primary repair* of the EAS is usually undertaken by obstetricians after vaginal delivery. In *sphincteroplasty*, the anal sphincter is laid open and the ends approximated and overlapped. The wound is usually left to heal without skin sutures. *Anterior rectal wall repair* with sphincteroplasty increases effective sphincter length. So does rectopexy in selected cases (Hiltunen and Matikainen, 1992).

The most common *sphincter encirclement* with muscle stimulation (dynamic anal myoplasty) is the graciloplasty. By programmed muscle stimulation, the gracilis becomes fatigue resistant with an increase in the percentage of type I fibres (Konsten et al, 1993). This surgery may be complicated by infection, short or long term, at the electrodes or in either wound site. Complicating local factors associated with anal repair include voiding difficulties and delayed healing due to infection.

Colostomy may be a last resort.

Physiotherapy complements all forms of reparative sphincter

Table 29.8 Aetiology of faecal incontinence

Trauma	*Congenital* – fistula, atresia, spinal lesions
Accidental – direct, spinal	
Surgical – haemorrhoidectomy	*Disease* – tumour, infection
anal dilation	
lateral sphincterotomy	*Incomplete emptying*
fistula	Overflow
Obstetric – complete / incomplete tears	Obstructed defaecation
Neuropathic	*Mechanical*
Obstetric	Anterior rectal wall prolapse
Straining	Rectal prolapse
Heavy lifting	Haemorrhoids
Impaired sensation	Solitary rectal ulcer
Urge incontinence (EAS)	
Passive incontinence (IAS)	*Motility*
Exaggerated RAIR response	Hypersensitivity – low compliance
IAS dysfunction	proctitis
Spinal stenosis	ulcerative colitis
Autonomic neuropathy (diabetes)	Giant rectal waves
Neurological disease (multiple sclerosis)	Irritable bowel syndrome
	Colorectal surgery
	(any combination of above)

Table 29.9 Pathogenesis and symptomatology of common aetiological factors of faecal incontinence

	Pathogenesis	Effect on muscles	Other effects on mechanism of continence	Symptoms
Obstetric trauma Pudendal nerve traction/compression neuropathy	Vaginal deliveries Long pushing stage Forceps delivery Large babies Cumulative damage **Straining at stool**	Haphazard denervation and reinnervation of levator ani and EAS →**DPS** IAS (autonomic damage) Denervated puborectalis → obtuse anorectal angle	RAIR activated by anterior rectal wall mucosal prolapse, associated with DPS **Rectal sensory blunting** Incomplete rectal emptying Prolonged RAIR with coughing ↑ IAP activities → **Faecal soiling**	**Faecal incontinence without patient's awareness** is due to IAS weakness Post-defaecatory soiling **Faecal loss with patient's awareness** is due to EAS weakness Rectal urgency and loss
Obstetric muscle tears Prevalence: 0.5–2% have 3rd degree tears (Kamm, 1994)	Primipara Occipitoposterior presentation May be combined with pudendal nerve neuropathy • Forceps • Large babies	Complete and incomplete tears of IAS/EAS (3rd degree) Perineal body damage Residual defects after primary repair	Levator neuropathy may be associated (see above)	Mild, moderate, severe faecal incontinence immediately post-partum Persistent symptoms Urge or passive faecal incontinence
Normal process of ageing	Changes at the climacteric (40–60 yrs) i.e. ↓ hormonal activity Symptom emergence due to decompensation of continence mechanism associated with life events or ageing *Motility changes* • Rectosigmoid motility • IBS } EAS hypo- • Diarrhoea } sensitivity in females	Obstructed defaecation • imbalance DPS • inco-ordination Neuropathy of ageing ↓ IAS pressure (resting pressure) ↓ EAS (squeeze pressure) ↓ Perianal, anal, rectal sensation ↓ Anal sampling ↓ EAS response to rectal distension	↓ Effect of oestrogen on anal mucosa? Ability of anal cushions to expand for closure, affected by lack of oestrogen?	Passive, urge, overflow faecal incontinence Post-defaecatory soiling Soiling with impact, effort

Bannister et al (1989); Barrett et al (1989); Duthie et al (1993); Gee and Durdey (1995); Houghton et al (1993); Kamm (1994); Laurberg and Swash (1989); Snooks et al (1985b, 1990); Sultan et al (1993); Meagher et al (1993); Womack et al (1986); Lubowski et al (1987).

Bold text indicates the most important factors.

surgery. Surrounding levator rehabilitation and specific defaecation retraining assist functional recovery at all levels of intervention.

Complicating factors in faecal incontinence in females include:

- increased colorectal motility (giant waves);
- irritable bowel syndrome is more common in women leading to heightened rectal sensitivity after diarrhoea and a decrease in defaecation threshold volume;
- non-compliant rectum or small colorectal reservoir or pouch;
- effect of decreased oestrogen on smooth muscle and anal mucosa(?);
- neuropathic FI induced by prolonged straining in obstructed defaecation(?);
- neuropathic FI induced by recurrent diarrhoea and straining to finish(?);
- anal gaping, caused by prolapsed rectal mucosa, may result in perianal irritation.

Biofeedback in Defaecation Disorders

'Biofeedback is a learning strategy derived from psychological learning theory' (Enck, 1993). It is based on Skinnerian operant conditioning, in which a correct response to a given stimulus is obtained after successive trials. The correct response is demonstrated via visual ± auditory feedback. Arhan et al (1994) considered that an adequate response is itself a recompense and a reinforcement factor. The first biofeedback paper for functional defaecation disorders was published in 1974.

Biofeedback to induce relaxation during psychotherapy was shown to help irritable bowel syndrome (IBS) patients symptomatically (Whitehead, 1985). Engel et al (1974) used a three-balloon system, as used in manometric testing, with visual feedback of rectoanal inhibitory responses, in the treatment of faecal incontinence. As the rectal volumes were decreased, progressively brisker IAS relaxation and EAS contractions occurred. This information was fed to the patient by visual biofeedback. Early use of transcutaneous EMG to measure EAS responses followed. Surface electrode EMG has become the most common form of biofeedback in the treatment of rectal outlet obstruction to measure EAS release. Until recently 'constipation' biofeedback was confined to the treatment of pelvic floor/ organ dyssynergia. Koutsomanis et al (1993, 1994) used biofeedback with patients suffering from slow-transit constipation. Park et al (1996) appear to have used biofeedback with two different forms of obstructed defaecation.

Aspects of biofeedback include the following:

- Physiological responses are measured and fed back, to alter muscle action.
- Objective measurements of rectal sensation and muscle activity are usually reported.
- Biofeedback only affects existing responses.
- Biofeedback adheres to a protocol.
- Long-term follow-up is necessary in evaluating the success of treatment.
- Cost may be considerable.

Faecal incontinence (FI)

Of interest historically or methodologically in the treatment of FI is the work of MacLeod (1987), Loening-Baucke (1990) and Miner et al (1990). Chiarioni et al (1993) considered the principles of muscle physiology to enhance the EAS endurance response. Arhan et al (1994) were the first to note that biofeedback could be developed as an educational tool. Sangwan et al (1995) concluded that following biofeedback, improvement in FI may be independent of anal resting and squeeze pressures. Improvement in rectal sensation appears to be the most commonly reported change.

Enck (1993) considered that the overall success of biofeedback used in 13 studies published up to 1993 was 79.8%.

Related pelvic floor dysfunction

Biofeedback in the treatment of anal pain was not shown to be successful (Grimaud et al, 1991). Paediatric use of biofeedback has centred on encopresis and faecal incontinence, often associated with congenital anal abnormalities.

Vaginal EMG biofeedback has been used as an adjunct in the treatment of the vulvar vestibulitis syndrome (Glazer et al, 1995). However, internal vaginal biofeedback may exacerbate vestibular or pudendal nerve pain. In physiotherapy, weight, pressure or EMG biofeedback is used commonly for pelvic floor muscle rehabilitation.

In patients with early or late stage dyssynergia, vaginal feedback may not be tolerated. Surface anal biofeedback for anismus is usually quite acceptable. In associated urogenital dysfunction, vaginal biofeedback may be unacceptable, as there is often a history of past sexual violation or abuse, which is a common aetiological factor in this condition.

Anorectal outlet obstruction

Biofeedback has been used widely on the EAS for anorectal outlet disorders since 1987, when the work of Bleijenberg and Kuipers and Weber et al was published. Females constitute the greatest proportion of subjects in most studies. The diagnosis of pelvic floor dyssynergia or anismus has included the use of manometry, EMG, defaecography and colon transit studies.

Feedback systems have generally used EMG surface electrodes (Bleijenberg and Kuipers, 1987; Kawimbe et al, 1991; Koutsomanis et al, 1993, 1994, 1995; Papachrysostomou and Smith, 1994; Park et al, 1996; Wexner et al, 1992). Ho et al (1996) used anal pressure biofeedback.

Table 29.10 outlines features common to most biofeedback

Table 29.10 Aspects of biofeedback

Faecal incontinence	Constipation
Setting and equipment	
• Home or clinic based • Manometric measurements, double/triple balloon systems, intra-anal electrodes • EMG (most common)	• Inpatient, home or clinic based • Manometric measurements, balloon expulsion, intra-anal electrodes • EMG (most common)
Patient criteria	
• All ages, sexes • Well motivated, no cognitive impairment • Neuropathic FI; encopresis, congenital disorders; post-surgery • Primary/secondary intervention	• Predominantly female • Anismus • Primary intervention
Modalities	
• Sensory training • Motor response training (EAS) • Co-ordination training (IAS and EAS) • All of the above	• Release of PR/EAS, modification of an existing response • Elicit a defaecation reflex? • Co-ordinated muscle instruction (Koutsomanis et al, 1995)
Outcomes	Outcomes diary to record:
• Improvement in rectal sensation most common • EAS activity ↑ but not always • IAS resting level little or no change • Dietary/medical management to alter bowel habits largely forgotten • Results similar to medical management alone or to well-structured behaviour modification • Multifactorial	• Effective straining • Frequency of bowel motions • ↓ laxative use • Other subjective symptomatic improvement • Placebo response from motivated therapist can't be ignored

studies. The studies varied as to whether conventional medical management, such as dietary and behaviour modification (e.g. timed emptying), had been used prior to biofeedback. In determining the success of biofeedback, a motivated therapist may have an immeasurable placebo effect.

The inter-relationship between rectus abdominus and puborectalis (PR) and the external anal sphincter (EAS) function has limited scientific support, although there is currently research activity to identify function. It has been hypothesized (Chiarelli and Markwell, 1992; Markwell and Mumme, 1991; Markwell and Sapsford, 1995b; Sapsford et al, 1996) that contraction of rectus abdominis in its inner range will be associated with a contraction of PR and EAS. Such a situation is desirable to maintain continence, but to allow relaxation of PR and EAS for expulsion of rectal contents, it is hypothesized that the rectus abdominis must be isometrically contracted in an outer range position. If such a synergistic muscle action is trained, it is believed that efficiency of evacuation will increase and the need to strain (and inherent problems associated with straining at stool) will decrease. Such a hypothesis has been trialed clinically over the past eight years (O'Neill et al, 1993) and is considered an integral component of treatment.

Three papers are of further interest. Koutsomanis et al (1994) differentiated between the two types of patients they treated: those who were ineffective strainers and those with pelvic floor dyssynergia. Papachrysostomou and Smith (1994) argue that biofeedback may influence the defaecation reflex, so that an improved conscious control of bowel function may follow. Koutsomanis et al (1995) reported on a controlled, randomized trial of standard biofeedback versus muscle training without a visual display, for intractable constipation. The results of this study suggest that focusing on retraining the co-ordination of rectus abdominis and puborectalis has beneficial effects on evacuation.

Park et al (1996) divided their patient cohort into two distinct types. Type A had a flattened anorectal angle, without a defined puborectalis indentation, but a closed anal canal. Type B patients had a clear puborectalis indentation, narrow anorectal angle and closed anal canal. Their success rate using biofeedback was 25% for type A and 86% for type B patients.

Physiological findings of type A patients showed greater perineal descent at rest and on straining and a higher incidence of significant rectocoele and intussusception than type B patients. These findings are suggestive of the lack of pubococcygeal and possibly lateral levator support seen in many patients with obstructed defaecation and commonly treated by physiotherapists. Functional outlet release is not usually achieved without combining levator support of the rectum with an isometric outer range contraction of rectus abdominis to release PR and EAS.

Enck (1993) traced the origins of biofeedback in defaecation disorders and differentiated its use clinically from that used in physical medicine. Traditional biofeedback must give way to specific combined abdominolevator muscle re-education which physiotherapy can provide. Optimally, physiotherapy should complement biofeedback. In considering the work of Koutsomanis et al (1995), Markwell and Mumme (1991), Markwell and Sapsford (1995b), Markwell et al (1993) and Sapsford et al (1996), we see the answer to the question 'Why physiotherapy?'.

The Role of Physiotherapy?

The striated musculature of the pelvic floor and the specific defaecation problems that arise are within the domain of physiotherapy management and rehabilitation. Deficits in afferent sensation and motor nerve conduction are treatable and preventable.

Physiotherapists are the ideal team members to undertake specific defaecation retraining and muscle rehabilitation. Pelvic floor muscle dysfunction is a unique situation. Anal sensation and pudendal nerve motor function may be affected by straining at stool. This may occur as a result of compression, ischaemia, fibrosis, stretch injury and the process of ageing, superimposed on the pathology of past straining (Engel and Kamm, 1994; Vaccaro et al, 1995).

Physiotherapists have the necessary skills in rehabilitation to enhance the function of reinnervated muscle. By muscle assessment and knowledge of integrated abdominopelvic floor patterns, aberrant muscle function may be isolated and specific muscle strengthened. Patterns may be learnt and introduced for specific function. Global factors, e.g. painful back problems, tight fascia, poor pelvic stabilization and posture correction, all fall into the physiotherapist's domain and all affect defaecation patterning. A recent study has shown that slumped sitting and rectus abdominis shortening, as a preferred posture and action on the toilet, correlated with the prevalence of dysfunctional defaecation. In that female population 15.9% strained at stool and 89.9% of the women who knew they did not strain were assessed to be correct. In contrast only 52.9% accurately reported that they strained. Questioning patients about straining is not sufficient in itself. Observation of posture and abdominal muscle palpation may be used as a clinical tool to determine those who actually strain at defaecation (Markwell et al, 1995).

The long-term effects of straining at stool are pelvi / perineal traction neuropathy with afferent disturbance and poor proprioception leading to levator ani and sphincter atrophy, dyskinesia, excretory organ sensory blunting and different forms of dysfunction, including pain.

Somatovisceral function with integrated smooth and striated muscle function is more effectively enhanced by physiotherapists because they deal with musculo-skeletal disorders than those using operant learning theory or treatment based on set protocols. Early intervention and education by physiotherapists may alter the natural progression of bowel dysfunction suffered by so many women.

Pain Syndromes

Pelvi / perineal and perianal pain is a frequent component of pelvic floor and pelvic organ dysfunction. Somatovisceral and viscerosomatic manifestations of pain are common.

Disabling pain may occur in the absence of inflammation, infection, trauma or malignancy. Pudendal neuralgia and the permutations within the areas innervated by the pelvic, pudendal and perineal nerves pose a multidisciplinary diagnostic and therapeutic challenge. Postural, traumatic and psychosexual factors may all be associated with these pain syndromes.

Chronic rectal, perianal and perineal pain may radiate widely from above the pubis to the labia, urethra, vagina, perineum and anterior and posterior thighs, calves and toes. Pain may peak in the fourth, fifth and sixth decades.

Visceral or orthopaedic surgery commonly precedes pain or is offered as a form of treatment (e.g. coccygectomy, hysterectomy and vaginal repair).

Colorectal investigation and classification of pelvi / pudendal pain syndromes with functional disorders of defaecation have been well developed (Wexner and Jorge, 1994). This author considers there are three 'non-organic' pain syndromes with a fourth, vulvar vestibulitis, displaying an inflammatory component. Long-term pelvic floor dyssynergia may predispose the patient to sympathetically maintained pain. A fifth syndrome, coccydynia, has an aetiology of trauma (see box).

Perianal and perineal pain syndromes

1. Proctalgia fugax
2. Pudendal nerve entrapment neuropathy
   - descending perineum syndrome
   - levator syndrome
3. Pelvic floor / pelvic organ dyssynergia
4. Sympathetically maintained pain:
   - vestibulitis
   - vulvodynia
5. Coccydynia; piriformis pain syndrome

Aetiology, characteristics and management of the different types of pain are covered in Table 29.11.

Dyspareunia is associated with sympathetically maintained pain and pelvic floor dyssynergia.

Two recent papers (Brasch et al, 1995; Infantino et al, 1994) have reported damage to the femoral nerve with resultant changes in sensation and pain, following hysterectomy, rectopexy and other abdominal surgery. Neuropathy is thought to be due to retractor pressure during surgery and is self-limiting. However, the onset and pain distribution may complicate pain diagnosis in these patients.

Gastroenterologists and gynaecologists often see pelvic pain attributable to the irritable bowel syndrome (IBS), while pelvic congestion may overlap with some symptoms associated with the descending perineum syndrome (DPS). IBS is often associated with difficult rectal evacuation and faecal incontinence. It is largely helped by relaxation techniques and a trial of antidepressant medication which has anticholinergic effects. Visceral pain perception is often altered. Increased venous pressure in compromised pelvic veins, while in the erect position, is due to gravity. Congestion pain is increased on bending forwards but, as with DPS pain, it may be relieved by lying down. Physiotherapeutic intervention is not indicated in these cases. Endometriotic tissue can also deposit in the rectovaginal septum and cause pain on defaecation.

Table 29.11 Aetiology, characteristics and management of different types of pain

Pain syndrome	Aetiology	Characteristics of pain	Physiotherapy	Other
Nerve entrapment compression/traction • Descending perineum syndrome (gravity related)	Pelvi/pudendal traction neuropathy Multiparous females Male symptoms related to heavy lifting, straining at stool, martial arts, selective overdevelopment of abdominal muscles	Nerve trunk pain (toothache, dragging) May have burning perineal pain Pain on palpation over pudendal nerve per vaginam Made worse by defaecation, straining at stool, prolonged standing, heavy lifting Relieved by lying down	**Muscle rehabilitation particularly pubococcygeus** Defaecation retraining Pain strategies • Lying down after defaecation • Restrict heavy lifting, impact activities	Colorectal management of associated structural defects Pain management
• Levator syndrome (positional pain)	Females, predominantly 4th, 5th, 6th decades Associated with past pelvi/perineal surgery (inhibition pain) Compression of an already irritated pudendal nerve • post-partum • non-relaxing pelvic floor	Often unilateral (left) May radiate widely Made worse by: sitting, defaecation, coitus, stress Pressure, discomfort, burning (paraesthesiae) Hypertonicity of puborectalis (pubococcygeus), ilio/ischiococcygeus, EAS Tenderness over muscle attachments to coccyx	Reverse muscle imbalance by musculotendinous stretches; specific muscle rehabilitation Rectal massage Use of heat to reduce resting anal pressure NMS to induce fatigue of hypertonic muscles? To improve P/C support **Defaecation retraining**	Pain management: • Medication • Pain blocks? • Sacral stimulation Nerve decompression?
Sympathetically maintained pain • Vulvar vestibulitis syndrome	Minor tissue injury, e.g. Pap smear, coitus, may result in prostaglandin sensitization of the nociceptive fibres 'Cross talk' between afferent nociceptive and efferent sympathetic nerves → self-sustaining pain loop Pain becomes autonomous	Affects reproductive age group Severe pain on vestibular touch or attempted vaginal entry Vestibular erythema May be associated with urethral symptoms	Maximize symptom relief Optimize positions for coitus **Destabilization of PF** Muscle rehabilitation (pubococcygeus) Defaecation retraining ↓ resting tone of lateral and sphincter muscles Pain strategies Electromyographic biofeedback?	Multidisciplinary approach Behavioural medicine to modify setting for pain-provoking behaviour Avoid triggers, e.g. infections, irritants, laser Medical management Vestibulectomy Perineoplasty
• Vulvodynia	Made worse by lying down	Increased resting tone of superficial PF and lateral levator plane		
Dyssynergic pain	Predominantly females Dissociation of PF function Non-relaxing pelvic floor Associated with sexual violation or abuse	Pain in PR or EAS or both Pain on voiding Pain on defaecation 'anismus' Dyspareunia – 'vaginismus'	Maximize the support afforded by PC **Defaecation and voiding retraining** Optimize coital positions and coital muscle action	Psycho and/or sex therapy

Proctalgia fugax	Distension or hypermotility of rectosigmoid colon → IAS hypertonia with superimposed activity of striated EAS and PR Increase in slow waves of IAS	Affects 8–14% of the population Fleeting severe pain Mid-line anorectal pain Non-radiating May last 3–4 minutes May accompany colorectal surgery	**Defaecation retraining / positioning** Contract / relax techniques to relax EAS / PR	Common complaint seen at all levels of intervention
Coccydynia	Females predominate Follows history of trauma or childbirth; trauma to sacrococcygeal joint Degenerative component Musculotendinous attachments may be disrupted at the anococcygeal raphe May be associated with any of the above syndromes	Pain on internal / external mobilization of the coccyx Pain on rising from a chair Sometimes associated with levator spasm	**Orthopaedic physiotherapy regimen**	Mobilization under anaesthesia Coccygectomy may further disrupt musculotendinous support
Orthopaedic conditions (piriformis syndrome)	Idiopathic Affects both sexes	Pain on and just after sitting Difficulty in climbing stairs / incline Dyspareunia	**Stretches** Exercise therapy, resisted abduction, resisted external rotation	

From Basson (1995), Broadhurst (1990), Devroede (1996b), Eckardt et al (1996), Glazer et al (1995), Kennedy (1995), Markwell and Mumme (1995).

It is suggested that the reader refer to the physiotherapy management in '*Moving in on Pain*' (Markwell and Mumme, 1995). Complicated feedback loops and control mechanisms are factors to consider in physiotherapy management to break the pain cycle.

Caution

If there is no obvious physical cause for exacerbation of pain during the course of physiotherapy treatment, refer the patient to her medical adviser to exclude other pathology, e.g. fungal, viral, infective or dysplasic changes.

Effective management depends on thorough clinical evaluation at each level of intervention. A multidisciplinary approach to diagnosis and treatment of patients allows a greater understanding of the underlying pathology and the classification and control of pain. There may be overlap between pain syndromes. Physiological elasticity and strength of the pelvic floor and visceral tissues in balanced interplay produce healthy co-ordination. Loss of co-ordinated urinary and rectal function accompany, to a great or lesser extent, the five pain syndromes listed.

Patients are encouraged to play an active part in their pain management and learn strategies to self-correct function, thereby controlling their pain independently. Education in the causative factors of pain exacerbation is essential.

References

Agachan F, Chen T, Pfeifer J et al (1996) A constipation scoring system to simplify evaluation and management of constipated patients. *Diseases of Colon and Rectum* **39**: 681–685.

Allen-Mersch TG, Henry MM and Nicholls RJ (1987) Natural history of anterior mucosal prolapse. *British Journal of Surgery* **74**: 679–682.

Arhan P, Faverdin C, Devroede G et al (1994) Biofeedback re-education of faecal continence in children. *International Journal of Colorectal Disease* **9**: 128–133.

Bannister JJ, Laurence WT, Smith A et al (1988) Urological abnormalities in young women with severe constipation. *Gut* **29**: 17–20.

Bannister JJ, Read NW, Donnelly TC and Sun WM (1989) External and internal anal sphincter responses to rectal distension in normal subjects and in patients with idiopathic faecal incontinence. *British Journal of Surgery* **76**: 617–621.

Barrett JA, Brocklehurst JC, Kiff ES et al (1989) Anal function in geriatric patients with faecal incontinence. *Gut* **30**: 1244–1251.

Bartolo DCC, Read NW, Jarratt JA et al (1983) Differences in anal sphincter function and clinical presentation in patients with pelvic floor descent. *Gastroenterology* **85**: 68–75.

Bartolo DCC, Roe Am, Virjee J and Mortensen NJMcC (1985) Evacuation proctography in obstructed defaecation and rectal intussusception. *British Journal of Surgery* 72 (Suppl): S111-S115.

Bartolo DCC, Devroede G, Kamm MA et al (1992) Symposium on constipation. *International Journal of Colorectal Disease* **7**: 47–67.

Bartram CI and Sultan AH (1995) Anal endosonography in faecal incontinence. *Gut* **37**: 4–6.

Bartram CI, Turnbull GK and Lennard-Jones JE (1988) Evacuation proctography: an investigation of rectal expulsion in 20 subjects without defecatory disturbance. *Gastrointestinal Radiology* **13**: 72–80.

Basson R (1995) Pathophysiology of lifelong vaginismus. *Canadian Journal of Human Sexuality* **4**: 183–189.

Bassotti G, Germani U and Morelli A (1995) Human colonic motility: physiological aspects. *International Journal of Colorectal Disease* **10**: 173–180.

Bennett EJ, Evans PR, Badcock CA et al (1996) Psychosocial and gender features of impaired gut transit in functional gastrointestinal disorders. *Journal of Gastroenterology and Hepatology* **11**(Suppl): A116.

Bentley E, Chandrasoma P, Cohen H et al (1985) Colitis cystica profunda: presenting with complete intestinal obstruction and recurrence. *Gastroenterology* **89**: 1157–1161.

Berman IR, Harris MS and Rabeler MB (1990) Delorme's transrectal excision of internal rectal prolapse. *Diseases of Colon and Rectum* **33**: 573–580.

Binnie NR, Papachrysostomou M, Clare N and Smith AN (1992) Solitary rectal ulcer: the place of biofeedback and surgery in the treatment of the syndrome. *World Journal of Surgery* **16**: 836–840.

Bleijenberg G and Kuijpers HC (1987) Treatment of spastic pelvic floor syndrome with biofeedback. *Diseases of Colon and Rectum* **30**: 108–111.

Brasch BC, Bufo AJ, Kreienberg PF and Johnson GP (1995) Femoral neuropathy secondary to the use of a self-retaining retractor. Report of three cases and review of the literature. *Diseases of Colon and Rectum* **38**: 1115–1118.

Bremmer S, Ahlback S, Uden R and Mellgren A (1995) Simultaneous defaecography and peritoneography in defaecation disorders. *Diseases of Colon and Rectum* **38**: 969–973.

Broadhurst N (1990) Piriformis syndrome and buttock pain. *Australian Family Physician* **19**: 1754.

Chiarelli P and Markwell S (1992) *Let's Get Things Moving*. Sydney: Gore and Osment.

Chiarioni G, Scattolini C, Bonfante F and Vantini I (1993) Liquid stool incontinence with severe urgency: anorectal function and effective biofeedback treatment. *Gut* **34**: 1576–1580.

Christensen J (1994) The motility of the colon. In: Johnson LR (ed) *Physiology of the Gastrointestinal Tract*, p. 991. New York: Raven Press.

Christensen J and Schulze-Delrieu K (1985) Nerves in the colon: discovery and rediscovery. *Gastroenterology* **89**: 222–223.

Devroede G (1996a) Psychophysiological approach of chronic idiopathic constipation. *Proceedings of a Conference on Controversies in Colon and Rectal Surgery*, Nijmegen.

Devroede G (1996b) Front and rear. *Proceedings of a Conference on Controversies in Colon and Rectal Surgery*, Nijmegen.

Drossman DA, Sandler RS, McKee DC and Lovitz AJ (1982) Bowel patterns among subjects not seeking health care. *Gastroenterology* **83**: 529–534.

Duthie GS, Miller R and Bartolo DCC (1993) Prolonged uncompensated rectoanal inhibition is responsible for stress faecal incontinence. *Proceedings of the British Society of Gastroenterology* **34**: S48.

Eckardt VF, Dodt O, Kanzler G and Bernhard G (1996) Anorectal function and morphology in patients with sporadic proctalgia fugax. *Diseases of Colon and Rectum* **39**: 755–762.

Enck P (1993) Biofeedback training in disordered defaecation. *Digestive Diseases and Sciences* **38**: 1953–1960.

Engel AF and Kamm MA (1994) The acute effect of straining on pelvic floor neurological function. *International Journal of Colorectal Disease* **9**: 8–12.

Engel AF, Nikoomansh P and Schuster MM (1974) Operant conditioning of rectosphincteric response in the treatment of faecal incontinence. *New England Journal of Medicine* **290**: 646–649.

Engel AF, Kamm MA, Bartram CI and Nicholls RJ (1995) Relationship of symptoms in faecal incontinence to specific sphincter abnormalities. *International Journal of Colorectal Disease* **10**: 152–155.

Farouk R and Bartolo DCC (1993) The clinical contribution of integrated laboratory and ambulatory anorectal physiology assessment in faecal incontinence. *International Journal of Colorectal Disease* **8**: 60–65.

Fowler CJ, Christmas TJ, Chapple RC et al (1988) Abnormal electromyographic activity of the urethral sphincter, voiding dysfunction and polycystic ovaries: a new syndrome. *British Medical Journal* **297**: 1436–1438.

Gantke B, Schafer A, Enck P and Lubke HJ (1993) Sonographic, manometric, and myographic evaluation of the anal sphincters morphology and function. *Diseases of Colon and Rectum* **36**: 1037–1041.

Gee AS and Durdey P (1995) Urge incontinence of faeces is a marker of severe external anal sphincter dysfunction. *British Journal of Surgery* **82**: 1179–1182.

Glazer HI, Rodke G, Swencionis C et al (1995) Treatment of vulvar vestibulitis syndrome with electromyographic biofeedback of pelvic floor musculature. *Journal of Reproductive Medicine* **40**: 283–290.

Grimaud JC, Bouvier M, Naudy B et al (1991) Manometric and radiologic investigations and biofeedback treatment of chronic idiopathic anal pain. *Diseases of Colon and Rectum* **34**: 690–695.

Hancock BD (1993) Haemorrhoids. In: Jones DJ and Irving MH (eds) *ABC of Colorectal Diseases*, pp. 23–25. London: BMJ Publishing.

Harris MS (1994) Evaluation and treatment of constipation. *Participate* **3**: 1–3.

Heaton KW, Emmett PM, Symes CL and Bradden FEM (1993) An explanation for gall stones in normal-weight women: slow intestinal transit. *Lancet* **341**: 8–10.

Henry MM, Parks AG and Swash M (1982) The pelvic floor musculature in the descending perineum syndrome. *British Journal of Surgery* **69**: 470–472.

Heyman MS (1996) MMPI testing in patients undergoing biofeedback. *Proceedings of a Conference on Controversies in Colon and Rectal Surgery*, Nijmegen.

Hiltunen D-M and Matikainen M (1992) Improvement of continence after abdominal rectopexy for rectal prolapse. *International Journal of Colorectal Disease* **7**: 8–10.

Ho Y-H, Tan M and Goh H-S (1996) Clinical and physiologic effects of biofeedback in outlet obstruction constipation. *Diseases of Colon and Rectum* **39**: 520–524.

Hock D, Lombard R, Jehaes C et al (1993) Colpocystodefecography. *Diseases of Colon and Rectum* **36**: 1015–1021.

Holley RL (1994) Enterocoele: a review. *Obstetrical and Gynecological Survey* **49**: 284–292.

Houghton LA, Wych J and Whorwell PJ (1993) Effect of acute diarrhoea on anorectal physiology in healthy volunteers. *Proceedings of the British Society of Gastroenterology* **34**: S3.

Houghton LA, Wych J and Whorwall PJ (1995) Acute diarrhoea induces rectal sensitivity in women but not men. *Gut* **37**: 270–273.

Hutson JM, Chow CW and Borg J (1996) Intractable constipation with a decrease in substance P-immuno-reactive fibres: is it a variant of intestinal neuronal dysplasia? *Journal of Paediatric Surgery* **31**: 580–583.

Infantino A, Fardin P, Pirone E et al (1994) Femoral nerve damage after abdominal rectopexy. *International Journal of Colorectal Disease* **9**: 32–34.

Janssen LWM and vanDijke CF (1994) Selection criteria for anterior rectal wall repair in symptomatic rectocele and anterior rectal wall prolapse. *Diseases of Colon and Rectum* **37**: 1100–1107.

Jorge JMN, Wexner SD, Ger GC et al (1992) Cinedefecography and electromyography in the diagnosis of nonrelaxing puborectalis syndrome. *Diseases of Colon and Rectum* **36**: 668–676.

Jorge JMN, Yong Y-K and Wexner SD (1994) Incidence and clinical significance of sigmoidoceles as determined by a new classification system. *Diseases of Colon and Rectum* **37**: 1112–1117.

Kamm MA (1994) Obstetric damage and faecal incontinence. *Lancet* **344**: 730–733.

Kawimbe BM, Papachrysostomou M, Binnie NR et al (1991) Outlet obstruction constipation (anismus) managed by biofeedback. *Gut* **32**: 1175–1179.

Kellow, JE (1990) Gastrointestinal motility – normal and abnormal. *Modern Medicine of Australia* **April**: 122–133.

Kennedy L (1995) *Vulvar Vestibulitis Syndrome*. Brisbane: Patient Education Material.

Konsten J, Baeten CG, Spaans F et al (1993) Follow-up of anal dynamic graciloplasty for fecal continence. *World Journal of Surgery* **17**: 404–408.

Koutsomanis D, Lemieux M-C, Lennard-Jones JE et al (1993) Symptomatic and objective benefits with biofeedback for intractable constipation. *Gut* **33**(Suppl 1): F263.

Koutsomanis D, Lennard-Jones JE and Kamm MA (1994) Prospective study of biofeedback treatment for patients with slow and normal transit constipation. *European Journal of Gastroenterology and Hepatology* **6**: 131–137.

Koutsomanis D, Lennard-Jones JE, Roy AJ and Kamm MA (1995) Controlled randomised trial of visual biofeedback versus muscle training without a visual display for intractable constipation. *Gut* **37**: 95–99.

Krishnamurthy S, Schuffler MD, Rohrmann CA et al (1984) Severe idiopathic constipation is associated with a distinctive abnormality of the colonic myentic plexus. *Gastroenterology* **88**: 26–34.

Kuijpers HC (1992) Treatment of complete rectal prolapse: to narrow, to wrap, to suspend, to fix, to encircle, to plicate or to resect? *World Journal of Surgery* **16**: 826–830.

Kuijpers HC, Schreve RH and Hoedemakers HTC (1986) Diagnosis of functional disorders of defecation causing the solitary rectal ulcer syndrome. *Diseases of Colon and Rectum* **29**: 126–129.

Lansman HH and Robertson EG (1992) Evolution of the pelvic floor. In: Benson JT (ed) *Female Pelvic Floor Disorders*, pp. 3–18. New York: W.W. Norton.

Laurberg S and Swash M (1989) Effects of aging on the anorectal sphincters and their innervation. *Diseases of Colon and Rectum* **32**: 737–742.

Lemieux M-C, Kamm MA and Fowler CJ (1993) Bowel dysfunction in young women with urinary retention. *Gut* **34**: 1397–1399.

Leroi AM, Bernier C, Watier A et al (1995) Prevalence of sexual abuse among patients with functional disorders of the lower gastrointestinal tract. *International Journal of Colorectal Disease* **10**: 200–206.

Loening-Baucke V (1990) Efficacy of biofeedback training in improving faecal incontinence and anorectal physiologic function. *Gut* **31**: 1395–1402.

Lubowski DZ, Nicholls RJ, Swash M and Jordan MJ (1987) Neural control of internal anal sphincter function. *British Journal of Surgery* **74**: 668–670.

MacDonald A, Carter K, Baxter JN et al (1993a) Patterns of colonic motility in patients with post-childbirth / hysterectomy constipation. *Gut* **34**(Suppl 4): W10.

MacDonald A, Baxter JN and Findlay IG (1993b) Ano-rectal manometry in patients with post-childbirth / hysterectomy constipation. *Gut* **34**(Suppl 4): F190.

MacLeod J (1987) Management of anal incontinence by biofeedback. *Gastroenterology* **93**: 291–294.

Margo J (1996) Anal incontinence worst among men. *Medical Observer* **March 1**: 31.

Markwell SJ and Mumme GA (1991) A role for physiotherapy in the management of patients with pelvic floor dysfunction and excretory disorders. *International Urogynecology Journal* **2**: 192.

Markwell SJ and Mumme GA (1995) A role for physiotherapy in perianal and perineal pain syndromes. In: Shacklock MO (ed) *Moving in on Pain*, pp. 145–152. Australia: Butterworth Heinemann.

Markwell SJ and Sapsford R (1995a) Physiotherapist, heal thyself. *Journal of the Australian Physiotherapists Association National Women's Health Group* **14**: 24.

Markwell SJ and Sapsford R (1995b) Physiotherapy management of obstructed defaecation. *Australian Journal of Physiotherapy* **41**: 279–283.

Markwell SJ, Mumme GA and O'Neill SM (1993) Proprioceptive retraining in pelvic floor dysfunction and excretory disorders. *Abstract International Continence Society Conference*, Rome, p. 132.

Markwell SJ, Sapsford R and Batistutta D (1995) To strain or not to strain – that is the question. Proceedings of the Australian Physiotherapy Association Conference, Sydney.

Meagher AP, Lubowski DZ and King DW (1993) The cough response of the anal sphincter. *International Journal of Colorectal Disease* **8**: 217–219.

Mellgren A, Johansson C, Dalk A et al (1994) Enterocele demonstrated by defaecography is associated with other pelvic floor disorders. *International Journal of Colorectal Disease* **9**: 121–124.

Milner P, Crave R, Kamm MA et al (1990) Vasoactive intestinal polypeptide levels in sigmoid colon in idiopathic constipation and diverticular disease. *Gastroenterology* **99**: 666–675.

Miner PB, Donnelly TC and Read NW (1990) Investigation of mode of action of biofeedback in treatment of fecal incontinence. *Digestive Diseases and Sciences* **35**: 1291–1298.

Mumme GA and Markwell SJ (1994) Rectal stabilisation improves bladder dysfunction in the descending perineum syndrome. *Abstracts of the International Continence Society Conference*, Prague, pp. 160–161.

O'Neill SM, Markwell SJ and Mumme GA (1993) The prevalence and management of bowel dysfunction in the climacteric: an Australian experience. Poster presentation, 7th International Congress on the Menopause, Stockholm.

Papachrysostomou M and Smith AN (1994) Effects of biofeedback on obstructive defecation – reconditioning of the defecation reflex? *Gut* **35**: 252–256.

Papachrysostomou M, Griffin TMJ, Ferrington C et al (1992) A method of computerised isotope dynamic proctography. *European Journal of Nuclear Medicine* **19**: 431–435.

Papachrysostomou M, Stevenson AJM, Ferrington C et al (1993) Evaluation of isotope proctography in constipated subjects. *International Journal of Colorectal Disease* **8**: 18–22.

Park UC, Choi SK, Piccirillo MF et al (1996) Patterns of anismus and the relation to biofeedback therapy. *Diseases of Colon and Rectum* **39**: 768–773.

Parks AG, Porter NH and Hardcastle JA (1966) The syndrome of the descending perineum. *Proceedings of the Royal Society of Medicine* **59**: 477–482.

Pemberton JH (1990) Anorectal and pelvic floor disorders: putting physiology into practice. *Journal of Gastroenterology and Hepatology* **5**(Suppl 1): 127–143.

Platell C, Scache D, Mumme G et al (1996) A long term follow-up of patients undergoing colectomy for chronic idiopathic constipation. *Australian and New Zealand Journal of Surgery* **66**: 525–529.

Preston DM and Lennard-Jones JE (1985) Anismus in chronic constipation. *Digestive Diseases and Sciences* **30**: 413–418.

Preston DM and Lennard-Jones JE (1986) Severe chronic constipation of young women: idiopathic slow transit constipation. *Gut* **27**: 41–48.

Preston DM, Lennard-Jones JE and Thomas BM (1985) Towards a radiologic definition of idiopathic megacolon. *Gastrointestinal Radiology* **10**: 167–169.

Prior A, Stanley K, Smith ARB and Read NW (1992) Effect of hysterectomy on anorectal and urethrovesical physiology. *Gut* **33**: 264–267.

Probert CSJ, Emmett PM and Heaton KW (1993) Some reasons why women have slower intestinal transit than men. *Proceedings of the British Society of Gastroenterology* **34**: S3.

Roig JV, Villoslada C, Lledo S et al (1995) Prevalence of pudendal neuropathy in fecal incontinence. Results of a prospective study. *Diseases of Colon and Rectum* *38*: 953–957.

Rutter KRP and Riddell RH (1975) The solitary ulcer syndrome of the rectum. *Clinics in Gastroenterology* **4**: 505–530.

Sangwan YP, Coller JA, Barrett RC et al (1995) Can manometric parameters predict response to biofeedback therapy in fecal incontinence? *Diseases of Colon and Rectum* **38**: 1021–1025.

Sangwan YP, Coller JA, Barrett RC et al (1996) Unilateral pudendal neuropathy. *Diseases of Colon and Rectum* **39**: 686–689.

Sapsford RR, Markwell SJ and Richardson CA (1996) Abdominal muscles and the anal sphincter: their interaction during defaecation. *Proceedings of the Australian Physiotherapy Association Congress*, Brisbane, pp. 103–104.

Schouten WR (1996) Treatment of anal fissure; is the answer NO? *Proceedings of Conference on Controversies in Colon and Rectal Surgery*, Nijmegen.

Schouten WR, ten Kate FJW, de Graaf EJR et al (1993) Visceral neuropathy in slow transit constipation: an immunohistochemical investigation with monoclonal antibodies against neurofilament. *Diseases of Colon and Rectum* **36**: 1112–1117.

Smith AN, Varma JS, Binnie NR et al (1990) Disordered colorectal motility in intractable constipation following hysterectomy. *British Journal of Surgery* **77**: 1361–1366.

Smith ARB (1994) Role of connective tissue and muscle in pelvic floor dysfunction. *Current Opinion in Obstetrics and Gynaecology* **6**: 317–319.

Snooks SJ, Barnes PRH, Swash, M and Henry MM (1985a) Damage to the innervation of the pelvic floor musculature in chronic constipation. *Gastroenterology* **89**: 977–981.

Snooks SJ, Henry MM and Swash M (1985b) Faecal incontinence due to external anal sphincter division in childbirth is associated with damage to the innervation of the pelvic floor musculature: a double pathology. *British Journal of Obstetrics and Gynaecology* **92**: 824–828.

Snooks SJ, Nicholls RJ, Henry MM and Swash M (1985c) Electrophysiological and manometric assessment of the pelvic floor in solitary rectal ulcer syndrome. *British Journal of Surgery* **72**: 131–133.

Snooks SJ, Swash M, Mathers SE and Henry MM (1990) Effect of vaginal delivery on the pelvic floor: a 5-year follow-up. *British Journal of Surgery* **77**: 1358–1360.

Spence-Jones C, Kamm MA, Henry MM and Hudson CN (1994) Bowel dysfunction: a pathogenic factor in uterovaginal prolapse and urinary stress incontinence. *British Journal of Obstetrics and Gynaecology* **101**: 147–152.

Sultan AH, Kamm MA, Hudson CN et al (1993) Anal-sphincter disruption during vaginal delivery. *New England Journal of Medicine* **329**: 1905–1911.

Taylor T, Smith AN and Fuller M (1990) Effects of hysterectomy on bowel and bladder function. *International Journal of Colorectal Disease* **5**: 228–231.

Thorpe AC, Williams NS, Badenoch DF et al (1993) Simultaneous dynamic electromyographic proctography and cystometrography. *British Journal of Surgery* **80**: 115–120.

Vaccaro CA, Wexner SD, Teoh TA et al (1995) Pudendal neuropathy is not related to physiologic pelvic outlet obstruction. *Diseases of Colon and Rectum* **38**: 630–633.

Van Laarhoven CJHN (1996) Solitary rectal ulcer syndrome: a mechanical lesion. *Proceedings of a Conference on Controversies in Colon and Rectal Surgery*, Nijmegen.

VanTets WJ and Kuijpers JHC (1995) Internal rectal intussusception – fact or fancy? *Diseases of Colon and Rectum* **38**: 1080–1083.

Wald A, Hinds JP and Caruana BJ (1989) Psychological and physiological characteristics of patients with severe idiopathic constipation. *Gastroenterology* **97**: 932–937.

Watier A, Devroede G, Suranceau A et al (1983) Constipation with colonic inertia. *Digestive Diseases and Sciences* **28**: 1025–1032.

Weber J, Ducrotte PH, Touchais JY et al (1987) Biofeedback training for constipation in adults and children. *Diseases of Colon and Rectum* **30**: 844–846.

Wexner SD and Jorge JM (1994) Colorectal physiological tests: use or abuse of technology? *European Journal of Surgery* **160**(3): 167–174.

Wexner SD, Cheape JD, Jorge JMN et al (1992) Prospective assessment of biofeedback for the treatment of paradoxical puborectalis contraction. *Diseases of Colon and Rectum* **35**: 145–150.

Whitehead WE (1985) Psychotherapy and biofeedback as the treatment for irritable bowel syndrome. In: Read NW (ed) *Irritable Bowel Syndrome*, pp. 245–266. London: Grune and Stratton.

Williams NS, Hughes SF and Stuchfield B (1994) Continent conduit for rectal evacuation in severe constipation. *Lancet* **343**: 1321–1324.

Wingate, DL (1993) The 'Rome Criteria of IBS'. In: Kumar D and Wingate D (eds) *An Illustrated Guide to Intestinal Motility*, 2nd edn., p. 584. Edinburgh: Churchill Livingstone.

Womack NR, Morrison JFB and Williams NS (1986) The role of pelvic floor denervation in the aetiology of idiopathic faecal incontinence. *British Journal of Surgery* **73**: 404–407.

Womack NR, Williams NS, Holmfield JHM and Morrison JFB (1987) Pressure and prolapse – the cause of solitary rectal ulceration. *Gut* **28**: 1228–1233.

Wood C, Maher P, Hill D and Sellwood T (1992) Hysterectomy: a time of change. *Medical Journal of Australia* **157**: 651–653.

Wynne JM, Myles JL, Jones I et al (1996) Disturbed anal sphincter function following vaginal delivery. *Gut* **39**: 120–124.

Yoshioka K, Matsui Y, Yamada O et al (1991) Physiologic and anatomic assessment of patients with rectocoele. *Diseases of Colon and Rectum* **34**: 704–708.

Further reading

Benson JT (ed) (1992) *Female Pelvic Floor Disorders*. New York: Norton Medical Books.

Henry MM and Swash M (eds) (1992) *Coloproctology and the Pelvic Floor*, 2nd edn. Oxford: Butterworth Heinemann.

Kumar D and Wingate D (1993) *An Illustrated Guide to Intestinal Motility*, 2nd edn. Edinburgh: Churchill Livingstone.

30

Physiotherapy Management of Pelvic Floor Dysfunction

SUE MARKWELL AND RUTH SAPSFORD

Urogenital Dysfunction
•
Anorectal Dysfunction

Physiotherapists who treat patients suffering from pelvic floor dysfunction need to be aware of the sensitivity of women with regard to these conditions. Urinary or faecal incontinence is often regarded as something to be ashamed of or as a regression to infancy, particularly among the older age groups. They are reluctant to seek help or discuss the problem with their doctors. Fortunately, the increase in female general practitioners has made it easier for women to raise the topic. Therefore, in assessing and treating these conditions, physiotherapists not only need to take their lead from the patient's attitude, but to realize that this area of health requires a different approach from that used in other musculoskeletal conditions.

Urogenital Dysfunction

Physiotherapists are responsible for accurate assessment and diagnosis prior to treatment. Medical referrals do not always provide enough information on which to base appropriate treatment and many women suffering pelvic floor dysfunction will refer themselves. Patient history and symptoms must be carefully sought. Symptoms include pelvic organ prolapse and urethrovesical and anorectal dysfunction.

Physiotherapy assessment

Physiotherapy assessment, as described, applies to all aspects of pelvic floor dysfunction. Assessments and treatments must be carried out in a private room, where questioning cannot be overheard and where there is no fear of intrusion by other staff. A 'Do Not Disturb' notice on the door is a good idea. Such areas are not easily come by in hospital physiotherapy departments. Even in a suitable room, during the physical examination the patient should be positioned facing away from the door.

A physiotherapy assessment should include:

- presenting symptoms in order of importance;
- relevant obstetric, medical, gynaecological and surgical history;
- investigations and previous and current treatment;
- details of activity levels, hormonal status and medications, both prescribed and over the counter;
- details of voiding dysfunction / incontinence;
- details from frequency / volume (F / V) chart, fluid intake;
- anorectal function and current management;
- objective assessment – defaecation pattern;
- objective PF muscle assessment;
  - external observation;
  - digital per vaginam muscle assessment;
  - digital per anum muscle assessment in some cases;
  - effect of coughing and straining on the vaginal wall and organ position.

A guide to pelvic floor assessment is to be found in Appendix 1 on p. 406. There are many assessment forms in use but this guide, which has been adapted from one prepared for physiotherapists who have little or no previous experience in treating pelvic floor dysfunction, may help you to compile your own assessment protocol.

This outlines a detailed assessment and completion takes a long time. Collection of data spread over two visits may be easier for the therapist and patient. However, before embarking on an assessment based on the guide, it is advisable to read the following explanations.

DEFAECATION

A simulated evacuation pattern. The patient sits, clothed, on a firm chair without back support and is asked to assume her normal defaecation position. Her lumbar spine position is noted. The investigator palpates the lateral abdominal wall at waist level and the lower abdominal wall suprapubically. The patient performs a simulated defaecatory action and is asked to report on perceived anal movement. The investigator notes changes in the abdominal wall, waist and the position of the spine. The options are:

- waist – widens, narrows or is static;
- lower abdomen – indrawn, bulges or is static;
- spine – posterior pelvic tilt, trunk sagging, normal lumbar curve, no change;
- anus – descends, lifts, bulges, tenses, flares, opens.

See details of a normal defaecation pattern in the anorectal section of this chapter.

PELVIC ORGAN PROLAPSE

If, on viewing the perineum, a prolapse protrudes from the vaginal introitus, there is little chance that muscle rehabilitation will change this. (The prolapse will be more obvious if viewed with the patient in standing.) Surgical repair is needed. However, improved muscle function will benefit most of these women. Depending on the extent of the prolapse and whether it can be reduced in lying, muscle rehabilitation can be conducted prior to surgical repair. Defaecation retraining may be particularly relevant.

PELVIC FLOOR MUSCLE ASSESSMENT

There are several ways in which pelvic floor muscle activity can be confirmed and tested. Some are more accurate than others. However, it is not always possible to use the best method.

The action of a combined PFM contraction, and the actions of the individual muscles were described in Chapter 7. There is no easy way to gain experience in assessing PFM, but watching a colleague do an assessment, and doing one under guidance, is very helpful. Torso models are used by some people, but they are of more value in overcoming apprehension than in getting a real feel of the muscle action.

Digital assessment It is inappropriate to digitally or even visually assess muscle or perineal activity in some patients. Girls and young adolescents should not be embarrassed by asking them to undress unless it is absolutely essential. Girls can be encouraged to feel the perineal movement through their underwear. This can be useful for others as well. Digital assessment of virgins and those with very atrophic vaginae is inappropriate. Don't examine during menstruation and wait until post-partum loss has ceased, to avoid risk of infection.

Notes

Prior to any assessment a thorough explanation of what is to be done and why this is necessary should be given to the patient and her *permission* sought to do this. Some institutions now ask patients to sign 'informed consent' forms. Others note verbal agreement on the chart. Find out the policy in your workplace. If the patient is reluctant or declines, record this too. Women who have been sexually assaulted/abused may decline. 'Implied consent' occurs when the patient willingly moves from a chair to the examination couch.

A waterproof underpad, a covering sheet, vinyl or latex gloves (sterile gloves are not necessary unless there is a greater risk of patient infection, e.g. early post-partum), a water-based lubricant, tissues and a suitable waste disposal bin are required. The patient is usually positioned in crook lying with a neutral lumbar spine, hips abducted and feet apart. Thorough hand washing is the best way to prevent transmission of infection and open skin wounds should be completely covered. Wash, dry and glove both hands before touching the perineal area.

Treat every patient with the same *universal precautions.* See Appendix 2 (p. 407) for guidelines on infection control. Remember hepatitis B is far more common than HIV. A follow-up blood test will confirm your own hepatitis B immunity after vaccination (see Chapter 9).

The internal examination covers the following.

1. The perineum, noting scars and skin condition. Excoriated skin indicates sustained wetness or soiling.
2. The vaginal introitus. Is it open? Is the mucosa reddened (post-menopausal)? Is there a cystocoele, prolapse of the cervix or rectocoele? (See Fig 27.5) Are vaginal mucosal rugae present?
3. Ask the patient to tighten her muscles and draw in and up around the introitus. There should be a closing of the opening and a lift towards the head. In patients with normal fascial integrity, the posterior vaginal wall can be seen to be drawn up and the urethral meatus is pulled dorsally as the anterior vaginal wall is lifted up. Any bulging down and protrusion indicates that an increase in intra-abdominal pressure (IAP) is forcing the perineum down.

4. Ask the patient to cough and observe any descent, bulging or urine loss.
5. Gently stretch apart the anal area, noting skin tags and haemorrhoids. As the patient draws the anus up and in and holds as long as possible, observe the skin puckering and any perineal lift.
6. Change to a clean pair of gloves.
7. Apply lubricant to the index finger of the examining hand. If the patient complains of allergies, use water.
8. Separate the labia and gently slide the palmar surface of the finger along the posterior vaginal wall to full finger length. If there is a prominent rectocoele work around this. Watch the patient's face for signs of discomfort while doing this.
9. Can you feel the cervix? It feels like a firmly closed ring. If you feel it, there is a degree of uterine prolapse.
10. Note any loose vaginal tissue (rectocoele), scar tissue, sensory awareness, sensitivity and pain and a full rectum.
11. While pressing posteriorly, ask the patient to 'draw in strongly around the vaginal opening and lift up towards your head'. Feel the anterior shift. This is the puborectalis. Assess the strength by noting the range of movement and the force with which the muscle moves and can hold against the palpating finger. Repeat three or four times and then hold (count the seconds for endurance) and feel the release. It may be extensive. Is the patient aware of the movement and the release?
12. Now palpate laterally to one side, still with the palmar surface of the index finger, in the region of 3–4 or 8–9 o'clock. The coccyx is at 6 o'clock. Note the vaginal width, muscle bulk, awareness, sensitivity and any pain. Ask the patient to draw up and in strongly towards her head. Repeat several times. Feel medial shift and elevation. This is the pubococcygeus. Assess strength, endurance, release and awareness. Repeat on the other side. Compare sides for atrophy and imbalance (this is very common). Sometimes no muscle activity is detected.
13. As the patient is tightening and holding her PF, observe her thorax, trunk and thighs. The chest should remain still with light upper chest breathing, the abdominal wall should not be actively or deliberately retracted or the pelvis tilted and gluteal and adductor movement should be minimal.
14. Now feel along the anterior vaginal wall. Is it slack? Does the bladder sag down (cystocoele)? Get the patient to lift the PF and feel the elevation of the bladder.
15. Ask the patient to cough. You may feel the bladder or the cervix press down or the anterior vaginal wall slide down.
16. Check the superficial perineal muscles at the introitus. It is probably easier to detect their contraction using two fingers, thus feeling a compression effect.

Having finished the internal assessment, ask the patient to roll onto her side, usually left lateral, facing away from you with her hips and knees flexed to 90°. Draw up the upper buttock and press on the ischial tuberosity. Estimate the position of the anus in relation to the bone. Is it 1 or 2 cm above? Now ask the patient to contract her anal sphincter strongly, draw up her pelvic floor and hold. Note anal skin puckering, hold and perineal lift. Next ask her to strain down hard as though about to empty the bowel (warn about possible wind loss). Note how far the anus descends. Is it lower than the ischial tuberosity, is there bulging or ballooning around the anus or perineum? In a normal perineum the anal verge should not descend beyond the level of the ischial tuberosities with hard straining.

If there is an anorectal problem you may need to examine the muscles per anum. Details of how to do this are outlined later in this chapter.

Now while the patient is wiping away the excess lubricant, dressing and handwashing, discard your gloves, wash and immediately record what you felt. One way to record data (atrophy, imbalance, pain and structural changes) is diagrammatically using a circle to represent the field assessed (Laycock, 1994a).

Short strong contractions are considered representative of *strength* and can be graded 0–5. Grades of the individual PFM could be interpreted thus:

Grade 0 – no movement palpable.
1 – minimal or very small muscle bulging on palpation.
2 – small range of movement, weak with brief hold.
3 – definite muscle movement, up to half range.
4 – firm muscle movement closing around finger, half to three-quarter range.
5 – very firm muscle pull which compresses finger, full range and strong hold.

Gradings of 2 and 3 are very difficult to assess reliably and some therapists prefer to use descriptive terminology. *Endurance*, measured in seconds, is the sustained activity in a muscle. It is considered to be submaximal activity, as there is usually a rapid decrease in maximal pelvic floor strength after three seconds (Santiesteban, 1988). Endurance can also be the number of repetitions of a particular action.

Remember that you are testing two different muscle actions. Most of the PF assessment methods described do not differentiate between the different actions of puborectalis and pubococcygeus. Differentiation occurs in function and this must be reflected in the assessment. Clinical experience indicates that it is possible to contract the puborectalis with minimal or reduced activity in other parts of the levator ani.

Testing in standing, as well as in lying, is also advocated by some therapists, as normal function requires holding against gravity (Laycock, 1994b). This test can be difficult.

Other ways of assessing the PF are used, but none of them, other than EMG, provides the detailed information that can be gained from a digital approach. Some physiotherapists will assess with index and middle fingers together and separate them to feel the medial shift of pubococcygeus.

Figure 30.1 (a) A PFX perineometer (Cardio Design, Sydney) which is used for biofeedback during pelvic floor exercises. Accurate quantification of squeeze pressure is not possible with this apparatus. (b) A Peritron vaginal perineometer (Cardio Design, Sydney) can provide an accurate, reproducible reading of vaginal squeeze pressure.

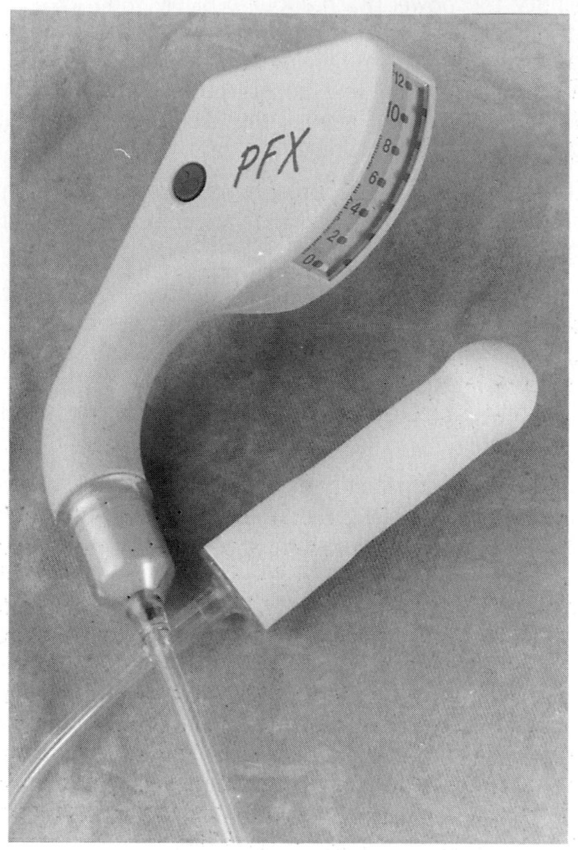

a

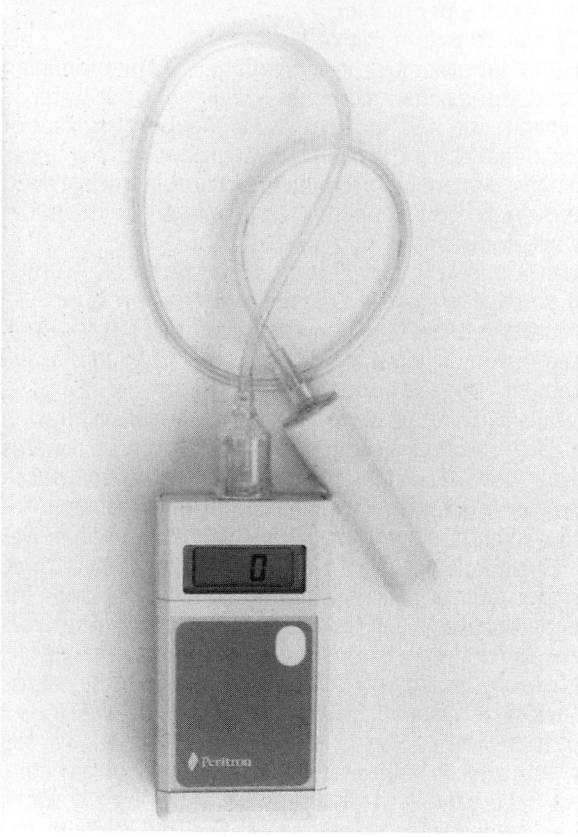

b

This does not allow such definition of atrophy as the index finger alone.

Perineometers Air-filled pressure probes are used to register vaginal pressure as an indication of PF strength. *The probe, covered by a condom, should always be inserted by the patient.* The first was developed by Kegel (1951). Patients must be able to initiate the correct muscle action, as increased IAP can register on the meter as the patient bears down. The Bourne perineometer (Doncast, Caterham, UK) has been available for a number of years and while it is reliable to record variations in pressure on one day, its day-to-day pressure recording is unreliable and could not be used to quantify strength (Salter et al, 1995). The PFX (Cardio Design, Australia) is a similar probe, designed for biofeedback, and is used with a reliable electronic meter, the Peritron (Cardio Design, Australia) (Fig. 30.1). There is no differentiation of individual muscle performance with a pressure probe. Due care must be taken with infection control with all such equipment. See Appendix 2 (p. 407) for guidelines on infection control.

Observation As with perinometers an indrawing movement in a cephalad direction at the vaginal introitus is an indication of a correct PFM contraction. It was shown that up to 27% of women were unable to contract the PF at the beginning of one study (Hesse et al, 1990) and in another, 25% of the subjects tended to bear down – a movement which could promote urine loss (Bump et al, 1991). A precise instruction is important.

Perineal palpation A hand held against the perineum can detect quite small degrees of perineal lift. This is a useful way for girls and others to detect the correct muscle action for themselves. It is more useful in detecting the incorrect bulging action which occurs in bearing down.

Stop test The patient is asked to stop or slow the flow of urine in mid-stream. This action probably reflects the strength of the periurethral and PF muscles as well as the intensity of the detrusor activity. It may take longer to inhibit a higher detrusor pressure. Greater urine volumes are not related to longer stop times. Stop test times are longer in multiparae compared with nulliparae, a mean of 4.4 seconds as compared with 1.96 seconds (Sampselle and DeLancey, 1992). For some people it may

Figure 30.2 Vaginal weights. Aquaflex (DePuy, UK) include two sizes of outer shells, to cater for small and larger vaginae. The 5 g and 10 g weights are added to the central spindle and placed inside the shell to create the desired mass. All these parts are autoclavable.

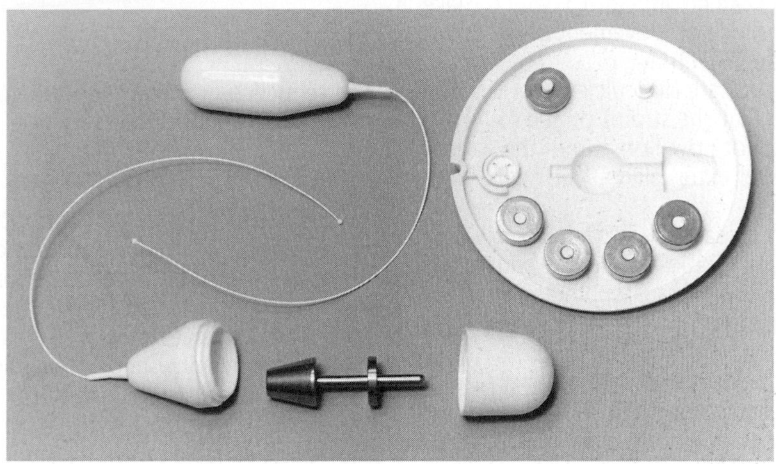

Figure 30.3 Vaginal weights. On the left, Femtone (Convatec, USA) are supplied in a set of five weights of increasing mass. They are for single patient use and cannot be autoclaved. On the right, one of a pair of Duo Balls (available from sex shops), is a cheap weight for the larger vagina. It must be used within a condom.

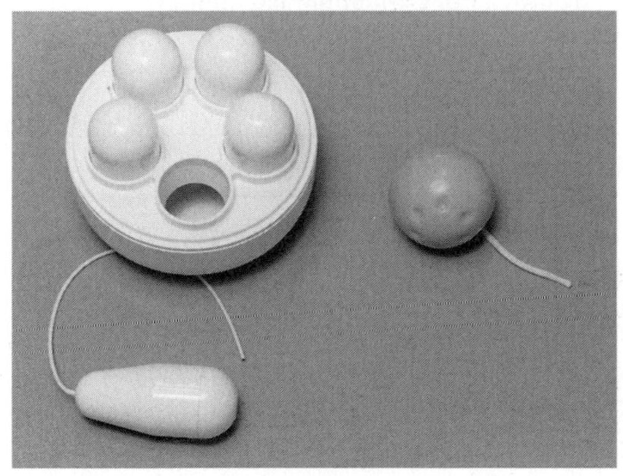

be difficult to reinitiate detrusor activity to empty the bladder after stopping the flow, so the value of this test is to give the patient the idea of a correct PFM action, not to quantify strength. It should not be done frequently.

Vaginal weights Weights, such as Femina Cones, of increasing mass were developed as a method of providing BFB and resistance for PFM. Figures 30.2 and 30.3 are examples of vaginal weights. They have been used to quantify 'resting strength' and 'active strength' (Plevnik, 1985). However, a large vaginal diameter, varying lubrication related to the menstrual cycle, a full rectum and positioning high in the vagina can render this method unreliable (Longmore, 1991).

Electromyography This is the most accurate method of objectively recording muscle activity when data are collected by fine wire or needle electrodes. External electrode placement on the perineum records superficial muscle activity. Surface electrodes are used intravaginally or intra-anally in some rehabilitation units as a biofeedback mechanism. Objective EMG data cannot be used to compare day-to-day progress, as electrode placement varies. Motor unit analysis, using needle electrodes, can be used on separate occasions to record changes in muscle, but is generally reserved to demonstrate denervation in research situations (Allen et al, 1990).

Assessment findings

Having observed the perineum and carried out a digital assessment, reflection on the findings and their relationship to the history provided is important before developing a treatment plan. This applies to all information from the frequency/volume chart as well. Some comments about the findings, based on clinical experience and the literature, are set out below.

- During digital assessment PF awareness and action are often increased dramatically by the feedback provided by touch, pressure and the repetition of contractions. The assessment session can be turned into a good exercising session using this tactile biofeedback.
- A puborectalis or pubococcygeus contraction palpated by the assessor may not be detected by the patient. Proprioception is deficient, yet the patient can respond to the request to 'lift the pelvic floor'.
- On palpation of pubococcygeus, reasonable muscle bulk can be detected, yet the patient is unable to voluntarily contract her muscle. It may respond reflexly on coughing (Bo et al, 1994).
- Unilateral atrophy and weakness of pubococcygeus are very common and digital assessment of this has been

shown to be accurate (Debus-Thiede et al, 1990). During digital palpation many patients can perceive the unilateral weakness that the investigator feels.

- Very weak muscle action can be difficult to detect. Make sure that what is being felt is not movement of the pelvis itself, such as posterior pelvic tilting.
- A large rectocoele can indicate difficult evacuation. The patient may be unaware that she strains or she may have strained in the past, but not now. Sometimes the patient uses digital support, either externally or per vaginam, to facilitate rectal emptying.
- A very firm posterior vaginal wall, in the absence of a history of surgery, generally indicates that the patient has built up a strong puborectalis and anal sphincter. This may result from prolonged defaecation straining or excessive 'sit-up' exercising.
- A strong anterior shift with weak or minimal 'lift' is another indication of defaecation straining or pelvic floor exercising with a posterior pelvic tilt, as in a car.
- A large excursion of perineal movement, observed externally or palpated during assessment of puborectalis, indicates lax fascial supporting tissues. This occurs in the descending perineum syndrome.
- Very large voided volumes (700 ml +) on a regular basis, during both day and night, indicate decreased bladder response to stretch and, in the long term, can lead to poor detrusor contractility and urinary retention.

Now a rehabilitation programme is needed for each person. Table 30.1 gives a guide as to what may be needed in each urethrovesical condition.

Treatment methods

The sequence in which physiotherapy treatment is carried out for pelvic floor dysfunction depends on individual needs. Most forms of dysfunction require muscle rehabilitation and/or functional training.

Advice is usually given to cease activities which aggravate the condition prior to rehabilitation, e.g. participation in sport and heavy lifting that triggers urine loss, smoking which aggravates cough-induced loss and straining at defaecation. While suggestions of alternative exercise options are easily provided (low-impact exercise, cycling, swimming), ceasing defaecation straining can be difficult. Advice regarding high-soluble, low-residue fibre intake, plenty of fluids and a more suitable position for defaecation is the first step. See the section on anorectal dysfunction for further details.

MUSCLE REHABILITATION

In the majority of patients the first treatment priority is improving muscle support. Pubococcygeus is the principal muscle requiring attention but before strengthening can begin, the patient must have an awareness of what she is doing, as visual cues are generally limited.

Table 30.1 Treatment outlines for urinary dysfunction and incontinence

Condition	Symptoms	Suggested management
Frequency	>8 voids/day	PFM rehab., bladder training, modify intake
Nocturia	2+ voids per night	PFM rehab., bladder training, modify intake and its timing Nocturnal polyuria – 2 hr midday rest, legs elevated
Hesitancy, strain, voiding dysfunction	Slow start, intermittent flow	Forward-lean voiding, PF release, adequate voiding time, voiding retraining
Urethral syndrome	Frequency, urgency, pain	PFM rehab., urge control, bladder and defaecation retraining, electrotherapy
Retention	Infections, 2nd large void after short interval	Forward-lean or squat voiding, voiding retraining, double void, self-catheterization
GSI	Small volume loss with ↑ IAP	PFM rehab., functional abdominal PF use, + or – defaecation retraining
Urgency, urge I, giggle I	Urgency, large loss, key in door, running water, unable to defer, perineal urge sensation	PFM rehab., urge control techniques, bladder training, functional abdominal PF use, relaxation, + or – defaecation retraining, electrotherapy
Overflow I	Continuous loss	Voiding retraining, self-catheterization
Reflex I	Sudden large loss, no warning	Self-catheterization
Nocturnal enuresis	Urine loss during sleep	Bladder training, urge control, enuresis alarm
Post-void loss	Loss after dressing	Voiding position, PFM rehab.

Muscle awareness This can be enhanced in a number of ways.

1. Recent clinical observation has demonstrated that a pubococcygeal contraction can be facilitated by a transversus abdominis contraction (Richardson and Jull, 1995) and this has been confirmed by EMG Studies (Sapsford et al, 1997a). In some women activation of transversus abdominis requires specific re-education and this may take some time.
2. Tactile input from the physiotherapist during assessment enables sensory and verbal feedback of a correct muscle action. This is often sufficient to enable progression to a strengthening programme.
3. Self-examination of external movement by mirror will have little value if pubococcygeal 'lift' is slight, but it will demonstrate bearing down – the wrong thing to do.
4. Self-digital assessment is recommended by a number of therapists. This usually necessitates lumbar flexion. Some women find this difficult or unacceptable. Use of two fingers vaginally with the instruction to 'feel the squeeze' feels little if muscles are very weak. Self-assessment using the thumb is more sensitive – each side is palpated to feel pubococcygeal medial shift and lift. It is easily carried out in shower or bath. Younger women are more likely to use digital feedback. Hand contact over the perineum is another way to detect perineal lift.
5. A vaginal weight is one of the best ways to provide feedback and enhance proprioception. A weight of appropriate diameter for the individual is required. Three sizes are needed – small for nulliparae and atrophied vaginae, large for post-partum when loss has ceased and moderate. It is not easy to obtain a supply of these, but more are becoming available, e.g. Duo balls, Femina Cones (Colgate Palmolive, UK), Femtone (Convatec, USA), steel ball bearings, Aquaflex (DePuy, UK) (see Figs 30.2, 30.3). The cheapest product is plasticine, often used with a steel ball bearing in the middle.

Precaution

All vaginal weights should be single patient use only, unless they are fully autoclavable. They should be decontaminated and sterilized before initial use and if necessary, be used within a new lubricated condom. However, some women are allergic to latex and the condom lubricant. Lightweight plastic freezer bags are an alternative. See Appendix 2 (p. 407) for infection control guidelines.

Instead of using weights in standing as initially advocated (Plevnik, 1985), the best way to commence use is in crook lying. The weight, within a condom, is inserted by the patient, like a tampon, to a full finger depth. The patient's head and shoulders are propped up with the lumbar spine flat. The lumbar spine should be kept straight or preferably have a normal lumbar curve. Grasping the end

Figure 30.4 An example of a neuromuscular stimulator, the Microscol with a fully autoclavable vaginal electrode. There are many types available. Supplied by Microsystems Electronics Pty Ltd., Stones Corner, Brisbane, Australia.

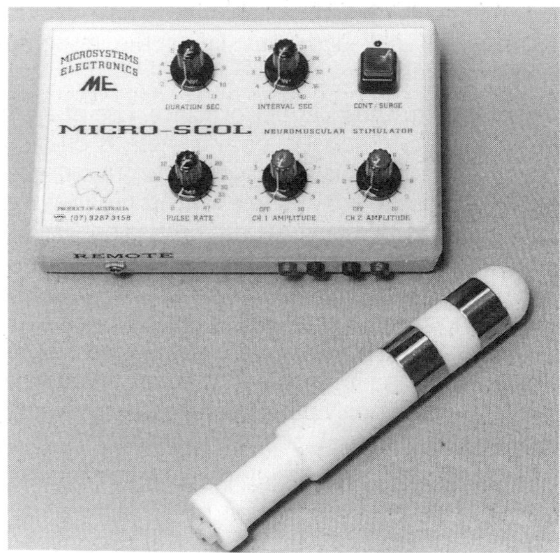

of the condom, she eases the tail of the weight or the condom outwards. When the weight is detected vaginally, she releases the finger tension as she 'lifts' the weight in a cephalad direction with her pubococcygeus and holds as long as possible

6. A Foley catheter, covered in a condom, can be used in a similar way to a weight and is useful for atrophied vaginae. Once inserted into the vagina, the balloon is inflated and tension is applied as for the weight.
7. Neuromuscular stimulation (NMS) using a vaginal electrode can be used to obtain a muscle contraction (Fig. 30.4). This may require the probe, inserted by the patient, to be used on each pubococcygeus, with the patient controlling the position and the current intensity. Palpation of the perineum can detect perineal lift which accompanies the muscle contraction (see Chapter 24).
8. Women with marked bilateral atrophy of the pubococcygeus, detected on palpation, may take a long time to respond to any of these methods and may not gain much strength. Iliococcygeus and ischiococcygeus may develop to compensate for the lack of pubococcygeus.

Re-education Having developed an awareness of the correct action, the re-education commences. Free exercise, biofeedback or NMS can be used in the process. Recent research confirms that a pubococcygeal lift is easier to activate and is more effective, by exercising with a normal lumbar curve, or in a fixed anterior pelvic tilt position (Sapsford et al, 1997b). Activation of transversus abdominis can be used to reinforce PFM contractions in most patients. Free exercise can be supervised with verbal enhancement provided by the physiotherapist or it can be home based with the patient responsible for her own programme. It takes a very disciplined patient to continue without further input from the therapist. A programme needs progressing as the patient improves and other measures are implemented, so continued contact is necessary.

During exercise the breath should not be held. This tends to increase the IAP and thus limits the response of pubococcygeus.

BFB in some form enhances performance. Use of a *vaginal weight* in lying, as described for awareness, is one way to provide feedback for daily exercising. Later the weight can be used in standing, but only some patients progress to this. *Self-digital BFB*, as for awareness, can be used on a daily basis at home. A *perineometer* is suggested by some physiotherapists. It is very important that the correct muscle action is performed and that the patient can perceive this before using a perineometer. The perineometer registers squeeze pressure and it is possible to create pressure using an increase in IAP or only puborectalis. Pubococcygeal 'lift' must be used.

NMS can be used as a biofeedback mechanism rather than as functional electrical stimulation for strengthening. It is sometimes used externally in this way (see Chapter 24). Its use should be restricted to the minimum time required to gain a reasonable muscle contraction. In functional electrical muscle stimulation used for strengthening, normal muscle recruitment order, of slow twitch first, is reversed and enhancement of strength is greater with voluntary effort once a reasonable contraction is achieved. Care should be taken that the patient does not use the machine to do the work, rather than doing it herself. If this is the case any improvement will soon fade when treatment ceases.

Having established a method to facilitate muscle activity, a decision has to be made on how to build up this function.

Exercise physiology Revision of pertinent exercise physiology may assist in formulating an exercise programme during muscle rehabilitation. In dealing with pelvic floor dysfunction, different muscle actions are required. Postural support for pelvic organs, a strong fast response to reinforce urethral closure under stress and rectal support during defaecation are all required. Pubococcygeus and puborectalis have predominantly slow-twitch fibres. There are no known studies that determined fibre content of iliococcygeus. As slow-twitch fibres tend to become fast acting with disuse, injury and ageing, the rehabilitation order should be slow-twitch function first, followed by maximal forceful contractions to increase strength and hypertrophy muscle and later fast repetitive contractions to build up fast fibre endurance.

Training in one type of activity does not improve function in another activity. *A muscle must be trained in the specific activity that is required in function* (McArdle et al, 1991).

Motivation to exercise It is much easier to 'have something done' than to 'have to do something'. Hence embarking on and continuing with an exercise programme requires motivation and self-discipline. Much has been written on this and how to achieve it. Regular professional input, some form of biofeedback and use of compliance diaries are among the methods used. If pain is a factor in a disorder, then compliance will generally be greater as the end – freedom from pain – justifies the means – exercise. So in planning you need the minimum to achieve the set goal and wherever possible you should combine exercise with function.

Endurance training Endurance is the ability to sustain muscle activity over a prolonged period. It depends on alternating slow-twitch fibre activity. In normal exercise slow-twitch fibres are recruited first with fast-twitch fibres coming in as more force and sustained strong activity are required. Training for endurance requires prolonged submaximal muscle holds. These can be done using a vaginal weight as biofeedback or without it. An example of an endurance programme is contained in the box.

Suggested endurance programme

Begin in supine and maintain a straight spine or normal lumbar curve.

PF lift and hold as long as possible.

Rest 5–7 seconds.

Repeat the above, hold and rest, three times (this is a set of four).

Rest 1–2 minutes.

Repeat the set of four.

Continue working in sets of four for 10–20 minutes, preferably in the morning. Increase the length of each hold as endurance improves – even up to 20–30 seconds. Do as many sets of four as possible at other times during the day, either in sitting or lying. Gradually substitute long submaximal transversus abdominis (TrA) holds for specific PF holds.

Strength training Strength is the maximal force generated by a muscle and it depends on the total cross-section of the fibres. Straplike muscles tend to generate low forces, but have a greater range of movement. Pennate muscles have a greater cross-sectional area and can generate greater force. Puborectalis is straplike, iliococcygeus has a pennate structure and pubococcygeus is a mixture of the two.

To develop strength, maximal force must be generated. A maximal contraction can only be maintained for a short time. Santiesteban (1988), in assessing PF strength using vaginal surface EMG, noted that one subject could sustain maximal force for seven seconds, but generally it was maintained for a shorter time, 3+ seconds.

Various authors have suggested different programmes to build up strength. Strengthening depends on the principle of overload, in which a muscle is exercised at a level above that of normal function. One example is suggested in the box.

Strengthening programme (DiNubile, 1991)

8–12 maximal contractions, sustained for 5–6 seconds each.

Do this series 3–4 times a day.

Train on 3–4 days a week.

Many physiotherapists believe that muscles should be worked daily, particularly when the training begins with very weak muscles.

Increasing the workload is difficult to apply directly to the PF. Femina Cones (Plevnik, 1985), which range from 10 to 90 g, have been used for this purpose. Once one cone can be retained for a set time in walking, a heavier cone is used in training. Other weights can be used similarly. Care must be taken that the weight is in the correct position within the vagina. In supine, traction can be applied to the tail of the weight to increase the workload. Patients can progress from lying to standing.

Strength development in the first 6–8 weeks of training is due to more effective recruitment of motor units. Further increases in strength, due to muscle hypertrophy, may take 5–6 months (Sale, 1988). Endurance can be gained in fast-twitch fibre activity, but this does not affect slow-twitch fibre endurance.

Fatigue and aching Estimation of the working potential for the given pathology and explaining this to the patient may save problems of fatigue. When working with a vaginal weight, the first sign of fatigue will be adductor shaking. The other sign is the inability to perform a previously performed exercise. The patient must heed the fatigue, as symptoms will worsen with overexercise. Generalized muscle aching in legs and back after exercising indicates that pubococcygeus is not being specifically activated.

Progression and maintenance Attendance for treatment varies with the patient's problem, attitude and understanding. Those who are able to contract their PFM and are well motivated may only require three or four treatment sessions spread over a two-month period. Long-term follow-up is advantageous. Some treatment centres use weekly biofeedback or class sessions to provide encouragement and supervised programmes. Digital muscle assessment is not necessary at every visit. It is important, though, to confirm a correct muscle action after the patient has been exercising for a period of time. If, however, the patient has difficulty with the programme more frequent sessions and palpation will be required.

Once a muscle has been re-educated and function improved, strength and endurance have to be maintained or function will deteriorate. A maintenance programme needs to be lifelong and easy to incorporate into daily living. Comparison with regular teeth cleaning or standing tall may be helpful. Improved function can be a great motivator. Abdominal drawing in and abdominal bracing once mastered provide a good PF response in most women. In bracing, the waist widens as the abdomen is drawn in a little. However, PF holds may be the best option in cases of significant pathology. Checking digitally during each abdominal pattern will confirm which action provides the best response. All three are easily done in regular working situations and can be used during regular fitness activities. Remembering and getting into the habit are the hardest parts.

FUNCTIONAL RETRAINING

PFM should provide ongoing organ support in normal activity and with increased load and should respond rapidly to stress (increase of IAP) situations. A voluntary contraction and hold is needed to provide stability when fascia is lengthened and to improve urethral closure. The muscle response is not automatic or at least not initially. Whether this response becomes automatic may depend on how the muscle is retrained, the degree of fascial laxity, the abdominal muscle work involved in the activity and the neural control. Research is needed into how to assess the co-ordinated response and the best way to retrain it.

Hence in all effort activities – sneeze, cough, lift, push, drag, nose blow – PF support is required. In occupations with heavy lifting, normal muscles are overloaded. In patients with pelvic floor dysfunction, normal loading is required on abnormal muscles. Alternative methods of achieving PF support are to strengthen and then utilize transversus abdominis and the obliques. *Abdominal drawing in* (transversus abdominis and internal obliques) activates anterior levator support, while *abdominal bracing* (external obliques and transversus with internal obliques) seems to activate posterolateral levator support. Studies by the authors are currently underway to confirm these clinical observations. Use during effort activities depends on individual need. Those with lax anterior tissues will find abdominal drawing in gives better support, while those with lax posterior support will benefit more from abdominal bracing. Both patterns must be taught and a combination is used to stabilize the trunk during heavy lifting.

Integrated functional patterns

Bracing for quick and sustained rises in intra-abdominal pressure

- This is the pattern used by weightlifters, furniture removers, martial arts devotees and wind instrument players.
- It is recruited to counter the downward impact on the pelvic floor and organs, e.g. sneeze, lift,

carry, drag, push (especially with inclines) and during impact activities (alighting from a bus or other high vehicle).

- Maintain a normal lumbar curve.
- Command: 'Make your waist wide and hold' (Kennedy, 1982). Muscle action: commencing with external obliques and adding transversus with internal obliques. Response: iliococcygeus, ischiococcygeus and then pubococcygeus.

Visceral interaction – sneeze

The sneezing pattern has been adapted from animal function, notably the cat. The cat's tail acts as the insertion for its levator muscles. The cat uses its tail as reinforced support during sneezing, i.e. it is wrapped around the body as the cat sits to sneeze. The cat braces, closes its glottis and uses its existing lung capacity before exhaling. As it releases the brace it creates a valve with the tongue moving down away from the roof of the mouth. The cat makes a well-supported sneeze and does not lose continence.

Many humans often make three errors – they inhale deeply on warning of a sneeze, they vocalize a sneeze and they recruit little or inappropriate abdomino-levator musculature. The consequent downward thrust is exerted predominantly on the pubococcygeus, with little lateral levator support for the viscera.

In learning to sneeze, brace and hold with a fixed diaphragm as the 'id' sound is made. This changes to 'choo' as the diaphragm forcibly expels the air. The timing of 'id' and 'choo' is variable.

Abdominal drawing in for coughing and lifting

- It should be recruited prior to raising the intra-abdominal pressure. It can be used as a preferred abdominopelvic floor pattern to bracing.
- Maintain a normal lumbar curve.
- Command: 'Draw in your abdomen at the bikini line, towards the lower back and hold' (Richardson and Jull, 1995). Muscle action: commencing with transversus and adding the obliques. Response: pubococcygeus, then iliococcygeus and ischiococcygeus.

Visceral interaction – cough

- Abdominal drawing in should occur before and be held during a cough/effort.
- The abdominopelvic floor coactivation is recruited before the diaphragm forces air up against a closed glottis, followed by sudden release of the glottis and expulsion of air.

These patterns facilitate trunk stability leading to improved pelvic floor function. From clinical observation, when a patient chooses to sit with a normal lumbar curve, rectus abdominis and puborectalis are no longer dominant abdomino-pelvic floor muscles.

Daily living presents many opportunities to incorporate muscle work around the home and at work. Muscle contraction, either PF or abdominal wall, must have been practised and be a familiar process before this can be done. When fitness activities are recommenced those that incorporate abdominal and PF activity, e.g. brisk walking, swimming, kick board work in the pool, should be chosen. The patient should grade into more vigorous activities. Abnormal fascial laxity will allow excessive organ movement if the generated IAP forces are great enough to overcome muscle support. Women with such problems should be advised not to return to high-impact, heavy gym or lifting activities. Incorporating voluntary PF or transversus abdominis activity during walking, jogging, etc. can give extra stability.

URGE CONTROL

Urgency to void occurs at any time but there are a number of situations, listed in the box, that women mention frequently.

Urge-provoking situations

On standing after quiet sitting

On rising from bed

While bending and moving

On homecoming – key in door

With the sound of running water

Entering a cold atmosphere

With anxiety

The urge generally occurs as a perineal sensation. Frequently there will be a loss of urine before reaching the toilet if the bladder is not quietened first. Some decrease in this urgency can occur with pelvic floor rehabilitation providing better bladder support. Lindstrom and Sudsuang (1989), in studies on cats, demonstrated inhibition of bladder activity on stimulation of the dorsal nerve of the penis and clitoris and afferent fibres from hip adductor muscles. Light pressure over the clitoris also produced inhibition. However, no such response occurred with stimulation of pelvic floor muscle afferents.

Women who suffer from urgency and urge incontinence can use several techniques, listed in the box, to inhibit the detrusor.

Methods of detrusor inhibition

Clitoral or perineal pressure by hand – young girls use this frequently.

Perineal pressure sitting on the edge of a hard seat, or folded towel.

Leg crossing in standing.

Strong gluteal contraction in standing.

It is important that the patient continues quiet breathing and does not increase IAP whilst controlling the urge. Once the bladder has quietened, in 10–15 seconds, the patient should stand carefully and walk to the toilet. However, the urge will recur as she approaches the toilet unless she can shift her mental focus away from the bladder. Counting every step en route to the toilet and breathing quietly can provide that focus. *Bladder Control: A Simple Self Help Guide* (Millard, 1987) gives a good outline of urge control and bladder training. A PFM or gluteal hold can be helpful in preventing urgency when turning on a tap or unlocking the door. If used to inhibit bladder activity, it must be initiated at the onset of the urge sensation otherwise detrusor activity will inhibit the urethral sphincter and other striated muscle activity. Some PFM strength and endurance is necessary for some of these techniques.

Mrs KT, a 49-year-old multipara, was referred to physiotherapy suffering from gradually worsening urinary incontinence. She had loss of urine on walking even short distances and needed to wear a panti-liner daily. She had been on combined hormone replacement therapy (HRT) and was just commencing cyclical use of progesterone. Urinary urgency and frequency had decreased since using HRT, but some urgency remained. She had a tendency to constipation, so was careful with her diet, consuming rye bread, 2–3 pieces of fruit and plenty of vegetables each day. She tended to get bloated at the end of the day. She practised pelvic floor exercises frequently, mostly in the car, but was unable to hold a contraction for long.

On examination, puborectalis was weak, with a 3–4 second wavering hold; right and left pubococcygeus, little lift and one-second hold. She tended to posterior pelvic tilt as she tried to hold the contraction. Transversus abdominis brought in a better pubococcygeal lift than did a voluntary pelvic floor contraction. Her evacuation pattern demonstrated a forward lean position with lumbar spine flexion and no abdominal bracing (waist widening).

Treatment consisted of pubococcygeal rehabilitation using a vaginal weight in lying, pelvic floor holds at other times in sitting and standing (always with a normal lumbar curve), urge control techniques, a corrected defaecation position and defaecation retraining and progressed to transversus abdominis strengthening as an exercise and also as a functional pattern for effort activities. Maintenance included abdominal drawing in, abdominal bracing and pelvic floor holds (some maximal five-second holds and some longer holds). Most of these were incorporated into fitness and general daily activities.

Bladder retraining

Bladder training aims to restore bladder capacity to near normal levels. Many people restrict fluid intake in an effort to control frequency and urine loss but increased fluid intake is often encouraged during treatment. Age, health status, activity levels and the weather should be taken into account when planning intake. It is often suggested that intake should be 1.5–2 litres of fluid a day. Renal function is adequately maintained if 1000 ml of urine is excreted in a day, so a large intake may not be necessary in the elderly. Patients with cardiac conditions should consult their doctors before increasing fluid intake.

Details of voided volumes and frequency are obtained from the frequency/volume chart. If voiding has become a habit and volumes are small (up to 100–150 ml) encouragement to defer and to cease 'just in case' voids can often be enough to begin to increase bladder capacity. Deferment for 2–3 minutes after the initial desire to void can gradually be extended. The bladder is trained to hold more urine. This may take three or more months.

Warning

If large bladder capacities, 600 ml and over, are a regular event, deferment of voiding should be discouraged. These people have a reduced bladder response to stretch and further stretch will worsen the condition. They should be encouraged to void approximately four-hourly even without a desire to void. At night, if they wake, they should not put off getting up to void. Long-term overstretching can lead to poor bladder contractility and incomplete emptying. This occurs in many elderly women.

More commonly, though, voiding is precipitated by a strong urge. Only after urge control methods have been practised and the patient knows that they work will she have the confidence to defer to increase capacity. No one is going to risk urine loss unnecessarily. It is important to set realistic goals. Many older people will never be able to defer, but reaching the toilet dry is a major achievement.

Some forms of bladder training aim at intervals of 3–4 hours between each void. This does not take into account varied fluid intake and activity patterns. Many women will consume several drinks between rising and with breakfast and follow this with household activities. Voiding in the morning tends to be more frequent, with larger intervals in the afternoon and during quiet periods. Urgency may never disappear, but it can be decreased and become controllable using the methods outlined.

Other treatment options are available. Oestrogen replacement, including vaginal oestrogen application, can be helpful. Medications such as oxybutinin, imipramine and propantheline are prescribed to quieten detrusor overactivity. These drugs have side effects of a dry mouth, dry eyes and decreased gastrointestinal motility and constipation and are contraindicated in narrow angle glaucoma. Electrotherapy – interferential and TENS – is said to be helpful, but studies are limited (see Chapter 24). Use of acupuncture has been reported in the literature. Severe intractable problems may eventually be treated surgically, using bladder augmentation procedures.

Mrs JG, aged 52 years, was referred to the physiotherapist by her GP, with a three-year history of urinary frequency with urge and bladder discomfort. It was gradually worsening. She voided from ½ to 2½-hourly during the day, with the longer interval being on 'good days'. Her micturition commenced without effort, but the flow tended to dribble and if she strained it did not improve. She had occasional stress incontinence with a sneeze. Nocturia was 0–1 times. She had to strain at times with defaecation, but evacuation was usually complete. She commented that she needed time to sit and relax to evacuate. She and her husband ran a business in a shopping complex in which they worked hard six days a week, in an attempt to recover from serious business problems.

On examination, puborectalis had good contraction (grade 4), with a hold of 3–4 seconds; right pubococcygeus had good bulk and strong lift (grade 5), with a 10-second hold which was slow to release; left had less bulk but good lift (grade 4), hold similar and slow to release. She had no awareness of muscle release.

On further questioning Mrs JG admitted that she was very busy and very stressed in her work environment, that she was better on her day at home and that she never sat on the toilet seat at work, always hovered above it. Her first void of the day was 500 ml and this was emptied without effort or discomfort. Day volumes were 25–150 ml.

Mrs JG was instructed to place paper on the toilet seat and to sit to void; to take time to fully release the pelvic floor muscles and to use the voiding retraining pattern, taking time to complete the void without straining. Emphasis was placed on pelvic floor release. Self-resisted hip abduction in sitting was used to facilitate adductor/PF release.

Within two weeks, day frequency was reduced, urine volumes increased and discomfort significantly improved. However, on stressful, busy days there was a tendency for the old hurried habits to return. Defaecation retraining was added later. Relaxation training was recommended, but business commitments restricted further treatment at that stage.

Voiding retraining

In patients whose pubococcygei or urethral sphincter do not relax prior to voiding, a change of voiding position and use of a specific abdominal pattern can facilitate bladder emptying. The pattern used includes a forward lean position, with a normal lumbar curve and the abdominal contents are allowed to fall forwards. The abdomen can then be pushed further forwards by diaphragmatic descent into a relaxed anterior abdominal wall. This pattern can be used to initiate micturition and also at the end to empty the bladder fully.

Uterovaginal Dysfunction

Muscle rehabilitation, activation of pelvic floor support during effort activities and defaecation retraining all have a part to play in cases of vaginal prolapse. The dragging discomfort, often experienced in the early stages of prolapse, can be helped in this way. In more obvious prolapse, surgery is generally required. However, if muscle strength is restored and functional retraining learnt prior to surgery, the repositioned organs have immediate support postoperatively.

Vaginal flatus can cause severe embarrassment. Weak pelvic floor muscles allow air to enter a capacious upper vagina. Its forced expulsion with increased IAP can result in audible release. While PF exercises should be practised, muscle patterns associated with defaecation retraining may enable expulsion of the air. If the problem is severe it may require surgery to narrow the vagina.

Other Interventions

Muscle rehabilitation and functional use of the pelvic floor generally do not improve fascial laxity, so alternative approaches may be needed. These may not be instituted by the physiotherapist, but knowledge of what is available is helpful. In cases of genuine stress incontinence, devices placed vaginally can be used to improve bladder neck support. Introl (Johnson and Johnson) and Continence Guard (Coloplast, Denmark) are two examples. Some women will use a lubricated tampon to support the bladder neck during an exercise session. Care must be taken that the vaginal mucosa is not abraded with too frequent tampon use and that the tampon is removed after exercising.

A urethral plug device (Avina, Convatec) has been developed to prevent leakage in cases of genuine stress incontinence. It is a single-use, soft flexible plastic 'bubble' with its own applicator.

In cases of uterovaginal prolapse a ring pessary can be used to support the upper vagina and cervix above the levator muscles. Figure 30.5 shows how this provides support. This may be used in older women who are unwilling or unfit to undergo surgery. The pessary will not stay in place if there is marked pubococcygeal muscle atrophy.

The use of catheters is necessary for some people. Self-catheterization, often referred to as intermittent clean self-catheterization (ICSC), has provided freedom for many people with urinary retention. No longer do they have to use a leg bag with an indwelling catheter. The clean, non-sterile procedure, in which the catheter is inserted only for long enough to empty the bladder, is carried out by the subject at 3–4-hourly intervals throughout the day and perhaps once at night, with little risk of infection. Indwelling catheters may be used with a valve, which allows intermittent emptying in the day and attachment to a collection bag at night.

In those cases where loss of urine cannot be controlled, a wide range of absorbent pads and pants are available which ensure comfort and containment. These allow the sufferer to socialize without embarrassment. Contact the nearest continence centre for more information on disposable and reusable absorbent aids.

Surgery Surgical repair is required in many cases of fascial laxity (see Chapter 27 for a brief outline of surgery). Even when the patient requires surgery, PFM strengthening prior to the operation develops the best possible supporting mechanism for the repositioned organs. Klarskov et al (1986) noted that operative results following surgery for stress incontinence were especially good in patients who had PFM training prior to surgery.

Recently collagen has been injected around the urethra to improve closure. While very effective, it is currently rather expensive and is not a permanent solution.

Figure 30.5 Illustration of a ring pessary in place in the vaginal fornices, above the supporting pelvic floor muscles. (Reproduced from *Illustrated Textbook of Gynaecology*, Mackay EV, Beischer NA, Pepperell RJ and Wood C (1992) 2nd edn, W.B. Saunders, with permission of Professor EV Mackay and the publisher.)

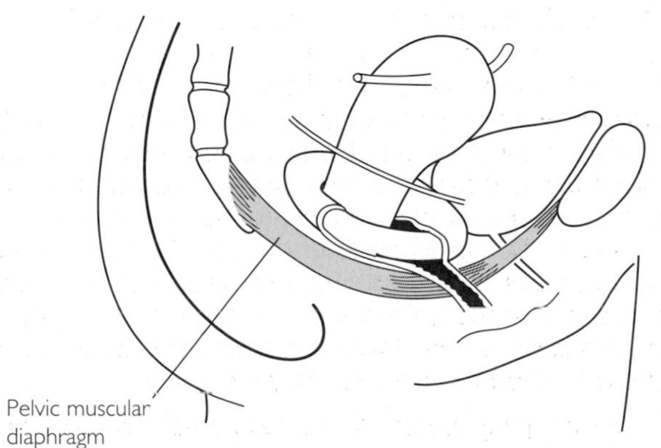

Enuresis alarms for bed wetting These aim to teach the bed wetter to wake to the sensation of a full bladder and to allow her to get up to void. As with other treatment for nocturnal enuresis, the impetus for change must come from the sufferer, not her mother. Hence treatment usually has to wait until the age of 7–8 years, though this treatment is also used for many adolescent girls.

There are two types of alarms. With the bell and pad alarm, the sensor pad is placed between two layers of sheeting and the alarm is placed at a distance from the bed. This alarm is usually hired. The body-worn alarm has a small sensor inserted in the underwear and the alarm is pinned to the clothing. This is reasonably cheap and is frequently purchased by the family.

Both alarms sound as soon as urine completes a circuit. The child wakes, stops the flow of urine, turns off the alarm, gets up to void the remainder, showers and dresses and helps to remake the bed. Initially the child may not wake and has to be woken by a parent. Early in the programme the whole family may be disturbed by the alarm, so treatment during the long school holidays may be preferable. The most satisfactory results from use of alarms come from good instruction and regular supervision and encouragement. It may take 2–3 months for the treatment to be effective. Sometimes alarm treatment is not effective at the first attempt.

For further details on suitability, management and access to alarms contact a continence clinic in your area or the Enuresis Resource and Information Centre in Bristol, UK.

Other treatment for bed wetting depends on the particular problem and includes urge control, bladder training and replacement of antidiuretic hormone at night (see Chapter 8).

Physiotherapy treatment outcomes

Many studies have looked at the benefits of pelvic floor exercise in the treatment of genuine stress incontinence. Exercise has often been combined with electrotherapy, use of vaginal weights and biofeedback. Many aspects of the studies varied. These included quantification of urine loss, verification of correct muscle action, pre- and post-treatment measurement of PFM strength, type of electrotherapy used, exercise programmes used, number of exercise sessions, length of overall programme and home exercise regimen.

Thus comparison between the studies is extremely difficult but an excellent review article has been written recently by Bo (1995). It seems that the optimum outcome from rehabilitation requires the exercise programme to continue for 5–6 months (Bo et al, 1989; Hesse et al, 1990). Bo and Talseth (1996) followed up their study subjects five years after an intensive exercise programme. The success rate of 60% was maintained after cessation of the formal treatment programme, with 70% still exercising at least once a week.

Different physiotherapists have advocated the use of electrotherapy in treatment programmes. Interferential therapy has had a reputation as being beneficial in the treatment of genuine stress incontinence and has been widely used (Mantle and Versi, 1991). Haig et al (1995) were unable to demonstrate a significant advantage in the use of interferential in addition to the exercise programme. However, the study subjects perceived a benefit from the use of an external 'machine'.

Improvement in muscle strength rather than endurance has generally been the aim of physiotherapists in the treatment of genuine stress incontinence. Laycock et al (1995), in a recent study, used two different muscle stimulation protocols, along with exercise and biofeedback. Chronic low-frequency stimulation (for endurance) was compared with short-term maximal intensity stimulation (for strength) and with exercise and biofeedback alone. The combined proportion of cured and improved was similar in each group. Stimulation at maximal intensity resulted in far greater strength yet that strength increase was not reflected in a greater improvement in function. Further analysis of strength versus endurance needs to be carried out.

Prevention

While the preceding section has covered assessment and treatment of established conditions, there is much that each woman can do to avoid problems and prevent deterioration. Learnt early in life, these steps become a life-long habit.

A regular fitness programme which incorporates the abdominals in pelvic and spinal stability during movement and hip extensor and adductor exercise can maintain good PFM strength and endurance. Other steps to be taken include:

- adequate fibre and fluid in the diet;
- abdomino/PF patterns during effort activities;
- avoidance of straining at defaecation;
- voiding only when necessary, not 'just in case';
- a few PF exercises on a regular basis.

These will all pay dividends throughout life for all women.

Anorectal Dysfunction

Anorectal dysfunction is not new to physiotherapists and early efforts were directed to faecal incontinence. Exercise therapy has been considered the 'Cinderella' of conservative medical management of faecal incontinence. Clinical progress has been slow and the results disappointing. Mills et al (1990), Fox et al (1991) and Farragher (1993) highlighted different aspects of physiotherapy management. Papachrysostomou et al (1994) looked at electrical stimulation of the pelvic floor and proctographic parameters. In 1995, Mills et al showed that there was significant diagnostic accuracy of the strength duration curve in demonstrating neuropathy of the external anal sphincter (EAS) for 'at risk' post-partum women. This application may facilitate early detection and encourage intervention. The quest for improved treatment methods to complement standard medical management of faecal incontinence led to the widespread use of behavioural training and biofeedback.

Until the late 1980s the effect of straining at stool on supporting structures and other pelvic organ function was not widely understood. Clinical and physiological research in the 1980s and 1990s paved the way for integrated management. Biofeedback was used in the treatment of anal outlet disorders to relieve constipation (Kuijpers and Bleijenberg, 1990).

In Australia, a fresh look at functional disorders and defaecation retraining was undertaken by a multidisciplinary team (Markwell et al, 1993). Successful collaboration with colorectal surgeons, physiotherapists and primary practitioners encouraged early involvement of other specialties.

The concept of total function has gained acceptance, as many specialties are involved with the pelvis, its muscles, soft tissue and its viscera. Gastrointestinal function is extremely complex and is still poorly understood. Many factors impinge on visceral function. Pharmacological agents directed at altering autonomic or neurotransmitter function are few and the effects of polypharmacy on gut function are many. The physiotherapist must understand that the following all affect gut function: inappropriate fluid and fibre intake; stress, hormonal and psychological factors; inflammatory and neurological diseases; surgical and obstetric history; present and past immobility and abuse states (sexual, eating, drug and alcohol). Pelvic visceral function relies on smooth muscle with intact autonomic pathways and complex striated muscle recruitment for appropriate sensation, retention and evacuation of contents.

It is strongly recommended that the physiotherapist reads *Let's Get Things Moving* (Chiarelli and Markwell, 1992) in conjunction with this chapter.

Who is qualified to analyse and teach?

The concept of visceral function and physiotherapy is challenging to the therapist, the patient and the medical personnel involved in the patient's care. The adoption of biofeedback (EMG and pressure) by the medical profession has shown that learning or relearning a specific task is required in certain anorectal conditions.

Physiotherapists are the ideal members of the team to analyse muscle dysfunction, correct specific deficiencies and teach co-ordinated function. As anorectal dysfunction is an area traditionally handled by the nursing and medical profession, the importance of the principles of rehabilitation and their mode of delivery must be understood and must be effective. Physiotherapy treatment for any condition calls for evaluation and ongoing re-evaluation of the primary dysfunction and progression of treatment. Attainable goals must be implemented. The patient must have a clear understanding of the expectations of treatment.

It may be difficult for patient and practitioner to appreciate the minimal size of the pelvic floor muscles and their complicated interaction. For example, pubococcygeus and puborectalis adjoin one another, may be an index finger in thickness and yet are able to reverse functional roles.

Appropriate teaching aids include models, X-rays, diagrams and handouts. Handouts should show basic anatomy, use colours to denote different pelvic floor and abdominal muscle integrated activity and give precise instructions on desired activities.

Defaecation

Defaecation is a complex physiological process dependent on co-ordinated smooth and striated muscle activity (see Chapter 7). It requires rectal support, anal outlet release and an effective abdominal expulsive effort. In normal defaecation, in most subjects, the rectum is emptied completely and this occurs without undue effort. At the appropriate time and place the subject sits or squats. A forward-leaning sitting position has been shown to lengthen the anal aperture and widen the anorectal angle, which puborectalis controls (Tagart, 1966). This can occur in squatting with a straight lumbar spine, with varying degrees of hip flexion (Fig. 30.6, 30.9).

When the woman is positioned effectively, relaxation of puborectalis, the external anal sphincter and the levator plate usually occurs. Increased IAP is used to initiate rectal emptying. Transversus abdominis (TrA) is the principal muscle in raising IAP. However in defaecation, the external obliques initiate the pressure rise, closely followed by the internal obliques and TrA, and then the diaphragm descends to a low level. This process resembles a 'bellows' action. As the IAP is maintained the pelvic floor descends 2–3 cm. As defaecation proceeds the raised IAP compresses the rectum against the coactivated supporting pubococcygeus (Lubowski et al, 1992). Activation of the external (and internal) obliques in abdominal bracing (Kennedy, 1982), seems to trigger contraction of iliococcygeus in particular. This elevation of the lateral levator plate further supports the rectum. Muscle slips from pubococcygeus contract to shorten the anus (funnelling).

In forward-lean sitting (Fig 30.9), gravity allows the anterior shift of abdominal contents. A downward pressure from the diaphragm will push the lower abdomen out and lengthen rectus abdominis (RA). TrA is the main visceral supporting muscle and takes the weight so that RA can move into outer range. By 'bulging' the abdomen, i.e. lengthening RA with an isometric hold in its outer range, puborectalis is able to release and anal shortening and widening occur (Sapsford et al, 1996) (Fig. 30.7). The anorectal angle must become obtuse (Fig. 30.8). Rectus abdominis working isometrically with the diaphragm further increases the compression to enhance expulsion.

Emptying may be assisted by colonic peristalsis. At the end of defaecation a closing reflex occurs in the internal and external anal sphincters, puborectalis and the levator plate. The anus assumes its closed attitude and the pelvic floor ascends to its normal position. Quick five-second repetitions of the pattern, allowing the anus to funnel and widen, may follow. Rapid repetitions are useful to empty fully (in the case of a megarectum), to check that nothing is present to cause a later urge to stool and to help discrimination of mucosal prolapse into the anus. The latter can give false messages of solid stool. This process is the 'trapdoor' function.

The body pattern which accompanies normal defaecation includes an upright or forward-lean sitting posture, with a normal lumbar curve. As the defaecatory effort is made, the waist widens laterally, the lower abdominal wall bulges forward and the lumbar spine does not lose its curve (Fig. 30.9). There is no spinal movement.

Anorectal muscle assessment

This assessment must only be conducted with a full understanding of the anatomy involved.

Figure 30.6 Squatting positions vary from East to West. Note the different lumbar spine positions, occuring with limited tendo-achilles extensibility. The flexed spine does not facilitate rectal emptying.

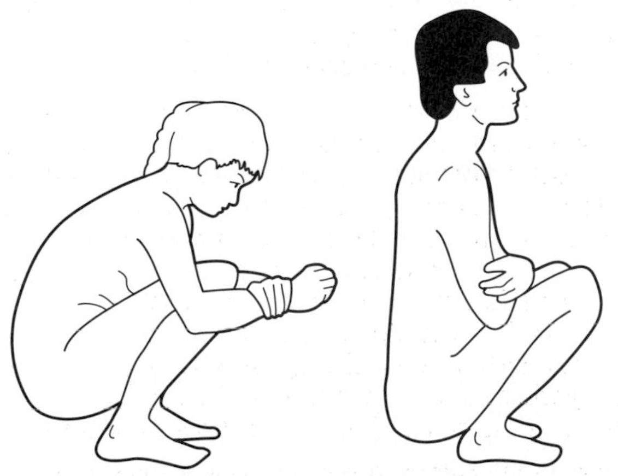

Figure 30.7 Diagrammatic representation of the anal sphincter and the pelvic floor at rest and during defaecation in normal subjects. The fine straight line indicates the level of the ischial tuberosities.

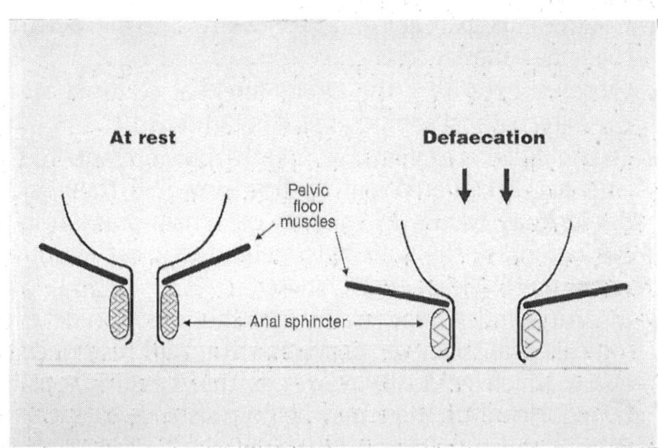

Figure 30.8 During defaecation the anorectal angle becomes obtuse and the anus shortens and widens. Anus closed (above) and during defaecation (below).

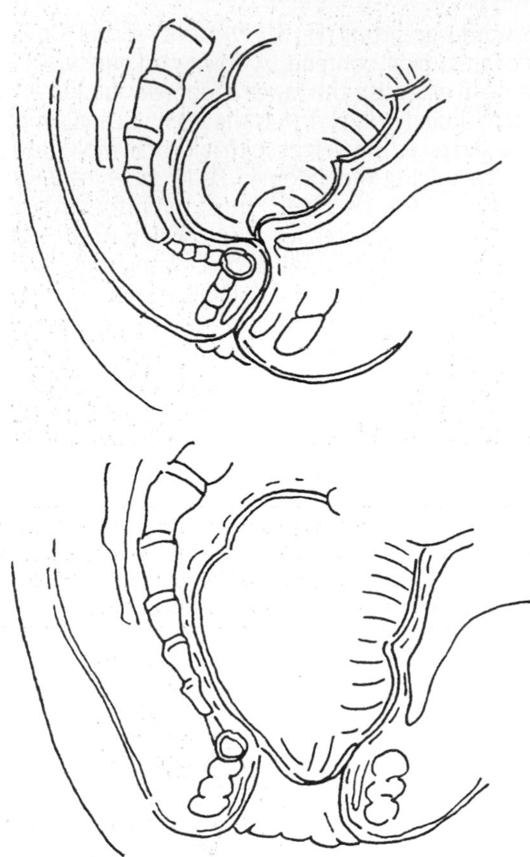

Figure 30.9 A forward-lean defaecation position, with bracing and lower abdominal bulging. The height of the subject determines the need for a foot stool. (Reproduced from *Australian Journal of Physiotherapy* (1995), **41**: 281 with permission of the Australian Physiotherapy Association.)

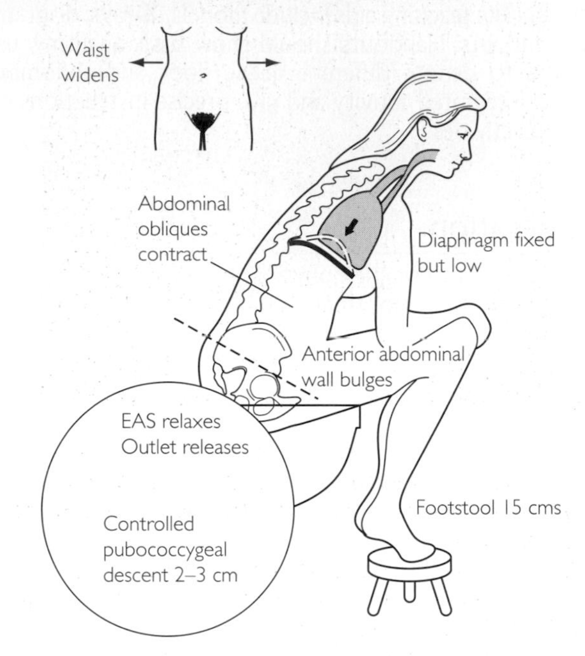

Figure 30.10 A simple diagram to record the findings of an anorectal muscle assessment.

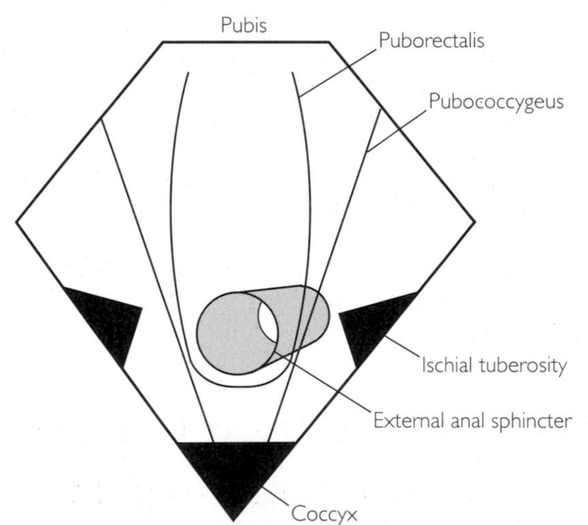

- The patient is comfortably positioned in left lateral, with knees drawn to the chest.
- A suitable covering preserves modesty.
- Clean gloves must be used even if rectal examination follows vaginal.
- Explain to the patient what is about to be done. No instruments will be used, only a gloved moistened index finger which will feel wet.
- Look for perineal descent at rest and on straining (see Fig. 23.1).
- Pull the anus apart at 9 and 3 o'clock to ascertain whether the anus gapes at rest.
- Observe externally the circumferential contraction of the external anal sphincter as it is tightened.
- To begin digital examination, gently apply pressure to the anus and ask the patient to 'bear down'. If there is no descent, as occurs in anismus or a high-pressure anal sphincter, ask the patient to bulge the lower abdomen forwards to release the sphincter.
- Insert the index finger slowly into the anus. A functional internal anal sphincter provides a constant resistance to entry, which gradually relaxes as the pressure is maintained. However, there may be no resistance to entry.
- Palpate the anus circumferentially, slowly and carefully, noting dehiscence (thinning or absence) of the muscle at the exterior or deeper in the funnel.
- Ask the patient to contract as the finger is moved slowly circumferentially. Muscle injury/tears are usually in the anterior quadrant.
- Explain that puborectalis is to be palpated. This may be felt as a strong bar posteriorly or may be obtuse and offer no resistance.
- Palpate posteriorly to locate the coccyx – note any pain on stretch or pressure on the muscle or coccyx.

Figure 30.11 Fascial stretch and poor muscle support allow marked descent on defaecation straining. This lack of support is an example of muscle imbalance in obstructed defaecation. Defaecograms show the anorectal angle at rest (a) and gross pelvic floor descent on straining and emptying (b).

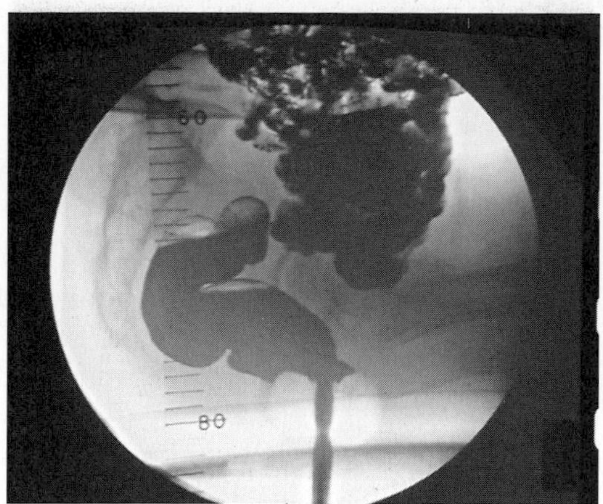

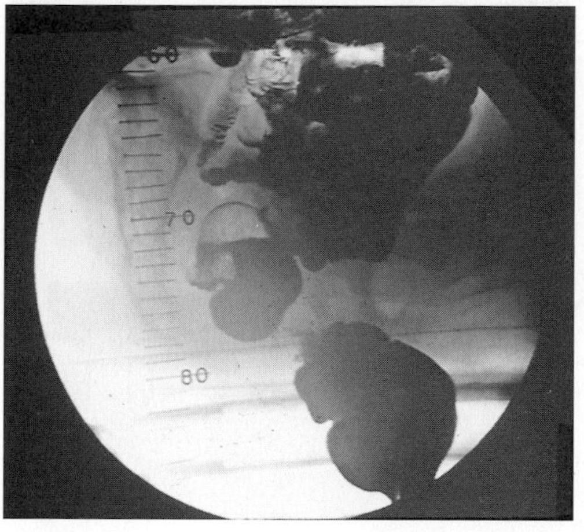

- Reassure the patient about the process. Explain the feeling of wanting to evacuate. Talk through each step of the examination.
- Puborectalis, pubococcygeus and iliococcygeus may all be palpated, though muscle identification is an acquired skill and individual variations occur.
- Palpate for atrophy, hypertrophy, imbalance and assess proprioception.
- Withdraw the examining finger carefully. Talk to the patient.
- Make the patient clean, comfortable, dry and cover her.
- Remove gloves and immediately wash hands.
- Write down the findings of the examination. These could be recorded on a diagram (Fig. 30.10).
- Withdraw to another room so that the patient can dress in privacy.
- Discuss the examination with the patient using diagrams to illustrate findings and function.

With experience, identification of levator deficiencies and dyskinesia can be made accurately per vaginam. Suspected anal sphincter defects still require anal examination.

Treatment of obstructed defaecation

ASSESSMENT FINDINGS AND TREATMENT PLANNING

Consider the following.

1. What muscles function normally?
2. Is the muscle capable of responding to conservative methods?
3. Is neuropathy severe?
4. Is NMS required?
5. Is there a reversal of muscle roles?
6. What muscle dysfunction must be prevented?
7. What order should be used for functional correction?
8. Can muscle rehabilitation improve *function* within the level of the patient's structural abnormality?

Figure 30.12 Poor defaecation pattern, resulting in perineal descent and inadequate release of the anal outlet. Note the abdominal retraction. (Reproduced from *Australian Journal of Physiotherapy* (1995), **41**: 281 with permission of the Australian Physiotherapy Association.)

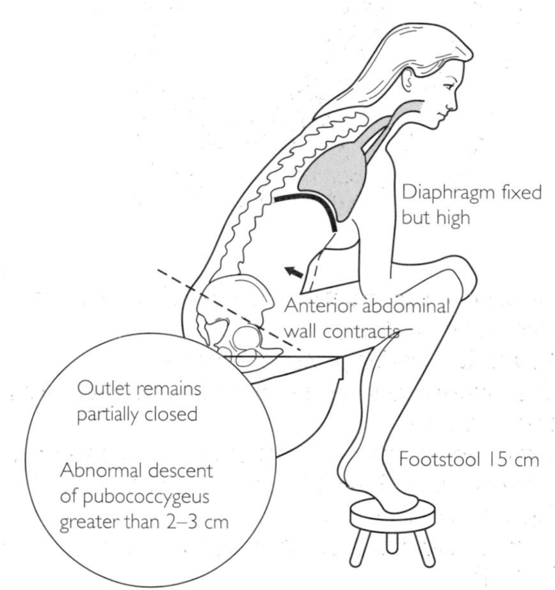

9. Could rehabilitation and retraining complement surgical intervention?

The supporting muscles, pubococcygeus, iliococcygeus and ischiococcygeus, are often inadequate, as a result of pelvic and pudendal nerve neuropathy (Fig. 30.11). Puborectalis often takes on a supporting role and loses its ability for co-ordinated release (Fig. 30.12). This process can also occur by selective abdominal muscle overdevelopment.

The basic aim of physiotherapy is to teach the patient to create an anal funnel and effectively empty the rectum, without compromising support. The effect of inappropriate muscle function (dyskinesia) will be to undermine organ

Figure 30.13 Diagrammatic representation of the anal sphincter and the pelvic floor during defaecation in subjects with patterns of imbalance and inco-ordination. The fine straight line indicates the level of the ischial tuberosities.

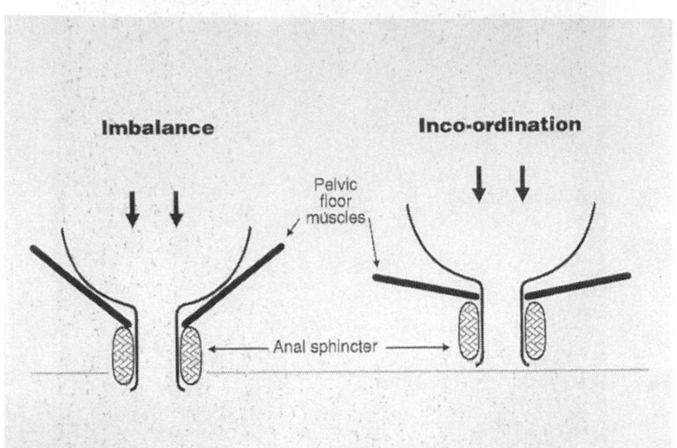

support and increase the mechanical derangements, e.g. the anterior rectal wall can become lax (rectocoele) as a result of straining at stool. Mechanical disorders may be categorized as those of *imbalance* and *inco-ordination* and must be treated as separate conditions (Figs 30.13, 30.14). An outline for the treatment of obstructed defaecation (imbalance and inco-ordination) is provided in Table 30.2.

Recent research has confirmed clinical observations that a co-activation occurs between specific abdominal and pelvic floor muscles. These findings have been instrumental in unlocking the key to pelvic organ and pelvic floor dysfunction (Markwell and Sapsford 1995, Richardson and Jull 1995, Sapsford et al 1996). Further research is in progress. As a result of these findings pelvic floor muscle rehabilitation can be approached in two ways. See Table 30.3. The particular approach used depends on the findings at assessment. Gross pathology requires very specific muscle activation, and in these cases direct pelvic floor rehabilitation must be the initial approach.

In training patients with anal outlet obstruction, it is important to increase IAP without increasing anal sphincter pressure. In response to this need a new method for treating patients has been devised. The training incorporates abdominal bracing together with lower abdominal bulging with a held breath (Markwell and Sapsford, 1995). During this pattern of simulated defaecation there is a lowering of anal sphincter activity towards the resting level. Defaecation retraining is outlined in Table 30.4. During recent research, significant increases in external oblique and rectus abdominis activity were noted during 'brace and bulge' as compared with bracing alone (Sapsford et al, 1996). This pattern has been shown to be extremely effective in clinical treatments. A randomized trial of biofeedback versus the muscle co-ordination retraining programme was shown to substantiate the clinical methods described here (Koutsomanis et al, 1995).

Steps in relearning the defaecation process

- Let the abdomen 'fall into your hands'.
- Bulge the anterior abdominal wall forward, i.e. as though you have swallowed a beach ball.
- Note that rectus abdominis (RA) must bulge, not retract. The ease with which this occurs will depend on the extensibility of RA.
- Should RA retract, the patient returns to the resting position and the process is repeated.
- Practise bracing before and hold during the bulge.
- Practise the pattern while seated on a firm chair.
- When brace and bulge has been mastered this is to be used as a *toilet technique only*.
- *Note*: Individual components of the pattern must be practised to maintain the pattern of recruitment. Individual components need checking, then the patient can learn to analyse and self-correct.

POSTURAL CONSIDERATIONS IN DEFAECATION RETRAINING

> The optimal sitting position involves bearing weight on the ischial tuberosities, the greater trochanters and the backs of the thighs. The trunk is held relatively straight so that the centre of gravity falls through the pelvis between the ischial tuberosities and greater trochanters (Sikorski, 1986, p. 149).

Toilet seats do not provide this support.

Subjects may choose to sit on or slump into the toilet:

- in a relaxed slumped position with lumbar flexion. In this position it is difficult to lengthen RA effectively and it can shorten, thus tightening puborectalis. Transversus abdominis may be more difficult to recruit in this position;
- leaning back with the centre of gravity behind the weight-bearing base, thus using abdominal muscles to hold them in equilibrium. RA is able to lengthen fully, but the body position is hard to maintain. Patients with anterior rectal wall mucosal prolapse often choose this position.

Before the ideal toilet position can be adopted tight fascial structures may require stretching in some patients. These tight structures prevent full forward movement of the trunk, while maintaining a lumbar curve, to allow the patient's arms to rest on her thighs (see Fig. 30.9).

WHAT HELPS AND WHAT HINDERS?

Various techniques can be used to improve the defaecation retraining. Some of these are included in Table 30.5.

At-risk women in the community are those who have trained to develop or maintain a 'flat abdomen' where

Figure 30.14 An inco-ordinated defaecation pattern (a) at rest and (b) on attempted evacuation. The anorectal angle does not relax and the contents cannot be released.

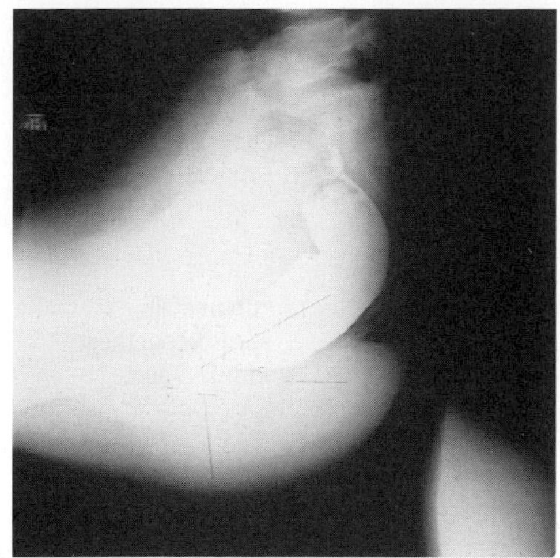

a

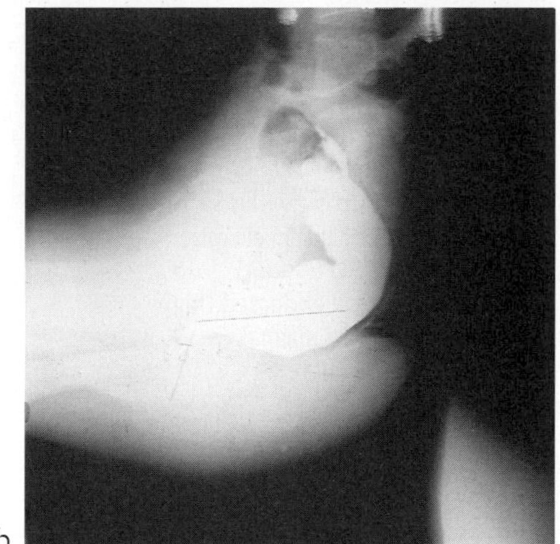

b

Table 30.2 Treatment plan for obstructed defaecation

	Imbalance – obstructed defaecation		Inco-ordination – 'anismus'
	• History • Physical examination • Per vaginam • ?Per rectum • Posture in sit / stand • Associated symptoms		• History • Physical examination • Per rectum • ?Per vaginam • Posture in sit / stand • Associated symptoms
Duration 3–4 months	Address major complaint first • PC rehabilitation • Dietary advice • Defaecation position • Bulging to release urethral and anal sphincters	Months 1–2	Address major complaint first • Defaecation position • Correct slumped sitting posture • Full defaecation retraining • Dietary advice
	Follow on with • Abdomino / PF patterns • ↑ Trunk stability • Complete defaecation retraining • Pain measures • Re-evaluate muscle rehab.	Months 3–4	Follow on with • Abdomino / PF patterns • PC rehab. if descent commencing • Pain measures • Maintenance
Review at 6 months	• Surgical intervention • Maintenance	Review frequently	• ? Refer for counselling

Table 30.3 Pelvic floor and abdominal approaches to rehabilitation of the pelvic floor muscles

Approach	Pubococcygeus (PC)	Iliococcygeus and ischiococcygeus	Puborectalis, external anal sphincter
Pelvic floor	PC lifts +/− weights NMS	Unilateral – lateral levator movements (tail wagging) Lift anus, direct tail bone towards knee, hold, release	Rectal lifts – lift up and to the front *Caution* – EAS squeezes may attenuate anal scar tissue
Abdominal	TrA – abdominal indrawing	Bracing – quick, sustained	Rectus abdominis work – posterior pelvic tilts, sit-ups

Table 30.4 Defaecation retraining

Position	Action	Primary muscle action	Pelvic muscle co-activation
Forward-lean sitting with feet plantarflexed and heels resting on the pedestal OR Forward-lean sitting with feet on 15 cm footstool and heels raised Hips flexed > 90° Forearms rest on abducted thighs Back is straight – maintain a normal lumbar curve	Specific abdominal muscle contraction to support levators	External obliques + TrA and IO	Iliococcygeus and ischiococcygeus. Pubococcygeus support
	Compress contents – *bracing* Open funnel – *bulging*	Rectus abdominis lengthening action Diaphragm then fixed	Puborectalis release, together with IAS and EAS

Table 30.5 Techniques to facilitate defaecation retraining

Pubococcygeus	Puborectalis	Lateral levators	External anal sphincter
How to enhance • Drawing up during coitus • Drawing in as a postural aid (TrA)	Why does it increase? • Posterior pelvic tilting • Habitual slumped sitting position • Sit-ups/crunches • Straining at stool	How to enhance • Correct lifting • Bracing • Martial arts preparation	Why does it increase? • Activities that enhance pubococcygeus • Subconscious tightening with clinical 'ismus' conditions
Negating factors • Impact activities • Coughing • Heavy lifting • Rowing machine • Netball • Basketball • Wind instrument use • Gymnastics • Singing • Vomiting • Straining at stool	How to decrease the overactivity • Practise 'bulging' as an exercise	Negating factors • Incorrect lifting • Poor martial arts techniques • Selective body building • Straining at stool	How does it decrease? • Recurrent diarrhoea • Obstructed defaecation – straining to empty (long term). • Alcoholism increases colon transit and leads to increased frequency

posterior pelvic tilting is especially encouraged, e.g. ballet. This can lead to an inco-ordinate defaecation pattern. Swimmers develop all abdominopelvic floor muscles. These elite athletes often sustain gross neuropathy during childbirth, as the musculature does not relax, or has limited extensibility, during the expulsive phase.

Mrs WA, a 70-year-old primipara, presented initially with stress urinary incontinence. She suffered from asthma. She had an extensive surgical history including a Manchester repair, an abdominal hysterectomy with left salpingo-oophorectomy, an anterior and posterior vaginal repair, a posterior vaginal repair, abdominoperineal repair of an enterocoele and a bladder neck suspension. Urodynamic investigation demonstrated genuine stress incontinence and urethral syndrome was diagnosed. Defaecography showed a low perineum at rest with no further descent on straining, non-release of the anorectal angle and little rectal motility. On initial physiotherapy contact she had a third-degree cystourethrocoele and admitted to a long history of straining at stool and use of hand support for defaecation. She chose to have further surgery in another city.

Two years later she was referred to physiotherapy with obstructed defaecation and genuine stress incontinence. Physiotherapy treatment progressed through defaecation retraining (position, brace and bulge) followed by pubococcygeal rehabilitation using a vaginal weight and integrated abdominopelvic floor patterns.

She was able to evacuate effectively without further structural damage and her stress incontinence resolved.

It is well documented that faecal incontinence can occur as a late-stage complication of obstructed defaecation and the evacuation straining that is required. This type of faecal incontinence has been attributed to pelvic floor denervation as a result of straining (Kiff et al, 1984).

Faecal incontinence

When the patient presents with uncontrolled loss of flatus, faecal soiling or frank faecal loss, a global approach to assessment and treatment must be taken. If medical assessment and investigations have not yet taken place, then a thorough understanding of the aetiology, pathogenesis and management must dictate how the patient is primarily managed and when to send her for secondary referral.

Global factors represent all information ascertained in history taking that affect visceral and pelvic floor function. They may include:

- cognition;
- diet, fluid intake, travel, poor toilet facilities;
- straining at defaecation;
- motility;
- medical history;
- medication;
- hormonal factors;
- obstetric and surgical history (for congenital and acquired conditions);
- results of physiological tests – ↑ or ↓ rectal compliance, rectal sensation, IAS and EAS pressures, incomplete and complete anal sphincter tears;
- mobility;
- local anorectal symptoms;
- pain.

Faecal incontinence can be divided into two types:

1. urge incontinence (when the subject is trying to 'hold on') indicates a defect of external anal sphincter and puborectalis function (Engel et al, 1995);
2. passive incontinence (when the subject is unaware of impending loss) indicates a defect of internal anal sphincter function (Engel et al, 1995).

- In cases of sphincter trauma medical investigation is the first intervention.
- Many patients will complain of soiling after emptying. This almost always indicates lack of rectal awareness with ineffective emptying, +/– an overstretched rectum which contracts poorly.
- One of the most common complaints is failure to, or difficulty in, cleaning the anus after emptying. This may indicate inappropriate abdominopelvic floor co-ordination during defaecation (poor support and ineffective opening). Emptying may be likened to squeezing a toothpaste tube in the middle and observing the residual ooze of paste, when the required amount has been applied to the brush.
- *Rectal sensation is the most important parameter to consider when planning treatment. 'Empty vessels don't leak'.*

Consistency of stool is very important. In mild or moderate cases attempts must be made to avoid flatulence-producing foods and achieve a soft bulky stool, which aids more complete emptying. Medication and dietary manipulation may have to be employed to regulate formed stool, should the patient's overall condition dictate (e.g. where there is little or no anal muscle). Rectal agents may be required to regulate emptying. Local oestrogen may be useful.

If soluble fibre supplements are suggested:

- small dosage is usual;
- extra fluid is required;
- space prescription medication and bulking agent to ensure effective medication absorption

The presence of incomplete internal and external anal tears combined with neuropathy will be more difficult to treat.

PHYSIOTHERAPY

Physiotherapy management of faecal incontinence is outlined in Table 30.6.

Physiotherapy plays a complementary role when surgery is required to repair sphincter trauma associated with childbirth and accidents. This may range from full pelvic floor rehabilitation and defaecation retraining prior to closure of a temporary stoma, to complementary therapy associated with operative repair of the sphincter. In some conditions associated with neuropathy, persistent rectal mucosal prolapse into the anus renders a 'forced opening' of an already compromised sphincter. Rehabilitation following surgery to remove the prolapse and plicate the sphincters is proving successful. This involves complex physiotherapy programmes using the normal methods of rehabilitation in combination with biofeedback.

BIOFEEDBACK (BFB)

This has been used in the treatment of faecal incontinence and obstructed anal outlet conditions (inco-ordination), e.g. anismus. It is based on operant psychological conditioning using anorectal pressure microtransducers, balloons, auditory and visual stimuli. It has been used with all ages and both sexes.

BFB requires costly equipment, suitable methods of decontamination and sterilization and the therapist's time. The patient is not given formal instruction in the muscle coordination required for effective defaecation retraining.

Table 30.6 Treatment plan for faecal incontinence

Neuropathic faecal incontinence	Trauma-induced faecal incontinence
• History • Physical examination – per vaginam and per rectum • Relevant investigations • Posture in sitting/standing • Associated symptoms, e.g. urinary incontinence • Address major complaint first	• History • Physical examination – per vaginam and per rectum • Refer for investigation
Treatment • Treat obstructed defaecation and descending perineum syndrome • Assist with correct usage of bulking/rectal agents for easy, timed emptying • Refer for investigation if first contact practitioner • ? Surgical intervention to lengthen anal canal • ? Biofeedback • ? Abdominal patterns for puborectalis	*Treatment* • Treat associated symptoms • Complement surgical intervention • Rehabilitate levator plate • *Do not exercise anal sphincter* – because of attenuation of muscle and scar tissue • ? Biofeedback

In the application to faecal incontinence, existing methods have improved rectal sensation and anal squeeze pressure but the IAS/EAS resting pressures have shown little quantitative improvement. In the future, complementary therapy of pelvic floor physiotherapy and pressure BFB (using microtransducers) will be used in selected cases.

Associated medical conditions

- Women in special situations must be considered. These might range from frank sexual abuse or rape to neurological conditions common in the community.
- Diabetes will manifest autonomic disturbance.
- Multiple sclerosis will present with complex urinary and defaecatory symptoms.
- Post-poliomyelitis patients, formerly thought to have lower motor neurone lesions limiting disability to atrophy and imbalance of the striated musculature, now have indications of smooth muscle involvement of the gut.
- Parkinsonian patients suffer from obstructed defaecation due to co-ordination difficulties.

However, lifestyle events, obstetric and surgical history suggest that pelvic floor dysfunction may be related, in the first instance, to vaginal delivery. All investigations and treatment should be directed to this, with the descending perineum syndrome and pudendal neuropathy being the common denominator on which specific clinical entities are superimposed.

Electrotherapy

1. From clinical experience, NMS is best reserved for those who do not respond to conservative measures.
2. This is not a first-line approach, except when gross neuropathy is present.
3. The vagina is the pelvic organ designed to accommodate penetration.
4. Vaginal applications are preferable to anal use when considering the levator plate.
5. Individual instruction may be given for pubococcygeus or puborectalis or combined muscle rehabilitation if required.
6. Anal stimulation should be used with care, as introduction of applicators may damage delicate or attenuated scar tissue and no gain is made.
7. Fatigue signs, similar to those that occur with the use of weights (adductor shaking and inability to repeat the exercise), can occur with NMS. With gross neuropathy this can occur after a very short time.

Mrs SM, a 64-year-old multipara (2), had a history of rectal prolapse and anal fistulae requiring extensive surgery. Following surgery she had faecal impaction for three weeks and had to be manually disimpacted. She was using Metamucil, Coloxyl and glycerin suppositories to manage her condition. She was referred to physiotherapy for pelvic floor exercise following post-anal repair.

On examination at physiotherapy, the anus was open at rest and the rectal lining was prolapsed. Muscle assessment: external anal sphincter, nil; puborectalis, weak; pubococcygeus, atrophied with poor proprioception and very weak contraction. There was right-sided anal pain on sitting.

Physiotherapy treatment included pubococcygeal rehabilitation using a vaginal catheter and then a vaginal weight; defaecation retraining; patterns for IAP increases; pain strategies and the use of a protective prosthesis to control pain. After rehabilitation there was no change in the anal gape or the anal sphincter function, but the patient was pain free and continent. Two years later she was still pain free and was faecally continent. She had avoided a colostomy and no longer needed her pain prosthesis. Functional continence has been maintained for five years and she leads a physically and socially active life.

The overall goal of anorectal physiotherapy is to improve the patient's condition, helping her to function normally within the limits of her disability. Only by understanding the nature of her complaint can she be helped to incorporate it into her life and improve her function.

References

Allen RE, Hosker GL, Smith ARB et al (1990) Pelvic floor damage and childbirth: a neurophysiological study. *British Journal of Obstetrics and Gynaecology* **97**: 770–779.

Bo K (1995) Pelvic muscle exercise for the treatment of stress urinary incontinence: an exercise physiology perspective. *International Urogynaecology Journal* **6**: 282–291.

Bo K and Talseth T (1996) Long term effect of pelvic floor muscle exercise 5 years after cessation of organised training. *Obstetrics and Gynecology* **87**: 261–265.

Bo K, Hagen R, Jorgensen et al (1989) The effect of two different pelvic floor muscle exercise programs in treatment of urinary stress incontinence in women. *Neurourology and Urodynamics* **8**: 355–356.

Bo K, Stien R, Kulseng-Hanssen S et al (1994) Clinical and urodynamic assessment of young nulliparous women with and without stress incontinence symptoms: a case control study. *Obstetrics and Gynecology* **84**: 1028–1032.

Bump RC, Hurt WG, Fantl JA et al (1991) Assessment of Kegel exercise performance after brief verbal instruction. *American Journal of Obstetrics and Gynecology* **165**: 322–329.

Chiarelli P and Markwell SJ (1992) *Let's Get Things Moving*. Sydney: Gore and Osment.

Debus-Thiede G, Hesse U, Maur B et al (1990) NMRI of the pelvic floor – a preliminary report. *Neurourology and Urodynamics* **9**: 392–393.

DiNubile NA (1991) Strength training. *Clinics in Sports Medicine* **10**: 33–62.

Engel AF, Kamm MA, Bartram CI and Nicholls RJ (1995) Relationship of symptoms in faecal incontinence to specific sphincter abnormalities. *International Journal of Colorectal Disease* **10**: 152–155.

Farragher D (1993) The asssessment and treatment of anorectal incontinence, a pudendal neuropathy. *Journal of Association of Chartered Physiotherapists in Obstetrics and Gynaecology* **72**: 7–9.

Fox J, Sylvestre L and Freeman JB (1991) Rectal incontinence: a team approach. *Physiotherapy* **77**: 665–672.

Haig L, Mantle J and Versi E (1995) Does interferential therapy (IFT) confer added benefit over a pelvic floor muscle exercise programme (PFMEP) for genuine stress incontinence. Abstract of the International Continence Society Conference, Sydney, pp. 36–37.

Hesse U, Schussler B, Frimberger J et al (1990) Effectiveness of a three step pelvic floor reeducation in the treatment of stress urinary incontinence: a clinical assessment. *Neurourology and Urodynamics* **9**: 397–398.

Kegel AH (1951) Physiologic therapy for urinary stress incontinence. *Journal of the American Medical Association* **146**: 915–917.

Kennedy B (1982) *Dynamic Back Care*. Sydney: Blake and Hargreaves.

Kiff ES, Barnes PRH and Swash M (1984) Evidence of pudendal neuropathy in patients with perineal descent and chronic straining at stool. *Gut* **25**: 1279–1282.

Klarskov P, Belving D, Bischoff N et al (1986) Pelvic floor exercise versus surgery for female urinary stress incontinence. *Urology International* **41**: 129–132.

Koutsomanis D, Lennard-Jones JE, Roy AJ and Kamm MA (1995) Controlled randomised trial of visual biofeedback versus muscle training without a visual display for intractable constipation. *Gut* **37**: 95–99.

Kuijpers HC and Bleijenberg G (1990) Assessment and treatment of obstructed defaecation. *Annals of Medicine* **22**: 405–411.

Laycock J (1994a) Female pelvic floor assessment: the Laycock ring of continence. *Australian Physiotherapy Association Women's Health Journal* **13**: 40–44.

Laycock J (1994b) Clinical evaluation of the pelvic floor. In: Schussler B, Laycock J, Norton P and Stanton S (eds) *Pelvic Floor Re-education*, pp. 42–48. London: Springer Verlag.

Laycock J, Knight S and Naylor D (1995) Prospective, randomised, controlled clinical trial to compare acute and chronic electrical stimulation in combination therapy for GSI. *Neurourology and Urodynamics* **14**: 425–426.

Lindstrom S and Sudsuang R (1989) Functionally specific bladder reflexes from pelvic and pudendal nerve branches: an experimental study in the cat. *Neurourology and Urodynamics* **6**: 393.

Longmore J (1991) The evaluation of existing systems used to measure pelvic floor muscle contractions. *Journal of Association of Chartered Physiotherapists in Obstetrics and Gynaecology* **70**: 8–10.

Lubowski DZ, King DW and Finlay IG (1992) Electromyography of the pubococcygeus muscle in patients with obstructed defaecation. *International Journal of Colorectal Disease* **7**: 184–187.

Mantle J and Versi E (1991) Physiotherapy for stress urinary incontinence: a national survey. *British Medical Journal* **302**: 753–755.

Markwell SJ and Sapsford RR (1995) Physiotherapy management of obstructed defaecation. *Australian Journal of Physiotherapy* **41**: 279–283.

Markwell SJ, Mumme GA and O'Neill SM (1993) Proprioceptive retraining in pelvic floor dysfunction and excretory disorders. Abstract of the International Continence Society Conference, Rome, pp. 132–133.

McArdle WD, Katch FI and Katch UL (1991) *Exercise Physiology – Energy, Nutrition and Human Performance*, 3rd edn, p. 465. Philadelphia: Lea and Febiger.

Millard RJ (1987) *Bladder Control: A Simple Self Help Guide*. Sydney: Williams and Wilkins.

Mills PM, Deakin M and Kiff ES (1990) Percutaneous electrical stimulation for ano-rectal incontinence. *Physiotherapy* **76**: 433–438.

Mills PM, Monk D, Deakin M et al (1995) The strength duration curve as a diagnostic test for the investigation of external anal sphincter (EAS) in women with anorectal incontinence. Proceedings of the World Conference of Physical Therapists, Washington, p. 1206.

Papachrysostomou MC, Smith AN and Stevenson AJM (1994) Does electrical stimulation of the pelvic floor alter the proctographic parameters in faecal incontinence? *European Journal of Gastroenterology and Hepatology* **6**: 139–144.

Plevnik S (1985) New method for testing and strengthening of pelvic floor muscles. *Neurourology and Urodynamics* **4**: 267–268.

Richardson CA and Jull GA (1995) Muscle control – pain control. What exercises would you prescribe? *Manual Therapy* **1**: 2–10.

Sale DG (1988) Cited in Bo K (1995) Pelvic floor exercise for the treatment of stress urinary incontinence: an exercise physiology perspective. *International Urogynecology Journal* **6**: 282–291.

Salter PM, Booth J and Rowe PJ (1995) An evaluation of the reliability of the Bourne perineometer. Proceedings World Confederation of Physical Therapists, Washington, p. 1207.

Sampselle CM and DeLancey JOL (1992) The urine stream interruption test and pelvic muscle function. *Nursing Research* **41**: 73–77.

Santiesteban AJ (1988) Electromyographic and dynamometric characteristics of female pelvic floor musculature. *Physical Therapy* **68**: 344–351.

Sapsford RR, Markwell SJ and Richardson CA (1996) Abdominal muscles and the anal sphincter: their interaction during defaecation. Proceedings of the National Congress of the Australian Physiotherapy Association, pp. 103–104.

Sapsford RR, Hodges PW, Richardson CA et al (1997a) Activation of pubococcygeus during a variety of isometric abdominal exercises. Conference Abstract. *International Continence Society, Yokohama*, 115.

Sapsford RR, Hodges PW, Richardson CA (1997b) Activation of the abdominal muscles is a normal response to contraction of the pelvic floor muscles. Conference Abstract. *International Continence Society, Yokohama*, 117.

Sikorski JM (1986) *Understanding Orthopaedics*, p. 149. Sydney: Butterworths.

Tagart REB (1966) The anal canal and rectum: their varying relationship and its effect on anal continence. *Diseases of Colon and Rectum* 9: 449–452.

Further reading

Zacharin RF (1985) *Pelvic Floor Anatomy and the Surgery of Pulsion Enterocoele*. New York: Springer Verlag.

Resources

Wherever possible the name and address of the manufacturer is supplied. Contact the manufacturer for local suppliers. In cases of multinational companies, contact the company in your country.

Avina Intra-urethral Plug, Convatec, USA. Contact Convatec suppliers in each country.

Aquaflex Weights, DePuy Healthcare, Millshaw House, Manor Mill Lane, Leeds LS11 9YY, UK.
Phone +44 532 706000 for suppliers.

Bourne Perineometer, Doncast Ltd, 56 Chaldon Common Rd, Chaldon, Caterham, Surrey CR3 5DD, UK.

Conveen Continence Guard, Coloplast A/S, Bronzevej 2–8, 3060 Espergaerde, Denmark. Contact the Coloplast agent in each country.

Duo Balls are available at any sex shop.

Enuresis Resource and Information Centre, 65 St Michael's Hill, Bristol BS2 8DZ, UK.

Femina Cones, Colgate Medical Ltd, 1 Fairacres Estate, Dedworth Rd, Windsor, Berkshire SL4 4LE, UK.

Femtone Weights, Convatec, USA. Contact Convatec suppliers in each country.

Introl, Johnson and Johnson Medical, PO Box 134, North Ryde, NSW 2113, Australia.
Phone +61 2 9878 9111, fax +61 2 9878 9222 for suppliers.

Microscol Neuromuscular Stimulator and Vaginal Electrode, Microsystems Electronics, 431 Logan Rd, Stones Corner, Brisbane, Australia 4120.
Phone +61 7 3394 8253, fax +61 7 3394 8223 for suppliers.

PFX and Peritron, Cardio Design Pty Ltd, PO Box 6407 BHBC, Baulkham Hills, NSW 2154, Australia.
Phone +61 2 9899 7463, fax +61 2 9899 2588 for suppliers.

Appendix 1 Guide to Assessment

(Modified from the assessment guide prepared by the Physiotherapy Women's Health Network Group, Brisbane.)

1. Presenting symptoms – list problems in order of importance, as perceived by patient.

2. History

(a) Medical – hypertension, cardiac disease, respiratory conditions, diabetes, hypothyroidism, MS, CVA, Parkinson's, dementia, irritable bowel syndrome, diverticulosis/itis, back pain.

(b) Obstetric – long active second stage, forceps, large babies, precipitate delivery, CS, prolonged epidural, episiotomy, tear – 2nd, 3rd, 4th degree, close pregnancies.

(c) Gynaecological conditions – endometriosis, abnormal cervical cells, vaginal infections, prolapse.

(d) Urogenital surgery – hysterectomy (abdominal, vaginal), vaginal repair (anterior, posterior), ovarian cystectomy, oophorectomy, tubal ligation, bladder neck suspension.

(e) Anorectal surgery – haemorrhoidectomy, rectocoele repair, sphincterotomy (release of tight anal sphincter), rectopexy (reattachment of rectum to sacrum).

(f) Relevant family history – nocturnal enuresis, poor connective tissue quality, joint hypermobility.

3. Investigations

(a) Urinary – microurine, urine culture, cystoscopy, IVP, urodynamics.

(b) Gynaecological – Papanicolaou smear (abnormal smear is possible contraindication for electrotherapy).

(c) Anorectal – barium enema, sigmoidoscopy, colonoscopy, anorectal physiology studies, EMG study, colon transit study, videoproctography.

4. Previous management and effect

(a) Medical – drugs.

(b) Surgery – effect.

(c) Physiotherapy – define modalities.

(d) Other – diet, acupuncture, herbal remedies.

5. Subjective assessment

(a) Fitness/obesity – activities.

(b) Hormonal status and influence – effect of menstrual cycle, lactation, peri/post-menopausal, hormone replacement therapy.

(c) Pain.

(d) Current medications – effects (see Table 28.3).

(e) Genuine stress incontinence (for definition see Chapter 28):

- urine loss on sneeze, cough, laugh, lift, run, rising from a chair, sexual activity;
- amount of loss – spot, wet pants, wet clothing. If more than a small amount with each event the cause may be detrusor instability triggered by ↑ IAP;
- midstream flow stop – note effect of attempted stop;
- urethral hypofunction – seepage when upright, often insensitive loss, greater loss with movement, dry in supine, often a factor in elderly, possible surgical scarring;
- aggravated by alpha-adrenergic blockers.

(f) Urgency and urge incontinence (for definition see Chapter 28):

- sensory urgency – mucosal hypersensitivity, incontinence less likely, infection, inflammation;
- motor urgency – detrusor overactivity, instability, urgency a perineal sensation.

Loss – large volume, wet legs, wet floor, frequency.

Triggers – key in door, running water, shower, sexual activity, supermarket freezer, moving and bending.

Ability to defer – <2 minutes, 2–5 minutes, >10 minutes.

Would you be wet if you didn't go to the toilet immediately?

Do you get wet as you try to undress?

Aggravated by caffeine, alcohol, fast-acting diuretics.

(g) Overflow incontinence (for definition see Chapter 28):

↓ detrusor contractility – hesitancy, slow to start, poor stream, strain to void, prolonged time to void, incomplete emptying, frequent small voids.

Frequent UTI.

Retention/overflow – detrusor acontractility, urethral obstruction (uncommon in women), distended palpable bladder, pain, continual dribble loss day and night, infection.

Refer for medical review – self-catheterization.

(h) Reflex incontinence (for definition see Chapter 28): in neurological conditions, self-catheterization.

(i) Nocturnal enuresis (for definition see Chapter 8).

(j) Fluid intake – amount of all fluids and type, note small (<600 ml) and large (>3 litre) intake.

(k) Frequency/volume chart – 3 days recommended but not often practical. Output greater than fluid intake except in hot weather. Note minimum, average and maximum volumes, occasions of loss, day/night ratio. Regular output > 6–700 ml indicates ↓ bladder sensitivity and overstretch. Do not defer.

(l) Anorectal function – frequency, awareness, urgency (can't defer five minutes), puts off urge, strain to empty, completeness of emptying, content consistency, pain (where and when), bleeding (must be investigated), bloating, alternating constipation/diarrhoea, soiling, incontinence, flatus control, aware/unaware of any loss.

Slow transit constipation – ↓ frequency/urge to empty, bloating (worse at end of day), pain, urinary symptoms. .

Obstructed defaecation – desire to empty, unable to do so completely with or without straining, digital assistance – external, internal or vaginal, dragging pain worse after defaecation.

(m) Diet – detail of daily food and fibre intake (cereal, bread, fruit, vegetables, bulking agents), laxatives.

6. Objective assessment

(a) Defaecation – position, simulated pattern, waist, lower abdomen, lumbar spine.

(b) Muscle assessment.

7. Treatment plan.

Appendix 2 Infection Control for Physiotherapists Working in Women's Health

It is the responsibility of all physiotherapists to be familiar with the guidelines for infection control which have been issued by their professional organization and their employer. Each person has a responsibility to adequately protect herself and the patients in her care.

Guidelines for Infection Control (Australian Physiotherapy Association 1995) and Infection Control in Office Practice: Medical, Dental and Allied Health (Australian National Council on AIDS 1994), or similar documents from other countries, should be studied by all physiotherapists. A very brief summary of procedures is contained below, but detail is insufficient for full working protocols.

1. *Universal precautions* – The underlying principle is to assume that all patients and staff are potentially infected with blood-borne pathogens. Precautions to prevent exposure must be taken for all patients.

2. *Protection from infection* – All physiotherapists should be vaccinated against hepatitis B. Instruments and equipment should be protected from the following contaminants: blood, faeces, urine, vaginal secretions, semen, saliva, sputum, all body fluids containing blood and peritoneal, amniotic, pleural, synovial and cerebrospinal fluids.

3. *Use of gloves* – Hands should be washed before gloves are put on and immediately they are removed. Gloves should be worn when contact with contaminants is likely and changed if punctured, between patients and between different body areas.

4. *Handwashing* – This is the most important and effective precaution in infection control. Wash hands before and after any significant patient care activities. Use a thorough washing technique. All cuts and abrasions should be covered in waterproof, occlusive dressings. Pay attention to skin care.

5. *Cleaning* – Containers and work areas should be kept clean. Clothing should be clean daily and changed if soiled by contaminants. Ventilation – ensure this is adequate, especially when working with disinfectants. Disposable items – use once only and dispose of appropriately.

6. *Cleaning of vaginal weights and catheters* – Many weights cannot be autoclaved so they must be for single patient use only. If used within a condom, decontamination with chemical agents must be carried out in accordance with guidelines, before and after use. Catheters (single patient use) must be covered with a condom to prevent accumulation of secretions. Written instructions for home use and cleaning should be provided to each patient.

7. *Vaginal and anal electrodes* – These must be single patient use unless totally autoclavable. Written instructions for home use should be supplied.

8. *Perineometers* – These should be used with a new condom, and preferably a double condom, on each occasion. Care must be taken on application and removal of the condoms and the instrument must be washed and decontaminated in chemical disinfectants, preferably by immersion, otherwise by wiping, after use and before storage. See guidelines for details. Written instructions for home use should be supplied.

9. *Ultrasound head and Interferential electrodes* – These should be decontaminated before and after use in cases of pelvic floor dysfunction. See guidelines for details.

31

Sexual Issues from 40 Years Onwards

JANE HOWARD AND YVONNE KIRKEGARD

Not all women in this age group will be sexually active, as some will be widowed, divorced, separated or not interested. A small percentage will be lesbians. In the years immediately preceding and following menopause the majority of women experience changes in sexual activity, with diminished sexual responsiveness and a decline in sexual interest (Fig. 31.1). Societal attitudes are negative towards sexual attractiveness in older women. Some women who do not enjoy sex see increasing age as the excuse they need to cease sexual activity. Hormonal and non-hormonal factors contribute to the development of psychosexual disorders at the menopause (Sarrell, 1990). Sex hormones exert both direct and indirect effects on neural activity in areas of the brain that subserve emotion and sexuality (Sherwin, 1994).

Relationship Issues and Partner's Sexual Function

The quality of a relationship has a profound effect on its sexual aspects and counselling may be beneficial for couples who have problems such as poor communication, violence, inequity or affairs. Medical problems and the treatment of medical conditions may also cause sexual dysfunction for the other partner.

The incidence of erectile dysfunction in men increases with age. Blood flow to the penis may be compromised by atherosclerosis, hypertension or diabetes and erections may be less hard than previously or may last for a shorter time. Diabetes, multiple sclerosis, chronic alcoholism and other conditions can damage the pelvic autonomic nervous system and impotence may occur.

Low libido in men is not common, but it may be caused by temporal lobe epilepsy, hypogonadism, depression and psychosis. However, research points to the quality of the existing marital and sexual relationship as being the most common cause of non-medical sexual dysfunction (Hawton et al, 1994).

Effects of the Menopause on Sexuality

Non-hormonal factors which influence sexual function at the time of the menopause include psychological reactions to being menopausal, sexual changes in the male partner, interpersonal conflicts and sociocultural attitudes towards sexual behaviour and attractiveness (Bachmann and Leiblum, 1991). Cross-sectional studies generally attest to decreased orgasmic ability, lowered coital frequency and reduced sexual interest during the two decades from 45–64 years (McCoy, 1992). Major studies of sexuality and ageing have found sex differences, with women reporting

Figure 31.1 Sequential changes in women's sexuality arising from menopausal hormone levels. (Reproduced from McCoy NL (1994) Survey research on the menopause and women's sexuality. In: Berg G and Hammar M (eds) *The Modern Management of the Menopause : A Perspective for the 21st Century*, pp. 581–587, with permission of NL McCoy and the publishers.)

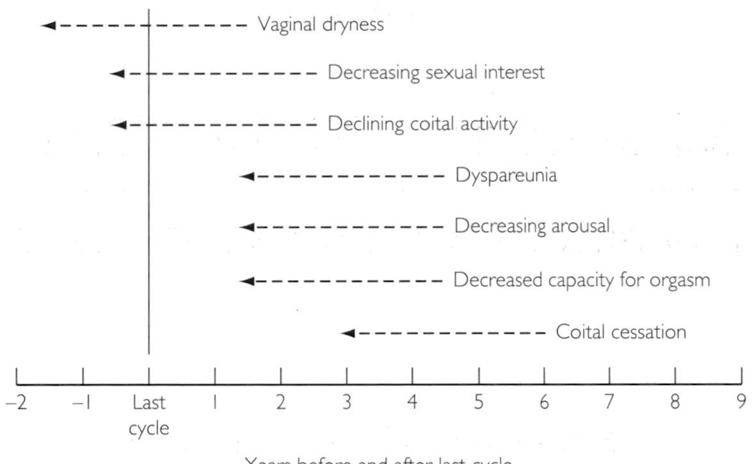

less sexual interest and less sexual intercourse. The earlier demise of male partners restricts sexual options for many women. After the early 50s the percentage of women reporting no interest in sex increases much more rapidly than it does for men (McCoy, 1992). Post-menopausal women are twice as likely to report a decrease in sexual interest (Morse, 1995).They are shown to have diminished or slower clitoral response, decreased vaginal secretion and weaker muscle contractions during orgasm. Labial engorgement and clitoral erection are diminished and fewer uterine contractions result in shorter orgasms.

Hormone effects on target organs

At the menopause the ovaries' production of oestrogen, progesterone and testosterone drops to very low levels. A lack of oestrogen often results in depression, anxiety and tiredness, which affect libido, and a dry sore vagina, which may cause dyspareunia (painful intercourse).

The thin atrophic skin of the vulva and vagina is more prone to splitting, causing a painful vaginal fissure. Inadequate lubrication with arousal and orgasm and post-coital bleeding can be directly linked to the atrophic changes of the vagina. With increasing age there is atrophy of pubococcygeus which may itself lead to dyspareunia. There is some evidence that oestrogen may also affect touch perception (Sarrell, 1990). Slowed, absent or adverse response to touch, loss of clitoral sensation and decreased capacity for orgasm may occur. Table 31.1 outlines the effects of lowered hormone levels on the sexual and reproductive anatomy of post-menopausal women.

If the woman has had damage to the pelvic floor in childbirth, her bladder and bowel symptoms may well be aggravated by oestrogen deficiency. Women with faecal soiling or urinary incontinence during intercourse are often very distressed and they avoid this sexual activity.

Hormone replacement therapy and sexual function

The effects of oestrogen replacement, which appear to be significant sexually, include prevention of genital atrophy, relief of dyspareunia, the enhancement of vaginal and vulval blood flow and the maintenance of sensory perception. Results of studies strongly suggest that testosterone and not oestrogen is of primary importance for libido or sexual desire in women (Burger et al, 1984; Cardozo et al, 1984). The addition of testosterone to the oestrogen replacement regimen is frequently successful in restoring libido and preventing lethargy and depression in both naturally and surgically menopausal women (Sherwin, 1994). Young women are usually given testosterone and oestrogen, in the form of subcutaneous implants, every six months. The use of testosterone replacement therapy in post-menopausal women is much more controversial, but it is occasionally used to treat low libido.

Sexuality Following Surgery

Oophorectomy

When oophorectomy and hysterectomy are performed in women under 50 years, the lack of oestrogen leads to dyspareunia, failed arousal and decreased libido, whilst the lack of testosterone leads to extreme tiredness and lack of

Table 31.1 Specific effects of lowered hormone levels on sexual and reproductive anatomy of post-menopausal women

Structure	Physical change	Effects
Vulva	Loss of subcutaneous fat	Shrinkage
Labia	Atrophic skin	Painful tissues
Clitoris		Decrease in clitoral sensitivity
Vagina	Pale Decreased lubrication Less elastic tissue Decrease in pH	Reduced vaginal size Narrowing of introitus Shortening of length Decreasing width Thinner and smoother walls Splitting of skin
Uterus	Shrinkage of endometrium Shrinkage of myometrium	Small and firm Decreased vascularity
Ovaries	Shrinkage	Small and impalpable
Fallopian tubes	Shrinkage	Small Decreased lubrication
Urinary tract	Urethral epithelium may thin Loss of elasticity	Urinary incontinence with orgasm Dysuria UTIs Stress incontinence is aggravated
Pelvic floor	Loss of muscle bulk (esp. pubococcygeus)	Weak and poorly supporting pelvic floor Dyspareunia Poor bowel emptying Faecal incontinence
Breasts	Dense stroma (interstitial tissue) replaced by fat	Decrease in size

Sources London and Hammond (1986), Judd (1987), and Masters and Johnson (1966).

libido. In women over 50 years of age the symptoms are often less severe.

Hysterectomy

Hysterectomy for a benign condition usually does not interfere with a woman's capacity to become sexually aroused. However, if she has relied on cervical pressure for arousal then this subtle feeling will no longer occur. Clitoral stimulation is usually similar before and after hysterectomy. The sensation of uterine contraction during orgasm is lacking, so it may feel different from that experienced prior to the operation.

When a woman has heavy bleeding, which restricts her sexual activity prior to hysterectomy, her sexual function may be improved after the operation. Loss of fertility and feelings of loss of femininity may result in loss of libido.

Hysterectomy for cancer

If the hysterectomy is performed because of cancer then the depression and anxiety associated with a life threat are likely to affect libido. After treatment, libido may return but sexual function may be altered. For example, after cancer surgery the woman may be left with a short vagina. This may be treated with plastic surgery to the vulva to increase vaginal length.

Radiotherapy

Radiotherapy for cancer of the cervix is likely to result in fibrosis and scarring of the vagina, which lead to difficult penetration and painful intercourse. Women are advised to use vaginal dilators at the time of treatment but frequently this does not prevent problems.

Mastectomy

Mastectomy is usually performed for a malignant condition so that depression and anxiety together with loss of libido are a common response to this life threat. A change in body image and perception of self as a sexual person is likely to occur. The reaction of the partner is crucial to the recovery of sexual activity in the relationship. Numbness or increased sensation in the scar may affect the capacity for sexual arousal.

By utilizing the advances in hormone replacement therapy and sexual counselling services, women are now able to address the sexual issues associated with the climacteric.

At this age the most profound change in sexuality is likely to be the menopause, which affects oestrogen, progesterone and testosterone production. Sexual desire levels are likely to drop and there are atrophic changes in the genitals, secondary to hormonal changes. The incidence of medical conditions increases with age. The illness itself or its treatment may interfere with sexuality. Surgical treatments to breasts and genitals are particularly likely to affect sexuality. The quality of the sexual relationship and the sexual function of the partner are important factors in continuing sexual activity for women.

References

Bachmann GA and Leiblum SR (1991) Sexuality in sexagenarian women. *Maturitas* 13: 43–50.

Burger HG, Hailes J, Menelaus et al (1984) The management of persistent menopausal symptoms with oestradiol-testosterone implants: clinical, lipid and hormonal results. *Maturitas* 6: 351–358.

Cardozo L, Gibb DMF, Tuck SM et al (1984) The effects of subcutaneous hormone implants during the climacteric. *Maturitas* 5: 177–184.

Hawton K, Gath D and Day A (1994) Sexual function in a community sample of middle-aged women with partners: effects of age, marital, socioeconomic, psychiatric, gynaecological and menopausal factors. *Archives of Sexual Behaviour* 23(4): 375–395.

Judd HL (1987) Menopause and post-menopause. In: Pernoll ML and Benson RC (eds) *Current Obstetric and Gynecologic Diagnosis and Treatment*, 6th edn, pp. 959–978. Norwalk: Appleton and Lange.

London SN and Hammond CB (1986) The climacteric. In: Danforth DN and Scott JR (eds) *Obstetrics and Gynecology*, 5th edn, pp. 905–926. Philadephia: J.B. Lippincott.

Masters WH and Johnson VE (1966) *Human Sexual Response*. Boston: Little, Brown.

McCoy NL (1992) Menopause and sexuality. In: Sitruck-Ware R and Utian WH (eds) *The Menopause and Hormonal Replacement Therapy: Facts and Controversies*, pp. 73–100. New York: Marcel Dekker.

Morse C (1995) Women's psychosexual well being during the menopausal transition – Melbourne midlife health study. Proceedings of the 5th Congress of the Australian Menopause Society, Hobart, Australia.

Sarrell, P (1990) Sexuality and menopause. *Obstetrics and Gynecology* 75: 26–31.

Sherwin BB (1994) Hormonal influences on sexuality in the postmenopause. In: Berg G and Hammar M (eds) *The Modern Management of the Menopause: A Perspective for the 21st Century*, pp. 589–598. London: Parthenon Publishing.

Further reading

Chiarelli P (1990) *Women's Waterworks: Curing Incontinence*. Rushcutter's Bay, NSW, Australia: Gore and Osment.

Farrell E and Westmore A (1993) *The HRT Handbook*. South Yarra, Victoria, Australia: Anne O'Donovan.

Gressor M (1993) *So You're Having a Hysterectomy*. Rushcutter's Bay, NSW, Australia: Gore and Osment.

Stoppard M (1994) *Menopause*. Ringwood, Victoria, Australia: Viking Penguin.

Sundquist K (1992) *Menopause: Make it Easy*. Rushcutter's Bay, NSW, Australia: Gore and Osment.

32

Osteoporosis

JUDY LARSEN

Osteoporosis is a condition characterized by an absolute decrease in bone mass. As a result bones can become thin or weak (less dense) and can be easily broken, often as a result of minimal trauma. Common sites of fracture are the spine, hip, wrist and ribs. Problems after fracture will vary but can include debilitating pain (post-spinal fracture) or loss of independence and subsequent institutionalization (post-hip fracture). Osteoporosis is often diagnosed after a fracture occurs. Recognizing those at risk of osteoporosis, including younger women, is a necessary clinical ability as the prevalence of the disease in the community increases. In clinical practice it is not only elderly women with the dowager's hump that need to be diagnosed but we must also consider athletes with a history of amenorrhoea, patients with anorexia nervosa, pre-menopausal women who have a number of risk factors and who may present with groin pain and generally 30% of the post-menopausal population (WHO, 1994).

As health practitioners our role in prevention and education is apparent. Treatment of osteoporosis is not complete without the current family history and the knowledge that it is the children and grandchildren of our patients with osteoporosis who may benefit most from lifestyle changes and preventive strategies.

Our role in treatment is varied and not always well documented. We have a significant role to play in pain reduction, maintenance of independence, exercise prescription and, perhaps the most important of all, the prevention of falls and thus the prevention of fractures. Recognizing those at risk and modifying treatment approaches is a skill we all have to master.

Pathophysiology

The cellular components of bone include osteoblasts and osteoclasts. Osteoblasts are responsible for the laying down of new bone while osteoclasts are responsible for bone resorption. The following is a brief synopsis of the process that occurs as our bones age and change according to different influences. Further reading is encouraged but the emphasis of this chapter will be on clinical relevance and practicalities.

Throughout its life bone can respond to external forces (or loads) such as the pull of tendon on bone and weight bearing. These forces can help to maintain bone mass or increase it in some circumstances. As a living tissue, bone material is constantly being turned over in a process called bone remodelling. In this process old bone is resorbed and new bone is formed. Many internal factors dictate the effectiveness of the remodelling process. These can include ageing, hormonal influences, metabolic variations and certain disease processes. Bone is most sensitive to mechanical loading during childhood. An increase in osteoblastic activity and thus in bone mass can result from the external forces (or loads) mentioned. Without these forces osteoclast activity (bone resorption) predominates and bone mass decreases (Norkin and Levangie, 1992). If the breakdown or resorption of bone (osteoclastic activity) exceeds the formation or laying down of bone (osteoblastic activity) then decreased bone density or osteopenia will occur. If this process continues unchecked it can lead to osteoporosis. Osteoporotic bone is more likely to fracture than bone of normal density.

Diagnosis and Investigations

There is a natural loss of bone associated with age which leads to a normal decline in bone mineral density. This loss is not clinically or medically problematic (Borner et al, 1988). There are a number of pathologies (Table 32.1) that can increase the rate of loss of bone and the risk of fracture.

Osteoporotic bones have a decreased density (mass per unit volume) compared to normal bone and as such are weaker and more likely to fracture with minimal trauma than normal bone. The presence of such fractures in combination with reduced bone mass has been used as the clinical marker for osteoporosis while reduced bone mass without fracture has been referred to as osteopenia. With the development of bone density measures a more accepted convention is to consider osteoporosis to be present when bone mineral density (BMD) falls to a level more than 2.5 standard deviations (SD) below the mean bone density at the same skeletal site in healthy young adults of the same gender and race. These people are at greater risk of developing a fracture (Borner et al, 1988). A normal bone density reading can be defined as BMD which falls within 1 SD of the young adult reference mean. Osteopenia or low bone mass can be defined as more than 1 SD below the young adult mean but less than 2.5 below this value. Severe osteoporosis (established osteoporosis) can be recognized as more than 2.5 SD below the young adult mean in the presence of one or more fragility fractures. These diagnostic categories are given in a report of a World Health Organization study group (WHO, 1994). Some variation will exist from country to country and recommended intervention will also vary (Fig. 32.1).

Measurement of bone mass/density

Bone densitometry makes it possible to quantify the risk of fracture in both the appendicular and axial skeleton. Technology is rapidly changing in the field of bone densitometry. Techniques used need to be safe in terms of radiation,

Table 32.1 Medical conditions associated with increased risk of osteoporosis

Endocrine disorders	Hyperparathyroidism Hyperthyroidism Premature menopause (including surgical) Amenorrhoea (>6 months)
Congenital disorders	Turner's syndrome Kleinfelter's syndrome
Gastrointestinal disorders	Post-gastrectomy
Other medical disorders	Anorexia nervosa Rheumatoid arthritis
Immobilizing disorders	Paralysis from any cause Bed rest
Medications	Long-term use of corticosteroids for asthma, RA, etc. Long-term use of aluminium-containing antacids Heparin
(The use of some medications will increase the risk of fracture due to increasing the risk of falling)	Neuroleptics Vasodilators Diuretics
Differential diagnosis	Other conditions that lead to low bone mass Multiple myeloma Lymphoma Leukaemia

Figure 32.1 This graph shows the definition of osteoporosis according to standard deviation units (SDU) above and below the young adult reference mean. This is not the distribution of osteoporosis in a given population.

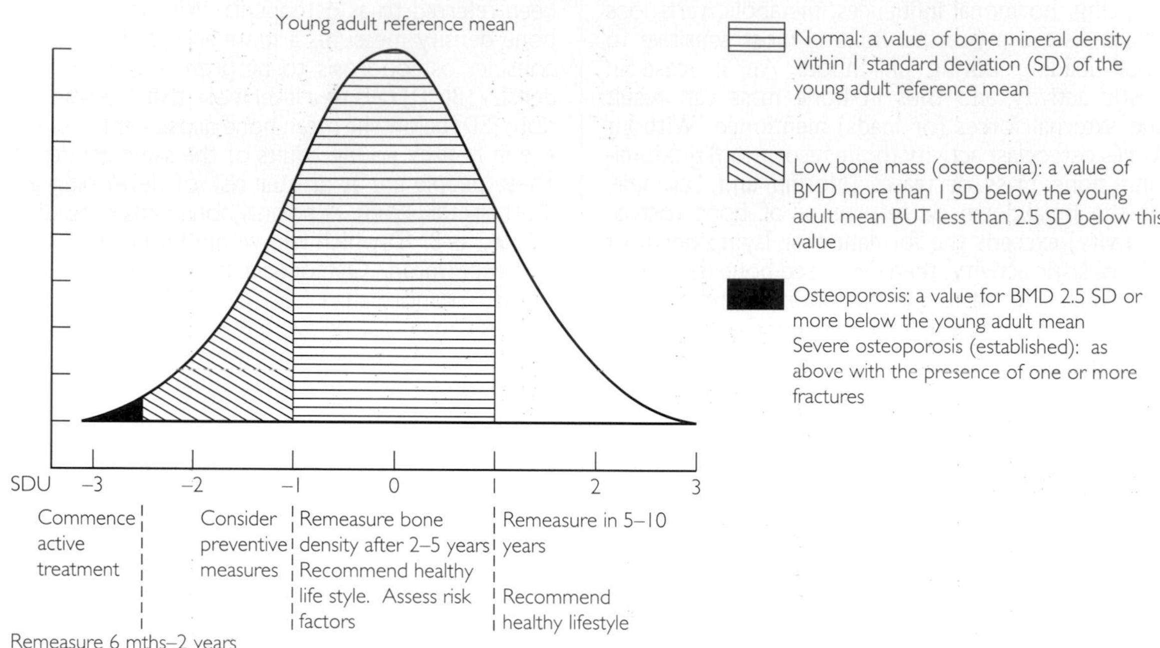

convenient, economically viable and have high repeatability. Patient comfort should be considered. Significant variation can exist between densitometry machines and patients should be encouraged to use the same densitometer in longitudinal follow-up studies.

Debate exists as to the need for mass screening of the 'at risk' population. If people are asymptomatic and are already modifying the main risk factors (including hormone replacement therapy (HRT), calcium and exercise) or they are unprepared to take these steps, there may be no need to undergo densitometry. If a woman is having difficulty making the decision to commence HRT or continuing with therapy then measurement of bone mass may serve to motivate her to accept or to continue with a prescribed therapy.

The major advantages and disadvantages of various techniques of measurement are listed in Table 32.2.

Dual energy X-ray absorptiometry (DEXA) is a commonly used technique. An example of a DEXA report for bone density screening is shown in Figure 32.2.

FREQUENCY OF MEASUREMENT

Bone density measurements may be made six-monthly or annually after therapeutic intervention has begun, particularly when patients are anticipated to be in rapid bone loss stage (early post-menopausal). Otherwise repeat densitometry at two or five years will be recommended according to the number of standard deviations below the race and gender-matched normal values of young adults and age-matched values. Health benefit subsidies and health insurance rebate on bone scans will vary and as such the cost to the patient will be a limiting factor when considering repeat densitometry.

Clinically, diagnosis of established osteoporosis is often made after presentation with a fracture that requires medical intervention, usually because of pain and alteration of functional capacity. An osteoporotic fracture is generally recognized as one that occurs as a result of minimal trauma as opposed to excessive trauma. Minimal trauma is considered to be a force the same as or less than that involved in falling from standing height or less (Kamien and Prince, 1986). Most fractures in older people are osteoporotic.

Often plain X-rays will be used to assess the fracture and may also show the presence of osteoporosis. By this stage 30% or more of bone density has already been lost. Bone densitometry will usually be suggested at this stage to give a 'benchmark' value for BMD if active treatment is to commence.

BIOCHEMICAL INVESTIGATIONS

Rate of bone loss can be assessed by a number of biochemical markers (Christiansen, 1994). These include plasma oestrogen, alkaline phosphatase, osteocalcin levels and the urinary secretion of hydroxyproline and calcium. Studies suggest that 'rapid losers' of bone as defined chemically have a 70–80% chance of being a rapid loser as defined by sequential bone mass measurements. More recent methods for estimating bone resorption (e.g. serum and urine deoxypyridinoline) and bone formation (e.g. serum bone specific alkaline phosphatase) have been developed

Table 32.2 Relative advantages and disadvantages of various bone density measurement techniques

Type of measurement	Time needed for scan	Sites that can be tested	Radiation dose	Cost	Disadvantages	Advantages
QCT (Quantitative computed tomography)	15–20 min	Multiple sites including hip and spine	Comparatively high	High cost	Precision and accuracy error	Trabecular bone can be examined separately from cortical bone
DXA (Dual energy X-ray absorptiometry)	10–20 min	Multiple sites including hip and spine	Low radiation	Relatively high cost	Possible accuracy error. Osteoarthritis of the spine and calcification in the area can affect interpretation	High precision
SPA (Single photon absorptiometry)	10–15 min	Appendicular sites only, e.g. forearm, heel	Low radiation	Low cost		Portability High accuracy
Conventional X-ray	<5 min	Multiple sites	High radiation		Relatively insensitive (bone loss is apparent when bone mass has decreased by 30–50%). Inappropriate as a screening test	Widespread availability. Detects fractures
Ultrasound		Multiple sites	None		Precision	The only technique that measures bone architecture. Currently used mainly as a research tool

Figure 32.2 Bone density readings for a healthy, 42-year-old, pre-menopausal Caucasian of slight build, moderate exercise habits, good calcium intake and moderate smoker. *Findings*: The average bone mineral density from L2 to L4 is 0.83 g cm^2. This is 79.3% of the age-matched reference range or 1.4 standard deviations below the mean. This is 71.7% of the young reference range or 2.12 standard deviations (T score) below the mean. This represents low bone-density or osteopenia.

DIAGNOSTIC IMAGING - C.T. X-ray Ultrasound & Nuclear Medicine

Name | *Ethnic* Caucasian
ID | *Height* 1615
Age 47 | *Sex* Female | *Weight* 60 kg

L H AP Spine 26/06/95 Sequence 1

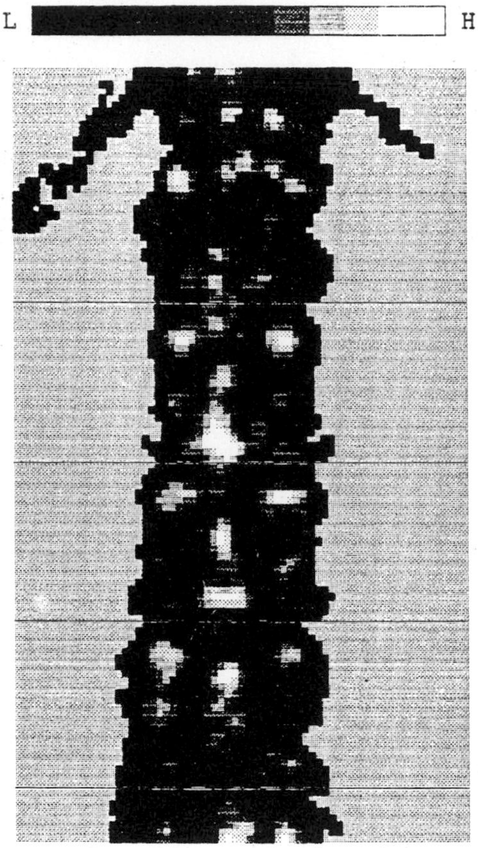

Bone image not for diagnosis

L2 - L4 Caucasian
Female N.Amer.Comb.

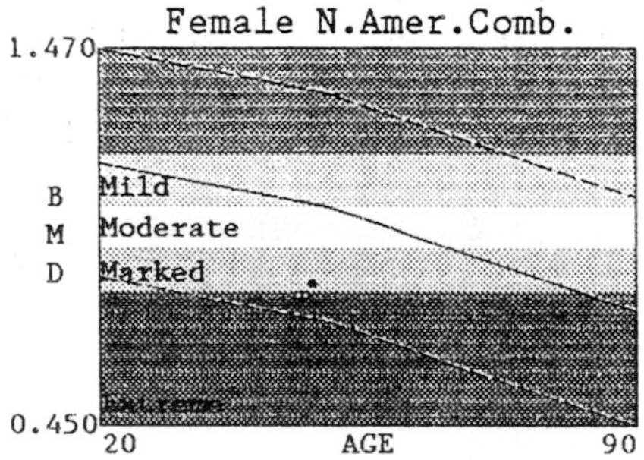

1.470 — 0.450 BMD; AGE 20 — 90; Mild, Moderate, Marked, Extreme

26/06/95 0.831
15/06/94 0.799
29/07/93 0.802

% Young Ref.	**71.7**
T - Score	**-2.12**
% Age Matched	**79.3**
Z - Score	**-1.40**

Change	%	%/Yr
Short	4.0	3.9
Long	3.7	1.9

	BMD g/cm^2	BMC g	LENGTH cm	AREA cm^2
L2	0.892	11.72	3.45	13.14
L3	0.826	11.80	3.45	14.28
L4	0.786	12.57	3.60	15.99
L2 - L4	**0.831**	**36.09**	**10.50**	**43.41**

STD CVs for L2-L4 BMD: 1.0 BMC: 1.5 See Guide for other CVs.
1.5 x 1.5 mm, 60 mm/s, 10.05 cm Rev. 2.5.2 / 1.1.4 Calib. 26/06/95

(Consensus Development Conference, 1993) and further tests are under investigation.

Estimation of bone loss based on biochemical markers alone or combined with bone mass measurements may help to identify women at menopause who are at risk of developing osteoporosis and assist with their choice of therapy and the monitoring of results (Audran, 1992). Sequential analysis of each individual is the most useful for diagnostic purposes.

Signs and Symptoms

There are a number of features (Fig. 32.3) that may be present in some patients which, along with the risk factors and other medical conditions (see Table 32.1), may help physiotherapists to identify patients at risk of osteoporosis. Many goals of physiotherapy treatment would have to be modified if the patient had osteoporosis. We need to consider any post-menopausal woman and young active sports woman as a possible osteoporotic candidate. Our assessment and screening processes should establish the presence of certain risk factors and symptoms and a decision on whether to modify treatment and/or refer the patient for medical advice needs to be made.

Summary of risk factors relating to physiotherapy assessment

- Gender
- Race
- Family history
- Age
- Low body weight
- Early menopause (including surgical)
- Loss of menstruation induced by anorexia
- Loss of menstruation induced by exercise
- Low physical activity levels and immobilization

Figure 32.3 Problems associated with osteoporosis.

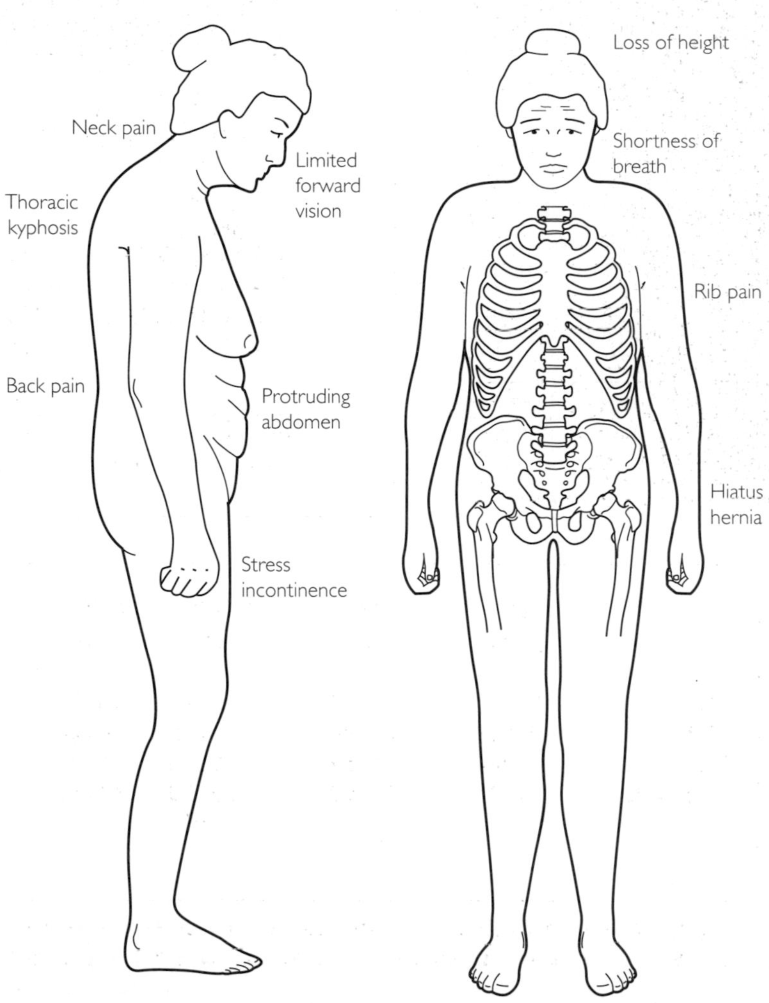

- Inadequate calcium intake or impaired calcium absorption
- Alcohol
- Caffeine
- Smoking
- Nullipara
- Glucocorticoid use
- Rheumatoid arthritis

Loss of height

A loss of 4 cm or more in height over 10 years seems to be associated with a significant decrease in bone mineral density and can be recommended as a clinical marker of osteoporosis (Sanila et al, 1994). The length of the long bones of the body, the arms and legs, remains unchanged and the loss of height occurs in the upper spine (Twomey, 1993). In some women there will be sudden collapse of the vertebra (compression fracture) but in others vertebral compression can occur over time without symptoms and result in reduction in height. One woman in eight loses 20% of her height between the ages of 50 and 70 (Llewellyn-Jones and Abraham, 1992) (Fig. 32.4). Sequential (yearly) height measurements would be a useful tool in all female patients with multiple risk fractures.

Pain

Osteoporotic bones, according to the literature, are rarely painful (Dixon and Woolf, 1989) prior to fracture or compression (Fig. 32.5). Patients may present with undiagnosed spinal fractures and resultant pain but, according to texts, rarely present for pain management prior to fracture. However, some patients who present with non-specific soft tissue type pain and no history of acute pain may have ligamentous strain due to postural changes (Fig. 32.5). Physiotherapists will often treat patients with non-specific back pain prior to fracture recognition and diagnosis of osteoporosis.

Figure 32.4 A woman can lose up to 20% of her height between the ages of 50 and 70 (Llewellyn-Jones and Abraham, 1992).

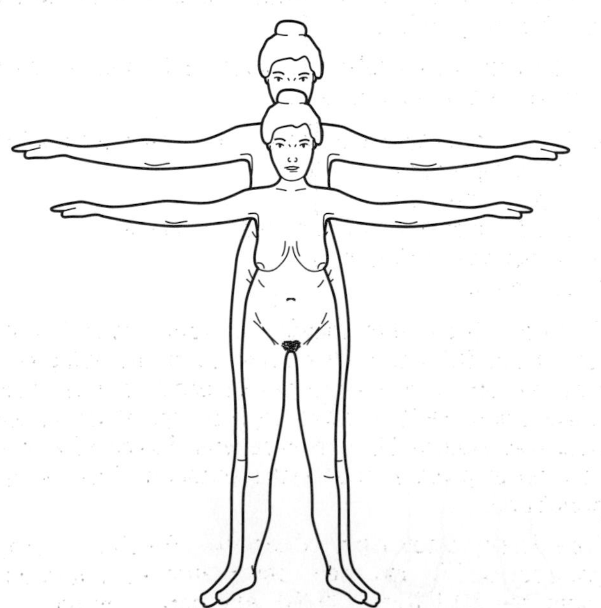

RIB PAIN

In established osteoporosis the distance between the bottom of the rib cage and the pelvis decreases. In severe cases pain may be experienced when the ribs contact the iliac crests. Postural assessment and extension exercises are encouraged. Sustained positions such as sitting to watch television should be carefully assessed to ensure further collapse is not encouraged by seating, etc. For some patients bracing or spinal orthoses may help relieve the pain of costal impingement on the pelvic bones.

Shortness of breath

As a result of the changes to posture and the shape of the thorax, there is less space for the lungs to expand and this can lead to shortness of breath. Postural exercises to maintain optimal position for lung function and breathing exercises and education to ensure good expansion can be helpful. An exercise programme that involves some level of aerobic work will assist in improving fitness levels. Caution with exercise prescription may be necessary and ensuring that patients understand the cause of the problem is essential. Shortness of breath is often directly related to cardiac or respiratory disease in the minds of some patients and fear of exercise will ensue.

Figure 32.5 An anterior wedge fracture of the vertebral body, often associated with osteoporosis. (Reproduced from Culham (1995) with permission.)

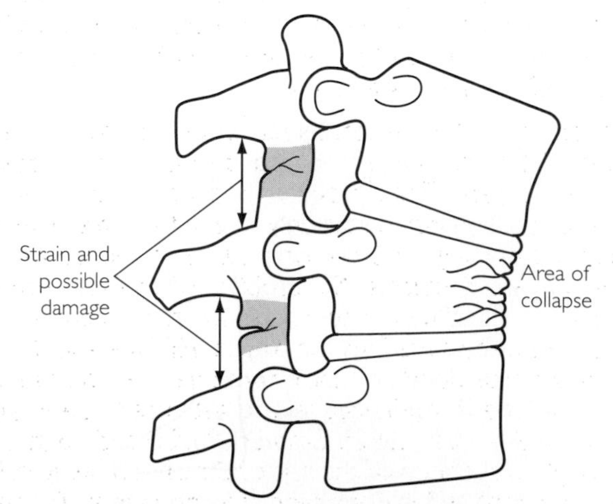

Hiatus hernia

Due to a decrease in abdominal volume, some patients will suffer from hiatus hernia and associated indigestion, heartburn or regurgitation. Posture can also aggravate this problem and stooping activities should be avoided or modified. Patients will often find sleeping on higher pillows to be helpful. If there are no medical contraindications the head of the bed can be raised an inch or two to relieve discomfort. Commercial indigestion preparations or antacids may be bought over the counter but patients should be encouraged to discuss these with their doctor to ensure there are no interactions with other medications. Patients must be aware that any preparation they take, traditional or alternative, should be discussed with the doctor or pharmacist for adverse effects or altered drug uptake. Antacids containing aluminium may be contraindicated for some patients.

Protuberant stomach

With the shortening of the crown–pubis height (Twomey, 1993) comes a bulging stomach and concertina-like skin folds (Dixon and Woolf, 1989). Patients may attempt abdominal strengthening programmes or resort to cosmetic 'corsetry'. The latter serves no real purpose other than psychological and in some patients will make indigestion problems worse. The former may in fact aggravate the situation and predispose the patient to future spinal fractures (Sinaki and Mikkelson, 1984). Education, including diagrammatic explanation of the anatomical reason for the 'pot belly' as well as postural exercises and, where appropriate, static abdominal exercises, may assist the patient physically as well as psychologically. Practicalities such as needing to shorten hemlines on a regular basis are a constant reminder of the progressive nature of this condition for some patients. Commercial cosmetic advice and guidance as to the most effective way to camouflage the offending stomach with suitably designed clothes can be motivating.

Stress incontinence

Increased abdominal pressure in these patients can lead to stress incontinence. Problems can also occur due to straining as a result of constipation provoked by medications, particularly calcium-based ones.

Assessment by the physiotherapist should always at least broach this topic in elderly men and women of the postmenopausal years. Embarrassment because of the use of an incontinence pad may be the only clue to these problems if direct questioning does not occur. Due to the nature of other medical problems, the problem of incontinence is often disregarded by the doctor or not mentioned by the patient. In many situations the patient will have adopted a 'nothing can be done' attitude or presume that you should 'accept a little incontinence as you get older' (Llewellyn-Jones and Abraham, 1992). Chapters 28, 30 and 36 give a thorough explanation of the role of the physiotherapist in the assessment and management of incontinence. The use of ill-fitting incontinence pads has been discussed as a possible cause of falls in older women. Correct education and fitting of these garments is essential.

Transparent skin

Studies have not been able to prove thin skin as a true predictor of osteoporosis. One study of older women with osteoporosis showed that 83% had transparent skin on the back of their hands as opposed to 13% with opaque skin (Notelovitz and Ware, 1982).

Clinically thin skin in those over the age of 60 may be suggestive of possible or existing osteopenia and risk factors should be assessed.

Dowager's hump

Severe kyphotic deformity of the spine resulting in a stooped or hunched posture can occur as a result of vertebral fractures. It should be noted that non-skeletal factors can also lead to kyphosis (Olney and Culham, 1995). Muscle weakness, habitual poor posture and poor self-esteem can all lead to an increased kyphotic posture. From a practical aspect, patients with a kyphotic deformity find clothes become ill fitting and sometimes uncomfortable.

Prevention

Prevention falls into two categories:

1. primary prevention;
2. secondary prevention.

Primary prevention implies identification of those at risk and secondary prevention is the treatment of those who have already had an osteoporotic fracture in order to prevent further problems.

We can consider the following factors in the prevention and management of osteoporosis:

1. hormone replacement therapy and other medications (see Chapter 26);
2. appropriate exercise;
3. an adequate intake of calcium and vitamins;
4. reduction of risk factors;
5. education.

Prevention is currently focused on women in their third, fourth and fifth decades with the aim of optimizing bone mass to cope with the decline that occurs at menopause (MacKinnon, 1988). As earlier reports suggested that peak bone mass occurred in women between 30 and 35 years of age, little emphasis was put on the education of the younger population.

Bone density is now reported to peak at 18–20 years of age (Sambrook, 1991) and then consolidation continues until about age 30 (Heaney, 1990). Appropriate exercise and diet in these early years may see optimum bone mass reached by our young adults. Education and identification of young adults and adolescents at risk is as important as and possibly will have greater long-term benefits than education and identification of post-menopausal women only.

A period of rapid bone loss begins at menopause. Women on average lose between a third and a half of their peak bone mass over their lifetime, while men lose less (Law et al, 1991). Men do get osteoporosis but a higher average bone density (at skeletal maturity men have 10–50% greater bone mass than women (WHO, 1994)) and a shorter life expectancy have until now meant that men do not tend to reach the fracture threshold until a greater age. Nor do men experience the rapid loss of bone mass associated with menopause. It is of growing concern that the rate of osteoporosis in men is rising rapidly but further discussion of this topic is beyond the scope of this book.

Appropriate management including exercise, diet and HRT may see a greater peak bone mass in young female adults and a less rapid decline in bone loss in menopausal women (Fig. 32.6).

Recognition and assessment of risk factors

A physiotherapist should be aware of risk factors that make some patients more likely to have or to develop osteoporosis. A 55-year-old woman of thin build presenting with compression fracture of L1 having fallen off the second rung of a ladder need not necessarily suggest to you a possible case of osteoporosis. The trauma involved is more than minimal (risk of falling increases with height above the ground) but on history taking you discover a poor childhood intake of dairy products, a previous smoker, a possible maternal family history and an early menopause (at age 45). The patient is currently on HRT to control 'flushes' but at less than the prescribed dosage. X-rays should be viewed carefully for obvious osteoporotic changes. Clinical reasoning should suggest to you an increased risk of osteoporosis and management modified accordingly. This should include education on risk factors and the decision as to whether abdominal exercises will progress from static to dynamic. The patient should be encouraged to discuss her risk factors with her doctor and further medical investigation may need to be considered.

Patients presenting for treatment with some medical conditions, e.g. rheumatoid arthritis, asthma with a long history of corticosteroid treatment or other conditions that could result in decreased bone mass (see Table 32.1), may also require clinical evaluation to rule out concomitant osteoporosis.

GENDER

There is a much greater risk of women developing osteoporosis than men. Suggested reasons for this include the fact that after menopause women have a period of rapid bone loss as a result of a sharp fall in oestrogen levels as ovarian function ceases. Up to 15% of bone can be lost

Figure 32.6 Peak bone mass showing possible changes to the graph with exercise and appropriate calcium intake in adolescent years and HRT in the early menopause. (a) Men. (b) Appropriate exercise and nutrition during childhood and adolescents will cause a higher peak bone mass. (c) This graph for the average woman shows an accelerated bone loss in the immediate post-menopausal years and a resulting drop in the graph. (d) A plot of the possible change to the graph with HRT and the slowing of the rapid stage of bone loss. (e) This line shows the effect that amenorrhoea in the adolescent and early adult years can have on peak bone mass. Where the graphs cross the fracture threshold is where the patient becomes at high risk of fracture. This point is seen as 2–2.5 (Nordin, 1994; WHO, 1994) standard deviations below the young adult reference mean. HRT extends the age at which women cross this fracture threshold. Because men have a higher initial peak bone mass and do not have a rapid drop in peak bone mass at menopause, they do not reach the fracture threshold until they are much older.

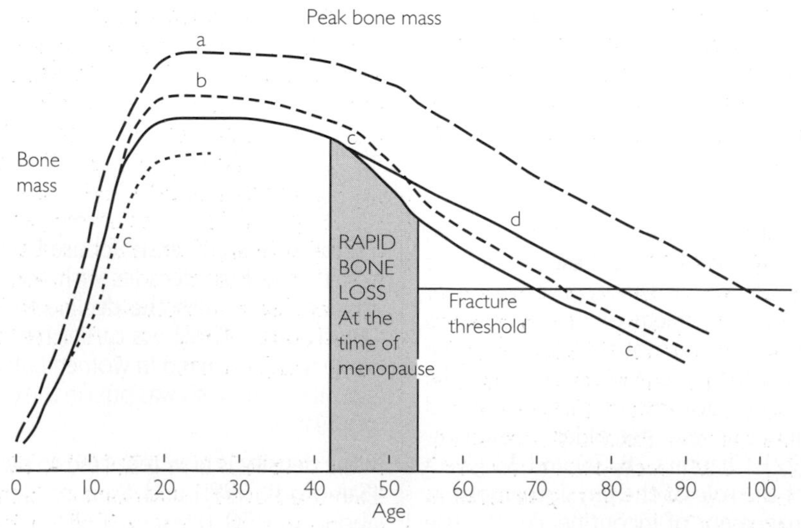

within 5–10 years of menopause (Seeman et al, 1991). Surgical removal of the ovaries can also result in rapid acceleration of loss of bone mineral content if hormone replacement therapy is not prescribed (Dixon, 1986). Men do not experience a similar rapid drop in testosterone which is responsible for bone mass in males. Also worth noting is that males tend to have a greater muscle mass than females and that this may be protective.

RACE

Osteoporosis is more common in white Caucasians and Asians and less common in blacks (Lindsay, 1987). This may be related to the fact that black people have greater bone mass than white people (Borner et al, 1988) and a greater muscle mass than whites.

FAMILY HISTORY

A highly significant percentage of individuals who suffer from osteoporosis will record the presence of kyphosis, height reduction and perhaps also hip fracture in the female members of their family (environmental factors as well as genetic may play a role) (Lindsay, 1987).

AGE

The incidence of osteoporosis and fracture increases with age. The incidence of Colles' and vertebral fractures in women increases soon after menopause. The incidence of Colles' fracture increases until age 65 and then plateaus but the incidence of vertebral fracture continues to rise. The incidence of hip fracture, however, increases slowly with age until late in life, when there is a substantial increase in occurrence (MacKinnon, 1988) after approximately 70 years. It is thought that the bone loss after menopause is mainly trabecular and this predisposes to fracture of the vertebrae and radius. (The distal radius and the vertebrae have high amounts of trabecular bone; the femur has both trabecular and cortical bone (MacKinnon, 1988).) It is also possible that fracture type may be related to the type of fall, the defensive responses used and protective structures (soft tissue padding) around the hip (Boonen et al, 1995). Age plays some role in these factors too.

LOW BODY WEIGHT (THIN BUILD)

Women who carry more fat tissue may have a protective benefit from the conversion of androgen to oestrogen which occurs in fat tissue (Drinkwater, 1995). As weight bearing is a force that can help to maintain or slow the loss of bone mass in some circumstances, those with low body weight may be disadvantaged. Recent studies have, however, looked at muscle mass as opposed to fat mass and suggest that the former has the greatest role to play in bone mineral density (Wegner et al, 1993).

EARLY MENOPAUSE

When menopause occurs early in a woman's life there is a longer period of time when her bones are not protected by oestrogen and this increases her chance of developing osteoporosis. An early menopause may also be a result of hysterectomy. Interestingly, a delayed puberty may predispose to low bone density in women (Seeman et al, 1991).

LOSS OF MENSTRUATION INDUCED BY ANOREXIA NERVOSA

Low oestrogen levels and the cessation of menstruation often result from the fast weight loss found in anorexics. There is often an associated low dietary calcium intake. When anorexia is associated with vigorous exercise (e.g. in order to achieve the lowest possible body fat to optimize sporting performance) the physiotherapist should educate and take certain precautions (see Exercise-induced loss of menstruation). Chapters 4 and 5 give further information on osteoporosis related to adolescent eating disorders and excessive exercise.

LOSS OF MENSTRUATION INDUCED BY EXERCISE

A number of inter-relating factors may exist in the female athlete including training intensity, low percentage body fat, low calorie intake and high protein intake. Amenorrhoeic athletes may have bone mineral densities 10% less than their eumenorrhoeic (normal) sedentary counterparts (Brown, 1995). There may be a high rate of stress fractures in this population.

Female athletes should be questioned as to their menstrual history and encouraged to seek further advice if their amenorrhoea lasts for longer than six months. They can be encouraged to alter their training programme to a point where menstruation returns. As compliance is often low with these patients when increased weight occurs and performance may suffer, they will often be treated by their doctor with hormone replacement therapy.

In sports-oriented physiotherapy practices the population at risk will be much younger than in general community practices. Care must be taken to identify those at risk in the amenorrhoeic population, to educate them and to encourage further medical intervention. Modification of treatment may be necessary in this 'at risk' population (Brown, 1995). The following sports are implicated in reduced or absent menstruation for over 20% of their female participants: gymnastics, light weight rowing, running, cycling and ballet (Wolman, 1994). Further reading on 'the female athlete triad,' which has three components: disordered eating, amenorrhea and osteoporosis, can be found in a *'Position Stand'* by the American College of Sports Medicine (Drinkwater and Johnson, 1997).

LOW PHYSICAL ACTIVITY AND IMMOBILIZATION

Decreased bone formation and increased bone resorption can occur due to the lack of gravitational and mechanical forces on bone. Immobilization can also lead to muscle weakness and decreased balance and co-ordination. The risk of falling may increase.

INADEQUATE CALCIUM INTAKE OR IMPAIRED CALCIUM ABSORPTION

Adequate dietary calcium is a requirement for normal healthy bones (Seeman et al, 1991). There seems to be a consensus that calcium is a prerequisite for bone growth and for reaching peak bone mass, but there is still debate as to its role in prevention and management of osteoporosis.

It is essential that patients realize that adequate or excessive calcium intake is not enough to prevent osteoporosis. Even when calcium intake is adequate, bone will not form unless a mechanical stress such as weight bearing is present and there is adequate oestrogen. To maintain a positive benefit calcium intake needs to be continued indefinitely (Law et al, 1991).

The importance of dietary calcium from birth should be stressed in relation to peak bone mass. Peak bone density seems to be associated with dietary calcium intake in childhood (Law et al, 1991). Modern trends to milk or lactose-free diets because of 'milk' allergies and lactose intolerance see many children reaching adolescence with significantly reduced calcium intake. Milk and milk products are also often seen to be fattening by an adolescent female population and tend to be avoided by our diet-conscious teenagers. The dietary use of low-fat milk products should be emphasized (Turner, 1991).

Calcium obtained from foods other than dairy can provide adequate dietary calcium but increased vigilance in ensuring adequate intake is essential. Low compliance of children and adolescents with the ingestion of non-dairy foods high in calcium may be a problem. The preferred source of calcium is through calcium-rich foods such as dairy products (National Institute of Health, 1994).

Debate exists over the benefit of supplements. If taken with adequate fluid, calcium provides few if any risks (Kamien and Prince, 1986). Calcium intake up to a total of 2000 mg per day appears to be safe in most individuals (NIH, 1994). One side effect rarely documented can be constipation. This can cause increased back pain and pelvic floor problems (stress incontinence) due to straining.

Daily calcium requirements vary according to age and reproductive phase and also from country to country (Table 32.3). Calcium uptake decreases with age as vitamin D (which enhances calcium absorption) becomes deficient due to insufficient vitamin D from diet (cod liver oil, fatty fish, vitamin D-fortified liquid dairy products), impaired renal synthesis of a major vitamin D metabolite and inadequate sunlight exposure (NIH, 1994). If a supplement is to be used or prescribed the least expensive form of calcium supplementation that provides the appropriate amount of elemental calcium is preferred (Lindsay, 1987).

Inefficient calcium absorption can occur for many reasons, including cortisone use, coeliac disease, in thyroid and liver disease or following gastrointestinal surgery (Witham and Davidson, 1994).

ALCOHOL

Excessive alcohol can decrease calcium absorption (Sambrook, 1991) and may depress bone formation and cause increased bone resorption (Seeman et al, 1991). People who abuse alcohol are also more likely to have fractures, possibly due to their greater likelihood of falling (Witham and Davidson, 1994). Moderate (1–2 glasses per day) alcohol intake does not appear to be deleterious (Sambrook, 1991).

CAFFEINE

Once considered a cause of increased urinary calcium loss, it has recently been suggested that caffeine has no detrimental effect at least in women with above average calcium intake (Heaney, 1990). Caffeine should be taken in moderation.

SMOKING

Metabolic products of tobacco decrease oestrogen production and increase oestrogen breakdown so that oestrogen taken by mouth or still produced in the body will be less effective (Seeman et al, 1991). Smokers have a greater tendency to be underweight which also increases their risk factor.

Pre-menopausal bone density is similar in smokers and non-smokers. Women who smoke tend to have an earlier menopause than their non-smoking counterparts. Thus the smoker is exposed to more time without oestrogen protection for her bones (Llewellyn-Jones and Abraham, 1992). Heavy smoking increases the risk of hip fracture at any age (Sambrook, 1991). A woman who stops smoking before the menopause will reduce her risk of hip fractures by about a quarter (Law et al, 1991).

Encouraging our adolescents and young adults to stop smoking will have many positive health benefits. Passive smokers do not escape. Women non-smokers who live in the same house as heavy smokers will also have an earlier menopause (Dixon and Woolf, 1989).

NULLIPARITY (NO PREGNANCIES)

Pregnancy increases the level of oestrogen circulating in the blood (Witham and Davidson, 1994). There may be a long-term protective value to bones after pregnancy.

CORTICOSTEROID USE

Long-term use of these drugs, as in certain medical conditions (e.g. asthma and rheumatoid arthritis), can increase the risk for osteoporosis through both the depression of bone formation and the acceleration of bone resorption (Seeman et al, 1991).

RHEUMATOID ARTHRITIS

Though not always listed as a risk factor, physiotherapists should always evaluate their rheumatoid arthritis patients

Table 32.3 Recommended daily allowance of calcium in Australia and America

Category	Age	Recommended daily intake of calcium (mg) (Mackerras, 1995) (Australian)	Category	Age (group)	Optimum calcium requirements in mg of calcium (NIH, 1994) (American)
Infants	0–6 months (breast fed)	300	Infants	Birth–6 months	400
	0–6 months (formula fed)	500		6 months–1 year	600
	6 months–1 year		Children	1–5 years	800
Children	1–3 yrs	700		6–10 years	800–1200
	4–7 yrs		Adolescents / young adults	11–24 years	1200–1500
Boys	8–11 yrs	800	Men	25–65 years	1000
	12–15 yrs	1200		Over 65 years	1500
	16–18 yrs	1000	Women	25–50 years	1000
Girls	8–11 yrs	900		Over 50 years (post-menopausal) on oestrogens	1000
				Not on oestrogens	1500
	12–15 yrs	1000		Over 65 years	1500
Men	19–64 yrs	800		Pregnant and nursing	1200–1500
	65+ yrs	1000			
Women	19–54 yrs (to menopause)	800			
	After menopause	1000			
	Pregnant (3rd trimester)	Add 300			
	Lactating	Add 500			

for coexisting osteoporosis. Osteoporosis is a common clinical problem in patients with rheumatoid arthritis (Sambrook and Reeve, 1988) but the reasoning for this is not well understood. There are two types of osteoporosis generally associated with rheumatoid arthritis. One is the juxta-articular osteoporosis associated with an individual joint. This is possibly related to decreased strength from limited resistance exercise and immobilization due to pain. The other is a generalized reduction in bone mass (Sambrook and Reeve, 1988).

LACTATION

Although not regarded as a risk factor for the majority of breast-feeding women, the effect of lactation on the bone of healthy women must be mentioned. During lactation, 160–300 mg per day of maternal calcium is lost through the production of breast milk. Acute bone loss occurs during the lactation period but is followed by rapid restoration of bone mass with weaning and the resumption of menses (NIH, 1994).

Education

Physiotherapists are educators. Our clinical skills in osteoporosis management are enhanced by our knowledge of pain, disability and our broad background in movement, physiology and medicine. We may be the health professional who spends the most time with the patient and so this time needs to be well spent. To treat a patient's pain and improve their mobility is important but our preventive role must encompass education and appropriate referral where necessary.

Informal education will occur during normal treatment sessions or class situations. Osteoporosis education should include information on:

1. risk factors;
2. the medical and pharmaceutical management including information on bone densitometry;
3. pain management including self-help techniques;
4. exercise;
5. nutritional information;
6. prevention of falls;
7. other professionals involved in the management of osteoporosis. How can they help?

Formal education programmes are available and physiotherapists should consider referring patients to these courses. Time constraints in a busy practice or institution will often limit the extent of education and the follow-through that is possible. Small-scale education programmes are also difficult to assess in terms of results and outcomes. One such formalized course is the Osteoporosis Prevention and Self-Management Course (OPSMC) which was developed in Australia by the Arthritis Foundation of Victoria (Witham and Davidson, 1993). It is based on the educational processes and format of the Arthritis Self-Management Course developed in 1979–80 by Kate Lorig, Senior Research Associate at the Department of Medicine, Stanford University (Lorig, 1990). The course uses a philosophy of self-help through empowerment as an approach to helping women make informed choices about osteoporosis prevention and management.

Most hospitals, community-based health organizations and centres and women's health units will have educational programmes for osteoporosis.

Most education courses are directed at the older post-menopausal women at risk of osteoporosis or with clinically diagnosed osteoporosis but younger women and adolescents who have a high risk factor for osteoporosis cannot be ignored. The daughters of patients with osteoporosis are often at increased risk of reduced bone mass (Seeman et al, 1989). Schools-based programmes, particularly those that are part of a 'health and fitness' curriculum, may assist in reaching the children of those at risk. Educational literature may be of some use. An active lifestyle including weight-bearing exercise, adequate intake of calcium and awareness about the importance of seeking advice should amenorrhoea persist for longer than six months should be encouraged.

Medical Management

The medical treatment of osteoporosis falls into two main categories: the prevention of osteoporosis and the treatment of established osteoporosis. Prevention is generally directed at slowing resorption while treatment is usually directed at the stimulation of bone formation. Hormone replacement therapy (HRT) is currently the treatment of choice in preventive medical management though new drugs are being evaluated all the time. HRT is also used in the treatment of established osteoporosis. Establishment of the treatment requirements may be facilitated by densitometry and biochemical investigations.

A distinction needs to be drawn between therapeutic and preventive regimes as the aetiology of bone formation and bone resorption is mediated by different physiological and chemical pathways so the pharmaceutical management will vary accordingly. Bone remodelling is cyclical and alterations in bone resorption will eventually affect bone formation. Drugs directed at either process will in turn affect the whole cycle. It is beyond the scope of this book to discuss the pharmaceutical pathways of various medications in depth. Few textbooks are available in this area and to keep up with current trends a review of the literature is probably the most effective means of further reading. The following is a summary of some of the current medications most commonly used in the medical management of osteoporosis.

Hormone replacement therapy

Bone loss occurs in most women in the years following menopause but the immediate post-menopausal bone loss is greatest. Oestrogens are effective in preventing loss of bone density when given at or near menopause but can still be effective in reducing bone loss over 10–15 years after menopause.

Some women will report quality of life improvements and a reduction in menopause-related symptoms including hot flushes, vaginal dryness, moodiness, insomnia and perspiration (Witham and Davidson, 1994). Some patients will not tolerate the side effects of breast tenderness or menstruation well. There may also be reduced risk of coronary heart disease (Seeman et al, 1991).

Oestrogen alone can increase the risk of endometrial cancer in those patients with an intact uterus. The use of progestogens in combination with oestrogen can minimize the risk of endometrial cancer (Seeman et al, 1991). Progestogens can be given either cyclically for a period of time each month or on a continual basis. Continual progestogens can avoid irregular bleeding that may occur (Consensus Development Conference, 1993). The oestrogen therapy itself should be continuous and long term.

POSSIBLE RISKS

An increased risk of breast cancer in long-term hormone replacement therapy patients has been both reported and denied in the literature. There is no consensus on this issue.

Neither a family history of breast cancer nor a personal history of previous breast cancer should be considered as an absolute contraindication to HRT. Each case should be assessed individually by experts in the field (MacLennan and Smith, 1995).

Current evidence suggests that if a woman is at risk of heart disease (e.g. she smokes or has high blood pressure, high cholesterol levels or a strong family history of heart disease) or osteoporosis (e.g. detected by a bone density test) then the beneficial effects of HRT on these diseases would outweigh even the worst suggested (but unproven) increase in risk of breast cancer (MacLennan and Smith, 1995). Patients at risk and in fact any woman should have regular breast examination and Pap smears.

Other concomitant conditions that need to be considered with extra caution when HRT is recommended are thrombosis or blood clotting disease and some types of liver disease.

With the many issues to be considered, compliance amongst HRT users is poor. Up to 50% of women may discontinue treatment within six months of commencement (MacLennan and Smith, 1995). Reasons for non-compliance include:

- fear of breast cancer;
- recurrent vaginal bleeding;
- personal beliefs;
- lack of knowledge or ignorance.

It should be remembered that oestrogen therapy is the only treatment that unequivocally reduces fractures in postmenopausal women (Consensus Development Conference, 1993).

Bisphosphonates

Bisphosphonates act by inhibiting bone resorption (Consensus Development Conference, 1993). In patients with post-menopausal osteoporosis orally administered bisphosphonates may reduce bone loss and the incidence of vertebral fractures. Their effect on non-vertebral fracture is yet to be assessed. It is thought that bisphosphonates are most useful in the first years of menopause and in glucocorticoid-mediated osteoporosis (Tilyard, 1993). Bisphosphonates are usually given to older patients with established vertebral osteoporosis.

Calcium

Adequate dietary calcium is a requirement for normal bones. The formation of peak bone mass in the late adolescent years suggests that calcium is an important dietary consideration for children and teenagers. Calcium supplements are widely recommended by specialists and should be considered by those who avoid dairy products. An increased calcium intake is not an adequate alternative to oestrogen therapy in prevention of menopausal bone loss (Seeman et al, 1991). Table 32.3 gives daily recommended calcium intakes.

Vitamin D

Adequate vitamin D is important in the elderly who are institutionalized, housebound or sunlight deprived (Consensus Development Conference, 1993). Correction of vitamin D deficiency can reduce hip and other non-vertebral fractures (O'Neill, 1997).

Vitamin D analogues

These can improve calcium absorption in postmenopausal osteoporosis and reduce vertebral and peripheral fracture rates.

Calcitonin

Calcitonin is an inhibitor of bone resorption. It can prevent perimenopausal trabecular bone loss (Consensus Development Conference, 1993) and is also used to prevent further bone loss in patients with established osteoporosis at femoral and vertebral sites. In patients with existing vertebral fractures it has been used for its analgesic effect (Tilyard, 1993). Its ability to reduce fracture rate in established osteoporosis is still being debated. The drug is given by injection or nasal spray and concomitant calcium therapy is necessary (Consensus Development Conference, 1993).

Fluoride (sodium fluoride)

Fluoride has been used in established osteoporosis for its stimulating effect on osteoblasts and its ability to increase cancellous bone mass (Tilyard, 1993). It is not a new drug in osteoporosis treatment but its use remains controversial. Up to one-third of patients do not respond to fluoride treatment (Seeman et al, 1991) and there are a number of side effects including synovitis, periostitis (inflammation of the periosteum) and gastritis (Kamien and Prince, 1986). Its usefulness in preventing fractures has not been established.

Anabolic steroids

Anabolic steroids can increase bone mass in some women with established osteoporosis (Seeman et al, 1991). Problems associated include huskiness of the voice, increased facial hair and liver dysfunction. Treatment with these steroids can reduce bone pain after vertebral crush fractures.

Other medical treatment

Other drugs that are less widely used or are being investigated for use in osteoporosis include parathyroid hormone, growth hormone, silicon-containing compounds and strontium salts.

Management of Acute Fractures

The most common fractures encountered are vertebral fractures, fractures of the proximal femur and the distal radius. Traditionally when these fractures occur in older people as a result of only minimal trauma, they are considered to be osteoporotic. Fractures of the proximal humerus and most pelvic fractures should also be included in this category.

Vertebral fractures

These are the most commonly occurring osteoporotic fractures though they are not associated with the same rate of mortality and high health-care costs as fractures to the proximal femur (hip). It is thought that excessive loss of trabecular bone occurs as a result of ovarian failure and results in vertebral fracture (Lindsay, 1987). The slower age-related loss of cortical bone is thought to influence the weakness of the femoral neck in the elderly. On densitometry many patients with hip fracture have vertebral bone mass measurements that are considered normal for the age group (Lindsay, 1987). Many vertebral fractures are initially undiagnosed due often to the minimal nature of the trauma involved in the fracture itself and the nature of the symptoms. The most frequently fractured vertebrae are the lower six thoracic vertebrae and all of the lumbar vertebrae.

SYMPTOMS

Most patients with vertebral crush fractures will present with acute pain at the fracture site, muscle spasm and protective guarding in local muscles, particularly the paravertebrals. Only a few patients will present with radicular pain that may result from nerve root irritation due to the nature of the fracture. Generally the posterior component of the vertebral body is preserved and as such neural compression is not generally associated with vertebral compression (Borenstein et al, 1995).

Pain may be increased by activity, inspiration or laughing. In some situations pain will not be relieved by traditional methods such as positioning, heat, ice and analgesics. For some patients the acute pain may diminish in a few days to a week, allowing gradual mobilization initially guided by discomfort and pain. For some pain will persist for longer and may result in extended periods of immobilization and bed rest. Some pain and therefore limitation to activity and exercise may last for 6–12 months. Extended periods of bed rest are to be avoided as the patient will become stiff, lose muscle tone, have decreased balance reactions, will risk complications associated with immobility (e.g. respiratory and circulatory problems) and will lose further bone density if immobilization lasts long enough.

TYPES OF VERTEBRAL FRACTURES

Compression In this type of fracture the entire vertebral body collapses. This can be a slow process that occurs over time.

Anterior wedge fractures Reduction of anterior height results when the anterior cortex collapses. Posterior height remains unchanged (see Fig. 32.5).

Biconcave fractures A concave deformity results after collapse of the superior or inferior endplate. Posterior and inferior heights may remain unchanged.

MANAGEMENT

Many patients will require bed rest or at least limitations to their activity. This is usually guided by pain. Extended periods of bed rest have the disadvantage of further detrimental effects on bone density and also on overall fitness, condition and psychological well-being. Some patients will be hospitalized at this stage. Need for this will vary and will be related to availability of home support services, the patient's ability to manage pain and their psychological state, their ability to mobilize for toileting, etc. and the amount of motivation they have from their doctor and caregivers. A patient is far more likely to mobilize 'through pain' or 'with pain' if the doctor has suggested that this is an important step in the rehabilitation process. If a patient is told not to move at all if there is pain they may well be in the same position six months later. Verbal cues to the patient are very important. 'Movement may hurt at first', 'Listen carefully to the pain – push limits sometimes and set limits at other times' are positive and reassuring comments. Comments such as 'Let pain be your guide' can lead to an avoidance of movement and progressive loss of function (McIndoe, 1995). It is possible that some patients will be more comfortable with a gentle mobility programme and sitting rather than bed rest. This is acceptable, even desirable, as long as the fracture is considered stable. Because of the compressive nature of many fractures they may never be considered unstable.

PHYSIOTHERAPY MANAGEMENT

Mobility and transfers Positions of comfort, individual to each patient, will need to be discussed. Often flexed positions will be more comfortable. Side lying with pillow support for the trunk and a pillow between the knees or crook lying with a pillow under the knees may be preferable. Purpose-designed mattress covers to decrease pressure and promote circulation may be useful. Where possible the mattress may need to be assessed for suitability. This is always related to individual preference, particularly in this population who may be reluctant to change a mattress. As soon as pain allows the patient must be encouraged to extend out of these positions into ones that encourage less flexion. The patient will need to be taught how to change positions in bed as well as transfer to chair and toilet with minimal stress and pain. Log rolling and sitting from side lying with hips in a flexed position and no trunk movement are important skills to minimize pain. Some will prefer moving off the bed backwards from prone (Fig. 32.7). Overhead monkey rings/trapeze may be useful for some but this technique and that of weight transferral on extended arms require good upper limb strength and scapular stability and may irritate paravertebral muscle spasm. They may be more helpful to some patients (lumbar fractures) and less helpful to others (thoracic fractures).

It is suggested that the patient stand out of bed for at least 10 minutes every hour (Luckert, 1994). This should be progressed daily if possible. The use of activity charts to record daily activity and exercise can be encouraging and motivational. The patient will be able to see progress over a period of time even if they are unaware of daily progression. Pain on a visual analogue scale of 0–10 and pain management techniques can also be mapped on this chart (Table 32.4).

A mobility aid may be necessary and will be chosen according to the patient's pain, tolerance and comorbid conditions (e.g. rheumatoid arthritis). A forearm support frame, a pick-up frame, a walking stick or even crutches can all offer confidence and support to the patient's efforts to mobilize. On occasions the use of frames and crutches may assist pain reduction by decreasing spinal loading. Without the use of such devices some patients will not achieve early mobilization. Any amount of mobilization should be encouraged and it can be useful to record distance or time so that gradual improvements in endurance are recognized and therefore motivational.

Pain management Collapse of the bone and stretching of the periosteum will result in acute pain and changing stresses on soft tissue structures and altered biomechanics will contribute to long-term chronic pain.

Figure 32.7 Patients will need to be taught to get in and out of bed with minimal pain. (a) Some will prefer going from side lying to sitting with a stiff back while others (b) may find moving off the bed backwards in prone helpful.

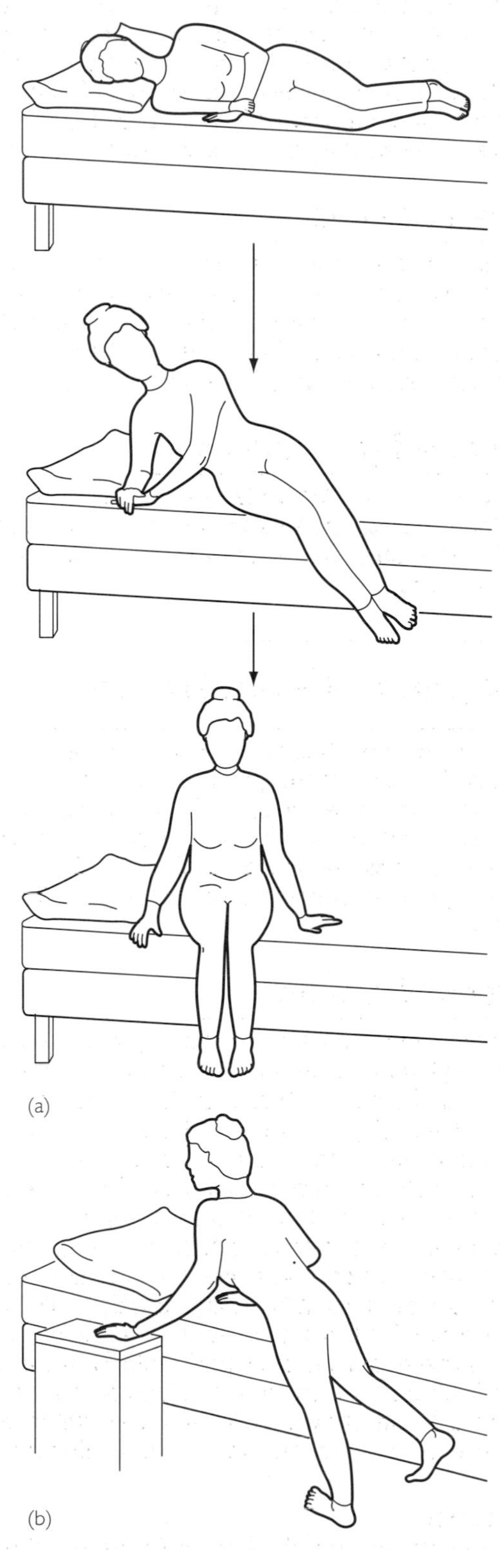

Table 32.4 Diary of activity, pain and medication

Date:		Sunday	Monday	Tuesday	Wednesday	Thursday	Friday	Saturday
Morning	Activity							
	Pain scale 0–10							
	Pain Relief							
Afternoon	Activity							
	Pain scale 0–10							
	Pain Relief							
Night	Activity							
	Pain scale 0–10							
	Pain Relief							

General comments

Achievements and gains:

Problems:

This week compared to last week:

Frustrations:

Codes:

Activity Wk = Walking (distance) around bedroom, house, shops, etc.
PE = Posture exercises (number according to your exercise sheet, repetitions)
RBE = Rubber band exercises (type of band and repetitions)
WE = Water exercises (intensity level – easy, moderate, hard (perceived exertion))
WT = Weight training (intensity, repetitions, weight)
Ae = Aerobics class (Intensity level – easy, moderate, hard (perceived exertion))

Other ____________________

Pain relief I = Ice
H = Heat
T = TENS
M = Medication (please specify)
O = Other
R = Rest in bed (list time)
B = Brace (list time without initially)

Pain Scale 0 = no pain, 10 = unbearable pain

Role of the physiotherapist The physiotherapist will need to bring many skills into the patient–therapist relationship that deals with acute and later chronic pain. An understanding of the relationship between pain and motivation and an understanding of the need to push gently yet not to lose the patient's confidence are both essential. The physiotherapist will spend considerable time with the patient and the patient often feels able to share their thoughts and concerns. Responding appropriately and giving correct verbal and tactile cues to promote early rehabilitation is important. The role of the physiotherapist will vary somewhat depending on the patient's situation in the health-care system. If they are 'employing' the physiotherapist and treatment does not meet their expectation then they may end the relationship. These are the realities of a commercial world. Patient expectations need to be considered.

Education for pain The patient will need some motivation and encouragement that their pain will in fact diminish. With some patients there can be no guarantee that their pain will totally disappear and some will have a residual level of disability. Patients should be encouraged to set some short-term realistic goals that are achievable and to have realistic longer term goals. As mentioned, pain and activity diaries can be useful to show the patient objectively that progress has in fact been made (see Table 32.4). These can also map for the patient the use of other pain management strategies such as medications and transcutaneous electrical nerve stimulation (TENS) and show a reduction of their use over time.

Ice Ice packs (Turner, 1991) or ice massage may be tolerated by some patients and can result in effective pain reduction for a few hours. Cold (as in ice packs) reduces the conduction of some pain nerves in the skin and can provide sensory stimulation that acts on the pain gate. Ice massage may act as a counterirritant (Low and Reed, 1990) and thus decrease the sensation of pain. Some patients will find ice of any kind unpleasant and as a result muscle spasm may increase. Increased stiffness may result from the cooling process (Low and Reed, 1990). Many patients are not willing to try ice as a treatment and they may associate it with pain to such an extent that the anticipated benefits are outweighed by the psychological stress (Palastanga, 1994).

Superficial heat Different forms of heat, even the simplest, can be useful in decreasing muscle spasm and pain. Afferent nerves stimulated by heat may have an analgesic effect by acting on the gate control mechanism and muscle spasm may also be reduced by superficial heat (Low and Reed, 1990). Electric heating pads, heated wheat products, hot water bottles and warm showers can be used but may be limited by the patient's ability to position themselves correctly and comfortably for the treatment.

Electrotherapy Pulsed shortwave can be used to reduce osteoporotic pain (Low and Reed, 1990). This may be as a result of a reduction in local swelling and inflammation or an increased rate of fibrin and collagen deposition. Pulsed ultrasound may be beneficial (Turner, 1991) either because of local thermal effects or an altered electrical activity in the nerves resulting in pain relief. Anecdotal reports suggest laser may be useful in some patients with localized pain.

Soft tissue manipulation Various forms of massage are mentioned in the literature as being useful. Effleurage and gentle muscle rolling techniques are suggested (Turner, 1991). It may be possible to decrease protective muscle spasm in the paraspinal muscles using these techniques and they may also help in the reduction of anxiety prior to exercise and mobilization. The massage can be incorporated into gentle passive and then active assisted movements of the trunk and limbs.

Spinal mobilization techniques As a result of pain and protective spasm, other segments of the spine will become stiff and immobile. This can increase pain and lack of function. Gentle mobilization techniques can be used to decrease these signs in the segments above and below the fracture. Many patients report that aquatic spinal mobilization assists in pain relief.

Transcutaneous electrical nerve stimulation Many patients will find that TENS offers significant pain relief and it can be effective in relieving the more chronic pain found in the older patient. Skin sensation should be assessed. Large stick-on electrodes can be used. TENS should be applied for at least 30 minutes and can be applied continuously or for a prescribed time. There is no apparent disadvantage in the use of this modality; as with all pain relief, there should be encouragement to progress which in this case means using it for progressively less time. Skin care is necessary, particularly in those patients who may have been on long-term steroids and whose skin is consequently very papery or transparent.

Bracing – spinal orthotics The literature is mixed in its view of braces. If the patient is getting adequate relief and able to commence early mobilization then the use of a brace may not be indicated. However, if the patient is slow to progress and pain is a problem or persists then a brace may be of benefit.

There is a range of suitable braces and corsets but all braces should be individually made or fitted. The type of brace will be dependent on the level of the fracture. Poor compliance is often related to ill-fitting devices. Braces generally help to stabilize and immobilize the spine to allow earlier mobility with less pain. The design of these devices is such that they restrict flexion and encourage neutral extension of the spine. Patients need to be educated that these appliances are an interim measure and that the body needs to reactivate its natural bracing mechanisms, including the back, neck and hip extensors and the abdominals, so that in time they will take over from the brace and better support the spine. Spinal bracing may lead to reduced use of the back extensor muscles and contribute to their increased weakness and loss of their stabilizing function (Culham, 1995). Abdominal strength may also quickly become reduced while wearing a brace (Vargo and Gerber, 1993). When prescribing a brace, the patient must be well educated to activate the extensors and the flexors either when the brace is removed or while it is on by drawing in their abdomen away from the support and isometrically activating multifidus (see Chapter 14). It is important that the therapist emphasizes stability of the spine and a tall posture without any exaggeration of the spinal curves.

Exercise The main problems faced by the patient are:

- pain;
- fear of movement;
- depression.

Goals for the physiotherapist include:

- To reduce or minimize pain during and after exercise;
- early mobilization;
- activation of the major trunk stabilizers;
- the maintenance of the patient–physiotherapist relationship.

In the initial phase pain and anxiety will severely limit the patient's desire to co-operate with any exercise programme. 'Movement' might be a better word than 'exercise', which frightens some people in pain (McIndoe, 1995).

Initial exercises during the acute phase will be directed at reduction of pain, maintenance of good circulation including prevention of pressure areas and good lung expansion. Pain will inhibit movement in all areas including the rib cage and chest expansion. The physiotherapist must be guided by the patient's pain tolerance, particularly to avoid further damage and also to maintain the patient's confidence in the physiotherapist. However, the reality is that the patient must move to prevent further bone loss, deterioration of other systems and an increased likelihood of falling. The patient–physiotherapist relationship may be a long one as pain can last for many months, significantly influencing movement and function.

Spinal extension exercises are commenced as early as possible though they may not be possible in the acute phase. An attempt to activate the muscles that extend the spine while in side lying may be a good compromise. The physiotherapist can place the fingers of one hand on the shelf of the sacrum and those of the other hand on the patient's occiput and can instruct the patient to imagine drawing these two points close together (Fig. 32.8). Such minimal contraction will help to maintain multifidus activation. In some cases these exercises themselves will assist in pain relief; in others little extension will be tolerated. A diary of exercises and pain scale can be kept to assure the patient that progress is slowly being made (see Table 32.4).

Initially static exercises are all the patient is capable of doing. These should progress to active exercises as soon as possible. Progression of the kyphotic deformity needs to be discouraged and spinal extensor exercises are the primary target. In most patients there will be weakness in other muscles, particularly the scapular stabilizers and shoulder extensors. Limited shoulder mobility in the sagittal plane has been demonstrated in the established osteoporotic population (Pearlmutter et al, 1995). A good exercise programme will look at all these muscle groups and other associated muscles and ensure strength and endurance in them all within the limits of pain. Patients are often concerned about their abdominal bulge or pot belly and need to be educated about the risk of dynamically exercising the abdominal flexors and predisposing themselves to future wedge fractures (Sinaki and Mikkelson, 1984). Static abdominal exercises need to be taught to the patient, particularly to train the transversus abdominis in its role as a stabilizer.

Figure 32.8 Facilitation of extension in side lying (see text).

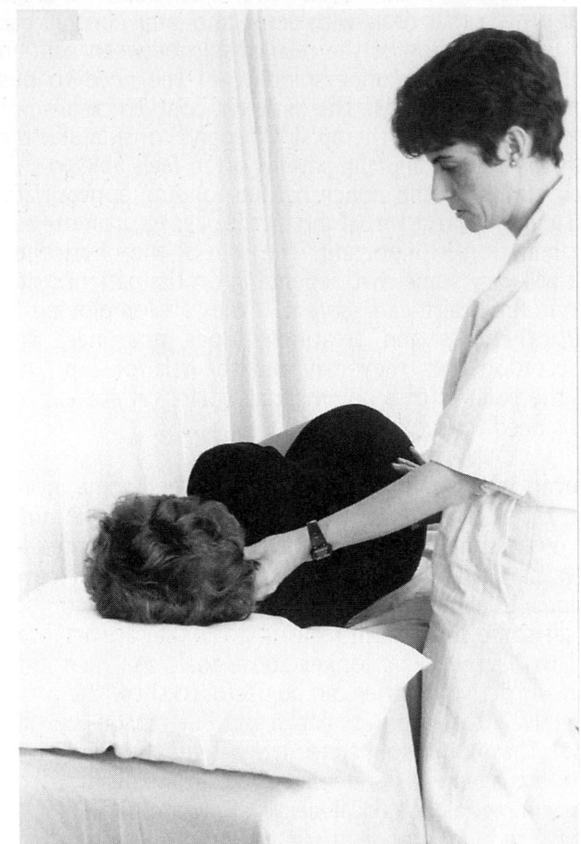

Extension may progress from side lying (Fig. 32.8) to supine if tolerated (Fig. 32.9). For some patients it may be more comfortable to begin extension in a chair (Fig. 32.10). Bridging will be difficult at first but should be encouraged as pain allows (Fig. 32.11a). In the bridging start position gentle rocking of the knees from side to side within pain limits will allow the beginning of functional rotation as an exercise (Fig. 32.11b). Rotation is often eliminated from exercise programmes for osteoporosis. It is, however, a functional movement (getting in and out of a car and bed) and should be re-educated slowly and with control.

Prone lying should be encouraged as soon as the patient is able to achieve the position. Hip extension from this position and extension of the head and shoulders should be

Figure 32.9 Extension exercises and postures in supine. (a) No pillow under head. Head can be gently pushed down into support and chin retracted. *Instruction*: 'Gently push the back of your head into the bed while pulling your chin down slightly against my finger.' *Inappropriate action*: Tilting the head back which will extend the cervical spine too far. *Handling*: Physiotherapist can facilitate under the mental protuberance of the mandible/chin. (b) Arms abducted to 90°, elbows at 90°. Push elbows back into bed. If the patient is unable to elevate the arms and keep the legs on the bed (as in e) without hyperextension of the lumbar spine then she can lie in crook lying and flex the elbows to 90°. (c) Alternate arm elevation. This can be used to mobilize the thoracic spine. The physiotherapist asks the patient to keep one scapula on the bed as she moves her opposite arm through range then as a progression, she can lift her ipsilateral scapula as she moves their arm through range, thus bringing in some rotation of the thoracic spine. (d) Bilateral arm elevation. *Instructions*: 'Lie on a firm surface with your arms above your head for a period of time so as to place your spine in a straight or slightly extended posture.' If possible the patient can push the arms and legs gently into the bed to activate the back, shoulder and hip extensors. (e) Arms elevated. A roll can be placed under the thoracic spine to increase thoracic extension if appropriate. In all the exercises above the knees can be flexed to a crook-lying position if the patient experiences pain rather than a simply a stretching sensation.

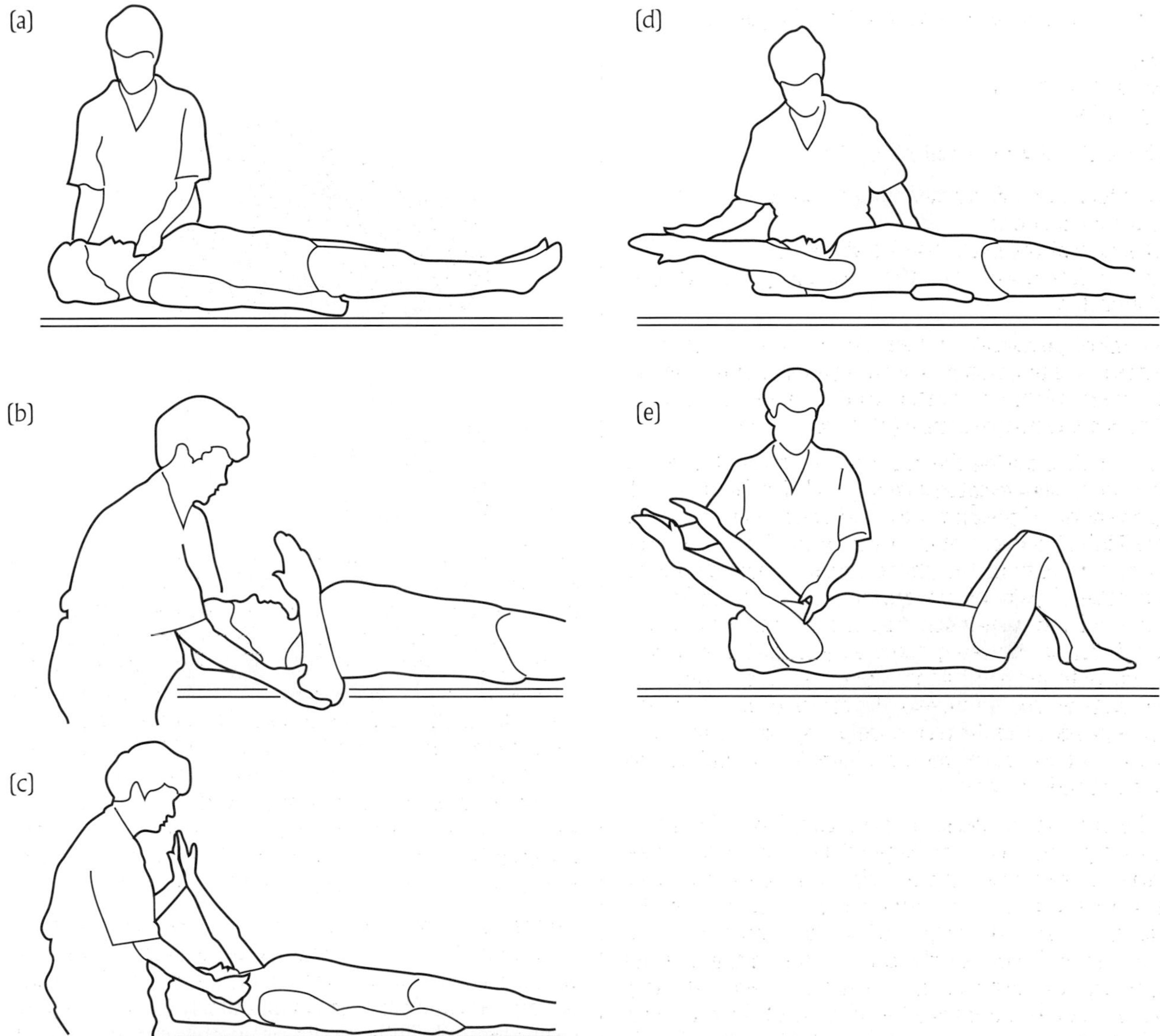

encouraged (Fig. 32.12). When pain and posture prevents extension in the prone position the patient may be able to stand in a safe and secure position and extend their leg, initially within a pain-free range.

Specific exercises designed to strengthen and stretch scapular musculature should be included as a component of an osteoporosis programme because limited shoulder mobility in the sagittal plane has been demonstrated in patients with established osteoporosis (Pearlmutter et al, 1995).

Exercise of peripheral musculature that can occur without increasing pain should be encouraged as early as tolerated. This will allow maintenance of flexibility, strength and endurance and hopefully slow deconditioning. Small hand weights and resistance bands may be encouraged.

Figure 32.10 Extension exercises (of neck and thoracic spine) and shoulder exercises may be more comfortable in a chair. These exercises can be continued but the patient should be encouraged to attempt the prone position as pain improves. (a) Chin tucks and spinal extension. Patient can aim to 'make herself taller'. Find a seat with a high back support (a car seat with head support may be appropriate). *Instructions*: 'Think that you have a string pulling up from the top of your head and making you 2 inches taller. Push the centre of the back of the head into the support while tucking the chin in. At the same time pull your shoulder blades down and together. Tilt your pelvis forward to make a slight hollow in the small of your back.' *Handling*: The physiotherapist can facilitate by holding a finger under the chin to encourage retraction. *Inappropriate action*: Levator scapulae and upper trapezius. Don't allow the cervical spine to extend. Starting position and action will depend on the kyphotic deformity present. (b) Thoracic extension and shoulder elevation in sitting. Have shoulder blades leaning gently on the back of a comfortable chair then elevate the arms as far as possible and extend the thoracic spine against the chair. *Inappropriate action*: Do not let the buttocks slide forward on the chair. (c) Neck extension and shoulder stretch (care taken not to extend the cervical spine too vigorously in rheumatoid patients). (d) Shoulder extension and scapular retraction, resisted by use of elastic/rubber tubing. Similarly, shoulder lateral rotation and rhomboids can be worked. Maintain contraction for 6–12 seconds. Physiotherapist can facilitate (a, on figure) scapular and thoracic control and (b, on figure) abdominal and trunk control.

a

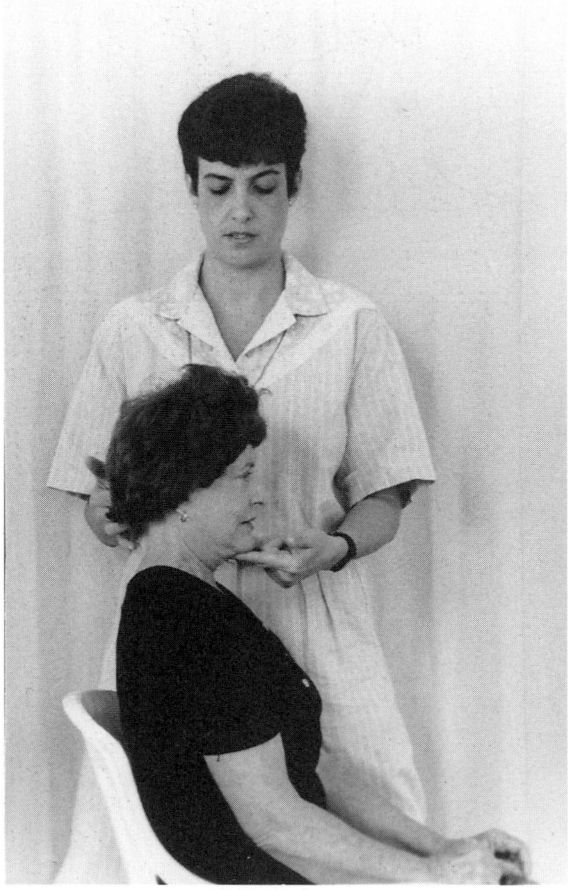

b

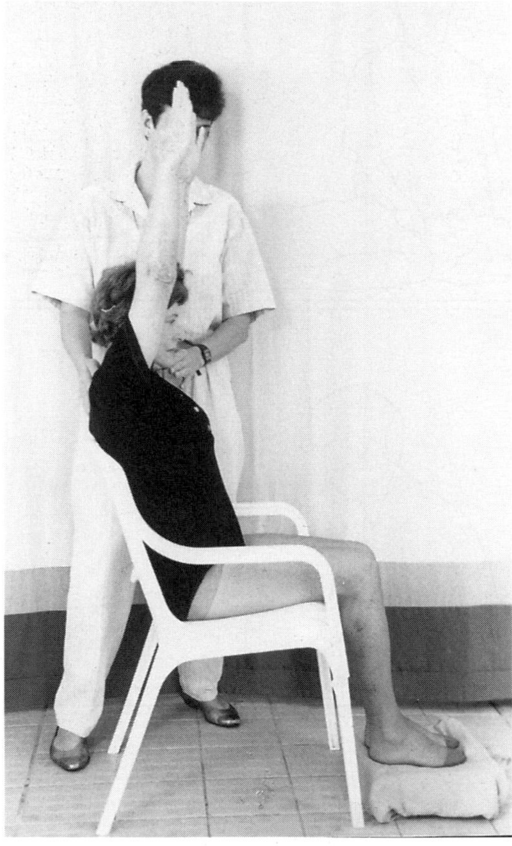

The existence of some comorbid conditions (e.g. rheumatoid arthritis) will require the combination of joint protection techniques with exercise prescription for osteoporosis.

Hydrotherapy Hydrotherapy should be considered as an early treatment option. Warmth and the effects of gravity reduction on pain will often allow early movement that the patient is unable to achieve on land. In some cases effort and diligence will inhibit pain and fun play and pleasure will facilitate movement (McIndoe, 1995). The hydrotherapy pool is often a less clinical environment which allows the patient to relax a little and yet still achieve both exercise and pain reduction. Hydrotherapy should be considered as soon as the patient can be transferred to the pool in a wheelchair and at this stage should be a hands-on treatment on a one-to-one basis. The main concern is that the patient may get significant pain relief and move too rapidly, causing later pain. Work for trunk stabilizers in the pool is essential. A full range of exercises for osteoporosis is included in the following pages. Patients' progression will initially be limited by their pain threshold and severity or number of fractures.

Hip fractures

Fractures of the hip are the most disabling and life-threatening consequence of osteoporosis (Notelovitz and Ware, 1982). Hip fractures are related to a one year mortality of 12–20%. Death from hip fractures is not a result of the fracture itself but rather the problems associated with immobilization and extended hospital or nursing home

Figure 32.10 Continued

c

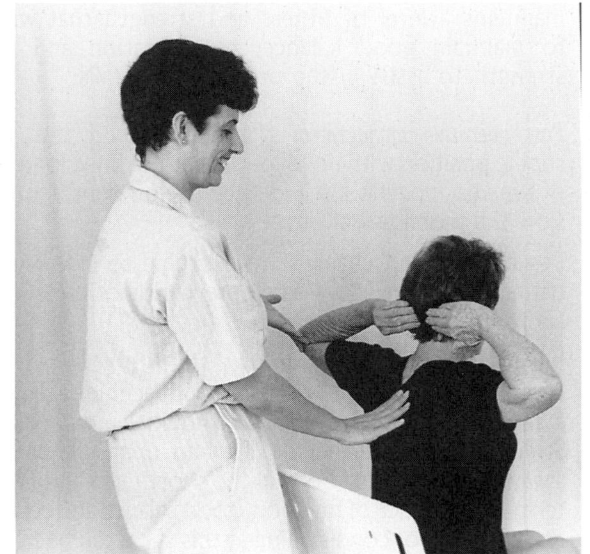

d

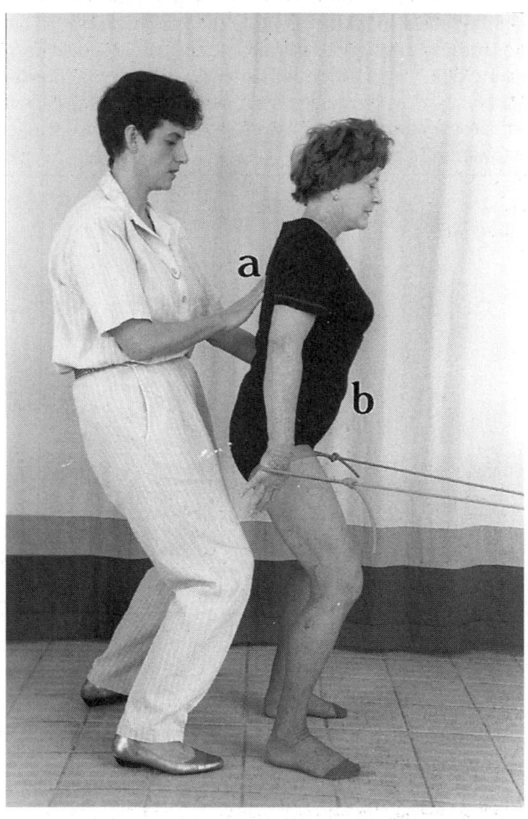

stay. Complications include pneumonia, thrombosis and fat embolism. Hip fractures are responsible for the primary costs arising from osteoporosis and this is related to the length of hospitalization and the nursing home admission for many patients. With surgical advances in the treatment of these fractures, the length of hospital stay has decreased but the growing aged population means that more fractures are presenting for admission. Length of hospital stay increases with age and the proportion discharged home decreases with age (Lord and Sinnett, 1986).

At the age of 50 a woman has a 15% chance of suffering a hip fracture in her subsequent life (Owen, personal communication). This risk increases with age.

TYPES OF FRACTURE AND SURGICAL INTERVENTION

The goal of management of hip fractures is to stabilize the fracture as early as possible and many hospitals aim to operate on hip fracture patients within 24–48 hours. Early intervention allows early mobilization and ambulation and the prevention of complications associated with immobility. It is noted that some countries with different financial structures for health care will be unable to achieve this surgical intervention. In these cases management is often bed rest and traction which was commonly the treatment used prior to access to advanced surgical procedure.

Where surgical intervention is appropriate, the anatomical position of the fracture will help to dictate the procedure used.

Intracapsular (cervical or subcapital) hip fracture These fractures will often be complicated by interruption to the blood supply to the femoral head. Because of this non-union and avascular necrosis are common complications. Surgical management with a hemiarthroplasty is the preferred treatment for displaced fractures in patients over the age of 85 and avoids such complications. In younger patients internal fixation may be the surgical option. In assessing final operative choice the pre-fracture activity levels and the general health of the patient as well as the amount of displacement and the degree of osteoporosis will be taken into account.

Extracapsular (pertrochanteric or basilar) There are fewer complications associated with interruption to the blood supply in this type of fracture. Surgical management is usually by internal fixation using a variety of pins, compression screws, nails and plates. Complications will include wound failure and medical problems such as pulmonary and cardiovascular complications. These are the most common fracture in this population.

Figure 32.11 (a) Bridging to assist bed mobility and promote gluteal extension. *Inappropriate action*: Overuse of hamstrings and not gluteal muscles. *Handling*: Facilitation can be given by gently touching the ASIS and asking the patient to lift her pelvis up towards your hand. (b) Gentle rotation or rocking can begin as pain allows. The patient should be in a comfortable crook-lying position and her feet should stay on the support. The physiotherapist can encourage the rotation by asking the patient to rotate her knees towards her hand, which is placed on the medial aspect of the knee towards the movement.

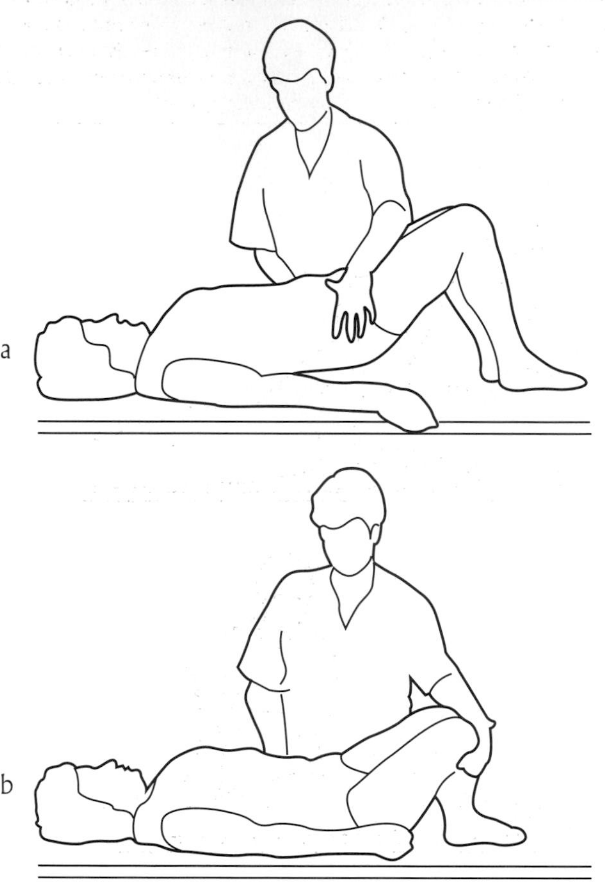

Subtrochanteric fractures Less common than the previous two categories, these fractures can occur through the femoral trochanter (avulsion) or between the trochanters (intertrochanteric). Non-union is rare as blood supply is good. Surgical management is often with intermedullary nail or other internal fixation.

Fractures at the site of an existing endoprosthesis such as total hip replacements are becoming more common and require difficult surgical procedures to revise original prostheses. The procedure is complicated by osteoporotic bones.

Physiotherapy management of hip fractures Improving range of movement of the affected hip joint and achieving early mobilization with a return to pain-free independent ambulation must be the overall goals of treatment. Prevention of complications related to immobilization is essential, particularly considering 30-day mortality rates of 7% (Owen, personal communication). That is, 7% of hip fracture patients will die within 30 days. As there is a high risk of patients with hip fractures refracturing their hips or falling again, it is important that the patient maintains a level of fitness and strength that will help to maintain good balance, co-ordination and muscle strength to assist in the prevention of falls.

Post-operative management Patients should rest in the supine position with no pillow under the knee for a period of time each day as hip and knee flexion contractures will slow the mobilization process.

Regular position changes from supine to side lying and sitting when allowed will assist prevention of pressure areas and ventilation.

Initially mobility in bed and with transfers should be discussed and supervised to ensure good technique. The use of a monkey bar above the bed should be demonstrated. Strength in the unaffected leg and upper limbs should always be considered both in the short term and for long-term maintenance of function, good balance and co-ordination. The loss of conditioning at this stage can be rapid and the patient should be encouraged to maintain as much muscle work as possible.

Exercises should include active assisted range of motion exercises for the hip and static quadriceps and gluteal exercises. A powder board or friction-free board is useful for mobilization and allows the patient to exercise when the physiotherapist is not present. This allows a shift from dependence on the therapist to self-management at a very basic level (McIndoe, 1995). Ankle and foot exercises including plantarflexion, dorsiflexion and circumduction should be encouraged hourly during waking hours to minimize risk of venous thrombosis. Upper limb exercises to maintain range of movement and strength should be encouraged, particularly if the patient is to have an extended time on crutches.

Early mobilization is necessary to prevent the secondary complications of immobilization. Protocols for mobilization will vary from surgeon to surgeon and will depend on surgical outcomes and the health status of the patient.

The use of appropriate mobility aids will assist early ambulation. Forearm support frames, pick-up frames and, for the more able patients, crutches can be used. Weight-bearing protocols will be as discussed with the surgeon but will usually progress from touch weight bearing to partial weight bearing and then full weight bearing over a period of six weeks to four months. Length of time spent on mobility aids will be a function of the success of the surgical stabilization (including radiographic examination) and will also be limited by pain and co-ordination, fear of movement, fear of falling, lack of motivation and depression.

Non-surgical management When surgical intervention is not possible due to the medical condition of the patient or possibly access to appropriate surgical care, then bed traction with immobilization is often the preferred treatment. Prevention of cardiorespiratory and circulatory complications is essential.

Figure 32.12 A progression of neck, back and shoulder extension exercises and postures in prone and four-point kneeling. (a) The patient is encouraged to lie prone as soon as pain allows. A pillow can be placed under the abdomen initially if lumbar lordosis causes pain. The patient is encouraged to maintain this position initially for a few minutes, progressing to 30 minutes or more. Progress to neck and shoulder extension (not shown). From the above starting position, the patient is encouraged to extend her neck while maintaining some chin retraction. *Handling*: The physiotherapist can place her hands over the scapula and thoracic spine to encourage lower trapezius and multifidus. (b) Scapular retraction and back extensor stabilization. The patient lies prone with the arms elevated. Initially the elbows can be flexed to approximately 80–90° then the exercise is progressed by having straight arms (shown). *Instructions*: 'Lift alternate arms (progressing to both arms) off the support.' (c) Patient can progress to a prone position on elbows. This position can initially be held for a few seconds but the time should be increased as pain permits. (d) Back extensor stabilizers with knee flexion. Patient is in prone lying and is asked to bend and straighten alternate knees. This can be progressed to bilateral knee flexion and then unilateral hip extension with knees flexed or extended. *Handling*: The physiotherapist can place her hand over the erector spinae and gluteal muscles to encourage activity in both. (e) Unilateral extension in four-point kneeling. The patient is assisted into four-point kneeling while maintaining slight flexion of the elbows, good scapula stability and control of the spine and pelvis. *Instructions*: 'Stretch one leg out behind while holding the shoulders and pelvis firm.' progress to knee bent. *Handling*: The physiotherapist can place one hand either on the gluteals to facilitate a contraction or on transverse abdominal muscles to promote stability. The other hand is on the posterior leg to guide the movement. If the patient is unable to achieve this position on land then it can be tried on a step or ramp in a hydrotherapy pool.

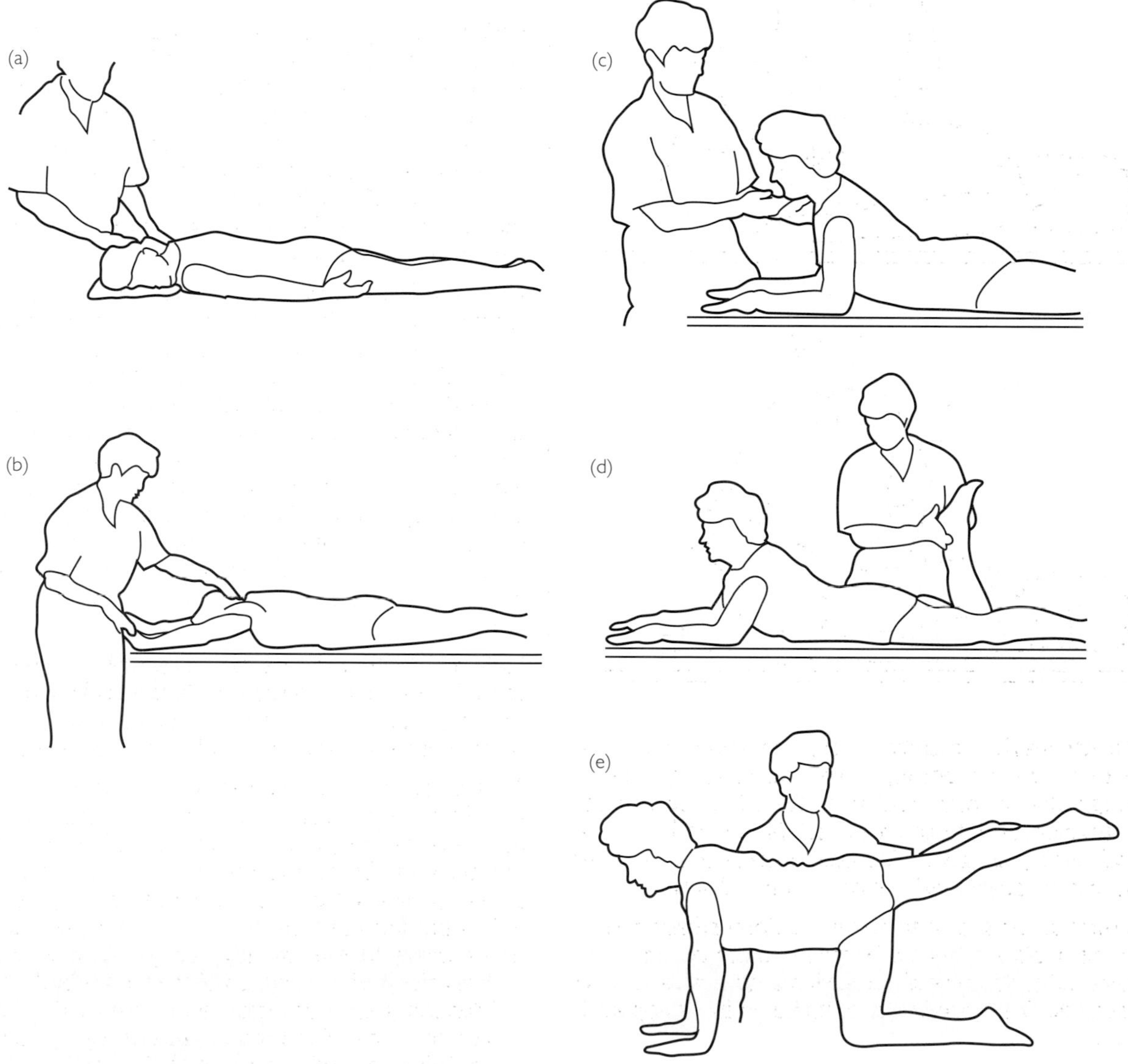

Hydrotherapy Hydrotherapy helps to accelerate the rehabilitation of elderly patients who have sustained fractured neck of femur (Skinner and Thomson, 1994). The fear of falling and decreasing confidence can inhibit the patient's progress, as can pain. In some patients who are slow to mobilize and respond to traditional orthopaedic intervention programmes, hydrotherapy can be a useful adjunct.

One-on-one treatment in a suitable pool can begin as soon as the wound is deemed safe to immerse. There are a variety of wound dressings that are widely used for this purpose. (The author has experience in taking total hip replacements into the pool on day 4 post-surgery.) Water temperatures that are thermoneutral (34–35°C) will assist in pain reduction due to both a sensory effect of the heat and a reduction of muscle spasm. Walking at determined depths to achieve specific weight bearing situations can be calculated (Harrison and Bulstrode, 1987). No mobility aid is necessary in the pool, but for those who have difficulty co-ordinating ambulatory aids, the pool can be a useful place to begin to practise using them. The reduced weight-bearing situation and the resulting reduction in pain will often see patients gain confidence in movement again. Programmes to improve balance, co-ordination, range of motion and strength can also be initiated in the pool (Fig. 32.13). Functional activities such as sit to stand, stairs and practising getting up from a fall are assisted by buoyancy and the patient can gain confidence in these movements. Fitness activities can begin in the pool relatively early in the rehabilitation programme. Compliance and motivation are often high because of pain reduction on immersion and because most hydrotherapy treatments develop a self-management approach, offer a social perspective and in fact are often enjoyable.

Distal radial fractures

PHYSIOTHERAPY MANAGEMENT

Patients presenting with distal forearm fractures (Colles') are rarely admitted to hospital and as such are not as great a financial problem to the community. Acute treatment is usually immobilization in plaster after reduction.

Static exercises of muscle groups around the elbow and wrist are commenced as directed by the orthopaedic surgeon. Posture should be assessed with plaster on and appropriate corrective exercises prescribed. Finger and shoulder exercises should be given as well as ensuring that normal activity levels will continue to maintain fitness and current bone mass. If the fracture is the result of a fall the patient may have lost confidence in mobility and performing everyday tasks. Considering that after a fall a patient has an increased risk of further falls, it is essential to commence fall prevention strategies.

Ensure that the patient has been screened for risk factors and possible osteoporosis if they have presented merely as a fracture. Education regarding exercise, calcium intake and reduction of risk factors is essential.

If the patient is unwilling to continue with any land exercise programme a hydrotherapy programme in either

Figure 32.13 (a) Active knee flexion and extension in sitting in the hydrotherapy pool. Initially no resistance device would be used. Progress by increasing the speed of the movement and adding devices that increase the surface area such as the Aquatoner (North Carolina, USA) (pictured) or Water Gator (Toronto, Australia). (b) Static standing balance can progress to the physiotherapist creating an external perturbation by using turbulence or the patient disturbing her own balance with shoulder flexion and extension, encouraging ankle, hip and knee balance strategies. *Instructions*: 'Keeping your elbows straight, pull your arms back and forward through the water in small range fast movements. Pull with your palms so once your hands are forward the palms should be turned over to lead the backward movement. Keep the rest of your body still by holding your stomach and buttocks tight.' Progress speed and add resistance devices such as gloves. Progress to doing on one leg and with eyes shut.

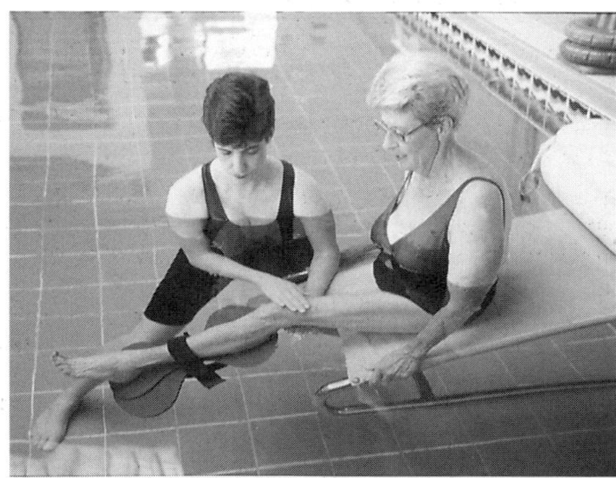

a

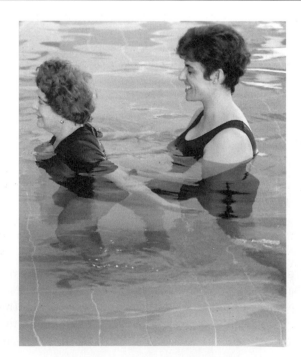

b

Figure 32.14 Devices are available that will allow the early mobilization in the pool of patients with plaster casts (Seal-Tight, Brisbane, Australia).

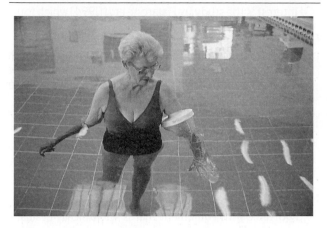

an individual or group session may be appropriate. An appliance is available to allow patients with plasters of Paris to both shower and perform pool activities while keeping their plaster dry (Seal-Tight, Brisbane, Australia) (Fig. 32.14). Fitness, range of shoulder movement, balance and co-ordination and falls prevention techniques can all begin in the hydrotherapy pool as soon as pain settles and thus prevent a long period of decreased mobility.

Following the removal of the plaster the objectives of physiotherapy are:

- to regain pain-free wrist and finger movement;
- to improve grip strength;
- to improve hand function;
- to ensure correct post-immobilization posture (scapular stabilizers, upper trapezius);
- to educate regarding osteoporosis management;
- to instigate fall prevention programme;
- to educate in lifestyle management.

General orthopaedic texts will further detail the treatment rationale for fractures of the distal radius.

Complications can occur and include reflex sympathetic dystrophy and shoulder hand syndrome.

Physiotherapy and Osteoporosis: Long-term Management

Physiotherapy-prescribed exercise, treatment and other management techniques for osteoporosis have the following goals.

- To maintain, slow the loss of or increase bone density in patients at risk of osteoporosis, those with diagnosed osteoporosis and no fracture or those with osteoporotic fracture.
- To reduce pain if it exists.
- To prevent spinal deformity and vertebral fractures.
- The prevention of falls and the maintenance of mobility and independence.
- Education.

Exercise to improve or maintain bone density for osteoporosis

Bone strength is a function of mechanical and structural properties. These can be modified in response to the mechanical forces or loads to which the bone has been exposed. Growing bone adapts to the load placed upon it by an enhanced bone mineral density.

Debate exists in the literature as to the benefit of exercise in maintaining or improving bone density in osteoporosis. Certainly exercise on its own without adequate oestrogen or calcium will not achieve bone mass improvements. Exercise in the immediate post-menopausal period must first overcome the rapid loss of bone mass as a result of the reduced oestrogen levels before it can influence bone mass. Exercise can have positive benefits. Nelson et al (1994) found that high-intensity strength training has a protective effect on the femoral neck and lumbar spine bone mineral density as well as promoting increased muscle mass, strength, dynamic balance and overall physical activity levels in post-menopausal women. It is suggested that these outcomes may mediate a reduction of the risk for future osteoporotic fractures. In contrast, traditional pharmacologic and nutritional approaches to the treatment or prevention of osteoporosis may be able to maintain or slow the loss of bone, but not improve balance, strength, muscle mass or physical activity levels.

Exercise that has the goal of maintaining or improving bone density in the post-menopausal woman falls into three categories:

1. weight-bearing exercise;
2. resistance exercise;
3. aerobic exercise.

WEIGHT-BEARING EXERCISE

Activities traditionally seen as weight bearing (e.g. walking) are important for developing bone and for the attainment of peak bone mass. As bone ages the effects of walking on bone accrual diminishes.

> In general, results from research examining walking intervention programs demonstrate that this activity, commonly prescribed for post-menopausal women, does not prevent bone loss. Other studies that include activities of higher intensity and the addition of muscle building exercises report a more positive skeletal response (Drinkwater, 1995).

Walking for 15–20 minutes a day three times a week is not enough to retard post-menopausal bone loss from the axial skeleton (Rutherford, 1990).

Problems with studies that looked at walking include difficulty in quantifying the intensity of walking exercise in a community setting and in monitoring compliance.

'A walking program may provide sufficient stimulation for bone formation in previously sedentary individuals but is unlikely to result in change in bone mass in persons with a more active lifestyle' (Culham, 1995).

When attempted, walking programmes should be safe and the patient assessed to ensure that they are not at greater risk of falling during their weight-bearing activity. Considering the principle of progressive overload, a level of activity needs to be prescribed that exceeds their normal loading (Drinkwater, 1995). Certainly a moderate level of exercise should be a progressive goal.

RESISTANCE EXERCISE

The concept that resistance training increases bone mineral density has been both supported in pre-menopausal (Gleeson et al, 1990) and post-menopausal women (Notelovitz et al, 1991) and refuted in pre-menopausal (Rockwell et al, 1990) and post-menopausal women (Moroz et al, 1989; Sinaki et al, 1989). There are also studies that suggest that the combination of resistance training and aerobic exercise is more beneficial to bone density than aerobic exercise alone (Rickli and McManus, 1990).

If a one-repetition maximum test (1-RM) is to be used as an assessment tool for establishing strength and strength gains some precautions must be taken. In a 1-RM test or whenever a maximal motor effort is performed, recruitment of non-target motor groups and altered body mechanics may occur. Guidelines to minimize this for each muscle group need to be developed and used, especially in testing older people (Skinner, 1993). A 1-RM test will be inappropriate in many cases.

The use of resistance training equipment for frail, aged patients with high risk of fracture or those with concomitant disease processes such as rheumatoid arthritis may not be appropriate. Strength of elderly subjects has improved in studies using light wrist and ankle weights and elastic bands (tube). It has been suggested that persons with spinal osteoporosis should lift no more than 10 lbs (Aisenbrey, 1987). An alternative way to provide resistance is through water exercise.

A 1991 study (Notelovitz et al, 1991) showed that a high-intensity, low-repetition muscle-strengthening programme in conjunction with oestrogen replacement therapy was more effective in increasing bone mineral density than oestrogen therapy alone. More recent studies have found that high-intensity, low-repetition exercise appears to be of most benefit to bone mass in post-menopausal women. Kerr et al (1994) found that peak strain is more important than the number of loading cycles in increasing bone density in early post-menopausal women. Another study shows that post-menopausal bone mass can be significantly increased by a strength regimen that uses high load/low repetition but not by an endurance regimen that uses low load/high repetition (Kerr et al, 1996). Further research is necessary.

Decreased muscle strength is seen as a risk factor contributing to falls. Women with osteoporosis have been shown to have deterioration in quadriceps muscle function (Stanley et al, 1994). Various studies have demonstrated that elderly patients can improve their strength with resistance training. Gains in strength can be accomplished only by overload, that is, muscular force exceeding that required by activities of daily living. The highest strength gains are achieved with few repetitions and a high resistance (Skinner, 1993).

Of interest is the study by Fiatarone et al (1994) which found that in strength-trained women spontaneous physical activity levels increased. In nursing home patients spontaneous physical activity increased by 28% after a 10-week strength-training programme. This increase in overall activity level related to strength training in older women is another modifiable risk factor for osteoporotic fractures (Sorock et al, 1988). The use of rubber tubing devices is discussed by Steinberg and Roettger (1993). Quantifying the resistance or force created using this type of apparatus has been a difficulty for physiotherapists. Steinberg and Roettger cited attempts to overcome this problem with 'Force deflection curves' for the particular type of tubing used in the book. It is important to compare equipment that is cheap, accessible and portable with equipment that is scientifically evaluated but not readily available to the frail aged either in their homes or in institutional care.

Resistance programmes should contain exercises that stress those parts of the skeleton most at risk (site specificity) and more significantly than normal daily activities (progressive overload). All the major muscle groups around the hip joint, the forearm and the spine should be considered. Bone densitometry may assist in exercise prescription by showing those areas most at risk of fracture. Exercises involving explosive, staccato or torsional movements should be avoided in those with diagnosed osteoporosis. Instructions from the physiotherapist should therefore include action words and statements such as 'slowly', 'gradually' and 'control the movement'.

Swimming has been mentioned in the literature with both positive (Snow-Harter and Marcus, 1991) and negligible effects on bone density (Nilsson and Westlin, 1971). Swimming is considered a non-weight-bearing activity and its positive effect on bone density may occur through loads created from high-intensity muscular activity. It is important to realize that men's bones are usually more dense than women's (mass per unit volume) and as such are less buoyant than women. Their energy expenditure in swimming is greater than that for women. Particularly as they get older, women will have less dense bones and often increased fat deposits. They can often swim with minimal effort and do not need to work as hard to keep themselves afloat. It is also very hard to assess intensity levels when swimming. Swimming may produce a more positive effect on bone density in women if resistance, surface area or drag are increased and the work of the hip muscles and back extensors maximized.

Care should be taken in prescribing swimming to patients without observing their style or checking their water safety. Swimming styles vary from individual to individual as much as posture does. Simple movement restrictions such as decreased neck rotation and kyphosis will alter swimming style. Movement deficiencies such as decreased shoulder range and changes in buoyancy with age will affect water safety.

Care must also be taken not to equate swimming with hydrotherapy or water exercise. Hydrotherapy and water exercise are generally individualized treatment or exercise programmes that are the result of a thorough physiotherapy assessment. Modified swimming may be a component of this programme but hydrotherapy is generally not simply swimming in a heated pool.

It is obvious from the literature that water exercise and hydrotherapy have not been adequately investigated for their BMD benefits, particularly in the frail, those with initial low density and those with pre-existing fractures. Resistance can be provided in the water and there is equipment available to measure this resistance (Aquanex, North Carolina, USA).

Most water studies have not adequately described the exercise intervention that was used, the programmes are largely unsupervised and the intensity often low. Individual differences in bone density in different regions of the body are not taken into account by individual prescription. As a result optimal results cannot be achieved. A recent study from Israel showed improved average BMD after water exercise programmes where water resistance was used as a bone-loading activity (Goldstein and Simkin, 1994). An improvement in lumbar spine density was also found in a Japanese study where post-menopausal women had been water exercising for 35.2 months or longer. The results of this study suggest that consistently participating in water exercise is an important factor in preventing bone loss and moreover, appears not only to indirectly improve awareness of daily physical activity but also to promote health and improve daily life (Tsukahara et al, 1994).

For those patients with already diminished bone density and mobility (possibly due to pain or other orthopaedic problems) hydrotherapy or a water exercise programme can at the very least be the start of a progressive resistance and weight-bearing programme and can include many useful exercises to increase fitness, balance, co-ordination and strength as part of a falls prevention programme.

AEROBIC EXERCISE

The positive effect of aerobic activity on bone density has been shown by Krall and Dawson-Hughes (1994) and Dalsky et al (1988) while others have reported no benefit (Cavanaugh and Cann, 1988; Prince et al, 1991). Physically fit women may have a better bone mineral density than their sedentary counterparts (Chow et al, 1986) and this would support including an aerobic component in an exercise programme for osteoporosis (Borner et al, 1988). The type of person who maintains a level of fitness may influence the outcome of such studies. As suggested by the literature, it is not the most important component and the emphasis should be on weight-bearing exercise and strength or resistance training.

Women who supplemented aerobic exercise with weight training of only one hour per week had higher spine densities than women who were sedentary or participating in aerobic exercise only. A submaximal stress test would be necessary for those patients who have not previously exercised.

OTHER CONSIDERATIONS

Initial bone mass measures Any accrual of bone mass appears to be dependent on the initial bone mass of the individual. Individuals with extremely low initial bone mass may have more to gain from exercise than those with moderately reduced bone mass (Forwood and Burr, 1993).

Site specificity The skeletal response to exercise is greatest at the site of maximum stress (Wolman, 1994), that is, it is site specific. In designing a programme for osteoporosis it is important to understand the principle of site specificity. Squeezing a tennis ball six times a day for 3–6 weeks improved radial bone density (Rutherford, 1990) while a bicycle ergometer study showed increased BMD in the spine but not in the femur (Bloomfield et al, 1993). A study by Kerr et al (1996) showed an increase in bone mass at the trochanteric and intertrochanteric sites but not at femoral neck sites after an exercise programme of low-repetition, high-load resistance exercises selected to work the ipsilateral forearm and hip region (the other side acted as the non-exercise control).

To ensure a benefit from exercise in a variety of sites, an exercise programme must therefore contain a variety of exercises and activities. Bone density studies will be a guide in prescribing exercises for the most at-risk areas. Relating exercise to sites of muscle insertion may be the basis of future exercise prescription. Bone scans may be necessary to adequately prescribe appropriate exercise.

Progressive overload It has proved difficult to quantify the intensity of the exercise required to elicit a training effect on bone mass. In order to effect change, the training stimulus must be greater than that habitually encountered (Skinner, 1993) and must slowly but consistently increase. This is called progressive overload and is as important in this group of patients as it is in sportspeople. In weight training it is relatively easy to apply this principle but in weight-bearing activities it is not as easily achieved. Running, jogging and stair climbing all put more stress on the skeleton than walking but the bones will eventually become habituated to the demands of these activities. It is not known if increasing frequency and/or duration of the exercise sessions can substitute for an increase in intensity (Drinkwater, 1990).

As with any exercise programme in an elderly population, it is important to emphasize a gradual introduction to the exercises to reduce the chance of fatigue and muscle soreness (Borner et al, 1988). An activity diary that lists what they are doing now is a good place from which to start. As compliance is a very important aspect of exercise for this population it is important not to overprescribe initially.

Individual differences It may be that in an inactive population (e.g. nursing home patients) the training stimulus (mechanical loading or activity) necessary to achieve a response in bone mineral content is minimal (Smith and Reddan, 1976; Smith et al, 1981). In a population with high levels of basal activity the training stimulus must be quite high to achieve a change in bone mass (Margulies et al,

1986; White et al, 1984). Thus basal activity levels must be assessed. Future studies may define a clinically assessable level of activity that we can use in prescribing activity and exercises. Each individual will also have a biological ceiling that determines the possible training effect. As this ceiling is approached gains in bone mass will slow and eventually plateau (Drinkwater, 1995).

Reversibility The change brought about by training diminishes if the stimulus is removed. Various studies have shown increases in BMD after five months, eight months and 12 months of appropriate exercise. Like other physiological systems, however, the skeleton 'detrains' when the training stimulus is removed (Drinkwater, 1990). It has been shown clearly that when women stop exercising their BMD returns to the pre-training levels (Dalsky et al, 1988). Thus commitment to exercise needs to be for life. Patients must not have the unreal expectation that they can exercise for a short period and achieve long-term effects on their bones.

Frequency and duration A study by Smith et al (1981) found that in older adults with severe bone loss improvements in bone mineral content is possible with a thrice-weekly (for 30 minutes) exercise programme (radial bone measurements were taken). In a study of nursing home patients BMD was increased after 30 minutes of exercise three times a week (Smith et al, 1981). The effect of increasing the frequency to 5–7 days is unknown (Drinkwater, 1990). Compliance would certainly become a problem in less active groups if we were to ask them to exercise this often. Some active women find that a combination of three days of aerobic exercise interspersed with three days of weight training provides the benefits of both yet allows each 'system' a rest period between training sessions (Drinkwater, 1990). Older women may again find compliance difficult with this programme.

Compliance Many studies over a long period have been unable to supervise exercise sessions and ensure compliance and intensity levels. Poor compliance with regular physical exercise in the untrained elderly is a major factor in explaining the lack of response to exercise treatment for the prevention of osteoporosis. The effect of exercise on bone mass may depend on the subject's motivation to exercise regularly (Preisinger et al, 1995). Strategies to increase compliance in a walking programme included establishing an exercise partner, varying the place and type of weight bearing to include a recreational component such as ballroom, square or line dancing and using an exercise videotape (Allen, 1994). Compliance can also be promoted by ensuring that injury levels are minimal by using good exercise practices.

Pain and previous fracture Both pain and previous fracture will affect exercise prescription. Weight lifted, distance walked or time spent exercising are just a few variables that would be affected if a patient were in pain.

Each patient will have limitations, both physical and medical, that may prevent them from achieving the most scientifically appropriate exercise programme. As physiotherapists, we are used to working within the capabilities of our patients' physical limitations. In the management of osteoporosis, however, there is a need to encourage and motivate the patient to progress with their programme towards a long-term goal of scientific adequacy. In the meantime we must set short-term goals that are realistic and achievable or the patients will feel demoralized and compliance will suffer.

Care must be taken to avoid overstressing bones that are already susceptible to fracture. Patients who have diagnosed osteoporosis should avoid exercise that requires twisting, explosive or staccato movements. Activities in this category include tennis, golf and bowling (MacKinnon, 1988). Rib and vertebral fractures have been known to occur after coughing, reaching out or bending to pick up an article. Extreme care must be taken at all times with patients in a high risk of fracture category.

Age There are three age groups that can be considered when looking at bone density studies.

Childhood and early adult years Active young women and athletes who participate in weight-bearing activities have higher bone mass at the lumbar spine and femoral neck than sedentary controls. Weight bearing is a key factor (Drinkwater, 1995). Strength or muscle mass may or may not play a role in enhancing bone mineral density in this group. The amenorrhoeics tend to be represented in this age group. Inadequate nutrition and interruption to the menses may lead to bone loss regardless of high exercise intensity.

The pre-menopausal woman It is probable that exercise can prevent or slow down bone loss in this group. There appears to be a positive correlation between muscle mass and strength and bone mineral density at this age. Site specificity is most important and bone mineral density measurements may assist exercise prescription.

The post-menopausal woman Bone loss accelerates in the years immediately after menopause (see Fig. 32.6). Initial bone mass levels, oestrogen levels, exercise intensity and site specificity are important. High-intensity activities and resistance or strength-training exercise appears to have a greater impact on bone mineral density than low-intensity exercise, including walking. Muscle mass and strength may play a role in bone mineral accrual at this age though fat mass is also important. In this age group the most positive benefit of exercise may be to slow bone loss as opposed to necessarily increasing it. Exercise alone cannot increase the loss of bone in post-menopausal osteoporosis. Fall prevention must be considered.

SUMMARY

It is known that weight-bearing activity is essential for the normal development and maintenance of healthy bone in children and young women and in some situations the maintenance of bone density in an older population. Increasing strength may also play a beneficial role in BMD. It is probable that less active or sedentary women may increase their bone density slightly by increasing their activity. Exercise cannot be recommended as a substitute for HRT at menopause (Drinkwater, 1995) or with the guarantee that it will necessarily increase or maintain bone density at that time. When prescribing for older women, a programme should include strength, flexibility and co-ordination activities which may help to decrease the incidence of osteoporotic fracture by lessening the risk of falling. An aerobic component can be included where possible.

Consensus does exist in relation to the effect of low levels of physical ability. We know that complete bed rest gives a negative calcium balance within a few days and a detectable reduction in bone density within a few weeks (Wolman, 1994). The non-exercising control group in many studies lost bone mass at a faster rate than the exercise groups. It may be better to direct our primary programmes to the reduction of other risk factors such as balance, strength and immobility. Active older people have significantly better co-ordination, balance and muscle strength than their sedentary peers (Drinkwater, 1990). Many of the medical profession are sceptical about the role of exercise in osteoporosis and do not promote activity levels that are anywhere near the levels suggested in the literature as being beneficial to osteoporosis or in simply maintaining bone density or maintaining balance and co-ordination skills that will assist in the prevention of falls. As physiotherapists, we need to respond to research and trends in science. We are unfortunately limited as a profession by the lack of adequate research in some areas of our clinical management of osteoporosis. In some situations the choice of a technique or modality must be based on the clinical outcome of reduced pain, improved function and mobility.

Although increases in the bone mass of the post-menopausal skeleton may be extremely modest, physical activity is important to preserve bone mass and muscle function. Detraining reduces any bone mass increase to pre-existing values so that long-term benefits are only retained with continuing exercise. Most importantly, the amount of bone gain that can be achieved appears dependent primarily on the initial bone mass, suggesting that individuals with extremely low initial bone mass may have more to gain from exercise than those with moderately reduced bone mass (Forwood and Burr, 1993).

The debate over some of the other interventions being used in the fight against osteoporosis is not only whether there is any benefit but what the side effects, cost and disadvantages are. Exercise has few if any disadvantages and many widely accepted advantages not only to bones but to many other body systems, e.g. in cardiac, respiratory, diabetic and many other conditions. The ethical dilemma for all health professionals may be in not prescribing some form of exercise to all patients rather than in overprescribing.

Techniques to reduce pain

The reduction of more established or chronic pain due to osteoporosis uses the same pain reduction techniques discussed in the section on vertebral fractures. Exercise itself will often help to relieve pain and has been regarded as the single most important strategy in the management of pain in older people (Herman and Scudds, 1995).

Hydrotherapy should be considered not only for acute patients but for those with ongoing pain and disability. Pain reduction in hydrotherapy can be due to a number of properties including the heat, the reduction of weight-bearing forces (unloading) and the reduction of muscle spasm. The combination of these benefits with gentle movement can overcome the fear and anxiety associated with exercise and pain. Often anxiety can reduce activity more than the impairment itself (Herman and Scudds, 1995). This treatment modality will also allow early commencement of a falls prevention programme and give significant psychological benefit to a patient with a chronic, painful disability.

Cognitive and behavioural strategies will be useful in the management of osteoporotic pain. A patient's response to pain can be shaped gradually over time by our own response to their pain. Attention should not be given only when a patient complains of pain. This can reinforce the 'illness' model. Rewards can be made for 'well behaviour' such as improved self-care or increased exercise (Herman and Scudds, 1995). The 'Let pain be your guide' model can in some situations lead to progressive loss of function as the patient avoids any movement that may lead to increased pain (McIndoe, 1995).

Rest is an important component of the rehabilitation programme but it can also be the reason why the programme fails to succeed. Too much rest can cause many problems. In the osteoporotic patient decreased strength, balance and co-ordination can all result from extended rest. The balance between rest and exercise is often a hard one to reach. Encouraging the patient to push to the edge of pain and yet to learn when to stop is not an easy task. Subjective assessment each day will hopefully see a gradual increase in exercise tolerance. Documenting this is important for the patient's psychological well-being. It is important that you have the support of all the health professionals working with the patient. Encouraging a patient to mobilize through pain can be difficult if other caregivers do not support your treatment plan. Communication is essential with all members of the team.

Relaxation therapy has long been recognized as a useful tool in the management of patients with chronic pain and it is one of the most effective and inexpensive treatments to reduce the subjective experience of pain and emotional distress (Herman and Scudds, 1995). Various relaxation techniques are available and patients should be encouraged to try different methods to find the style that suits them.

Thus modalities for the treatment of osteoporotic pain include:

- education for pain;
- TENS;
- soft tissue manipulation;
- spinal mobilization techniques;
- hydrotherapy techniques including mobilization and other manual therapy;
- exercise;
- ice;
- heat;
- electrotherapy;
- bracing and spinal orthotics;
- cognitive and behavioural strategies;
- relaxation.

Prevention of vertebral fractures and spinal deformity

The goals of reducing the risk of vertebral fracture and prevention of spinal deformity are achieved through the following methods.

- Postural assessment and appropriate correction and exercise.
- Exercise to maintain bone density (see previous section on exercise).
- Fall prevention.
- Education (see section on prevention).

POSTURAL ASSESSMENT, CORRECTION AND EXERCISE

Encouraging correct posture in osteoporosis is important in a number of ways. We may retard the correct alignment of the skeleton to enhance the benefit of mechanical strain on bone remodelling. We can prevent, where possible, the development of kyphosis and associated symptoms (e.g. shortness of breath). We may assist pain management by posture correction in cases where pain is due to stretching of connective tissue.

The alteration of the spine and its curves in osteoporosis will be somewhat dependent on the existing fractures and their type and position. An increase in thoracic kyphosis and a compensatory increase in lumbar lordosis will tend to occur with mid-thoracic fractures. Thoracolumbar kyphosis or total kyphotic curvature of the spine tends to result from thoracolumbar or lumbar fractures.

In the non-osteoporotic person, preferred standing posture in the sagittal plane is most commonly described as one in which a plumbline dropped from the ear lobe will fall through the shoulder joint, mid-way through the trunk, through the greater trochanter, slightly anterior to a mid-line through the knee and slightly anteriorly to the lateral malleolus (Olney and Culham, 1995). If this plumbline moves forward of this optimal position (as in osteoporosis) then the forces of gravity, weight bearing, heavy breasts and other flexion forces may put undue pressure on the anterior portion of the vertebral bodies, thus increasing the deformity and in some cases the pain. The strength of the back extensors and other supportive structures around the spine and scapular may help to counteract these forces.

Postural re-education and correction of muscular imbalance are important for all clients regardless of age in order to normalize mechanical forces that stimulate increased bone mass, that is, tensile forces from muscular action and axial compression from weight bearing. Improved biomechanics to assist bone mass accrual may therefore be considered a beneficial side effect of postural correction and dynamic stabilization exercise for the trunk and the limb girdles. For example, progressive resistive exercise causing hypertrophy in previously weak hip abductor muscles and correction of Trendelenburg weight bearing may positively affect bone mass in the proximal femur, given the bony insertion of gluteus medius and minimus on the greater trochanter (Brown, 1995).

Significantly more vertebral compression fractures occur in patients with post-menopausal osteoporosis who follow a dynamic flexion exercise programme compared with those using extension exercises or static abdominals. Extension and isometric abdominal exercises seem to be more appropriate for patients with post-menopausal osteoporosis. In a study where flexion exercises and extension exercises were compared in post-menopausal patients with back pain, wedging and compression fractures before and after intervention were recorded. In the group performing extension exercises, 16% of subjects had further wedge or compression fractures at the end of the study. In the flexion exercise group 89% had further fractures and in the group that had combined flexion and extension exercises 53% of the subjects had further fractures. The control group which did not exercise had 67% further fractures (Sinaki and Mikkelson, 1984). Extension exercises and static abdominal exercises (Fig. 32.15) should be prescribed and dynamic abdominal exercises or sustained flexed postures avoided (Fig. 32.16).

Back extension exercises to encourage both strength (stability) and later mobility are initially prescribed in side lying. When tolerated, these exercises can be done in supine (see Fig. 32.9). A progression can occur (as the patient tolerates) to chair exercises (see Fig. 32.10) and prone (see Fig. 32.12). Some patients with severe pain or multiple fractures will not be able to achieve prone lying for weeks while others will have no difficulty. Postural adjustments will need to be made for each individual and the position of their fracture and pain. To prevent accentuation of the compensatory lumbar lordosis in patients with thoracic kyphosis, a pillow can be placed under the stomach during prone exercise.

Exercises that address scapular strength and scapulothoracic mobility (Fig. 32.17) should be emphasized. In women with osteoporosis there can be reduced range of movement of the shoulder in the sagittal plane. Limited shoulder flexion in these patients may be the result of an altered starting position of the scapula due to kyphosis (Pearlmutter et al, 1995). As thoracic kyphosis increases there may be gradual lengthening of the structures having attachment to the cervical spine and scapula, for example, the levator scapula and rhomboid muscles and the suprascapular nerves (Olney and Culham, 1995).

Figure 32.15 Progression of exercises using leg loading for strength and endurance of abdominals during pelvic and lumbar stability work. (a) In supine with both legs bent, feet on the support, the patient is instructed to push her lower back into the bed and slowly move bent leg forward and backward through a small range. This should be held for 6–10 seconds then returned to the starting position. (b) This can be progressed to slowly extending the leg right out while still maintaining position of lower back. *Handling*: The physiotherapist can place one hand under the patient's lower back to facilitate good pelvic control and one hand on the heel of the foot to facilitate the extension of the leg. (c) Progress to doing the same leg movement with the support leg taken off the support.

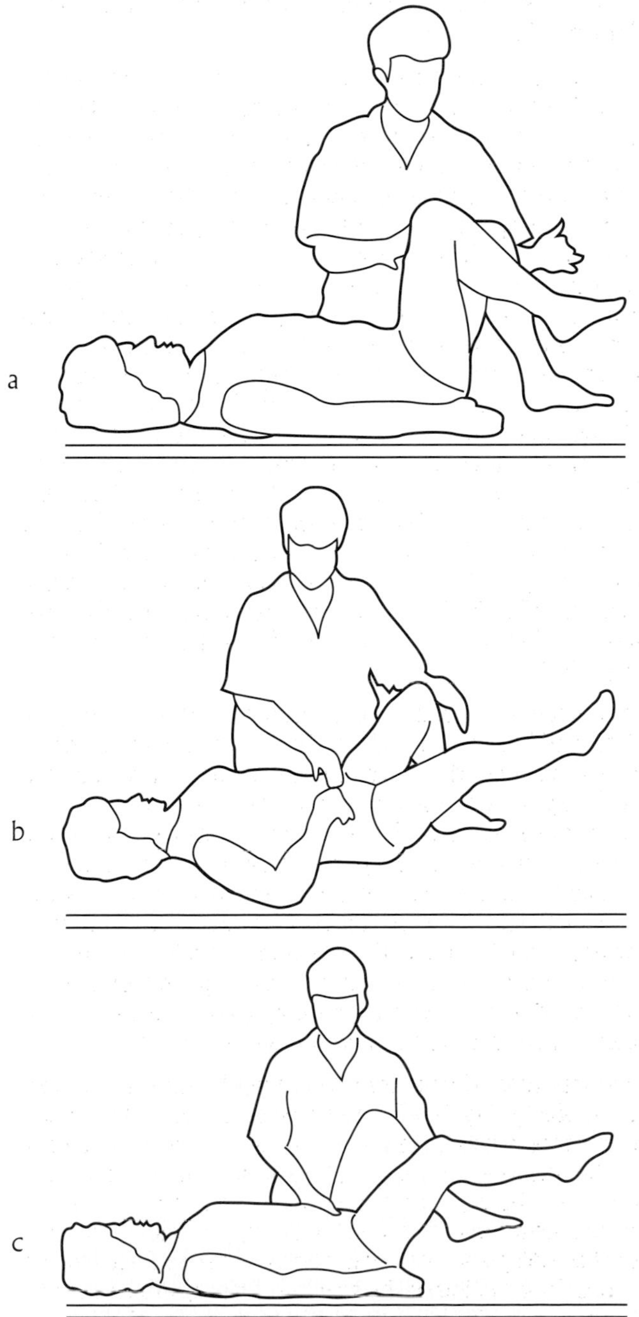

Figure 32.16 (a) Avoid dynamic abdominal sit-ups. (b, c) Avoid prolonged flexion activities and habitual flexion postures that put stress on anterior aspects of the vertebral column and could lead to further wedging and compression fractures. (d) Avoid sitting in a 'C' shaped posture.

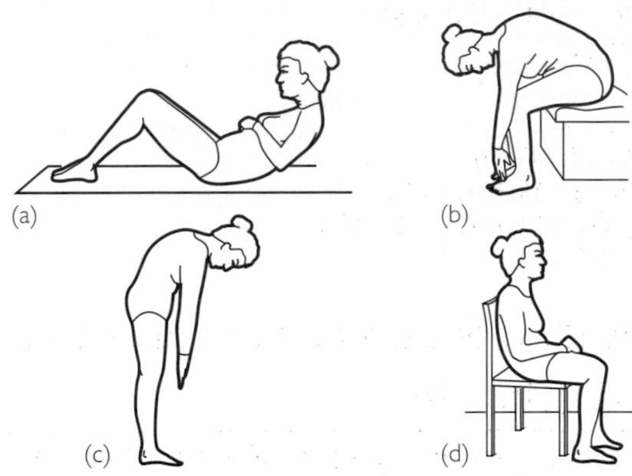

Assessment of sitting, standing and lying postures should be made. The use of a lumbar roll in the sitting position is useful for those with reduced lordosis. Arm rests can help to align the spine by moving the weight of the head back over the spine in forward head postures (Fig. 32.18). Neck retraction exercises (see Fig. 32.10c) are often pain relieving and also help to correct forward head postures.

The use of braces has been discussed in acute management of vertebral fractures. They may also have a place in the long-term management of patients with severe pain and disability. Another form of posture training device has been described (Kaplan and Sinaki, 1993) in which a weight is attached to a pouch that hangs below the scapula and is attached to shoulder straps. If used properly, it promotes extension of the shoulders and a proprioceptive reinforcement to improved posture.

Strapping has also been used as a proprioceptive device to stimulate extension of the spine and retraction of the shoulders. Tolerance and skin allergies or fragility should be considered.

Postural bras, including some sports bras, may also be useful in encouraging improved posture and if well fitted, may relieve pain (Fig. 32.19).

Lifting techniques should be discussed so as to avoid pain, minimize stress on the vertebrae and prevent future fractures. Patients with vertebral fractures should be discouraged from lifting heavy weights. If pain exists a 'pick-up stick' (assistive device for picking things up off the floor) may be useful. This will also protect the anterior wall of the vertebrae. The major issue for physiotherapists in the prevention of hip fractures is the prevention of falls and fall-related fractures.

Prevention of falls and the maintenance of mobility and independence

Preventive measures aimed at promoting, maintaining and increasing bone density tend to be directed to the at-risk

Figure 32.17 (a) The patient stands in a relaxed position and is then asked to bring the shoulder blades down and together towards the mid-line. She is encouraged to hold the position for 6–10 seconds and learn to maintain this posture during activity. *Handling*: The physiotherapist places her hands over the inferior angle and medial border of the scapula to facilitate the movement. (b) Sitting with the arms abducted to 90°, the elbows at 90° and the hands resting on either side of a door frame or other solid object if possible. The patient is asked to pull her scapula towards the mid-line. While holding that scapula position, the patient is asked to move her arms slowly up and down the door frame (30–130° abduction) while holding shoulder blades still. When she feels the shoulder blades move, return to starting position (see Pearlmutter et al (1995) for more information). *Inappropriate action*: Overactivity of levator scapulae.

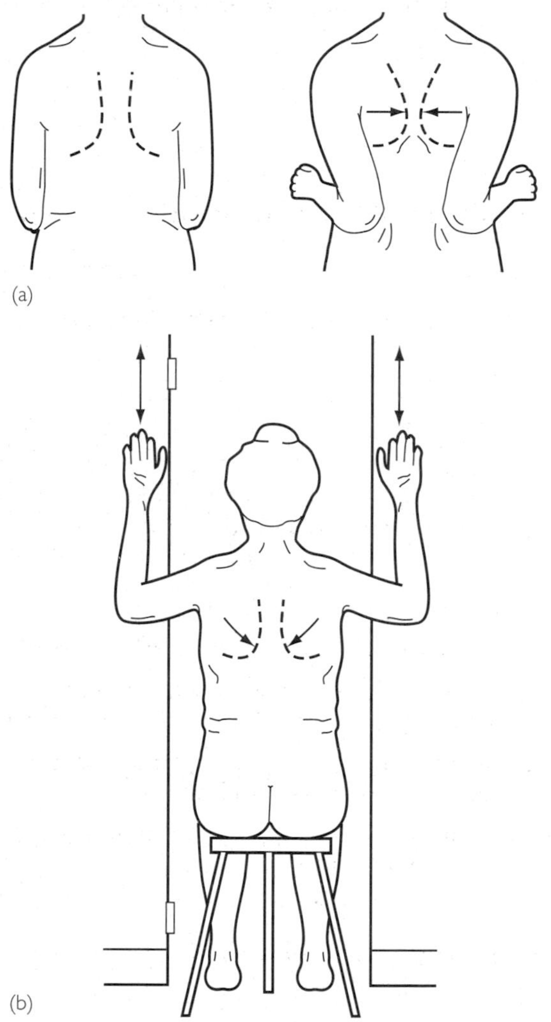

Figure 32.18 (a) A chair with no arm supports may encourage a forward flexed posture. (b) A more erect posture is encouraged by suitable arm rests.

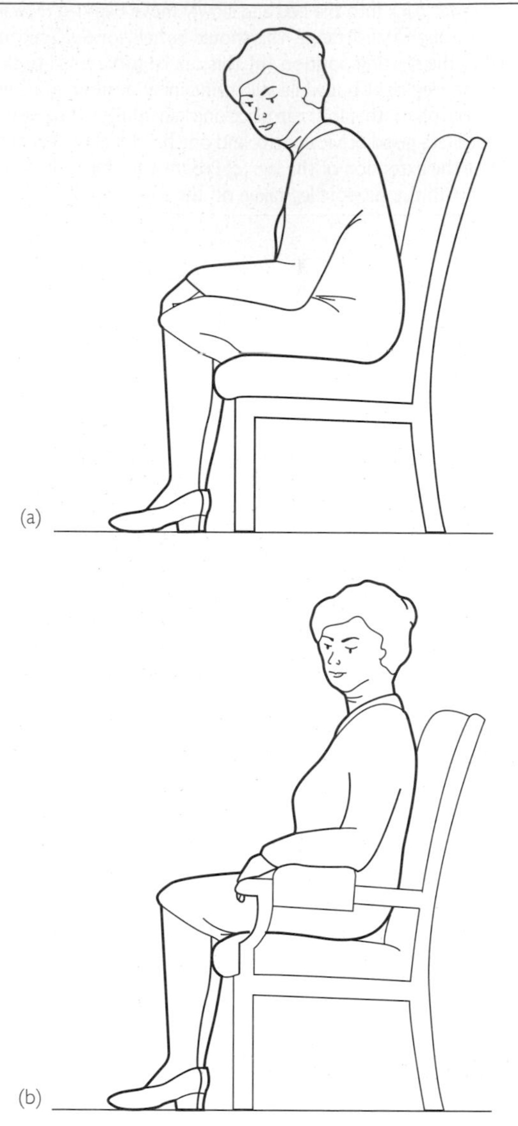

pre- and perimenopausal woman and sometimes to her adolescent relatives. We must also consider the rapidly ageing population and those who will have escaped education and medical intervention to maintain their bone density at a level that can withstand minimal trauma and thus avoid fracture.

Approximately one-third of older people living in the community have falls each year (Lord et al, 1994). Not all falls will result in fractures but as the person ages the risk of falling increases. One percent of falls result in hip fracture and 5% result in other fracture (Conforti, 1995). Falls may cause loss of confidence in ambulation skills and may lead to withdrawal and inactivity (Vandervoort et al, 1990). Falls are often the result of a number of contributing factors rather than one specific factor and the risk of falls increases with the number of risk factors present (Tinetti et al, 1988). The physiotherapist is often in an excellent position to assess risk factors and monitor risk factor modification over time and should consider developing a questionnaire to identify those at risk of falling because of deficits that may be treated through physiotherapy (Speechley and Tinetti, 1990).

Why it is that some falls result in fractures and others do not has been the subject of investigation. The type of fall, the strength of the bone, the amount of protection offered by soft tissue over the hip (Greenspan et al, 1994) and the type of gait and changes in gait speed (Cummings and Nevitt, 1989) may all play some role.

Figure 32.19 There are various postural bras commercially available. They may help to improve posture and decrease pain.

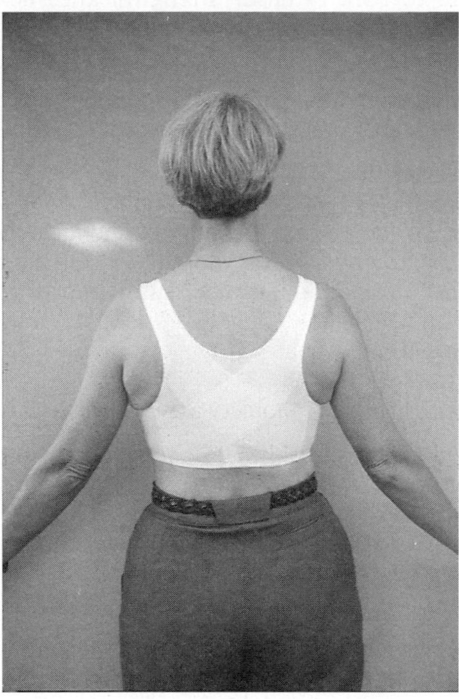

There is a tendency in the literature to describe two major categories of risk factors. Intrinsic factors are usually pathological or physiological and can include those changes that occur with age. Extrinsic factors are usually environmental hazards. One study suggested that as age increases, extrinsic factors have less importance as a cause of falls and that after the age of 75 there was little point in modifying environmental factors as falls after this age were more often associated with intrinsic factors (Morfitt, 1983).

Risk factors for falling

Intrinsic factors

- Musculoskeletal conditions

  Muscle weakness

  Foot problems: pain, bunions

  Deformities: flexion deformity at the hip, knee or ankle, thoracic kyphosis

  Osteoporosis, previous fractures

  Arthritis

- Neurological conditions

  Sensory impairment including visual, proprioceptive and vestibular systems

  Cerebrovascular accident

  Parkinson's disease

  Impairment of balance and co-ordination

  Increased sway

  Decreased reaction times

  Gait problems, including forward centre of gravity

- Medication

  Polypharmacy (four or more drugs)

  Sedatives

  Alcohol

  Psychotropic drugs

- General health and other conditions

  Illness

  Deconditioning, e.g. after immobilization

  Pain

  Depression

  Dementia

  Sleep problems and fatigue

Extrinsic factors

- Surfaces: slippery, wet, uneven, stairs, grab rails
- Obstacles: children's toys, low furniture, scatter rugs, pets, electrical leads, low steps and ledges
- Lighting: no lighting at night (often to conserve money) or inadequate lighting
- Clothing: too long, inappropriate, ill-fitting continence pads or glasses
- Footwear: size, type, sole

(See Steinmetz and Hobson (1994) for further reading)

Modification of intrinsic and extrinsic factors may play a role in a falls prevention programme. Health-care workers are often available to do such assessments but few intervention programmes will fund the broad-based services necessary to assess and observe at-risk individuals in their own home as well as the clinical assessment needed to identify intrinsic risk factors. Education of the patient or their relatives is of primary concern and the physiotherapist may at best be able to discuss with the patient the most likely modifiable risk factors. Consensus as to the most identifiable and alterable of risks does not exist. Not every patient with weak quadriceps will fall. A study by Campbell et al (1990) showed over 1000 loose rugs as possible hazards in the homes of those being assessed but only five of these rugs were at fault in ensuing falls. In fact, the study found that household objects in an uncluttered environment were the cause of the majority of falls (Campbell et al, 1990). Altering a familiar environment does have its risks to an older person who is reliant on memories and habit, but small changes can be made over time to minimize confusion. Encouraging someone to increase their muscle strength can do little harm if done correctly and will in fact have other benefits. As preventive therapists, we need to proceed with caution rather than err on the side of statistical outcomes and deny education and information in possible risk reduction areas.

A recent study by Lord et al (1994) looked at the most useful tests (muscle strength, tactile sensitivity, visual field dependence (roll vection) and body sway) for identifying fallers in an institutional setting and found that these tests were also useful in identifying community-based ambulatory patients who suffer from falls.

There is evidence that a general slowing of sensory, integrative and motor processes controlling posture is associated with ageing. It is unlikely that any one system alone is responsible for the increased frequency of falls in the elderly (Vandervoort et al, 1990).

Prescribing an exercise programme to increase strength and improve balance and co-ordination (Tinetti et al, 1988), assessing and treating visual disorders (Lord et al, 1994) and assessing medications and their effect on various measures (e.g. balance and co-ordination) may be the basis for falls prevention. The physiotherapist can play an active role in such a programme. One option may be to adapt the Sensory Motor Stimulation Program developed by Janda and Vavrova to this population.

The area of falls prevention is growing. We have little research to support our treatment strategies yet have an underlying knowledge and belief that above all we must keep these patients mobile and agile.

Institutionalization of our elderly because of inability to cope with daily functional activities, pain or pathology (e.g. fracture after a fall) is an enormous cost to our health system. Maintaining the elderly at home or in low-care community-based settings has to be a goal of our practical management of patients with osteoporosis or the population at risk.

PHYSIOTHERAPY MANAGEMENT: FALLS PREVENTION

Identifying those patients at risk of falling is an area being investigated by many health practitioner groups. It is not clear which risk factors are most indicative of future fallers. Many of us will not have the luxury of working purely in prevention and as such will need to recognize in our existing patients the risk factors that may make them more likely to fall.

Assessment

Muscle strength: Hip flexion and extension, grip (may correlate to back extensor strength), knee flexion and extension, ankle flexion and extension.

Range of movement: Neck extension (may limit visual field), shoulder, hip, knee, ankle (important for ankle strategy for postural control (Daleiden, 1990)), elbow.

Gait assessment

- Centre of gravity in forward walking
- Timed up and go (as a measure of functional mobility – see Connelly and Vandervoort (1995) for more details. For Get Up and Go test, see Mathias et al (1986)
- Sway on walking
- Decreased step height
- Step test
- Appropriate use of mobility aids

Balance and transfer skills: Sit to stand, on and off the toilet or bed, in and out of car, bath and shower transfers, moving around the kitchen, up and down stairs, reaching, standing sway, single leg stance and sway. Ankle, hip and stepping strategies (see Daleiden, 1990). Protective responses.

Continence: Frequency, urgency and incontinence can all stress women with poor mobility, both in the day and with frequent rising at night. See Chapters 30 and 36 for continence management.

Foot pathology or problems

- Pain
- Range of movement (see above)
- Deformities. These may be correctable with education, orthosis, shoes, etc.
- Uncut nails (may curve over toe)
- Sensation
- Shoes: too big, small, in need of repair, inappropriate. Sporting shoes with very effective non-slip, flared soles can in fact grip the floor and increase the effort needed to clear the foot from the ground
- High heels become less appropriate, particularly if centre of gravity is already forward
- Refer to a podiatrist where necessary

Vision: Does the patient wear glasses? Are they clean? Are they their own prescription? When were they last tested? Do they fit properly? Discuss with appropriate health professional.

Medications: Polypharmacia and drug type (discuss with doctor).

Sleep and fatigue: There is little in the literature that relates either of these to falls but there is little doubt that sleeping patterns change as ageing occurs. Confusional states and fatigue may play a role in some falls. Education and simple advice may be beneficial.

Management

Strength exercises: These will often need to be home based so free weights or rubber tubing can be useful. Putty can be used for hand strength. There is no absolute consensus as to whether the training principle of progressive overload mentioned earlier, and as cited in any good exercise texts, is totally applicable to the older patient. There is suggestion that submaximal effort will see strength gains in this type of patient (Agre et al, 1988). A research report by Koch et al (1994) gives a practical and realistic programme to follow.

Range of movement: Stretching exercises as appropriate.

Gait training: Discuss stride length, body rotation, swing-through phase. Patients will often be unaware of changes that have occurred in their gait as they aged and are able to partially correct them if they are made aware.

Balance and co-ordination: Task-specific activities where possible (Daleiden, 1990). Weight transfer activities as highlighted in individual's assessment (see Daleiden, (1990) for more information on weight transfer as a treatment). Progressive balance exercises (see Koch et al (1994) for further information).

Hydrotherapy: Will be useful for some patients. The partial elimination of gravity allows those with movement inhibition and the fear of falling to exercise in a relatively safe and non-threatening environment. Balance and co-ordination have been shown to improve in patients who participated in water exercise programmes (Lord et al, 1993). Individual hydrotherapy with prescription according to assessment could have an even greater outcome. Extrinsic perturbations on land to evoke ankle, hip and stepping strategies are often stressful to the patient. In the hydrotherapy pool eliminating the fear of falling can allow extrinsic and volitional perturbations to encourage repetition of postural adjustments that may motivate a patient who has a fear of movement due to pain or falling. Visual input can also be eliminated without increasing the patient's fear. With the resistance of the water and appropriate equipment, strength training can commence in the pool.

Foot problems: Manage as appropriate.

Education

All of the above areas may need to be discussed in a group education session as opposed to a clinical treatment session, depending on funding and services available. The principles of osteoporosis education should be taught on the premise that it is never too late to make positive changes. Literature is widely available for all aspects of osteoporosis and it should be used. Refer to the education section earlier in the chapter. Lorig (1990) has helpful suggestions for planning an education programme.

Guidelines for Physiotherapy Management of the Osteoporotic Patient

It is important in this population to approach assessment with caution. The patient will often be in pain and an assessment that increases their pain will not promote a good therapist–patient relationship. Often the assessment will need to be performed over a number of treatment sessions. Patient expectations are important and if the patient is expecting pain relief, that needs to be a primary goal of your treatment. Patients who are in a private system will not choose to continue treatment if their expectations are not met in some way. Educating the patient to have realistic expectations is an important component of management.

Assessment

MUSCULOSKELETAL

- Strength of major or associated muscle groups (limited by pain and anxiety)
- Joint range
- Scans and X-rays
- Posture assessment. Start with those postures that cause the most pain, progress in time to habitual postures

RISK FACTORS

Refer to earlier section for a more detailed discussion of risk factors.

CURRENT ACTIVITY LEVELS

What exercise / activity are you currently doing? What level were you doing prior to this injury / problem?

BALANCE AND CO-ORDINATION

- Sway
- Timed up and go
- Reaction time

CURRENT PAIN LEVELS

A visual analogue scale (VAS) can be used, usually on a scale of 0–10 with 0 being no pain and 10 being the worst pain imaginable.

MOBILITY ANALYSIS

Gait analysis, posture, assistive devices used.

CARDIOVASCULAR

Submaximal stress test if treatment likely to progress to a level of exercise that will promote cardiovascular fitness.

GOALS

- To decrease pain
- To improve or maintain mobility
- To decrease risk of fracture by falls prevention
- To increase fitness endurance
- To improve and maintain quality of life (including avoidance of institutional care)
- To improve or maintain bone density (according to available scientific research)

Pain management

- Soft tissue manipulation, spinal mobilization techniques (avoid fracture site)
- Hydrotherapy
- Posture correction and exercise (include sleeping posture)
- Bracing and supportive devices (spinal orthotics, bras, taping)
- Heat: home techniques (heat pad, water bottle, wheat products, shower)
- Electrotherapy: TENS, other
- Ice massage / packs
- Mobility analysis and aids
- Education for pain
- Assistive devices: pick-up devices, toe-drying devices

Exercise prescription (land and water)

Warm up, warm down. Flexibility and range of movement.

POSTURAL EXERCISES

- Neck extension / retraction
- Back extensors: static or dynamic
- Scapula stability
- Static abdominals (Fig. 32.20)
- Major hip, knee and ankle muscle groups
- Water exercise

RESISTANCE EXERCISES

Major muscles of hip, knee, ankle, spine and forearm. High-intensity, low-repetition where possible. Machines / rubber bands / free weights / bicycle / water exercises.

WEIGHT BEARING

As tolerated. Walk / line dance / square dance / steps.

AEROBIC

As tolerated, start slowly. Respect needs of concomitant conditions.

AVOID

- Pain, although some discomfort may be expected
- dynamic abdominals
- habitual postures that encourage flexion
- dependency on braces, pain medications
- explosive, staccato and rotational or torsional movements
- lifting weights greater than 10 kg in established osteoporosis may not be appropriate

REMEMBER

Training principles, particularly progressive overload.

Figure 32.20 Vertical suspension (spinal unloading) in a neutral position is often successful at relieving pain from vertebral fracture. Once pain has been relieved, gentle mobilization activities, such as striding or hip abduction / adduction, can begin while in this 'unloaded' position.

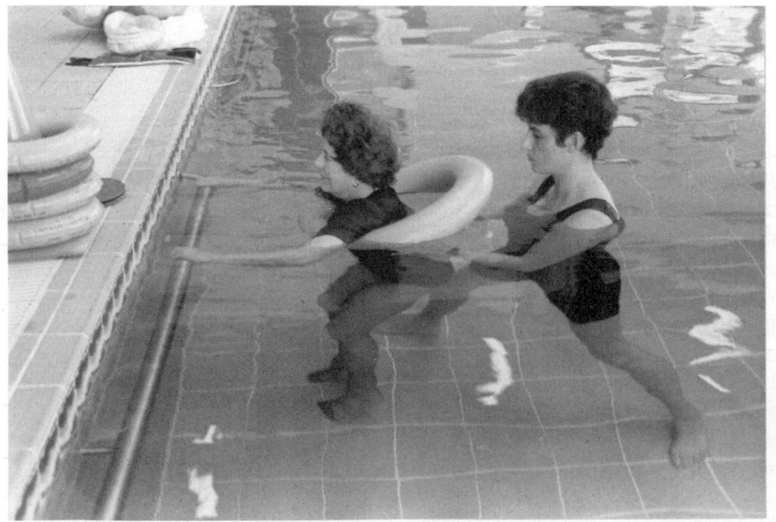

Education

- Exercises
- Calcium and diet
- Hormone replacement therapy
- Falls prevention
- Risk factor modification

Compliance

- START WITH WHAT YOU CAN DO NOW AND BUILD UP
- Set short-term achievable goals
- Set long-term achievable goals
- Respect for pain
- Exercise should be enjoyable, pain free, varied and appropriate to age group
- Exercise with a friend

A 51-year-old petite, fit, female Caucasian presents as an outpatient six weeks after an anterior wedge fracture of L2 after falling off the bottom rung of a ladder. Initial medical treatment was two weeks hospitalization in an orthopaedic ward, oral analgesia, home in a rigid lumbar support.

Prior treatment

- Foot and ankle exercises (circulation)
- Breathing exercises
- Mobility assessment and education – mobility around bed
  – transfers
  – gait training with and without aids
- Ice
- Heat packs
- Exercises in supine – knee to chest
  – hip abduction/adduction
  – alternate hip and knee flexion/extension

On Examination

C/o constant pain L2 and surrounding area, pain 8 on 0–10 pain scale. Pain on sit to stand, prolonged sitting or standing or lying, stairs, in and out of the car. Patient anxious and fearful of movement. Unable to lie in prone. Stiffness, unable to bend to pull up clothes, shoes. Position of comfort side lying with hips and knees flexed. Unable to walk without pain – maximum distance possible 10–20 metres. Putting on weight (often a concern of a slim patient). Gait stiff and restricted, no rotation, short step length, minimal hip extension. Muscle spasm from T12 to L4. No leg pain, no pins and needles, no apparent wasting (grade 3–4 all major muscle groups around hips and knees – hip extension caused increased pain).

Posture assessment: Kyphotic, flattened lumbar spine, arms at rest well forward of mid-line. Bed posture discussed and suggestions for improvement made. Other postures including chair to be assessed as pain lessens and patient tolerance increases.

History (significant points)

- Post-menopausal
- HRT at less than prescribed dose
- No children
- Previously casual smoker
- Small build
- No bone scan
- Moderate exercise history
- Drinks milk in beverages only. No other real calcium intake

Evaluation

Patient has a number of risk factors for osteoporosis. Fall from bottom rung of a ladder not excessive trauma though not regarded as minimal. Suggest patient discuss possible bone density analysis with doctor. Restrict abdominal exercises to static ones until further medical data available.

Aim: to decrease pain and increase mobility. Modality of hydrotherapy chosen because:

- circumferential heat will help to decrease muscle spasm and pain;
- decreased effect of gravity will decrease loading on lumbar spine and decrease pain;
- fear of movement may be decreased by warmth, buoyancy;
- Unable to lie in prone on land but in supine float can palpate and mobilize back above and below injury.

Initial treatment

Hydrotherapy screening and precautions checked. Vertical suspension for approximately five minutes (placed in position of comfort to relieve pain). Vertical suspension with mobility (while exercising in this position avoid pain at all times) (Fig. 32.20).

Exercises in vertical suspension:

- Hip abduction/adduction × 10 reps slowly
- Alternate high stepping × 10 reps slowly

- Striding (straight leg forward, other leg back and keep swapping legs) × 10 (see Fig. 32.20)
- Knees to chest to neutral position × 10

Assess pain: Patient c/o no pain then repeat cycle.

- Supine float (with postural neck support, hip and knee supports) seaweeding gently with stabilization at fracture site
- Supine float with specific joint mobilizations grade i–ii of T1–12 and L3–5 avoiding pain (Fig 32.21)
- Supine float with soft tissue mobilization of paraspinal muscles and scapula

Assess pain: Patient c/o no pain continue.

- Supine float with sculling
- Supine float with bilateral hip abduction/adduction (ankles supported in small rings)
- Walk forward in chest deep water × 3 widths (15 metres)
- Standing, set abdominals, gluteals, scapula while doing double arm swing (small fast movements)
- Avoid pain

On completion of treatment advise patient of possible increase in pain on exiting pool and need to increase fluid intake to compensate for physiological changes following immersion.

Treatment 2

Pain 5–6 (on a 0–10 pain scale), increased pain 4–6 hours after treatment but last two nights has slept best yet since injury. Repeat treatment while increasing repetitions of vertical suspension exercises to 20 and walking to five widths.

Treatment 3

Pain 5 (on 0–10 pain scale), patient feeling more mobile, pain less on sit to stand, getting out of bed easier. Repeat treatment with following additions:

- Vertical suspension with lumbar extension as tolerated
- Supine float with shoulder and arm destabilization for static abdominals
- Modified Bad Ragaz for static trunk side flexion
- Supported in corner with pillow and hip float, pull-downs using hip extensors through small range against resistance of small floats
- Kicking and sculling to work back extensors
- Standing holding rail/side of pool doing hip abduction/adduction and hip flexion/extension (small range/fast movements)
- Squat to stand at pool side
- Land exercises: gluteals, quadriceps, hamstrings, scapula stability, hip and knee rotation in crook lying, prone lying if tolerated. Avoid pain

Treatment 4 and 5

Pain 4 and not constant, walking tolerance improved. Additional exercises in water:

Figure 32.21 While in appropriate postural flotation supports (Peppertown, Brisbane, Australia) gentle spinal stabilization and soft tissue techniques can commence. From this position 'destabilizing' stability exercises can be initiated.

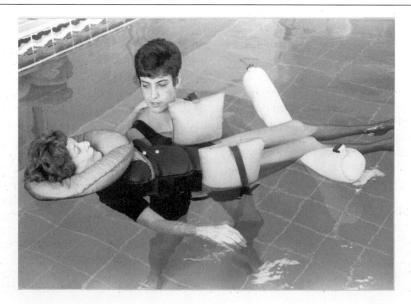

- Elastic tube exercises for shoulder extensors and scapula stability
- Jump to the wall for static abdominal contraction (ensure hips do not flex more than 90 °)
- Double arm swing with resistance for back and shoulder work and for balance and co-ordination (see Fig. 32.14b)
- Knee flexion and extension in sitting to encourage quadriceps strength (see Fig. 32.14a)
- 'Crutch walking' for scapula stability (set scapular, hold on to two small floats and push into water till elbows nearly extended, swing arms alternately, maintain tight abdominals and gluteals throughout exercise)

Additional exercises on land:

- Prone lying with alternate hip extension
- Prone lying with alternate arm extension
- Shoulder extension
- Scapula stability
- Introduce elastic tubing for resistance and small free weights as tolerated

Patient subsequently assessed with Bone Densitometry Report which showed osteoporosis of the hip and spine. Local medical officer ensured HRT dose was adequate and specialist endocrinologist appointment made.

Treatment progressed to including education on:

- Exercise (including site specificity, progressive overload, reversibility, avoidance of dynamic abdominals)
- Calcium intake
- Posture correction

Home programme established including resistance exercises, walking programme, water exercise, general fitness. Individual treatment as pain demanded.

With increasing life expectancy, more and more women will present for treatment of osteoporosis. Hopefully health promotion will alert many women to the potential problem of osteoporosis and they will seek prophylactic management routines to avoid such adverse outcomes. Physiotherapists play a very important role in education and management.

Questions on Osteoporosis

Question 1

A 65-year-old post-menopausal woman presents with osteoarthritic pain in her knees. She would like an exercise programme to increase her bone mineral density (she has had previous physiotherapy for her knees and does not want further treatment). Densitometry has shown slight decrease on age-matched controls. She walks three times a week for 20 minutes at a comfortable intensity but her knees hurt her for 24–48 hours afterwards. What general management strategies would you give her regarding exercise for osteoporosis?

- Assessment including muscle strength, range of movement, gait analysis, timed up and go, shoes, submaximal exercise testing if appropriate.
- Review scan for areas of significant bone loss.
- Discuss inability to prescribe exercises that can guarantee a positive effect on bone mineral density because of individual variables. Discuss the fact that current exercise levels are unlikely to improve bone density but may play a role in slowing bone loss. Discuss other benefits of exercise, including falls prevention.
- Suggest techniques to reduce pain resulting from walking, including self-management techniques (ice, heat, specific exercise, etc.).
- Explain progressive overload, site specificity, reversibility, frequency (30 min, 3 times / week) and intensity.
- Suggest inclusion of some resistance exercise in addition to or in place of some walking activity. Rubber tubing may be useful initially. Is a gym programme a possibility in the future?
- Discuss the role of falls prevention and the type of exercise that may be suitable. Suggest hydrotherapy as an option for initial resistance exercise, falls prevention, variety, etc.
- Swimming or water aerobics to improve cardiovascular fitness. An exercise bike with resistance may not aggravate her knees.
- Discuss compliance issues including boredom, lack of variety, pain. Can she exercise with a friend or join a local group? Draw up an activity chart.
- Check major educational principles and risk factors including HRT status, calcium intake, smoking, etc.

Question 2

A 55-year-old woman seeks treatment for acute low back pain that has not settled 10 days after injury after slipping on a wet floor (minimal trauma). She has had some physiotherapy but there has been no relief from pain. What questions should you ask to ascertain her risk of having osteoporosis?

All risk factors should be checked, particularly her gynaecological history including number of children, menstrual history, time of menopause, calcium history, exercise background, family history and general medical background including long-term medications. Observe stature and posture. Check smoking and alcohol history. There is no consensus as to the number of risk factors that need to be present to constitute a definite risk. Communicating with the medical practitioner and being conservative where necessary, particularly with manipulative and mobilizing techniques, are sensible steps. Further tests may include

X-ray to check fracture and osteoporosis status and bone densitometry if fracture is present.

References

Aisenbrey JA (1987) Exercise in the prevention and management of osteoporosis. *Physical Therapy* **67**: 1100–1104.

Agre JC, Pierce LE, Raab DM et al (1988) Light resistance and stretching exercise in elderly women: effect upon stength. *Archives of Physical and Medical Rehabilitation* **69**: 273–276.

Allen SH (1994) Exercise considerations for postmenopausal women with osteoporosis. *Arthritis Care and Research* **7**: 205–214.

Audran M (1992) Epidemiology, etiology, and diagnosis of osteoporosis. *Current Opinion in Rheumatology* **4**: 394–401.

Bloomfield SA, Williams NI, Lamb DR et al (1993) Non-weightbearing exercise may increase lumbar spine bone mineral density in healthy post-menopausal women. *American Journal of Physical and Medical Rehabilitation* **72**: 204–209.

Boonen S, Aerssens J, Breeman S et al (1995) Fractures of the proximal femur: implications of age related decline in muscle function. *Journal of Orthopaedic Rheumatology* **8**: 127–133.

Borenstein DG, Wiesel SW and Boden SD (1995) *Low Back Pain: Medical Diagnosis and Comprehensive Management*, 2nd edn. Philadelphia: W.B. Saunders.

Borner JA, Dilworth BB and Sullivan KM (1988) Exercise and osteoporosis: a critique of the literature. *Physiotherapy Canada* **40**: 146–155.

Brown AM (1995) The effects of exercise on bone mass: implications for manipulative therapy. *Journal of Manual and Manipulative Therapy* **3**: 3–8.

Campbell AJ, Borrie MJ, Spears GF et al (1990) Circumstances and consequences of falls experienced by a community population 70 years and over during a prospective study. *Age and Ageing* **19**: 136–141.

Cavanaugh DJ and Cann CE (1988) Brisk walking does not stop bone loss in post-menopausal women. *Bone* **9**: 201–204.

Chow RK, Harrison JE, Brown CF et al (1986) Physical fitness effect on bone mass in post-menopausal women. *Archives of Physical and Medical Rehabilitation* **67**: 231–234.

Christiansen C (1994) Postmenopausal bone loss and the risk of osteoporosis. *Osteoporosis International* **4**(Suppl 1): 47–51.

Conforti D (1995) How to investigate falls in the elderly. *Modern Medicine Australia* **2**: 138–140.

Connelly DM and Vandervoort AA (1995) Improvement in knee extensor strength of institutionalised elderly women after exercise with ankle weights. *Physiotherapy Canada* **47**: 15–23.

Consensus Development Conference (1993) Diagnosis, prophylaxis, and treatment of osteoporosis. *American Journal of Medicine* **94**: 646–650.

Culham EG (1995) Osteoporosis and osteoporotic fractures. In: Pickles B, Compton A, Simpson JM et al (eds) *Physiotherapy with Older People*, pp. 213–230. London: W.B. Saunders.

Cummings SR and Nevitt MC (1989) A hypothesis: the causes of hip fracture. *Journal of Gerontology* **44**: M107–M111.

Daleiden S (1990) Weight shifting as a treatment for balance deficits: a literature review. *Physiotherapy Canada* **42**: 81–87.

Dalsky GP, Stocke KS, Ensani AA et al (1988) Weight-bearing exercise training and lumbar bone mineral content in postmenopausal women. *Annals of Internal Medicine* **108**: 824–828.

Dixon A and Woolf A (1989) *Avoiding Osteoporosis*, p. 151. London: McDonald.

Drinkwater BL (1990) Physical exercise and bone health. *Journal of the American Medical Women's Association* **45**: 91–96.

Drinkwater BL (1995) ACSM position stand on osteoporosis and exercise. *Medicine in Science of Sports and Exercise* **27**: 1–7.

Drinkwater BL and Johnson M (1997) Position stand: The female triad. *Medicine and Science in Sports and Exercise* **29**: 1–9.

Fiatarone MA, O'Neill C, Ryan N et al (1994) A randomised controlled trial of exercise and nutrition for physical frailty in the oldest old. *New England Journal of Medicine* **330**: 1769–1775.

Forwood MR and Burr DM (1993) Physical activity and bone mass: exercises in futility? *Bone and Mineral* **21**: 89–112.

Gleeson PB, Protas EJ, LeBlanc AD et al (1990) Effects of weight lifting on bone mineral density in premenopausal women. *Journal of Bone and Mineral Research* **5**: 153–158.

Goldstein E and Simkin A (1994) The influence of weight-bearing water exercises on bone density of post-menopausal women. In: Lidor R, Ben-Sira D and Artzi Z (eds) *Physical Activity in the Life Cycle*, pp. 232–234. Netanya (Israel): The Zinman College of Physical Education at the Wingate Institution.

Greenspan SL, Myers ER, Maitland LA et al (1994) Fall severity and bone mineral density as risk factors for hip fracture in ambulatory elderly. *Journal of the American Medical Association* **271**: 128–133.

Harrison RA and Bulstrode SJ (1987) Percentage weight-bearing during partial immersion in the hydrotherapy pool. *Physiothery Practice* **3**: 60–63.

Heaney RP (1990) Calcium intake and bone health throughout life. *Journal of the American Medical Women's Association* **45**: 80–86.

Herman E and Scudds R (1995) Pain. In: Pickles B, Compton A, Simpson JM et al (eds) *Physiotherapy with Older People*, pp. 289–305. London: W.B. Saunders.

Kamien M and Prince R (1986) Osteoporosis is a preventable condition. *Australian Family Physician* **15**: 1305–1307.

Kaplan RS and Sinaki M (1993) Posture training support: preliminary report on a series of patients with diminished symptomatic complications of osteoporosis. *Mayo Clinic Proceedings* **68**: 1171–1176.

Kerr D, Prince RL, Morton A et al (1994) Does high resistance weight training have a greater effect on bone mass than low resistance weight training? *Journal of Bone and Mineral Research* **9** (Suppl 1): S152.

Kerr D, Morton A, Dick I and Prince R (1996) Exercise effects on bone mass in post-menopausal women are site-specific and load-dependent. *Journal of Bone and Mineral Research* **11**: 218–225.

Koch M, Gottschalk M, Baker DI et al (1994) An impairment and disability assessment and treatment protocol for community-living elderly persons. *Physical Therapy* **74**: 286–294.

Krall EA and Dawson-Hughes B (1994) Walking is related to bone density and rate of bone loss. *American Journal of Physical and Medical Rehabilitation* **96**: 20–26.

Law MR, Wald NJ and Meade TW (1991) Strategies for prevention of osteoporosis and hip fracture. *British Medical Journal* **303**: 453–459.

Lindsay R (1987) Prevention of osteoporosis. *Clinical Orthopaedics* **222**: 44–59.

Llewellyn-Jones D and Abraham S (1992) *Everywoman's Middle Years*, pp. 174. Melbourne: Ashwood House Medical.

Lord SR and Sinnett PF (1986) Femoral neck fractures: admissions, bed use, outcomes and projections. *Medical Journal of Australia* **145**: 493–496.

Lord SR, Mitchell D and Williams P (1993) Effect of water exercise on balance and related factors in older people. *Australian Journal of Physiotherapy* **39**: 217–222.

Lord SR, Ward JA, Williams P et al (1994) Physiological factors associated with falls in older community dwelling women. *Journal of the American Geriatric Society* **42**: 1110–1117.

Lord SR, Sambrook PN, Gilbert C et al (1994) Postural stability, falls and fractures in the elderly: results from Dubbo Osteoporosis Epidemiology Study. *Medical Journal of Australia* **160**: 684–691.

Lorig K (1990) *The Arthritis Self-Management Leader's Manual.* Stanford: Stanford Arthritis Center.

Low J and Reed A (1990) Electrotherapy Explained: *Principles and Practice.* London: Butterworth and Heinemann.

Luckert BP (1994) Vertebral compression fractures: how to manage pain, avoid disability. *Geriatrics* **49**: 22–26.

Mackerras D (1995) Calcium intake and osteoporosis. *Australian Journal of Nutrition and Dietetics* **52**: S21–S25.

MacKinnon JL (1988) Osteoporosis: a review. *Physical Therapy* **68**: 1533–1541.

MacLennan AH and Smith M (1995) Hormone replacement therapy and breast cancer: what are the facts? *Medical Journal of Australia* **163**: 483–485.

Margulies JY, Simkin A, Leichter I et al (1986) Effect of intense physical activity on the bone-mineral content in the lower limbs of young adults. *Journal of Bone and Joint Surgery* **68A**: 1090–1093.

Mathias S, Nayak USL and Isaacs B (1986) Balance in elderly patients: the 'Get-up and Go' test. *Archives of Physical and Medical Rehabilitation* **67**: 387–389.

McIndoe R (1995) Moving out of pain: hands-on or hands-off. In: Shacklock M (ed) *Moving in on Pain*, pp. 153–160. Sydney: Butterworth Heinemann.

Morfitt JM (1983) Falls in old people at home: intrinsic versus environmental factors in causation. *Public Health* **91**: 115–120.

Moroz D, Sale D and Webber C (1989) The effect of intensive training on axial and appendicular bone mineral in normal post-menopausal women. *Journal of Bone and Mineral Research* **4**: S233.

National Institute of Health (NIH) (1994) Consensus Statement. *Optimum Calcium Uptake* **12**(4): 1–31.

Nelson ME, Fiatarone MA, Morganti CM et al (1994) Effects of high intensity strength training on multiple risk factors for osteoporotic fractures. A randomised controlled trial. *Journal of the American Medical Association* **272**: 1909–1914.

Nilsson BE and Westlin NE (1971) Bone density in athletes. *Clinical Orthopaedics* **77**: 179–182.

Nordin BE (1994) Guidelines for bone densitometry. *The Medical Journal of Australia* **160**: 517–520.

Norkin CC and Levangie PK (1992) *Joint Structure and Function: A Comprehensive Analysis.* Philadelphia: FA Davis Co.

Notelovitz M and Ware M (1982) *Stand Tall: A Woman's Guide to Preventing Osteoporosis.* Melbourne: Schwartz and Wilkinson.

Notelovitz M, Martin D, Tesar R et al (1991) Oestrogen therapy and variable resistance weight training increases bone mineral in surgically menopausal women. *Journal of Bone and Mineral Research* **6**: 583–590.

Olney SJ and Culham EG (1995) Changes in posture and gait. In: Pickles B, Compton A, Simpson JM et al (eds) *Physiotherapy with Older People*, pp. 81–94. London: W.B. Saunders.

O'Neill S (1997) Consensus statement: The prevention and management of osteoporosis. *Journal of the Australian Medical Association* **167** (Suppl. P): S4–S15.

Palastanga NP (1994) Heat and cold. In: Wells PE, Frampton V and Bowsher D (eds) *Pain Management by Physiotherapy*, 2nd edn, pp. 177–186. London: Butterworth Heinemann.

Pearlmutter LL, Bode BY, Wilkinson WE et al (1995) Shoulder range of motion in patients with osteoporosis. *Arthritis Care Research* **8**: 194–198.

Preisinger E, Alacamlioglu Y, Pils K et al (1995) Therapeutic exercise in the prevention of bone loss: a controlled trial with women after menopause. *American Journal of Physical and Medical Rehabilitation* **74**: 120–123.

Prince RL, Smith M, Dick IM et al (1991) Prevention of postmenopausal osteoporosis: a comparative study of exercise, calcium supplementation and hormone replacement therapy. *New England Journal of Medicine* **325**: 1189–1195.

Rickli RE and McManus BG (1990) Effects of exercise on bone mineral content in post-menopausal women. *Res Q Exerc Sport* **61**: 243–245.

Rockwell JC, Sorenson AM, Baker S et al (1990) Weight training decreases vertebral bone density in pre-menopausal women: a prospective study. *Journal of Clinical Endocrinology and Metabolism* **71**: 988–993.

Rutherford OM (1990) The role of exercise in prevention of osteoporosis. *Physiotherapy* **76**: 522–526.

Sambrook P (1991) Osteoporosis: significance, diagnosis, prevention and management. *Modern Medicine Australia* **8**: 22–32.

Sambrook P and Reeve J (1988) Bone disease in rheumatoid arthritis. *Clinical Science* **74**: 225–230.

Sanila M, Kotaniemi A, Viikare J and Isomake H (1994) Height loss rate as a marker of osteoporosis in post-menopausal women with rheumatoid arthritis. *Clinical Rheumatology* **13**(2): 256–260.

Seeman E, Hopper J, Bach L et al (1989) Reduced bone mass in daughters of women with osteoporosis. *New England Journal of Medicine* **320**: 554–558.

Seeman E, Eisman J, Gutteridge D et al (1991) Osteoporosis: its causes, prevention and treatment. *Modern Medicine Australia* **8**: 37–41.

Sinaki M and Mikkelson BA (1984) Postmenopausal spinal osteoporosis: flexion versus extension exercises. *Archives of Physical and Medical Rehabilitation* **65**: 593–596.

Sinaki M, Wahner HW, Offord KP et al (1989) Efficacy of nonloading exercises in prevention of vertebral bone loss in post-menopausal women: a controlled trial. *Clinical Proceedings* **64**: 762.

Skinner JS (1993) *Exercise Testing and Exercise Prescription for Special Cases – Theoretical Basis and Clinical Application*, 2nd edn, pp. 132–137. Philadelphia: Lea and Febiger.

Skinner AT and Thomson AM (1994) Hydrotherapy. In: Wells PE, Frampton V and Bowsher (eds) *Pain Management by Physiotherapy*, 2nd edn, pp. 228–237. London: Butterworth and Heinemann.

Smith EL and Reddan W (1976) Physical activity – a modality for bone accretion in the aged. *American Journal of Roentgenology* **126**: 1297.

Smith EL, Reddan JW and Smith PE (1981) Physical activity and calcium modalities for bone mineral increase in aged women. *Medical Science of Sports and Exercise* **13**: 60–64.

Snow-Harter C and Marcus R (1991) Exercise, bone mineral density, and osteoporosis. *Exercise and Sport Science Review* **19**: 351–388.

Sorock GS, Bush TL, Golden AL et al (1988) Physical activity and fracture risk in free living elderly cohort. *Journal of Gerontology* **43**: M134–M139.

Speechley M and Tinetti M (1990) Assessment of risk and prevention of falls among elderly persons: role of the physiotherapist. *Physiotherapy Canada* **42**: 75–79.

Stanley SN, Marshall RN, Tilyard MW et al (1994) Skeletal muscle mechanics in osteoporotic and non-osteoporotic post-menopausal women. *European Journal of Applied Physiology and Occupational Physiology* **65**: 450–455.

Steinberg FU and Roettger RF (1993) Exercise prevention and therapy in osteoporosis. In: Avioli LV (ed) *The Osteoporotic Syndrome: Detection, Prevention and Treatment*, 3rd edn, pp. 171–207. New York: Wiley-Liss.

Steinmetz HM and Hobson JG (1994) Prevention of falls among the community-dwelling elderly: an overview. *Physical and Occupational Therapy in Geriatrics* **12**(4): 13–29.

Tilyard M (1993) Bone preservation in women. *Patient Management* **17**: 25–27.

Tinetti ME, Speechley M and Ginter SF (1988) Risk factors for falls among elderly persons living in the community. *New England Journal Medicine* **319**: 1701–1709.

Tsukahara N, Toda A, Goto J and Ezawa I (1994) Cross-sectional and longitudinal studies on the effect of water exercise in controlling bone loss in Japanese post-menopausal women. *Journal of Nutritional Science and Vitaminology (Tokyo)* **40**: 37–42.

Turner P (1991) Osteoporotic back pain – its prevention and treatment. *Physiotherapy* **77**: 642–645.

Twomey L (1993) Physical activity and ageing bones. *Patient Management* **17**: 31–34.

Vandervoort A, Hill K, Sandrin M et al (1990) Mobility impairment and falling in the elderly. *Physiotherapy Canada* **42**: 99–107.

Vargo M and Gerber L (1993) Exercise strategies for osteoporosis. *Bulletin on the Rheumatic Diseases* **42**: 6–9.

Wegner M, Snow-Harter C, Robinson T et al (1993) Lean mass, not fat mass, independently predicts whole body mineral density in post-menopausal women. *Medical Science of Sports and Exercise* **25**: S854.

White MK, Martin RB, Yeater RA et al (1984) The effects of exercise on the bones of post-menopausal women. *International Orthopaedics* **7**: 209.

Witham B and Davidson J (1993) The osteoporosis prevention and self-management course. *Health Promotion Journal of Australia* **3**: 9–10.

Witham B and Davidson J (1994) *The Osteoporosis Handbook*, 3rd edn, p. 89. Victoria: The Arthritis Foundation of Victoria.

Wolman RL (1994) Osteoporosis and exercise. *British Medical Journal* **30**(9): 400–403.

WHO (1994) *Assessment of Fracture Risk and Its Appli#ation to Screening for Post-menopausal Osteoporosis: Report of a WHO Study Group*, pp. 129. Geneva: World Health Organization.

33

Rehabilitation after Breast Cancer

ROBYN BOX

Breast cancer will affect up to one in 13 women during their lifetime (Kelsey and Gammon, 1991; Kissin, 1994) and it is estimated that one in 25 female deaths in Australia is due to breast cancer (Australian Cancer Society, 1994). Disease-free survival after diagnosis and treatment of breast cancer has been reported as between 63% to 74% at 10 years, with an overall survival rate of 63–86% (Jacobsen et al, 1995; Winchester and Cox, 1992). Therefore it has become the focus of research to optimize the quality of care and survival of women diagnosed with breast cancer.

The management of breast cancer involves a multimodal approach using the appropriate combination of surgical excision, radiotherapy, chemotherapy and hormone therapy. The combination of surgical excision and adjuvant therapy for each individual woman diagnosed with breast cancer is dependent upon her clinical presentation, the staging of the breast cancer and her informed choice of the treatment options available. Physiotherapists are part of the multidisciplinary team and have a considerable role to play in assisting the recovery of women after treatment for breast cancer. To actively contribute to the care of women undergoing treatment, it is important that physiotherapists have an understanding of the detection and diagnosis of breast cancer and its management. This knowledge allows the physiotherapist to anticipate and recognize potential problems early, facilitating the appropriate intervention or referral.

The Diagnosis of Breast Cancer

Women with breast cancer most often present after finding a lump in their breast or a lesion has been identified in a screening mammogram. Other less common clinical manifestations include changes in the nipple, breast shape or the skin over the breast and breast pain. While the causes of breast cancer remain unknown, a number of factors have been associated with its increased incidence (Table 33.1).

Additional investigative procedures such as:

- breast ultrasound
- fine-needle aspiration biopsy or cytology (FNAB/FNAC):
- needle core biopsy (NCB) or
- open excision biopsy with or without frozen section

may be performed to confirm the diagnosis of breast cancer and assist in the planning of optimal treatment combinations.

Staging of breast cancer

Treatment planning after the diagnosis of breast cancer is assisted by the 'staging' of the disease. This term refers to the classification of patients according to the extent of their disease and is determined from the results of clinical examination, radiological and laboratory investigations. Breast

Table 33.1 Risk factors for breast cancer

Risk factor	High risk group
Age	> 40 years, particularly > 50 years
Country	Western
Socioeconomic status	High
Race	Western
Nulliparous	Yes
Age at first pregnancy	⩾ 30 years
Pre-menopausal oophorectomy	No
Age at menopause	Late
Age at menarche	Early
Weight	Obese
History of breast cancer	Yes
History of epithelial atypia	Yes
Family history	Yes
Radiation to chest	Large doses

From Clark (1991), Kelsey and Gammon (1991), Kissin (1994).

cancer is classified using the recognized 'TNM system' which identifies the tumour size (T), lymph node involvement (N) and presence of secondary tumours or metastases (M) (Harris et al, 1992) (Table 33.2).

The precise tumour size will be confirmed by surgical excision. Histological examination of the (surgically) excised tissue indicates the type of cancer and involvement of axillary lymph nodes. Positive lymph nodes suggest the possibility of the spread of breast cancer to other sites and systemic treatment is recommended. Further investigations such as chest X-rays, bone and liver scans as well as specific blood tests may be performed to determine the presence of metastatic disease which, if found, will require systemic treatment. Adjuvant systemic treatment may also be required in the presence of negative lymph nodes in some cancer types.

Types of breast cancer

The breast is made up of glandular tissue organized into a number of lobes. The lobes are connected by fibrous tissue and separated by fatty tissue. Each lobe consists of a number of lobules connected by areolar tissue, blood vessels and ducts. These ducts unite and form larger ducts, which converge toward the areola and nipple. Lymph channels permeate the breast and may drain to the axillary or internal mammary lymph nodes (Fig. 33.1a).

Cancer cells may form in any part of the breast tissue, with the ducts and lobules being the most common sites. The different types of breast cancer and characteristics of their presentation are summarized in Table 33.3.

Table 33.2 Staging of breast cancer using TNM classification system

TNM classification	Clinical stage	Description
T_1, N_0, M_0	I	Tumour ≤2 cm, confined to the breast, no lymph node or metastatic involvement
T_{0-2}, N_{0-1}, M_0	IIA	No primary tumour to tumour ≤5 cm, no or only ipsilateral moveable axillary lymph node involvement, no metastases
T_{2-3}, N_{0-1}, M_0	IIB	Tumour >2 cm, no or only ipsilateral moveable axillary lymph node involvement, no metastases
T_{0-1}, N_2, M_0 or T_{2-3}, N_{1-2}, M_0	IIIA*	No primary tumour to tumour ≤2 cm, adherent ipsilateral axillary lymph node involvement, no metastases *or* tumour ≥2 cm, ipsilateral axillary lymph node involvement, no metastases
T_4, any N, M_0 or any T, N_3, M_0	IIIB*	Any size tumour extending into chest wall, any level of lymph node involvement, no metastases *or* any size tumour with ipsilateral internal mammary lymph node involvement, no metastases
Any T, any N, M_1	IV*	Any tumour, any level of lymph node involvement, metastases

From Clark (1991), Denton (1991), Harris et al (1992), Kissin (1994).
* Early detection with breast self-examination and screening has increased the number of women presenting with early-stage breast cancer.

Primary Management of Breast Cancer

The optimal management of a woman with breast cancer is decided after the interpretation of her clinical, radiological and histological results. The histological results may be obtained from the FNAB, NCB or tissue obtained from surgical excision of the lump, surrounding tissue or axillary lymph nodes. The combination of surgery, radiotherapy, chemotherapy and hormone therapy for any woman with breast cancer is dependent upon a number of factors which include:

- histological type of breast cancer, including oestrogen receptor status;
- size of the tumour;
- stage of breast cancer;
- grade of the tumour;
- multifocality / multicentricity;

Figure 33.1 Anatomical structure of the breast and axilla. (a) Diagrammatic representation of the female breast. (b) Surgical anatomy of the breast.

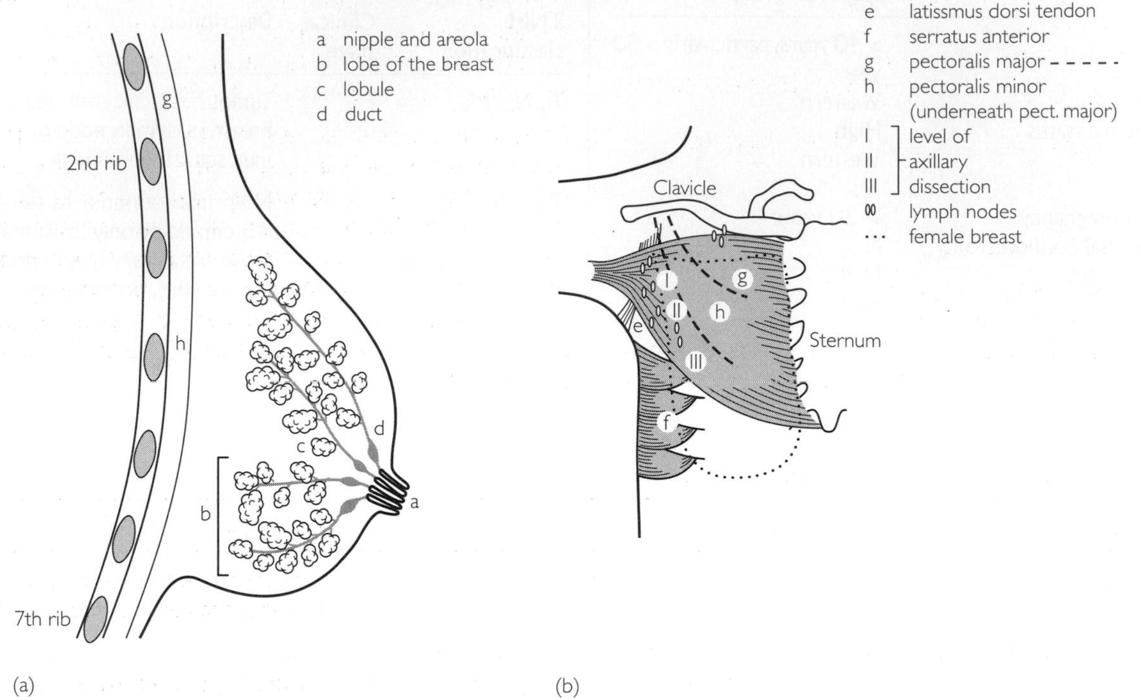

Table 33.3 Common types of breast cancer

Type	Histological features	Clinical notes
Ductal carcinoma *in situ*+	Proliferation of cells with a malignant appearance within the ducts, no invasion into surrounding tissue	Often extensive lesions Possible precursor to invasive carcinoma of the breast Extremely low rate of axillary lymph node involvement
Invasive breast cancer	Most are adenocarcinomas	
Invasive ductal	No special histologic features	75% of breast cancers
Tubular++	Tubule formation	2% of breast cancers, incidence is increasing with breast screening Infrequent metastases
Medullary++	Poorly differentiated nuclei within a defined border with lymphocytes and plasma cell infiltration	5–7% of breast cancers, decreasing with breast screening Favourable prognosis if all histological features present
Mucinous++	Extracellular mucin accumulates around tumour cell clusters	3% of breast cancers Slow growing Favourable prognosis
Invasive lobular	Linear small cells growing around the ducts and lobules	*5–10% of breast cancers *Ill-defined thickening on palpation
Paget's disease		Erosion of the nipple with redness or roughness Tingling, itching or discomfort around nipple Occurs in 1 in 50 breast cancers

From Frykberg and Bland (1994), Harris et al (1992), Hughes (1993), Kissin (1994).
\+ Lobular carcinoma *in situ* is a precursor / marker for the potential development of cancer in either breast
++ All are subgroups of invasive ductal carcinoma.

- presence of lymphatic or vascular invasion within the surrounding breast tissue;
- tumour location within the breast;
- patient preference;
- pre- or post-menopausal status;
- past history of breast cancer in the ipsilateral or contralateral breast;
- previous surgery, radiotherapy or chemotherapy.

Surgical procedures

A number of surgical procedures (Table 33.4) may be performed depending upon the clinical presentation and histological results. During the last 5–10 years the early detection of breast cancer through screening programmes, together with the results of clinical trials, have changed the types of surgical procedures performed. Previously the emphasis was to remove as much of the breast and surrounding tissue as possible to control the disease. More recently, the emphasis has turned to breast conservation with radiotherapy for smaller cancers.

Some tumours are not suitable for breast conservation and a modified radical mastectomy (MRM) will be performed. Post-operatively women require a breast prosthesis or may undergo early or late breast reconstruction (Table 33.4). The more radical surgical procedures are reserved for the exceptional cases of more advanced breast cancer. They are often used as a palliative procedure to control locally advanced disease to improve quality of life.

Table 33.4 Summary of surgical procedures for breast cancer

Surgical procedure	Description	Indications
Breast biopsy (lumpectomy)	Excision of breast lump	All histological analysis prior to planning definitive surgical procedure
Breast conservation (wide local excision; quadrantectomy; tylectomy; partial mastectomy)	Excision of tumour and surrounding breast tissue to give an adequate surgical margin from cancer cells Axillary dissection performed in conjunction	I, IIA Radiotherapy to remaining breast tissue recommended for invasive tumours
Axillary dissection	Removal of axillary lymph nodes Level I – dissection of contents between latissimus dorsi muscle, axillary vein and lateral border of pectoralis minor muscle Level II – as for level I plus tissue from beneath pectoralis minor Level III – as for I & II plus division and resection of pectoralis minor muscle (see Fig. 33.1)	All – some controversy over extent of axillary dissection required Provides information to accurately stage breast cancer Recommended for all invasive tumours
Simple mastectomy	Excision of all the breast tissue	IIA, IIB, IIIA Patient choice
Modified radical mastectomy (Patey)	Excision of all the breast tissue, axillary dissection and pectoralis minor muscle	II, III Patient choice
Radical mastectomy (Halsted)	As for modified radical mastectomy with the excision of pectoralis major muscle	IIIB IV
Extended radical mastectomy	As for radical mastectomy with the excision of the underlying chest wall (ribs); a split skin graft is required to cover the surgical defect on the chest wall	IV
Breast reconstruction (implants or myocutaneous flap)	1. Surgical implant (saline) with or without prior use of tissue expanders or 2. Skin and muscle flap (latissimus dorsi, rectus abdominis or gluteal muscle) with or without intact blood supply is used to reconstruct the breast, nipple reconstruction or prosthesis required	Patient choice after mastectomy

From Clark (1991), Denton (1991), Kissin (1994), Osteen and Smith (1990), Veronesi et al (1981).

Radiotherapy

Radiotherapy involves the application of external electron beams to the breast tissue to assist in the local control of breast cancer. It is used as routine treatment in conjunction with breast conservation surgery. In addition, it may be used following mastectomy if local invasion of the skin or muscle is detected. In rare instances, radiotherapy may be used as the primary treatment choice in fungating breast cancer. The axilla region is not irradiated if surgical dissection has occurred except in the rare case of insufficient clearance of positive lymph nodes. The total dose of radiotherapy is given as a number of smaller daily doses over 4–6 weeks to minimize the potential side effects of:

- lethargy;
- skin reaction which may be irritating and painful;
- breast lymphoedema and fibrosis;
- fibrosis resulting in a tightening of the skin and muscles on the anterior chest wall.

Booster doses to the tumour bed may be required for some women at the end of their initial treatment dose.

Chemotherapy

The role of chemotherapy in the management of breast cancer is to eradicate micrometastases and treat metastatic disease. Combinations of chemotherapy agents tend to be used in a cyclical pattern (one dose every 2–4 weeks) to minimize the side effects of treatment. Many women still suffer from side effects which may include:

- nausea and vomiting;
- lethargy;
- hair loss;
- bone marrow depression with decreased red and white blood cell formation resulting in immunosuppression.

Hormone therapy

As breast cancer may be influenced by female hormones (oestrogen and progesterone), endocrine, or hormone, therapy may be used. Its most common use is for postmenopausal women with oestrogen receptor-positive tumours who may or may not have lymph node involvement. Hormone therapy aims to reduce the effect of oestrogen on any residual microscopic breast cancer cells in an attempt to reduce tumour growth. The most common agent is Nolvadex (tamoxifen) but ablation of the ovaries (chemical, surgical or by irradiation) may also be used to reduce the available oestrogen in some women. The possible long-term effects of reduced oestrogen in pre-menopausal women with breast cancer has made the role of hormone therapy in this group of patients less clear.

Morbidity of primary breast cancer management

The aim of breast cancer treatment is to eradicate local disease and control the development of disease, thus enhancing the survival of the women so diagnosed. However, there are many potential problems that may occur in women who have been treated for breast cancer. Attempts are made to minimize the incidence of these problems with good surgical technique and post-operative care while using the appropriate doses of adjuvant therapies. However, the problems that may arise in some women include the following.

- Decreased shoulder movement and function secondary to:
  1. axillary dissection;
  2. more radical procedures; or
  3. fibrosis after radiotherapy.
- Wound infection and delayed wound healing in the early post-operative period.
- Seroma development on the anterior chest or axilla after wound drains are removed. Needle aspirations may be required for some women.
- Lymphoedema of the arm and/or breast secondary to the surgical removal of or radiation damage to the axillary lymph nodes and remaining breast tissue.
- Neural disorders including:
  1. sensory disturbances in medial upper arm due to dissection of intercostobrachial nerve;
  2. neuralgia; or
  3. nerve entrapment in the arm.
- Fibrosis of the skin and muscle of the chest wall after radiotherapy.
- Psychological effects resulting from the woman's concern about surgical procedure, diagnosis, recurrence or spread, life-threatening crisis of diagnosis, lifestyle changes during the treatment period.
- Local recurrence or metastatic spread of breast cancer.

The physiotherapist plays a significant role in the identification, prevention and/or management of many of these problems. Physiotherapists also assist in the support of women before, during and after the treatment and follow-up period for breast cancer.

Physiotherapist's Role in the Management of Breast Cancer

Physiotherapy has been recommended to improve the physical recovery of women after breast cancer surgery (Gutman et al, 1990; Wingate et al, 1989) but it tends not to be used for all women in clinical practice. Reasons for its lack of use include:

- poor recognition of the role and benefits of early physiotherapy intervention with this group of patients by some physiotherapists and other health professionals;

- limited access to physiotherapy services due to decreased resources, geographical location or costs.

The physiotherapist provides appropriate exercise prescription and assists in the education of women after breast cancer surgery to facilitate their:

- recovery of shoulder range of movement (ROM) and physical function of the operated arm; and
- awareness of lymphoedema, its prevention and early detection

while providing support as part of the multidisciplinary team. A planned approach to the physiotherapy management of women after breast cancer surgery with the ability to individualize exercise and education programmes is essential to ensure optimal quality of care and best practice.

Aims of physiotherapy management

The aims of physiotherapy management of women undergoing treatment for breast cancer are that patients should:

- regain their preoperative shoulder ROM and function within three months of surgery;
- maintain their ROM over time after surgery;
- obtain knowledge of lymphoedema, its prevention and an awareness of its early signs;
- not have their wound drainage or length of hospital stay adversely affected by the commencement of shoulder movement;
- minimize the effect of the development of secondary complications on their ultimate physical recovery.

Physiotherapy management care plan

The physiotherapy management care plan (PMCP) outlined in Figure 33.2 has been developed from the literature and extensive clinical practice. Using this PMCP, the aims outlined above have been achieved with ROM being decreased at day 5 and one month after surgery but maintained at preoperative levels from three months post-operatively (Box and Reul-Hirche, 1995a). Complications or problems that may develop during the post-operative period that need to be identified by physiotherapists for the appropriate intervention and modification are summarized in Table 33.5.

POST-OPERATIVE PRESENTATION

After surgery for breast cancer a woman will present with:

- an incision(s) which will be dependent upon the procedure performed;
- pressure dressings over the operative site;
- wound drains from the breast and axilla which will be monitored and recorded until the wound drainage is reduced to <20–30 ml in a 24-hour period;
- an intravenous line until her oral intake is normal;
- a donor site for the split skin graft if radical surgery has been performed.

Breast cancer surgery is performed under a general anaesthetic but most women are able to mobilize within 6–8 hours and are allowed to eat normally (as tolerated) after four hours. It is associated with a low incidence of the normal potential problems of surgery and the emphasis in the post-operative period is aimed at upper limb ROM, function and lymphoedema prevention. Patients with other medical conditions would need the appropriate physiotherapy intervention to prevent post-operative complications.

In the immediate post-operative period the operated arm is often rested on one pillow for comfort and the woman should be instructed in gentle active elbow and hand exercises. These preliminary exercises aim to facilitate the muscle pump in the arm, promoting venous and lymph drainage to establish new lymph channels through the tissue planes. Reassurance is often required for the sensory changes in the upper arm and the prevention of lymphoedema.

SHOULDER RANGE OF MOVEMENT AND FUNCTION

The commencement of shoulder movements after axillary dissection for breast cancer remains controversial and is dependent upon each surgeon's preference and protocol. The differences in opinion centre around the issues of wound drainage, seromas, shoulder stiffness, complications and length of hospital stay. Some authors recommend early movement to minimize shoulder dysfunction (Pollard et al, 1976) while others argue for delayed movement to minimize complications (Flew, 1979). Rodier et al (1987) found that in the immediate post-operative period there was no difference in the amount of wound drainage (WD) or length of stay (LOS) when early or delayed physiotherapy was used following mastectomy. In contrast, Lotze et al (1981) found that WD, LOS and incidence of wound complications were greater in women who had early shoulder movement after a MRM and this was supported by Dawson et al (1989). These authors found that the WD volume was 15% greater in women who had early shoulder movement but there was no significant difference in shoulder movement at two weeks when the women were discharged from hospital. The removal of drains may be dependent upon the amount of drainage in a 24-hour period (Tadych and Donegan, 1987), but Parikh et al (1992) found that there was no difference in the incidence or size of seromas requiring needle aspiration with early or late removal of drains after MRM.

Wingate (1985) found that women who received physiotherapy from day one post-operatively had better outcomes in terms of shoulder ROM and function but there was some increase in arm swelling. However, at three months post-operatively, the amount of swelling was below the accepted level for minimal oedema. These findings were repeated in a later study by Wingate et al (1989) but the issue of arm swelling was unresolved. This second study combined retrospective and prospective data while using the non-operative side for comparison. Another problem with the studies by Wingate and co-workers (1985 and 1989) is that the identification of lymphoedema was from only two points on the

Figure 33.2 Physiotherapy Management Care Plan

PATIENT ATTENDS PRE-ADMISSION CLINIC/ADMITTED TO WARD

PREOPERATIVE VISIT BY PHYSIOTHERAPIST

Assessment – shoulder ROM
– functional questionnaire
– limb size

Education – post-operative presentation and exercises
– preliminary lymphoedema education

DAILY POST-OPERATIVE VISITS

Hand/elbow exercises – commences immediately

Shoulder movement – if no axillary dissection has been performed, commenced immediately post-operatively and progressed within discomfort to full ROM
– if axillary dissection has been performed, commenced at surgeon's request or when wound drainage is <100ml/24 hours or there is a marked decrease in drainage over 24-hour period,
– restricted to ≤100° for first 2 days of movement and then gradually increase ROM using a limit of a discomfort rating of 3/10

Lymphoedema prevention education progressed as appropriate for each woman

DISCHARGE FROM HOSPITAL

Instruct in home programme and limitation of activities initially

Remeasure shoulder ROM, functional questionnaire and limb size

BREAST CLINIC APPOINTMENT

Review home programme and activity levels, progress exercises

Lymphoedema prevention education and pamphlet

1 MONTH

Progress exercises and stretches

Discuss exercise progressions for next month

Advice for functional activity progressions

Lymphoedema prevention education

Remeasure shoulder ROM, functional questionnaire and limb size

2 MONTHS

Assess effects of adjuvant therapies and modify or progress exercises/stretches

Advice for return to preoperative function and activity levels

FOLLOW-UP AT 3, 6, 12, 18, 24 MONTHS

Assess progress with remeasurement of ROM, functional activity questionnaire and limb size

Provide instruction or modification of exercises as appropriate

ROM = range of movement

arm. Clinical experience has shown that most of the early swelling occurs in the upper arm and axillary region which would not have been detected by their measurements.

Gutman et al (1990) found that women who underwent wide local excision and axillary dissection (WLE+AD) with radiotherapy obtained their pre-operative ROM faster

Table 33.5 Potential complications or problems that may interfere with physical recovery

Complication or problem	Definition	Physiotherapy intervention
Seroma	Collection of serous fluid around the incision line. Sometimes the collection may be blood and is referred to as a haematoma	Heaviness and discomfort associated with the fluid build-up often restricts exercise ability. Needle aspiration may be required and referral to surgeon is necessary
Wound infection	Bacterial infection of the incision and surrounding tissue. Antibiotic therapy and needle aspiration may be required	Recognition of signs of local infection is important to facilitate referral to surgeon. Exercises may need to be modified until the infection settles
Radiotherapy reaction	Redness and tightness in the irradiated skin may occur during treatment and often increases once it is finished. Contraction of soft tissues may cause discomfort	Adequate ROM is required for radiotherapy treatment but further progress may be hampered. Emphasis on prolonged stretching of the anterior chest wall and axilla is required
Lethargy	Tiredness associated with radiotherapy and chemotherapy treatment	Limits the woman's ability to exercise. Emphasis on ROM gaining and maintaining exercises during treatment, with increased intensity when treatment finished
Cording	Formation of fibrous band(s) running from the axilla to the wrist and associated with varying degrees of discomfort and pain. Usually exacerbated by reaching with an extended elbow. It is unclear if these bands are fibrosed lymph or blood vessels	This condition can seriously impair the ROM recovery. Additional exercises to stretch the 'cords' are required. Modification of other exercises to maximize shoulder ROM recovery without exacerbating pain associated with the cording (see Figure 33.3)
Neural disturbances	Ranges from sensory loss in the upper arm and axilla to neuralgic pain and muscle weakness	Reassurance of sensory loss is important. Appropriate intervention for pain relief, ROM and muscle activity are important
Lymphoedema	Protein-rich fluid build-up in the operated arm. If severe, it may impede exercise ability and progression to full recovery	Its early recognition and intervention are essential. See section on lymphoedema in this chapter and Chapter 35 for more information
Non-adherence to exercise programme	Cessation of exercise programme early in the post-operative period	The pre-operative and early post-operative period must stress the importance of continued exercise for at least three months after surgery to optimize long-term recovery

than those who had a MRM but all regained normal ROM within three months post-operatively. These authors recommend that while both groups require physiotherapy, the group with MRM required more intensive and longer treatment. In a pilot study by Hladiuk et al (1992) the recovery of women after breast cancer surgery was monitored for 12 months. These authors suggest that women who had poor recovery tended to have had a mastectomy, more lymph nodes removed, more positive lymph nodes and were less compliant with the exercise programme at one month after surgery. The clinical data from the PMCP outlined in Box and Reul-Hirche (1995a) did not concur with these points. Factors influencing recovery of ROM using the PMCP varied for different movements but included:

- slower ROM recovery for older patients;
- a loss of ROM at six months post-operatively tended to occur in those women with a history of previous shoulder problems;
- development of post-operative seroma was associated with less reduction in shoulder ROM in the early post-operative period (i.e. vigorous early movement);
- development of cording (Fig. 33.3) reduced ROM in the first two months after surgery but this was not evident at six months.

The principles of exercise after breast cancer surgery are:

- assisted movements initially;
- slow and rhythmical;
- sustained movements and stretches incorporated after 14–21 days;
- limiting point is discomfort (not pain);
- care with the vigour of the exercises performed to minimize interference with the regeneration of lymphatic channels;
- scar massage may be required to facilitate exercise ability;
- continued for 6–12 months post-operatively as the soft

Figure 33.3 Cording. Fibrous band in elbow (a), area of pain distribution (shaded), fibrous band in axilla (b).

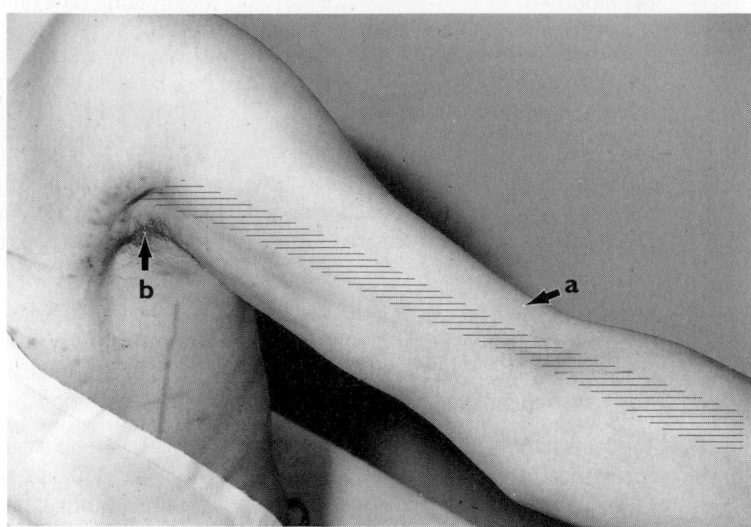

tissues tend to continue to remodel and contract during this period;
- gradual progression of the type, duration and repetition of the exercises with the development of warm-up and warm-down with the specific exercises.

The exercise instruction should place emphasis on regaining all of the movements of the shoulder. Particular attention should be directed to the physiological movements of abduction, flexion, extension, internal and external rotation as well as their functional movement combinations to ensure full recovery.

A 38-year-old woman, married with two young children, had a modified radical mastectomy for stage IIB breast cancer two weeks ago. She has had an uncomplicated post-operative recovery and is due to commence radiotherapy next week. Her ROM when reassessed today was:

- abduction 125° (170°)
- flexion 140° (175°)
- extension 35° (40°)
- internal rotation 65° (70°)
- external rotation 90° (100°)

indicating good progress so far. Although her limb circumferential measurements are unchanged, she is particularly concerned about lymphoedema. Her concern has arisen because she has an aunt who developed it after breast cancer surgery and her mother has swollen legs since her surgery for ovarian cancer five years ago.

Physiotherapy management

The exercise programme should be reviewed and progressed to incorporate sustained stretches. Gradual return to normal level of activities over the next 2–4 weeks is encouraged. Education about lymphoedema, its causes and precautions for its prevention/early detection should be continued. With her family history the patient may wish to be prepared in detail about lymphoedema.

The STRETCH (Strength Through Recreation Exercise Togetherness Care Health) Programme was developed to assist with the recovery of women after breast cancer surgery (Gaskin et al, 1989). It involves attendance at an eight-week programme which provides exercise and education within each two-hour session. Enrolment may occur at any time after eight weeks after surgery and it complements the early PMCP very well to optimize the physical recovery of women after breast cancer surgery (Box and Reul-Hirche, 1995b).

LYMPHOEDEMA EDUCATION AND PREVENTION

Secondary lymphoedema has been reported to occur in 14–62.5% of women after treatment for breast cancer (Kissin et al, 1986; Nikkanen et al, 1978; Zeissler et al, 1972) and often presents after the compromised lymphatic system has been overloaded (see Chapter 35). Risk factors for the development of secondary lymphoedema after breast cancer treatment have been identified and are summarized in Table 33.6.

During the pre- and post-operative period the physiotherapist should enhance a woman's understanding of her risk of lymphoedema without increasing her anxiety. Explanation of the cause and her individual risk should be complemented by education on the precautions to minimize its occurrence. All women 'at risk' of developing lymphoedema should also be informed on the signs of its early presentation and advised where to seek assistance for its management. The earlier lymphoedema is detected and managed, the better are the results of efforts to control it. The

Table 33.6 Risk factors for lymphoedema development after breast cancer treatment

Risk factor	Higher risk
Surgical removal of lymph nodes	Higher level of axillary dissection and more lymph nodes removed
Positive lymph nodes	Greater number
Wound infection and seromas	Post-operative development
Post-operative shoulder movement	Unskilled early movement that may increase scarring and interfere with the regeneration of lymphatic channels
Wound drainage	Large early post-operative wound drainage
Irradiation	To axilla (increased further if surgical removal of lymph nodes) and/or breast
Overloading the compromised lymphatic system	Activities that increase demand on the lymphatic system*

From Zeissler et al (1972), Kissin et al (1986), Yeoh et al (1986), Tadych and Donegan (1987), Ryttov et al (1988) and Foldi et al (1989).
* See Chapter 35.

education provided by physiotherapists about care of the 'at-risk' arm is outlined in the box.

Avoid:
1. overuse
2. prolonged lifting and carrying of heavy objects
3. trauma from household and hygiene activities. If trauma does occur, clean and take care of the wound until it has healed. Seek early medical attention if signs of infection occur (redness, swelling, increased warmth)
4. wearing tight jewellery or clothing
5. poor skin condition by using moisturizers and refraining from excessive sun exposure
6. blood pressure readings, venepuncture or intravenous lines on that arm

Do:
1. wear a compression garment and move the arm frequently during aircraft flights and long journeys by train, car or bus
2. be aware of early signs of lymphoedema such as swelling in the back of the hand, between the knuckles, back of upper arm or axilla
3. note if rings, watch band, shirt sleeve, bra or waistband become tighter.

Seek attention early while the swelling is mild.

The initial management of lymphoedema may involve combinations of elevation, exercise, massage to promote axilloaxillary and axilloinguinal lymphatic anastomoses and a compression garment. If the swelling continues to progress complex physical therapy is usually required. The reader is referred to Chapter 35 where lymphoedema and its management are discussed in detail with the rationale for the precautions of the 'at-risk' or affected arm.

It is important to remember that women undergoing treatment for breast cancer have faced a number of psychological and emotional challenges. The introduction of more detail on lymphoedema and their individual risk must be gradual and progressive to avoid increasing their anxiety. Many women prefer a brief explanation supplemented by written material with further education at a later stage in their recovery.

PALLIATIVE AND TERMINAL CARE

It has been mentioned that breast cancer screening has led to the earlier presentation and changes in the management of breast cancer. However, some women will present with stage III and IV breast cancer that may require surgery to remove the local disease. Adjuvant therapy may be palliative and often only undertaken for symptomatic relief of metastases. The physiotherapist's role during the early post-operative period will be similar to that outlined previously but may change after the confirmation of more advanced disease. The psychological impact of the diagnosis of advanced breast cancer may be devastating and most women will travel through a normal grief reaction. Behaviours and emotions consistent with the stages of denial, anger, bargaining, depression and acceptance necessitate a change in the physiotherapist's approach. Goal setting with the patient is imperative, remembering that listening and talking are effective therapy tools. As the systemic spread of the breast cancer progresses the physiotherapist may assist in maintaining the mobility and independence of the woman for as long as possible and contribute to her physical comforts to provide an acceptable quality of life during the terminal phases of her disease.

A 45-year-old woman has been referred to physiotherapy for management of her low back pain and reduced mobility. She had a radical mastectomy performed four weeks ago for advanced breast cancer and is currently receiving radiotherapy for lumbar spine metastases. She has limited shoulder movement and there is swelling of her upper arm following a wound infection post-operatively. Her split skin graft has taken but the edges remain slightly infected.

Physiotherapy management

Techniques and strategies that could be used in this woman's treatment include:

- transcutaneous nerve stimulation for pain relief (care with skin reaction to radiotherapy)
- positioning and support
- assisted arm movements and stretches
- relaxation techniques
- elevation of the arm
- massage to the posterior chest towards the opposite axilla and down the trunk to the ipsilateral inguinal region (refer to Chapter 35) to stimulate the superficial lymphatic drainage
- education as appropriate
- involvement of her partner in these assisted activities.

Summary

This chapter has provided an overview of breast cancer and its management. Physiotherapists need to determine the individual surgeon's preference for post-operative care. The physiotherapy management of women undergoing surgery for breast cancer must strike a balance between regaining shoulder ROM and function without increasing the risk for lymphoedema in order to maximize the quality of life. The involvement of physiotherapists to regain shoulder ROM and function is supported by the literature. The programme must ensure that the exercise prescription does not compromise wound drainage and healing nor contribute to the risk of lymphoedema. The involvement of physiotherapists in the multi-disciplinary team is necessary to facilitate the optimal recovery of women surviving the diagnosis of breast cancer.

ACKNOWLEDGEMENTS

I wish to thank Dr Cherrill Hirst for her review and comments in the preparation of this chapter.

References

Australian Cancer Society Breast Cancer Consensus Report (1994) Management of newly diagnosed early breast cancer and a national approach to breast cancer control. *Cancer Forum* **18** (2): 72–76.

Box R and Reul-Hirche H (1995a) Results of a quality improvement project evaluating a physiotherapy programme for women after breast cancer surgery. *Proceedings of the 22nd Annual Scientific Meeting of the Clinical Oncological Society of Australia*, p. 69.

Box R and Reul-Hirche H (1995b) An evaluation of the STRETCH Programme for women recovering from breast cancer surgery. *Proceedings of the 22nd Annual Scientific Meeting of the Clinical Oncological Society of Australia*, p. 101.

Clark A (1991) What is breast cancer and how is it treated? A surgeon's experience of breast cancer. In: Fallowfield L (ed) *Breast Cancer*, pp. 1–16. London: Tavistock/ Routledge.

Dawson I, Stam L, Heslinga J and Kalsbeek H (1989) Effect of shoulder immobilization on wound seroma and shoulder dysfunction following modified radical mastectomy: a randomised prospective clinical trial. *British Journal of Surgery* **76**(3): 311–312.

Denton S (1991) Nursing patients with breast cancer. In: Tiffany R and Borley D (eds) *Oncology for Nurses and Health Care Professionals*, 2nd edn, Vol 3 Cancer Nursing, pp. 309–339. London: Harper Collins Academic.

Flew T (1979) Wound drainage following radical mastectomy: the effect of restriction of shoulder movement. *British Journal of Surgery* **66**: 302–305.

Foldi E, Foldi M and Clodius L (1989) The lymphoedema chaos: a lancet. *Annals of Plastic Surgery* **22**: 505–515

Frykberg ER and Bland KI (1994) Management of *in situ* and minimally invasive breast carcinoma. *World Journal of Surgery* **18**: 45–57.

Gaskin T, LoBuglio A, Kelly P et al (1989) The rehabilitative program for patients with breast cancer. *Southern Medical Journal* **82**(4): 467–469.

Gutman H, Kersz T, Barzilai T et al (1990) Achievements of physical therapy in patients after modified radical mastectomy compared with quadrantectomy, axillary dissection and radiation for carcinoma of the breast. *Archives of Surgery* **125**: 389–391.

Harris JR, Lippman ME, Veronesi U and Willett W (1992) Breast cancer. *New England Journal of Medicine* **327** (6): 390–398.

Hladiuk M, Huchcroft S, Temple W and Schurr BE (1992) Arm function after axillary dissection for breast cancer: a pilot study to provide parameter estimates. *Journal of Surgical Oncology* **50**: 47–52.

Hughes LE (1993) Paget's disease and other malignancies of the female breast. *Surgery* **11**(9): 489–492.

Jacobsen JA, Danforth DN, Cowan KH et al (1995) Ten-year results of a comparison of conservation with mastectomy in the treatment of stage I and II breast cancer. *New England Journal of Medicine* **332** (14): 907–911.

Kelsey JL and Gammon MD (1991) The epidemiology of breast cancer. *CA – A Cancer Journal for Clinicians* **41** (3): 146–165.

Kissin MW (1994) The breast. In: Williamson RCN and Waxman BP (eds) *Scott: An Aid to Clinical Surgery*, 5th edn, pp. 189–203. London: Churchill Livingstone.

Kissin MW, Querci della Rovere G, Easton D and Westbury G (1986) Risk of lymphoedema following the treatment of breast cancer. *British Journal of Surgery* **73**(7): 580–584.

Lotze M, Duncan M, Gerber L et al (1981) Early versus delayed shoulder motion following axillary dissection. *Annals of Surgery* **193**(3): 288–295.

Nikkanen TAV, Vanharanta H and Helenius-Reunanen H (1978) Swelling of the upper extremity, function and muscle strength of the shoulder joint following mastectomy combined with radiotherapy. *Annals of Clinical Research* **10**: 273–279.

Osteen RT and Smith BL (1990) Results of conservative surgery and radiation therapy for breast cancer. *Surgery Clinics of North America* **70**(5): 1005–1021.

Parikh H, Badwe R, Ash C et al (1992) Early drain removal following modified radical mastectomy: a randomised trial. *Journal of Surgical Oncology* **51**: 266–269.

Pollard R, Callum K, Altman D and Bates T (1976) Shoulder movement following mastectomy. *Clinical Oncology* **2**: 243–249.

Rodier J, Gadonneix P, Dauplat J et al (1987) Influence of the timing of physiotherapy upon the lymphatic complications of axillary dissection for breast cancer. *International Surgery* **72**(1): 166–169.

Ryttov N, Holm N, Qvist N and Blichert-Toft M (1988) Influence of adjuvant irradiation on the development of late arm lymphoedema and impaired shoulder mobility after mastectomy for carcinoma of the breast. *Acta Oncologica* **27**(6a): 667–670.

Tadych K and Donegan W (1987) Post mastectomy seromas and wound drainage. *Surgery, Gynecology and Obstetrics* **165**: 483–487.

Veronesi U, Saccozzi R, Del Vecchi M et al (1981) Comparing radical mastectomy with quadrantectomy, axillary dissection and radiotherapy in patients with small cancers of the breast. *New England Journal of Medicine* **305**(1): 6–11.

Winchester DP and Cox JD (1992) Standards for breast-conservation treatment. *CA – A Cancer Journal for Clinicians* **42**(3): 134–162.

Wingate L (1985) Efficacy of physical therapy for patients who have undergone mastectomies: a prospective study. *Physical Therapy* **65**(6): 896–900.

Wingate L, Croghan I, Natarjan N et al (1989) Rehabilitation of the mastectomy patient: a randomised, blind prospective study. *Archives of Physical Medicine and Rehabilitation* **70**(1): 21–24.

Yeoh E, Denham J, Davies S and Spittle M (1986) Primary breast cancer: complications of axillary management. *Acta Radiologica et Oncologica* **25**(2): 105–108.

Zeissler RH, Rose GB and Nelson PA (1972) Postmastectomy lymphoedema: late results of treatment in 385 patients. *Archives of Physical Medicine and Rehabilitation* **53**: 159–166.

Further reading

Aitken RJ, Gaze MN, Rodger A et al (1989) Arm morbidity within a trial of mastectomy and either nodal sample with selective radiotherapy or axillary clearance. *British Journal of Surgery* **76**(6): 568–571.

Beatty JD, Robinson GV, Zaia JA et al (1983) A prospective analysis of nosocomial wound infection after mastectomy. *Archives of Surgery* **118**: 1421–1424.

Chatterton P (1988) Physiotherapy for the terminally ill. *Physiotherapy* **74**(1): 42–46.

Clodius L (1977) *Lymphedema*, pp. 147–155. Stuttgart: Georg Thieme.

Donegan WL and Spratt JS (1995) *Cancer of the Breast*, 4th edn. Philadelphia: W.B. Saunders.

Dowden RV (1991) Selection criteria for successful immediate breast reconstruction. *Plastic and Reconstructive Surgery* **88**(4): 628–634.

Fallowfield LJ and Hall A (1991) Psychosocial and sexual impact of diagnosis and treatment of breast cancer. *British Medical Bulletin* **47**(2): 388–399.

Foldi M (1977) Physiology and pathophysiology of lymph flow. In: Clodius L (ed) *Lymphedema*, pp. 1–11. Stuttgart: Georg Thieme.

Keramopoulos A, Tsionou C, Minaretzis D et al (1993) Arm morbidity following treatment of breast cancer with total axillary dissection: a multivariate approach. *Oncology* **50**: 445–449.

Kinne DW (1993) Controversies in primary breast cancer management. *American Journal of Surgery* **166**: 502–508.

Moore MP and Kinne DW (1994) Patient selection for conservation surgery versus mastectomy: Memorial Hospital Breast Service Experience. *World Journal of Surgery* **18**: 58–62.

National Health and Medical Research Council (1995) *Clinical Practice Guidelines: The Management of Early Breast Cancer.* Sydney: National Breast Cancer Centre Publications.

National Health and Medical Research Council (1995) *A Consumer's Guide: Early Breast Cancer.* Sydney: National Breast Cancer Centre Publications.

Senofsky GM, Moffat FL, Davis K et al (1991) Total axillary lymphadenectomy in the management of breast cancer. *Archives of Surgery* **126**: 1336–1342.

Vinton AL, Traverso W and Jolly PC (1991) Wound complications after modified radical mastectomy compared with tylectomy with axillary lymph node dissection. *American Journal of Surgery* **161**: 584–588.

Watson M, Greer S, Blake S and Shrapnell K (1984) Reaction to a diagnosis of breast cancer. *Cancer* **53**(9): 2008–2012.

Wazer D, DiPetrillo T, Schmidt-Ullrich R et al (1992) Factors influencing cosmetic outcome and complication risk after conservative surgery and radiotherapy for early-stage breast carcinoma. *Journal of Clinical Oncology* **10**(3): 356–363.

34

Physiotherapy and Gynaecological Surgery

ROBYN SHARPE

Physiotherapists who have worked in acute surgical wards will be familiar with many facets of management of gynaecological surgical patients. Particular aspects related to pelvic surgery are dealt with in this chapter. Indications for gynaecological surgery include menorrhagia, malignancy, prolapse, dyspareunia, incontinence and infertility. The surgical approach can be either abdominal or vaginal and sometimes both. Laparoscopic surgery is becoming more common and sometimes this is combined with a vaginal approach, as in a laparoscopic-assisted vaginal hysterectomy (see Chapter 27). The position of the patient during surgery may be supine for abdominal approach and lithotomy for perineal surgery. Left lateral is used in perianal surgery. The use of a knee-chest position is decreasing. Details of the common surgical procedures and indications for them are outlined in Tables 27.5 and 27.6.

Physiotherapy Management

Physiotherapy management of gynaecological surgical patients covers those aspects which apply to other abdominal surgery:

- prevention of respiratory and circulatory complications,
- facilitation of mobilization;
- education about back care and ergonomics;
- abdominal muscle strengthening.

In addition PF rehabilitation and associated functional activity is considered of prime importance for patients with prolapse or incontinence and is useful for other gynaecological conditions. To provide optimum care, PT management should commence pre-operatively. Assessment, education and treatment, if necessary, enable the patient to cope more effectively with post-operative demands.

Pre-operative Management

Pre-operative education can be given individually or in groups, before admission (multidisciplinary pre-admission clinics) or on the eve of surgery and may involve instruction as well as treatment. As with any surgery, certain patients have a higher risk of post-operative complications. Patients with respiratory conditions, e.g. asthma, emphysema or bronchiectasis will require pre-operative treatment to optimize their recovery. This may be done on an outpatient basis or during a pre-operative admission work-up. Smokers are strongly encouraged to cease smoking at least 48 hours prior to surgery, preferably earlier. Cessation of smoking at least six weeks prior to surgery is necessary to avoid smoking-induced post-operative respiratory complications (Hall et al, 1996).

Opinion is divided as to the value of routine respiratory physiotherapy treatment for low-risk patients. For the healthy non-smoker under 60 years undergoing elective abdominal surgery, Condie et al (1993) reported that the incidence of chest infection for non-smoking patients was low, namely 5%. Other studies, including Hall et al (1996), found atelectasis to be more prevalent than infection and quoted a 14% respiratory complication rate for patients undergoing abdominal surgery. There is a need for further research, especially with gynaecological surgery, into the role of routine respiratory physiotherapy post-operatively.

Gynaecology / oncology patients need to be considered as a separate entity, as surgery is more complex. All patients undergoing gynaecological surgery need to be assessed as to their risk status. Age, medical history, smoking, weight and general health are considered and the patient treated as required.

The issues for these patients are similar to those for abdominal surgery patients, so a brief summary will be provided here.

A pre-operative PT programme for each patient should:

- assess for risk factors;
- educate as to what to expect post-operatively;
- teach post-operative skills;
- give an overview of the recovery course.

Pre-operative programme

Relevant details of the patient's records include:

- respiratory, cardiac and vascular pathology;
- relevant medical history;
- pathology and X-ray results.

Subjective assessment should cover:

- physical and emotional well-being;
- pre-existing respiratory or circulatory problems;
- pelvic organ function, e.g. constipation or obstructed defaecation, urinary frequency, urgency or incontinence.

Orthopaedic conditions may require particular nursing care. Obstructed defaecation will be helped by pre-operative instruction on positioning and defaecation retraining (see Chapter 30). Urge control techniques can be useful for urinary urgency and urge incontinence (see Chapter 30).

Assessment and treatment

A standard respiratory and circulatory assessment is carried out. (For specific details about appropriate physiotherapy procedures refer to Ellis and Alison (1993), Webber and Pryor (1993).)

RESPIRATORY

Smoking, obesity and pre-existing respiratory disease all compromise the patient post-operatively (Webber and Pryor, 1993). Effective deep breathing, use of active cycle breathing techniques (ACBT) and a supported huff and cough will assist in keeping airways clear. Deep breaths, with an inspiratory hold at the end, followed by a good huff enables clearance of the upper airways. Use of ACBT-facilitated inspiration, peak expiratory pressure (PEP) masks and incentive spirometry will assist clearance of retained secretions. These may be used pre-operatively on an outpatient or inpatient basis (Webber and Pryor, 1993).

CIRCULATORY

The risk of deep venous thrombosis (DVT) post-gynaecological surgery may be increased in those patients maintained in the lithotomy position for a long time. Antiembolic stockings are ordered by some surgeons. Pre-operative exercise sessions which increase venous return will enhance post-operative co-operation. Many surgeons use subcutaneous anticoagulant therapy for surgical patients as a preventive measure for DVT (Crandon and Koutts, 1983). Early mobilization may also aid in the prevention of DVT and pulmonary embolism (Ellis and Alison, 1993; Webber and Pryor, 1993). Patel et al (1996) found a high incidence (55%) of DVT following laparoscopic surgery for cholecystectomy. The median duration of pneumo-perineum was 80 min (range 40–160 min). Clinically, gynaecological surgery does not seem to have the same rate of DVT. Further research in this area is warranted.

Post-operative DVT is more frequent in patients operated on for malignant diseases than for other disorders. Indeed, there is mounting evidence that thrombotic abnormalities may precede cancer diagnosis by months or even years (Donati, 1994, 1995).

Researchers have found that *on admission* patients with uterine malignancy had an incidence of nearly 12% of pulmonary embolism and almost 7% of DVT. The use of subcutaneous heparin was found to reduce these figures (Graf et al, 1996). The role of prophylactic exercises and early mobilization in reducing the risk was not looked at. It would appear that both these measures, being readily available as the physiotherapist is already involved in the management of the post-operative patient, have an important role in reducing the risks.

Netzer et al (1996) approached the subject from a different perspective. They found abnormal abdominal ultrasound findings in 65% of subjects with DVT, with 10% being clinically significant for malignancy. Their recommendation is for routine abdominal ultrasound for all patients with confirmed DVT.

MOBILITY

An explanation of mobility techniques will enable more comfortable post-operative mobilization. Moving across the bed, transfers from supine to sitting on the side of the bed, getting out of a chair and crawling back into bed can be helpful in minimizing stress on the abdominal incision (see Chapter 19).

STRENGTHENING

Pelvic floor rehabilitation may have been provided for some patients pre-operatively. All patients undergoing gynaecological surgery will benefit from PF exercises and instruction in the functional use of the pelvic floor. Instruction in defaecation dynamics can be very beneficial for post-operative function.

Abdominal muscle-strengthening exercises taught pre-operatively enable easier activation post-operatively. Lumbar spine instability, prevention of back strain and restoration of muscle function following surgery can all be assisted by exercises. Abdominal drawing in (Richardson and Jull, 1995) can be taught in different positions. Pelvic rocking assists in relieving backache and pain associated with wind.

Psychological Aspects

The impact of gynaecological surgery on the patient is different from that of other surgery such as cholecystectomy. Women react in various ways to the removal of reproductive organs. It is important for all health professionals not to assume how the patient will feel. Patients of all ages may have concerns about their sexuality and return to intimacy.

Often the physiotherapist is the person in whom the patient confides her fears and concerns. This may be due to the time required for physiotherapy pre-operative assessment or discussion on pelvic floor function and the tactile nature of the treatment, which allow the woman to feel more comfortable with the physiotherapist. The physiotherapist should be able to give a clear explanation of physical changes and what to expect. More complex issues of self-esteem, body image and relationships may be better dealt with by a counsellor specializing in this field (Corney et al, 1993). Referral to a social worker or psychiatrist is appropriate for some women.

Diagnosis and treatment of gynaecological cancers has profound psychosocial implications, in addition to the obvious biological ones. Women are confronted with the issues of having cancer and treatments which may impact adversely on body image, sexuality and relationships, in addition to the possibility of imposed infertility and/or menopause.

Patients having surgery for malignancy require reassurance and emotional support. However, responsibility for imparting to the patient information concerning the condition and counselling does not lie with the physiotherapist. Most hospitals utilize a team approach and the appropriate person in that team should be contacted if the patient is requesting information inappropriately from the physiotherapist. It is essential that the physiotherapist knows the current status and information level of the patient, in order not to disclose information inadvertently.

Pre-operative Instructions – Individual or Class?

Whilst it is desirable for some patients, e.g. those with co-morbidities, language difficulties or psychological problems, to receive individual instruction pre-operatively, many patients benefit from pre-operative information given in a class setting. They gain support from other women undergoing similar procedures and usually have more time to institute pre-operative changes such as ceasing smoking and practising the exercises taught. The physiotherapist is able to give more detailed information to a larger group than would normally be possible on an individual basis. All patients attending a class should still be seen on hospital admission by the physiotherapist to allow for respiratory assessment at the time of surgery and a review of the exercises taught in class. Pelvic floor, bladder control and defaecation information is more thoroughly taught in a class situation than individual education time would allow for. However, if a patient then indicates she lacks pelvic floor awareness or has a continence problem, she may benefit from treatment as an outpatient, prior to surgery, to improve her condition.

A pilot project comparing the effectiveness of a pre-operative class education with individual pre-operative education is currently being undertaken by the author. Interim subjective data, based on patient satisfaction surveys done post-operatively, suggest that class patients feel better prepared for their surgery and more involved in their own care than those who did not attend class.

Following pre-operative assessment and treatment, a plan for individual post-operative care is made. Patients at greater risk of complications (pre-existing conditions or prolonged surgery) can be targeted with earlier and more frequent post-operative treatment.

Post-operative Management – Abdominal Surgery

Day of operation

It is preferable to see the patient, albeit briefly, in the immediate post-operative hours. Post-operative checking includes:

- *operation notes.* These will provide accurate information regarding the procedure performed and will enable the physiotherapist to provide timely and effective treat-

ment, taking into account the type, severity and outcome of surgery;
- *state of consciousness* – asleep, drowsy, rousable, alert;
- *pain level.* If the patient appears to be in pain at rest, adequate analgesia should be sought from the nursing staff. If the patient has a patient-controlled analgesic (PCA) device, she should be encouraged to use it prior to treatment. Harbourne (1995) has found analgesia required for physiotherapy treatment is higher than that required when the patient is at rest;
- *analgesia* – epidural, patient-controlled analgesia, IM narcotics;
- *wound site* – see Chapter 27;
- *attachments.* Post-operatively the patient usually has an IV line and an IDC *in situ.* Depending on the surgery, she may also have an epidural line, drain tubes from the abdomen, central venous lines, arterial lines, infusion lines for analgesia or insulin and occasionally nasogastric tubes and total parenteral nutrition lines. Additional monitoring equipment may be used if the patient is classed as high dependency. This may include pulse oximetry, ECG and BP monitoring on a continuous basis;
- *position.* The patient is usually supine on return from theatre. She can be assessed in this position for calf tenderness and wound condition and her chest auscultated.

CONSENT

The patient's co-operation is sought and her consent for treatment obtained, usually verbally.

TREATMENT

This is usually brief on the day of surgery. The emphasis is on respiratory and circulatory function. Careful auscultation of the chest can be achieved in supine. Upper, anterior and anterolateral segments of the lungs can be listened to and, if air entry is decreased, the posterior segments may be auscultated by carefully rolling the patient into side lying.

Calf circulation can be checked by Homan's test, palpation and observation.

Treatment consists of assisting and encouraging deep breaths and inspiratory holds, supported huff/cough and lower limb exercises. The patient may be drowsy but usually is able to be roused sufficiently to practise deep breathing and circulatory exercises. Supported coughing is done after five deep breaths with inspiratory holds. The physiotherapist may need to assist in supporting the wound, with hands, pillow or towel. The patient is encouraged to repeat these exercises hourly and nursing staff will also need to reinforce this with the patient.

If the patient has a moist cough, measures are taken to assist in the removal of the secretions. Vertical and high abdominal incisions make it more painful for the patient to move and cough. This needs to be considered when treating the patient, with regard to support and pain relief. If the patient has retained secretions, ACBT will assist their removal with less discomfort to the patient.

Day one

By now the patient will be more alert and have good pain control, sufficient to make it possible to sit out of bed, though this may only be for 10 minutes on the first day. There are fewer respiratory complications if a patient sits out early and mobilizes as soon as possible. The patient should be shown how to, and assisted in, rolling into side lying and pushing up into sitting (see Fig. 19.22). Use of an overbed ring should be minimized as the patient may become reliant on it for moving in the bed and then have difficulty managing at home. Some patients report aching shoulders and sore abdomens after overusing the ring. Physiotherapy treatment can be timed to coincide with the patient sitting out to enable a more thorough assessment of respiratory function to be made. Depending on the surgery, the patient should be able to perform effective deep breathing exercises and supported coughing and do calf stretches in this position (see Fig. 19.25). She is to be encouraged to continue deep breathing hourly and lower limb circulatory exercises quarter-hourly. Unilateral upper limb movements assist in chest expansion and are also encouraged hourly. Luttrell (1996) found the increased venous flow in calf and femoral veins continued for only 10–15 min after plantar/dorsiflexion exercises. Patients should therefore be encouraged to do plantar/dorsiflexion exercises every 15 min.

Wind can be a problem for many women, particularly following major surgery where the bowel has been handled, e.g. total abdominal hysterectomy (TAH) and tumour debulking surgery. In addition to pelvic rocking and abdominal drawing in, abdominal massage in the direction of the large bowel and early mobilizing all assist in the relief of 'wind' or 'gas' pains. All patients will benefit from a written information booklet to reinforce the points covered in pre-operative education (Haslett and Jennings, 1992).

Day two

By day two, the patient is able to ambulate short distances with assistance, continue day one exercise and commence pelvic rocking. Rocking assists in relieving backache resulting from prolonged lying. Abdominal drawing in as for strengthening can assist in relieving wind pain. On this day epidural or patient-controlled analgesia may be ceased and intermittent intramuscular or oral analgesia commenced. Thus the patient may perceive more pain than she has previously. Care is required not to tire the patient, nor cause her unnecessary distress. Treatment may be timed to follow 20 minutes after IM analgesia (e.g. pethidine). The patient may find it more difficult to cough effectively, once continuous analgesia has ceased.

Sit the patient forward or sit her on the side of the bed with foot support. A towel binder or a pillow held firmly against the wound will provide abdominal support for coughing (see Fig. 19.25).

Some patients find it difficult to breathe deeply and maintain basal expansion of their lungs after surgery. Incentive spirometry may be useful to encourage the patient to continue breathing exercises independently between treatments. Hall et al (1991, 1993) have shown that instruction in deep breathing with inspiratory holds is more cost effective than using incentive spirometers. However, careful instruction plus the device is helpful for many patients in encouraging them to continue to do the exercises independently.

If IM narcotics are used, care must be taken in walking the patient too soon after the drug is given to avoid dizziness or fainting.

Day three onwards

From day three onwards, as drains, IVs, IDC or SPC, etc. are progressively removed, the patient's level of activity can be increased. Longer periods of sitting out are encouraged, as are walks around the ward. Previous exercises are continued. Post-operative stays are becoming shorter and treatment outlined for later may have to be compressed into three days. Patients often have sutures removed in a community setting.

Around day five / six, staples or sutures are usually removed and abdominal drawing in may be commenced in standing. Pelvic floor exercises are commenced once the urethral catheter is removed, with the patient commencing with five repetitions of five-second holds (or less if need be), four or five times per day and gradually increasing (refer to Chapter 30).

Post-operative Complications

These are the same as occur with other abdominal surgery and include bleeding, DVT, respiratory problems, paralytic ileus, urinary tract infection and wound infection (see also Chapter 27).

Post-discharge Advice

Before leaving hospital, the patient should be educated about recuperation at home. Depending on the indication for and the type of surgery and doctor's advice, she should be informed as to when to return to work, exercise, housework, driving and leisure activities. The patient should be encouraged to commence a daily walking programme, starting slowly and building up until she can walk briskly for 30–40 minutes three times per week by six weeks post-surgery. Abdominal exercises should also be continued twice a day for this period. The medical adviser gives guidelines about driving. Generally it should be avoided until sudden, forceful and twisting movements no longer cause pain. This may be for 4–6 weeks.

Activities of high impact such as tennis, netball, running, etc. are best avoided for 10–12 weeks post-operatively. Less vigorous activity, e.g. low-impact aerobics or swimming, may be commenced after six weeks, after the post-operative checkup with the surgeon. Many patients with pelvic floor laxity should never return to high-impact or heavy strengthening activities and should be encouraged to restrict heavy lifting.

Posture and back care education needs to be constantly reinforced during hospitalization and post-discharge advice is reinforced by written information.

Correct lifting and bending techniques are taught to prevent undue strain on the abdominal wall and incision during the recuperative phase.

Generally the patient is instructed to lift only light objects (around 1 kg) for six weeks, with no heavy lifting before 8–10 weeks. Those who have had bladder neck suspensions must restrict lifting to a greater extent. Those women who work in the caring professions, especially in nursing homes, need longer before returning to that type of lifting. Lighter duties, initially, should be recommended. For women undergoing pelvic floor surgery the need to contract the pelvic floor during lifting and all activities which increase intra-abdominal pressure must be emphasized (see Chapter 30). Advice about the optimal defaecation position and pattern, and urinary urge control techniques (Chapter 30) should be included.

Post-operative Management – Vaginal Surgery

Much of the preceding section also applies here, but recovery from vaginal surgery does differ.

Day of surgery

On the day of surgery, the patient usually has a vaginal pack *in situ* to absorb post-operative wound ooze. This can cause low backache in many women due to intrapelvic pressure. Heat and gentle pelvic rocking in side lying can help alleviate the pain. Usually the vaginal pack is removed 24 hours post-operatively.

Respiratory and circulatory exercises are performed as they are for abdominal surgery. Support for coughing is given by holding a pad on the perineum. From clinical experience, many patients also find that pressure applied to the pubis assists when coughing.

Day one

On day one the patient should be sitting out of bed and may walk short distances by the end of the day. As with all surgery, some patients experience severe nausea post-operatively and this may limit mobility. Respiratory and circulatory exercises are continued hourly. Patients without abdominal incisions should have little difficulty with deep breathing. However, smokers may involuntarily trigger a cough with a deep breath and be reluctant to do breathing exercises for this reason.

Patients who have had a vaginal hysterectomy or posterior vaginal repair will probably have their IDC removed on day one or two. This depends on the surgeon's instruction. Patients with a bladder neck suspension, vaginal urethroplasty or anterior vaginal repair may have an indwelling catheter or suprapubic catheter for 3–5 days.

Apart from commencing abdominal drawing in exercises and pelvic rocking on day two, the major rehabilitation following vaginal surgery is pelvic floor retraining. After removal of the IDC, the patient undergoes a 'trial of void'. This involves measuring every urine output following removal of the catheter, for a period of 8–10 hours. After this time a catheter is passed and the residual volume of urine is measured. If it is below the level prescribed by the surgeon, frequently <100 ml, the patient has 'passed' her trial of void. If the residue is greater than the amount specified, the IDC is reinserted. Repeat trials are conducted and if unsuccessful, the patient is taught self-catheterization which she then continues at home. Trial of void is repeated at intervals until voiding is satisfactory. Bladder neck suspension surgery is responsible for most of the post-operative voiding difficulty.

Physiotherapists can assist patients during their trial of void. By careful positioning on the toilet, i.e. use of a foot stool to increase hip/knee flexion and pelvic floor support and sphincter release, the patient can often void more effectively (see Chapter 30).

Most patients go home around day three to seven, depending on the type of surgery and their ability to void (Farrer, 1991).

Post-discharge

Post discharge advice for patients undergoing vaginal surgery is similar to that given to abdominal surgery patients. Lifting, however, is restricted to light loads (e.g. 1–2 kg, progressing to 3 kg) for 12 weeks for patients who have had anterior and/or posterior repairs and bladder neck suspensions. Similar restrictions are placed on high-impact activities, e.g. running, tennis, netball. This is to minimize stress on the newly repaired pelvic floor. Women whose work involves heavy lifting are taught to tighten their pelvic floor and abdominal wall and prepare to lift. The same restrictions about high-impact activities, heavy lifting and defaecation straining apply in both abdominal and vaginal surgery (see Chapter 30).

Ideally, all patients undergoing gynaecological surgery should see the physiotherapist at the six-week post-operative medical check-up, to assess for rate of recovery and treat any ongoing problems, e.g. pelvic floor dysfunction.

Relaxation

Gynaecological surgery, whether for cancer or correction of menstrual or continence problems, is a very stressful procedure. Issues of fertility, lifespan, sexual function and feelings of 'wholeness' are interwoven with apprehension about a hospital stay, time away from family, absence from work, disfigurement, pain and all the other concerns and fears associated with the surgery. Many of these women will have had symptoms which interfered with their everyday functioning for months or years, e.g. heavy bleeding, urinary incontinence, prolapse, dysmenorrhoea, and will be less than well when they enter hospital.

Relaxation can offer these patients one way to deal with the stress of illness and surgery and cope better with the hospital admission. Sommers (1993) states '. . . the mind and body, although two entities, work as one unified whole, and cannot be separated'. Reduction in stress and anxiety may help patients cope better with post-operative pain.

The optimal time to teach relaxation is in a class situation, prior to admission to hospital. Further practice at home and suggestions for incorporating relaxation into activities of daily living enable the patient to prepare mentally and physically for her surgery. Handouts reinforce teaching.

Methods

Reciprocal relaxation is a very effective way of teaching the patient how to differentiate between a tense body and a body at ease (Mitchell, 1988). (For further reading refer to Chapter 18.) Once the patient is familiar and comfortable with this method, other ways of relaxing may be introduced, e.g. visualization, music, meditation. It is useful to have a supply of relaxation tapes and portable tape players to loan inpatients who are particularly stressed by their experience.

Referral to other agencies such as relaxation centres or women's health centres is appropriate for women with ongoing stressors.

Support Groups

In the field of gynaecology/oncology, support groups run at the hospital or in the community provide ongoing assistance to cope with the diagnosis and treatments required. 'Look Good, Feel Better' programmes assist women with cancer to adapt to the side effects of treatments such as hair loss and skin changes, as well as to cope with stress and anxiety. Many countries run similar programmes.

Lymphoedema

Patients who have pelvic or groin node dissection during surgery for malignant diseases may have problems post-operatively with lymphoedema in their lower limbs, lower abdomen and / or groin. This is due to the reduced transport capacity of the lymph system. Patients need to be informed after such surgery of the small risk of lymphoedema developing and to note any signs of heaviness or increased size in their legs, pubic area or vulva. The risk of lymphoedema is present from the immediate post-operative period and is lifelong. It appears that only a small percentage of women actually develop it, but very little information is available in the literature on lower limb lymphoedema (Logan, 1995).

If such symptoms are noticed, the patient is advised to contact her doctor and physiotherapist as soon as possible. Prompt intervention can reduce the severity of this problem and enable the patient to manage the lymphoedema and not be too severely restricted by it.

Treatment involves massage, exercise, compression and skin care (for further reading see Chapter 35). If the patient does not live near the treating hospital, she should be referred to the appropriate community resource with facilities to manage this problem, e.g. domiciliary services, local hospital, private physiotherapist.

All aspects of physiotherapy management are enhanced by written information. Provision of the physiotherapist's name and contact phone number for patients to access, if necessary, can be reassuring.

Mrs MF, a 38-year-old mother of two young children, presented to her GP with a six-month history of post-coital bleeding. This, plus an abnormal Pap smear, resulted in referral for colposcopy, which confirmed stage IB cancer of the cervix.

Mrs MF did not return for surgery, preferring to try alternative treatment. One year after her initial symptoms, she re-presented for surgery and radical hysterectomy with pelvic and para-aortic lymphadenectomy were performed. Advanced disease was evident at the time of surgery with 24/35 nodes positive for malignancy.

Pre-operative assessment confirmed that Mrs MF had smoked 25/day for the past 10 years, had stress incontinence when coughing and was moderately obese at 93 kg. She was taught how to use incentive spirometry in addition to routine respiratory and circulatory exercises. Pelvic floor exercises were taught and support when coughing encouraged. Because of the removal of her lymph nodes, her lower limbs were measured for a baseline against which to measure post-operative changes.

Post-operatively, Mrs MF was febrile to 38.5°C for 48 hours. Pre-operative chest X-ray had not shown any abnormal features, but a film 36 hours post-op. showed R lower lobe atelectasis and consolidation. This was despite immediate post-operative physiotherapy intervention. Incentive spirometry use was poor – 500 ml. The patient was mobilized on day 1, with limitations from L lower limb motor loss induced by epidural pain relief. She was sat out of bed t.d.s. from day 1. Physiotherapy continued b.d. until the patient was mobilizing independently on day 3. Frequent sitting out, demand ventilation exercises, ACTB and mobilization continued daily. By day 3 her respiratory signs had resolved, AE was normal and she was afebrile. She was mobilized freely after removal of the epidural and resolution of L leg motor loss. Her post-op course continued normally until day 6 when she complained of tightness in her R thigh and genital area.

Remeasurement of her lower limbs showed an increase of 3–4 cm at each 50, 60 and 70 cm measurement mark. Mrs MF was given an information leaflet on lymphoedema precautions and was educated as to exercise, self-massage and the need to keep her legs elevated when sitting for any length of time. As she was remaining to commence her radiotherapy treatment, daily massage and exercise continued for the rest of her admission. Firm bike pants were recommended to be worn during day and night if these felt comfortable.

By discharge on day 11, her legs showed a decrease of >2.5 cm at each mark and the patient reported feeling much more comfortable. Genital swelling had also decreased significantly.

Pelvic floor exercises were continued throughout her admission. Abdominal exercises were commenced on day 1, with static work, progressing to forward-leaning transversus abdominis training and postural training. Back care and ergonomic advice were ongoing throughout her hospital stay, commencing with good sitting and walking postures, through to education for a return to normal activity and daily exercise. A follow-up outpatient appointment was made to reassess her lymphoedema at six weeks post-op.

Despite radiotherapy, further surgery and chemotherapy, Mrs MF died from her disease $2^1/_2$ years after her initial symptoms appeared. The five-year survival rate of cancer of the cervix stage I is 86%, when comparing the proportion of potentially cured patients with the matched population (Sondik et al, 1985).

Post-operative treatment of patients undergoing gynaecological surgery is frequently part of a general hospital roster. However, it may not be until these patients are considered as a specific group that a comprehensive programme, as outlined here, is available to them. Physiotherapists working in the area of women's health can enhance the care of these women by encouraging the development of such programmes.

References

Condie E, Hack K and Ross A (1993) An investigation of the value of routine provision of post-operative chest physiotherapy in non-smoking patients undergoing elective abdominal surgery. *Physiotherapy* **79**: 547–552.

Corney RH, Crowther ME, Everett H et al (1993) Psychosexual dysfunction in women with gynaecological cancer following radical pelvic surgery. *British Journal of Gynaecologic Oncology* **100**: 745–746.

Crandon AJ and Koutts J (1983) Incidence of post-operative deep vein thrombosis in gynaecological oncology. *Australian and New Zealand Journal of Obstetrics and Gynaecology* **23**: 216–219.

Donati MB (1994) Cancer and thrombosis. *Haemostasis* **24**: 128–131.

Donati MB (1995) Cancer and thrombosis: from Phlegmasia alba dolens to transgenic mice. *Thrombosis and Haemostasis* **74**: 278–281.

Ellis E and Alison J (eds) (1993) *Key Issues in Cardiorespiratory Physiotherapy*, pp. 115–123. Oxford: Butterworth Heinemann.

Farrer H (1991) *Gynaecological Care*, 2nd edn, pp. 192–99. Melbourne: Churchill Livingstone.

Graf AH, Graf B, Truan H and Staudach A (1996) Risk and prevention of thromboembolism complications in gynecologic malignancies. *Gynakologisch-Geburtshilfliche Rundschau* **36**: 37–39.

Hall JC, Tarala R, Harris J et al (1991) Incentive spirometry versus routine chest physiotherapy for prevention of pulmonary complications after abdominal surgery. *Lancet* **337**: 953–956.

Hall JC, Tapper J and Tarala R (1993) The cost-efficiency of incentive spirometry after abdominal surgery. *Australian and New Zealand Journal of Surgery* **63**: 356–359.

Hall JC, Tarala R, Tapper J and Hall JL (1996) Prevention of respiratory complications after abdominal surgery: a randomised clinical trial. *British Medical Journal* **312**: 148–152.

Harbourne NG (1995). A study investigating the effects of post operative physiotherapy on pain levels of patients receiving different types of pain control following lower abdominal-gynaecological surgery: a pilot study. University of Queensland, 4th year Physiotherapy Honours thesis.

Haslett S and Jennings M (1992) *Hysterectomy and Vaginal Repair*, 3rd edn, pp. 1–28. Beaconsfield: Beaconsfield Publishers.

Logan VB (1995) Incidence and prevalence of lymphoedema: a literature review. *Journal of Clinical Nursing* **4**: 213–219.

Luttrel N (1996) *The Effect of Ankle Plantar Flexion and Dorsiflexion on Venous Blood Flow Velocity in Postsurgical Patients*. Honours thesis, Department of Physiotherapy, University of Queensland.

Mitchell L (1988) *Simple Relaxation*, 2nd edn. London: John Murray.

Netzer P, Lazarevic V and Hammer B (1996) Value of abdominal ultrasonography in deep venous thrombosis. Retrospective study of 104 patients. *Schweizerische Medizinische Wochenschrift-Supplementum* **79**: 58S–63S.

Patel MI, Hardman DTA, Nicholl D et al (1996) The incidence of deep venous thrombosis after laparoscopic cholecystectomy. *Medical Journal of Australia* **164**: 652–656.

Richardson CA and Jull GA (1995) An historical perspective on the development of clinical techniques to evaluate and treat the active stabilizing system of the lumbar spine. *Australian Journal of Physiotherapy Monograph* **1**: 5–13.

Sommers S (1993) Stress and Illness and the Mind Body Connection. *A Discussion Paper*. Melbourne: Monash University.

Sondik EJ, Young JL, Horm JW and Gloeckler LA (1985) Annual cancer statistics review. Cited in Berek JS and Hacker NF (1994) *Practical Gynecologic Oncology*, 2nd edn, p. 181. Baltimore: Williams and Wilkins.

Webber BA and Pryor JA (1993) *Physiotherapy for Respiratory and Cardiac Problems*, pp. 237–244. Edinburgh: Churchill Livingstone.

Further reading

Ellis E and Alison J (eds) (1993) *Key Issues in Cardiorespiratory Physiotherapy*. Oxford: Butterworth Heinemann.

Farrer H (1991) *Gynaecological Care*, 2nd edn. Melbourne: Churchill Livingstone.

Mitchell L (1988) *Simple Relaxation*, 2nd edn. London: John Murray.

Webber BA and Pryor JA (1993) *Physiotherapy for Respiratory and Cardiac Problems*. Edinburgh: Churchill Livingstone.

35

Physiotherapy Management of Lymphoedema

HILDEGARD REUL-HIRCHE

Lymphoedema is difficult to classify, as it does not fall exclusively into the area of women's health or oncology. Although the majority of lymphoedema patients are women it can also affect children and men.

This chapter is designed to raise awareness and provide an understanding of the treatment of lymphoedema by:

- defining lymphoedema;
- outlining the anatomy and physiology / pathophysiology;
- examining assessment and treatment.

The literature indicates that optimum treatment outcomes result when therapy is provided by a physiotherapist skilled in management of lymphoedema. However, it is important for all physiotherapists to be able to identify and treat the condition as well as assess and educate patients who are at risk of developing it (Földi et al, 1985; Mason, 1993).

Definition, Prevalence and Incidence of Lymphoedema

There is general agreement that lymphoedema is a condition in which the lymphatic load exceeds the transport capacity of the lymphatic system. As a result of this inadequacy, oedema occurs. Olszewski (1991, p. 348) defines lymphoedema as 'a progressive disorder characterized by impairment of the lymph flow from the tissues to the blood circulation due to damage of lymphatics'. Piller (1994) notes that the International Society for Lymphology extends the definition to a high-protein oedema caused by less than normal transport capacity and tissue proteolytic capacity of the lymphatic system. This is supported further by Földi et al (1989) who concisely describe it as a quantitative problem between the lymphatic load and the lymphatic transport capacity.

The prevalence of lymphoedema varies. Secondary lymphoedema has a higher incidence than primary lymphoedema. Regionally, there is a higher incidence in arm than leg. The expressions 'primary' and 'secondary' refer to the cause of the oedema. Primary lymphoedema is considered to be a developmental disorder, whereas secondary lymphoedema is an acquired deficiency of the lymphatic system.

Many workers report that the combination of surgery and irradiation increases the incidence of lymphoedema (Axelrod and Osborne, 1989; Casley-Smith and Casley-Smith, 1986a). Földi and Földi (1991a) consider that every tenth woman will be affected with breast cancer and that one in 25 of those women who were treated with axillary dissection or radiation will develop lymphoedema at some stage of their lives. The National Health and Medical Research Council (NH&MRC) Australia states that the incidence of lymphoedema after the axilla has been treated with either surgery or radium is one in 20. This may increase to one in five or even one in three if both surgery and radium therapy are applied (NH&MRC, 1995). The incidence of lymphoedema after total hysterectomy is reported as being approximately one in four women (Földi and Földi, 1991a).

All the above data refer to secondary lymphoedema. Few predictions have been made for primary lymphoedema. Petlund (1990) reports that 45.2% of all cases of chronic lymphoedema are of primary origin.

As yet, there is no cure available for lymphoedema but the condition can be managed very successfully. So that the diagnosis and treatment of lymphoedema can be fully understood, it is important to review the relevant anatomy and physiology. As an introduction it is interesting to note the history of the discovery of the lymphatic system.

History of the Discovery of the Lymphatic System

The lymphatic system has been known since the time of Hippocrates (460–377 BC). However, over the next two millennia study of this system was ignored, presumably due to the influence of the church with its opposition to the study of anatomy.

Investigation of the lymphatic system re-commenced during the Renaissance in the 17th century. At that time, Gaspare Aselli and Jean Pecquet described parts of the lymphatic system and Thomas Bartholin and Olof Rudbeck developed an overview of the smaller previous discoveries, helping to consolidate information on the lymphatic system. Bartholin named all the newly investigated vessels 'vasa lymphatica' and the fluid 'lympha' from the Latin word *limpidus*, meaning clear.

The integrity of the lymphatic system was elaborated further by the contribution of Cruickshank (1789), Mascani (1787) and later Sappey (1810–1890) who injected quicksilver to display the lymphatics of human beings and animals. Sappey illustrated the findings by copperplate engravings, which were published in 1885. Henri Rouviere (1876–1952) developed the anatomical details even further and his *Anatomy of the Human Lymphatic System* is still in use today.

During the 1860s Carl Ludwig identified the forces which govern the fluid transfer from blood to tissue. Further, the work of Ernst Starling in the 1890s showed that both the hydrostatic and the colloid osmotic pressure in the blood and in tissue fluid are important for the fluid exchange. Starling's work provided a great step in understanding and the hypothesis developed is known today as the Law of the Capillaries.

In the latter half of the 20th century a number of scientists from various nations were integral in furthering the understanding of the lymphatic system and its function. Földi, Kubik, Clodius and Casley-Smith have contributed significantly to this research.

Anatomy of the Lymphatic System

The lymphatic system may be considered as a one-way drainage system from the tissue back to the blood circulation. It is divided into a superficial system, which drains the skin and subcutis, and a deep system, with its drainage starting at the muscle fascia. The treatment of lymphoedema concentrates on the stimulation of the superficial lymphatic system.

The superficial lymphatic system begins in the skin and takes the form of blind-ending, fingerlike protrusions, which are interconnected through a capillary mesh. They have the appearance of three-dimensional fingers of a glove and are referred to as *initial lymphatics* although they may also be called *lymph capillaries* (Bringezu and Schreiner, 1991a).

The vessel wall of the initial lymphatic consists of single-layered endothelial cells, mostly without any basal membrane. These endothelial cells partially overlap, forming an opening or junction. These junctions are often referred to as *swinging flaps*. Anchoring filaments are attached to the outside of the two overlapping cells. These support the endothelial cells in their action as inlet valves by allowing the inner cell to open only towards the inside. When the total tissue pressure is low, fluid filters in through the junctions by pressing the inner endothelial cell towards the inside. This action is depicted in Figure 35.1.

After the initial lymphatic has been filled with fluid from the interstitium, the increased pressure closes the junction by pressing the 'flap' against the outside cell. At this point the fluid is clear and is called lymph. The varying total tissue pressure, caused by external influences such as muscle contraction, movement, respiration or pulsation of adjacent blood vessels, pushes the lymph into the valveless, interconnected capillary mesh (Kubik, 1991). The whole body is covered by this near valveless lymphatic system and on this superficial level the lymph can be moved in any direction. This is an important factor for treatment and will be discussed later in the chapter.

Figure 35.1 Filling and emptying of initial lymphatic. 1. Start of filling. 2. Progression of filling. 3–5 Emptying phase. 6. Beginning of filling phase. 7. Initial lymphatic plexus. 8. Efferent precollector. (Reproduced from Bringezu and Schreiner (1991) with permission.)

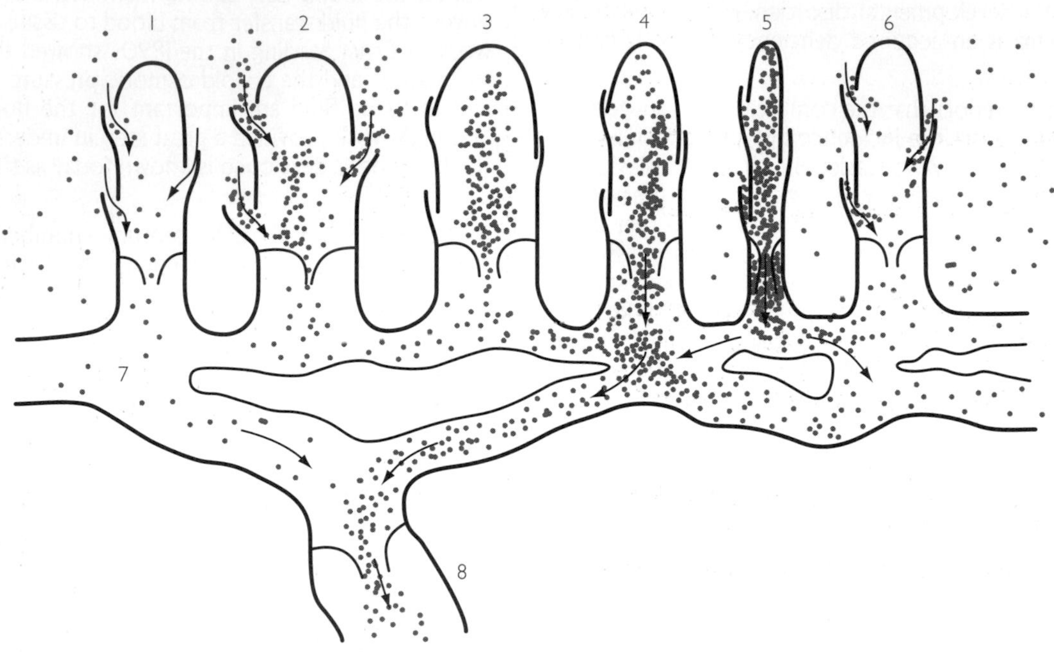

From the capillary mesh of the initial lymphatics, the lymph passes through the *precollectors* into the *collecting lymphatics.* These are the larger lymph vessels which have valves and direct the lymph towards the regional lymph nodes. The section between two valves is called a *lymphangion.* The structure of the larger lymph vessels resembles that of blood vessels with adventitia, media and intima layers but only on the thoracic duct, the largest lymphatic vessel in the body, can these layers be differentiated easily. The media contains smooth muscle with more muscle fibres present in the middle of the lymphangion than in the vessel wall close to the valves.

The valves passively prevent the backflow of the incoming lymph. During normal flow both proximal and distal valves are slightly open to ensure continuous flow. With increased lymph flow, the vessel wall of the lymphangion is stretched and this elicits a wall contraction, which pushes the lymph in the direction of the regional lymph nodes. During maximal wall contraction the lymphangion is emptied and the process starts again. This active process is called the *lymphangiomotoric* (Castenholz, 1991) and details are shown in Figure 35.2. The frequency of the emptying mechanism is dependent on the lymphatic load. (Lymphatic load is discussed in the section on physiology, p. 479).

The next step in the journey of the lymph from the tissue to the venous blood circulation involves the lymphangions guiding the lymph to the *lymph nodes.* The human body can contain up to 600–700 lymph nodes, but there is considerable individual variation (Kubik, 1991).

The functions of the lymph nodes are best described as:

- filtration – a protective function to prevent any damaging material from reaching the blood circulation;
- production of lymphocytes to support the immune system;
- regulation of the amount of lymph fluid;
- regulation of the amount of protein in the lymph fluid.

Such regulation can involve both the storage and release of lymph fluid and / or protein.

Although lymph vessels can regenerate, lymph nodes cannot. Thus any patient who has lymph nodes removed or scarred is at risk of developing lymphoedema for the duration of their life. The more superficial lymph nodes, in particular the axillary and inguinal lymph nodes, are most important in the treatment of lymphoedema.

From the lymph nodes the lymph travels in the *lymph trunks,* which have the same structure as lymphangions but are larger. Eventually these trunks lead back to the venous blood circulation, with most of them connecting into the largest lymph trunk – the *thoracic duct.*

The thoracic duct has its origin between the level of L2 and T10, where it forms a sac-like extension called the *cisterna chyle.* It ascends with the aorta through the diaphragm and enters into the junction of the left internal jugular and subclavian veins. Through the addition of lipids from the intestine, the lymph in the thoracic duct changes from clear fluid into a milk-like substance, called *chyle.*

The thoracic duct delivers the lymph from three-quarters of the body to the venous blood circulation, from:

Figure 35.2 The different action phases of a lymphangion. 1. Continuous flow of 'normal' lymphatic load (both valves open). 2. Increased lymph flow with extension of vessel wall. 3. Start of active emptying phase through wall contraction. 4. Maximal wall contraction with emptying towards proximal, distal valve closed. (Reproduced from Bringezu and Schreiner (1991) with permission.)

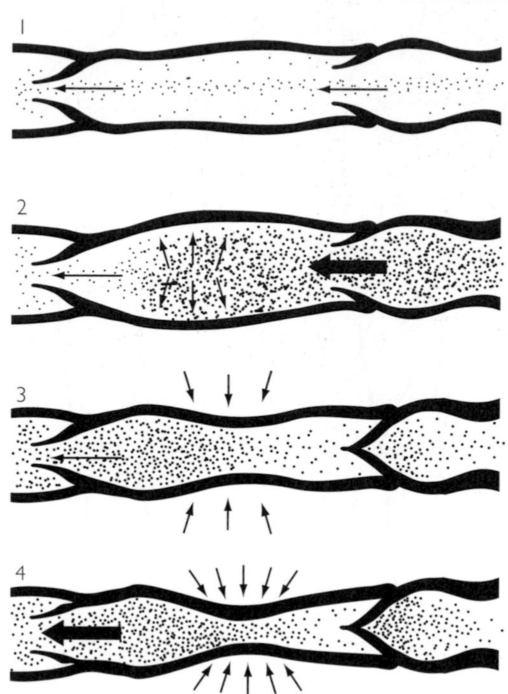

Figure 35.3 Areas drained by right lymphatic duct (shaded) and thoracic duct.

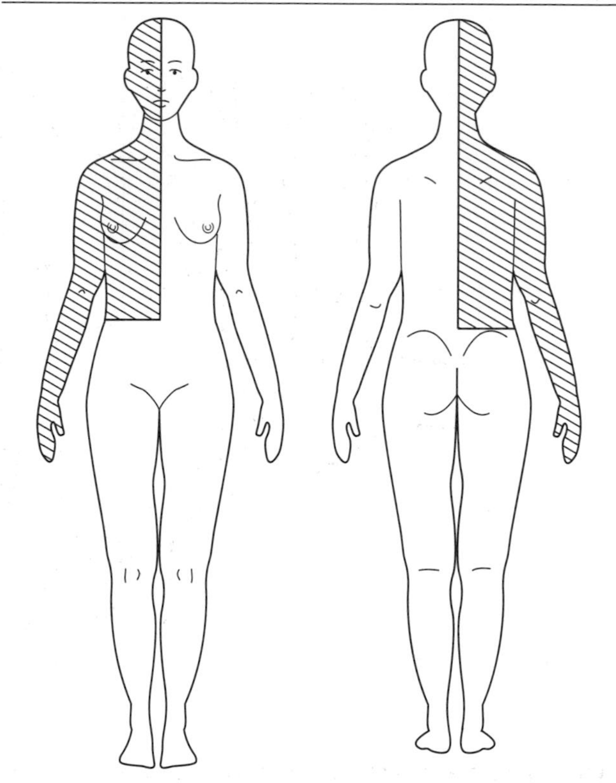

- both legs;
- the lower half of the body;
- the left side of the head and neck;
- the left upper half of the body;
- the left arm.

The smaller right lymphatic duct returns the lymph back to the venous blood circulation at the junction of the right internal jugular and right subclavian veins. It carries the lymph from:

- the right side of the head and neck;
- the right upper half of the body;
- the right arm (Adair and Guyton, 1985) (Fig. 35.3).

A critical point in the journey of the lymph occurs at the regional lymph nodes, where the lymph leaves the superficial system and proceeds deeper into the body. For the trunk, the regional lymph nodes are the *axillary* and *inguinal* lymph nodes. As the lymph nodes are situated on the trunk extremity border, they drain not only the trunk but also the adjacent limb.

Lymphatic watersheds divide the trunk in four quadrants, also called *lymphatic territories*. The watersheds are the dividing line for the direction of the valves in the collecting lymphatics. The valves direct the lymph flow towards the regional lymph nodes. The significance of the watersheds is most apparent when drainage to the lymph nodes is interrupted and swelling occurs in both the limb and the adjacent quadrant. As the initial lymphatics are interconnected they can overcome the watersheds and allow drainage from one quadrant to the next. This is extremely important in the treatment of lymphoedema.

The body possesses two main watersheds: the *vertical watershed*, which divides the trunk into halves, and the *transverse* or *horizontal watershed*, which starts from the level of the umbilicus and ascends along the ribs to the level of L2, thus dividing the trunk further into four basic quadrants: two upper or thoracic and two lower or abdominal. (Fig. 35.4).

Anastomoses are another structure of the lymphatic system which help to overcome an interruption in the lymphatic flow. Some of the vertical and diagonal lymph collectors of a quadrant meet with collectors from the opposite quadrant at the watershed. At this point the direction of the lymphatic drainage changes, e.g. for the upper trunk the drainage directions from the vertical watershed go towards left and right axillary lymph nodes. In the case of interruption, e.g. swelling in one of the quadrants, the cutaneous lymphatics allow drainage from one quadrant to another, thus overcoming the watershed (Manestar, 1991).

The axilloaxillary anastomosis or interaxillary connection connects left and right axilla not only anteriorly, but also on the posterior chest wall by crossing the vertical watershed. The axilloinguinal anastomosis connects axillary and inguinal lymph nodes on the same side of the body by crossing the transverse watershed. The suprapubic

Figure 35.4 Basic illustration of watersheds and anastomoses.

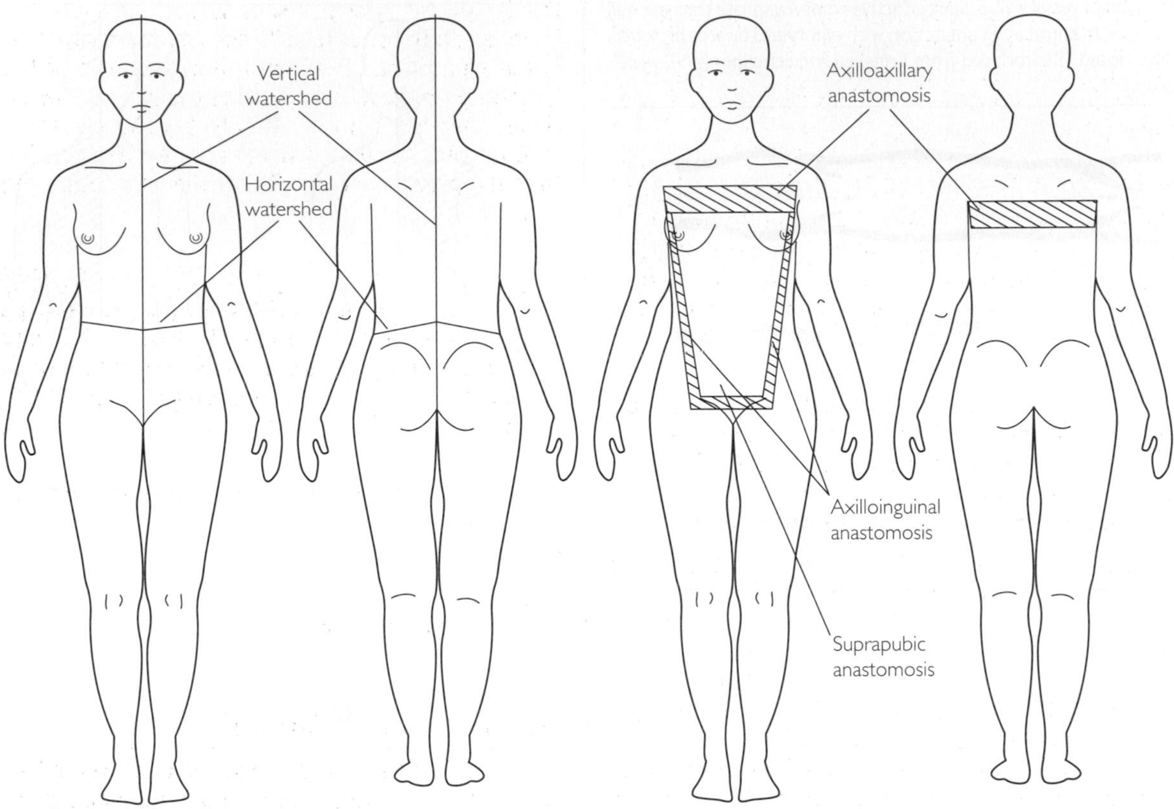

anastomosis connects the left and right lower quadrant, as shown in Figure 35.4. This drainage possibility is of extreme importance in the treatment of lymphodema.

Summary

The lymphatic system consists of **initial lymphatics,** which are interconnected and lead the lymph into the **precollectors.** From there it continues into **collectors,** which contain **valves,** through **lymph nodes** into the **lymph trunks,** the largest being the **thoratic duct,** which ends in the venous blood circulation. The watersheds are the dividing line for the direction of the valves towards the regional lymph nodes with the **anastomoses** forming the connections between them.

Physiology and Pathophysiology

The lymphatic system not only has a significant role in the immune system, but also an equally important transport function. The most important part of this function is the transportation of large particles, especially protein. Similarly, other substances which can no longer be absorbed by the blood capillaries need the lymphatic system as a transport vehicle to leave the interstitial tissue and return to the venous blood circulation. These include lymphocytes, granulocytes, monocytes and erythrocytes, as well as bacteria, cancerous cells and cell debris (after trauma) (Bringezu and Schreiner, 1991b).

To understand the physiology of the lymphatic system, a quick revision of terms should be helpful.

Diffusion

When two salt solutions of differing concentrations are overlayed in one container, salt will migrate to the less concentrated solution, while water will seek the more concentrated solution. After a while the two solutions will reach an equilibrium state. The process is called diffusion.

Osmosis

If two different salt solutions are divided by a semipermeable membrane which is impermeable to larger salt molecules, water will travel from the less concentrated to the more concentrated solution. This is called osmosis.

Osmotic pressure

Osmotic pressure arises in the chamber with the more concentrated solution and it represents the energy by which the salt attracts the water.

Filtration

Filtration is the reversal of osmotic pressure. This can be achieved by applying pressure from outside to the more concentrated solution, thereby overcoming the osmotic pressure and reversing the process.

Colloid osmotic pressure and ultrafiltration

If the above example is applied to a protein solution the osmotic pressure will be termed colloid osmotic pressure and the process of filtration will be called ultrafiltration (Földi and Földi, 1991c)

In the human blood circulation the capillary wall acts like a fully permeable membrane for all small molecules dissolved in the blood. There is no hindrance to diffusion from the capillary into the interstitial tissue and back, but the capillary wall is mostly impermeable to protein molecules.

At the arterial end of the blood capillary, the blood capillary pressure (blood pressure) is higher than the colloid osmotic pressure of the blood plasma. On the venous side, the blood capillary pressure is lower than the colloid osmotic pressure of the blood plasma, resulting in ultrafiltration on the arterial side and reabsorption (ultrafiltration in the opposite direction) on the venous side. Ultrafiltration is a process directed to the outside, while reabsorption is the opposite, directed to the inside. However, some proteins leave the blood capillaries for the interstitial tissue, thereby causing the colloid osmotic pressure to vary. The pressures within the interstitium fluctuate and hence influence ultrafiltration.

In summary, four forces act on each arterial and venous capillary:

1. the colloid osmotic pressure of the blood plasma;
2. the pressure of the blood capillary (blood pressure);
3. the colloid osmotic pressure in the interstitium;
4. the interstitial pressure.

On the arterial as well as on the venous side, the blood capillary pressure tries to free the fluid from the protein molecules and press it into the interstitium, but this is reduced (or raised) by the interstitial pressure. The colloid osmotic pressure of the blood plasma, which tries to hold the fluid, is reduced by the colloid osmotic pressure in the interstitium (Földi and Földi, 1991b).

Approximately 20 litres of fluid leave the blood vessels over 24 hours and 80–90% is reabsorbed. The remaining fluid, which amounts to 2–4 litres over 24 hours, contains the larger protein molecules. As they cannot pass through the capillary wall this fluid returns, as lymph, to the venous blood circulation via the lymphatic system (Bringezu and Schreiner, 1991b).

If an *imbalance* occurs in the four forces mentioned, oedema will occur. For example, if the blood capillary pressure is raised the ultrafiltration is increased. On the other hand, if the colloid osmotic pressure of the blood plasma is reduced the reabsorption is diminished. In such situations the lymphatic system responds with an increase in the lymphangiomotoric. To fulfil the *transport capacity,* which is the highest possible lymph flow per unit of time, the lymphangiomotoric can increase the lymph flow up to 10 times. Therefore a normal healthy lymphatic system is able to control an increased water and protein load for some time and prevent oedema. This is the *lymphatic safety valve factor.*

As long as the transport capacity is higher than the lymphatic load no oedema will occur. If the lymphatic load exceeds the lymphatic transport capacity, oedema will be present (Földi et al (1989).

Földi et al (1989) distinguish three forms of lymph vascular insufficiency:

1. dynamic;
2. mechanical;
3. safety valve (see Table 35.1).

Dynamic insufficiency

The term 'dynamic insufficiency' is used where lymphatic vessels, although normal in anatomy and function, are overwhelmed by the lymphatic load, as in a high-flow oedema. Depending on the cause, it can either be high or low in protein. High-flow, low-protein oedema can be caused by raised blood capillary pressure, low colloid osmotic pressure of the blood plasma or low interstitial pressure, while injuries to blood vessels and vitamin deficiencies can lead to high-flow, high-protein oedema.

Mechanical insufficiency

The reduction of the lymphatic transport capacity due to impairment of the lymphatic system constitutes a mechanical insufficiency and is the cause of a low-flow, high-protein oedema.

Safety valve insufficiency

This term is used when a reduced transport capacity is further compromised by an increased lymphatic load. For example, after axillary clearance (reduced transport capacity) an infection occurs (increased lymphatic load), causing tissue necrosis leading to chronic inflammation and hence to an increased lymphatic load. This results in a low-flow, high-protein oedema.

Of the three lymph vascular insufficiencies outlined above, only the mechanical and safety valve are low-flow, high-protein oedemas, or lymphoedemas, and as such can be treated with complex physical therapy.

Table 35.1 Lymph vascular insufficiencies

Dynamic insufficiency	TC normal, LL ↑	High/low-protein oedema
Mechanical insufficiency	TC ↓, LL normal	High-protein oedema
Safety valve insufficiency	TC ↓, LL ↑	High-protein oedema

Key: TC= transport capacity; LL= lymphatic load.

Dynamic insufficiency is beyond physical treatment, as the lymphatic system is not impaired.

Summary

Four forces influence ultrafiltration (process directed to the outside) and reabsorption (process directed to the inside) between arterial and venous capillary. These are the colloid osmotic pressure of the blood plasma, the pressure of the blood capillary, the colloid osmotic pressure in the interstitium and the interstitial pressure. If these forces are unbalanced oedema can occur. Prior to the development of oedema the body would first react with an increase in lymphangiomotoric to fulfil the transport capacity. The lymphangiomotoric can increase up to 10-fold. This is the maximum lymph flow per unit of time and enables the prevention of oedema in the short term.

Specific Causes of Lymphoedema

All lymphoedemas can be divided into primary and secondary lymphoedema by considering the inherent and acquired pathology of the condition.

Primary lymphoedema – the lymphoedema of unknown cause

Primary lymphoedema is a developmental disorder in which the main pathological mechanisms might be:

- *aplasia* – the initial or collecting lymphatics have not been developed and are missing;
- *hypoplasia* – the number of lymph collectors is reduced and/or the diameter of the lymph vessel is smaller than normal;
- *hyperplasia* – the lymph vessels can be compared to varicose veins. They are enlarged and therefore the valves are unable to perform their function and a normal lymph flow is not possible.

Without investigation the cause of the primary lymphoedema will not be clear. Primary lymphoedema is more common in women than men. It also develops more often in legs than arms.

Primary lymphoedema is also grouped according to the time of onset:

- *connatal* – lymphoedema is present at birth and belongs to the familial (i.e. genetically caused) lymphoedema, often called Milroy's or Nonne-Milroy's disease;
- *lymphoedema praecox* – presents before the age of 17. This is the most common form of primary lymphoedema;
- *lymphoedema tarda* – appears after the age of 35.

> With all primary lymphoedema it is of extreme importance that the possibility of a malignancy is excluded

Secondary lymphoedema – lymphoedema of known cause

Secondary lymphoedema is easily diagnosed by taking a detailed case history, as it is caused by damage to a normally functioning lymphatic system. Such damage can be caused by the following.

SURGERY AND/OR RADIUM TREATMENT

The most common cause of secondary lymphoedema is the removal of lymph nodes as part of the surgical treatment for cancer. If the lymph nodes have not been removed but have received radiation they may stop functioning due to chronic inflammation, fibrosis and scarring. Research shows that the combination of surgery and radiotherapy increases the risk of lymphoedema threefold compared with surgery alone (Casley-Smith and Casley-Smith, 1994a).

VARICOSE VEIN STRIPPING

As lymphatic vessels lie close to the venous system, during an operation to cut or strip varicose veins the lymphatic vessels may be destroyed or damaged.

LIPOSUCTION

During the process of liposuction not only are the fat cells removed, but the fine small lymphatic lymph vessels can be removed as well.

TRAUMA

Any extensive superficial trauma, where large skin areas are affected, could destroy the superficial lymphatics, e.g. large abrasions, injuries or burns.

TUMOUR

A tumour, benign or malignant, can block the lymphatic flow by obstructing or infiltrating a lymph vessel and/or lymph nodes.

INFECTION

An infection of the lymph vessels and lymph nodes caused by virus, fungus, bacteria or parasites can cause impairment of the lymphatic system and subsequent lymphoedema. During an acute inflammation the affected lymph vessel is unable to fulfil its transport function. The vessel wall becomes oedematous, stops pulsating and the lymph coagulates inside the inflamed vessel. The infected vessel does not heal, but becomes fibrosclerotic and stops functioning. If a large number of lymph vessels are affected in this way then a secondary lymphoedema could result (Földi and Földi, 1991a).

FILARITIC LYMPHOEDEMA

Filariasis is caused by worms which are transmitted by mosquitoes. It occurs in India, Malaysia, Indonesia and Papua New Guinea, mainly during the rainy season. The worms enter the lymphatic system and proceed to the larger lymphatic vessel, growing to a length of up to 20 cm and a diameter of 1–2 mm. They are a near-perfect parasite consisting of proteins similar to those of the human body. Thus a minimal immune reaction occurs and the worms may not cause problems until they die, 5–10 years after the original infiltration. At that point severe local inflammation occurs with the release of many foreign proteins from the dead worms causing fibrosis, ultimately leading to lymphoedema (Casley-Smith and Casley-Smith, 1994a).

CHRONIC VENOUS INSUFFICIENCY

Lymphoedema can also result from chronic venous insufficiency (Clodius, 1977).

Lipoedema

Allied with the causes of secondary lymphoedema is the specific condition of lipoedema. In lipoedema a pathological amount of fat cells occur, particularly from the hip to ankle. The patient is often obese, but weight reduction will not reduce the fat cells from the bottom half of the body.

Lipoedema is not a lymphoedema, but due to the underlying causes the affected person often acquires the condition. In the normal individual the lymph vessels occur in an almost straight line, whereas in the patient suffering from lipoedema the lymphatic vessels have a corkscrew pattern. The fat cells have pushed the lymph vessels aside so the lymphatic transport capacity is reduced.

Although there is no lymphoedema involved in the beginning stages of lipoedema, the patient often develops the combination of lipolymphoedema later in life. Once lymphoedema has developed the previously unaffected dorsum of the foot may be involved and swelling will occur.

Women are predominantly affected by lipoedema and its symptoms are:

- symmetrical distribution, e.g. both legs enlarged from iliac crest to ankle;
- foot is not involved;
- large fat deposits medial to knee;
- palpation can be very painful;
- bruise easily;
- mattress-like tissue;
- occasionally the arm is involved, but only from elbow to wrist.

Summary of the causes of secondary lymphoedema

- Surgery and/or radium treatment
- Varicose vein stripping
- Liposuction
- Infection
- Trauma
- Filariasis
- Chronic venous insufficiency

Factors Inhibiting the Development of Lymphoedema

Four compensatory mechanisms may occur to overcome blockage and/or damage to the lymphatic system and thus inhibit the development of lymphoedema and these are laid out in Table 35.2.

Table 35.2 Factors inhibiting the development of lymphoedema

Lympholymphatic anastomosis	New anastomoses develop between the neighbouring lymphatic vessels around the blocked area
Collateral lymphatic circulation	The surviving lymphatics dilate and form a collateral circulation, e.g. cephalic or deltoid lymph vessel in the case of axillary dissection, which bypasses the axilla and drains into the supraclavicular lymph nodes
Lymphovenous anastomosis	The lymphatic vessel drains into a nearby vein
The phagocytic system	Monocytes migrate from the blood vessels into the interstitium and change into macrophages (scavenger cells) and reduce the amount of protein

Furthermore, if a lymphatic vessel is cut the ends can be united by sprouting from the stump of the vessel. This results in a narrow, thin-walled growth which tries to connect with the vessel on the other side of the wound. These new growths are at first solid endothelial protrusions, which then develop a lumen, but both the sprouting and the remodelling are greatly limited by the formation of scars. A scar thicker than 1 mm will prevent the union of the two sprouting lymphatic vessels (Clodius, 1977).

With all these compensatory factors, the question arises as to why a patient is under lifelong risk of developing lymphoedema. Table 35.3 lists the factors that can singularly or in combination result in the development of lymphoedema at any time in an at-risk patient.

The System of Grading

In 1985 during the Xth International Congress of Lymphology the International Society for Lymphology (Casley-Smith, 1994) decided to develop a common grading for lymphoedema.

Grade 1

Swelling in the limb will consist of a protein-rich fluid stasis without any tissue changes. The swollen limb will be soft and there is pitting oedema. The swelling will reduce with elevation and will often disappear overnight. This describes a **grade 1** lymphoedema, which Földi and Földi (1991a) call the *reversible stage*. As long as the lymph fluid is removed, the tissue returns to its normal state.

Table 35.3 Factors which can contribute to development of lymphoedema in an at-risk patient

Reduced transport capacity	When the transport capacity has been reduced, the remaining lymphatic vessels have to work harder
Age	The transport capacity is reduced with ageing
Increased pressure in the vessel	The lymphatic vessel wall is normally permeable to lymph fluid. With reduced transport capacity, pressure is increased and more lymph fluid trickles into the vessel wall and forms a protein-rich ring around the lymphatic vessel. This will eventually become fibrotic and will stop the lymphangiomotoric
Valve insufficiency	If the pressure is greatly increased the vessel will be so enlarged that as a result the valves become insufficient

Grade 2

If no intervention is undertaken, e.g. in the form of complex physical therapy, the swelling will persist. The lymphoedema has then progressed to **grade 2** or, as Földi and Földi call it, the *spontaneous irreversible stage*. The tissue is no longer pitting and elevation does not reduce the swelling. The high concentration of protein has encouraged fibrosis through fibroblasts and the tissue becomes hard. The macrophages act and with the lysis of proteins, they store fat and change into fat cells.

Casley-Smith and Casley-Smith (1986b) state 'The effects of oedema can themselves lead to more oedema'. This means that the excess fibrosis will hinder the flow of fluid and protein into the initial vessel and hamper the entrance of the macrophages. The filling of the initial lymphatics and the lymph transport into the collecting lymphatics will also be reduced. The anchoring filaments can loosen and the initial lymphatics collapse, resulting in increased lymphoedema. With reduced oxygen pressure all of the cell functions are reduced, including the immune response, and this greatly increases the possibility of an infection. Also the stagnant protein causes a chronic inflammation, which causes cell death. With this cell death a vicious circle starts, as it increases the chronic inflammation and the lymphoedema increases.

EXTENSION / COMPLICATION OF GRADE 2

If this cycle is not disrupted and the patient develops frequent infections, the lymphoedema could slowly progress and develop into *elephantiasis*. If an infection occurs it causes an acute hyperaemia, resulting in increased ultrafiltration and lymphatic fluid load. The blood vessels also become more permeable to protein. The end result of all these effects is a safety valve insufficiency. At this stage the volume is further increased, the arm / leg resembles that of an elephant with skin changes occurring. The skin gets hard and scaly and wart-like protrusions might appear.

Grading of lymphoedema according to the International Society for Lymphology

Grade 1

- Pitting oedema (reversible stage)
- Reduces with elevation overnight
- No fibrotic changes

Grade 2

- Non-pitting (spontaneous irreversible stage)
- No reduction with elevation, fibrotic changes

Grade 2 extension complication

- Elephantiasis
- Increased volume, skin changes, frequent bouts of infection

Each grade has subgroups of mild, moderate and severe.

General Management of Lymphoedema

Assessment and treatment

Greater understanding of lymphoedema and an increased awareness of the treatment modalities over the last few years have given the impression that this is a new condition. However, in 1892 Alexander Ritter von Winiwarter (Germany) wrote the book *Die Elephantiasis* describing methods of treating lymphoedema with physical therapy. He used elevation, compression and light massage in combination as a therapeutic tool, but unfortunately his treatment regime was not used widely and was forgotten.

Dr Emil Vodder and his wife Estrid developed 'manual lymphatic drainage' in France between 1932 and 1936. This involved stimulating swollen cervical lymph nodes with gentle circular motion to clear chronic colds and skin conditions. Professor Michael Földi developed the Vodder technique further and with his wife Dr Ethel Földi, started the 'Fachklinik für Lymphologie' in Hinterzarten, Germany. Today the treatment is known worldwide.

In Australia the Adelaide Lymphoedema Clinic was established in 1987 by physiotherapist Michael Mason. Drs Judith and John Casley-Smith commenced teaching the treatment of lymphoedema in 1990 in Adelaide, in association with the Lymphoedema Association of Australia and the University of Adelaide.

Generally present-day treatment owes its origin to the techniques developed by Vodder and Földi. Treatment is determined on a case-by-case basis by the physiotherapist, after a thorough assessment to establish both cause and type of lymphoedema and define appropriate treatment.

ASSESSMENT

The diagnosis and treatment can involve a multidisciplinary approach. It is important that both the patient and the physiotherapist have contact with the referring medical practitioner throughout the treatment. There is agreement that a diagnosis can be made by history plus clinical examination and that investigations with invasive tests are not routinely necessary (Casley-Smith and Casley-Smith, 1994b; Földi and Földi, 1991c). In some European countries, especially Germany, the patient will have been examined by a specialist before being referred to the physiotherapist for treatment.

However, physiotherapists are often the first contact practitioners and therefore have to be alert to the signs which require further investigation and a thorough assessment. This is especially so when dealing with primary lymphoedema. It is necessary to differentiate between lymphoedema and other conditions with associated swelling, such as cardiac or renal failure. Subjective statements such as 'the swelling started in one leg/arm' and 'one leg/arm is still more prominent' point to lymphoedema. If the patient reports that both limbs started to swell at the same time and that there has been no difference between the degree of swelling then the possibility of cardiac or renal failure must be further investigated and referral back to the medical practitioner is imperative.

The use of a specifically designed lymphoedema assessment form is very helpful when the physiotherapist is the first contact practitioner. One such form, developed by a group of Brisbane physiotherapists with a special interest in the treatment of lymphoedema, offers a guide for a thorough assessment (Table 35.4). The initial assessment of a lymphoedema patient involves a full appraisal of their history. Following assessment, an exploration of treatment possibilities for each patient is undertaken. The treatment is lengthy and places time demands on both the patient and the physiotherapist with daily treatment, 5–6 times a week, of one hour or more. Therefore cost can be a major factor. The patient must be informed about the intensity of the treatment and be able to wear a compression garment at the end of the intensive treatment phase. Otherwise within a month the lymphoedematous limb will return to its previous swollen state (Swedborg, 1980, 1984).

Measurement

With all measurements to identify and monitor lymphoedema, it is important to remember that there may be normal differences between size of limbs, due to dominance and muscle bulk. A pivotal aspect of the assessment and treatment of lymphoedema is the measurement procedure. As detailed earlier, pre-operative measurements provide a good base to judge any increase in arm/leg circumference. Sequential, periodic measuring and monitoring gives an insight into the severity of the lymphoedema and the progress of the treatment. There are a number of methods that may be used to assess the severity of lymphoedema. These include circumferential measurements, volume by formula calculation, plethysmography (water displacement method) and more recently bioimpedance analysis.

CIRCUMFERENTIAL MEASUREMENTS

These measures are the easiest way to measure and monitor a limb. They can be performed with or without a measuring board, which offers exact reference points for repeated measurements. With the limb extended on the measuring board points are marked on the limb with the help of a set square (Fig. 35.5). These begin at the mid hand/foot, followed by the narrowest part of wrist/ankle and then every 10 cm beginning at the next 10 cm mark. For example, if the

Table 35.4 Example of lymphoedema assessment form (*additional comments are in italics to assist in the completion of the assessment*)

LYMPHOEDEMA ASSESSMENT Date

Name:

Address: D.O.B

Phone:

Diagnosis:

Dominance:

Carer: Yes / No (*Is carer willing and able to assist with self-management?*)

Area affected:

GP:

Specialist:

MEDICAL HISTORY

Date / place of operation: (*Applicable only for secondary lymphoedema*)

Surgeon:

Procedure:

Number of L / N removed:

Number of L / N metastatic:

Post-op problems (infect / seromas, etc): (*Any post-op problems may increase the risk of lymphoedema*)

Chemotherapy date:

Radiotherapy date: (*Knowledge of extent of radium treatment is important as treated area can be scarred, so drainage will be impaired*)

Length of treatment:

X-ray:

Other investigations: (*Lymphoscintigram, CT scan*)

Other surgery:

Other medical problems: (*Incl. arterial / venous / renal*)

Med:

SUBJECTIVE ASSESSMENT

History of oedema

Date of onset:

Cause: (*e.g. trauma, infections, overuse*)

Site:

Infections:

Behaviour of oedema: (*Fluctuating, stable*)

Reducing factors: (*Elevation, rest, compression*)

Previous treatment:

Sequential / non-sequential pump:

Garments:

Overseas travel: (*Filariasis*)

Table 35.4 Continued

Pain behaviour / description

Area = record on body chart

Pain scale (0–10) record on body chart

Description: *(More often described as heaviness and tightness, rather than pain, but pain is possible and the cause needs to be established)*

P ↑:

P ↓:

Night pain:

AM – PM: *(Pain behaviour during day)*

Sensory changes:

Pins / needles / numbness:

Activities of daily living – problems

Work / hobbies

LEG

Shoes

Washing

ARM

Bra

Shower

Cleaning / housework

OBJECTIVE ASSESSMENT

Height :

Weight: *(Obesity = increased risk of lymphoedema)*

Type of lymphoedema:

Grade of lymphoedema:

Skin condition:

Nail condition:

Scars: *(Record on body chart)*

Burns:

Telangiectasis: *(Permanent dilation of pre-existing blood vessels)*

Collateral veins:

Photos: *(Pre- and post-treatment, anterior, posterior and lateral views)*

Arterial pulse:

Neural tension:

Cording: *(For details see Chapter 33 on breast cancer)*

Skinfold: *(Different skinfold thickness on either side of trunk)*

Stemmer sign: *(Skinfold difference of fingers / toes of affected and unaffected limb, record as positive or negative)*

Table 35.4 Continued

Measurements:

Circumference: *(Refer to text)*
Plethysmography: *(Refer to text)*

ROM:

shoulder / hip

elbow / knee

wrist / ankle

Strength / muscle wasting:

Posture:

Functional assessment, if necessary:

SUMMARY

1. Physiotherapy diagnosis / code
2. Patient's functional goals and expectations / hobbies
3. Therapist's prognosis / anticipated outcome
4. Patient / therapist contract
5. Treatment plan

OUTCOMES – POST-TREATMENT

Patient satisfaction / cosmetic consideration:

Patient's goals achieved:

Measurements / reduction in %:

Function / goals achieved:

Pain reduction:

ROM / strength:

SUMMARY – POST-TREATMENT

Problems solved:

Problems unsolved:

Future management=Home programme:

Review date:

Developed by Brisbane physiotherapists who have a special interest in the treatment of lymphoedema (adapted by author)

narrowest part of the ankle is 16 cm, the next stroke mark is at 20 cm, then 30, 40, etc. If no measuring board is available the measurements can start on a bony prominence and the limb will be marked every 10 cm.

With both procedures, a tape measure is then used either above or below the pen stroke to measure the circumference of the limb. There is no one correct way of measuring the limb, but the chosen method must be recorded and be reproducible.

The circumferential measurements are recorded on a separate chart. It is necessary to measure both limbs and therefore it is helpful to record the different limb measurements in different colours, e.g. unaffected limb red, affected limb black, for easier comparison later. The circumferential measurements are then summed to provide an overall limb size.

Another form of measurement includes the application of simple geometric principles. These measurements assume that the limb is a series of 'cones' or 'cylinder' segments (Bunce et al, 1994; Casley-Smith, 1994). Bunce et al (1994) use circumferential measurements taken in 10 cm segments from the ulnar styloid process to a distance of 40 cm from the wrist. The volume of the limb is then calculated using the formula:

Figure 35.5 The use of a measuring board to mark the limb for circumferential measurements.

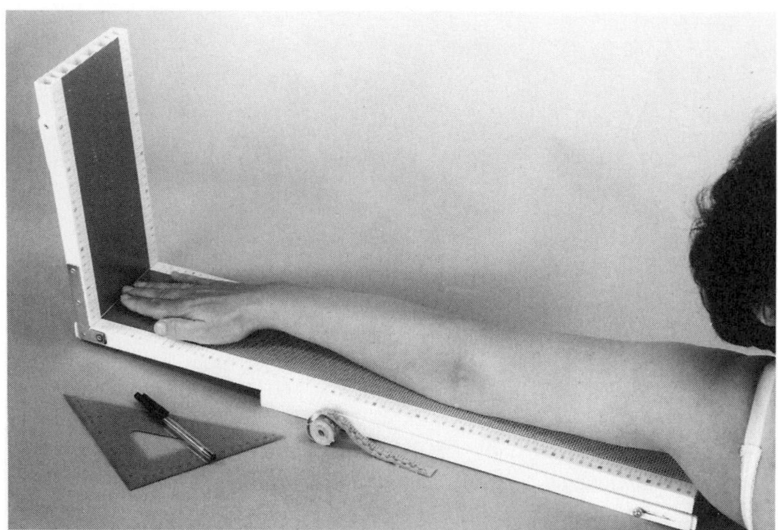

$$\text{Volume} = \Pi(\text{circumference}/2\Pi)^2\, h$$

where the circumference = the mean of the two adjacent circumferences and h = height (distance between the two circumferential measurements, in this case 10 cm).

The total limb volume is calculated as the sum of the volumes of the individual 'cylindrical' segments (Bunce et al, 1994).

The differences between limbs can be calculated by subtracting the affected limb from the unaffected limb and comparing the reduction (change over time). This is applicable for unilateral lymphoedema, but in primary lymphoedema the 'unaffected' limb may also be swollen. Therefore, it is more appropriate to calculate the reduction of the affected limb against itself rather than compare it to the unaffected side. This also applies to bilateral secondary lymphoedema.

Calculation for difference of limbs in percentage (Brennan, 1991)

$$\frac{\text{Lymphoedematous limb (cm or ml)} - \text{Normal limb (cm or ml)} \times 100}{\text{Normal limb (cm or ml)}}$$

Calculation for a unilateral limb expressed in percentage reduction

$$\frac{(\text{Final volume} - \text{initial volume}) \times 100}{\text{Initial volume}}$$

Initial volume stands for the volume at the start of the treatment and final volume for the volume at the end of the intense treatment phase. The same calculations can be applied by using the total circumferential measurements (Casley-Smith and Casley-Smith, 1994d). The reader is referred to Casley-Smith (1994) for further information.

PLETHYSMOGRAPHY OR VOLUMETRY

Phlethysmography is often used in addition to circumferential measurement. The limb is immersed in a plastic tank of suitable size, which is filled with water. The water displaced during the immersion of the limb is measured and the results compared to the unaffected limb. It ought to be noted that the volume of the dominant limb is usually up to 50–69 ml larger than the non-dominant limb (Petlund, 1991).

TONOMETRY

A tonometer (Fig. 35.6) measures the compressibility and elasticity of the limb. A swollen and/or fibrotic limb is relatively incompressible compared to a slightly swollen or a treated limb, which has had the fluid and/or fibrosis reduced. Therefore measurements are again taken on both limbs at the same position to establish baseline values for later comparison (Piller, 1994).

BIO-IMPEDANCE MEASUREMENTS

Bioelectrial impedance analysis (BIA) is a fast, easy, non-invasive method used to measure body composition. It is an instrument which measures the impedance or resistance of the body tissues to the flow of alternating currents and allows predictions of the intracellular and extracellular fluid (Ward et al, 1992). These authors suggest that multifrequency BIA with spectroscopy may be more appropriate for use in the identification and monitoring of lymphoedema.

Signs of possible malignancies

During assessment and treatment it is not uncommon for malignancies to be identified. The following symptoms

Figure 35.6 The use of a tonometer. (Reproduced from Mason (1995) with permission.)

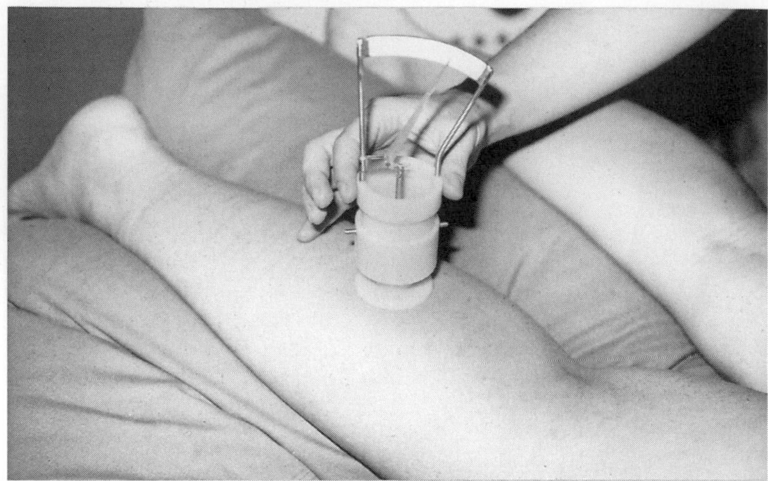

could be caused by malignancy and need further investigation by the medical practitioner.

Signs of possible malignancies

- Sudden start of lymphoedema
- Quick and constant progression
- Reduction of neck–acromion distance
- Protrusion and/or lumps in the supraclavicular fossa
- Lumps in other areas
- Skin changes

POSSIBLE SKIN CHANGES ASSOCIATED WITH MALIGNANCY

- *Lymphangiosis carcinomatosa.* This is a reddish discoloration on the skin and can be distinguished from an infection by carefully questioning the patient regarding the development of the condition. In contrast to an infection, which develops fast and the patient is unwell, lymphangiosis carcinomatosa develops slowly without influence on well-being.
- *Angiosarcoma* (Stewart-Treves syndrome). It is clinically like the Kaposi sarcoma. The patient has blue patches, which are easily distinguished from haematoma by questioning.
- *Collateral vein.* This might point to a thrombosis, a malignancy or a radiogenic fibrosis which can compromise the vein.
- *Lymphocysts.* These are dilated initial lymphatics which are visible as small blisters.
- *Lymphfistulae.* The fistula exists between lymph vessels and skin.
- *Open wounds.* These could be radiogenic ulcers or tumour.
- *Unbearable pain.*
- *Paralysis* in lymphoedematous limb (Gültig et al, 1991).

Treatment modalities for lymphoedema aim to reduce oedema caused by the malfunction of the lymphatic system. The majority of patients receive complex physical therapy as the primary form of treatment. Intermittent compression devices and laser provide additional avenues of treatment.

Complex physical therapy

Complex physical therapy is still a relatively new treatment in many countries outside continental Europe. It is important to apply the treatment correctly and completely for optimal success.

The four aspects of this treatment, all equally important, are integrated. As an example, the manual lymphatic drainage will not achieve a great reduction without the bandaging and the bandaging alone will not optimally reduce the lymphoedema. The four aspects are:

1. manual lymphatic drainage / self-massage;
2. bandaging and compression / garments;
3. skin care;
4. exercises.

MANUAL LYMPHATIC DRAINAGE

This term originally referred to the massage technique developed by Dr Emil Vodder, but it is nowadays often used for any lymphatic massage. Manual lymphatic drainage is a very light massage technique and should never be unpleasant or painful for the patient.

The purpose of manual lymphatic drainage is to:

- increase the formation of lymph;
- increase the movement of lymph and tissue fluid;

- increase the lymphangiomotoric;
- increase the lymph time volume in the impaired lymphatic vessel;
- soften fibrotic areas.

Principles of manual lymphatic drainage A number of massage techniques have been developed. The most widely used are the Vodder and Földi treatment in Europe and in Australia, the Casley-Smith treatment. All have the same principles.

- Movements are slow, as the lymph is a sluggish moving fluid.
- Optimal massage pressure is important, as a too strong massage could compress the superficial lymphatics and thus block the lymph flow;
- The whole body needs to be treated, especially the trunk to create a reservoir into which the fluid from the limb can drain.
- The lymph nodes need to be stimulated. They have to be freed of the stored lymph fluid, so that the fluid from the limb can be reabsorbed.
- Anastomoses have to be opened and new pathways across the watersheds need to be created.
- Quadrants adjacent to the lymphoedematous limb must be treated.
- The limb is treated proximal to distal.
- Scars need to be taken into account as lymphatic capillaries are unable to form through scar tissue thicker than 0.5–1 mm.

Contraindications for manual lymphatic drainage

- Malignancy is a relative contraindication and should be discussed with the treating medical practitioner.
- Any acute inflammation.
- Chronic cardiac failure. If more fluid is pushed into the body it might overload the cardiovascular system even more.

Treatment regimen A considerable degree of practical training is necessary to enable the physiotherapist to apply the massage techniques correctly and successfully.

A full treatment course involves daily treatment for up to four weeks or longer in severe cases. The daily treatment involves lymphatic drainage, renewal of the bandages, exercises and skin care. During this intense treatment period self-management is taught, so that the patient is able to maintain the achieved reduction.

The self-management includes:

- self-massage, daily for the first six months after the intense treatment phase to help the lymphoedema to stabilize. A carer (spouse, relative, friend) could assist with the lymphatic massage. After the lymphoedema has stabilized, 2–4 times a week might be enough to keep the lymphoedema under control;
- specific exercises;
- wearing of compression (garment or bandages) 23/24 hours;
- ideally at night the limb should be bandaged. If the patient is unable to apply the bandages a slightly lighter garment (reduced pressure) should be worn. After a period of 6–12 months, if the limb has stabilized, the patient should be reassessed regarding the need for continued night compression. The decision depends on the severity of the lymphoedema, general health and ability of the patient;
- education about care and monitoring of limb size;
- awareness of activities and lifestyles that might exacerbate the lymphoedema.

Patient progress is monitored by reviews at one week, six weeks, six months and one year after the initial treatment phase. Ideally patients should continue to be reviewed half yearly. Baseline and subsequent measurement of limb circumference and/or volume are essential in determining the outcome and efficacy of the intense treatment phase and the self-management.

BANDAGING AND COMPRESSION GARMENTS

Bandages are necessary to provide suitable compression to maintain the reduction achieved by the manual lymphatic drainage. They are adjustable to the slowly reducing circumference of the limb and therefore are used during the intense treatment stage. Following this, compression garments are used to maintain the reduction.

The purpose of bandaging is to:

- increase total tissue pressure;
- create a resting and a working pressure;
- maintain reduction achieved through manual lymphatic drainage;
- soften fibrotic areas through special padding.

Principles

- On the first day of treatment the bandages are only applied up to the knee/elbow.
- At the start of treatment the bandages are applied with light pressure which increases as the treatment progresses.
- Bandages are applied with slightly higher pressure distally than proximally.
- The amount of pressure applied can be varied by increasing or decreasing the overlap of the bandage or by applying an extra bandage over the ones already applied.
- Circulation needs to be checked at the completion of the bandaging. At the beginning of treatment the patient needs to be informed of what action to take if the circulation is compromised.

Contraindications for compression

- Chronic cardiac failure
- Arterial insufficiency

Bandaging procedure If the fingers/toes are swollen and the sign of Stemmer (refer to assessment form) is positive the digits should be bandaged.

- *Gauze bandages* are applied on the fingers/toes with low pressure. The tips of the fingers must not be covered so circulation can be checked.
- The first layer of limb bandaging consists of a *fine cotton stocking* used on the skin for hygiene. It will soak up any sweat and will protect from the synthetic material used in the next layer.
- The second layer consists of padding, in the form of *synthetic 'cotton wool'* or *low-density foam*. The function of this layer is to equal out any bony prominences or deep skinfolds and create a cylindrical form. Failure to achieve this results in increased pressures over such features. This is often further supported by foam pieces around the malleoli, the dorsum/palm of the hand and the anterior lower leg.
- Extra foam padding is used under the bandages to avoid increased pressure from the bandages during movement. In the leg it is needed over the popliteal fossa and on the arm in the cubital fossa.
- *Chipbags* are used to soften hard, fibrotic areas. A chipbag can easily be made out of a piece of fine cotton sleeve filled with high-density foam bits and taped together at the ends. Its size depends on the fibrotic area it has to cover. The chipbag is then placed over this area and under the bandages and will give variable pressure with movement. This will help to break the fibrosis down.
- The third layer involves *low-stretch bandages* to apply pressure on the limb. The low-stretch bandages give a low resting pressure (pressure from outside, with rest) and an excellent working pressure (pressure from within, during muscle activity).

It is important for bandages to be applied evenly, with their pressure higher distally and decreasing slightly proximally. The ends of the bandages are always secured with tape and never with clips, to exclude any chance of skin injury (Fig. 35.7).

COMPRESSION GARMENT

After the lymphoedema has been reduced through manual lymphatic drainage and bandaging, it is necessary for the patient to wear a compression garment to maintain the reduction. As mentioned earlier, without compression, the limb will have accumulated fluid to its former size within a month (Swedborg, 1984). During the wearing of a compression garment the fibrotic tissue can be further reduced.

A custom-made garment is always preferable but not always feasible. Depending on the manufacturer and the specific requirements, the cost of a custom-made garment could be 1.5–6 times the price of a ready-made one. A well-fitting garment is essential and it should:

- fit without folds anywhere, at rest and with movement;
- not cut in during elbow/knee flexion and extension;
- be long enough to cover the limb up to the axilla/groin without cutting in.

The patient should be able to apply the garment independently.

Two garments are required (one to wash and one to wear). Most garments have a lifespan of 4–6 months. There are many different garments available, depending on the

Figure 35.7 Bandaging materials A. Foam. B. Low-stretch bandages. C. Padding. D. Chipbag. E. Tape. F. Finger bandages. G. Cotton stockings. H. Scissors.

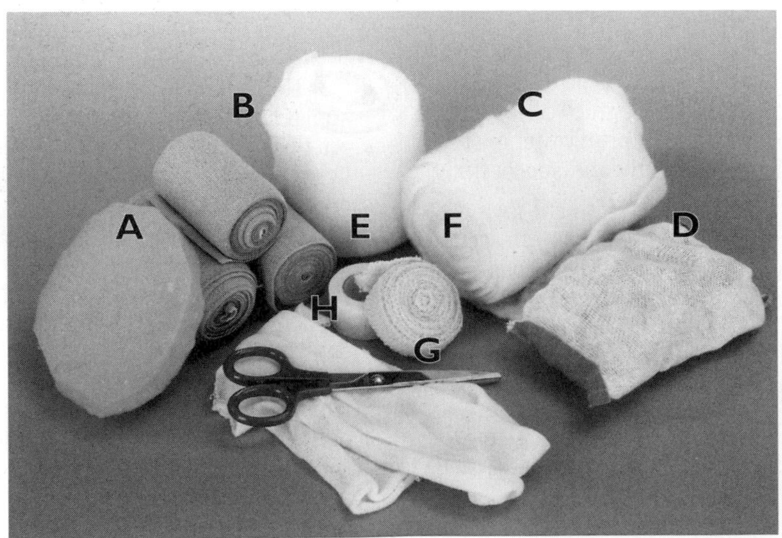

Figure 35.8 Arm bandages.

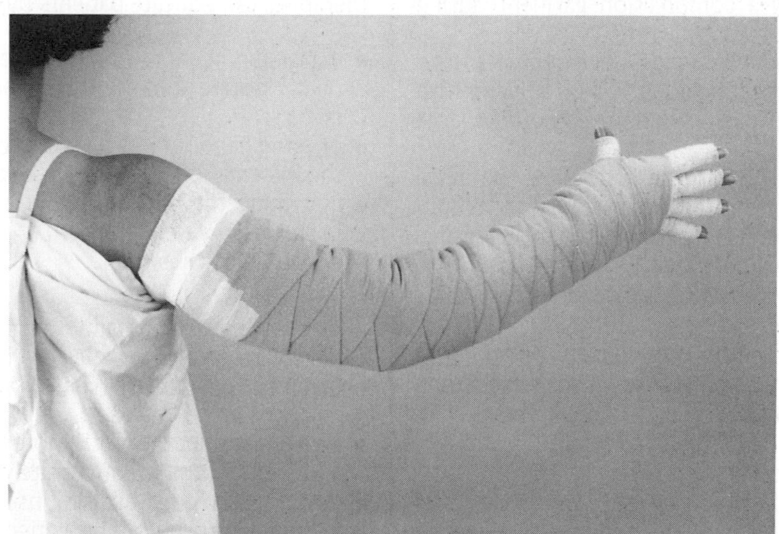

patient's requirements. For example, the arm sleeve might include a gauntlet, to cover the arm from hand to axilla, or extend from the wrist to axilla with a separate glove for the hand.

The pressures used in the compression garments are divided into classes with different classification between manufacturers. The compression for an average lymphoedematous arm sleeve is 25–40 mmHg, depending on manufacturer. For mild leg lymphoedema the stocking should have a pressure of 30–40 mmHg and 40–60 mmHg is required for severe leg lymphoedema. If severe lower leg swelling exists, the combination of a normal stocking and a calf-length stocking on top during active hours might work very well.

Again, the bandaging and the compression garment need to be adjusted to the individual needs of each patient. Figures 35.8 and 35.9 illustrate bandaging of the arm and leg respectively.

SKIN CARE

The skin of the lymphoedematous limb has the tendency to be dry, so regular application of an unperfumed moisturizer is recommended. Any tinea or other fungal infections need prompt attention, as the condition leaves small openings in the skin which increase the risk of infection. Scrupulous personal hygiene is also required to reduce this risk.

EXERCISES

Muscle activity as well as passive movement enhances the entry into and the flow of the fluid within the initial lymphatic system. The purpose of exercise is to:

- increase lymph flow;
- address any postural or muscle weakness;
- maintain full range of movement of the joints in the affected limb.

Figure 35.9 Leg bandages.

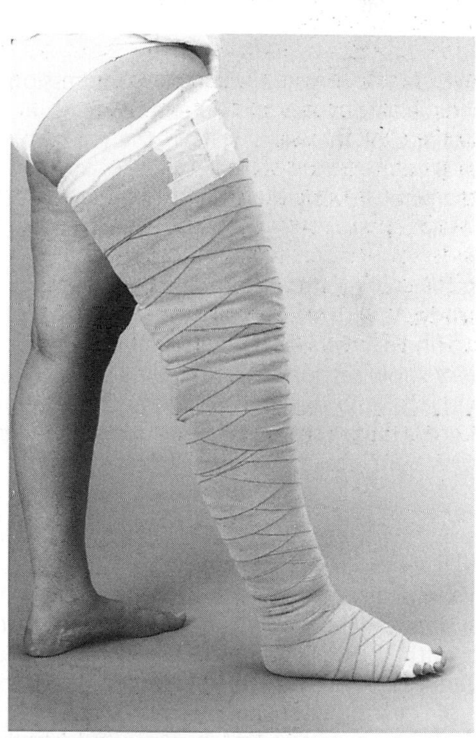

Principles

- Each exercise programme should be designed individually by the physiotherapist, taking into account the patient's age, daily activities and her level of fitness, as well as any other musculoskeletal problems (Mason, 1995).

- While exercising during the intensive treatment phase, bandages must be worn. In the follow-up phase bandages are replaced by a compression garment during exercises.
- Like the manual lymphatic drainage, the exercises should start with the trunk, then include the limb starting with the proximal muscle groups, concentrating on the large muscles.
- For maximal benefit it is important to allow the initial lymphatics to fill (approximately five seconds) and empty (approximately one second). Therefore the exercise programme should be conducted with a contraction phase of one second and a relaxation phase of five seconds (Piller et al, 1992).
- The exercise regimen should include deep breathing as the negative intrathoracic pressure enhances the lymph flow in the thoracic duct.

HYDROTHERAPY

Although the effect of hydrotherapy on the lymphoedematous limb has not been researched, the knowledge of the physical characteristics of water suggests it is an ideal exercise environment. The buoyancy of the water will reduce the heaviness of the limb and exercising will be easier.

- The hydrostatic pressure will apply compression on the lymphoedematous area and act as a sleeve.
- The warmth of the water will aid the relaxation of the muscles.
- The temperature should not exceed approximately 30–31°C.

The possibility of group work or individual swimming gives some variety. As with other exercises, it is necessary for each patient to find her own level of activity. It is advisable to start with a very short session to avoid fatigue and to rest afterwards with the limb elevated. As the hydrostatic pressure acts as a sleeve during swimming, it is important to apply the garment straight after the hydrotherapy session.

EDUCATION

The physiotherapy profession is responsible for educating patients about lymphoedema, even if they have been referred with a totally unrelated condition. The main aim of education should be focused on those patients at risk of developing lymphoedema. Although lymph vessels have compensatory mechanisms, the lymph nodes do not regrow and the risk of developing the condition is lifelong.

Often patients may believe that they have to be careful for a short period only and become careless after six months to one year. It is not uncommon for lymphoedema to occur up to 30 years after an axillary dissection. Every lymph node dissection leads to reduced lymph transport capacity even without the evidence of oedema. This has been shown by lymphscintigraphy (Földi and Földi, 1991a).

As in all therapy, patients who understand the reason behind a request will always be more compliant. Physiotherapists can educate patients by:

- explaining in small 'portions', for example why the lymphatic system is impaired and what happens if an infection occurs;
- offering handouts, as patients are often overwhelmed by the information and unable to take it all in;
- informing the patients about support groups, e.g. the Lymphoedema Association;
- encouraging questions.

The following list contains the main precautions for the patient with an arm or a leg at risk of developing lymphoedema or with already established lymphoedema.

- The patient should not ignore any increase in limb size and seek treatment immediately.
- Any trauma, cuts, bruises, insect bites or sport injuries should be avoided. The patient has to be particularly careful with pets to avoid scratches.
- Any cuts or skin damage need immediate attention. The area should be cleaned and antiseptic cream applied immediately. If the abrasion becomes even slightly red a doctor should be consulted without delay.
- Medical opinion should be sought for any redness of the skin, which could be the start of an infection.
- Sunburn should be avoided.
- The patient should be careful when cutting nails.
- The limb should be kept spotlessly clean. When drying, the patient needs to be gentle but thorough.
- Bras and pants should not leave indentations. After the garment has been removed no marks should be visible.
- Exercise is important, but overexercising must be avoided. The limb should not ache from fatigue but if this occurs the limb should be elevated.
- If travelling by air or during long car and bus journeys, a compression garment must be used on the 'at-risk' limb or extra compression in the form of a bandage should be applied over the compression garment. There is a high proportion of lymphoedema which has commenced or has been made worse during flying. The exact cause is unknown, but it is assumed that the reduced cabin pressure has an influence. If prolonged sitting was the only cause then long bus and car journeys would have the same effect. However, reports of the development of lymphoedema after long bus journeys are far fewer than incidences after flying (Brennan, 1991; Casley-Smith and Casley-Smith, 1996).
- Hair removal needs to be undertaken with a well-maintained electrical razor.
- Skin needs to be supple and well moisturized, so it needs to be moisturized regularly.
- A well-balanced diet is important. Lymphoedema is a high-protein oedema but a reduction of protein intake will only increase the problem.
- Research has shown that obesity increases the risk of development of lymphoedema, therefore the maintenance of a healthy body weight is important.

SPECIFIC PRECAUTIONS FOR AT-RISK ARM LYMPHOEDEMA

- Blood pressure readings should never be taken on the affected arm (the blood pressure cuff compresses the already impaired lymphatic system).
- Venous puncture is not permitted on the affected arm. Although the procedure is undertaken with sterile instruments, it still involves compression to allow easier access to the vein.
- While undertaking activities such as washing up, gardening or sewing, protection should be used, such as gloves and thimbles.
- Heavy loads should not be carried with the at-risk arm.
- Pads under bra straps might be necessary, especially with patients who have large breasts / prostheses.

SPECIFIC PRECAUTIONS FOR AT-RISK LEG LYMPHOEDEMA

- Injections should not be given in the leg.
- During activities such as bush walking, protective clothing and boots should be worn.
- High heels and standing for long periods should be avoided.
- Patients with primary leg lymphoedema should remember that the other leg is also at risk, e.g. it may also have an abnormal lymph drainage.

It is important to explain to the patient that all these precautions do not mean a total change in lifestyle. Patients are often under the impression that previous hobbies are not possible any longer and this can lead to depression. It is important to stress that more precautions are necessary and that the length of time the patient is able to participate in these activities has to be monitored and adjusted. Similar principles apply to housework, particularly cleaning, and the patient is advised to spread the chores over the whole week.

Other Treatment Modalities

Intermittent compression devices

Compression devices have been used extensively over the last 10–15 years. The one-chamber pump used to be common but today it has been replaced by the sequential compression pump.

An inflatable plastic sleeve is fitted to the limb, enclosing the hand / foot. The sleeve then inflates and compresses the limb in a set cycle with variable compression. The sequential pumps have multiple small chambers which inflate and deflate in a sequence. The ideal pressure is a maximum of 45 mmHg for high-protein oedema and 15 mmHg for low-protein oedema (Casley-Smith and Casley-Smith, 1994c).

Research has shown that the one-chamber pump just 'pushed' the tissue fluid to the proximal part of the limb, but left the protein behind and this attracted the fluid again. The small amounts of protein which were transported towards the body remained at the proximal end of the limb and slowly gathered a fibrotic ring around them. This made the normal transport of lymph from the limb into the trunk even harder and in the end increased the severity of the lymphoedema.

The pump should not be allowed to become part of a passive treatment. The body needs to be prepared with manual lympatic drainage to create a reservoir for the fluid to drain into, prior to pump usage.

While the intermittent compression device is applied the patient has to continuously drain the proximal part of the limb. Appropriately used, the compression pump can be very helpful in softening hard, fibrotic areas.

The International Congress for Lymphology in 1993 came to a general agreement that the pump should never be used alone and that the trunk must be prepared before applying the machine (Casley-Smith and Casley-Smith, 1994c).

The greatest complication during leg treatment occurs if the trunk has not been prepared and genital swelling occurs.

Laser

Laser therapy for lymphoedema shows great promise. It is thought that the regeneration of lymphatic vessels can be aided with the use of laser by increasing the diameter and improving the contractility of the vessel. Treatment by laser can aid in the removal of stagnant protein and increases the macrophage activity. Thelander (1994) used a scanning laser (helium neon and infrared laser) to reduce chronic post-mastectomy lymphoedema. Application was over the medial and lateral aspects of the forearm and upper arm. Any proximal trunk swelling was treated concurrently. Significant reduction was achieved over the treated areas, rendering them smaller and softer.

Medication

Diuretics and benzopyrones are two medications which are often mentioned in connection with the treatment of lymphoedema.

DIURETICS

Diuretics are often prescribed for lymphoedema, in many cases as a lifelong therapy. However, as the underlying cause of lymphoedema is increased protein stagnation, the removal of water increases the protein concentration even further and the lymphoedematous limb will, in the long term, became even more fibrotic (Földi et al, 1989).

BENZOPYRONES

The benzopyrones (Loedema) are also called coumarins. This medication stimulates the macrophages to act as scavenger cells on the stagnating protein cells. Initially it was thought that benzopyrones would increase the lymph flow or help to open the collateral lymphatics faster, but their action lies only in the increased proteolysis (Piller, 1991). After reports of increased hepatotoxicity the medication has been withdrawn from sale locally, pending further investigation.

Surgery

The International Society for Lymphology (Adelaide, 1985) concluded that conservative treatment should always be tried before surgery is considered. The reasons given were that surgery always involves risk and conservative treatment is usually cheaper.

Surgery can be divided into three categories:

1. procedures to improve lymph drainage;
2. debulking of lymphoedematous tissue;
3. ligating of hypertrophied lymph vessels to stop reflux.

PROCEDURES TO IMPROVE LYMPH DRAINAGE

Many different materials have been used to create new lymphatics, such as silk threads, silver and Teflon wicks and even fishing lines. The problem has been the inability of the artificial vessels to pump the lymph away against gravity. Creation of a lymphovenous anastomosis was also unsuccessful. Fibrotic tissue developed as a result of surgery and added extra risks. The overall results initially were good for six months and then deteriorated with very poor outcomes in the long term.

DEBULKING OF LYMPHOEDEMATOUS TISSUE

Debulking involves the excision of the lymphoedematous tissue down to the deep fascia and then covering it with a split skin graft. This has produced unacceptable hyperkeratosis of the graft.

LIGATING OF HYPERTROPHIED LYMPH VESSELS TO STOP REFLUX

Some patients with hypertrophied lymphatics suffer from reflux. If this occurs in the abdomen, chyle can accumulate in the scrotum and/or legs. Surgery has been proposed to the lymph vessels in the form of lymph vessel ligation (Morgan, 1994).

General Patient Management

Diet and obesity

As the lymphoedema patient gains an understanding of the condition, misguided changes in diet, especially reduced protein and fluid intake, often occur. The patient needs guidance and reassurance that a well-balanced diet and good fluid intake are essential for her well-being and that it will be beneficial for the lymphoedema as well. In the extreme case, reduced protein intake could lead to hypoproteinaemia which would only reduce the effective reabsorbing pressure and with this the lymphoedema would increase.

The obese patient needs advice on weight reduction and this is best done through referral to a dietitian. It has been shown that obesity increases the risk of development of lymphoedema and also reduces the effect of treatment if lymphoedema is present. Bertelli et al (1992) found that women who had developed arm lymphoedema after surgery and had gained weight between surgery and admission for lymphoedema treatment achieved only a 13% reduction compared to the patient group without weight gain, who achieved a 25% reduction.

Obesity is also a predisposing factor for the development of lymphangiosarcoma in chronic lymphoedema.

Management of the Palliative Care Patient

The term 'palliative care' generally denotes 'relieving without cure'. With patients in the palliative care stage, particularly in the terminal stage, the treatment aim might have to change.

The foremost aim is to improve the quality of life. Comfort is more important than long-term reduction of the lymphoedematous limb. The treatment plan needs to be adjusted according to the patient's:

- present state of health;
- emotional status;
- support from family and friends (if the treatment is to be carried out in an outpatient setting);
- acceptance, e.g. does she want treatment?

The treatment plan may be limited if the patient is unable to:

- come to an outpatient facility for daily treatment;
- tolerate a full four-week programme;
- tolerate full bandaging;
- stay in the required position for the duration of treatment, e.g. unable to lie prone.

Modification of the ideal management for lymphoedema for the palliative patient might include the following.

- Reduction of the length of treatment. Depending on health status, one or two weeks treatment might be enough to decrease swelling sufficiently to increase quality of life.
- The use of single or a double-layered elastic tubing or antiembolic stockings can provide good support, if pressure bandaging cannot be tolerated.
- The treatment position can be changed to make the treatment more comfortable, e.g. side lying or sitting.

It should not be forgotten that body contact and the light, rhythmic technique of manual lymphatic drainage will have a relaxing effect and with this an influence on pain.

Summary

This chapter has discussed the definition of lymphoedema. The anatomy and physiology have been outlined and the assessment and treatment have been examined. The key points are as follows.

- Lymphoedema is a progressive disorder, characterized by:
  1. collection of excessive tissue protein;
  2. swelling;
  3. chronic inflammation;
  4. fibrosis.
- The lymphatic system can be seen as a one-way pathway from the tissues to the venous blood circulation.
- The anatomy of the lymphatic system includes initial lymphatics, precollectors and collectors, which contain valves. The lymphangion is the section between two valves. The lymph travels through the lymph nodes into lymph trunks, eventually ending in the venous blood circulation. The watershed, which is the dividing line for the direction of the lymph flow, divides the body into four quadrants. With the help of the initial lymphatics the watersheds can be overcome. This and the anastomosis, which forms the connection between the quadrants, are extremely important for treatment.
- The insufficiency of the lymphatic system is divided into dynamic, mechanical and safety valve insufficiency.
- Lymphoedema is categorized into primary and secondary lymphoedema and classed according to the severity into two grades.
- General management of lymphoedema involves a thorough assessment to establish cause and type of lymphoedema and create a treatment plan, which needs to be discussed with the patient.
- The treatment consists primarily of complex physical therapy, which includes manual lymphatic drainage, bandaging initially and later compression garments, skin care and exercises. These four aspects are of equal importance and need to be addressed. Laser, intermittent compression devices and self-massage have an important role to play, especially as complex physical therapy is time consuming and therefore expensive.
- Education is of great importance, especially for patients who are at risk of developing lymphoedema.

A 42-year-old woman presented with right arm swelling. Her history revealed a right modified radical mastectomy four years previously, with no post-operative complications. She had six weeks of radiotherapy after the operation, without any problems. She was not given any advice regarding the prevention of lymphoedema and she was unaware of the need for any precautions for her arm. Four years after the operation she worked intensively in her garden for almost one week. Slight swelling in her right arm was noticed at the end of the day. When her arm had been slightly swollen previously she found that elevation and rest reduced the swelling. During her week of gardening her arms received a lot of minor scratches and an infection started in her right arm. Unfortunately the patient was not aware of the seriousness and delayed the visit to her doctor by 24 hours, when the swelling in her right arm was quite noticeable. The infection was treated with antibiotics and settled after two courses. However, the swelling did not reduce and she was referred by her medical practitioner to a physiotherapist specializing in the treatment of lymphoedema. At this time her rings were too tight to wear on her right hand and so was the wristband of her watch. Her general health was fine and beside tamoxifen, she took no other medication regularly.

The subjective assessment showed that the sign of Stemmer was positive and the dorsum of her hand showed pitting oedema. The right arm was visibly swollen with the swelling mostly a grade 2. The sum of her measurements showed a difference of 23.4 cm between the affected and unaffected arms. The range of motion of her shoulder, elbow and wrist joint was normal. Her posture was rounded with thoracic hyperkyphosis and hyperextended cervical spine.

At the end of the initial assessment an explanation of the cause of the lymphoedema was given and treatment options discussed. A course of complex physical therapy was suggested and the details were explained. The patient agreed.

As lymphoedema involves not only the swelling of the limb but the adjacent quadrant as well, manual lymphatic drainage involved the following sequence.

1. *Stimulation of the cervical lymph nodes.*
2. *Activation of the contralateral axilla lymph nodes.*
3. *Activation of the ipsilateral inguinal lymph nodes.*
4. *The axilloaxillary anastomosis was opened to create a pathway to the left axilla.*
5. *The axilloinguinal anastomosis was opened to create a pathway to the right groin.*
6. *The contralateral quadrant was cleared to the left axilla.*
7. *The right quadrant was cleared into the left quadrant.*
8. *This involved the anterior and posterior aspect of the trunk.*
9. *After the trunk has been sufficiently prepared the treatment continued on the proximal right arm and slowly progressed distally.*
10. *The fingers were the last part treated.*

In a severe arm lymphoedema, it might take 1–2 weeks of trunk massage before progressing to the arm.

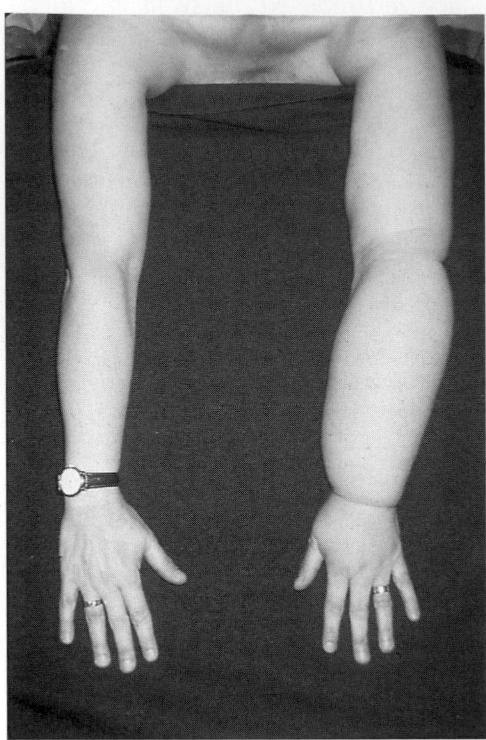

Figure 35.10 Pre-treatment arm lymphoedema.

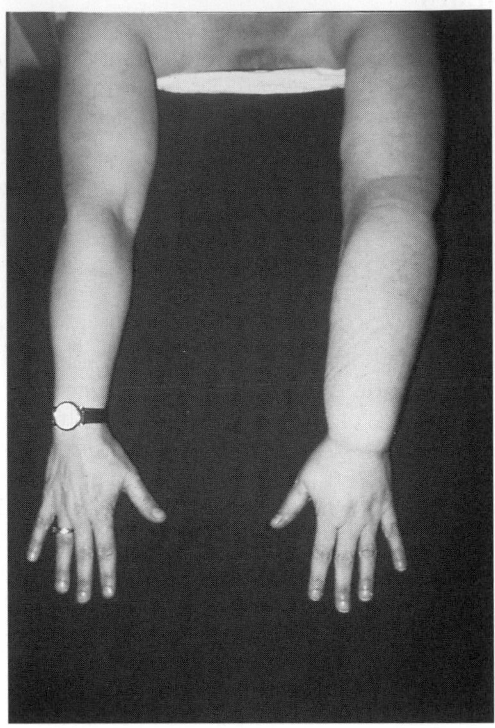

Figure 35.11 Post-treatment arm lymphoedema.

After the massage the arm was bandaged, including the fingers. The bandages were left in place until the next day's treatment.

The patient was given an exercise programme, which she undertook daily. During the treatment phase education, postural advice and self-massage were addressed.

Over the four-week duration of the treatment programme the arm circumference reduced by 78%. At the conclusion of the intensive treatment phase a custom-made compression garment, which included the fingers, was worn during the day. At night the patient bandaged the arm. After the lymphoedema had stabilized she was able to wear a lighter garment at night instead of the bandaging.

She continued with her self-management and showed further reduction during the reviews (one week, six weeks, six months, one year) after the treatment. Figures 35.10 and 35.11 illustrate the change in lymphoedema before and after the treatment period.

ACKNOWLEDGEMENT

I would like to thank Julie Arthur (Australian Catholic University) for her invaluable help with editing and Robyn Box and Elaine Unkles for their professional advice.

References

Adair T and Guyton A (1985) Introduction to the lymphatic system. In: Johnston M (ed) *Experimental Biology of the Lymphatic Circulation*, pp. 1–5. Amsterdam: Elsevier.

Axelrod D and Osborne M (1989) The swollen extremity. In: Witte R (ed) *Manual of Oncologic Therapeutics 1989/1990*, pp. 565–568. Philadelphia: J.B. Lippincott.

Bertelli G, Ventorini M, Forno G et al (1992) An analysis of prognostic factors in response to conservative treatment of post-mastectomy lymphoedema. *Surgery, Gynecology and Obstetrics* **175: 455–460.**

Brennan M (1991) Lymphoedema following the surgical treatment of breast cancer: a review of pathophysiology and treatment. *Journal of Pain Symptom Management* **7**: 110–116.

Bringezu G and Schreiner O (1991a) Topography der Lymphgefässverläufe. In: Bringezu G and Schreiner O (eds) *Die Therapieform Manuelle Lymphdrainage*, 3rd edn, pp. 73–77. Lübeck: Ebert Verlag.

Bringezu G and Schreiner O (1991b) Das Lymphgefässystem. In: Bringezu G and Schreiner O (eds) *Die Therapieform Manuelle Lymphdrainage*, 3rd edn, pp. 54–57. Lübeck: Ebert Verlag.

Bunce I, Mirolo B, Hennessy J et al (1994) Post-mastectomy lymphoedema treatment and measurement. *Medical Journal of Australia* **161**: 125–128.

Casley-Smith JR (1994) Measuring and representing peripheral oedema and its alterations. *Lymphology* **27**: 56–70.

Casley-Smith JR and Casley-Smith J (1986a) The incidence of high-protein oedema. In: Casley-Smith JR and Casley-Smith J (eds) *High-Protein Oedemas and the Benzo-Pyrones*, pp. 158–161. Sydney: J.B. Lippincott.

Casley-Smith JR and Casley-Smith J (1986b) Modes of action of the benzo-pyrones. In: Casley-Smith JR and Casley-Smith J (eds) *High-Protein Oedemas and the Benzo-Pyrones*, pp. 269–338. Sydney: J.B. Lippincott.

Casley-Smith J and Casley-Smith JR (1994a) Aetiologies of lymphoedema. In: *Modern Treatment for Lymphoedema*, pp. 67–70. Adelaide: The Lymphoedema Association of Australia.

Casley-Smith J and Casley-Smith JR (1994b) Diagnosis of lymphoedema: clinical. In: *Modern Treatment for Lymphoedema*, pp. 71–75. Adelaide: The Lymphoedema Association of Australia.

Casley-Smith J and Casley-Smith JR (1994c) Other physical therapy for lymphoedema: pumps, heating, etc. In: *Modern Treatment for Lymphoedema*, pp. 200–206. Adelaide: The Lymphoedema Association of Australia.

Casley-Smith J and Casley-Smith JR (1994d) Measuring and representing lymphoedema. In: *Modern Treatment for Lymphoedema*, pp. 90–98. Adelaide: The Lymphoedema Association of Australia.

Casley-Smith JR and Casley-Smith J (1996) Lymphoedema initiated by aircraft flights. *Aviation Space and Environmental Medicine* **69**: 52–56.

Castenholz A (1991) Structure of initial and collecting lymphatic vessels. In: Olszewski W (ed) *Lymph Stasis: Pathophysiology, Diagnosis and Treatment*, pp. 33–36. Boca Raton: CRC Press.

Clodius L (1977) Secondary arm lymphoedema. In: Clodius L (ed) *Lymphedema*, pp. 147–163. Stuttgart: Georg Thieme.

Földi E and Földi M (1991a) Das Lymphödem. In: Földi M and Kubik S (eds) *Lehrbuch der Lymphologie für Mediziner und Physiotherapeuten*, 2nd edn, pp. 231–246. Stuttgart: Gustav Fischer Verlag.

Földi E and Földi M (1991b) Physiologie und Pathophysiologie des Lymphgefässystems. In: Földi M and Kubik S (eds) *Lehrbuch der Lymphologie für Mediziner und Physiotherapeuten*, 2nd edn, pp. 185–228. Stuttgart: Gustav Fischer Verlag.

Földi M and Földi E (1991c) *Lymphoedema: A Guide For Patients and Therapists*, pp. 21–26. Victoria: Lymphoedema Association of Victoria.

Földi E, Földi M and Weissleder H (1985) Conservative treatment of lymphoedema of the limbs. *Angiology* **36**: 179.

Földi E, Földi M and Clodius L (1989) The lymphoedema chaos: a lancet. *Annals of Plastic Surgery* **22**: 505–515.

Gültig O, Knauer A, Pritschow H et al (1991) Praktische Hinweise fur Physiotherapeuten In: Földi M and Kubik S (eds) *Lehrbuch der Lymphologie für Mediziner und Physiotherapeuten*, 2nd edn, pp. 419–430. Stuttgart: Gustav Fischer Verlag.

Kubik S (1991) Anatomie des Lymphgefässystems. In: Földi M and Kubik S (eds) *Lehrbuch der Lymphologie für Mediziner und Physiotherapeuten*, 2nd edn, pp. 1–18. Stuttgart: Gustav Fischer Verlag.

Manestar M (1991) Oberflächliches Lymphsystem In: Földi M and Kubik S (eds) *Lehrbuch der Lymphologie für Mediziner und Physiotherapeuten*, 2nd edn, pp. 107–108. Stuttgart: Gustav Fischer Verlag.

Mason M (1993) The treatment of lymphoedema by complex physical therapy. *Australian Physiotherapy Journal* **39**: 41–45.

Mason M (1995). *Living with Lymphoedema. A Handbook for Patients*, pp. 20–23. Adelaide: Norwood, Lymphoedema Clinic.

Morgan RG (1994) Surgery and microsurgery for lymphoedema. In: *Modern Treatment for Lymphoedema*, pp. 226–227. Adelaide: The Lymphoedema Association of Australia.

National Health and Medical Research Council (1995) *Management of Early Breast Cancer, Clinical Practice Guidelines*, pp. 56–57. Canberra: Australian Government Publishing.

Olszewski W (1991) Clinical picture of lymphoedema. In: Olszewski W (ed) *Lymph Stasis: Pathophysiology, Diagnosis and Treatment*, p. 348. Boca Raton: CRC Press.

Petlund C (1990) The prevalence or incidence of chronic lymphoedema in a western European country. In: Nishi M, Uchino S and Yabuki S (eds) *Progress in Lymphology, XII*, pp. 91–95. Amsterdam: Elsevier.

Petlund C (1991) Volumetry of limbs. In: Olszewski W (ed) *Lymph Stasis: Pathophysiology, Diagnosis and Treatment*, pp. 444–450. Boca Raton: CRC Press.

Piller N (1991) Pharmacological treatment of lymph stasis In: Olszewski W (ed) *Lymph Stasis: Pathophysiology, Diagnosis and Treatment*, pp. 502–520. Boca Raton: CRC Press.

Piller N (1994) The management and treatment of lymphoedemas. *Australian Physiotherapy Association National Women's Health Group Journal* **13**: 17.

Piller N, Swedborg I and Norrefalk JR (1992) Lymphoedema rehabilitation programme. *The European Journal of Lymphology* **3**: 57–71.

Swedborg I (1980) Effectiveness of combined methods of physiotherapy for post-mastectomy lymphoedema. *Scandinavian Journal of Rehabilitation Medicine* **12**: 77.

Swedborg I (1984) Effects of treatment with an elastic sleeve and intermittent pneumatic compression in post-mastectomy patients with lymphoedema of the arm. *Scandinavian Journal of Rehabilitation Medicine* **16**: 35–41.

Thelander A (1994) Laser therapy for lymphoedema. *Australian Physiotherapy Association National Women's Health Group Journal* **13**: 26–30.

Ward L, Bunce I, Cornish B et al (1992) Multi-frequency bioelectrical impedance augments the diagnosis and management of lymphoedema in post-mastectomy patients. *European Journal of Clinical Investigation* **22**: 751–757.

Further reading

Bringezu G and Schreiner O (1991) *Die Therapieform Manuelle Lymphdrainage*. Lübeck: Ebert Verlag (only available in the German language).

Casley-Smith JR and Casley-Smith J (1986) *High-Protein Oedemas and the Benzo-Pyrones*. Sydney: J.B. Lippincott.

Casley-Smith J and Casley-Smith JR (1994) *Modern Treatment for Lymphoedema*. The Lymphoedema Association of Australia, c/o The Henry Thomas Laboratory (Microcirculation Research), University of Adelaide, Adelaide, SA 5005, Australia.

Clodius L (ed) (1977) *Lymphedema*. Stuttgart: Georg Thieme.

Földi M and Casley-Smith JR (eds) (1983) *Lymphangiology*. Stuttgart: F.K. Schattauer Verlag.

Földi M and Földi E (1991) *Lymphoedema: A Guide For Patients and Therapists*. English translation published in 1993 by the Lymphoedema Association of Victoria, 50 St George Rd, Upper Beaconsfield, Victoria 3167, Australia.

Földi M and Kubik S (eds) (1991) *Lehrbuch der Lymphologie*. Stuttgart: Gustav Fischer Verlag (only available in the German language).

Kurz I (1986) *Introduction to Dr. Vodder's Manual Lymph Drainage. Volume 2*: Therapy. Heidelberg: Karl F. Haug.

Kurz I (1987) *Textbook of Dr. Vodder's Manual Lymph Drainage. Volume 3: Therapy II (Treatment Manual)*. Heidelberg: Karl F. Hauf.

Mason M (1995) *Living with Lymphoedema. A Handbook for Patients*. Adelaide Lymphoedema Clinic, 90 Fullarton Road, Norwood, South Australia 5067.

Olszewski W (ed) (1991) *Lymph Stasis: Pathophysiology, Diagnosis and Treatment*. Boca Raton: CRC Press.

Wittlinger H and Wittlinger G (1990) *Textbook of Dr. Vodder's Manual Lymph Drainage. Volume 1: Basic Course*. Heidelberg: Karl F. Haug.

36

The Aged

YVONNE KIRKEGARD, RUTH SAPSFORD, JANE HOWARD AND SUE MARKWELL

Musculoskeletal System
•
Alzheimer's Disease and Dementia
•
Urogenital Ageing
•
Sexual Issues for Women over 60 Years
•
Bowel Dysfunction in the Ageing Women

The average life-span of women has been increasing for the past 2000 years. Currently, in industrialized Western society, 95% of women live to experience the menopause and 60% live to the age of 75 years (Cope, 1976; Speroff et al, 1994).

Women can now expect to live one-third of their lives after the menopause. The problems of the post-menopausal period, by virtue of the older population size alone, have achieved the status of a major public health concern (Diczfalusy, 1986).

The number of 'older' women is increasing in both the developed and developing countries, due both to a decline in mortality and the control of fertility (Diczfalusy, 1986). As well as this, the older population in general is getting older (Hazzard, 1986).

In industrialized countries the male to female ratio is 75:100 in the 60–69 age group and approximately 50:100 in the 80 and over group (Diczfalusy, 1986).

The disorders that are common to this age group are osteoporosis, atherosclerotic cardiovascular disease, musculoskeletal disorders and urogenital ageing.

Musculoskeletal System

The muscles weaken, the subcutaneous fat disappears and the vertebral column caves in with a resultant increase in the thoracic kyphosis and a flattening of the lumbar lordosis. The rib cage comes to rest on the pelvic crest, the height of the body decreases, but the arm span remains the same.

Osteoporosis is a major health problem in most 'ageing' Western societies. It is a condition characterized by a reduction in bone density, which predisposes to fractures with minimal trauma. These lead to considerable distress, disability and substantial costs to the health-care system. Falls are increasingly recognized as an important contributing factor in fractures (Lord and Castell, 1994).

From age 55–60 onwards, both men and women lose bone steadily at the rate of about 1% per year. In women, there is added to this a 15% bone loss within 5–10 years after the menopause. The incidence of fractures rises with age in both sexes, but the rate in men is half that in women (Grill and Martin, 1995).

The Dubbo study (Lord et al, 1994) concluded that the lifetime risk of an osteoporotic fracture in a person aged 60 is 56% for females and 29% for males. The most common sites for osteoporotic fractures include vertebrae, hip and forearm.

Physiological changes associated with advancing age in the musculoskeletal system

Muscle strength (lean body mass) decreases due to loss in both size and number of myocytes, a decrease in the pro-

Figure 36.1 Projected size of the world population age 60 and older. (Reproduced from Diczfalusy (1986) with permission.)

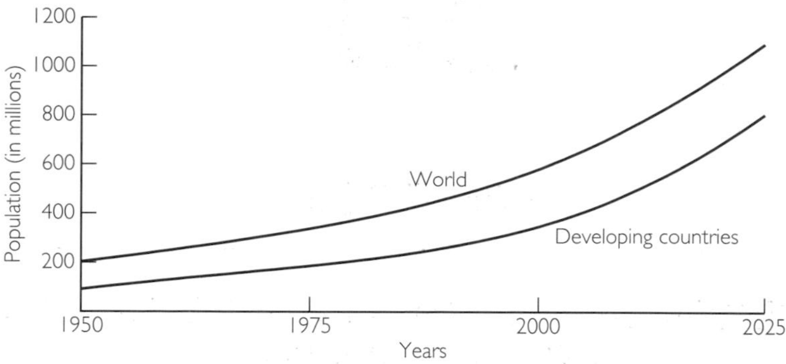

Figure 36.2 Pictorial representation of woman at different ages. (Reproduced from Evers and Heineman (1990) with permission.)

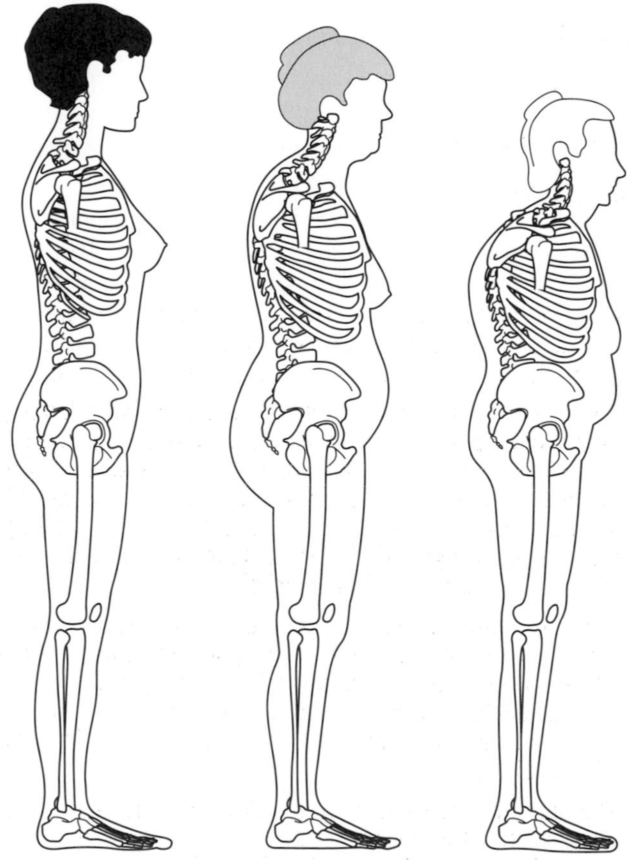

portion of type 2 fibres and progressive disuse. Replacement of muscle fibres with fatty tissue also contributes to the decrease in muscle mass (Tideiksaar, 1989a). At this age there is muscle weakness and decreased endurance, degenerative bone, joint and tendon problems and impaired balance and neuromuscular co-ordination (Skinner, 1987).

Physical limitations are widespread among elderly women. In the United States, approximately 20% of non-institutionalized individuals aged 65 years and over may experience difficulty in walking and as many as 10% have trouble getting out of chairs and beds (National Center for Health Statistics, 1987). Deficiencies in balance, mobility, musculoskeletal strength and flexibility contribute to loss of independence, increased risk of injury and greater rates of institutionalization.

Nguyen et al (1993) have shown that bone mineral density, body sway (a predictor of the rate of falling over) and muscle strength are independent predictors of fracture incidents. There is now good evidence that intervention in older people to improve bone density and quadriceps strength or to decrease postural sway may decrease fracture risk quite considerably.

Exercise in the elderly

PHYSICAL TRAINING

Fiatorone et al (1994) demonstrated that high-intensity resistance training improves muscle strength and size amongst frail and sedentary 72–98-year-old men and women. A dramatic improvement in strength among extremely sedentary men and women aged between 86 and 96 years was also shown. They concluded that the musculoskeletal system retains its responsiveness to training in elderly persons, resulting in improved functional mobility (Fiatorone et al, 1990).

A progressive exercise programme among older women (mean age 62.5 years) resulted in improvements in reaction time, neuromuscular control, body sway and muscle strength (Lord and Castell, 1994). Relatively short-term longitudinal studies have shown exercise programmes to have positive effects on bone mass in the older age group (Aloia et al, 1989; Krolner et al, 1983).

Falls in the elderly

Falls increase with age, are common in the elderly (Tideiksaar, 1989b) and from the age of 65 women fall more frequently than men.

Figure 36.3 Decreases in height after the 40th year. (Reproduced from Evers and Heineman (1990) with permission.)

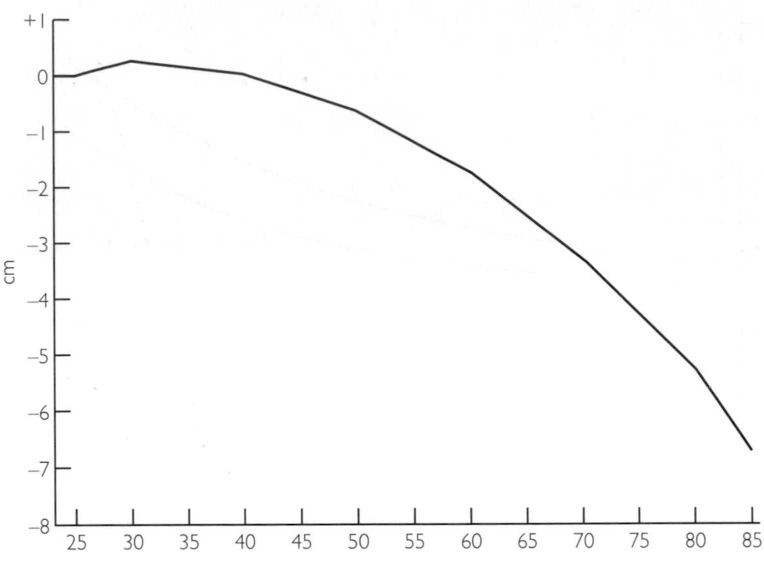

Some risk factors for injurious falls

Age
Female sex
Impaired performance of central processing speed
Decreased vision
Decreased mobility
Decreased muscle strength in lower limbs
Increased postural sway
(Birge, 1995; Tideiksaar, 1989a)

Impaired performance of central processing speed results in an increase in reaction time to avoid a perceived hazard.

Postural sway (a predictor of the rate of falling over) is more common in females than in males. Body sway increases with age in both sexes. People who fall have more sway than non-fallers (Tideiksaar, 1989a).

HIP FRACTURE

Over 95% of hip fractures follow a fall. With hip fractures there is a very good correlation between the change in bone mass (osteoporosis) with age and the observed incidence of hip fracture. About the age of 70 this relationship deteriorates and some other age-related factor becomes the dominant determinant of hip fracture risk and a good candidate for that is the change in central processing speed (Birge, 1995).

In older women the rate of hip fracture is 10 times greater above 84 than at 65–74 years (Tideiksaar, 1989b).

The older faller is unable to defend herself from injury due to defective central processing. A minor fall and osteoporotic bones will result in a hip fracture (Birge, 1995).

Alzheimer's Disease and Dementia

Alzheimer's disease accounts for most cases of dementia. Jorm et al (1987) have established that dementia prevalence increases with age according to an exponential model, with rates doubling every five years. Women have significantly higher rates of Alzheimer's disease than men.

Age-specific incidence of dementia increases more rapidly in women than it does in men. There is a consistent female to male predominance of Alzheimer's disease. The ratio is very similar to the difference in injurious falls and hip fractures between women and men (Birge, 1995). Birge suggests that the age-related changes in central processing speed (reaction time) is an expression of clinical dementia.

Paganini-Hill and Henderson (1994) showed that women who used oestrogen were less likely to have died from Alzheimer's disease than those who had not taken oestrogen. The risk of Alzheimer's and related dementia was decreased significantly with increasing oestrogen dose and with increasing duration of oestrogen use. This study suggests that the increased incidence of Alzheimer's disease in older women may be due to oestrogen deficiency and that oestrogen replacement may be useful for preventing or delaying the onset of this dementia.

Figure 36.4 Increase in the numbers of hip fractures with age. (Reproduced from Evers and Heineman (1990) with permission.)

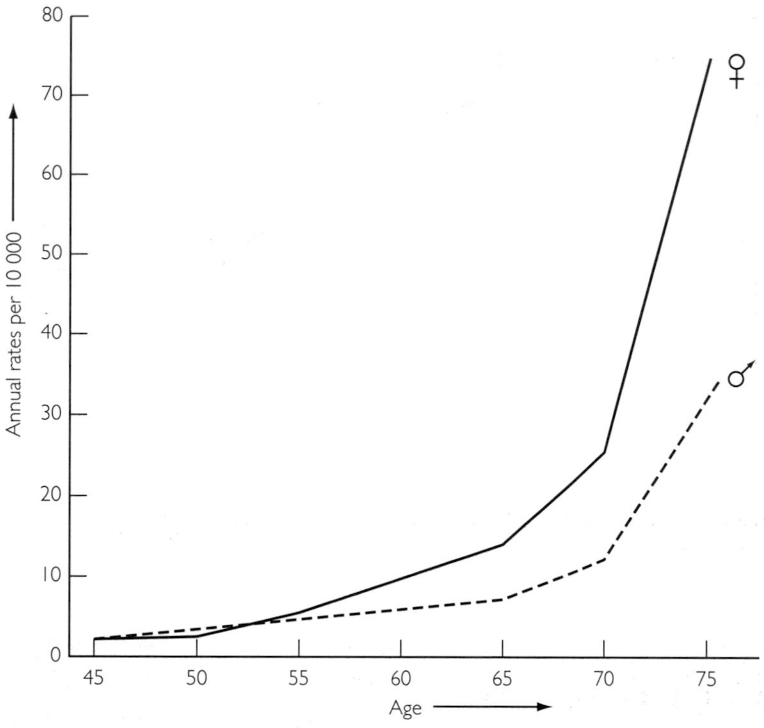

Figure 36.5 Estimated and observed prevalance of dementia by age, for baseline population. (Reproduced from Jorm et al (1987) with permission.)

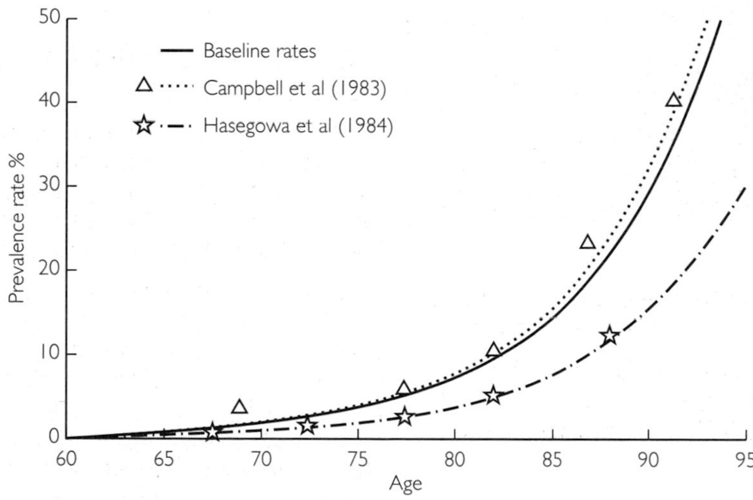

Urogenital Ageing

Urogenital age-related changes can cause distressing problems in women. Some years after the menopause up to 50% of women in this age group have symptoms from the urogenital mucosae and urinary symptoms (Iosif and Bekassy, 1984). The genital and urinary tracts are intimately associated and share a common embryology. Oestrogen receptors have been identified in the vagina, bladder, trigone and urethra (Iosif et al, 1981). However, oestrogen receptors have not been found in pelvic floor muscle fibres (Bernstein et al, 1995) though they may be present in the surrounding connective tissue. Age-related urogenital problems are outlined in the flow chart below.

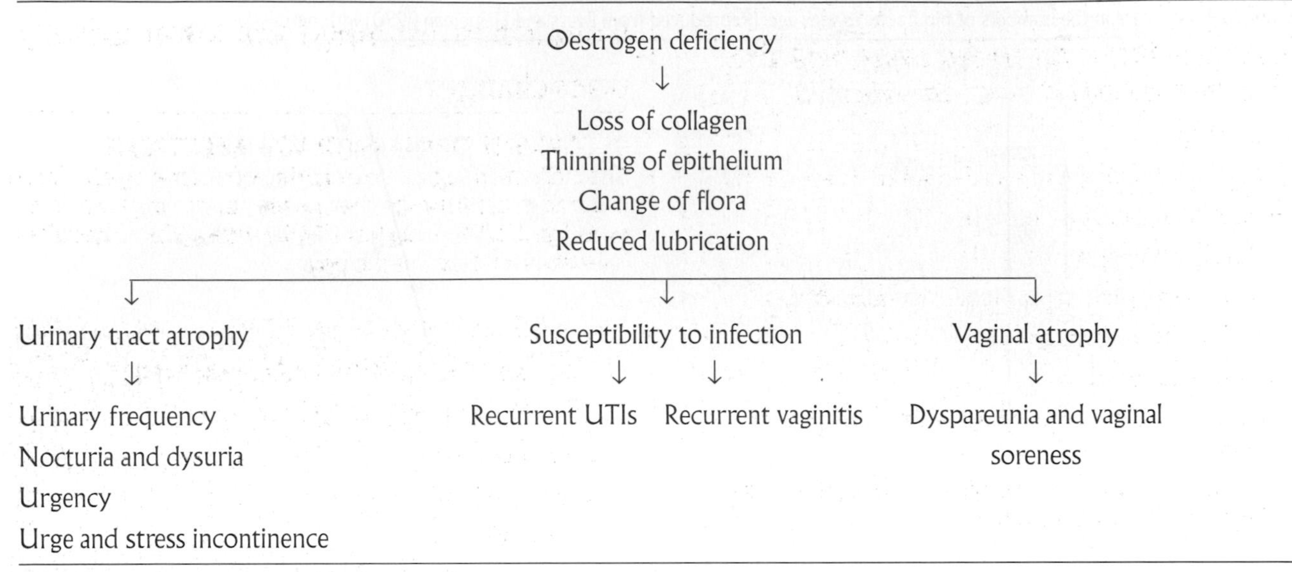

(after Pigne, 1994)

Vaginal changes

Senile changes in the vagina are listed in the box, followed by a description of some of the conditions which result from those changes.

> **Senile changes of the vagina**
>
> Reduced mucosal thickness
> Loss of glycogen content
> Leucocytic invasion
> Increase in vaginal pH
> Reduced vaginal blood flow

RECURRENT VAGINITIS

The predominant flora in the pre-menopausal vagina are the lactobacilli. Acid vaginal fluid (pH 3.8–4.5) as occurs pre-menopausally favours their growth. An increase in pH favours adherence and overgrowth of other bacteria at the expense of lactobacilli. In post-menopausal women the vaginal epithelium is thinner and the pH is increased. There is an increased susceptibility to infection with faecal flora e.g. *E. coli* and streptococci (Iosif, 1992; Tsai et al, 1987).

GENITAL ATROPHY

Lack of oestrogen affects both the vulva and the vagina, causing a thinner and smoother vaginal wall and vulval skin. Eventually in some women there is narrowing of the introitus to a marked degree. Associated symptoms include discomfort, burning, vaginal dryness, itching, discharge or dyspareunia. Replacement of oestrogen, either locally or systemically, is effective in reversing vaginal atrophy and increasing lubrication (Erikssen and Rasmussen, 1992; Smith et al, 1993).

GENITAL TRACT PROLAPSE

Prolapse of the bladder neck, the uterus and the posterior vaginal wall can be aggravated by age changes in connective tissue, smooth muscle and decreased PFM support. Loss of general fitness, obesity and constipation also contribute. Management includes use of a ring pessary or surgery. The role of physiotherapy has been discussed in Chapter 30.

Changes in urine production

In the elderly, urine volumes produced during the night hours equal the day urine volumes, whereas in younger people the day : night proportion is 2 : 1. This increased diuresis, with increased voiding, can lead to sleep problems (Asplund and Aberg, 1992). Certain pathological conditions also lead to increased urine production at night. These include cardiac oedema (increased venous return occurs in supine), diabetes and chronic renal failure. Nocturia >2–3 times a night is considered pathological. The physiological changes in the lower urinary tract and changes in bladder function with ageing are listed in the boxes.

Age-related changes affecting the lower urinary tract in women

↓ collagen

Loss of smooth muscle in the submucosa

Atrophy of skeletal muscle

Detrusor hypertrophy

↓ oestrogen leading to urogenital atrophy

↓ blood flow through vascular tissues

↓ urethral length

Loss of protective glycosaminoglycan layer of the bladder

↓ production of or response to ADH, leading to larger night urine volumes

Changes in bladder function with ageing

Earlier first desire to void

↓ capacity

↓ urethral closure

↓ urine flow rate, due to lower detrusor contraction speed

↑ residual urine

Tendency for detrusor to fail on initiation of voiding (Malone-Lee and Wahedna, 1993)

↓ ability to voluntarily suppress or initiate detrusor contraction

Bladder function is further compromised by several factors. Drugs prescribed for non-urological medical conditions can affect lower urinary tract function and may have some effect, either beneficial or adverse, on incontinence. The most common drugs involved are diuretics, calcium channel blockers and tricyclic antidepressants (Gormley et al, 1993) (see Table 28.3). Other factors are listed in the box.

Factors further affecting bladder function

Medications affecting the lower urinary tract

Disease processes in other organs

↓ fluid intake

Faecal impaction

Changes in environment/functional status

Conditions resulting from lower urinary tract changes

RECURRENT URINARY TRACT INFECTIONS

The increase in vaginal colonization of Gram-negative faecal organisms predisposes the woman to urinary tract infections (Iosif, 1992; Tsai et al, 1987). Factors which precipitate infections are listed in the box.

Causes of UTI in older women

↓ urethral closing pressure

Low fluid intake

↓ urethral length

↑ residual urine

Changes in bladder epithelium

(after Pigne, 1994)

Oestrogen replacement restores the vaginal, urethral and trigonal epithelium and leads to reappearance of the normal acid, lactobacilli-dominated, pre-menopausal flora. Oestrogen therapy is helpful before any other therapy, such as pelvic floor rehabilitation, medications and surgery, is considered (Pigne, 1994).

Conditions associated with urethrovesical dysfunction and their causes are listed in Tables 1 and 2 in Chapter 28. However, there are extra aspects of these problems which occur in the elderly and aged that require further comment here.

URINARY DYSFUNCTION

- *Frequency* – may be due to incomplete emptying. Those on weight reduction programmes frequently have a large fluid intake, assessed at over 1800 ml in elderly women (Saito et al, 1993).
- *Urgency* – decreased cortical and mid-brain perfusion affects inhibitory function.
- *Nocturia* – may be due to increased venous return of fluid from dependent oedema or poor ADH response, as well as other factors.
- *Incomplete bladder emptying* – due to an unsustained detrusor contraction. Voiding a second time after standing and moving or with water running can decrease residual urine.

URINARY INCONTINENCE

It is important to restate that incontinence is a symptom. This, along with confusion and falls, constitutes a common symptom of illness in the elderly. Thus incontinence must be investigated medically and not given 'bandaid' treatment for, with appropriate treatment of the illness, incontinence may resolve. Transient incontinence can occur with pneumonia, UTI, normal pressure hydrocephalus and some drugs, as well as in many other conditions.

The incidence of urinary incontinence in the elderly and old increases with age and is different in the community and institutions. Nursing home residents are said to have a 50–60% incidence (Fonda, 1985; Ouslander, 1990). In one survey this was the single major disability in a proportion (14.3%) of those institutionalized (Fonda, 1985). In community-dwelling women over 65 years, incontinence occurs in 11.6–19% of the population (Pagano et al, 1992; Thomas et al, 1980) and increases to 28% for those near 80 years.

Costs related to urinary incontinence are tremendous. In the early 1990s, 2% of the total health budget in Sweden was spent on incontinence, half of this in the elderly (Geirsson et al, 1993). Annual costs in USA are said to be in the billions of dollars.

Detrusor instability and urge incontinence In women over 75 years with urinary symptoms, 75–85% have detrusor instability (Malone-Lee, 1994). This instability is manifest as:

- urine loss and urgency, which may be provoked by a spontaneous detrusor contraction or by an increase in IAP;
- uninhibited detrusor overactivity with a decreased perception of fullness and insensitive urine loss – the subject is unaware that loss is about to occur (Geirsson et al, 1993).

There is a high incidence of detrusor instability in Parkinson's disease and other upper motor neurone lesions. Urge incontinence in the elderly is strongly associated with decreased perfusion of the cortex and mid-brain (Griffiths et al, 1990). The tendency of the detrusor contraction to fail soon after initiation of voiding can also occur in the presence of detrusor overactivity. So even though the patient has a strong urge to void there can be large residual volumes of urine.

Stress incontinence This occurs in 46% of elderly women presenting for treatment of incontinence. The mechanism of stress incontinence which appears for the first time in this age group is frequently urethral hypofunction and in many women this is combined with urge incontinence (McGuire, 1990). There is a continual seepage of urine in the upright position.

Post-micturition loss A few ml of urine may be lost while dressing after voiding. It may be related to a cystocoele or poor support of the bladder base. In both cases urine pools below the bladder outlet. To overcome this the subject may strain at the end of voiding in an attempt to completely empty the bladder.

Many elderly and old women are well motivated to work at exercise and bladder training to improve their dysfunction. Quality of life, rather than quantity, is a very important factor. Dementia or dependence on high levels of home support services generally mean that the subject is unable to co-operate in self-help type interventions, such as exercise and bladder training. Timed or prompted voiding and use of protective garments will be useful in these cases.

Treatments for urinary dysfunction in the elderly can vary from those used in younger women. Table 36.1 outlines some of the variations.

Treatment outcomes

Improvement in muscle strength after exercise has been reported in old people. The benefits of pelvic floor exercise in the elderly and aged are reflected in improved urinary control and are illustrated by the following examples.

Harrison (1987) showed decreased urinary frequency, nocturia and incontinent episodes in a group of women attending senior citizens fitness classes, after three months of pelvic floor exercises. In the old old (mean age 86.6 years) PF exercises taught using anal or perianal EMG with visual computer feedback resulted in a 67% decrease in episodes of incontinence (Woolner and Ouslander, 1992). Improvement in 63% and cure in 25% was noted in a group of incontinent men and women, with a mean age of 74.8 years, after four months of conservative treatment. The programme included advice, oestrogen, PF exercise and bladder training. The improvement was sustained at a 12-month follow-up (Fonda et al, 1994). Many other studies have included the elderly and old and reinforce the benefits of

Table 36.1 Treatment outlines for conditions of urinary dysfunction in the elderly and aged

Condition	Treatment
Frequency	PF exercise, systemic or vaginal oestrogen. If incomplete emptying – voiding retraining, double void, self-catheterization
Nocturia	PF exercise, systemic or vaginal oestrogen. If large night volumes – modify intake timing, rest for 2 hours with legs elevated in middle of day
Incomplete emptying	Double void, voiding retraining, self-catheterization.
Post-voiding loss	PF exercise
Stress incontinence (hypofunction)	PF exercise, vaginal oestrogen, systemic oestrogen + α-adrenergic agonist
Urge incontinence	PF exercise, urge control, bladder retraining, systemic oestrogen
Nocturnal enuresis	If large night volumes, use alarm to wake and void

Treatments recommended in older women may vary from those used in younger women.

exercise in a co-operative, non-demented, yet often frail population.

Sexual Issues for Women over 60 years

Social, psychological and biological factors influence sexual function in older women. Societal attitudes are negative and often older women who do enjoy sex are seen as perverted. Personal attitudes are important, as is the health of both partners. Several studies have shown that sexual activity and interest decline with age (Pfeiffer and Davis, 1972; Rockstein and Sussman, 1979). The effect of ageing on sexual response is outlined in the box. The fall in sexual interest in women is greater than that seen in men (Kinsey et al, 1953). Sexual activity in older women is highest in married women, but women's interest in sex is unaffected by marriage. The earlier demise of male partners restricts sexual options for many women.

The effect of ageing on sexual response

Frequency of intercourse is less

Sexual arousal takes longer

Lubrication is less

Clitoral and labial engorgement is less

Orgasm is less intense with fewer muscle contractions

Resolution is faster

Many chronic illnesses affect sexual function. Heart disease, diabetes and hypertension may have an impact on sexual response. Many drugs also have an effect on sexual interest and response, e.g. antidepressants, antihypertensives and antipsychotic drugs. Cancer surgery may damage personal perceptions of sexual attractiveness.

The lack of ovarian hormonal influences on the genitals may result in loss of libido and painful intercourse. Vaginal discomfort can be helped with lubricants or local or systemic HRT.

However, the capacity for female orgasm is lifelong in a healthy woman and health workers should promote sexual activity as being natural and healthy.

Bowel Dysfunction in the Ageing Woman

Faecal incontinence, like urinary incontinence, though rarely fatal, may bring about social death (Tallis, 1993). Faecal incontinence is one of the several bowel disorders that commonly present at the climacteric or beyond (O'Neill et al, 1993). Life events, age-related changes and lifestyle are all cumulative in their aetiology and pathogenesis. Other disorders causing distress in the older woman include decreased colorectal motility (constipation), obstructed defaecation and faecal impaction. These symptoms may range from nuisance value to causing social withdrawal. They may be life threatening, e.g. mortality associated with straining at stool with the added cardiovascular risk in females at this time. However, the vast majority of healthy and active aged enjoy normal bowel function.

Faecal impaction and overflow incontinence are found in the very young and the elderly. Musculoskeletal changes reflect the 'transient' ability to effectively position the body and co-ordinate to evacuate – 'toilet training' is required at the two extremes of life.

Physiotherapy management requires a thorough understanding of the physiological changes with normal ageing. Treatment must be modified to reflect the physical, cognitive and environmental changes of the patient.

Constipation

In successful ageing, colon transit time (CTT) is not symptomatically decreased. However, colon motility fluctuates widely over a 24-hour period. The following age-related physiological and behavioural factors may affect colon motility (see Table 36.2). Institutionalized living may present a polarized symptom picture.

CAUSES OF CONSTIPATION IN THE ELDERLY

Decreased colorectal motility

1. Modified and decreased fibre and fluid intake
2. Redundant / megacolon / megarectum
3. Irritable bowel syndrome
4. Endocrine – ↓ oestrogen, dehydration, hypothyroidism
5. Metabolic – ↓ fluid in ageing colons
6. Neurological – somatic, autonomic, enteric
7. Psychological – depression, stress, confusion, dementia
8. Polypharmacy – opioids, antidepressants, diuretics, anticholinergics, iron, antacids, selected cholesterol-lowering agents, selected antihypertensives
9. Mechanical obstruction – diverticulosis, adhesions and strictures (benign neoplasms), colorectal malignancies, anorectal conditions
10. Immobility – cognitive, neurological, orthopaedic
11. Multiple factors
12. Aggregate of minor ailments

Obstructed defaecation

Age-related changes – disuse or denervation

1. Poor defaecation pattern
2. Descending perineum syndrome
- Destabilization of pelvic floor – S234 nerve root and somatic nerve neuropathy
- Lack of organ support

Table 36.2 The effect of ageing on colon motility

Factor	Effect	Age related
Sleep Daytime naps	Depresses colon motility Greatly reduce motility	Sleep patterns change with age and level of activity
Morning awakening	↑ segmental colonic contractions ↑ defaecatory stimulus on wakening	Non-propagating segmental contractions ↓ with age (pelvic colon stasis) Immobility over time may inhibit urge to evacuate
Ingestion of food	↑ motility minutes after eating – may last hours. More sustained in distal colon	Effects of poor mastication, anorexia, etc. Faecal impaction inhibits rectal urge
Caloric content	Fat is main stimulus. Large quantities of carbohydrate have a similar response. Protein inhibits motility	Diet planning. Food preparation may be impaired. Timing of food types important
Normal activity/inactivity	Exercise has been shown to have conflicting responses on CTT. ↑ gastrocolic reflex	**Immobility delays CTT up to 7–14 days.** ↓ gastrocolic reflex leads to ↓ urge to empty
Metabolic changes	Electrolyte disturbances ↓ water content of colon	↓ stool bulk (pebbles)

Physiological changes, particularly as a result of immobility, have a greater effect on CTT than dietary variation and lack of exercise. (Adapted from Bassotti et al, 1995.)

- Rectoanal prolapse
- Megarectum
- ↑ rectal compliance
- ↓ rectal sensation
- ↓ rectoanal inhibitory reflex
- IAS/EAS pressure changes

Faecal impaction

- Terminal reservoir syndrome
- Combination with any of the above – stool soft, hard or liquid – may result in incontinence

Faecal incontinence

- Overflow (frequent soiling – small amounts)
- Post-defaecatory soiling
- Diarrhoea
- Neuropathic – associated with descending perineum syndrome – urge or passive.
- Undiagnosed IAS/EAS muscle trauma associated with childbirth
- Dementia
- Multiple factors, e.g. any combination of the above.

PREVALENCE OF FAECAL INCONTINENCE

This is difficult to determine accurately. Barrett and Kiff (1993) suggested that rates differed widely among the elderly living at home and those in nursing homes. Independent risk factors in a community-based study, with a 2.2% prevalence of faecal incontinence, were shown to be female sex, age, poor general health and limited physical activity (Nelson et al, 1995). In contrast Lubowski (1996) found that 20% of Australian men and only 11% of women in the general community complained of faecal incontinence. Rates were similar both under and over 65 years. Mild symptoms predominate in males. As in females, decreased rectal sensation and pelvic floor denervation are common causes in the male.

Most irritable bowel syndrome sufferers who also have faecal incontinence are female. However, Barrett and Kiff (1993) consider faecal impaction and its sequelae to be the most common cause of faecal incontinence in the aged. Poor toilet access may be as important as physical and cognitive changes at this time.

There are changes in the anal sphincter with ageing which may affect continence. They are listed in the box. Figure 36.6 illustrates anal sphincter musculature in a normal subject.

The ageing anal sphincter

EAS thickness – male>female

IAS no gender difference

EAS becomes thinner with age

IAS becomes thicker with age

EAS thickness inversely correlates with IAS thickness

Sum of IAS/EAS reflects tonic activity (Papachrysostomou et al, 1993)

Before a physiotherapy programme may be initiated, an understanding of the sensory, motor and proprioceptive changes of the ageing anorectum must be considered.

Effective management is multifactorial and must not be directed to the anal sphincter alone (Chapter 30). The box gives an explanation of the changes occurring with disuse or denervation. Figure 36.7 illustrates problems resulting from neuropathy.

Physiological aspects of neuropathic faecal incontinence

Sensory	↓ rectal sensation (↓ PF proprioception)
	Absent RAIR
	Profound loss of sensation in megarectum and faecal impaction
	Perianal sensory deficits affect 'sampling process'
Motor	↓ EAS strength
	Destabilization of the pelvic floor
	Loss of anorectal angle
	Disuse/denervation → ↓ reflex contractions of EAS with ↑ IAP
Mechanical/ *other*	↓ oestrogen related to onset of symptoms
	Prolapsed rectal mucosa into anus
	Irritable bowel syndrome
	↓ rectal compliance (radiation scarring)
	↓ Cognition with CVA, dementia Neurogenic with spinal stenosis
	(Varma et al, 1988; Barrett et al, 1989)

Figure 36.6 Normal anal sphincters demonstrated by anal endosonography.

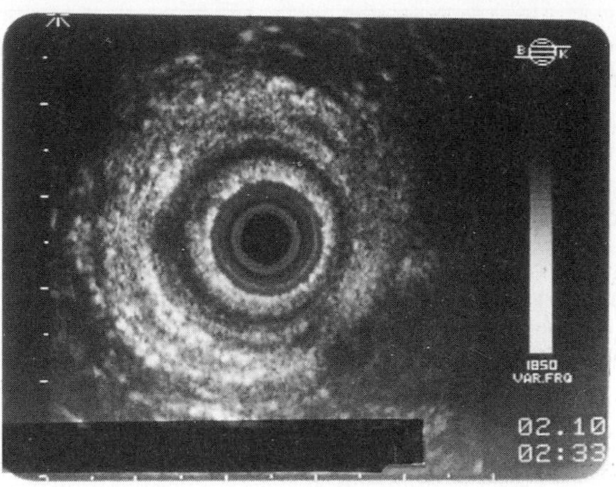

Neurological conditions are concomitant with age and lifestyle related bowel dysfunction described earlier. Table 36.3 outlines the symptoms and physiotherapy management indicated in these conditions.

The role of surgery is based on functional outcome and alleviation of pain. Surgery is designed to improve structure and this is combined with physiotherapy to enhance mechanical factors. Successful outcome depends on both (Markwell and Mumme, 1995).

Functional anorectal surgery in the elderly

Faecal incontinence:

- Age makes no difference to outcomes of sphincter repairs for trauma.
- Graciloplasty more effective for traumatic than neuropathic faecal incontinence.
- Bilateral pudendal neuropathy compounds.

Figure 36.7 (a) Low perineum at rest; (b) total loss of anorectal angle on straining. The patient presented with obstructed defaecation and faecal incontinence due to gross neuropathy.

a

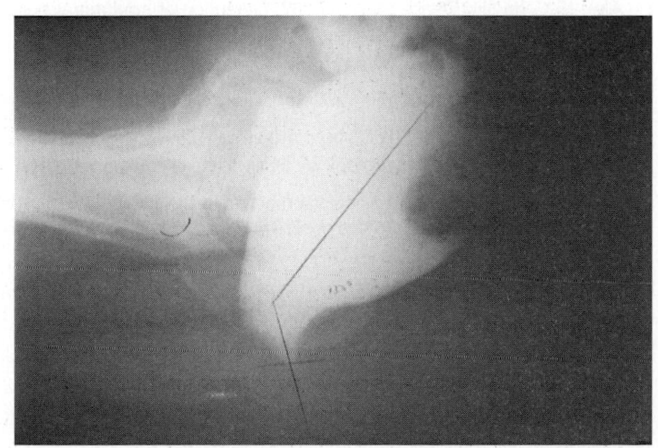

b

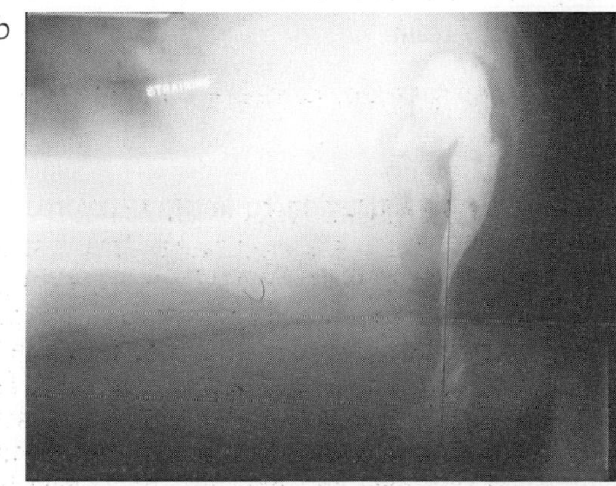

Table 36.3 Neurological conditions affecting bowel function

Disease	Presenting symptoms	Gastrointestinal pathology	Treatment
Multiple sclerosis (Waldron et al, 1993)	Constipation Faecal incontinence	Slow CTT distally Outlet obstruction ↓ EAS pressure PF destabilization	Dietary modification Regulating medication Physiotherapy for imbalance
Diabetes (Rogers et al, 1988)	Recurrent diarrhoea Faecal incontinence Rectal stasis	Diabetic peripheral neuropathy of PF Sensorimotor deficit of anorectum	As above. Physiotherapy for imbalance
Parkinson's disease (Ashraf et al, 1994)	Obstructed defaecation	Pressure manometry of EAS + EMG of EAS/PR correlates with 'off period' changes Return to normal function	Sphincter/levator inco-ordination due to 'on-off' response Often associated with bladder dysfunction Physiotherapy for inco-ordination

Obstructed defaecation:

- Minor to major surgery for obstructed defaecation is determined by age and medical status.
- Mucosal banding.
- Peranal Delorme procedure for rectal prolapse +/− sphincter plication (Mumme GA, personal communication).
- Resection of redundant segments of colon +/− rectopexy.

Peranal Delorme procedures are combined with physiotherapy for maximum effectiveness. This form of rectal stabilization plus functional physiotherapy has been shown to improve mixed urinary incontinence and voiding dysfunction (Mumme and Markwell, 1994).

Bowel function in the mobile aged may be managed on an outpatient basis with dietary modification, bulking agents and functional physiotherapy. This may include selective biofeedback to complement surgery. In residential care a team approach of dietary, medical, nursing and behavioural (timed evacuation) programmes will be established. Defaecation retraining, selective rehabilitation and mobility assistance complete the physiotherapist's contribution.

Management

Multidisciplinary team

- History
- Investigations
- Skin care
- Dietary modification
- Regimen of oral medication to improve colorectal and rectoanal function
- Rectal medication for terminal reservoir syndrome
- ↑ mobility
- Behavioural therapy – dementia
- Physiotherapy
- Biofeedback
- Surgery
- Maintenance programme

Warning

Care must be taken with the administration of bulking agents in the elderly. Allow two hours between bulking agent ingestion and the taking of prescription medication, for maximum absorption.

Cognitive change, reduced mobility and polypharmacy at this time are reflected in altered bowel function.

As women age they generally have more time to devote to themselves and to reflect upon what they want from the rest of their lives. In those who are free of disease, disturbances of function, as described in this chapter, can adversely affect the quality of life and limit activities. Hence women in this age bracket are well motivated to comply with treatment and maintenance programmes implemented by the physiotherapist.

References

Aloia JF, Cohn SH, Ostuni JA et al (1989) Prevention of involutional bone loss by exercise. *Annals of Internal Medicine* **89**: 356–358.

Ashraf W, Wszloek ZK, Pfeiffer RF et al (1994) Variations in anorectal function in relation to on-off fluctuations in Parkinson's disease. *Gastroenterology* **107**(4): 1232.

Asplund R and Aberg HE (1992) Micturition habits in older people. *Scandanavian Journal of Urology and Nephrology* **26**: 345–349.

Barrett JA and Kiff ES (1993) Anorectal function in the elderly. In: Henry MM and Swash M (eds) *Coloproctology and the Pelvic Floor*, 2nd edn, pp. 470–476. Oxford: Butterworth Heinemann.

Barrett JA, Brocklehurst JC, Kiff ES et al (1989) Anal function in geriatric patients with faecal incontinence. *Gut* **30**: 1244–1251.

Bassotti G, German U and Morrelli A (1995) Human colonic motility: physiological aspects. *International Journal of Colorectal Disease* **10**: 173–180.

Bernstein I, Balslev E, Bodker A et al (1995) Estrogen receptors in the human levator ani muscles. *Neurourology and Urodynamics* **14**: 520–521.

Birge SJ (1995) Role of oestrogen in the treatment and prevention of falls, fractures and dementia. Proceedings of the 5th Congress of the Australian Menopause Society, Hobart, Australia.

Cope E (1976) Physical changes associated with the post-menopausal years. In: Campbell S (ed) *The Management of the Menopause and Post-Menopausal Years*, p. 33. Baltimore: University Press.

Diczfalusy E (1986) Menopause, developing countries and the 21st century. *Acta Obstetrica et Gynecologica* **45**(Suppl): 134–411.

Erikssen PS and Rasmussen H (1992) Low-dose 17-beta oestradiol vaginal tablets in the treatment of atrophic vaginitis: a double-blind placebo controlled study. *European Journal of Obstetrics, Gynaecology and Reproductive Biology* **44**: 137–144.

Evers JLH and Heineman MJ (1990) Gynaecology of old age. In: Evers JLH and Heineman MJ (eds) *Gynaecology: A Clinical Atlas*, pp. 146–166. Ontwerpers: Koninklijke Smeets Offset, Organon.

Fiatorone MA, Marks EC, Ryan ND et al (1990) High intensity strength training in nonagenarians: effects on skeletal muscle. *Journal of the American Medical Association* **262**: 3029–3034.

Fiatorone MA, O'Neill EF, Ryan ND et al (1994) Exercise training and nutritional supplementation for physical frailty in very elderly people. *New England Journal of Medicine* **330**: 1669–1675.

Fonda D (1985) Urinary incontinence in the elderly: its prevalence and cost implications. *Proceedings of the 20th Annual Conference of the Australian Association of Gerentology*, p. 51.

Fonda D, Woodward M, D'Astoli M et al (1994) The continued success of conservative management for established urinary incontinence in older people. *Australian Journal of Ageing* **13**: 12–16.

Geirsson G, Fall M and Lindstrom S (1993) Subtypes of overactive bladder in old age. *Age and Ageing* **22**: 125–131.

Gormley EA, Griffiths DJ, McCracken PN et al (1993) Polypharmacy and its effect on urinary incontinence in a geriatric population. *British Journal of Urology* **71**: 265–269.

Griffiths DJ, McCracken PN, Harrison GM et al (1990) Geriatric urge incontinence: basic dysfunction and contributory factors. *Neurourology and Urodynamics* **9**: 406–407.

Grill V and Martin TJ (1995) Metabolic bone diseases. *Medical Journal of Australia* **163**: 38–41.

Harrison SM (1987) Micturition disorders in senior citizens fitness groups. *Proceedings of the World Confederation of Physical Therapists Congress*, Sydney, pp. 1031–1035.

Hazzard WR (1986) Biological basis of the sex differential in longevity. *Journal of the American Geriatric Society* **35**: 455–471.

Iosif C (1992) Effects of protracted administration of estriol on the lower urogenital tract in post-menopausal women. *Archives of Gynecology and Obstetrics* **251**: 115–120.

Iosif C and Bekassy Z (1984) Prevalence of genito-urinary symptoms in the later menopause. *Acta Obstetrica et Gynecologica Scandinavica* **63**: 257–260.

Iosif C, Batra SC, Ek A et al (1981) Estrogen receptors in the human female lower urinary tract. *American Journal of Obstetrics and Gynecology* **14**: 817–820.

Jorm AF, Korten AE and Henderson AS (1987) The prevalence of dementia: a quantitative integration of the literature. *Acta Psychiatrica Scandinavica* **76**: 465–479.

Kinsey AC, Pomeroy WB, Martin CE et al (1953) *Sexual Behaviour in the Human Female*. Philadelphia: W.B. Saunders.

Krolner B, Toft B, Nielsen SP et al (1983) Physical exercise as prophylaxis against involutional vertebral bone loss: a controlled trial. *Clinical Science* **6**: 541–547.

Lord S and Castell S (1994) Effect of exercise on balance, strength and reaction time in older people. *Australian Journal of Physiotherapy* **40**: 83–88.

Lord S, Sambrook PN, Gilbert C et al (1994) Postural stability, falls and fractures in the elderly: results from the Dubbo Osteoporosis Epidemiology Study. *Medical Journal of Australia* **160**: 684–691.

Lubowski DZ (1996) Cited in Margo JA Anal incontinence worst among men. *Medical Observer* March 1: 31.

Malone-Lee J (1994) Recent developments in urinary incontinence in late life. *Physiotherapy* **80**: 133–134.

Malone-Lee J and Wahedna I (1993) Characterisation of detrusor contractile function in relation to old age. *British Journal of Urology* **72**: 873–880.

Markwell SJ and Mumme GA (1995) A role for physiotherapy in perianal and perineal pain syndromes. In: Shacklock MO (ed) *Moving in on Pain*, pp. 145–152. Sydney: Butterworth Heinemann.

McGuire EJ (1990) Identifying and managing stress incontinence in the elderly. *Geriatrics* **45**: 44–52.

Mumme GA and Markwell SJ (1994) Rectal stabilisation improves bladder dysfunction in the descending perineum syndrome. Abstract. International Continence Society Conference, Prague, pp. 160–161.

National Center for Health Statistics (1987) *Ageing in the 80's: Functional Limitations of Individuals age 65 and over.* Washington DC: USI HHS.

Nelson R, Norton N, Cantley E et al (1995) Community based prevalence of anal incontinence. *Journal of the American Medical Association* **274**(7): 559–561.

Nguyen T, Sambrook PN, Kelly P et al (1993) Prediction of osteoporotic fractures by postural instability and bone density. *British Medical Journal* **307**: 1111–1115.

O'Neill SM, Markwell SJ and Mumme GA (1993) Prevalence and management of bowel dysfunction in the climacteric: an Australian experience. International Congress on the Menopause, Stockholm, poster 263.

Ouslander JG (1990) Urinary incontinence in nursing homes. *Journal of the American Geriatric Society* **38**: 289–291.

Paganini-Hill A and Henderson VW (1994) Estrogen deficiency and risk of Alzheimer's disease in women. *American Journal of Epidemiology* **140**(3): 256–261.

Pagano F, Artibani W and Cisternino A (1992) Epidemiological research on the prevalence of urinary incontinence in the area covered by national health authority no. 2. *Neurourology and Urodynamics* **11**: 355–357.

Papachrysostomou M, Pye SD, Wild SR et al (1993) Anal endosonography in asymptomatic subjects. *Scandanavian Journal of Gastroenterology* **28**: 551–556.

Pfeiffer E and Davis GC (1972) Determinants of sexual behaviour in middle and old age. *Journal of the American Geriatric Society* **20**: 151–158.

Pigne A (1994) Video 'The pathophysiology, clinical aspects and roles of oestrogen in urogenital ageing'. Australian Menopause Society.

Rockstein M and Sussman M (1979) *Biology of Ageing*. Belmont, California: Wadsworth.

Rogers J, Levy DM, Henry MM et al (1988) Pelvic floor neuropathy: a comparative study of diabetes mellitus and idiopathic faecal incontinence. *Gut* **29**: 756–761.

Saito M, Kondo A, Kato T et al (1993) Frequency-volume charts: comparison of frequency between elderly and adult patients. *British Journal of Urology* **72**: 38–41.

Skinner JS (1987) *Exercise Testing and Exercise Prescription for Special Cases: Theoretical Basis and Clinical Application*, pp. 67–75. Phildelphia: Lea and Febiger.

Smith P, Heimer G, Lindskog M et al (1993) Oestradiol-releasing vaginal ring for the treatment of post-menopausal urogenital atrophy. *Maturitas* **16**: 145–154.

Speroff L, Glass RH and Kase NG (1994) Menopause and postmenopausal hormone therapy. In: Speroff L, Glass RH and Kase NG (eds) Clinical Gynaecologic Endocrinology and Infertility, pp. 583–649. Baltimore: Williams and Wilkins.

Tallis R (1993) Foreword. In: Barrett JA (ed) *Faecal Incontinence and Related Problems in the Older Adult*, p. v. London: Edward Arnold.

Thomas TM, Plymat KR, Blannin J et al (1980) Prevalence of urinary incontinence. *British Medical Journal* **281**: 1243–1245.

Tideiksaar R (1989a) Normal aging changes and the risk of falling. In: Tideiksaar R (ed) Falling in Old Age, pp. 11–19. New York: Springer.

Tideiksaar R (1989b) An overview of the problem: prevalence of falls in the elderly. In: Tideiksaar R (ed) Falling in Old Age, pp. 1–9. New York: Springer.

Tsai C, Semmens J, Lam F et al (1987) Vaginal physiology in post-menopausal women: pH value, transvaginal electropotential difference and estimated blood flow. *Southern Medical Journal* **80**: 987–990.

Varma JS, Bradnoch J, Smith RG et al (1988) Constipation in the elderly: a physiologic study. *Diseases of Colon and Rectum* **31**(2): 111–115.

Waldron DJ, Horgan PG, Patel FR et al (1993) Multiple sclerosis: assessment of colonic and anorectal function in the presence of faecal incontinence. *International Journal of Colorectal Disease* **8**: 220–224.

Woolner BF and Ouslander JG (1992) Experience with biofeedback for incontinence and related urinary symptoms in the old old. *Neurourology and Urodynamics* 11: 425–426.

Further reading

Barrett JA (1993) *Faecal Incontinence and Related Problems in the Older Adult.* London: Edward Arnold.

Index

Note:
1. The entries and qualifiers *women* and *physiotherapy* are largely omitted from this index as they would be ubiquitous
2. Pages numbers in **bold** indicate tables; and in *italics* indicate figures. There are frequently also textual references on these pages.